Family
Nurse
Practitioner

CERTIFICATION REVIEW

Family Nurse Practitioner

CERTIFICATION REVIEW

Second Edition

Pamela S. Kidd, RN, ARNP, BC, PhD, FAAN

Professor and Associate Dean for Graduate Programs and Research
Community Health Services Clinic: Family Nurse Practitioner
Arizona State University College of Nursing
Tempe, Arizona

Denise L. Robinson, RN, ARNP, BC, PhD

Professor
Northern Kentucky University
Director, MSN Programs
Health Point Family Care, Inc.: Family Nurse Practitioner
Highland Heights, Kentucky

Cheryl Pope Kish, RNC, WHNP, EdD

Professor, Coordinator Graduate Programs in Health Sciences, and Director FNP Program
Nurse Practitioner Student Health Services
Georgia College & State University
Milledgeville, Georgia

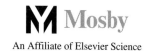

An Affiliate of Elsevier Science

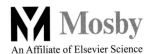

An Affiliate of Elsevier Science

11830 Westline Industrial Drive
St. Louis, Missouri 63146

NOTICE

Nursing is an ever-changing field. Standard safety precautions must be followed, but as new research and clinical experience broaden our knowledge, changes in treatment and drug therapy may become necessary or appropriate. Readers are advised to check the most current product information provided by the manufacturer of each drug to be administered to verify the recommended dose, the method and duration of administration, and contraindications. It is the responsibility of the licensed prescriber, relying on experience and knowledge of the patient, to determine dosages and the best treatment for each individual patient. Neither the publisher nor the editor assumes any liability for any injury and/or damage to persons or property arising from this publication.

Previous edition copyrighted 1999.

Library of Congress Cataloging-in-Publication Data

Family nurse practitioner certification review / [edited by] Pamela S. Kidd, Denise L. Robinson, Cheryl P. Kish.–2nd ed.
       p. ; cm.
    Includes bibliographical references and index.
    ISBN 0-323-01976-5
    1. Family nursing–Examinations, questions, etc. 2. Nurse practitioners–Examinations, questions, etc. I. Kidd, Pamela Stinson. II. Robinson, Denise L. III. Kish, Cheryl Pope.
    [DNLM: 1. Family Practice–Examination Questions. 2. Nurse Practitioners–Examination Questions. WY 18.2 F198 2003]
RT120.F34 F353 2003
610.73′076–dc21   2002026469

Vice President and Publishing Director, Nursing: Sally Schrefer
Executive Publisher: Barbara Nelson Cullen
Developmental Editor: Victoria Bruno
Publishing Services Manager: Catherine Jackson
Project Manager: Clay S. Broeker
Designer: Amy Buxton

KI/MVY

Printed in the United States of America

Last digit is the print number: 9   8   7   6   5   4   3   2   1

This book is dedicated to my family, who make me smile and remember what is important in life. It is also dedicated to my parents, who always believed in me, even if they didn't always know what it was that I did for a living. A special thanks to my colleagues Cheryl and Denise, who never dropped the ball and slept and played as little as I did to get the job done!
PSK

This book is dedicated to my family, who are proud and supportive of my efforts. Their love and belief in my abilities have always helped me to grow throughout the years. Cheryl, your test-writing skills inspired us both. Pam, your organization and dedication are unsurpassed. The teamwork made the process almost easy! Thanks.
DLR

This book is dedicated to my family, who take pride in my work and bring me special joy every day, and especially to my granddaughter Elizabeth, the newest "sunshine in my life." To Pam and Denise, thanks for sharing a place on your team with me—it was a special place to be and to create!
CPK

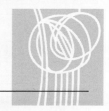

Reviewers

Phyllis Adams, EdD, RN, FNP
University of Texas at Arlington School of Nursing
Arlington, Texas
Diamond Hill Clinics of JPS Health Network
Fort Worth, Texas

Genell Hilton, MS, CRNP, CCRN
Clinical Faculty
School of Nursing
University of Maryland
Baltimore, Maryland

Joan A. Osborne, BSN, MS, RN-CS, FNP
Director of Nursing
Correctional Health Services, Inc.
Verona, New Jersey

Valerie K. Sabol, RN, MSN, ACNP-C
Nurse Practitioner/Clinical Instructor
School of Nursing
University of Maryland
Baltimore, Maryland

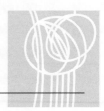

Preface

This book was developed to meet the needs of family nurse practitioners (FNPs) preparing to take the national certification examinations. As nurse practitioners, we were frustrated as we tried to prepare for the examinations because there were few comprehensive preparation books. Most review books are not structured to reflect the FNP's approach to practice (context), based on the Subjective, Objective, Assessment, Plan, Evaluate (SOAPE) format. We found the existing review books to be limited in both content and context.

With these two issues in mind, we wrote this review book to provide greater depth (content) and to develop a format that accommodates preparing for both the Academy of Nurse Practitioners (Academy) and the test blueprint of the American Nurses Credentialing Center (ANCC) FNP exams. The SOAPE approach used for both the chapter content and the test questions reflects all components of the Academy's domains (assessment, diagnosis, plan, and evaluation) and the ANCC format (history taking, physical examination, diagnosis, management, and evaluation) for acute and chronic illness. Tables are used to cluster wellness content across the lifespan. Major changes in the second edition include the following:

- Topics organized alphabetically to make it easier for the user to find topic areas.
- Topics that relate across the lifespan (e.g. immunizations) are organized in the same chapter using subheadings to facilitate comparisons and support retention of learning.
- Inclusion of a chapter on advanced assessment techniques and maneuvers to condense frequently tested information in one area
- Increased emphasis placed on pathophysiology in the chapters
- Inclusion of many more topics to reflect current practice
- Use of the Internet to increase the number of questions we could include with the book

- Use of national guidelines where appropriate for each condition

At the end of each chapter are test questions pertaining to the specific content reviewed. In addition to these post-section questions, there is a comprehensive examination (Sample Examination) that reflect the actual length of the certification examinations. Twenty-five pretest items are also included to mimic the setup of the actual examination. Test questions related to the clinical topics are classified according to the SOAPE format. This approach allows you to examine the type of item you are having the most difficulty processing and to focus your study efforts. The rationale for each correct answer is provided. Additional review questions are included in both the book and on the website, organized by system, to facilitate a focused review. Questions are also included about the major issues impacting practice by the FNP; these reflect the issues tested on the certification examinations. Information about the difficulty and discrimination levels of the national certification examinations is confidential and is not released to the public. We have made every effort to construct sample examinations that reflect the national examination, based on the published information from both testing agencies. However, the actual test blueprints are not published; only information about the testing categories is available. Therefore the exact weight placed on a given problem area or domain is not known and the weight placed on content areas within the sample examinations may not be representative of the actual examinations. However, we are confident that the major areas are addressed here. We renewed our certification by retesting to help us make this book as useful as possible in preparing for the exams. No book—not even this one—can replace confidence in yourself and your abilities. Go for it!

Pamela S. Kidd
Denise L. Robinson
Cheryl Pope Kish

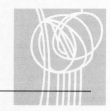

Acknowledgments

We thank our colleagues across the nation who helped create the foundation for the second edition of this book. Thanks also to the students who expect the best from us—their standards always raise the bar. We thank our clients who reinforce the essentials daily and help us to separate the "must know" from the "nice to know."

Special thanks to Deborah Knight Williams, MSN, ARNP, SANE, LNC, Clinical Forensic Nurse Specialist and Family Nurse Practitioner at the University of Louisville, who contributed test questions on scoliosis, seizures, meningitis, multiple sclerosis, and tinnitus as part of an independent study she completed while attending Northern Kentucky University.

Pamela S. Kidd
Denise L. Robinson
Cheryl Pope Kish

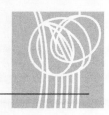

Contents

PART II

CLIENT WELLNESS

PART III

ISSUES

PART IV

ADDITIONAL SYSTEM REVIEW QUESTIONS

PART V

SAMPLE EXAMINATION QUESTIONS

APPENDIX

GENERAL ASSESSMENT AND COMMON PRESENTING PROBLEMS AND SYMPTOMS

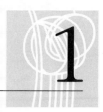

Test-Taking Guidelines

USING THIS BOOK AS A STUDY AID

The beauty of a book such as *Family Nurse Practitioner Certification Review* is that the content, relevant to the family nurse practitioner (FNP) practice, has been collected across the life span, reduced to essential information, and formatted to support a test matrix (Subjective, Objective, Assessment, Plan, Evaluate [SOAPE]). The book provides a comprehensive review in an easy-to-find format. Test questions address key principles and common application of these principles.

The review questions in this book were constructed to reflect the nursing process. Each question addresses assessment, analysis/diagnosis, implementation/plan, or evaluation. It is helpful to make note of which types of items you miss more frequently so that you can anticipate those particular types on the exam, slow down, and answer it carefully. *Assessment* items require the test taker to collect information of value. *Analysis/diagnosis* items require the test taker to deduce and synthesize from collected information. *Implementation/plan* items require the test taker to manage a situation. *Evaluation* items require the test taker to examine outcomes for their value.

Recognize that exam questions are written to reflect different types of knowledge levels and require different types of thinking. Many questions require recall. These are *fact-oriented questions*. The answer is clear if you know the question area. Mnemonic devices assist recall. You may use these in studying and in testing. *Comprehension-level questions* require you to understand a condition or situation to choose the answer. *Application* questions ask you to analyze a situation and then select the best of several plausible options. Clues (such as the first step or the priority action) are provided in the item stem to help you select the best option.

HOW TO APPROACH THE EXAMINATION

1. *Assess your knowledge.* Complete practice questions before the examination. Spend your time wisely. Concentrate review on areas in which you perform inconsistently or poorly during practice sessions.
2. *Believe in yourself.* Speak of *when* you are certified, not *if* you pass the test.
3. *Determine whether you study better independently or with others.* Form a study group if this will help you.
4. *Develop "flash cards" to help you remember difficult concepts or memorize material, for example, screening guidelines.*
5. *Establish a schedule for reviewing.* Determine the amount of content you need to review and the amount of time you have before the testing date, and "dose" your study periods.
6. *Rest and eat a light meal before the examination.*
7. *Budget your time.* If taking a "pencil and paper" test, divide the total time allowed for the test by the number of items on the test–for example, 60 minutes divided by 30 items is 2 minutes per item. Keep this number in mind as you work through the test. If an item is taking too much time, move on and return to it later.
8. *Read each item carefully before going on to the answer options.* Identify key words in the item stem. This includes whether it is asking for a negative or wrong response.
9. *Try answering the question before reading the options.* Then read all the answer options completely before choosing.
10. *Eliminate the options that are obviously wrong.*
11. *Make sure that the selected option relates grammatically to the item stem.* For example, if the item asks for one action, do not select an option that includes two actions.
12. *Answer every question.*
13. *Do not change your answer unless you have a good reason for doing so.* Most first impressions are accurate if you have read the item carefully.
14. *If you need to guess, guess logically.* The longest option is usually correct. Avoid options with all-inclusive terms

such as *never* and *always*. Correct options tend to be in the middle.

These guidelines are your "rules of the road." You cannot guarantee that you will arrive at your destination safely (in this case, pass the certification examination). However, the probability of success should be greater than if you did not use these guidelines, and you can approach the exam confidently and strategically.

Assessment Review

Assessment is the foundation on which a diagnosis is made. Although much of the material in this chapter is basic, it is frequently tested to ensure that the exam candidate can discriminate assessment findings among conditions and across the life span. Information in this chapter appears throughout the book as it is relevant to the specific condition being addressed. Review questions are provided at the end of the chapter to reinforce and review learning.

HISTORY TAKING

Components of the history are relevant to review because some aspects of the history have greater importance when discriminating among possible diagnoses. The ability to discriminate plausible diagnoses based on data collected through the history is an expectation of the family nurse practitioner (FNP). The following components are included in a comprehensive history:

I. Comprehensive history: adult
  A. Date
  B. Identifying data (demographics)
  C. Source of referral (if appropriate)
  D. Source of history
  E. Chief complaints (use client's own words)
  F. Present illness; primary symptom analysis
    1. Location
    2. Quality
    3. Severity
    4. Timing
    5. Setting
    6. Relieving/aggravating factors
    7. Associated symptoms
    8. Pain assessment (if appropriate)
      a. P = provoke
      b. Q = quality
      c. R = radiation
      d. S = severity
      e. T = timing
  G. Past history
    1. General state of health
    2. Childhood illness
    3. Adult illness
    4. Mental health illness
    5. Injuries
    6. Hospitalizations
  H. Current history
    1. Allergies
    2. Immunizations
    3. Screening tests as appropriate for age, gender, or ethnicity
    4. Environmental exposures
    5. Occupation
    6. Use of safety measures
    7. Exercise/leisure activities
    8. Complementary therapies (yoga, acupuncture, tai chi)
    9. Sleep patterns
    10. Diet and dietary supplements
    11. Medications
    12. Tobacco, drugs, alcohol, botanicals and other supplements
  I. Family history
  J. Psychosocial history
  K. Review of systems
    1. General
    2. Skin
    3. Head
    4. Eyes
    5. Ears
    6. Nose and sinuses
    7. Mouth and throat
    8. Neck
    9. Breasts
    10. Respiratory
    11. Cardiac
    12. Gastrointestinal
    13. Urinary

14. Genitoreproductive
15. Peripheral vascular
16. Musculoskeletal
17. Neurologic
18. Hematologic
19. Endocrine
20. Psychiatric
II. Comprehensive history: child
   A. Identifying data
   B. Chief complaints
   C. Present illness
   D. Past history
     1. Birth history
     2. Prenatal
     3. Neonatal
   E. Feeding history
     1. Breastfeeding
     2. Eating habits
   F. Growth and development
     1. Physical growth
     2. Developmental milestones
   G. Social development
     1. Sleep
     2. Toileting
     3. Speech
     4. Habits
     5. Discipline
     6. School
     7. Sexuality
     8. Personality
   H. Childhood illness
   I. Injuries
   J. Hospitalizations
   K. Current health status
     1. Allergies
     2. Immunizations
     3. Screening procedures
   L. Family history
   M. Review of systems as with adult client

HEALTH EDUCATION MODEL (PLISSIT)

Health education is gaining greater prominence within the anticipatory guidance aspect of the FNP role. This is because unhealthy lifestyles contribute the most to conditions discussed in this book and covered on the exam. The PLISSIT model is a frequently used framework for identifying at what stage health education is provided and what range of education is capable of being provided. (Originally designed for sexuality education, this model is appropriate for all health information.)

P (permission) = establishes with client permission to address a particular concern or health issue
LI (limited information) = provides specific but not detailed information, dispels myths, stimulates curiosity
SS (specific suggestions) = interventions are directed toward solving problems and creating a plan; includes client's ideas about the problem and goals for change
IT (intensive therapy) = specialists in topic area are involved and a customized plan is developed for change/problem solving

PHYSICAL EXAMINATION BASICS

The following tables organize basic assessment data and review how to interpret the information. This information frequently appears on exams as answer options for multiple choice questions that require the exam candidate to analyze assessment data.

Percussion

TONE/SAMPLE LOCATION	INTENSITY	PITCH	DURATION
Flat (thigh)	Soft	High	Short
Dull (liver)	Medium	Medium	Medium
Resonance (lung)	Loud	Low	Long
Hyperresonance (COPD/ emphysematous lung)	Very loud	Lower	Longer
Tympany (gastric area)	Loud	High	Short

*COPD, Chronic obstructive pulmonary disease.

Auscultation of Lungs

TERM	DEFINITION	CONDITION
Egophony	"Ee" to "aa" changes	Pneumonia, pleural effusion
Whispered pectoriloquy	Clearer transmission of whispered sound	Pneumonia, pleural effusion
Bronchophony	Clearer transmission of all voice sounds	Pneumonia, pleural effusion
Crackles	Sound produced when deflated airways are reinflated during inspiration	Pneumonia, CHF, pulmonary fibrosis
Wheezes	Musical sound produced by air passing through narrowed bronchus	Asthma, foreign body aspiration, tumor

CHF, Congestive heart failure.

Assessment of Cranial Nerves

NERVE	NAME	ASSESSMENT
Cranial nerve I	Olfactory	Smell
Cranial nerve II	Optic	Vision
Cranial nerve III	Oculomotor	Papillary constriction, EOMs
Cranial nerve IV	Trochlear	EOMs
Cranial nerve V	Trigeminal	Motor—jaw clenching, sensory—cotton ball to forehead, cheek, and jaw areas
Cranial nerve VI	Abducens	EOMs
Cranial nerve VII	Facial	Grin
Cranial nerve VIII	Acoustic	Hearing and balance
Cranial nerve IX	Glossopharyngeal	Sensory/taste, motor/swallow
Cranial nerve X	Vagus	Swallow, say "ah," rise of uvula
Cranial nerve XI	Spinal accessory	Shrug shoulders, turn neck
Cranial nerve XII	Hypoglossal	Stick out tongue

EOM, Extraocular movement.

Deep Tendon Reflexes

REFLEX	SPINAL SEGMENT ASSESSED
Biceps	Cervical 5 and 6
Supinator (brachioradialis)	Cervical 5 and 6
Triceps	Cervical 6, 7, 8
Knee	Lumbar 2, 3, 4
Ankle	Lumbar 5, sacral 1, 2
Abdominal reflex (upper)	Thoracic 8, 9, 10
Abdominal reflex (lower)	Thoracic 10, 11, 12
Plantar	Lumbar 4, 5, sacral 1, 2

Extraocular Movements

DIRECTION	CRANIAL NERVE
Looking down and to the right	Third cranial nerve OD, fourth cranial nerve OS
Looking down and to the left	Fourth cranial nerve OD, third cranial nerve OS
Looking up and to the right	Third cranial nerve OU
Looking up and to the left	Third cranial nerve OU
Looking to the right (lateral)	Sixth cranial nerve OD, third cranial nerve OS
Looking to the left (lateral)	Third cranial nerve OD, sixth cranial nerve OS

OD, Right eye; *OS*, left eye; *OU*, each eye.

Special Assessment Techniques

Extraocular movements (EOMs) are discussed separately because their execution is needed to assess the integrity of three of the cranial nerves.

MANEUVERS

Maneuvers are used extensively to confirm or to disconfirm a diagnosis. They may be found on the test by name, requiring the exam candidate to know the maneuver, how to execute it, and when it should be used, or the maneuver may be described and the exam candidate must name the maneuver.

CONVERSIONS

- To convert centigrade to Fahrenheit: (9/5 × Temperature) + 32
- To convert Fahrenheit to centigrade: (Temperature − 32) × 5/9
- 1 kg = 2.2 pounds

Maneuver and Objective Signs Summary Chart

NAME OF TEST	DIAGNOSTIC FOR:	HOW TO PERFORM
Adam's position	Screening test for scoliosis	Forward bend position
Allergic shiner	Allergic rhinitis	Darkening of skin below eyes
Anterior drawer test	ACL injury/stability	90 degrees of flexion of knee with anteriorly directed force applied to proximal tibia
Auspitz's sign	Suggests psoriasis	Positive when slight scratching or curetting of lesion reveals punctuate bleeding points within the lesion
Barlow test	Developmental dysplasia of hip	Infant supine with pelvis on flat surface; adduct and internally rotate hips; palpable clunk confirms hip dislocation
Bell's phenomenon	Bell's palsy	Exaggerated upward curve of the eyelid with lid closure
Brudzinski's sign	Meningeal irritation	When client is supine, passive flexion of the neck elicits flexion of hips and neck
Chadwick's sign	Indication of pregnancy	Blue, soft cervix
Chandelier's sign	Inflammatory process	Cervix tenderness when in motion
Cullen's sign	Blood in peritoneal cavity	Bluish discoloration around umbilicus
CVA tenderness	Pyelonephritis	Tenderness over costovertebral angle with direct fist percussion
Fukuda's test	Labyrinth disease	Client walks in place with eyes closed; a positive sign occurs when the client rotates toward the diseased labyrinth
Galeazzi sign	Developmental dysplasia of hip	Child supine with knees fully adducted and held together; test is positive if one femur is shorter than the other
Gowers' sign	Generalized muscle weakness— muscular dystrophy	Client maneuvers to a position supported by both arms and legs, pushes off the floor to rest hands on knees, then pushes upright
Homans' sign	Indication of DVT	Pain upon dorsiflexion of toes
Hoover's sign	Malingering or back pain	Examiner places hands under both heels, asks client to raise affected leg; if pain is real, the heel on the other leg will push into the examiner's hand
Iliopsoas	Peritoneal irritation	Psoas muscle pain with active hip flexion or passive extension
Kernig's sign	Meningeal irritation	When the client is supine with hip and knee flexed toward abdomen, extension of knee elicits neck pain
Lachman's test	ACL stability/injury	Performed at 30 degrees of flexion with anteriorly directed force to the proximal tibia while the opposite hand stabilizes the thigh
Magnuson's test	Nonorganic physical signs/ malingering	Mark areas that were tender; return to the marked areas later in exam to see if pain can be reproduced
McMurray's test	Meniscal problems	The leg in flexion is moved from valgus, external rotation, to varus, internal rotation; alternatively, the knee can be extended during the maneuver; a palpable click or joint line pain is positive
Murphy's sign	Cholecystitis	Temporary inspiratory arrest with palpation of right subcostal margin
Obturator sign	Peritoneal irritation	Pain with internal/external rotation of flexed thigh from 90 degree hip/knee flexion position
Ortolani's test	Developmental dysplasia of hip	Infant supine with pelvis on flat surface; abduct and externally rotate hip; middle finger should be over the greater trochanter; a palpable clunk confirms reduction of the dislocated hip
Patrick's test	Degenerative hip joint disease	Client is in a supine position, position the heel of the right foot on the knee of the left leg; lower the right leg toward the examination table by placing moderate manual pressure on the right knee; repeat on opposite leg
Phalen's test	Carpal tunnel syndrome	Flex wrists maximally and hold for 60 seconds; results are positive if carpal tunnel symptoms are reproduced
Posterior drawer test	PCL injury/stability	PCL deficiency results in a posterior sag (Godfrey sag) in the resting position—90 degrees flexion; posteriorly directed force produces the posterior drawer test to determine extent of laxity
Rebound tenderness	Peritoneal irritation	Increased pain on release of deep palpation

Rinne test	Hearing: air conduction is greater than bone conduction	Tuning fork is placed first on the mastoid bone; client detects sound; once sound is no longer heard, tuning fork is placed in front of the ear canal, where it should be heard
Rollover test	Evaluate elevated BP during pregnancy	Measure BP in left lateral; roll to supine; take BP again; retake BP in 5 minutes in supine position; positive test is an increase of more than 20 mm Hg at 5-minute reading
Romberg's test	Cerebellar functioning	Feet together, eyes closed; maintain balance; a positive Romberg's test is the inability to maintain balance
Straight leg raise	Nerve root irritation	Can be done sitting or supine; when sitting, both hip and knee are flexed at 90 degrees; slowly extend the knee; while supine, flex hip to 80 degrees; a positive test for either sitting or lying is pain that radiates down the leg at 30 degrees of flexion or less
Tinel's sign	Carpal tunnel syndrome	Tap at the volar surface of the wrist; results are positive if reproduces symptoms or tingling into median nerve distribution
Varus/valgus	Collateral ligament test	Valgus: full extension with pressure against lateral knee (tests MCL) Varus: full extension with pressure against medial knee (LCL)
Waddell's sign	Nonorganic physical signs	Tenderness that is nonanatomic or superficial, distraction, regionalization (inappropriate location of pain from normal neuroanatomy), overreaction
Weber's test	Hearing localization	Place the tuning fork on the forehead or in center of head; have client identify on which side it can best be heard

ACL, Anterior cruciate ligament; *CVA,* costovertebral angle; *DVT,* deep vein thrombosis; *PCL,* posterior cruciate ligament; *BP,* blood pressure; *MCL,* medial collateral ligament; *LCL,* lateral collateral ligament.

Review Questions

1. When percussing the chest of a client with chronic obstructive pulmonary disease (COPD), the nurse practitioner would expect to hear:
  a. A flat sound
  b. A tympanic sound
  c. A dull sound
  d. A hyperresonant sound

2. In assessing a client with a possible foreign body aspiration, the nurse practitioner would expect to find:
  a. "E" to "a" changes
  b. Clearer transmission of whispered sound
  c. Wheezes
  d. Crackles

3. When assessing a client with pneumonia, the nurse practitioner would expect to find all of the following *except:*
  a. Resonance on percussion
  b. Wheezes
  c. Crackles
  d. "E" to "a" changes with spoken sound

4. If a client can perform all extraocular movements, which cranial nerves are intact?
  a. II, IV, VII
  b. III, IV, VI
  c. II, III, V
  d. V, VI, VII

5. If a client has a biceps reflex, which spinal nerves are intact?
  a. Cervical 6, 7, 8
  b. Lumbar 2, 3, 4
  c. Cervical 5, 6
  d. Lumbar 5

6. When performing a pelvic exam, the nurse practitioner notes a bluish, soft cervix. This should be charted as a positive:
  a. Chadwick's sign
  b. Chandelier's sign
  c. Cullen's sign
  d. Brudzinski's sign

7. To assess for the presence of degenerative joint disease of the hip, the nurse practitioner should perform:
  a. Ortolani's test
  b. Hoover's test
  c. Lachman's test
  d. Patrick's test

8. A client weighs 126 pounds. The client's weight in kilograms is approximately:
  a. 277
  b. 57
  c. 25
  d. 630

Answers and Rationale

1. *Answer:* d (assessment).
  Rationale: Flat sounds indicate tissue, such as in the thigh area. Dull sounds indicate density and tissue such as that found in the liver. Tympanic sounds indicate air, but reflect a hollow reservoir such as the stomach. Hyperresonant sounds occur with trapped air as occurs in COPD.

2. *Answer:* c (assessment).

Rationale: Pneumonia and pleural effusions are associated with "e" to "a" changes (egophony) and whispered pectoriloquy. Crackles occur in pneumonia, congestive heart failure (CHF), and pulmonary fibrosis. Wheezes indicate an obstruction to airflow that may be produced by a narrowing of the bronchi (asthma) or a foreign body.

3. *Answer:* b (assessment).

Rationale: Pneumonia produces mucus and decreased air movement. On percussion there will still be resonance where air is moving. The alveoli are "sticky" and, when opening because of air movement, produce a crackling sound. Egophony ("e" to "a" changes) occur because of consolidation. Wheezes should not occur unless there is an obstruction.

4. *Answer:* b (analysis/diagnosis).

Rationale: Cranial nerve II is optic and produces vision. Cranial nerve III (oculomotor) is involved with EOMs. Cranial nerve IV (trochlear) produces EOMs. Cranial nerve V (trigeminal) supports jaw clenching and sensation to the face. Cranial nerve VI (abducens) produces EOMs. Cranial nerve VII (facial) allows grinning.

5. *Answer:* c (analysis/diagnosis).

Rationale: Triceps are related to cervical nerves 6, 7, 8. Knee reflex is associated with the spinal lumbar nerves 2, 3, 4. Lumbar nerve 5 is associated with an ankle reflex.

6. *Answer:* a (analysis/diagnosis).

Rationale: Chadwick's sign is an indication of pregnancy. Chandelier's sign is tenderness on movement of the cervix and indicates inflammation. Cullen's sign is discoloration around the umbilicus and indicates blood in the peritoneal cavity. Brudzinski's sign is flexion of the hips with passive flexion of the neck and indicates meningeal irritation.

7. *Answer:* d (assessment).

Rationale: Ortolani's test is positive in developmental dysplasia of the hip. A clunk occurs on abduction and external rotation of the hip. Hoover's test assesses malingering with back pain and involves harder pushing of one heel in the examiner's hand when the client raises the other leg. Lachman's test is used to assess anterior cruciate ligament (ACL) stability and requires force to be placed on the proximal tibia while the thigh is stabilized by the examiner's hand.

8. *Answer:* b (analysis/diagnosis).

Rationale: The conversion is 1 kg = 2.2 lb; 126 divided by 2.2 = 57.27, or 57 kg.

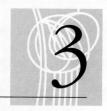

Common Presenting Problems and Symptoms

ABDOMINAL PAIN *Denise Robinson*

OVERVIEW
Definition

Pain that originates in the abdominal area.

Incidence

- Accounts for 5% of all emergency department (ED) visits and is the most frequently described reason for ambulatory visits within general adult and family practice settings.
- In 50% of patients with abdominal pain, no cause is identified.
- Most common causes are medical, not surgical. Surgical causes account for less than 15% of cases.

Pathophysiology

Common pathogenic mechanisms underlying acute (surgical) abdominal pain include perforation (hollow viscus), obstruction (intestinal, sigmoid volvulus), ischemia (mesenteric infarction), inflammation (diverticulitis with perforation, peritonitis), and hemorrhage (abdominal aneurysm, ulcers, ectopic pregnancy).

Nonemergency causes may include hepatitis, cholecystitis, gastritis, nephrolithiasis, pneumonia, hernia, pyelonephritis, endometriosis, and colon carcinoma. Pain impulses originate within the abdominal cavity and are transmitted via the autonomic and anterior/lateral spinothalamic tracts. Three major causes of pain exist. They are the following:

- Colic
- Ischemia
- Peritoneal inflammation

ASSESSMENT: SUBJECTIVE/HISTORY

It is important to quickly determine the acuity level; consider the worst possibilities first and then systematically exclude them from the differential. Assess for immediate surgery by checking vital signs and orthostatics. Palpate the abdomen. If the client has a boardlike abdomen with guarding, contact a surgeon immediately. If not in immediate danger, proceed with a more detailed history and physical.

History of Present Illness

- Location at onset and at present
- Radiation
- Aggravating factors (movement, coughing, respiration)
- Mitigating factors (position, lying still, vomiting, antacids, food)
- Mode of onset with progression (better, same, worse)
- Abruptness of onset, duration, and character (intermittent, steady, colicky)
- Previous similar episodes of the pain
- Severity (rated on a 1 to 10 scale); **remember older people tend to under-report pain;** to determine pain level in children, use visual analogue scale for pain or the "oucher" (Wong "smiley face") scale
- Last bowel movement; stools: tarry or bloody
- Urinary pattern (frequency, urgency, flank or back pain)

Women. Regardless of age, inquire about the following:
- Vaginal bleeding (including last normal menses)
- Sexual history
- Obstetric history
- Ectopic risk factors
- Pelvic inflammatory disease (PID)
- Intrauterine contraceptive device (IUD)
- Previous ectopic pregnancy, history of tubal surgery
- Infertility treatment

Men. Ask men about the following:
- Urologic history: hesitancy, nocturia, low urinary volume, lower abdominal distention
- Sexual history

Children. Question child, parent, or both about general indicators of illness, including the following:
- Activity level
- Appetite and food intake
- History of recent infection, current infections, and presence of fever
- Stool patterns

Symptoms

Anorexia, nausea, vomiting, and diarrhea are nonspecific symptoms but are significant in the presence of abdominal pain. The onset of pain before vomiting or diarrhea favors a diagnosis of acute abdomen. Patients with an acute abdomen usually have no desire for food.

Clients with an acute abdomen often have a paralytic ileus, so it is important to determine whether the common and often subjective report of constipation is really obstipation (absence of both stool and flatus). True obstipation is strongly suggestive of a mechanical bowel obstruction, especially when accompanied by progressively increasing abdominal distention or repeated vomiting.

Past Medical History

Ask about the following:
- Previous abdominal surgery
- Cardiovascular disease: hypertension (HTN)
- Analgesic use (acute or chronic)
- Alcohol use
- Other substance abuse (tobacco or recreational drugs)
- Weight change
- Past illness
- Risk factors such as recent travel (travel history may direct the examiner to the possibility of gastroenteritis or dysentery), environmental exposure, or immunologic suppression
- Medications
- Allergies
- Previous surgery, especially abdominal or gynecologic operations, is a common predisposing factor in bowel obstruction caused by adhesions.

Family History

Appendicitis, aortic aneurysm (20% chance in first degree relatives, especially men).

Psychosocial History

- Social history indicating intimate partner violence
- In female clients, menstrual and obstetric histories to rule out ectopic pregnancy, mittelschmerz, and endometriosis

Medication History

- Anticoagulant therapy has been implicated in the development of abdominal hematomas.

- Oral contraceptives have been associated with hepatic adenomas and with mesenteric infarction.
- Corticosteroids may mask the symptoms of advanced peritonitis.
- Nonsteroidal antiinflammatory drugs (NSAIDs) can lead to peptic ulcer disease.

Review of Systems

A complete review of systems should be performed (as allowed by the client's condition). Special attention should be given to cardiac, pulmonary, gynecologic, and genitourinary systems because abdominal pain may originate from these systems (e.g., angina, basal pneumonia, PID, pyelonephritis).

Children
- Weight loss
- Growth and developmental delay
- Fever
- Rash

ASSESSMENT: OBJECTIVE/ PHYSICAL EXAMINATION
Physical Examination

Perform a complete history and physical examination when possible. Important areas to stress include the following:
- Vital signs with orthostatics
- General observation: check for lymphadenopathy if concerned about mononucleosis and splenic rupture, note gait
- Cardiopulmonary system
- Abdominal, rectal, and pelvic examinations
  - Inspect abnormal pulsations, scars, character of skin, color, and temperature
  - Auscultate bruits, bowel sounds, character of sounds
  - Percuss for abdominal distention, shifting dullness in ascites
  - Palpate abdomen while observing for facial grimacing, involuntary guarding, organomegaly, or abnormal masses; measure abdomen if distention is present.

Special maneuvers to perform during the physical examination are shown in the maneuver table in Chapter 2.

Pediatric Abdominal Examination
- As much as possible, examine the young child while he or she is seated with the parent.
- Place the child's hand over your hand during palpation.
- Normal abdomen is rounded and scaphoid in children who are school-aged and younger.
- Attempts to elicit psoas and obturator signs in the young child are seldom helpful.

A

- Have child jump up and down to provide a clear indicator of the degree of abdominal pain.
- Use gentle percussion instead of the usual test for rebound tenderness.
- Palpate liver and spleen in all children, and the kidney in neonates.
- Examine the inguinal canal for hernias.

Diagnostic Procedures

History and physical examination alone can diagnose approximately 65% of acute surgical abdomen cases. However, supplemental examinations are necessary for diagnosis or exclusion of nonsurgical abdominal pain. Laboratory tests for all clients with severe abdominal pain include the following:

- Complete blood count (CBC) with differential, erythrocyte sedimentation rate (ESR)
- Urinalysis
- Stool sample for occult blood

Other tests that may be ordered depending on history and physical include the following:

- Renal and liver function tests (LFTs) (alanine aminotransferase [ALT], aspartate aminotransferase [AST], and alkaline phosphatase) amylase, chemistry
- Serum pregnancy test in women if the possibility of pregnancy exists (a necessity for women of childbearing age).
- Chest radiograph to rule out conditions that may mimic an acute abdomen, such as basal pneumonia or pleural effusion.
- Flat and upright radiograph films of abdomen to detect the presence of free air (perforated viscus), necessary before operation.
- Ultrasound to evaluate asymptomatic aortic aneurysm, gallstones.

DIAGNOSIS

Conditions to be considered in differential diagnosis of abdominal pain are shown in Table 3-1. The five big indicators that help identify those patients who need a surgical consult are:

- Fever
- Increased white blood cell (WBC) count

- Tachycardia
- Peritoneal signs
- Advanced age

The most common causes of acute abdominal pain are presented by age group in Table 3-2. If the patient has an appendix, appendicitis should be one of the first diagnoses considered for abdominal pain.

THERAPEUTIC PLAN

- Clients with minimal symptoms may be managed initially with clear liquids and analgesics (after surgical consultation).
- Therapy for moderate to severe pain and vomiting includes intravenous (IV) fluids, nasogastric suction, and correction of electrolyte imbalance. Antibiotics should be considered if the client has fever. Histamine (H_2) blockers may be indicated for the relief of gastritis and colicky pain.
- Advise client to avoid spicy or gas-producing foods.
- Refer client to physician or surgeon when appropriate.

Prevention

There is no prevention for abdominal pain.

EVALUATION/FOLLOW-UP

Advise adult client to return immediately if any of the following occur:

- Pain gets worse or is isolated in one area only
- Bloody emesis or stool
- Dizziness or syncope
- Abdomen becomes swollen
- Elevated temperature (>102° F orally)
- Difficulty passing urine
- Shortness of breath

Advise parent of **pediatric client** to return immediately if the child experiences any of the following:

- Pain increases or is isolated in one specific area only
- Bloody vomit or stool
- Walking bent over or holding the abdomen, or refuses to walk
- Pain in the testicle or scrotum

TABLE **3-1** Differential Diagnosis With Abdominal Pain

DIFFERENTIAL DIAGNOSIS	SYMPTOMS
SIGNIFICANT VOMITING OR DIARRHEA	
Bowel obstruction	No flatus, abdominal distention, vomiting, bowel sounds diminished or absent or with peristaltic rushes, abdominal radiograph shows air
Gastroenteritis	Crampy, diffuse abdominal pain that follows or coincides with a bout of diarrhea; cramping occurs primarily after meals
Gastroparesis	Epigastric fullness, reflux or vomiting of gastric contents may occur
Pregnancy	Morning sickness (i.e., nausea and vomiting) common during the first 12 weeks of pregnancy
Volvulus	See "Constipation" later in this table

Continued

TABLE **3-1** Differential Diagnosis With Abdominal Pain—cont'd

HEMATEMESIS OR MELENA

Aortic enteric fistula	Massive hematemesis or hematochezia
Diverticular disease	Acute abdominal pain and fever, LLQ tenderness and mass, increased WBC count, N/V are frequent; constipation or loose stools may be present
Malignancy	May be asymptomatic, may have dark or black stools
Polyps	May be asymptomatic, may have dark or black stools
Ulcers	Heartburn indigestion, RUQ pain with variable relationship to meals; in older patients the first sign may be peritonitis caused by perforation or anemia; melena, improved with antacids
Varices	Vomiting red emesis (hematemesis)

SYNCOPE

Aortic aneurysm	Tearing abdominal pain, severe middle to lower back pain; may radiate to genitals, sacrum or flank; pulsatile middle to upper abdominal mass, lower extremity ischemia
Ectopic pregnancy	Late or missed menses, breast tenderness, unexplained weight gain, lower quadrant abdominal pain, vaginal spotting, positive HCGa
Gastroenteritis	As "Significant Vomiting or Diarrhea" previously in this table
GI bleed	Vomiting of dark red or black emesis, black or bloody stools
Myocardial infarction	Gastritis, heartburn, nausea, diaphoresis, chest pain, arm numbness, SOB, fatigue; just doesn't feel right, worse with exercise

DYSURIA, URGENCY, FREQUENCY, OR HEMATURIA

Pyelonephritis	Fever, chills, flank pain and tenderness, and urgency, dysuria, and frequency
Renal colic	Severe flank pain, hematuria

CONSTIPATION

Bowel ischemia	Crampy, generalized or periumbilical pain, often severe
Bowel obstruction	No flatus, abdominal distention, vomiting, bowel sounds diminished or absent or with peristaltic rushes, abdominal radiograph shows free air
Diverticular disease	See "Hematemesis or Melena" previously in this table
Volvulus (occurs when the sigmoid twists around its base)	Severe, crampy abdominal pain; intractable retching with emesis; more common in adults than children; mean age at presentation is 8 years; predisposing factors in adults are institutionalization, chronic constipation and laxative abuse; Hirschsprung's disease and neurologic disorders are also predisposing factors; radiograph reveals an omega loop; surgery is most effective treatment method

RECTAL PAIN

Ovarian cyst	Vague local pressure, heaviness, cramping on affected side
Prostatitis	Fever, urgency, nocturia, perineal or suprapubic pain, low back pain, and fatigue

MISCELLANEOUS TOPICS NOT CATEGORIZED BY SYMPTOMS

Cholecystitis	RUQ pain, radiation to right shoulder, postprandial pain, especially after fatty food
Appendicitis	Diffuse abdominal pain, migration to RLQ, nausea is common, emesis follows the onset of pain; in **pregnant women,** the pain may not be in the classic RLQ—get obstetrical consultation, especially in second and third trimester for right-sided abdominal pain; progression of pain usually occurs over 36-48 hr.

Most common diagnoses are in bold type.

Data from American College of Emergency Physicians (1994). Clinical policy for the initial approach to patients with chief complaint of nontraumatic abdominal pain. *Annals of Emergency Medicine 23*(4), 906-922.

LLQ, Left lower quadrant; *WBC,* white blood cell; *N/V,* nausea/vomiting; *RUQ,* right upper quadrant; *GI,* gastrointestinal; *HCG,* human chorionic gonadotropin; *SOB,* shortness of breath; *RLQ,* right lower quadrant.

TABLE **3-2** Most Common Causes of Acute Abdominal Pain

AGE (YR)	COMMON	LESS COMMON
0-1	Intussusception Incarcerated hernias Gastroenteritis Hernia	Appendicitis Testicular torsion
2-5	Appendicitis Constipation Gastroenteritis Pneumonia	Intussusception UTI Testicular torsion
6-11	Appendicitis Pneumonia Constipation Gastroenteritis UTI	Intussusception Testicular torsion Incarcerated inguinal Hernia
12-21	Appendicitis Testicular torsion PID Mittelschmerz Pregnancy Ectopic pregnancy	UTI Pneumonia Constipation

Data from Finelli, L. (1991). Evaluation of the child with acute abdominal pain. *Journal of Pediatric Health Care, 5*(5), 251–256.

PID, Pelvic inflammatory disease; *UTI,* urinary tract infection.

- Abdomen becomes swollen or tender to the touch
- Difficulty urinating
- Shortness of breath

Follow up abdominal pain in 1 week, or sooner if the client has fever or prostrating pain. If no problems in 1 week, follow up in 1 month and then 6 months.

COMPLICATIONS

The most serious complication is missing the need for acute surgical intervention and consequently exacerbating the underlying cause of abdominal pain. Examples include the following:

- Rupture of appendix or diverticula with development of peritonitis
- Rupture of abdominal aortic aneurysm
- Perforation of peptic ulcer
- Symptoms of tachycardia or hypotension, suggesting a serious illness requiring a rapid assessment and disposition

REFERENCES

A one-antibiotic regimen for ruptured appendix. (1992). *Emergency Medicine, 24*(2), 742.

Acosta, R. Goldman, H., Crain, E. (2001). Computed tomography with rectal contrast in children with suspected appendicitis. *Academic Emergency Medicine, 8*(5), 446-447.

American College of Emergency Physicians. (1994). Clinical policy for the initial approach to patients with a chief complaint of nontraumatic acute abdominal pain. *Annals of Emergency Medicine, 23*(4), 906-922.

Burkhardt, C. (1992). Guidelines for the rapid assessment of abdominal pain indicative of acute surgical abdomen. *Nurse Practitioner, 17*(6), 43-46.

Finelli, L. (1991). Evaluation of the child with acute abdominal pain. *Journal of Pediatric Health Care, 5*(5), 251-256.

Mead, M. (1996). Detecting appendicitis. *Practice Nurse, 11*(7), 486-487.

Rice, P. (1996). Abdominal pain: predicting who will need an operation. *Emergency Medicine,* April, 14-25.

Robinson, D. (2000). Abdominal pain. In D. Robinson, P. Kidd, & K. Rogers (Eds.). *Primary care across the Lifespan* (pp. 309-330). St. Louis: Mosby.

Rothrock, S. (1996). When appendicitis isn't "classic." *Emergency Medicine, 28*(3), 108-124.

Stone, R. (1996). Primary care diagnosis of acute abdominal pain. *Nurse Practitioner, 21*(12), 19-40.

Review Questions

1. Which of the following tests should be performed first in clients with abdominal pain?
   a. Upper gastrointestinal (GI) series
   b. Colonoscopy
   c. Screen for *Helicobacter pylori*
   d. CBC and ESR

2. True obstipation is strongly suggestive of a mechanical bowel obstruction, especially when accompanied by which of the following?
   a. Pain after vomiting
   b. Diarrhea
   c. Increasing abdominal distention and repeated vomiting
   d. Nausea

3. If the client's presenting symptom is vague abdominal pain, with no abdominal tenderness or systemic symptoms, what should the nurse practitioner (NP) do?
   a. Consult with the surgeon right away.
   b. Reassess the client in 3 to 4 hours.
   c. Order needed laboratory tests.
   d. Send the client home.

4. Which of the following symptoms indicates the need for urgent surgical consultation?
   a. Achy pain at the umbilicus
   b. Abdominal pain followed by vomiting
   c. Temperature of 97.8° F
   d. Diarrhea after eating ice cream

5. Which of the following is an appropriate test to check for peritoneal irritation?
   a. Epigastric sign
   b. Tinel's sign
   c. Obturator sign
   d. Patrick's sign

6. While performing an abdominal examination for reported abdominal pain, you note a pause in inspiration. The client reports increased pain. You would note this as which of the following?

- **a.** A positive Murphy's sign
- **b.** A positive Phalen's maneuver
- **c.** Evidence of malingering
- **d.** A negative McBurney's sign

Answers and Rationales

1. *Answer:* **d** (analysis/diagnosis)
Rationale: Initial tests for abdominal pain include tests to rule out acute abdomen, such as CBC, ESR, stool for guaiac, chemistry. If the history and physical, and the first line tests are positive, a more thorough workup is performed (Robinson, 2000).

2. *Answer:* **c** (analysis/diagnosis)
Rationale: True obstipation is suggested when abdominal distention and repeated vomiting are present (Burkhardt, 1992).

3. *Answer:* **b** (implementation/plan)
Rationale: If there are no systemic symptoms and no abdominal pain on examination, the client can be reevaluated to determine progression of the illness (Mead, 1996).

4. *Answer:* **b** (assessment)
Rationale: Pain that is followed by vomiting is more indicative of a surgical abdomen. A normal temperature is 97.8° F and does not indicate a fever. Pain that is located at the umbilicus is less likely to be organic. Diarrhea after eating ice cream describes lactose intolerance (Stone, 1996).

5. *Answer:* **c** (assessment)
Rationale: Obturator signs indicate inflammation of the peritoneum. Tinel's sign is used for carpal tunnel syndrome; Patrick's sign indicates osteoarthritis of the hip. Epigastric sign is not a clinical test (Stone, 1996).

6. *Answer:* **a** (assessment)
Rationale: A positive Murphy's sign is described as a pause on inspiration caused by pain over the gallbladder. Phalen's maneuver is related to carpal tunnel syndrome. McBurney's point is located over the left lower quadrant and is related to appendicitis (Robinson, 2000).

ABDOMINAL PAIN RECURRENT IN CHILDREN *Denise Robinson*

OVERVIEW
Definition

Chronic or recurrent abdominal pain (RAP) in children is defined as abdominal pain lasting more than 3 months duration.

Incidence

- 10-15% of school aged children have RAP
- Occurs in 2 peaks:
  - First peak occurs between 5 and 7 years of age, equal frequency in boys and girls, occurs in 5-8% of children
  - Second peak between 8 and 12 years of age, more prevalent in girls with approximate prevalence of 25%

Pathophysiology

Some evidence suggests that abnormal bowel motility, constipation, and lactose intolerance may play a role. Others suggest that it may be an increased sensitivity of some children to visceral sensations (Stein, 2001). In most children, the causes are multifactorial and complex. About 10% have organic disease. Indicators of organic disease include the following:

- Pain further away from umbilicus
- Fever
- Weight loss
- Changes in bowel function or blood in stools
- Anemia
- Dysuria
- Elevated ESR
- Pain awakening child at night (Stein, 2001)

ASSESSMENT: SUBJECTIVE/HISTORY
History of Present Illness

Use questions delineated in the general abdominal pain section.

Symptoms

- Vague, crampy like abdominal pain, no radiation
- No constitutional symptoms such as weight loss, changes in bowel habit
- Functioning well at home and school

Aggravating Factors. Dairy products may increase pain.

Relieving Factors. The child may rest or sit quietly until pains go away.

Past Medical History

Past medical history is non-contributory.

Medication History

- Antibiotics (bacterial overgrowth)
- Acne medications (esophagitis)
- Tricyclic antidepressants (constipation)

Family History

- Irritable bowel syndrome (IBS)
- Peptic ulcer disease (PUD), pancreatitis or biliary disease
- Migraines

Psychosocial History

- The client may have a dysfunctional family interaction.
- Determine if symptoms of depression or anxiety are present.

ASSESSMENT: OBJECTIVE/PHYSICAL EXAMINATION

To identify RAP, use the same procedure described in *Abdominal Pain*.

DIAGNOSTIC PROCEDURES

RAP is a diagnosis of exclusion, so tests are done to rule out organic diseases. Initial tests should include the following:

- CBC, ESR
- Urine analysis (U/A) and culture
- Stool examination for ova and parasites and blood

Second line tests might include ultrasound (U/S) of abdomen and screening for *H. pylori*. Further tests can be ordered depending on the outcome of these tests. In RAP, the tests are all normal.

DIAGNOSIS

The differential diagnoses include the following:

- Acute abdomen
- PUD (night pain or pain on awakening)
- Constipation (pain in the evening or during dinner)
- Abdominal migraines (episodic nausea, abdominal pain, and significant emesis)
- Irritable bowel disease (pain in lower abdomen, cramping after meals and with activity, decrease in food intake, weight loss)
- IBS (intestinal dysmotility with diarrhea or constipation; pain in left lower quadrant [LLQ]; infrequent before late adolescence)

THERAPEUTIC PLAN
Nonpharmacologic Treatment

- Client should keep a prospective symptom diary (frequency of pain, related events, responses to intervention for 3-7 days).
- Client should increase fiber.
- Client should decrease ingestion of excessive undigested carbohydrates such as frequent juice intake.
- NP should provide reassurance to client that no organic causes have been found.
- NP should encourage client to continue normal activities (i.e., attend school).

Pharmacologic Treatment

- Client should take a fiber supplement (5 g/day); fiber tablets can be used in children more than 10 years old, and for those less than 10 there are fiber powders that can be mixed with juice.
- Empiric trials of antidepressants, antispasmodics, or anxiolytics are not appropriate.
- Trial of H_2-blocker may be appropriate if history and physical suggest a peptic origin.
- Bowel retraining may be appropriate if constipation is determined to be the cause.

Client Education/Prevention

- Reassure parents and child that there is no organic cause of RAP.
- Make sure parents and child are not made to think it is all in his/her head or that the client is crazy.
- Ensure continued follow-up as needed if pain continues.
- Facilitate discussion of ways to prevent constipation.
- Teach relaxation techniques to control feelings or sensations in different parts of the child's body.
- Discuss with parents and child when to seek medical attention.

EVALUATION/FOLLOW-UP

- Follow client every 2 weeks until improvement is seen in abdominal pain; close follow-up is important so the child and family do not feel abandoned.
- Of all clients experiencing abdominal pain, one third have pain that resolves spontaneously, one third continue to have recurrent pain, and one third develop other pain syndromes in adolescence and adulthood such as IBS or headaches.

COMPLICATIONS

There is no organic cause for RAP. Children with functional abdominal pain are likely to become adults with abdominal pain, although the symptoms may change in nature.

REFERENCES

Lake, A. (2001). Chronic abdominal pain in childhood: diagnosis and management. *American Family Physician.* Available online: http://www.aafp.org/afp/990401ap/1823.html. Accessed July 1, 2002.

Latimer, C., Bijur, P., & Gallagher, E. (2001). Validity and reliability of a visual analog scale to measure acute abdominal pain. *Academic Emergency Medicine, 8*(5), 484.

Rice, P. (1996). Abdominal pain: Predicting who will need an operation. *Emergency Medicine,* April, 14-25.

Robinson, D. (2000). Abdominal pain. In D. Robinson, P. Kidd, & K. Rogers (Eds.). *Primary care across the lifespan* (pp. 3-13), St. Louis: Mosby.

Sharfuddin, A., Gleason, W., & Odita, J. (2001). An 11 year old girl with chronic abdominal pain. *Clinical Pediatrics, 40*(4), 213-217.

Stein, M. (2001). Recurrent abdominal pain. *Pediatrics, 107*(4), 935-939.

Review Questions

1. Carly is a 10-year-old girl with complaints of abdominal pain. Which of the following historical data is consistent with a diagnosis of RAP?

a. Pain awakens Carly at night.
b. Carly has lost 5 pounds since the pain has started.
c. Carly has not missed any school because of the pain.
d. Vomiting is common when Carly gets the pain.

2. During the physical assessment, which of the comments made by Carly in response to palpation of her abdomen is consistent with the diagnosis of RAP?

a. "When you touch over my bone (suprapubic) it really hurts."
b. "It hurts the most when you tap on my side."
c. "It does not hurt when you press around my belly button."
d. "It makes me short of breath when you touch my tummy."

3. Which of the following comments by Steve, an 8-year-old diagnosed with RAP, indicates attainment of a realistic treatment goal?

a. "I hardly feel the pain anymore."
b. "I have a bowel movement every 5 days."
c. "I stay home from school whenever I get any abdominal pain."
d. "Now that I have gotten better, I don't have abdominal pain at night anymore."

4. Which of the following empiric drug choices is most appropriate for Carrie, an 11-year-old with RAP?

a. Naproxen (Naprosyn) 250 mg PO bid
b. Dicyclomine (Bentyl) 10 mg qid
c. Docusate sodium (Colace) 50 mg QD
d. Calcium polycarbophil (FiberCon) 1 tab 1-4×/day

5. The purpose of keeping an abdominal pain journal for 3-7 days is which of the following?

a. Monitor for fiber intake.
b. Determine the psychologic component to the pain.
c. Identify the patterns of the abdominal pain.
d. Monitor for fluid intake.

Answers and Rationales

1. *Answer:* **c** (assessment)
Rationale: RAP is a functional disorder and typically does not cause pain at night, weight loss, or vomiting with the pain. Those are symptoms typical of an organic problem. Most children with RAP function well at school and home despite the abdominal pain (Stein, 2001).

2. *Answer:* **c** (assessment)
Rationale: The history and physical of a client with RAP is usually normal. Flank pain is indicative of kidney problems; severe pain indicates an acute abdomen or organic problem. Dyspnea may be seen with pneumonia or organic causes of abdominal pain (Stein, 2001).

3. *Answer:* **a** (evaluation)
Rationale: If the plan of care is effective, the patient experiences the abdominal pain less frequently. In RAP, the pain should not occur at night—that is more indicative of an organic problem. The child with RAP should be encouraged to continue his or her normal activities. Staying home from school is not usually part of the plan of care. Constipation can exacerbate RAP, so a bowel movement (BM) every 5 days does not indicate that the plan of care has been followed (Lake, 2001).

4. *Answer:* **d** (implementation/plan)
Rationale: Increasing fiber in children with RAP has been shown to decrease abdominal pain. The use of pain medicine and antispasmodics should not be empiric choices for treatment. Although Colace may relieve constipation, the use of increased fiber is a better choice to treat the abdominal pain (Stein, 2001).

5. *Answer:* **c** (analysis/diagnosis)
Rationale: The use of an abdominal pain journal helps identify the extent of pain, determine patterns of pain, and actions that seem to relieve the pain. It serves as the basis for diagnosis of RAP (Lake, 2001).

ABDOMINAL AND DYSFUNCTIONAL UTERINE BLEEDING *Cheryl Kish*

OVERVIEW

Definition

Abnormal uterine bleeding represents a wide range of menstrual disturbances and clinical complaints related to the periodicity and amount of menstrual flow experienced by women as part of the process of menstruation (Box 3-1). Dysfunctional uterine bleeding (DUB) refers to abnormal uterine bleeding that has no demonstrable pathologic cause. Dysfunctional bleeding represents disordered balance in hormones during the menstrual cycle under the control of the hypothalamic–pituitary–ovarian (HPO) axis. Box 3-1 provides descriptions of abnormal uterine bleeding.

Incidence

Abnormal uterine bleeding accounts for 10%-15% of gynecologic client visits. Only 25% are found to have an anatomic or organic cause for the bleeding; in 75% of cases, the bleeding is categorized as dysfunctional because no demonstrable pathology is found. Dysfunctional

A

Box 3-1 Descriptions of Abnormal Uterine Bleeding

MENORRHAGIA (HYPERMENORRHEA)

Menorrhagia is a heavy or prolonged menses.

Examples

Examples of causes of menorrhagia include complications of pregnancy such as spontaneous abortion; blood dyscrasias in adolescents; leiomyomas; adenomyosis; endometrial polyps; anovulation.

HYPOMENORRHEA

Hypomenorrhea is a decreased duration and amount of menstrual flow; spotting at regular intervals.

METRORRHAGIA

Metrorrhagia is menstrual bleeding at irregular intervals; characteristics of flow can be normal.

MENOMETRORRHAGIA

Menometrorrhagia is frequent, excessive, and prolonged bleeding that occurs at irregular intervals.

POLYMENORRHEA

Polymenorrhea is bleeding that occurs too frequently; menstrual interval less than every 21 days.

Example

An example of a condition that causes polymenorrhea is a luteal phase defect.

OLIGOMENORRHEA

Oligomenorrhea is a decrease in the number of bleeding episodes; a menstrual interval greater than every 35 days.

AMENORRHEA (SECONDARY)

Secondary amenorrhea is an absence of menses for 6 months or longer in a woman with previously regular cycles.

POSTCOITAL BLEEDING

Postcoital bleeding is bleeding following the act of coitus.

Examples

Conditions that cause postcoital bleeding include cervical polyps and cervicitis.

INTERMENSTRUAL BLEEDING

Intermenstrual bleeding is spotting between normal periods.

Examples

Conditions that cause intermenstrual bleeding include cervical pathologic causes and breakthrough bleeding resulting from use of hormonal contraceptives.

---

bleeding occurs most commonly at either end of the reproductive cycle, most commonly because of anovulation. Teens account for 20% of those with dysfunctional bleeding; 50% of cases occur in perimenopausal women. An exact incidence is not available.

Pathophysiology

Normally, physiologic shedding of the uterine endometrium occurs monthly from the age of menarche (11-14 years) to menopause (45-55 years). This process is directed by the HPO axis and a complicated hormonal feedback loop. If these processes fail to occur in the proper sequence, dysfunctional uterine bleeding occurs. There is a wide variation for normal cycles; the following are the normally expected characteristics of normal menses:

- Frequency: every 28 days ± 2 (<21 days or >35 days considered abnormal)
- Duration: 4 days ± 2
- Amount of flow: 40 ml ±20; 80% of blood loss occurs in the first 48 hours (>80 ml total considered abnormal)

It is common for menses to be anovulatory and irregular for the first 20 cycles after menarche as the HPO axis matures. Again, at the end of the reproductive cycle, women become anovulatory, this time because of ovarian

failure, and dysfunctional bleeding is common. Otherwise, throughout a woman's menstrual experience, her own cycle characteristics, including amount of flow, serve as her standard for judging normalcy.

An important part of evaluating abnormal or dysfunctional uterine bleeding is determining if cycles are ovulatory or anovulatory. Table 3-3 compares the two.

ASSESSMENT: SUBJECTIVE/HISTORY

Because the diagnosis of abnormal uterine bleeding is one of exclusion, the value of a comprehensive history cannot be overemphasized. Because the cause of abnormal bleeding varies across the lifespan, noting the woman's age and the common risk factors is important to guide the history (Table 3-4).

History of Present Illness

Ask the woman to describe the duration and pattern of her symptoms. How frequently does she have this bleeding pattern? Is it a recent phenomenon or does it occur with most or all cycles? Has this pattern occurred since menarche? (New onset symptoms suggest a different pathology than a pattern existing since menarche.) Are there coincident or associated symptoms such as pain, postcoital bleeding, or dyspareunia? If bleeding is excessive, how many pads or tampons is she using in 24 hours

TABLE **3-3** Comparison of Ovulatory and Anovulatory Menstrual Cycles

OVULATORY CYCLES	ANOVULATORY CYCLES
Occur in a regular pattern	Have an unpredictable pattern
Often associated with dysmenorrhea	Not associated with dysmenorrhea
Associated with biphasic basal body temperature curve secondary to progesterone	Associated with monophasic basal body temperature curve
Positive LH on LH predictor kit secondary to LH surge	No LH surge
Molimina: premenstrual symptoms—breast tenderness, pelvic fullness, bloating, and mood changes	Absence of molimina symptoms
Mittelschmerz (transient pain associated with ovulation)	No mittelschmerz
Preovulatory cervical mucous clear with spinnbarkeit of 6 cm; postovulatory cervical mucous thick	Cervical mucous is relatively unchanging throughout the monthly cycle
Serum progesterone at midluteal phase 10 ng/ml; confirms ovulation	Serum progesterone at midluteal phase low

LH, Luteinizing hormone.

TABLE **3-4** Causes of Abnormal Uterine Bleeding by Age Group

<14 YEARS OLD	14-25 YEARS OLD	25-35 YEARS OLD	35-45 YEARS OLD	>45 YEARS OLD
Blood dyscrasias	Pregnancy	Pregnancy	Pregnancy	Hormone replacement therapy
Foreign bodies	Anovulation	Hormonal contraceptive use	Anovulation	Endometrial hyperplasia
Vaginitis	Hormonal contraceptive use	Cervicitis/STD	Endometrial hyperplasia	Polyps
Vaginal trauma	Cervicitis/STD	Anovulation	Fibroids	Endometrial cancer
Pregnancy	Psychologic (anorexia, bulimia, stress, excess exercise)	Vaginal trauma	Adenomyosis	Fibroids
	Vaginal trauma	Foreign bodies	Endometriosis	Coital injury related to atrophic vaginitis
	Foreign bodies	Fibroids	Endometrial cancer	Hypothyroidism and other systemic diseases
		Endometrial hyperplasia	Hormonal contraceptive use	
		Hypothyroidism and other systemic diseases	Cervical polyps	
			Hypothyroidism and other systemic disease	

STD, Sexually transmitted disease.

and what degree of saturation is occurring? To what extent does she leak through onto under clothes? Is she expelling clots or fragments of tissue? Could she be pregnant? When was her last menstrual period (LMP)? Are there symptoms of menopause? Are there signs of molimina, suggesting an ovulatory menstrual pattern? Has there been sexual abuse or insertion of a foreign body?

Past Medical History

Ask her to compare the current symptoms with her normal menstrual pattern. At what age did she start menstruating? Ask her to describe her usual cycles and characteristics of her usual menses. Ask about birth control now and in the past. Inquire about previous pregnancies and

their outcomes. Determine if there is a history of liver disease, renal disease, diabetes mellitus (DM), thyroid disease, blood dyscrasias, coagulation defects, surgical or dental procedures associated with heavy bleeding, anorexia or bulimia, or galactorrhea. Do her gums bleed with tooth brushing?

Identify all current medications, including prescription, over-the-counter (OTC), herbs, and supplements. Ask specifically about anticoagulants, heavy aspirin or NSAID use, oral contraception, depomedroxyprogesterone acetate (DMPA), levonorgestrel implants (Norplant), thyroid replacement or suppression, steroids, amphetamines, marijuana, or chemotherapy. Inquire about current weight in comparison with past weight; has there been recent gain or loss? Ask about date and results of last Pap smear. Inquire about previous sexually transmitted diseases (STDs) or PID and treatment.

Family History

Inquire about family history of leiomyoma and mother's age at menopause. Ask about family history of thyroid disease or DM, either of which in a woman may cause abnormal uterine bleeding.

Psychosocial History

Ask about mental illness, anorexia nervosa, and bulimia nervosa. Ask about exercise pattern because heavy exercise is associated with anovulation. Determine the last sexual act, whether voluntary or abusive.

Diet History

Complete a 24-hour diet recall especially in cases in which there is obesity or suspicion of an eating disorder or anemia.

ASSESSMENT: OBJECTIVE/PHYSICAL EXAMINATION
Physical Examination

A problem-focused physical examination, noting evidence of trauma, should be done with attention to the following components:

- Note vital signs. In cases of heavy or prolonged bleeding, assess for orthostatic effects. Take blood pressure (BP) while client is sitting, standing, and lying.
- Note weight, height, and body mass.
- Perform a skin inspection. Note acne, petechiae, bruising, and pallor. (Twenty percent of teens have abnormal bleeding related to blood dyscrasias, such as Von Willebrand's disease, discovered at menarche.)
- Note hair distribution pattern. (Hirsutism may indicate polycystic ovary syndrome [PCOS].)
- Examine heart and lungs.
- Examine thyroid. Check for nodules or diffuse enlargement. (Hypothyroidism often causes hypermenorrhea; hyperthyroidism often is associated with hypomenorrhea or irregular menses.)
- Examine breasts. Note Tanner stage. Note galactorrhea. Note color changes associated with pregnancy.
- Examine abdomen. Note tenderness, guarding, distention, and organomegaly. Note changes associated with pregnancy.
- Examine perineum. Note Tanner stage.
- Perform a pelvic examination. Note trauma to vaginal tissue. Assess cervix for lesions, erosion, cervical motion tenderness (CMT), and polyps. Note if os is closed or dilated. Note discharge or bleeding from cervical os.
- Perform a bimanual examination. Note size, contour, position, and tenderness of uterus. Assess adnexa for tenderness and masses.
- Perform a rectal examination. Rule out hemorrhoids or polyps as cause of bleeding.

Diagnostic Procedures

Dysfunctional uterine bleeding is a diagnosis of exclusion. The diagnosis is often used presumptively; expensive and invasive testing to rule out an organic cause is often not ordered until after medication treatment has failed. The most significant differential to consider is whether the presenting problem appears to be ovulatory or anovulatory. **If the problem is severe enough to require emergent intervention, the client should be referred immediately.**

The following diagnostic testing is appropriate in assessing abnormal uterine bleeding:

- CBC and differential should be done in all cases of menorrhagia to determine blood loss and platelet adequacy as well as presence of infection.
- Serum human chorionic gonadotropin (HCG) should be done on all women of childbearing age to rule out pregnancy-related bleeding.
- Other tests to perform if indicated by history and physical findings are LFTs, thyroid-stimulating hormone (TSH) levels, follicle-stimulating hormone (FSH) levels, coagulation studies, blood chemistry, Pap smear, cervical cultures, adrenal studies, and hormonal assays (progesterone, androgens, prolactin, gonadotropins).
- Perform an endometrial biopsy; this is appropriate for women more than 35 years old or at risk of endometrial cancer (oligomenorrhea, chronic anovulation) to rule out carcinoma or endometrial hyperplasia. The biopsy can be done as an office procedure with a pipelle to aspirate tissue. The procedure takes 30 to 45 seconds and causes some uterine cramping. Ibuprofen 600 mg to 800 mg PO 30 to 60 minutes before the procedure minimizes cramping.
- Ultrasonography is useful for identifying leiomyomas, polyps, or adnexal masses and measuring thickness of the endometrial stripe.
- Consider referral for a hysteroscopy or sonohysteroscopy (involves instillation of fluid into endometrial cavity to affect visualization).
- If systemic disease is suspected as a cause, perform appropriate testing. In cases of heavy bleeding in an adolescent girl, consider coagulation defects or blood dyscrasias and perform these tests: bleeding time, prothrombin time, and partial thromboplastin.

A

Box 3-2   Differential Diagnosis: Abnormal Uterine Bleeding

PREGNANCY COMPLICATIONS
Ectopic Pregnancy
Trophoblastic disease
Placenta previa
Spontaneous abortion

GENITAL TRACT INFECTIONS
Cervicitis
Endometritis

GENITAL TRACT TRAUMA
Laceration or abrasion
Sexual abuse or assault
Foreign body

GENITAL TRACT MALIGNANCY
Cervical cancer
Ovarian cancer
Endometrial cancer

PSYCHOSOCIAL FACTORS
Anorexia nervosa
Bulimia nervosa
Stress
Excessive exercise

GENITAL TRACT BENIGN LESIONS
Cervical polyps
Endometrial polyps

Leiomyoma
Endometriosis
Adenomyosis

SYSTEMIC DISEASE
Liver disease
Renal disease
Hyperprolactinemia
Adrenal disease
Blood discrasias
Coagulation defects
Polycystic ovary syndrome

MEDICATIONS/CONTRACEPTIVES
IUD
OCPs
HRT
DMPA
Lunelle
Norplant
Anticoagulants
Digitalis
Amphetamines
Marijuana

IUD, Intrauterine contraceptive device; *OCP*, oral contraceptive pill; *HRT*, hormone replacement therapy; *DMPA*, depomedroxyprogesterone acetate.

DIAGNOSIS

The differential diagnosis should consider the common causes of abnormal uterine bleeding for the client's age group (Box 3-2). **Pregnancy must always be considered, even with a history of reliable contraception and in many cases of denial of sexual activity where woman may be fearful of disclosure.**

THERAPEUTIC PLAN

Treatment depends on specific cause. Goals of treatment include control of acute bleeding episodes, restoration of normal menstrual patterns, and detection and treatment of any potentially damaging conditions.

Pharmacologic Treatment

If bleeding is severe, refer the woman to an emergency unit or obtain gynecologic consultation with hospitalization for IV conjugated estrogens, possibly a dilatation and curettage. Fluid and blood replacement may be necessary to stabilize the client. Various oral regimens of estrogen and progesterone follow for at least 3 months to prevent recurrence.

Treatment of nonemergent bleeding episodes depends on age and cause. Oral contraception can be used to control bleeding. The initial withdrawal menses may be heavy. Therapy is considered for 3 cycles. If contraception is desired, the oral contraceptive pills (OCPs) can be continued beyond that time. If the woman does not desire contraception, medroxyprogesterone acetate (MPA) 10 mg/day for 10 days each month or norethindrone 5 to 10 mg once to 3 times daily organizes the endometrial lining. Withdrawal of the progestin results in regular bleeding patterns. Progestin therapy can be extended to 14 or 21 days to achieve satisfactory cycling. Iron replacement may be needed for anemic individuals.

NSAIDs, which are prostaglandin inhibitors, especially mefenamic acid (Ponstel 500 mg tid), Naproxen (275 mg every 6 hours), meclofenamate (100 mg tid), and ibuprofen (400 mg every 6 hours), reduce blood loss by 20% to 30% and menstrual symptoms. Ideally, to prevent menorrhagia, these drugs are started 3 days before or at the onset of menses and continued 3 to 5 days.

Other drugs that can be used to decrease menstrual bleeding have high side effect profiles and cost, and generally require consultation or referral. These include danazol and GnRH agonists.

Hormone contraceptives can be used to help regulate menstrual patterns. **All bleeding after menopause is considered to be cancer until proven otherwise.**

Endometrial biopsy is essential for diagnosis. Cyclic or continuous combined hormone replacement therapy may be used to treat DUB in these individuals.

If systemic disease is identified as a cause of abnormal uterine bleeding, treatment of the underlying cause may solve the menstrual problems.

Nonpharmacologic Treatment

A menstrual diary can be a helpful adjunct to assessing abnormal uterine bleeding. In addition, it provides an opportunity for watchful waiting since some causes of DUB self-correct over one to two cycles, spontaneously resolving without intervention.

Pelvic examination may be deferred in very young teens who have classic symptoms of anovulatory cycles soon after menarche on the following conditions: normal hematocrit, not sexually active, and are reliable for follow-up care.

For women with menorrhagia who have no desire for future fertility, surgical treatment options are available when medical treatment fails. Short-term response may be achieved with dilatation and curettage. Endometrial ablation with laser or electrocautery is another option. In some cases, such as cervical cancer or leiomyomas, hysterectomy may be the option of choice. Clearly, these procedures are invasive and require the consent of a fully informed woman.

Client Education

- Explain the menstrual cycle and what factors may be causing the abnormal uterine bleeding.
- Pay particular attention to the adolescent's concerns about the effects of DUB on her lifestyle, including social engagements. Be prepared to deal with her concerns about hormone treatment and her parents' concerns about prescribed birth control for DUB. Provide reassurance to the girl and her parents that anovulatory and irregular periods are common for up to 20 months after menarche.
- Advise appropriately when extreme exercise, stress, or dietary patterns are contributing to abnormal uterine bleeding. For example, weight management for under- or overweight clients, relaxation techniques for stress.
- Teach women who are experiencing menorrhagia how to increase iron in their daily diets to minimize the risk of anemia.
- Educate clients about medications.
- Advise women to avoid increased activity during days of heaviest menstrual flow; to appreciate that prolonged standing and up-right positions increases flow; to avoid hot tubs during heavy flow; and to avoid aspirin for 1 week before expected menses.
- Advise women to change tampons every 2 hours to decrease potential for toxic shock syndrome (TSS). Teach women about the importance of good handwashing during menstrual hygiene. Review the facts about TSS. Box 3-3 provides summary information about TSS for the provider.
- Stress importance of follow-up as recommended, including annual Pap smears.
- Reinforce safe sexual practices.
- Because this may be the initial pelvic examination for the adolescent or young woman, provide anticipatory guidance related to the examination; use models or diagrams and equipment to explain the procedure. Allow the client to use a mirror to view her anatomy if desired. Be sure to interview the teen in private but

---

BOX 3-3 Summary Information about Toxic Shock Syndrome

Risk of TSS increases with use of tampons and diaphragms. Usually begins within 5 days of menstrual period in women who have used tampons. Nonmenstrual cases also occur.

Toxins causing TSS are produced by often asymptomatic *Staphylococcus aureus.*

Three conditions are required for TSS to occur:
   Colonization by bacteria
   Production of toxins
   Portal of entry

Symptoms include high fever (>38.9° C or 102° F); myalgia; nausea, vomiting and diarrhea; diffuse, sunburnlike rash; hypotension; agitation; confusion; erythema of pharynx, vulva, vagina, and conjunctiva; and desquamation of palms and soles 1-2 weeks after onset. Rash is absent on portions of body covered by tight clothing.

Mortality 5%-10%, often associated with organ failure or adult respiratory distress. Renal or cardiac insufficiency may occur.

Treatment involves supportive care, fluid replacement, removal of contaminated item, antibiotic therapy with beta lactamase-resistant antistaphylococcal agent, and management of cardiac or renal insufficiency.

Women diagnosed with TSS should not use tampons or diaphragms in the future.

Information from Smith, R. (1997). *Gynecology in primary care.* Baltimore: Williams & Wilkins; Tierney, L.M., McPhee, S.J., & Papadakis, M.A. (2001). *Current medical diagnosis and treatment.* New York: Lange Medical Books/McGraw-Hill.
TSS, Toxic shock syndrome.

allow support person to be present for examination if the client desires. Be cautious about confidentiality with adolescent client accompanied by a parent.

Referral

Women who are hemodynamically unstable because of excessive menstrual bleeding should be referred to either an ED or a gynecologist. Those with an uncertain diagnosis and those unresponsive to treatment should be referred.

Prevention

In general, there is no way to prevent most cases of abnormal uterine bleeding.

EVALUATION/FOLLOW-UP

The recommended follow-up for abnormal bleeding depends on its cause and the treatment modality prescribed.

COMPLICATIONS

Clearly, abnormal uterine bleeding affects the quality of women's lives because of its unpredictability and disruptive inconvenience. Women with menorrhagia are at risk for hypovolemic shock with its inherent sequela and potential threat to life. Those who use tampons are at risk for toxic shock syndrome.

DUB patterns that involve irregular periods complicate attempts to become pregnant or make accidental pregnancy a greater risk. Anovulatory cycles that are allowed to continue place women at risk of endometrial cancer and osteoporosis.

REFERENCES

Hawkins, J. W., Roberto-Nichols, D. M., & Stanley-Haney, J. L. (1997). *Protocols for nurse practitioners in gynecologic settings.* New York: Tiresias.

Hillard, P. J. (1999). *Diagnosing and controlling abnormal uterine bleeding.* Contemporary Adolescent Gynecology. (Continuing Education Program–National Association of Nurse Practitioners in Reproductive Health.) Montvale, NJ: Medical Economics.

Mehring, P. (1997). Uterine bleeding: Evaluating this common complaint. *Advance for Nurse Practitioners, 5*(11), 27-32.

Oriel, K. A. & Schrager, S. (1999). Abnormal uterine bleeding. *American Family Physician, 60*(5), 1371-1382.

Schnare, S. M. (2000). *Abnormal and dysfunctional uterine bleeding.* Women's Health Care in the New Millenium Conference. National Association of Nurse Practitioners in Women's Health. October 11-14, 2000, Albuquerque, New Mexico.

Smith, C. B. (1998). Pinpointing the cause of abnormal uterine bleeding. *Women's Health in Primary Care, 1*(10), 835-844.

Smith, M. A. & Shimp, L. A. (2000). *20 common problems in women's health care.* New York: McGraw-Hill.

Smith, R. (1997). *Gynecology in primary care.* Baltimore: Williams & Wilkins.

Tierney, L. M., McPhee, S. J., & Papadakis, M. A. (2001). *Current medical diagnosis and treatment.* New York: Lange Medical Books/McGraw-Hill.

Review Questions

1. Mrs. Kimbell is a 54-year-old woman, who presents with vaginal bleeding of several days' duration. She is concerned because her LMP was nearly 2 years ago. She asks, "Why is this happening now?" This presentation is consistent with a diagnosis of which of the following?
- **a.** Uterine fibroids
- **b.** Perimenopause
- **c.** Endometrial cancer
- **d.** Luteal dysfunction

2. Which of the following laboratory studies should be done on any woman with excessive vaginal bleeding?
- **a.** Serum HCG
- **b.** FSH
- **c.** Hematocrit and hemoglobin (Hgb)
- **d.** TSH

3. Which of the following must be included in the physical examination of a 38-year-old woman who reports contact bleeding?
- **a.** Uterine biopsy
- **b.** Papanicolaou smear
- **c.** Palpation of thyroid
- **d.** IUD string visualization

4. Beverly, age 13, is brought into the clinic by her mother, who is concerned about the girl's irregular periods. She reports that Beverly started menstruating a year ago and has had periods only every few months. History is unremarkable and physical examination is normal. Which action is most appropriate?
- **a.** Schedule Beverly for an immediate bone age assessment.
- **b.** Order a serum chemistry, thyroid profile, FSH levels, and dehydroepiandrosterone (DHEA) levels.
- **c.** Refer Beverly to a gynecologist that specializes in adolescent health.
- **d.** Reassure them both that irregular periods are common in the initial 20 months.

5. Which of the following findings on examination is consistent with a diagnosis of toxic shock syndrome in 16-year-old Meredith?
- **a.** Fever, sunburnlike rash, hypotension, and watery diarrhea
- **b.** Purulent vaginal discharge, palpitations, agitation, and injected conjunctiva
- **c.** Severe uterine cramping, chills, lethargy, and icteric sclera
- **d.** Subnormal temperature, strawberry tongue, adenopathy, and pelvic pain

6. Sally presents with sudden onset of severe uterine cramping, backache, and excessive bright red uterine bleeding. Her LMP was 2 months ago. Examination reveals a slightly enlarged uterus and a dilated cervical os. Which diagnosis is suspected?

a. Threatened abortion
b. Chlamydia cervicitis
c. Leiomyoma
d. Cervical polyps

7. Which of the following women should definitely have an endometrial biopsy as part of her evaluation of excessive uterine bleeding?

   a. A 16-year-old with a history of gonorrhea.
   b. A 31-year-old who uses a diaphragm for contraception.
   c. A 34-year-old who takes thyroid hormone daily.
   d. A 50-year-old with menopausal symptoms.

8. Charlene complains of a sudden change in her menstrual pattern; her periods, which were once regular, now occur every 40 to 45 days. Given this description, the family NP offers the following description in her notes:

   a. Hypomenorrhea
   b. Metrorrhagia
   c. Oligomenorrhea
   d. Amenorrhea

9. Petra, age 38, complains of pelvic pressure and backache and says that her menses have become heavier in the last 6 months. Examination reveals a 12-week size uterus with irregular contour. These factors are consistent with a diagnosis of which of the following?

   a. Missed abortion
   b. Uterine fibroid
   c. Cervical stenosis
   d. Luteal phase deficiency

10. The NP is treating 22-year-old Nancy for dysfunctional bleeding. The NP ruled out an anatomic cause and treated Nancy for 7 days with a high dose estrogen and progesterone. Appropriate management now includes which of the following?

   a. Low-dose oral contraceptives
   b. Four more weeks of high dose estrogen and progesterone
   c. Hysteroscopy
   d. NSAIDs

Answers and Rationales

1. *Answer:* **c** (assessment)
   Rationale: Postmenopausal bleeding should be considered to be endometrial cancer until proven otherwise (Oriel & Schrager, 1999).

2. *Answer:* **a** (assessment)
   Rationale: Pregnancy must always be ruled out as a cause of abnormal uterine bleeding in women of reproductive age (Smith, 1997).

3. *Answer:* **b** (analysis/diagnosis)
   Rationale: Contact bleeding, also known as postcoital bleeding, is often associated with cervical abnormalities: erosion, polyps, and cancer. Pap smear, the gold standard for screening cervical cancer, should be done (Smith, 1998).

4. *Answer:* **d** (implementation/plan)
   Rationale: Reassurance is appropriate for this young woman and her mother. Because of anovulatory cycles during the first 1 to 2 years of menses, irregular periods are common (Hillard, 1999).

5. *Answer:* **a** (assessment)
   Rationale: High fever, sunburnlike rash, confusion, nausea, vomiting, watery diarrhea, and hypotension are all classic symptoms of toxic shock syndrome (Smith, 1997).

6. *Answer:* **a** (analysis/diagnosis)
   Rationale: An enlarged uterus, cramping, excess bleeding with a LMP 2 months previously, and a dilated cervical os are clinical findings consistent with a diagnosis of a threatened abortion (Smith, 1998).

7. *Answer:* **d** (implementation/plan)
   Rationale: As women age, their risk for endometrial carcinoma increases. An endometrial biopsy is an appropriate diagnostic test in a 50-year-old with dysfunctional uterine bleeding (Oriel & Schrager, 1999).

8. *Answer:* **c** (assessment)
   Rationale: Oligomenorrhea is the description for a menstrual interval >35 days (Smith, 1997).

9. *Answer:* **b** (analysis/diagnosis)
   Rationale: An enlarged uterus with an irregular contour and a history of pelvic fullness, backache, and menorrhagia are consistent clinical features of fibroids (Oriel & Schrager, 1999).

10. *Answer:* **a** (implementation/plan)
   Rationale: Low dose OCPs for 3 months after acute management with high dose estrogen and progesterone is an appropriate management strategy. If the client desires contraception, the OCPs are continued; if not, oral progesterone 10 mg/day each month is prescribed (Smith, 1998).

ACNE VULGARIS   *Denise Robinson*

OVERVIEW
Definition

Acne is a chronic follicular eruption at the pilosebaceous unit that begins as a comedone. Papules, pustules, and cysts develop if an inflammatory reaction occurs. Other disorders have been labeled acne, such as neonatal acne and steroid acne. These disorders, better labeled acneiform, originate with inflammation, skipping the comedone stage.

Incidence

Acne vulgaris affects nearly 17 million people in the United States. The peak onset is at puberty. Boys are affected more than girls; nearly 100% of boys have acne by age 16. The prevalence decreases in adulthood; it is 8% among those 25 to 34 years old and 3% among adults 35 to 44 years old. Acne vulgaris usually improves during pregnancy; however, exacerbations may also occur.

Pathophysiology

The exact pathogenesis of acne is still not completely understood. The cause is multifactorial and is most influenced by the following factors:

- Excessive sebum production: The rate of sebum production is determined genetically. The production of sebum is increased by the presence of androgens.
- Comedogenesis: The follicle canal becomes blocked by the sebum, resulting in the formation of comedones. These may be open comedones, or blackheads, and closed comedones, or whiteheads. Comedogenesis occurs in sebaceous follicles only.
- *Propionibacterium* acnes: The presence of *P.* acnes causes the inflammatory aspects of acne. This bacterium is benign and resides on the skin at all times.

Factors Increasing Susceptibility

Lithium, isoniazid, and phenytoin are some of the most common drugs that cause drug-induced acne.

Protective Factors

- Age (rare over 44 years of age)
- Female gender

NOTE: *Dirty skin does not contribute to acne.*

ASSESSMENT: SUBJECTIVE/HISTORY
Symptoms

Clients usually complain of a combination of both black and white comedones with inflammation characterized by periodic "flare-ups."

Past Medical History

Determine the timing of the onset of pubertal changes in relationship to the increase in acne. Females with cystic acne should be assessed for hirsutism and a history of irregular menses to rule out polycystic ovary disease.

Medication History

Oral and injectable steroids, both prescribed and illicit, should be noted.

Family History

Ask about parental and sibling history of acne.

Dietary History

Dietary habits do not contribute to acne.

Home Treatments

Ask about type of soap used, frequency of face washing, OTC treatments tried, and use of cosmetics.

Work History

Is the client working in a fast food restaurant around hot grease?

Psychosocial History

Is the acne of concern to the client? Does the client's appearance inhibit social interactions?

ASSESSMENT: OBJECTIVE/PHYSICAL EXAMINATION
Physical Examination

A problem-oriented physical assessment should be conducted, with attention to the skin on the face, chest, neck, and upper back.

- Adolescents: Assess pubertal stage and hirsutism in females with cystic acne.
- Skin: Assess the severity of the lesions. Assess for scarring.
- Determine the grade of the acne.
  - Grade I: Pure comedonal acne
  - Grade II: Mild papular acne
  - Grade II to III: Papulopustular and cystic acne
  - Grade III to IV: Persistent pustulocystic acne
  - Grade V: Pustulocystic nodular acne

Diagnostic Procedures

No diagnostic tests are indicated.

DIAGNOSIS

Differential diagnosis includes the following:

- Acneiform lesions, such as drug-induced acne
- Neonatal acne
- Acne conglobata
- Rosacea

THERAPEUTIC PLAN
Nonpharmacologic Treatment

Wash face bid with mild soap (e.g., Ivory, Dove). Do not rub skin vigorously.

Pharmacologic Treatment

Treatment options depend on the severity of the acne lesions. Understanding the pathogenesis is the key to choosing the proper treatment. Treatment may need to be long-term to avoid exacerbations.

Topical Treatment
Pure Comedonal Acne (Grade I). Several formulations of tretinoin (Retin-A) exist, with cream (0.025%, 0.05%, or 0.1%) being the most mild, followed by gel (0.01% or 0.025%) and liquid (0.05%). To avoid overdrying the skin, the treatment should be initiated on an every-other-day basis.

Mild Papular Acne (Grade II). Benzoyl peroxide is available only as a 5% or 10% gel by prescription. Begin treatment slowly, with every-other-day application to avoid overdrying of the skin.

Papulopustular Acne (Grades II-III). Combination therapy is with tretinoin and benzoyl peroxide, each applied once daily, or with tretinoin and a topical antibiotic, especially in inflammatory acne. Topical clindamycin (1%) is available in solution, lotion, and gel formulations.

Systemic and Combination Treatments

Papulopustural and Cystic Acne (Grade III or IV). More severe acne may require systemic therapy with oral antibiotics. The first-line choice is most commonly tetracycline, 500 to 1000 mg/day, decreased gradually to a goal of 250 mg/day or every other day. Erythromycin, minocycline, doxycycline, and occasionally trimethoprim-sulfamethoxazole may also be prescribed.

Females with Mild to Moderate Acne. These clients may respond well to topical treatment and the addition of an OCP. OCPs reduce endogenous androgen production and decrease the bioavailability of circulating androgens. Research has demonstrated that combination OCPs containing levonorgestrel, gestodene, and desogestrel as the progestin component have decreased acne in women. However, few studies have compared different formulations of pills with each other.

Severe Cystic Acne with Scarring (Pustulocystic Nodular) (Grade V). Refer client to dermatology for isotretinoin (Accutane), 1 mg/kg daily for 5 months. Get consent form for all females before beginning therapy. Perform pregnancy test before initiation.

Client Education

- Wash the skin bid with a gentle soap.
- Use a moisturizer unless skin is extremely oily.
- All cosmetics should be removed nightly.
- Instruct the client not to pick at lesions.
- Warn the client that improvement will not be noted until after 4 to 6 weeks of treatment.
- Sunscreen and sun protection must be used with tretinoin, oral tetracycline, doxycycline, and isotretinoin. The sunscreen should be oil free.
- Tretinoin should be applied with the three-dot method. Dispense a pea-sized amount on the finger, divide it into three smaller dots, and rub it into the affected area.
- Women of childbearing age must be using an effective contraceptive method 1 month before starting isotretinoin, when taking isotretinoin, and for 1 month after discontinuation.
- Cholesterol and triglyceride levels must be monitored during isotretinoin treatment.
- Clients receiving isotretinoin should be advised to avoid excessive alcohol consumption.

Referral

- Clients in need of isotretinoin treatment
- Females with cystic acne, irregular menses, and hirsutism, for hormonal evaluation
- Clients with significant depressive symptoms as a result of the acne

Prevention

Avoid scarring by not manipulating lesions.

EVALUATION/FOLLOW-UP

Reevaluate at 4 to 6 weeks and consider combination treatments. Assess for satisfaction with medication and for problems with skin irritation. Note the number and types of lesions present. Consider combination treatment if current treatment is not decreasing the lesions.

COMPLICATIONS

Scarring and permanent body image problems are possible.

REFERENCES

Berger, T. (2001). Skin, hair, and nails. In L. Tierney, S. McPhee, & M. Papadakis, (Eds.), *Current medical diagnosis.* McGraw-Hill, NY.

Berson, D.S., & Shalita, A.R. (1995). The treatment of acne: The role of combination therapies. *Journal of the American Academy of Dermatology, 32,* S31-S41.

Hurwitz, S. (1995). Acne treatment for the '90s. *Contemporary Pediatrics, 12*(8), 19-32.

Kaminer, M.S., & Gilchrest, B.A. (1995). The many faces of acne. *Journal of the American Academy of Dermatology, 32,* S6-S14.

Leyden, J.J. (1995). New understandings of the pathogenesis of acne. *Journal of the American Academy of Dermatology, 32,* S15-S25.

Peters, S. (1997). Saving face: Treating adolescents affected by acne vulgaris. *ADVANCE for Nurse Practitioners, 5*(3), 43-46, 49, 64.

Usatine R., Quan M., Strick R. (1998). Acne vulgaris: a treatment update. *Hospital Practice 33*(2), 111-117.

Review Questions

1. Acne vulgaris can be differentiated from acneiform causes of acne by the presence of which of the following?

   a. Inflammatory pustules
   b. Comedones
   c. Cystic lesions
   d. Scarring

2. Which of the following instructions should be given to a client using tretinoin (Retin-A) for treating acne?

   a. Apply generously to affected area.
   b. Apply sunscreen to affected area.

A

   c. Monitor for unusual hair growth.
   d. Use birth control.

3. Which of the following medication changes is the most effective for the client with very dry skin and continued inflammatory acne after 6 weeks with topical tretinoin cream?
   a. Discontinue the topical tretinoin and initiate topical antibiotic cream.
   b. Initiate therapy with systemic isotretinoin.
   c. Change the treatment to topical tretinoin gel.
   d. Continue the topical tretinoin at night with the addition of a topical antibiotic in the morning.

4. Which of the following is the recommended phone triage for an adolescent reporting severe burning sensations after 2 weeks of treatment with tretinoin cream twice daily?
   a. Discontinue treatment immediately and schedule office visit for allergic reaction.
   b. Decrease the use of the medication to once daily.
   c. Encourage the adolescent to apply the medication immediately after washing the face with a mild soap.
   d. Change the prescription to a gel formulation to decrease irritation.

5. The NP would like to prescribe Accutane for a 17-year-old female patient. Before considering this course of therapy, the NP should do which of the following?
   a. Perform a pregnancy test.
   b. Determine if the client has been on Accutane before.
   c. Perform a baseline CBC.
   d. Instruct the patient not to take tetracycline with the drug.

Answers and Rationales

1. **Answer: b** (analysis/diagnosis)
   Rationale: True acne vulgaris is characterized by an eruption of the pilosebaceous unit (the sebaceous gland and hair follicles) that begins as a comedone.

2. **Answer: b** (implementation/plan)
   Rationale: Tretinoin should not be confused with isotretinoin. Isotretinoin is teratogenic. Tretinoin should be applied sparingly because of its drying effect. Sunscreen should be used because of a higher likelihood of sunburn during use.

3. **Answer: d** (evaluation)
   Rationale: Combination therapy with tretinoin and topical antibiotic formulations are highly effective in the treatment of inflammatory acne.

4. **Answer: b** (evaluation)
   Rationale: Topical tretinoin can be highly irritating to the skin, so therapy should begin with daily or every-other-day application. Cream formulations are less irritating than gel formulations. The tretinoin should be applied 20 to 30 minutes after washing with a mild soap to decrease irritation to the skin.

5. **Answer: a** (implementation/plan)
   Rationale: Accutane is a teratogenic drug. It is imperative that pregnancy be ruled out before starting therapy and that contraceptives be used 1 month before and 1 month discontinuing therapy.

ADDISON'S DISEASE   *Pamela Kidd*

OVERVIEW
Definition

Addison's disease is a condition caused by an insufficient amount of adrenocorticotropic hormone (ACTH) resulting from a primary or secondary dysfunction of the adrenal cortex.

Incidence

- Found in 4 per 100,000 of the population.
- Can occur among all age groups.
- Appears most commonly between the ages of 30 and 50 years.
- Autoimmune destruction of the adrenals most commonly occurs before age 15.
- Adrenal hemorrhage in children is usually caused by meningococcal and pseudomonas septicemia.

Pathophysiology

The destruction of the adrenal cortex leads to a deficiency in glucocorticoids (e.g., cortisol) and mineralocorticoids (e.g., aldosterone). In Addison's disease, 90% of the adrenal cortex must be destroyed before the disease manifests itself. The lack of cortisol causes a decreased gluconeogenesis and liver glycogen and an increased insulin sensitivity with resulting hypoglycemia. The decrease in aldosterone results in hyponatremia and hyperkalemia. Most cases are related to autoimmune destruction of the adrenals. The remaining cases are due to tuberculosis, fungal infections, metastases to the adrenal glands, adrenal hemorrhage, surgical procedure of bilateral adrenalectomy, cytomegalovirus infection, acquired immunodeficiency syndrome (AIDS), and medications such as ketoconazole, aminoglutethimide, metyrapone, trilostane, mitotane, suramin, RU 486, etomidate, rifampin, and phenytoin. In adults, adrenal hemorrhage can occur as a result of anticoagulant therapy and spontaneous coagulopathy.

ASSESSMENT: SUBJECTIVE/HISTORY
Most Common Symptoms

- Adults most commonly complain of weakness, fatigue, and weight loss. Other possibilities include anorexia, nausea, vomiting, abdominal discomfort, diarrhea, dizziness, and salt craving.

- Children may experience fatigue, weakness, failure to gain weight or loss of weight, salt craving, and vomiting.

Associated Symptoms

- Hyperpigmentation of the skin and mucous membranes may give clients the appearance of having a deep suntan. This symptom only appears if ACTH is elevated.
- Pain may occur in the abdomen, back, or flank areas.
- Mental changes such as depression, apathy, and confusion often occur.

Past Medical History

- Hypoglycemia
- Hypotension
- Amenorrhea, primary ovulatory failure
- Recent surgery or trauma

Medication History

Ask about recent use of ketoconazole, aminoglutethimide, metyrapone, trilostane, mitotane, suramin, RU 486, etomidate, rifampin, or phenytoin.

Family History

Inquire about autoimmune disorders.

Dietary History

- Salt cravings
- Weight loss

Psychosocial History

- Depression
- Apathy
- Confusion
- Decreased libido

ASSESSMENT: OBJECTIVE/PHYSICAL EXAMINATION
Physical Examination

A complete physical examination should be performed with particular attention to the following:
- Vital signs (orthostatic hypotension)
- Weight (loss of weight)
- Cardiovascular (tachycardia)
- Musculoskeletal (muscle wasting, weakness)
- Skin (hyperpigmentation of buccal mucosa, pressure areas: knuckles, elbows, creases of hands, areolae, and new scars)
- Hair distribution (women: loss of axillary or pubic hair)

Diagnostic Procedures

The best screening tool for Addison's disease is the ACTH stimulation test. Perform the following steps:
1. Draw baseline serum cortisol, ACTH, and aldosterone levels.
2. Inject synthetic ACTH (Cortrosyn 0.25 mg) intravenously.
3. Measure cortisol levels at 30 and 60 minutes after injection.

Interpretation. A typical response to ACTH stimulation is a minimum 10 mg/dL rise in cortisol levels above baseline and a maximum 18 mg/dL rise in cortisol levels at 60 minutes. An individual with primary adrenal insufficiency exhibits no response to ACTH stimulation. With secondary adrenal insufficiency, the response may be normal or blunted to the ACTH stimulation.

Chemistry Profile. Chemistry results may reveal hyponatremia, hypoglycemia, or hyperkalemia.

DIAGNOSIS

The differential diagnosis includes the following:
- Depression
- Anorexia nervosa
- Myasthenia gravis
- Tuberculosis
- AIDS
- Salt-losing nephritis
- Gastrointestinal disease (related to symptoms of nausea, vomiting, abdominal pain, and diarrhea)

THERAPEUTIC PLAN
Nonpharmacologic Treatment

Not applicable.

Pharmacologic Treatment. In primary adrenal insufficiency, cortisol and mineralocorticoids must be replaced. Cortisol is replaced with hydrocortisone 20 to 30 mg daily. Mineralocorticoids are replaced with fludrocortisone 0.05 to 2 mg daily. In secondary adrenal insufficiency, cortisol only is replaced.

CLIENT EDUCATION

- Signs and symptoms of adrenal insufficiency
- Self-injection of hydrocortisone for occasions when client is unable to take oral medications
- Emergency kit of hydrocortisone
- Medic-Alert bracelet or necklace
- Family included in education
- Lifelong need for replacement therapy
- Diet with liberal sodium intake (3000 mg/day)

Referral

Refer to a physician or endocrinologist for evaluation and treatment.

Prevention

Treat all infections immediately and vigorously. Increase dose of cortisol. Anticipate need for increased cortisol during times of stress (e.g., surgery).

EVALUATION/FOLLOW-UP

Monitor electrolytes every 3 to 4 months during the first year of therapy.

COMPLICATIONS

Death without replacement of cortisol and mineral corticoids.

REFERENCES

Barker, L.R., Burton, J.R., & Zieve, P.D. (1995). *Principles of ambulatory medicine.* Baltimore: Williams & Wilkins.

Brosnan, C., & Gowing, N. (1996). Addison's disease. *British Medical Journal, 312,* 1085-1087.

Davis-Martin, S. (1996). Disorders of the adrenal glands. *Journal of the American Academy of Nurse Practitioners, 8,* 323-326.

Gance-Cleveland, B. (2001). Addison's Disease. In D. Robinson, P. Kidd, & K. Rogers (Eds.), *Primary care across the lifespan.* Mosby: St. Louis.

Gumowski, J., & Loughran, M. (1996). Diseases of the adrenal gland. *Nursing Clinics of North America, 31,* 747-768.

Hay, W., Groothius, J., Hayward, A., & Levin, M. (1997). *Current pediatric diagnosis and treatment.* Norwalk, CT: Appleton & Lange.

Loriaux, T. (1996). Endocrine assessment: Red flags for those on the front lines. *Nursing Clinics of North America, 31,* 695-712.

Price, S., & Wilson, L. (1997). *Pathophysiology: Clinical concepts of disease processes.* St. Louis: Mosby.

Rusterholtz, A. (1996). Interpretation of diagnostic laboratory tests in selected endocrine disorders. *Nursing Clinics of North America, 31,* 715-724.

Review Questions

1. Which of the following statements indicates the client understands information provided about Addison's Disease?
   a. "I need to follow a no added salt (NAS) diet."
   b. "I have a life-long disease."
   c. "I need to decrease my cortisol dose in times of stress."
   d. "I can occasionally skip my medicine."

2. The most common causes of Addison's disease in children are which of the following?
   a. AIDS/syphilis
   b. Tuberculosis/bronchitis
   c. Adrenal hemorrhage/surgery
   d. Autoimmune process/genetic

3. Systems most commonly affected by Addison's disease include which of the following?
   a. Cardiovascular, ophthalmic, musculoskeletal
   b. Musculoskeletal, skin, ophthalmic
   c. Musculoskeletal, cardiovascular, skin
   d. Cardiovascular, skin, neurologic

4. A client with Addison's disease caused by a primary insufficiency typically responds to the ACTH stimulation test with which of the following?
   a. Cortisol levels at baseline 5 mg/dL; 30 minutes after injection 10 mg/dL; 60 minutes after injection 15 mg/dL
   b. Cortisol levels at baseline 5 mg/dL; 30 minutes after injection 5 mg/dL; 60 minutes after injection 5 mg/dL
   c. Cortisol levels at baseline 5 mg/dL; 30 minutes after injection 30 mg/dL; 60 minutes after injection 50 mg/dL
   d. Cortisol levels at baseline 5 mg/dL; 30 minutes after injection 10 mg/dL; 60 minutes after injection 30 mg/dL

5. A 27-year-old man reports to the NP. He has experienced nausea, weight loss, and fatigue. Which of the following would *not* be included in the differential diagnosis?
   a. Adrenal insufficiency
   b. IBS
   c. AIDS
   d. Tuberculosis

Answers and Rationales

1. *Answer:* **b** (evaluation)
   Rationale: In Addison's disease, life-long replacement therapy is required. Failure to take medication daily or to increase the amount of cortisol during times of stress can result in electrolyte abnormalities and death. A diet with liberal salt intake is needed for sodium replacement.

2. *Answer:* **d** (assessment)
   Rationale: The leading causes of Addison's disease today are hereditary enzyme defects with congenital adrenal hyperplasia and loss of adrenal function resulting from autoimmune destruction of the glands (Gance-Cleveland, B. 2001).

3. *Answer:* **c** (analysis/diagnosis)
   Rationale: Postural hypotension, muscle wasting, and hyperpigmentation of the skin are the most common physical findings (Gance-Cleveland, B. 2001).

4. *Answer:* **b** (analysis/diagnosis)
   Rationale: In Addison's disease, cortisol levels are low and do not rise in response to ACTH.

5. *Answer:* **b** (analysis/diagnosis)
   Rationale: A person with IBS usually does not have weight loss.

ALLERGIC RHINITIS *Denise Robinson*

OVERVIEW
Definition
Rhinitis is a hyperfunction of the nose that results in rhinorrhea and nasal obstruction. Allergic rhinitis often has a seasonal component or specific inciting agents such as animals or dust.

Incidence
- Affects 1 in 5 adults and children in the United States.
- Affects more than 40 million people in the United States.
- Prevalence may be as high as 40%.
- Direct and indirect costs total $2.4 billion.

Pathophysiology
Atrophic patients produce excessive amounts of immunoglobulin E (IgE) antibodies. IgE binds to high affinity receptors on the surface of mast cells and basophils, thus serving as an allergen receptor. With reexposure, there is binding of the allergen to the mast cell surface IgE, which triggers a cascade of cell activation. The inhaled allergen rapidly initiates release of chemical mediators from mast cells (e.g., histamine, prostaglandin D, and leukotriene C4). These mediators cause variable degrees of vasodilation and edema (nasal congestion), increased mucous secretion and cellular recruitment (rhinorrhea) and increased capillary and mucosal permeability. The mediators also probably disturb the balanced nervous control of nasal function, leading to direct and reflex vascular dilation and hypersecretion. The sneezing threshold falls. After continued daily allergen exposure, lesser quantities of the specific allergen cause severe nasal symptoms. Similar mechanisms lead to the tearing and itching of the eye associated with allergic rhinitis (Zeiger & Schatz, 1998).

Allergic rhinitis and asthma both have an inherited tendency to develop IgE immune responses. Cross-sectional epidemiologic data studies have shown that asthma and allergic rhinitis frequently coexist. Rhinitis is diagnosed in up to 78% of patients with asthma, and asthma is diagnosed in up to 58% of patients with rhinitis. In the general population of patients with both diseases, allergic rhinitis may be a significant risk factor for asthma (Yawn & Ledgerwood, 2001).

ASSESSMENT: SUBJECTIVE/HISTORY
Symptoms
- Headache
- Sensation of facial pressure around eyes
- Itching of eye, tearing
- Sneezing
- Post nasal drip
- Recurrent head colds

- Stuffy head
- Chronic sinusitis
- Chronic cough
- Plugged or itching ears
- Diminished smell and taste
- Sleep disturbances including sleep apnea

History
- Ask about onset, triggers, exposure.
- Ask about onset, duration, and progression of symptoms.
- Ask about self treatment: use of antihistamines, nasal sprays.
- Investigate possibility of seasonal allergic rhinitis, including the following:
  - Ragweed: mid-August until the first frost
  - Tree pollen: March to May
  - Grass pollen: May to early June
- Perennial allergic rhinitis
- Dust mites
- Mold
- Animal dander or saliva
- Cockroach antigen

Aggravating Factors
- Dietary (e.g., maternal or infant diet)
- Hygiene hypothesis
- Increased exposure to indoor allergens
- Environmental pollution
- More sedentary lifestyle

Past Medical History
- Ask about frequent sinus infections.
- Ask about persistent otitis media in children.

Medications
Ask about OTC medications.

Psychosocial History
Ask about smoking.

Family History
Adults with a family history of allergic rhinitis have a two- to sixfold risk of developing rhinitis compared with adults without a family history.

ASSESSMENT: OBJECTIVE/PHYSICAL EXAMINATION
Physical Examination
- Take vital signs. Temperature should be normal; pulse and BP may be elevated if sympathomimetic drugs were used.

- Pay special attention to head, eyes, ears, nose, throat (HEENT), and chest.
- Check eyes for allergic shiners, tearing of eyes, conjunctival injection, and lid edema.
- Check ears to rule out otitis media, and to check for serous otitis.
- Check nares. Nasal mucosa is often pale blue and boggy with a clear mucous discharge and edematous turbinates.
- Check pharynx for tonsillar enlargement and inflammation, and lymphoid hyperplasia in poster oropharynx (cobblestoning). May also see mouth breathing.
- Check face for sinus tenderness and sinus transillumination.
- Check neck for lymphadenopathy.
- Check heart for abnormal sounds.
- Check lungs to rule out concurrent asthma or lower airway infection.

Diagnostic Procedures

Diagnosis is generally based on history and examination. However, if allergic rhinitis is suspected and immunotherapy is being considered, skin testing is necessary because treatment depends on accurate evaluation of allergen sensitivities. Spirometry is appropriate in all patients with long standing and severe allergic rhinitis and in patients who commonly cough following exercise, laughing, or exposure to cold air, or who develop a chronic cough after a viral respiratory tract infection.

DIAGNOSIS

Diagnosis of allergic rhinitis is based on the following:
- History
- Nature of presenting complaints
- Onset of symptoms
- Pattern of symptoms
- Duration

Differential diagnoses include the following:
- Upper respiratory infection (URI)
- Sinusitis
- Otitis media
- Nasal abnormalities such as polyps, septal deviations

THERAPEUTIC PLAN
Nonpharmacologic Treatment

- Lifestyle/environment control
- Identify triggers, avoid/control causes

Pharmacologic Treatment

- Antihistamines
  - Block H_1 receptors
  - Relieve sneezing, itching and rhinorrhea
  - First line therapy
  - Can be used with topical corticosteroids

- First generation products cause drowsiness in 10-40% of users (diphenhydramine, chlorpheniramine)
- Second generation usually nonsedative (Fexofenadine, cetirizine, loratadine)

- Oral decongestants
  - Sympathomimetic agents
  - Relieve symptoms of nasal congestion
  - May cause systemic side effects
  - Use in patients with HTN, coronary artery disease, DM, benign prostatic hyperplasia, thyroid disease

- Topical decongestants
  - Act rapidly and effectively to relieve nasal congestion
  - Can cause rebound effect
  - Limit course of therapy to 3 to 5 days

- Intranasal corticosteroids (beclomethasone, budesonide, fluticasone)
  - Preventive use: reduce congestion, sneezing, rhinorrhea, pruritus, and cough
  - Must be used qd in the absence of symptoms
  - Some authors believe that these products are less expensive and more effective than second generation antihistamines

- Oral corticosteroids
  - Antiinflammatory agent
  - Reduces severe symptoms and reduces polyps
  - 3 to 7 day course of therapy to achieve symptom control

- Mast cell stabilizer:
- Intranasal cromolyn sodium
  - Topical antiinflammatory agent
  - Relieves sneezing, rhinorrhea, nasal congestion, nasal pruritus
  - Given 2 to 4 times qd

- Ocular antiallergic/antiinflammatory drugs
  - There are NSAIDs available for eye discomfort, such as ketorolac trometanmine (Acular)
  - Mast cell stabilizer: Nedocromil sodium (Alocril) for treatment of allergic conjunctivitis
  - Antihistamine/mast cell stabilizer: olopatadine (Patanol)
  - Some eye medications can be used with contact lenses (remove contacts for 10 minutes and reinsert), and others cannot.

Immunotherapy

When the history and physical examination indicate perennial rhinitis, screening tests for various allergens should be done. These tests indicate IgE mediated reactions to specific allergens and are necessary if immunotherapy is being considered.

Immunotherapy involves injecting the patient with increasing doses of the specific allergen that is causing the allergic reaction. These injections are usually done over an extended period.

Client Education/Prevention

- Teach about allergic rhinitis and how to control it.
- Discuss morbidities and complications.
- Teach types of medications, how they work and side effects.
- Teach self-management skills to improve compliance.
- Teach allergen avoidance.
  - Limit exposure to molds, pollens and dusts in the home.
  - Close windows and use air conditioner.
  - Wear face mask for mowing the grass or doing factory work that produces dust.
  - Vacuum rather than sweep; vacuum furniture at least two times per week.
  - Use disposable bags in the vacuum cleaner.
  - Use a humidifier if the air is too dry or a dehumidifier if the air is too moist. Keep humidity below 50%.
  - Dust house daily with a moist cloth.
  - Do not allow anyone to smoke in the house.
  - Clean curtains monthly.
  - Encase mattress, box springs, and pillows in plastic or allergen impermeable material.
  - Install air filters.
  - Keep closet doors shut.
  - Remove feather pillows, woolen blankets; replace with synthetic.

Prevention in Children

- Breastfeeding can help prevent the development of allergic rhinitis in those families with atopic history.
- Delay the introduction of solid foods until after 4 months of age.
- Avoid exposure to tobacco smoke in the home.
- Do not allow children to sleep with furry toys in their beds.
- Toys should be vacuumed, tumble dried, or put in deep freeze overnight to reduce mites.

EVALUATION/FOLLOW-UP

If response to treatment is poor, refer to allergist or ear, nose, and throat specialist. Consider an anatomic or secondary disorder.

COMPLICATIONS

- Asthma
- Frequent sinusitis
- Headaches

REFERENCES

Cornell, S. (1997). Allergic rhinitis in children: it's nothing to sneeze at. *Advanced Nurse Practitioner, 5*(2), 30-32.

Lemanske, R. (1998). A review of current guidelines for allergic rhinitis and asthma. *Journal of allergic clinical immunology, 101*(2), S392-S396.

McConlogue, O., Shaughnessy, L. (2000). Allergic rhinitis. In D. Robinson, P. Kidd, K. Rogers (Eds.), *Primary care across the lifespan*, St. Louis: Mosby.

Stempel, D. (2001). Intranasal corticosteroids for first line treatment of allergic rhinitis: what's the evidence? *Formulary, 36*, 276-293.

Yawn, B., & Ledgerwood, G. (2001). Allergic rhinitis and asthma: a clinical practice update. Available online: http://www.aafp.org/videocme/asthma/ara/credits.htm

Zeiger, R., & Schatz, M. (1998). Rhinitis. In J. Stein (Ed). *Internal medicine*, (5th ed.). St. Louis: Mosby.

Review Questions

1. Steve, is a 35-year-old male with complaints of sneezing and runny nose. Which of the following historical data is consistent with a diagnosis of allergic rhinitis?
- **a.** "All of my family has similar symptoms."
- **b.** "I was out mowing the grass yesterday."
- **c.** "My throat is scratchy."
- **d.** "The cough is keeping me awake at night."

2. Which finding during the physical assessment is consistent with the diagnosis of allergic rhinitis?
- **a.** Erythematous nasal mucosa
- **b.** Pale, boggy nasal mucosa
- **c.** Yellow green nasal discharge
- **d.** Wheezes anterior and posterior

3. Which of the following drug choices is the most appropriate first choice for allergic rhinitis?
- **a.** Oral corticosteroid dose pak
- **b.** Topical decongestant
- **c.** Oral decongestant
- **d.** Antihistamine

4. The NP provides instruction about pharmacologic therapy for allergic rhinitis. Which comment by the patient indicates a need for further instruction?
- **a.** "I can use this decongestant nose spray for as long as I have these symptoms."
- **b.** "I need to be careful when I take diphenhydramine (Benadryl) because it might make me sleepy."
- **c.** "I still need to limit my exposure to pollens and dust."
- **d.** "If the diphenhydramine makes me too sleepy, I will check on the non-sedating antihistamines."

5. Which of the following is most helpful in terms of preventing allergic rhinitis?
- **a.** Avoid the offending agents.
- **b.** Take an antihistamine before a known exposure to allergen.

   c. No smoking in the house.
   d. Dust daily with a moist cloth.

6. Which of the following medications is most appropriate for an over-the-road trucker who has severe allergic rhinitis?
   a. Diphenhydramine (Benadryl)
   b. Intranasal corticosteroids
   c. Oral corticosteroids
   d. Topical decongestant

7. Intranasal corticosteroids work primarily through what mechanism in allergic rhinitis?
   a. Act rapidly to relieve nasal congestion
   b. Mast cell stabilizer
   c. Antiinflammatory agent
   d. Blocks H_1 receptors

8. Sylvia complains of having ragweed allergies. What time of the year does she need to take prophylactic medication to help decrease her symptoms?
   a. Winter
   b. Spring
   c. Summer
   d. Fall

Answers and Rationales

1. Answer: b (assessment)
   Rationale: Symptoms of allergic rhinitis tend to get worse when contact is made with the allergen. Mowing the grass provides access to pollens. Symptoms in the family tend to be caused by a viral illness, as would a scratchy throat and cough (McConlogue & O'Shaughnessy, 2000).

2. Answer: b (assessment)
   Rationale: The usual symptoms of allergic rhinitis include pale, boggy nasal mucosa, tearing/watering eyes, sneezing, clear nasal discharge. A common cold has erythematous nasal mucosa, yellow/green nasal discharge and systemic symptoms (Yawn & Ledgerwood, 2001).

3. Answer: d (implementation/plan)
   Rationale: The first line treatment for allergic rhinitis is an antihistamine. A topical decongestant can only be used on a time-limited basis, and an oral decongestant has limited success in controlling symptoms. A steroid dose pak should be reserved for that patient with severe symptoms.

4. Answer: a (evaluation)
   Rationale: The use of a topical nasal decongestant spray can only be used on a time-limited basis because of the problem of rebound congestion that occurs with longer use (Yawn & Ledgerwood, 2001).

5. Answer: a (implementation/plan)
   Rationale: The most effective way to prevent allergic rhinitis is to avoid the offending allergens. All answers do help decrease allergic rhinitis; however, avoiding the allergen is most effective (Yawn & Ledgerwood, 2001).

6. Answer: b (implementation/plan)
   Rationale: A sedating antihistamine should be avoided for patients who drive or operate heavy machinery. Intranasal corticosteroids are a better choice because they are effective in reducing most of the symptoms of allergic rhinitis (Yawn & Ledgerwood, 2001).

7. Answer: c (implementation/plan)
   Rationale: Corticosteroids are potent antiinflammatory agents (Stempel, 2001).

8. Answer: d (evaluation)
   Rationale: Ragweed is most prevalent from August 1 through the first frost (McConlough & O'Shaughnessy, 2000).

ALOPECIA *Pamela Kidd*

OVERVIEW
Definition

Alopecia is hair loss from any part of the body where hair normally grows. There are two classifications: scarring (cicatricial) and nonscarring (noncicatricial).

Incidence

Alopecia areata has a lifetime incidence rate of 2%, with the same rate in males as in females. One third to one half of all cases occur by the age of 20. Relapses are frequent. As males age over age 20, percentage of hair loss corresponds to the age group. For example, 35% of males older than age 35 experience some degree of alopecia (Proctor, 1999).

Pathophysiology

The initial event is usually abnormal sensitivity to the male sex hormones. Hormones allow the hair follicle to be perceived as a foreign body by the immune system. The hair follicle can also be destroyed by physical agents and infection.

   Factors Increasing Susceptibility. Genetic predisposition for some types of balding (androgenetic/pattern baldness).

   Protective Factors. No protective factors have been identified.

ASSESSMENT: SUBJECTIVE/HISTORY
Symptoms

Ask about onset, duration, severity, and pattern of loss. Listen to complaints of thin hair; 50% or more of hair can be lost without obvious visual detection (Berger, 2001). Assess for physical agents (dyes, curlers, straightening agents, hot combs). Assess for increased stress levels (surgery, infection, newly diagnosed disease).

Past Medical History

Assess for systemic disease and autoimmune disorders. Assess for treatment of these disorders as well. Ask about pregnancy and postpregnancy correlations, and crash diets. One form of alopecia, telogen effluvium, is characterized by hair follicles in a "resting phase" poststress. The symptom of telogen effluvium is a large number of hairs with white "tips" or "bulbs" coming out when combing the hair (>150).

Medication History

Assess OCP use, levonorgestrel (Norplant) and medroxyprogesterone (DepoProvera) in females. Drug-induced alopecia is common. Drugs associated with hair loss are vitamin A, retinoids, antimiotic agents, anticoagulants, antithyroid agents, allopurinol, indomethacin, amphetamines, salicylates, propranolol, levodopa, and chemotherapy.

Family History

Assess baldness patterns in both males and females within the family.

Dietary History

Dietary history is applicable only in that a nutritious diet supports both skin, hair, and nail growth. Ensure adequate iron intake.

ASSESSMENT: OBJECTIVE/PHYSICAL EXAMINATION
Physical Examination

Conduct a problem-focused physical examination. Determine if source is scarring or nonscarring. Scarring forms follow specific patterns; nonscarring tends to cause general loss of hair. Assess scalp for inflammation, scaling, and fungal infection (using Wood's lamp, a fluorescent glow will appear if fungal agent is present). Check for evidence of scratching (may indicate parasitic infection).

Diagnostic Procedures

Biopsy can be useful in determining cause of scarring (nonreversible) alopecia. Take specimen from active border and not from scarred area. Biopsies to perform are the following:

- KOH culture of hair follicle to rule out fungal infection
- Iron level to rule out telogen effluvium. Iron deficiency produces this disorder.

Perform assays as needed to rule out autoimmune process or systemic disease (e.g. antinuclear antibody [ANA] titer for connective tissue disorders).

DIAGNOSIS

- Telogen effluvium: associated with stressful event, low iron levels
- Androgenetic alopecia: symmetrical beginning at front of scalp, older client with family history of baldness, in females associated with overproduction of androgens
- Tinea capitis: more likely in children; scalp pruritus is present.
- Positive KOH and Wood's Lamp
- Alopecia areata: consists of patches of tiny hairs (2 mm to 3 mm in length); can progress to all scalp hair (alopecia totalis) or all body hair (alopecia universalis); associated with autoimmune disease, pernicious anemia, Addison's disease

THERAPEUTIC PLAN
Nonpharmacologic Treatment

Scarring forms of alopecia are not reversible. Nonscarring forms are treated by correcting the underlying condition. In drug-induced alopecia, the agent should be removed or replaced with alternative drug. Treatment process is frequently trial and error with no one agent producing the final result. Restoration of hair requires drug therapy.

Pharmacologic Treatment

See Table 3-5.

TABLE **3-5** Pharmacologic Treatment of Alopecia

CONDITION	AGENT/DOSE	COMMENTS
Alopecia areata	Triamcinolone acetonide intralesional (Aristocort), 2.5-10 mg/ml vial; inject 0.1 ml at 1-2 cm intervals, not to exceed 30 mg/month dose	Not recommended for children
	Anthralin (Drithoscalp) 0.25% to .50% ointment, apply to lesions sparingly	May irritate skin or stain hair; not recommended for children
Androgenetic alopecia	Topical minoxidil (Rogaine) (50mg/ml, available OTC), apply 1 ml to scalp bid	Chest pain, dizziness, tachycardia possible
	Finasteride (Propecia) 1 mg qd PO	Used only in males

OTC, Over the counter.

Client Education

- Instruct about cause if known and treat underlying condition if possible.
- Instruct about medication for hair regrowth in non-scarring alopecia.
- Avoid alkaline (caustic) shampoo.
- Comb hair, avoid brushing.
- Give advice on hairpieces and hair transplants.

Referral

Refer to dermatologist for intralesional injections.

Prevention

- Client should practice good hair hygiene.
- Provide preventive care to identify chronic/autoimmune illness early.
- Assess scalp and hair each visit for clients using medications associated with hair loss.

EVALUATION/FOLLOW-UP

Client should return every month to monitor hair regrowth for several months, then on an as-needed basis.

COMPLICATIONS

Compromised self-image is a possible complication.

REFERENCES

Berger, T. (2001). Skin, hair, and nails. In L. Tierney, S. McPhee, & M. Papadakis, (Eds.), *Current medical diagnosis and treatment.* McGraw-Hill: New York.

Johnsen, D.A. (2001) Alopecia. D. Robinson, P. Kidd, & K. Rogers, (Eds.), *Primary care across the lifespan.* Mosby: St. Louis.

Proctor, P. (1999). Hair raising: Latest news on male-pattern baldness. *ADVANCE for Nurse Practitioners, 7*(4), 39-40, 42, 83.

Review Questions

1. What data supports the diagnosis of alopecia?
   - a. Positive KOH test of hair follicle
   - b. Use of tretinoin for acne
   - c. Male client, age 55
   - d. Daily hair washing

2. Assessment of a client reveals a general loss of hair without scaling and with hairs of normal length. The NP's diagnosis is which of the following?
   - a. Alopecia areata
   - b. Androgenetic alopecia
   - c. Tinea capitis
   - d. Scarring alopecia

3. Which of the following statements indicates the client understands treatment for his or her alopecia?
   - a. "I will brush my hair once a day."
   - b. "I will avoid alkaline shampoos."
   - c. "I will wash my hair once a week."
   - d. "I will apply topical minoxidil every other day."

4. An NP develops a treatment plan for a female client with alopecia. The plan may include *except* which of the following?
   - a. referral to a dermatologist
   - b. Finasteride 1 mg PO qd
   - c. use of nonalkaline shampoo
   - d. consideration of hair pieces

Answers and Rationales

1. **Answer: b** (analysis/diagnosis)
   Rationale: Several drugs are associated with alopecia; retinoids are one class. Positive KOH indicates tinea capitis. Age is not a predisposing factor in either gender. Use of dyes, curlers, or straightening agents may damage hair, but daily washing is not associated with alopecia.

2. **Answer: b** (assessment)
   Rationale: Alopecia areata is a condition with patches of tiny hairs. Scarring alopecia has a specific, not general, pattern. Tinea capitis is associated with scaling and itching.

3. **Answer: b** (evaluation)
   Rationale: Combing, not brushing is best to decrease hair loss. Alkaline shampoos should be avoided. They are caustic to hair follicles. Topical minoxidil is used bid. Good hygiene means washing hair when dirty or oily; it should not be based on a specific number of times a week.

4. **Answer: b** (implementation/plan)
   Rationale: Finasteride is contraindicated in females. Non-alkaline shampoos are less caustic. Hair pieces may be used to improve body image. Referral to a dermatologist may be indicated.

ALZHEIMER'S DISEASE *Pamela Kidd*

OVERVIEW
Definition

Alzheimer's disease (AD) is a slow progressive deterioration of the brain leading to death. AD is marked by changes in behavior and personality and by an irreversible decline in intellectual abilities. Problems with memory are the hallmark of AD.

Incidence

Approximatley 6 to 8% of all persons older than age 65 have AD. The prevalence doubles every 5 years after age 60. Approximately 30% of persons older than age 85 and 50% older than age 90 have AD. Two to four million Americans are affected at any one time. Costs reach almost $100 billion per year.

Pathophysiology

Cells in the hippocampus and cerebral cortex are destroyed, which leads to problems with memory, language, and reasoning. Amyloid plaques and neurofibrillary tangles appear to be related to cell destruction.

Amyloid (Neuritic) plaques are thought to either initiate or be an early finding in a slow multi-step process that leads to brain cell malfunction. Beta-amyloid may be toxic to neurons, disrupt potassium channels, reduce choline levels, and/or a combination of these effects. Neurofibrillary tangles result as Tau (a protein) twists into paired helical filaments and microtubules that carry nutrients collapse.

Factors Increasing Susceptibility

- Aging
- Presence of Down syndrome
- Family history of AD
- Severe head injury with loss of consciousness
- Low level of education and/or occupation
- Female sex

Potentially Protective Factors

- Postmenopausal estrogen replacement therapy
- Long-term use of nonsteroidal antiinflammatory drugs
- Cigarette smoking
- Higher education and occupation

ASSESSMENT/SUBJECTIVE/HISTORY
Description of Most Common Symptoms

Difficulty with the following:
- Learning and retaining new information
- Performing complex tasks
- Reasoning ability
- Deteriorating spatial ability and orientation (e.g., getting lost in familiar places)
- Difficulty with language (e.g. finding words)
- Changes in behavior or dress
- Failing to arrive at the right time for appointments
- Difficulty discussing current events
- Demonstrating agitation, mood disturbances, and/or psychotic symptoms such as hallucinations; symptoms increase in severity as the disease progresses

Associated Symptoms

- Decline in functional ability and the ability to manage personal affairs
- Depression

History of Cognitive Decline

Obtain the history from the client *and* a reliable informant. Preferable to include more than one informant. Interview the client alone first and tell the client that others will be interviewed. Interview the informants apart from the client and be aware of possible questionable motives.

Obtain a detailed description of the chief complaint including (1) when symptoms began, (2) if symptoms had an abrupt or gradual onset or occurred in a stepwise or continuous progression, and (3) whether they are worsening, fluctuating, or improving.

Ask if there are signs of confusion, delirium, or dysphoric mood (e.g., depression)

Past Medical History

- Ask about relevant systemic diseases, psychiatric disorders, head trauma, and other neurologic disorders.
- Ask about alcohol and other substance abuse and exposure to environmental toxins (e.g., occupational toxins).
- Ask about infectious or metabolic illness such as pneumonia, urinary tract infection (UTI), diabetes, or acute or chronic renal disease.

Medication History

Ask about prescription and nonprescription drugs.

Family History

Ask about family history of early and late-onset AD, Down syndrome, Huntington's disease, or other genetic conditions leading to dementia.

Psychosocial History

- Ask about education, literacy, socioeconomic, ethnic, and cultural background.
- Ask about recent life events and social support. (May affect risk for dementia and performance on mental status exams.)

ASSESSMENT: OBJECTIVE/PHYSICAL EXAMINATION

Physical Examination

- Do a brief neurologic examination.
- Assess for life threatening or rapidly progressing symptoms such as mass lesions, vascular lesions, and infections.
- Measure blood pressure and pulse, supine and standing.
- Assess vision and hearing.
- Evaluate for evidence of cardiac failure, poor respiratory function, or problems with mobility or balance.
- Assess for caregiver abuse or neglect.

Functional Assessment. Conduct a functional assessment (see Functional Assessment later in this chapter).

Mental Status Assessment

- Assess abstract reasoning and judgment (e.g., ask client what he or she would do if there was a fire in the home).
- Administer a mental status examination. (NOTE: Clients with increased education may perform at a higher level and may not score as impaired during early stages of AD.)

Diagnostic Procedures

If the client demonstrates delirium, depression, impairment in multiple domains that represents a decline from previous levels, and/or confounding factors such as lower education:

Obtain: CBC, sedimentation rate, comprehensive metabolic profile, LFTs, U/A, TSH levels, vitamin B_{12} levels, rapid protein reagin (RPR) or venereal disease research laboratory (VDRL), and human immunodeficiency virus (HIV) if indicated by risk factors.

If indicated by the history and physical examination, obtain an electrocardiogram, chest radiograph, or psychiatric evaluation.

Consult physician regarding: computed tomography (CT) scan or magnetic resonance imaging (MRI) to exclude mass lesions, assess vascular changes, and determine regional atrophy; positron emission tomography, electroencephalogram to exclude Creutzfeldt-Jakob or epilepsy; or lumbar puncture with rapidly progressing symptoms that indicate inflammation.

DIAGNOSIS

The most common differential diagnoses related to AD are vascular dementia, AIDS-related dementia, diffuse Lewy body disease, and Parkinson's, Pick's, Creutzfeldt-Jakob, and Huntington's diseases. See Box 3-4. The major differences between AD and vascular dementia (VD) are the following (Fletcher & Damagaard, 1998):

- VD has sudden onset.
- VD has step-wise deterioration.
- VD is accompanied by history of falls or unsteady gait.
- VD is associated with personality and mood changes.

BOX 3-4   Diagnostic Criteria for Dementia of the Alzheimer's Type

A. The development of multiple cognitive deficits manifested by both:
   1. Memory impairment (impaired ability to learn new information or to recall previously learned information)
   2. One (or more) of the following cognitive disturbances
      a. Aphasia (language disturbance)
      b. Apraxia (impaired ability to carry out motor activities despite intact motor function)
      c. Agnosia (failure to recognize or identify objects despite intact sensory function)
      d. Disturbance in executive functioning (i.e., planning, organizing, sequencing, abstracting)
B. The cognitive deficits in Criteria A1 and A2 each cause significant impairment in social or occupational functioning and represent a significant decline from a previous level of functioning.
C. The course is characterized by gradual onset and continuing cognitive decline.

D. The cognitive deficits in Criteria A1 and A2 are not caused by any of the following:
   1. Other central nervous system conditions that cause progressive deficits in memory and cognition (e.g., cerebrovascular disease, Parkinson's disease, Huntington's disease, subdural hematoma, normal-pressure hydrocephalus, brain tumor)
   2. Systemic conditions that are known to cause dementia (e.g., hypothyroidism, vitamin B_{12} or folic acid deficiency, niacin deficiency, hypercalcemia, neurosyphilis, HIV infection)
   3. The deficits do not occur exclusively during the course of a delirium
   4. The disturbance is not better accounted for by another Axis I disorder (e.g., Major Depressive Disorder, Schizophrenia)

Data from American Psychiatric Association (1994). *Diagnostic and statistical manual for mental disorders.* (4th ed.). Washington, DC: Author.

THERAPEUTIC PLAN
Pharmacologic Treatment

Provide cholinesterase inhibitors, which prevent degradation of endogenously released acetylcholine, to improve memory. These agents temporarily improve cognition or delay decline. Cholinesterase inhibitors include the following:

- Tacrine hydrochloride (Cognex)
  - Improves cognitive functioning in 20% to 30% of persons with AD in the mild to moderate stage.
  - Start with 10 mg qid (increase to maximum of 40 mg qid).
  - Obtain baseline ALT before initiating and every week for 16 weeks. Modify dose according to manufacturer's directions if elevations are greater than 2 times the upper limits of normal.
  - Take with meals to decrease GI irritation.
  - Treat for a minimum of 3 months to assess therapeutic response.
- Donepezil hydrochloride (Aricept)
  - Donepezil has a longer duration of action than tacrine and a greater specificity for brain tissue.
  - Start with 5 mg qd and increase if needed to 10 mg qd after 1 month.
  - Side effects of nausea, vomiting, and diarrhea are increased with a more rapid increase in dose.
  - Prescribe hs with or without food.

NOTE: *Administer baseline and follow-up mental status and functional status examinations to provide a quantitative comparison of functioning. Other medications in clinical trials with inconclusive evidence include the following:*

- Estrogen, NSAIDs, ginkgo biloba, vitamin B_{12}, selegiline, vitamins E and C
- Antidepressants
  - Consider antidepressant medication in clients with depressive symptoms even if they fail to meet criteria for a depressive syndrome.
  - Refer clients with suicidal ideation and signs of major depressive symptoms to geropsychiatry.
  - Selective serotonin reuptake inhibitors (SSRIs) (fluoxetine, paroxetine and sertraline) are considered first-line by many specialists.
  - Tricyclic antidepressants can cause significant anticholinergic activity and orthostatic hypotension or cardiac conduction abnormalities. *Do not prescribe.* They are contraindicated in AD because lack of acetylcholine is the presumed pathologic cause of AD. All medications with anticholinergic activity should be avoided. Check before prescribing.
  - Monoamine oxidase inhibitors (MAOIs) can cause postural hypotension and have complex drug and food interactions.

Nonpharmacologic Treatment

The goal is to maintain normal activities as long as possible with attention to safety. Suggest an exercise routine to continue safe ambulation as long as possible. Supervise walks and use door locks or electronic guards to prevent wandering in the later stages of AD. Keep client active during the day to foster sleep at night.

Evaluate activities for safety issues to prevent injuries (e.g. the use of power tools that may cause injury with memory loss [putting one's hand in the area of the blade without shutting off electricity]).

Discuss driving issues early and help patient and family decide when driving a car should be stopped. Examine your state laws regarding AD driving. Patients with advanced dementia should not drive.

Encourage patients to maintain social and intellectual activities as tolerated.

Help caregivers establish a routine to maintain predictability. Stimulate memory through clocks, calendars, written lists, newspapers, radios, and television. Too much stimulation in the environment often increases confusion.

Finger foods may be helpful in maintaining nutrition during the later stages.

Client Education

- Help clients understand the disease process and management regime according to their tolerance for knowledge.
- Assist them in putting their personal affairs in order during the mild cognitive impairment phase.
- Establish and maintain a close working relationship with caregivers.
- Establish a health maintenance program for caregivers.
- Help caregivers establish medical and legal advance directives. Suggest that a trusted family member co-sign any important financial transactions and pay bills.
- Help families anticipate long-term care placement and encourage them to make arrangements in advance.
- Inform caregivers of community resources. Encourage attendance at support groups and to secure information from national AD centers.

Referral/Consultation

- Refer patients with major depression, psychosis, and/or violent behavior to geropsychiatry.
- Consider clinical psychologists for care givers with adjustment problems not helped by support groups.
- Refer to social workers for assistance in securing community resources.
- Consider enlisting physical therapists to assist with physical activity and occupational therapists for strategies to maximize functioning.
- Consult with geriatrician or geriatric psychiatrists regarding pharmaceutical management of mild agitation or aggression.

A

- Consult with neurologist regarding patients with parkinsonism type symptoms, focal neurologic signs, rapid progression, or abnormal neuroimaging findings.
- Consult with neuropsychologists to clarify uncertainties in diagnosis and the degree and type of impairment.

Prevention

There is not enough data to support that prevention of AD is possible. The role of vitamin E, C, and Ginkgo biloba in preventing AD is under investigation.

EVALUATION/FOLLOW-UP

- Schedule patient surveillance and health maintenance visits every 3 to 6 months; more often as needed for problems.
- The goal of care for the client is to maintain the highest possible level of wellness for the longest possible time. This entails helping the patient complete the grieving process, complete personal affairs, avoid excess disability, live in a supportive environment, and die with dignity and with the highest possible physical and emotional comfort.
- The goal of care for the family is to help them provide the highest level of physical and emotional care to the client while maintaining their own personal health and well-being, maintaining a positive relationship with the client, experiencing satisfaction with their caregiving role, and successfully completing the grieving process.

REFERENCES

Alzheimer's Association. (1997). *ADVANCES In Alzheimer's research, 7,* 1A-4A, 1-7.

American Psychiatric Association. (1994). *Diagnostic and statistical manual of mental disorders.* (4th ed). Washington, DC: Author.

Buckwalter, K., & Hall, G. (1996). Alzheimer's disease. In McBride, A., & Austin, J. *Psychiatric mental health nursing: Integrating the behavioral and biological sciences,* (pp. 348-392). Philadelphia: W.B. Saunders.

Fletcher, K., & Damgaard, P. (1998). A Glimmer of Hope: Alzheimer's Disease, Present and Future Issues. *ADVANCE for Nurse Practitioners.* 6(6), 49-52, 84.

Knapp, M., Knopman, D., Solomon, P., Pendlebury, W., Davis, C., & Gracon, S. (1994). A 30-week randomized controlled trial of high-dose tacrine in patients with Alzheimer's Disease. *Journal of the American Medical Association, 271,* 985-991.

McKhann, G., Drachman, M., Folstein, M., Katzman, R., Price, D., & Stadlan, E. (1984). Clinical diagnosis of Alzheimer's disease: Report of the NINCDS-ARDRA Work Group under the auspices of Department of Health and Human Services Task Force on Alzheimer's disease. *Neurology, 34,* 939-944.

National Institutes on Aging, National Institutes of Health (1995). *Progress report on Alzheimer's Disease.* (NIH Publication No. 95-3994). Rockville, MD: Author.

Pfeffer, R., Kurosaki, T., Harrah, C., Chance, J., & Filos, S. (1992). Measurement of functional activities of older adults in the community. *Journal of Gerontology, 37,* 323-329.

Roberts, K. (2000). Alzheimer's Disease and related disorders. In D. Robinson, P. Kidd, K. Rogers (Eds.), *Primary care across the lifespan.* St. Louis: Mosby.

Small, G.W., Rabins, P.V., Barry, P.P., Buckholz, N.S., DeKosky, S.T., Ferris, S.H., et al. (1997). Diagnosis and treatment of Alzheimer Disease and related disorders: General consensus statement of the American Association of Geriatric Psychiatry, the Alzheimer's Association, and the American Geriatric Society. *Journal of the American Medical Association, 278*(16), 1363-1372.

U.S. Department of Health and Human Services. (1996). *Early identification of Alzheimer's Disease and related dementias.* (AHCPR Publication No-97-0703). Rockville, MD: Author.

U.S. Department of Health and Human Services. (1997). Quick reference guide for clinicians: Early identification of Alzheimer's disease and related dementias. *American Academy of Nurse Practitioners, 9,* 85-87.

Review Questions

1. The single most important source of information in the diagnosis of AD is which of the following?

- **a.** Neurologic examination
- **b.** CT or MRI
- **c.** Mental status examination
- **d.** Clinical history

2. All the following support the diagnosis of AD except the fact that the client:

- **a.** Forgets where she put things.
- **b.** Is unable to balance her checkbook.
- **c.** Got lost driving home from the grocery store.
- **d.** Cries almost every day.

3. All the following tests are included in a recommended battery of laboratory tests to exclude occult causes of dementia except which of the following?

- **a.** CBC
- **b.** Blood glucose
- **c.** ESR
- **d.** Full thyroid profile

4. Results of a client's initial testing demonstrated abnormal mental status, impaired functional ability, and absence of depression. What is the next step?

- **a.** Reassure the client and family and have them return in 6 months.
- **b.** Refer for a second opinion.
- **c.** Conduct a battery of laboratory and radiologic tests to rule out medical conditions.
- **d.** Refer for a neuropsychologic evaluation.

A

5. When administering the Mini-Mental State Examination, what elements in the client's history should be used in interpreting the results of the test?
   a. Family history of AD
   b. Past history of concussion
   c. Estrogen replacement therapy
   d. Teaching occupation

6. Successful therapy with tacrine or donepezil is indicated by which of the following?
   a. Cessation of the progressive course of AD
   b. Improvements in memory and functional status for an undetermined period of time
   c. Remission of AD
   d. Functional but no mental improvement

7. The best approach for eliciting a history in a client with potential AD is to do which of the following?
   a. Interview the client with family member or friend present.
   b. Obtain client history from a reliable informant.
   c. Interview client and family member or friend independently.
   d. Depend on client interview and observe the client.

Answers and Rationales

1. ***Answer:*** **d** (analysis/diagnosis)
   Rationale: The clinical history demonstrates the symptoms and progression that is characteristic of AD.

2. ***Answer:*** **d** (assessment)
   Rationale: Although depression may coexist with dementia, sadness that leads to daily tears is indicative of a depressed state. The depression must be addressed before the possibility of dementia can be fully addressed.

3. ***Answer:*** **d** (analysis/diagnosis)
   Rationale: A TSH level is recommended as the screening test to include in the test battery for occult causes of dementia.

4. ***Answer:*** **c** (implementation/plan)
   Rationale: 1996 AHCPR guidelines recommend that if results from the mental and functional assessment are abnormal, the client is likely to have a dementing illness. The client should be clinically evaluated.

5. ***Answer:*** **d** (analysis/diagnosis)
   Rationale: It is important to look for cultural and/or educational biases that might influence results. A high educational level increases the likelihood that a cognitively impaired person will test as unimpaired.

6. ***Answer:*** **b** (evaluation)
   Rationale: Because of more effective utilization of acetylcholine, clients experience improvements in cognition or at least a slowing of the decline. The medications do not alter the progressive course of the disease, and functioning eventually declines. Clients may function at a higher level for a longer period of time.

7. ***Answer:*** **c** (assessment)
   Rationale: It is best to interview the client and another person. Tell client that you will be interviewing others but always interview the client first. Beware of possible negative motives when interviewing others. Interviewing several family members or friends is the best option but is not always feasible. Interviewing both together may agitate the client and put the informant in an uncomfortable position in which he or she may not be honest.

AMBLYOPIA   *Denise Robinson*

OVERVIEW
Definition

Amblyopia is secondary vision loss related to disease of the visual pathways. It is a reduction in central visual acuity (VA) caused by sensory deprivation of a well formed retinal image that occurs with or without a visible organic lesion commensurate with the degree of visual loss (Eisenbaum, 1999). It is typically associated with strabismus or other refractive disorders, which act by impeding visual development at the cortical level. Commonly it is know as "lazy eye."

Incidence

- Visual problems affect 5% to 10% of children.
- Of children older than 6 years, 3% have strabismus.
- Of those, as many as 40% subsequently develop amblyopia. It is the leading cause of monocular vision loss in people between the ages of 20 and 70 (Broderick, 1998).
- Amblyopia is the leading cause of preventable blindness in the United States. It affects approximately 4% of the children born each year in the United States.

Pathophysiology

The ability to focus a visual image on the central retina develops at about 2 to 3 months of age. To get the most sharply delineated image, all rays of light must converge on the macula. If the retinal image is distorted in one eye because of refractive difference between the eyes or strabismus, the cortical image is too dissimilar to permit binocular resolution. The brain quickly learns to suppress the poorer image from the affected eye to allow for clear vision. Because cortical visual development depends on continuous stimuli, neurodevelopment is impeded in the visual cortex corresponding to the suppressed eye. The result can be permanent visual impairment in an otherwise normal eye (Broderick, 1998).

ASSESSMENT: SUBJECTIVE/HISTORY

Amblyopia is usually asymptomatic and is detected through screening programs only.

Symptoms

- Crossed eyes
- Head tilt (to minimize diplopia)
- Eyes that misalign

Past Medical History

Prematurity, cerebral palsy, hydrocephalus, congenital cataracts, colobomas, and retinoblastoma are possible indicators of amblyopia.

Family History

- Strabismus, eye deviations, cataracts
- Previous eye surgery in family members, patching therapy, glasses and eye muscle surgery

Medications

Not applicable.

Psychosocial History

Not applicable.

Aggravating Factors

Illness or fatigue may make visual problem worse.

ASSESSMENT: OBJECTIVE/PHYSICAL EXAMINATION

Physical Examination

- Screening for visual problem is essential at every well child visit.
- Ideally the infant or child should be awake and alert.
- Observe for assumed head tilt.
- Observe the eyes, including the eyelids, for size, shape, symmetry, and general appearance.
- Observe as to whether the infant or child will follow an object or the examiner's face.
- Assess the red reflex for color, brightness, and symmetry. The room should be slightly darkened, and the ophthalmoscope should be set on +1 diopter.
- Assess for pupillary reflex in infants and children older than 2 months. The pupils should constrict and remain constricted as a light is moved from one pupil to another.
- Assess the Hirschberg corneal reflex test or corneal light reflex. The reflection of light from each cornea should be symmetrical and in the center of each pupil. In the presence of strabismus, the reflected light appears off center for the affected eye.
- Assess for extraocular movements.
- Assess an older infant or child by the cover/uncover test at a distance and at close range. One eye is covered by the examiner, who looks for movement in the contralateral eye. The covered eye is then uncovered, assessing for movement in that eye. Repeat the same sequence on the other eye. The cover/uncover test differentiates phoria from tropias.
- Assess for VA of each eye and both eyes together.

Diagnostic Procedures

None needed.

DIAGNOSIS

The diagnosis of amblyopia is made by clinical inspection and eye examination.

THERAPEUTIC PLAN

Nonpharmacologic Treatment

Treatment for amblyopia consists of treating the cause (e.g., strabismus, refractive error). Initial treatment of the underlying causes of amblyopia must be individualized. Corrective lenses, surgery, or other therapies may be needed.

In unilateral cases, force use of the impaired eye. The "good" eye is occluded, usually with an adhesive patch. The patch is removed for several hours each day so the good eye does not develop amblyopia.

Pharmacologic Treatment

A mydriatic such as atropine can be used to blur the vision in the "good" eye of children if a patch is not tolerated.

Client Education/Prevention

The child needs to wear a patch until vision is normalized. The treatment is age dependent. The younger the child, the faster the normalization of vision is seen.

Parents should know that non-compliance is the most frequent reason for failure of amblyopia therapy. Other factors include age at time of treatment, severity of amblyopia and other eye conditions.

Children should have eye screening incorporated into all well visits (see Table 3-6 for normal development of vision and eye movements).

Referral

Any child with abnormal anatomy, fixation, ocular misalignment, asymmetric or abnormal red reflexes, nystagmus, or failure to achieve 20/40 in each eye should undergo a more complete visual evaluation (Mills, 1999).

Children who are premature, with a family history of childhood vision problems or with other increased risks should have an early referral.

TABLE **3-6** Normal Vision, Eye Movements, and Screening for Children

AGE	NORMAL VISION AND EYE MOVEMENTS	PEDIATRIC SCREENING
Birth (term)	Fixation Poor following Intermittent strabismus frequently present VA 20/400 to 20/600	External (penlight) examination for surface abnormalities Ocular alignment (corneal reflexes) Ophthalmoscopy for red reflexes
1 month	Horizontal following to midline Normal alignment VA 20/300	Same
2 months	Vertical following begins Normal alignment VA 20/200	Same
3 months	Good horizontal and vertical following Normal alignment VA 20/100 Accommodation begins Binocularity detectable	Same
6 months	VA 20/20 to 20/30 Binocularity well developed Consistent synchronized eye movements	Ability to fix and follow light, face, or small toy As above + pupillary examination
3-4 years	Visual capabilities undergo refinement Color vision and depth perception are fully established	VA by picture chart or tumbling E as above + ocular motility and alignment (ocular movements, cover test and corneal reflections) Examination of retina and optic nerve
5-6 years	Acuity 20/20, no color blindness	VA by Snellen Same examination as above

VA, Visual acuity.
Data from Mills, M. (1999). *American Family Physician, 60,* 907–918, and Broderick, P. (1998). *American Family Physician,* Available online: http://www.aafp.org/afp/98090/ap/broderic.html.

EVALUATION/FOLLOW-UP

Frequent vision checks and observation are necessary for clients who have occlusion therapy to monitor treatment. It is important to monitor the good eye to ensure it does not also develop amblyopia.

Children need to continue therapy until vision in the affected eye is normalized or until no further improvement is seen.

COMPLICATIONS

- By 10 years of age, it is not known if amblyopia treatment can affect the eyes, so there is a window for which therapy is effective. It is currently believed that the sensitive period for amblyopia is younger than 10 years of age.
- Amblyopia is detrimental to childhood development, educational achievement, and self esteem.
- Amblyopia causes vision loss in the affected eye: monocular vision loss.
- Causes impairment of depth perception, peripheral vision and contrast sensitivity.

- The most common reason for failure of amblyopia therapy is noncompliance.

REFERENCES

Bane, M., & Beauchamp, G. (2001). Update on vision screening. *Review of Ophthalmology,* March 2001.
Broderick, P. (1998, September). Pediatric vision screening for the family physician. *American Family Physician.* Available online: http://www.aafp.org/afp/980901ap/broderic. html.
Eisenbaum, A. (1999). Eye. In W. Hay, A. Hayward, M. Levin, J. Sondheimer, (Eds.), *Current pediatric diagnosis and treatment,* (14th ed, pp. 360-383). Stamford, CT: Appleton & Lange.
Lempert, P. (2001). Prevention may be the best way to deal with amblyopia. *Ophthalmology Times, 26*(7): 60.
Mills, M. (1999). The eye in childhood. *American Family Physician, 60,* 907-918. Available online: http://www.afp.org/afp. 99091ap/907.html
Moseley, M., & Fielder, A. (2001). Improvement in amblyopic eye function and contralateral eye disease: evidence of residual plasticity. *Lancet, 357,* 902-904.
Talsma, J., & Donahue, S. (2001). Screening urged for kids 2 and older. *Ophthalmology Times, 26*(4), 1.

Review Questions

1. What is the most common visual disorder associated with amblyopia?

- **a.** Strabismus
- **b.** Glaucoma
- **c.** Eye trauma
- **d.** Late night reading with poor light

2. Which of the following historical data in a child is consistent with a diagnosis of amblyopia?

- **a.** Child has to sit close to the board to see.
- **b.** Child sees better up close than far away.
- **c.** Child tilts her head all the time to see better.
- **d.** Child has tearing and tenderness at the inner canthus of eye.

3. Treatment measures for amblyopia include all but which of the following?

- **a.** Surgery
- **b.** Patching
- **c.** Eye drops
- **d.** Watchful waiting

4. The NP provides instruction about the nonpharmacologic treatment for amblyopia. Which comment by the mother indicates a need for further instruction?

- **a.** "Steve can take the patch off when it bothers him."
- **b.** "Susie can remove the patch for 2 hours before bed time."
- **c.** "Mya must wear the patch all the time except during bathing and before bed."
- **d.** "The adhesive of the patch fits on the lens of Kim's glasses."

5. Which of the following children should have a prompt referral to an ophthalmologist?

- **a.** Sara, a 6-year-old who has 20/30 vision
- **b.** Stacey, a 12-year-old who has 20/20 vision
- **c.** Erin, an 8-year-old with V/A on Snellen's chart: 20/40 left eye, 20/60 right eye
- **d.** Cody, a 3-month-old with flat nasal bridge

6. Which of the following physical examination data are consistent with diagnosis of amblyopia?

- **a.** Three-month-old child, red reflex present both eyes
- **b.** Seven-year-old child, VA on Snellen's chart of 20/30 left eye, 20/35 right eye
- **c.** Three-year-old with corneal light reflex in different positions on the cornea of each eye
- **d.** Six-year-old with no movement of eye during cover/uncover test

7. Which of the following is the appropriate way to check for alignment of the eyes in a 3-month-old?

- **a.** Red reflex test
- **b.** Hirschberg corneal reflex test
- **c.** Cover/uncover
- **d.** Funduscopic examination

8. When is ocular alignment present in children?

- **a.** Newborn
- **b.** One month
- **c.** Twelve months
- **d.** Eighteen months

Answers and Rationales

1. *Answer:* **a** (analysis/diagnosis)

Rationale: Strabismus is the most common cause of amblyopia (Broderick, 1998).

2. *Answer:* **c** (assessment)

Rationale: A child who tilts his or her head is doing so to minimize diplopia. This is common with vertical strabismus (Broderick, 1998). Answers a and b discuss myopia and hyperopia. Answer d is indicative of dacryostenosis.

3. *Answer:* **d** (implementation/plan)

Rationale: Watchful waiting is not appropriate. In most cases amblyopia is more easily treated the earlier it is found. All other options are possible treatments for amblyopia (Mills, 1999).

4. *Answer:* **a** (evaluation)

Rationale: The most common reason for unsuccessful treatment is noncompliance. The patch should be left in place except for 1 to 2 waking hours (Broderick, 1998).

5. *Answer:* **c** (implementation/plan)

Rationale: All but answer c are normal findings. Answer c is an abnormal finding and merits a prompt referral to an ophthalmologist (Broderick, 1998).

6. *Answer:* **c** (assessment)

Rationale: The Hirschberg corneal reflex test is indicative of strabismus and amblyopia. When the test is done, the light should be centered within the pupil and the pupils should be symmetric in each eye (Mills, 1999).

7. *Answer:* **b** (assessment)

Rationale: Both the Hirschberg corneal reflex test and the cover/uncover check for alignment are appropriate. However, a 3-month-old cannot cooperate, so this test is appropriate for children ages 5 years or older. The red reflex test checks for opacity of the cornea and cataract, among others. A funduscopic examination involves looking at the retina, the optic disc, and the macula (Mills, 1999).

8. *Answer:* **b** (analysis/diagnosis)

Rationale: Normal alignment is expected in children by the age of 1 month (Mills, 1999).

AMENORRHEA *Cheryl Kish*

OVERVIEW
Definition

Amenorrhea refers to the absence of menstruation in a woman despite appropriate menstrual age and developmental characteristics (i.e., a woman of childbearing age). Amenorrhea is categorized as physiologic or functional, primary, or secondary.

- Physiologic or functional amenorrhea refers to expected absence of menstruation associated with normal life transitions: before menarche, during pregnancy and lactation, and after menopause. A particular type of functional amenorrhea is associated with hysterectomy.
- Primary amenorrhea refers to a lack of menarche by age 14 with an absence of secondary sexual characteristics, or by age 16 regardless of development of secondary sexual characteristics.
- Secondary amenorrhea describes menses absent for 6 months in women who have previously menstruated. In those women with oligomenorrhea (menses occurring at intervals greater than 35 days), loss of previously established periods for a 12-month interval defines secondary amenorrhea.

Incidence

Secondary amenorrhea occurs in approximately 5% of women during their reproductive years. The incidence is more common in competitive athletes; for example, the incidence in ballet dancers is 37% to 44%; in runners the rate is 5% to 26%. Primary amenorrhea is infrequent (0.1% to 2.5% of all women of reproductive age).

Pathophysiology

Menarche generally occurs between the ages of 11 to 14 years; the mean age in the United States is 12.7 years. Menopause, the natural end of menstruation, occurs between 44 to 55 years of age, with an average of 51.5 years. Between those intervals, normal menstrual periods require a mature, intact HPO axis, functional ovaries, functional endometrium, and an unobstructed outflow tract. Disruption of any of these requirements may cause amenorrhea.

The most common causes of secondary amenorrhea are pregnancy, lactation, and disorders of the HPO axis, including effects of excessive stress, exercise, weight loss, or malnutrition. Less common causes include the following:

- Medication use: antipsychotics (phenothiazides, haloperidol), antidepressants (tricyclics, MAOIs), antihypertensives (calcium channel blockers, methyldopa), marijuana, hormonal contraceptives (OCPs, medroxyprogesterone [DepoProvera], levonorgestrel [Norplant], MPA and estradiol cypionate injectable suspension [Lunelle]), digitalis, and chemotherapeutic agents
- Chronic anovulation including polycystic ovary disease
- Asherman's syndrome: endometrial adhesions secondary to overzealous curettage, endometritis, or radiation
- Adrenal disease (congenital adrenal hyperplasia, Cushing's disease)
- Ovarian failure (persistent corpus luteum cysts, premature ovarian failure, autoimmune disease-related, radiation)
- Hyperprolactinemia (30%)

Primary amenorrhea can be pathophysiologically classified by physical examination with focus on secondary sexual characteristics. This type of amenorrhea is often related to the following:

- Gonadal dysgenesis or chromosomal abnormality affecting ovarian function (e.g., Turner's syndrome, s 45 XO karyotype), presents with primary amenorrhea, short stature, delayed puberty
- Mullerian anomalies (congenital absence of uterus and upper portion of vagina)
- Hypothalamic/pituitary disorders
- Constitutional delays related to HPO immaturity (short stature: 5 feet tall at age 14).

ASSESSMENT: SUBJECTIVE/HISTORY
History of Present Illness

A careful menstrual, sexual, and pregnancy history should include the following:

- Chronology of development of secondary sexual characteristics
- Past and current methods of contraception
- Recent medications (including illicit drugs)
- Any signs and symptoms of menopause
- Any chronic or acute illnesses
- Sources of emotional stress
- Present weight and weight 1 year ago
- Amount of daily exercise

Symptoms

Clients should be questioned regarding breast discharge, hirsutism, male pattern baldness, deepening of voice, and signs and symptoms of hypothyroidism or type 1 diabetes. Also to be noted are severe fluctuations in weight and excessive exercising (e.g., long-distance running, gymnastics, especially when training began before onset of puberty).

Past Medical History

Question client about any history of hypothyroidism, autoimmune disease, diabetes, Crohn's disease, galactorrhea, pituitary disease, fibroids, or endometriosis. Ask about diagnosed congenital anomalies. Ask about treatment for childhood cancer and head injury.

Medication History

Inquire about medication use with emphasis on those drugs known to be associated with amenorrhea.

Family History

Inquire about maternal and female sibling history of menarche.

Diet History

Complete a 24-hour recall for clients who are overweight or severely underweight. Ask about a history of anorexia or bulimia.

ASSESSMENT: OBJECTIVE/PHYSICAL EXAMINATION

Physical Examination

Examination should focus on neck (thyroid), breasts (assessing for discharge), and complete pelvic examination looking at mucosa, hymen, size of uterus, and adnexa. Abnormalities of the outflow tract should be noted. Baseline vital signs, including weight and body mass should be obtained. Tanner staging should be documented. Characteristics of androgen–estrogen imbalance should be noted. Visual field testing may help rule out pituitary adenoma.

Diagnostic Procedures

The first-line test for any report of amenorrhea should be a pregnancy test. This should be a priority despite a history of reliable contraception. **Pregnancy is the number one cause of secondary amenorrhea.** In addition, ruling out pregnancy is important to allay anxiety, and avoids unnecessary testing and exposure of the embryo to imaging or medical treatment.

If the client is not pregnant, then TSH and prolactin levels should be drawn. Increased TSH raises the index of suspicion for hypothyroidism. Increased prolactin could be caused by a pituitary adenoma and should be followed with an evaluation of the sella turcica with radiograph examination of the pituitary region. Normal prolactin level is less than 20 ng/mL.

If both TSH and prolactin levels are normal, assess estrogen status and competence of reproductive tract with the progesterone challenge test. Administer MPA (Provera)10 mg/day for 5 days. A positive result is demonstrated by any withdrawal bleeding 2 to 7 days after medication is discontinued. A positive result means that the HPO axis is intact and that the amenorrhea is likely caused by anovulation.

If no withdrawal bleeding occurs, a combination OCP is then initiated (or estrogen, 1.25 mg days 1 through 21, with medroxyprogesterone, 5 to 10 mg on days 16 through 21). Withdrawal bleeding excludes anatomic causes, including outflow tract abnormality or uterine problems. If normal anatomy has been found on physical examination, refer client for hysteroscopy to rule out Asherman's syndrome, especially if client has a history suggestive of Asherman's (p. 45). If questions remain about normalcy of anatomy, refer.

Clients with prolonged amenorrhea and signs of androgen excess should be referred for endometrial biopsy before initiating withdrawal bleeding. Endometrial biopsy also is appropriate for any women with prolonged duration of unopposed estrogen, amenorrhea lasting longer than 12 months, or with a 3-month history of abnormal uterine bleeding.

Clients with menopausal symptoms may be evaluated for ovarian failure; ovarian failure is considered premature if it occurs in women younger than 40 years of age. A FSH level greater than 40 indicates ovarian failure.

DIAGNOSIS

Irregular menses are not uncommon early in menarche. Differential diagnosis includes the following:

- Pregnancy
- Pituitary tumor
- Menopause
- Excessive dieting
- Excessive exercise
- Use of hormonal contraceptive methods
- Changes in lifestyle (e.g., stress)
- Thyroid disease (usually hypothyroidism)
- Polycystic ovary
- Eating disorders
- Premature ovarian failure or ovarian dysfunction
- Primary amenorrhea

THERAPEUTIC PLAN

Only 20% of patients discovered to have primary amenorrhea have a treatable condition. Goals of treatment include (1) initiation of pubertal changes if needed, (2) maintenance of estrogen status, and (3) initiation of menarche. In clients with outflow tract abnormalities, surgical correction may be possible. Referral to a specialist is appropriate for all clients with suspected primary amenorrhea.

Management of secondary amenorrhea depends on the woman's desire for fertility. Those who desire pregnancy should be referred to an infertility specialist. For women not seeking pregnancy, goals include restoring estrogen status if needed and treating the underlying cause of the amenorrhea. For women with sufficient estrogen levels, a withdrawal bleed 4 to 6 times per year avoids endometrial hyperplasia and the subsequent risk of endometrial cancer and dysfunctional bleeding patterns. This can be accomplished with MPA (Provera) 10 mg/day for the first 10 days of the month, or with OCPs if there are no contraindications. For women with deficient estrogen levels, estrogen replacement therapy is appropriate; OCPs or estrogen and progesterone (with intact uterus) may be of value.

If amenorrhea is due to systemic disease, treatment of that disease is indicated.

Client Education

- Educate woman about the evaluation required to identify the cause of amenorrhea, that it may be lengthy and extensive.
- Support adolescent and her parents through the evaluation process for primary amenorrhea, providing education and subspecialty referral appropriately.
- Educate young women about how nutrition and exercise affect menstrual cycles. Teach good nutrition and recommend 2 days off from exercise weekly or to decrease exercise time. Encourage weight gain for significantly underweight women (less than 22% body fat is associated with amenorrhea).

Prevention

Some cases of secondary amenorrhea are preventable by avoiding medications and life behaviors that are contributory and by avoiding pregnancy. However, amenorrhea generally is not considered a preventable disorder.

EVALUATION/FOLLOW-UP

Perform evaluation as indicated by diagnosis. Consult with specialists as needed to manage the evaluation of women with amenorrhea or refer. Failure to develop normally is inherently stressful for young women and their parents. Emotional support throughout the difficult days of evaluation and uncertainty is of inestimable value. In some cases, clients seek care prematurely because of comparison with the developmental timetable in friends or family members. Education about normal puberty and development of secondary sexual characteristics is an important role for NPs, whether in one-on-one sessions or in groups. If pregnancy is determined to be the cause of amenorrhea, schedule the woman for prenatal care. Annual follow-up of women being treated for amenorrhea is appropriate.

COMPLICATIONS

Women with chronic anovulation with adequate estrogen are at increased risk for endometrial cancer from the unopposed estrogen. Competitive athletes with exercise-induced anovulation/amenorrhea are at risk for osteoporosis. Polycystic ovary disease, a state of chronic or persistent anovulation, is associated with increased risk of cardiovascular disease secondary to androgen excess and hyperinsulinemia.

REFERENCES

Cash, J.C., & Glass, C.A. (2000). *Family practice guidelines.* Philadelphia: Lippincott.

Hawkins, J. W., Roberto-Nichols, D. M., & Stanley-Haney, J. L. (Eds.). (1997). *Protocols for nurse practitioners in gynecologic settings,* (5th ed.). New York: Tiresias Press.

Meredith, P.V., & Horan, N.M. (2000). *Adult primary care.* Philadelphia: W.B. Saunders.

Smith, M.A., & Shimp, L.A. (2000). *20 common problems in women's health care.* New York: McGraw-Hill.

Smith, R.P. (1997). *Gynecology in primary care.* Baltimore: Williams & Wilkins.

Tierney, C.M., McPhee, S.J., & Papadakis, M.A. (2001). *Current medical diagnosis and treatment.* New York: Lange Medical Books/McGraw-Hill.

Youngkin, E.Q., & Davis, M.S. (1998). *Women's health: A Primary care clinical guide.* Stamford, CT: Appleton & Lange.

Review Questions

1. A 45-year-old woman, mother of two, comes to the clinic reporting amenorrhea for the preceding 3 months. Before this, her menses had been becoming irregular, occurring anywhere between 21 and 36 days apart. She reports fatigue and constipation along with "mood swings." First-line testing includes which of the following?

   a. TSH and prolactin levels
   b. FSH and luteinizing hormone (LH) levels
   c. CBC count with differential
   d. HCG level

2. A 23-year-old woman with previously normal menses who reports amenorrhea with an increase in acne, increased muscle mass, decreased breast size, deepening of voice, and temporal balding should do which of the following?

   a. Respond to the progesterone challenge and have withdrawal bleeding.
   b. Have elevated prolactin levels, indicating galactorrhea.
   c. Have elevated FSH levels, indicating ovarian failure.
   d. Be evaluated by a physician before initiation of withdrawal bleeding.

3. A 39-year-old woman with amenorrhea who has an elevated TSH should do which of the following?

   a. Be sent for a thyroid scan
   b. Be started on a thyroid replacement regimen
   c. Begin propylthiouracil (PTU) to decrease the amount of circulating thyroid hormone
   d. be sent to have a CT scan to evaluate for a pituitary-secreting tumor.

4. A 13-year-old girl started menstruating 11 months ago. Physical examination shows that she is Tanner stage III. She reports that she has a regular period for a couple of months, followed by a month or two without menstruating. She is currently menstruating. What does the NP do?

    a. Suggest checking FSH level to evaluate ovarian function.
    b. Suggest keeping a menstrual calendar to evaluate cycles.
    c. Obtain urine for a pregnancy test.
    d. Check TSH and prolactin levels.

5. Amenorrhea is the most common side effect of which medication?

    a. Levothyroxine (Synthroid)
    b. Beta-blockers
    c. Levonorgestrel (Norplant)
    d. Medroxyprogesterone (Depo-Provera)

6. Women with a diagnosis of chronic anovulation should be regulated with hormones for which of the following reasons?

    a. They are at higher risk for endometrial cancer.
    b. They will have an increasingly difficult time becoming pregnant if they are not "primed" with estrogen on a regular basis.
    c. They are at higher risk for heart disease.
    d. They have an increased risk for development of endometriosis and fibroid tumors.

7. Which finding in a 16-year-old is most consistent with a diagnosis of secondary amenorrhea?

    a. Underweight by 3 pounds
    b. History of slight scoliosis
    c. History of brain injury in childhood auto accident
    d. Both mother and older sister have experienced amenorrhea

8. Which of the following girls is *least* likely to have amenorrhea?

    a. One with history of congenital dislocated hips
    b. A ballet dancer
    c. One with history of bulimia
    d. A long-distance swimmer

9. Edy, an adolescent, is to undergo a progesterone challenge test as part of an evaluation of her amenorrhea. The NP provides anticipatory guidance about the test. Which comment by Edy or her mother indicates a need for further teaching?

    a. "I will take a hormone pill for 5 days as part of this test."
    b. "I should have some bleeding within 1 week after my last dose of the medicine for the test."
    c. "We can expect Edy to bleed heavily if she has a positive test."
    d. "Withdrawal bleeding will show that Edy does not have structural problems causing her amenorrhea."

10. Mrs. Milgrim, age 38, presents with concerns about an absence of menstrual periods for the last 5 months. She wonders about menopause because she has begun to have hot flashes. Her mother had an "early menopause." Examination findings raise a high index of suspicion that Mrs. Milgrim is experiencing premature ovarian failure. Which test confirms that diagnosis?

    a. Elevated FSH.
    b. Elevated LH.
    c. Low serum progesterone.
    d. Low DHEA levels.

Answers and Rationales

1. *Answer:* **d** (analysis/diagnosis)
    Rationale: The most common cause of amenorrhea in women of childbearing years is pregnancy. Women in the perimenopausal period may incorrectly believe that they are unable to become pregnant and become lax in their use of birth control. Further testing should take place only after pregnancy is ruled out (Smith, 1997)

2. *Answer:* **d** (implementation/plan)
    Rationale: These features of androgen excess that may indicate polycystic ovarian disease should be evaluated by a physician before initiation of hormone therapy. Because these symptoms are a change in her normal status, a more serious condition must be ruled out (Tierney et al., 2001).

3. *Answer:* **b** (implementation/plan)
    Rationale: Hypothyroidism is a fairly common cause of amenorrhea and with treatment should result in regular menstrual cycles. PTU is the treatment for hyperthyroidism. A thyroid scan is not necessary if the client responds to replacement therapy, and neither is a CT scan (Cash & Glass, 2000).

4. *Answer:* **b** (implementation/plan)
    Rationale: Irregular menstrual cycles are common for the first year or two as a result of irregular ovulatory cycles or anovulation. It is not necessary to do further testing as long as she continues to menstruate at least once every 6 months (Youngkin & Davis, 1998).

5. *Answer:* **d** (evaluation)
    Rationale: One of the side effects of medroxyprogesterone (Depo-Provera) is irregular menstrual cycles, often including amenorrhea. Levonorgestrel (Norplant) may cause breakthrough bleeding. Neither levothyroxine (Synthroid) nor beta-blockers are known to cause amenorrhea (Hawkins, Roberto-Nichols, & Stanley-Haney, 1997).

6. *Answer:* **a** (plan/implementation)
    Rationale: Although anovulatory women may have a difficult time becoming pregnant, "priming" them with low-dose estrogen does not increase their fertility. Withdrawal bleeding indicates sufficient estrogen to prevent osteoporosis and heart disease, which may occur from a decrease in estrogen production. They are also at no greater risk for development of endometriosis and uterine fibroids. However, unopposed estrogen may predispose these women toward endometrial cancer; therefore hormonal regulation is necessary.

7. *Answer:* **c** (assessment)
    Rationale: History of significant head injury is correlated with a diagnosis of amenorrhea (Tierney, et al, 2001).

8. *Answer:* **a** (assessment)
    Rationale: Excessive exercise required by ballet dancers and long-distance swimmers and malnutrition experienced by a person with a history of bulimia are associated with amenor-

rhea; a history of congenital dislocation of the hips is not an associated factor (Tierney, et al, 2001).

9. Answer: c (evaluation)
   Rationale: Heavy bleeding is not required for a positive test result; withdrawal bleeding indicating a positive response to the progesterone challenge test can be uterine spotting only (Smith & Shimp, 2000).

10. Answer: a (analysis/diagnosis)
   Rationale: Although the LH level may be elevated in premature ovarian failure, it is the FSH level greater than 40 that indicates ovarian failure (Cash & Glass, 2000).

ANEMIA *Pamela Kidd*

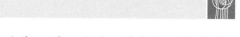

OVERVIEW
Definition

Anemia is a condition in which the concentration of Hgb or the number or volume of red blood cells (RBCs) is reduced to a below-normal value. Anemia may be caused by impaired production of RBCs, increased destruction of RBCs, or rapid loss of RBCs.

Incidence

- Anemia occurs most frequently in young children, women of reproductive age, and older adults.
- Iron deficiency is the most common cause.
- The prevalence of iron deficiency is currently estimated to be approximately 3% for children 1 to 5 years old.
- A low Hgb level is present in about 9% of women 15 to 44 years old and is especially common during pregnancy.
- The prevalence of anemia in persons older than 65 years is 2.3% in males and 5.5% in females.
- Sickle cell anemia affects more than 70,000 blacks, with one third between 2 and 16 years old.

Pathophysiology

The physiologic defects caused by anemia are a decrease in the oxygen-carrying capacity of the blood and a reduction in the oxygen available to the tissues. The signs and symptoms of anemia are a result of failure to oxygenate tissues and the degree of acuity (gradual onset of anemia allows time for compensatory mechanisms to increase oxygenation). Anemias can be classified either by causal (etiologic) mechanisms or by RBC morphology. On an etiologic basis, anemia results from the following:
- Acute or chronic hemorrhage
- An increased loss or destruction of RBCs
- Production of abnormal Hgb, leading to anemia and tissue damage from vascular blockage by trapped, abnormal RBCs; RBCs assume crescent shape when oxygen tension is lowered (sickle cell)
- Impaired Hgb and RBC formation (nutritional, bone marrow infiltration, chronic disease)

The morphologic classification of anemia includes the following:
- Normocytic/normochromic (blood loss, hemolytic anemia, chronic disease, bone marrow infiltration)
- Microcytic/hypochromic (iron deficiency, lead, thalassemias)
- Macrocytic/normochromic (vitamin B_{12} or folate deficiency, drugs, bone marrow failure)

Refer to Box 3-5 for classification of anemias.

Factors Increasing Susceptibility. In neonates, the most common causes of anemia include blood loss, isoimmunization, congenital infection, and congenital hemolytic anemia.

In infants ages 3 to 6 months, anemia is usually caused by congenital disorders of Hgb synthesis or Hgb structure. Nutritional iron deficiency is almost never seen in an otherwise healthy term infant. Prematurity predisposes toward early development of iron deficiency.

In older infants or toddlers, nutritional iron deficiency may be seen in those who switched to whole cow's milk.

Ethnicity
- Hgb S and Hgb C are more common in blacks.
- Beta-thalassemia is more common in people of Mediterranean background.
- Alpha-thalassemia is more common among blacks and Asians.

Protective Factors
- Nutritious diet
- Genetic profile

ASSESSMENT: SUBJECTIVE/HISTORY
Symptoms
- Irritability, mood disturbances
- Dyspnea (particularly exertional)
- Fatigue, weakness
- Palpitations
- Dizziness
- Headache
- Edema
- Jaundice (particularly during neonatal period secondary to hyperbilirubinemia)
- Bleeding
- Any recent weight gain or loss
- Anorexia
- Nausea or vomiting
- Decreased intake

BOX 3-5 Classification of Anemia

MICROCYTIC/HYPOCHROMIC ANEMIA (DEFICIENT ERYTHROPOIESIS)

Microcytic anemias are produced by inadequate iron intake, increased iron requirement, decreased iron absorption and/or inadequate iron transport.

Iron deficiency anemia is caused by increased physiologic requirements, decreased intake of iron, or chronic blood loss.

Lead ingestion leads to increased aminolevulinic acid, which leads to deficient Hgb synthesis.

Thalassemias are genetically caused, related to deficient synthesis of one or more of the polypeptide chains of Hgb. Iron intake may be fine, but transport of iron becomes the problem.

- Thalassemia major: Lack of b-chain synthesis, intramedullary hemolysis
- Thalassemia minor: Heterozygous state
- Thalassemia alpha: Deletion of one or more alpha-chain genes

NORMOCYTIC/NORMOCHROMIC ANEMIA

Normocytic anemia is reduced survival of circulating RBCs caused by their intrinsic defect, or extrinsic defects such as destruction in the circulation (intravascular) or within the phagocytic cells of the liver, spleen, or bone marrow (extravascular).

Intrinsic RBC Defects

- Congenital spherocytosis is abnormality of RBC membranes as a result of spectrin deficiency.

- In G6PD deficiency, a deficient enzyme concentration does not allow detoxification of oxygen free radicals by the reduced form of nicotinamide adenine dinucleotide, precipitating hemolysis.
- Hemoglobinopathies include Hgb SS and Hgb C (sickle cell).

Extrinsic RBC Defects

- Immune mediated
- Hemolytic disease of the neonate (ABO incompatibility)

Anemia of chronic disease may be caused by the following:

- Chronic infection
- Osteomyelitis
- Tuberculosis
- Pyelonephritis
- Chronic inflammatory disorders (rheumatoid arthritis, SLE, IBD)

MACROCYTIC ANEMIA

Abnormally large but inefficient RBCs are produced.

- Aplastic anemia/Fanconi's anemia: Causes include idiopathic, hepatitis, chemicals, and pregnancy.
- Vitamin B_{12}/folate deficiency: Causes include inadequate intake, malabsorption, and increased body requirements.
- Hemolysis (excessive RBC destruction)

RBC, Red blood cell; *G6PD,* glucose-6-phosphate dehydrogenase; *Hgb,* hemoglobin; *SLE,* systemic lupus erythematosus; *IBD,* irritable bowel disease.

- Diarrhea
- Bone pain

Past Medical History

- Anemia with previous pregnancies
- Infection
- Heart murmur
- Chronic illness
- Drug use
- Past viral infections
- Environmental exposures at home and in the workplace (lead, chemicals, and heavy metals)

Medication History

Anticonvulsants and chemotherapy increase risk of anemias.

Family History

- Ethnic origin
- Travel

- History of gallstones or splenectomy in other family members (may indicate blood dyscrasia)

Dietary History

- Decreased iron, folate, vitamin B_{12}, or vitamin E
- Alcohol ingestion
- Pica (craving for unusual substances such as clay or ice suggests iron deficiency)
- Formula type and amount, use of cow's milk

ASSESSMENT: OBJECTIVE/PHYSICAL EXAMINATION

Physical Examination

Perform a complete physical examination with increased attention to the following:

- Vital signs, weight, height

In mild anemia (Hgb 10 to 14 g/dL) and even moderate anemia (6 to 10 g/dL), few clinical manifestations may be seen. Most commonly, palpitations and dyspnea are the first symptoms seen. In severe anemia (Hgb less than 6 g/dL), the following may be seen:

- *General:* sensitivity to cold, weight loss, lethargy, mood changes (indication of vitamin B_{12}, folate, or iron deficiency)
- *Skin:* jaundice, bleeding, pallor, petechiae, purpura
- Mouth: glossitis (indication of vitamin B_{12}, folate, or iron deficiency), angular stomatitis
- *Eyes:* eyelid edema, retinal hemorrhage, color blindness (indication of vitamin B_{12}, folate, or iron deficiency)
- *Respiratory:* tachypnea
- *Cardiovascular:* tachycardia, systolic ejection murmur, or gallop; angina; myocardial infarction; congestive heart failure
- *Abdominal:* hepatosplenomegaly (most common in hemolytic anemia) or other masses, lymphadenopathy, anorexia
- *Musculoskeletal:* bone pain
- *Neurologic:* headache, vertigo, irritability, depression, impaired thought processes, tremors, peripheral loss of sensation, ataxia, loss of taste and smell (most common with vitamin B_{12} deficiency)
- In infants: iron deficiency anemia common symptoms are pallor, tachycardia, and fatigue

Diagnostic Procedures

- CBC count, including all indexes, mean cell volume (MCV), mean corpuscular Hgb (MCH), mean corpuscular Hgb concentration (MCHC)

- Hgb
- Hematocrit (percentage of packed RBCs in the blood)
- Peripheral blood smear (size [anisocytosis, microcytes, macrocytes], inclusions [basophilic stippling, Howell-Jolly bodies, polychromasia])
- Absolute reticulocyte count (Reflects state of erythroid activity of bone marrow [normal 0.5% to 1.5%])
- Bone marrow (evaluates number of RBC precursors and maturation; rules out infiltration)
- Direct and indirect bilirubin
- Levels of lactate dehydrogenase (LDH), AST, uric acid, total iron, vitamin B_{12}, vitamin E, folic acid
- Direct and indirect Coombs' test
- Total iron-binding capacity (TIBC)
- Ferritin
- Free erythrocyte protoporphyrin
- Serum methylmalonic acid (elevated in vitamin B_{12} deficiency)

NOTE: *Results of serum testing are falsely low (when an anemia does not exist), in cases of hemodilution (e.g., pregnancy, heart failure). Results may be artificially higher than actually exists when the client is dehydrated.*

A translation of pertinent laboratory results is located in Box 3-6.

DIAGNOSIS

The client's Hgb and hematocrit should be compared with a set of standards appropriate for age. The corpuscular MCV and reticulocyte count should be analyzed to suggest a potential cause of the anemia.

BOX 3-6 Translation of Pertinent Laboratory Results

PERIPHERAL BLOOD SMEAR
- Hypochromic microcytosis *indicates iron deficiency or thalassemia.*
- Fragmented red blood cells *indicates traumatic hemolysis.*
- Hypersegmented neutrophils *indicates vitamin B_{12} or folic acid deficiency.*
- Nucleated red blood cells *indicates autoimmune hemolysis, thalassemia, vitamin B_{12} and folate deficiency.*
- Anisocytes and poikilocytes *indicate vitamin B_{12} deficiency.*
- Echinocytes *indicates renal failure, iron deficiency.*
- Acanthocytes *indicates liver disease.*
- Low white blood cell count, low platelet count, blasts *indicate aplastic anemia, leukemia.*

ABSOLUTE RETICULOCYTE COUNT
- Low absolute reticulocyte count *indicates anemias of chronic disease, iron, vitamin B_{12}, folate deficiency, aplastic anemia.*

- High absolute reticulocyte count *indicates autoimmune or traumatic hemolysis, sickle cell anemia, Rh isoimmunization, G6PD deficiency.*

SERUM FERRITIN LEVEL
- Twelve mcg/L *indicates iron deficiency anemia.*

HEMATOCRIT
- <40% *indicates anemia in male.*
- <37% *indicates anemia in female.*

HEMOGLOBIN
- <14 g/dL *indicates anemia in male.*
- <12 g/dL *indicates anemia in female.*

RED BLOOD CELL MASS
- $<4.5 \times 10^{12}$ *indicates anemia in male.*
- $<4.0 \times 10^{12}$ *indicates anemia in female.*

G6PD, Glucose-6-phosphate dehydrogenase; *Rh,* rhodium.

Differential diagnosis includes the following:

- Autoimmune pancytopenia
- Marrow infiltration with a solid tumor
- Marrow suppression caused by drug toxins or infections
- Bleeding colitis
- Osteomyelitis
- Pyelonephritis
- Blood loss
- Hemolysis
- Chronic inflammatory bowel disease (IBD)
- Rheumatoid arthritis
- systemic lupus erythematosus (SLE)
- Leukemia
- Age-specific diagnosis located in Box 3-7

THERAPEUTIC PLAN
Nonpharmacologic Treatment

Diet with meat and dairy products for vitamin B_{12} and folate deficiency. If client is vegan or strict vegetarian, consider oral B_{12} supplements.

Advise legumes, leafy green vegetables, fruits, and liver to treat folate deficiency.

Pharmacologic Treatment

- Client should take 50 to 60 mg of elemental iron (300 mg ferrous sulfate tablet provides 60 mg of elemental iron). Do not take with milk (precipitates). Metabolization is enhanced with orange juice. Ingestion with meals decreases GI effects, but also decreases absorption. Therapy is discontinued when ferritin level is greater than 50 mcg/L.

- For vitamin B_{12} deficiency, administer 1000 mcg cyanocobalamin or hydroxocobalamin subcutaneously weekly.
- A viable alternative to subcutaneous administration may be 2 mg of oral cyanocobalamin (Blackweel & Hendrix, 2001).
- Prescribe folic acid 1.0 mg PO for folate deficiency.
- Recombinant human erythropoietin (RrHuEPO) intravenously or subcutaneously 50 to 100 U/kg three times a week is used to treat anemia of renal failure.
- Oral prednisone (up to 100 mg) is used for treating for autoimmune hemolytic anemia.
- The goal of treatment is to eradicate the anemia and its cause.

Client Education
Iron Deficiency Anemia

- Identify causes of low iron and needed treatment plan.
- Teach family about diet high in iron and about side effects of iron therapy (e.g., constipation).

Sickle Cell Anemia

- Identify causes of sickle cell crisis and disease process.
- Teach family awareness of precipitating factors:
  - Cold exposure
  - Decreased fluid intake
  - Exercise at high altitude
  - Overexertion, emotional or physical stress
  - Increased blood viscosity
  - Viral or bacterial infections
  - Surgery, blood loss

BOX 3-7   Age-Specific Diagnosis of Anemia

NEWBORN
- Blood loss
- Hemolysis

INFANT
- Iron deficiency anemia
- GI bleeding
- Thalassemia
- Sickle cell anemia
- Lead exposure
- Spherocytosis

TODDLER AND SCHOOL-AGE CHILD
- Fanconi's anemia
- Aplastic anemia
- Anemia of chronic G6PD deficiency
- Transient erythroblastopenia after illness

ADOLESCENT
- Iron deficiency anemia
- Aplastic anemia
- Autoimmune hemolysis
- Sickle cell anemia

ADULT
- Folic acid deficiency
- Pernicious anemia
- Iron deficiency anemia
- Autoimmune hemolysis
- Aplastic anemia

PREGNANT FEMALE
- Acute blood loss
- Iron deficiency anemia
- Folic acid deficiency

GI, Gastrointestinal; *G6PD,* glucose-6-phosphate dehydrogenase.

- Explain need for routine health care.
- Provide psychosocial support.
- Provide prenatal counseling.

Pernicious Anemia
- Explain etiology and nature of disease.
- Explain need for lifelong B_{12} replacement.
- Review side effects of B_{12} injection.

Referral

Recommend referral to hematologist for multidisciplinary approach and pain management if needed for sickle cell anemia.

Prevention

- Prenatal and genetic counseling for genetically linked anemias and Rh isoimmunization
- Nutritious diet

EVALUATION/FOLLOW-UP

Evaluation of treatment response is discussed in the following sections.

Iron Deficiency Anemia

- In infants reticulocyte count should be increased in 2 to 3 days. Hgb is rechecked in 2 to 3 weeks, at which time indices should have returned to normal. Iron therapy is continued for 2 to 3 months after Hgb levels have returned to normal to replenish iron stores.
- In adults recheck absolute reticulocyte count in 10 days; if it has returned to normal, iron dosage is correct. Continue iron 3 months after return of normal Hgb to replenish iron stores. Recheck CBC count.

Pernicious Anemia

- Follow-up older adults and clients with cardiac conditions in 48 hours (a rapid increase in RBC production can lead to hypovolemia).
- Consider iron supplementation.
- Check initial hematologic response in 4 to 6 weeks, then every 6 months for hematocrit, with stool check for occult blood (incidence of gastric cancer increases with pernicious anemia).

Folic Acid Deficiency

- Repeat Hgb measurement and hematocrit in 2 to 4 weeks (should expect increase of 2 points in Hgb within 1 month).
- Refer if anemia is severe.

COMPLICATIONS

- Hypovolemic shock
- Permanent neurologic damage
- Cardiac dysrhythmias

REFERENCES

Blackwell, S., & Hendrix, P. (2001a). Common Anemias: What lies beneath. *Clinician Reviews. 11*(3), 53-62.

Blackwell, S., & Hendrix, P. (2001b). Less common anemias: Beyond iron deficiency. *Clinician Reviews. 11*(4), 57-65.

Cunningham, F., McDonald, P., Gant, N., Levens, K., Gilstrap, L., Hankins, G., & Clark, S. (1997). Hematological disorders. In *Williams obstetrics* (20th ed., pp. 1173-1189). Norwalk, CT: Appleton & Lange.

Kalinyak, K. (1997). Anemias. In R. Arceci (Ed.), *Hematology/oncology/stem cell transplant handbook* (2nd ed., pp. 87-116). Cincinnati: Hematology Oncology Division of Children's Hospital Medical Center.

Lane, P., Nuss, R., & Ambruso, D. (1995). Hematologic disorders. In W. Hay, J. Groothuis, A. Hayward, & M. Levin (Eds.), *Current pediatric diagnosis and treatment* (pp. 819-839). Norwalk, CT: Appleton & Lange.

Mitus, A., & Rosenthal, D. (1995). History and physical examination of relevance to the hematologist. In R. Handlin, S. Lux, & T. Stossel (Eds.), *Blood: Principles and practice of hematology* (pp. 3-19). Philadelphia: J. B. Lippincott.

Review Questions

1. The most common presenting symptoms in childhood iron deficiency anemia include which of the following?
- **a.** Fever, pallor, and pain
- **b.** Pallor, lymphadenopathy, and night sweats
- **c.** Weight loss, pallor, and fever
- **d.** Pallor, tachycardia, fatigue, and poor dietary intake

2. Risk factors for development of anemia include all the following *except:*
- **a.** Family history of anemia
- **b.** History of pica
- **c.** Hyperbilirubinemia in the neonatal period
- **d.** Sibling with a history of hepatitis.

3. In which of the following clients would you suspect vitamin B_{12} deficiency?
- **a.** Male, 36 years old, with 2-week history of pallor, fatigue, and anorexia
- **b.** Female, 60 years old, with a beefy, red, smooth tongue
- **c.** Male, 70 years old, with a 2- to 3-month history of fatigue, anorexia, and black, tarry stools
- **d.** Female, 30 years old, with history of 330 pg/ml serum vitamin B_{12} level

4. Which of the following would be *inaccurate* information to provide to a client being treated with iron supplement for iron deficiency anemia?
- **a.** Constipation is common.
- **b.** Milk enhances absorption.
- **c.** Efficacy of therapy can be determined within 10 days.
- **d.** Take one tablet each day.

5. Signs and symptoms of folate deficiency are similar to those of Vitamin B_{12} deficiency *except* there is no:

    a. Neurologic involvement
    b. Glossitis
    c. Color blindness
    d. Mood changes

6. Which response indicates improvement in a client diagnosed with sickle cell anemia?

    a. Increase in WBC count
    b. Increase in serum ferritin level
    c. Decrease in serum methylmalonic acid
    d. Decrease in reticulocyte count

7. A client with anemia related to sickle cell disease exhibits which of the following?

    a. Macrocytic anemia
    b. Microcytic/hypochromic anemia
    c. Normocytic/normochromic anemia
    d. Hypersegmented neutrophils on the peripheral blood smear

8. A pregnant client has a Hgb level of 11 g/dL. Based on this result the nurse practitioner should consider which of the following?

    a. It is a normal finding due to hemodilution.
    b. A work up for folic acid deficiency is indicated.
    c. A work up for iron deficiency anemia is indicated.
    d. Exploring sources of potential blood loss is indicated.

Answers and Rationales

1. *Answer:* **d** (assessment)
    Rationale: Pallor, tachycardia, fatigue, and poor dietary intake are symptoms most commonly seen in children during the course of iron deficiency anemia. These symptoms reflect iron deficiency, which is always caused by nutritional deficits of iron in young children who consume a diet high in unfortified cow's milk.

2. *Answer:* **d** (assessment)
    Rationale: Risk factors in development of anemia include a positive family history, a known history of pica, and hyperbilirubinemia in the neonatal period. Risk factors do not include a sibling with hepatitis.

3. *Answer:* **b** (assessment)
    Rationale: The objective assessment of a 60-year-old woman with the beefy, red, smooth tongue points to vitamin B_{12} deficiency. For the 36-year-old man, sudden onset of symptoms leads one to suspect blood loss; for the 70-year-old, one suspects blood loss through the GI tract. The 30-year-old woman's serum vitamin concentration is elevated, not decreased.

4. *Answer:* **b** (implementation/plan)
    Rationale: Iron absorption is decreased with both food and milk products. It does produce constipation, is dosed once a day, and will elevate the absolute reticulocyte count in 7 to 10 days (Blackwell & Hendrix, 2001A).

5. *Answer:* **a** (analysis/diagnosis)
    Rationale: Symptoms and signs related to Vitamin B_{12} and folic acid deficiency are very similar. They may coexist. However, correcting folic acid alleviates the anemia but does not alleviate neurologic symptoms. The neurologic symptoms are caused by a deficiency in vitamin B_{12}. To distinguish between the two anemias, a methylmalonic acid level is obtained. This value is elevated in vitamin B_{12} deficiency but not in folate deficiency (Blackwell & Hendrix, 2001B).

6. *Answer:* **d** (evaluation)
    Rationale: In sickle cell anemia, the reticulocyte count is high; therefore a return to normal (decrease) indicates a favorable response to therapy and avoidance of precipitating factors. Increased WBCs indicate leukemia or infection. Increased serum ferritin is present in iron deficiency anemia. Decreased serum methylmalonic acid is present in vitamin B_{12} deficiency.

7. *Answer:* **c** (analysis/diagnosis)
    Rationale: Normocytic/normochromic is due to decreased survival of circulating RBCs. Macrocytic anemia is related to abnormally large but inefficient RBCs. Microcytic/ hypochromic represents inadequate intake or transport of iron. Hypersegmented neutrophils are common in Vitamin B_{12} deficiency.

8. *Answer:* **a** (analysis/diagnosis)
    Rationale: A normal Hgb level for females is 12 g/dL. Hemodilution and falsely low levels (not indicative of anemia) are common in pregnancy. Hgb level alone is not a sensitive or specific marker of anemia.

ANXIETY   *Denise Robinson*

OVERVIEW
Definition

Anxiety is the fundamental emotion that is thought to be the motivating factor from which other emotions, such as anger and guilt, flow. It is an uncomfortable feeling of apprehension and/or fear usually accompanied by psychologic, physiologic, and behavioral symptoms. The symptoms of anxiety alert the individual to real or perceived threats to self or significant others and motivates the individual to take action to relieve the unpleasant feelings. The source of the anxiety is frequently unknown to the person who is experiencing it and is referred to as *generalized* or *diffuse.* Although anxiety is essential for human survival, excessive high and persistent levels interfere with health and life. Anxiety is considered pathologic when the anxiety reaction is out of proportion to the actual experience of the threat, and impaired social or intellectual functioning and psychosomatic symptoms occur.

Types of Anxiety

- Generalized anxiety disorder (GAD)
- Panic disorder
- Phobias
- Posttraumatic stress disorder
- Obsessive-compulsive disorder

Incidence

- Lifetime prevalence of 4% to 6% in general population (Gliatto, 2000)
- Most prevalent psychiatric disorder in the United States, affecting 19 million each year
- More common in women than in men
- Median age of onset is early 20s
- Correlation between cardiac problems, hypoglycemia, and seizure disorders, and individuals who suffer from anxiety
- Accounts for nearly one third of the nation's total mental health care costs in 1990, at approximately $46.6 billion
- Lifetime prevalence of panic disorder between 1.5% and 3%
- Anxiety in children approximately 6% prevalence

Etiology

There are four basic theoretic perspectives to understanding anxiety:

- In psychoanalytic (Freudian) theory, anxiety reflects a conflict between the demands of one's instinctual drives (the id), the realistic perception of the specific situation (the ego), and the moralistic controlling conscience (the superego). Anxiety signals the ego of an unconscious impulse reflecting hidden psychologic conflict.
- According to learning-behavioral theory, anxiety is a learned response to a stimulus that is perceived as painful or uncomfortable. The individual learns to reduce anxiety by avoiding the uncomfortable stimulus.
- The biochemical theory states that anxiety is the uncomfortable feeling caused by a perceived danger and accompanied by physiologic symptoms that prepares the individual for the "fight or flight" response. Primarily, these symptoms are due to cardiovascular and neuroendocrine system stimulation. As the production of norepinephrine increases in humans, so does the level of anxiety.
- Interpersonal theory views all human behavior as a response to our relationship with significant others in our life. Anxiety is the emotional discomfort that results when our expectations of others are not met and our interpersonal security is threatened. Coping mechanisms are learned as a child and then become integrated into the personality of the adult.

Pathophysiology

Neuroregulators have been implicated as the cause of anxiety. These include neurotransmitters, (norepinephrine, dopamine, and serotonin) neuromodulators, endorphins and neurohormones, antidiuretic hormones, angiotensin II and somatostatin.

Patients who experience anxiety have an excessive autonomic reaction with an increased reaction of catecholamines (sympathetic response). Decreased gamma-aminobutyric acid (GABA) causes a central nervous system (CNS) hyperactivity (GABA inhibits CNS activity). An increased serotonin level causes anxiety; increased dopaminergic activity is also associated with anxiety. The hyperactive center is in the temporal cerebral cortex. The locus ceruleus is the center of nonadrenergic neurons; it becomes hyperactive in anxiety states. Conditioned learning may also play a role in the development of anxiety disorders.

Protective Factors. Defense mechanisms and coping behaviors learned early in life relieve the discomfort of anxiety and provide a sense of protection. Examples of individual coping behaviors include the following:

ADAPTIVE	MALADAPTIVE
Prayer	Drugs and/or alcohol
Exercise	Abuse
Relaxation techniques	Excessive eating
Problem solving	Social isolation
	Self-injury

As the level of anxiety increases, the use of the following ego defense mechanisms may become necessary:

- Compensation: Emphasizing a perceived asset in an attempt to overcome feelings of insecurity.
- Denial: Refusing to accept an unpleasant situation as reality based.
- Displacement: Transferring a feeling from the original person or experience to a more neutral one.
- Dissociation: Breaking off certain aspects of one's personality from one's consciousness.
- Identification: Transferring to oneself the attributes of another person.
- Intellectualization: Separating a painful feeling from the experience by the use of excessive reasoning.
- Projection: Transferring one's unacceptable ideas or feelings to another person.
- Rationalization: Using excuses or substituting acceptable reasons to justify unacceptable thoughts or behavior.

A

- Reaction formation: Behavior that is the opposite of one's true, unacceptable feelings.
- Regression: Reverting to an earlier personality developmental level of functioning.
- Repression: Dismissing any undesirable thoughts, feelings, or desires from conscious awareness.
- Sublimation: Expressing unacceptable desires in a more socially acceptable manner.

Coping resources include individual abilities, social support, economic resources, motivation, defensive techniques, health, and high self-esteem.

Factors Increasing Susceptibility
- Anxiety levels exceed coping abilities.
- Coping mechanisms are maladaptive.
- Abnormal levels of norepinephrine and blood lactate are thought to be causative factors.

Anxiety is considered pathologic when any of the following occur:
- The anxiety reaction exceeds the severity or the duration of the threat.
- Impairment in social or intellectual functioning occurs.
- Concurrent psychosomatic problems, such as colitis, exist.

Common Causal Factors
- Developmental crisis
  - Separation of a child from the parent to attend school
  - Growth and sexual development
  - Changes in relationships and roles
  - Aging
- Threats to safety and security
  - Assault and abuse
  - Natural disasters
  - Loss
  - Death of loved one
  - Divorce
  - Major illness and disability
  - Retirement
- Threats to self-esteem and integrity
- Guilt

ASSESSMENT: SUBJECTIVE/HISTORY
Symptoms
- Selective inattention and hesitation
- Diminished problem solving ability
- Rapid speech with frequent change of topic
- Muscle tension and restlessness
- Tachycardia, dyspnea, and hyperventilation
- Fear of loss and impending doom
- Chest pain and feeling of choking, shortness of breath
- Feelings of apprehension, dread, guilt
- Clammy hands
- Dry mouth
- Sweating
- Urinary frequency
- Trouble swallowing
- Exaggerated startle response

Associated Symptoms
- Restlessness and irritability
- Difficulty sleeping/awakening frequently during the night
- Significant changes in eating (anorexia, overeating)
- Chronic fatigue
- Acting out behaviors: violence, truancy, alcohol, drug abuse
- Somatic complaints: stomachache, nausea/vomiting, headache

Characteristics of Anxiety by Level
1. Mild anxiety/normal state of alertness
   - Enhanced perception and concentration
   - Increased motivation and problem solving
2. Moderate anxiety/narrowed focus of perception
   - Selective inattention and hesitation
   - Diminished problem solving
   - Rapid speech with frequent change of topic
   - Muscle tension and restlessness
3. Severe anxiety/severely limited cognitive and perceptual ability
   - Loss of ability to concentrate or problem solve
   - Fear of loss of control and impending doom
   - Continued increase in vital signs with hyperventilation and tachycardia
   - Headache, dizziness
   - Trembling and purposeless movement
   - Urinary frequency, nausea
4. Panic anxiety/greatly impaired perception
   - Inability to reason or problem solve
   - Inability to function safely by self
   - Incoherent speech
   - Chest pain and feeling of choking
   - Incontinence
   - Fear of dying
   - Restlessness and irritability
5. Other symptoms
   - Difficulty sleeping (awakening frequently during the night or awakening in the early morning)
   - Significant changes in eating (anorexia, overeating)
   - Chronic fatigue
   - Feelings of apprehension, guilt, dread
   - Acting out behaviors (anger that may be directly or indirectly expressed, violence, truancy, alcohol and drug abuse)
   - Somatic complaints (stomach ache, nausea and vomiting, headache)

History of Current Illness

- Attempt to identify the precipitating factor or event as perceived by the client.
- Determine the client's perception of when the problem started and its duration.
- Determine the client's coping behaviors and support systems.
- Ask about similar symptoms in the past.
- Other questions that may be helpful to ask include the following:
  - Would you describe yourself as a nervous person, a worrier?
  - Have you ever had a sudden onset of rapid heartbeat, a rush of intense fear, anxiety or nervousness?
  - Some people have fears like heights, flying, or bugs. Do you have any strong fears?
  - Some people are bothered by doing something over and over that they can't resist. Has anything like that been a problem for you?
  - Have you ever experienced a traumatic event in which you thought your life was in danger, or someone else's life was in danger? What happened?

Past Medical History

Most persons with anxiety have a long history of symptoms, especially during stress.

Medications

Some medications can cause anxiety symptoms, such as the following:
- Amphetamines
- Diet aids
- Pseudoephedrine
- Medications, foods, and drink with caffeine
- Withdrawal from some medications, especially sedatives
- Steroids
- Thyroxine
- Theophylline
- SSRIs

Family History

High incidence of anxiety occurring in other family members is indicative of anxiety disorder.

Psychosocial History

Inquire about recent life changes, both positive and negative, including the following:
- Marriage or divorce
- Birth of a child
- Loss
- Job loss, change or promotion
- Entering school
- Change in residence
- Alcohol use (the most commonly used OTC drug to treat anxiety; consider CAGE screening test for alcohol dependence)
- Smoking
- Drug use

ASSESSMENT: OBJECTIVE/PHYSICAL EXAMINATION

Physical Examination

Patients with GAD present with a wide variety of complaints. There may be no indication that GAD is the cause.

A complete physical examination should be made with particular attention to the cardiovascular and neuroendocrine systems. Complete a mental status examination, observing the following:
- Behavior and appearance
- Level of consciousness, cognitive functioning, and memory
- Thought processes, concentration, speech patterns
- Insight
- Suicidal or homicidal ideation

Several assessment tools exist to assist in this examination. They include the Mini-Mental State Examination and the Short Portable Mental Status Questionnaire.
- Primary care evaluation of mental disorders (Prime MD; screening test for the five most common psychiatric disorders)
- Hamilton Anxiety Scale
- Zung Anxiety Scale

Diagnostic Procedures

Laboratory tests primarily ordered to rule out physiologic causes for the presenting symptoms usually include the following:
- ECG
- CBC count with differential and electrolytes
- Thyroid function
- Liver function profile
- Urinalysis with drug screen
- Chest x-ray examination

DIAGNOSIS

Medical conditions need to be ruled out before GAD can be diagnosed. Neurologic and endocrine diseases are the most frequent medical causes of anxiety. Others causes that, although uncommon, must be ruled out include the following:
- Mitral valve prolapse
- Carcinoid syndrome
- Pheochromocytoma
- IBS
- Gastritis
- Vitamin B_{12} deficiency
- Perimenopause
- Substance abuse

Diagnostic Criteria for GAD

Excessive anxiety and worry (apprehensive expectation) occurring more days than not for at least 6 months, about a number of events or activities (e.g., at school or work). The person finds it difficult to control the worry.

The anxiety and worry are associated with three or more of the following symptoms (Only one item is required in children):

- Restlessness or feeling keyed up or on edge
- Being easily fatigued
- Difficulty concentrating or mind going blank
- Irritability
- Muscle tension
- Sleep disturbance

The anxiety, worry, or physical symptoms cause clinically significant distress or impairment in social, occupational or other important areas of functioning (APA, 1994).

Other Psychiatric Disorders

At this point, several other abnormal anxiety syndromes must be ruled out, including the following:

- Panic disorder is characterized by sudden, intense, unpredictable anxiety attacks and is manifested by severe debilitating physical and emotional symptoms associated with a sense of fear and impending doom. Onset usually occurs in late adolescence or mid-30s. Family history may reveal panic disorder, major depression, or alcohol abuse.
- Posttraumatic stress disorder is the recurrent re-experiencing of a traumatic event and the feelings associated with that previous experience. Examples include natural disasters, rape, major injury events, and military combat. Beside the symptoms of severe anxiety, substance abuse and depression are frequently seen as a means of dealing with the emotional pain.
- Phobia is an anxiety disorder characterized by irrational fear of specific places or situations (agoraphobia), appearing inept in the company of others (social phobia), or fear of a specific object or thing (specific phobia).
- Depression is a persistently low mood. The usual age of onset is the mid-20s. Symptoms include lack of appetite and insomnia. Family history may reveal depression or alcohol abuse.
- Obsessive-compulsive disorder involves recurring, intrusive thoughts or actions.
- Somatization disorder involves chronic, multiple physical complaints that involve several organ systems.

THERAPEUTIC PLAN

Pharmacologic Treatment

Antianxiety Agents. Benzodiazepines (lorazepam [Ativan], alprazolam [Xanax])

- These drugs are short acting
- Numerous side effects include drowsiness, light headedness, and confusion.
- Should not be administered for long periods.
- Elderly patients are vulnerable to these drugs.
- Do not use with comorbid substance abuse.
- Multiple drug interactions exist. Do not take with ketoconazole and itraconazole; increased CNS depression with alcohol, pain medications, sedatives, muscle relaxants, or antihistamines
- Benzodiazepines are psychologically and physiologically addicting; if given for long periods of time, increasingly higher doses are required.
  - If benzodiazepines are discontinued abruptly, withdrawal symptoms can occur, which may not appear for a week following the last dose.

Nonbenzodiazepine antianxiety agent (buspirone [BuSpar]).

- Nonbenzodiazepines have a slower onset. May take 2 to 3 weeks before benefit seen.
- These drugs are contraindicated in those using MAOIs.
- Buspirone (BuSpar) is not effective for acute crises because of its delayed onset of action.
- Side effects include dizziness, nausea, headache, nervousness, light-headedness, and excitement.

Antidepressants

- Antidepressants are sometimes prescribed when depression is an integral factor in the anxiety.
- The antidepressants may worsen anxiety initially before achieving their full antidepressant effect.

Tricyclic antidepressants (amitriptyline, clomipramine, desipramine)

- SSRIs (citalopram, fluoxetine, paroxetine)
- Other agents: serotonin 2A antagonist (Nefazodone)
- Serotonin-norepinephrine reuptake inhibitor (Venlafaxine)
- MAOIs (not first line treatment)

Psychologic Modalities

For mild anxiety, nonpharmacologic treatments should be the initial treatment.

- Relaxation techniques
- Biofeedback
- Cognitive therapy

For generalized moderate anxiety, assist the client in problem solving to facilitate the identification of stressors and effective coping skills. Various relaxation techniques, such as exercise and rest, guided imagery, and other stress reduction techniques, can be used in combination with medication or alone. If the client is experiencing a higher level of anxiety (severe or panic), crisis intervention techniques are used. The initial focus is to relieve symptoms and ensure safety. The following techniques are used:

- The client must not be left alone.
- Provide a quiet, safe environment.
- Assess for suicidal or homicidal ideation.
- Permit expression of feelings but do not ask for detailed explanations.
- Assess support systems and coping mechanisms.
- Evaluate the need for medication and hospitalization.

The broad treatment modalities for anxiety include cognitive therapy, individual psychotherapy, behavior therapy, and group/family therapy.

Client Education

- Stress reduction exercises
- Deep breathing, exercise
- Effective coping behaviors
- Appropriate use of medication
- Availability of various treatment resources
- Options for treatment
- Avoidance of foods that contain stimulants

Referral

Seek consultation with a mental health specialist when any of the following occur:

- Psychotic paranoid thought processes
- Panic level of anxiety
- Suicidal/homicidal ideation
- Escalation of symptoms to the point of refusal of treatment
- No response to standard treatment
- Comorbid psychiatric diagnoses

Refer to Alcoholics Anonymous or Narcotics Anonymous if alcohol or drug abuse is a contributing factor.

EVALUATION/FOLLOW-UP

Follow-up weekly to evaluate the client's response. Progress is made when the client accomplishes the following:

- Is compliant with the treatment plan.
- Is able to recognize early signs of own anxiety response.
- Is able to recognize current life stressors that trigger an anxiety response.
- Attempts to eliminate maladaptive coping behaviors.
- Implements adaptive coping behaviors.

Prevention

No known prevention.

COMPLICATIONS

Inability to function within society, necessitating social service support.

REFERENCES

American Psychiatric Association (1994). *Diagnostic and statistical manual of mental disorders (DSM-IV)* (4th ed.). Washington, DC: Author.

Anxiety and antidepressant drugs. (1993, January). *The Harvard Mental Health Letter*, p. 6.

Aquilera, D.C., & Messick, J.M. (1990). *Crisis intervention theory and methodology.* St. Louis: Mosby.

Aromando, L. (1995). *Mental health and psychiatric nursing* (2nd ed., pp. 18-25). Springhouse, PA: Springhouse.

Burgess, A.N. (1997). *Psychiatric nursing promoting mental health* (pp. 78-89, 202-221). Norwalk, CT: Appleton & Lange.

Gliatto, M. (2000). Generalized anxiety disorder. *American Family Physician, 62,* 1591-1600, 1602.

Kushner, P. & Stahl, S. (2000). Generalized anxiety disorder. *American Academy of Family Physicians.* Retrieved July 13, 2002, from http://www.aafp.org/come/videocme/805.html

King, P. (2000). Anxiety. In D. Robinson, P. Kidd, & K Rogers. (Eds.), *Primary care across the lifespan,* St. Louis: Mosby, 75-84.

Saeed, S. & Bruce, T. (1998). Panic disorder: effective treatment options. *American Family Physician.* Available online: http://www.aafp.org/afp/980515ap/saeed.html.

Wilson, B.A., Shannon, M.T., & Stang, C.L. (1997). *Nurses drug book.* Norwalk, CT: Appleton & Lange.

Review Questions

1. If the patient has a diagnosis of GAD, what complaints is the NP likely to find in the history?

- **a.** Slowed, tired muscles
- **b.** Dry mouth, palpitations
- **c.** Constipation
- **d.** Intolerance to cold

2. Ruth is a 25-year-old college student who reports that when she must take an examination, she experiences inability to problem solve, rapid heartbeat with palpitations and faintness, and increased respirations. You assess her as having which of the following?

- **a.** Panic attack
- **b.** Attention-seeking behavior
- **c.** Posttraumatic stress disorder
- **d.** Hypoglycemia

3. To decrease the severe anxiety level being manifested by Martha who was in an automobile crash with her boyfriend, Bill, the nurse practitioner should do which of the following?

- **a.** Remain with Martha.
- **b.** Question Martha about the automobile crash.

A

   c. Reassure Martha that Bill is going to be okay.
   d. Tell Martha that her family is on their way to the hospital.

4. GAD must be differentiated from panic disorder. Compared with GAD, panic disorder is associated with which of the following?
   a. Constantly recurring thoughts
   b. Symptoms of anxiety characterized by flashbacks
   c. Fear of a situation, object or activity
   d. Intense fear accompanied by somatic symptoms

5. The rationale for using cognitive therapy for a client who has anxiety is which of the following?
   a. Help the client to view worries more realistically.
   b. Help the client avoid dealing with the cause of the worry.
   c. Increase the client's sensitivity to danger signals.
   d. Justify the extent of the client's concerns.

6. A client who has been treated for 2 months with a benzodiazepine telephones and complains of sweating, tremors, and inability to sleep. Based on an evaluation of the symptoms, which of the following applies to the client?
   a. The client probably stopped taking the medication abruptly and is having withdrawal symptoms.
   b. The client requires an increase in medication dosage because of exacerbation in anxiety symptoms.
   c. The client has built up a tolerance to the medication and needs an increase in the dosage.
   d. The client is experiencing common side effects of the drug and needs the dosage slightly altered.

7. When evaluating a client's coping skills, which of the following would be considered a maladaptive coping behavior?
   a. Daily prayer
   b. Social isolation
   c. Exercise
   d. Relaxation techniques

8. You are planning to start Darla on a medication for her GAD. She is currently in cognitive therapy. Her history is significant for positive family history of psychiatric disorders, and her own past medical history reveals alcohol and nicotine dependence. Which of the following drugs would not be a good choice for Darla as first line therapy?
   a. Buspirone (Buspar)
   b. Fluoxetine (Prozac)

   c. Alpazolam (Xanax)
   d. Nefazodone (Serzone)

Answers and Rationales

1. *Answer:* **b** (assessment)
   Rationale: Symptoms of anxiety include palpitations, nausea, vomiting, diarrhea, sweating, trembling, and dizziness (Gliatto, 2000).

2. *Answer:* **a** (analysis/diagnosis)
   Rationale: Symptoms of panic attacks include diaphoresis, dyspnea, dizziness, faintness and palpitations (King, 2000).

3. *Answer:* **a** (implementation/plan)
   Rationale: The presence of the NP can provide a sense of security and a link with reality (Aromando, 1995).

4. *Answer:* **d** (analysis/diagnosis)
   Rationale: Symptoms of panic attacks include diaphoresis, dyspnea, dizziness, faintness and palpitations (King, 2000).

5. *Answer:* **a** (implementation/plan)
   Rationale: Cognitive therapy helps clients to limit cognitive distortions by viewing their worries more realistically, helping them to develop more effective plans to manage the anxiety. Avoidance is not an effective way to solve problems. Patients with anxiety do not need to be more sensitized to danger signals, nor do they need to rationalize the rightness of their reactions (Gliatto, 2000).

6. *Answer:* **a** (evaluation)
   Rationale: Benzodiazepines are addicting; if benzodiazepines are discontinued abruptly, withdrawal can occur (Wilson, Shannon, & Stang, 1997).

7. *Answer:* **b** (evaluation)
   Rationale: Social isolation does not relieve the discomfort of anxiety or provide a sense of protection (Burgess, 1997).

8. *Answer:* **c** (implementation/plan)
   Rationale: Benzodiazepines should be avoided in those who have a history of substance abuse (Gliatto, 2000).

APHTHOUS ULCERS (CANKER SORES)   *Denise Robinson*

OVERVIEW
Definition

An aphthous ulcer is a superficial ulceration of the mucous membranes of the mouth and lips.

Occasional Aphthae. Single lesions occur at intervals of months or years. They usually heal without complications.

Acute Multiple Aphthae. These are associated with gastrointestinal disorders. An acute episode may last for weeks. Lesions develop sequentially at different sites in the mouth.

Chronic Recurrent Aphthae. One or more lesions are always present for years. They can also be classified as minor, major and herpetiform.
   • Minor: Generally located on labial or buccal mucosa, the soft palate and the floor of the mouth. They tend to be less than 1 cm in diameter and shallow.
   • Major: Are larger and involve deeper ulceration. They are also more likely to scar with healing.
   • Herpetiform: These ulcers are more numerous and vesicular in morphology.

Incidence

- Twenty percent to 50% of adults affected
- More commonly affects young adults
- More common in females than males
- Familial tendencies
- More common during the winter and spring months

Pathophysiology

The pathophysiology is poorly understood. Histologically, apthae contain a mononuclear infiltrate with a fibrin coating (McBride, 2000). Patients with recurrent aphthae may have alteration of local cell mediated immunity. Systemic T and B cell responses have been reported as altered in patients with recurrent apthae.

Common Pathogens. These ulcers were once thought to be caused by the herpes simplex virus, but the actual cause is not known.

ASSESSMENT: SUBJECTIVE/HISTORY
Symptoms

- Burning sensation 1 to 48 hours before eruption of ulcer
- Pain
- Swelling
- Redness

Past Medical History

- Allergies to chocolate, nuts, tomatoes, or other foods
- Autoimmune disease
- Recent trauma
- Drugs: Possible reaction
- Stressors: Physical or emotional

Medication History

- Antibiotics
- Steroids (especially inhaled)

Family History

- History of the same
- Autoimmune diseases

Psychosocial History

Inquire about recent life stressors.

Dietary History

Ask about possible recent decrease in oral intake as a result of pain.

Protective Factors

- Practice good oral hygiene.
- Avoid oral exposure to others with same.
- Smoking offers a somewhat protective effect against recurrent aphthae.

Aggravating Factors

- Stress
- Physical or chemical trauma
- Food sensitivity
- Infection

ASSESSMENT: OBJECTIVE/PHYSICAL EXAMINATION
Physical Examination

A problem-oriented examination should be conducted with particular attention to the following:

- Examine general appearance: Does the client look ill?
- Determine hydration status: May become dehydrated because of decreased oral intake.
- Oral membrane characteristic lesions (lesions found on buccal or labial mucosa, pharynx or lateral tongue):
  - One or more lesions
  - Small size: less than 10 mm
  - Superficial, shallow, and oval
  - Light yellow to gray fibrinoid center
  - Red ridges
- Examine skin for lesions in other locations (e.g., hands, feet, buttocks, genitals).
- Patients with benign aphthous ulcers have no other findings such as fever, adenopathy, GI symptoms, or other skin or mucus membrane symptoms.

Diagnostic Procedures

Perform incisional biopsy of the lesion if (1) you are unsure of the cause of the lesion or (2) the lesion becomes larger or changes to a color that is inconsistent with previous aphthous ulcers.

If lesions are larger and slow to heal, perform Tzank staining if available. If ulcers are large and slow to heal, check HIV status.

DIAGNOSIS

Differential diagnosis may include the following:

Viral

- Herpes simplex virus (vascular lesions, positive Tzank stain)
- Cytomegalovirus (immunocompromised patient, biopsy results positive for multinucleated giant cells)
- Treponemal
- Syphilis (risk factors, other skin lesions, positive RPR/fluorescent treponemal antibody [FTA])

Drug Allergies

Autoimmune

- Behçet's disease (genital ulceration, uveitis, retinitis)
- IBD (recurrent bloody or mucous diarrhea, other GI ulcerations)
- Reiter's syndrome (uveitis, conjunctivitis, human leukocyte antigen [HLA] B27 arthritis)
- Lupus erythematosus (malar rash, positive ANA)

Miscellaneous

- Squamous cell carcinoma (chronicity, head/neck adenopathy, positive biopsy)
- Cyclic Neutropenia (periodic fever, neutropenia) (McBride, 2000)

THERAPEUTIC PLAN

Pharmacologic Treatment

Topical Steroids

- Triamcinolone acetonide 0.1%
- Fluocinonide ointment 0.05% in an adhesive base (Orabase Plain) applied to lesions 3 times a day

Mouth Coating

- Mixture of diphenhydramine (Benadryl) suspension (5 mg/ml) and Maalox or Mylanta in equal parts
- Viscous lidocaine (Xylocaine) 15 ml swished in mouth every 4 hours for clients older than 12 years; 3 to 5 ml for children 5 to 12 years old

Mouth Rinse

- Use tetracycline 250 mg capsule opened and the powder mixed in 30 to 50 ml of water, 3 to 4 times a day for 5 to 7 days. Tetracycline tends to abort the lesions and prevent secondary infections. This should not be used during pregnancy.
- Use chloraseptic mouthwash every 2 hours for children older than 6 years.
  For patients infected with HIV who have severe aphthous ulcers, thalidomide (Thalomide) is an immune agent used for severe pain with eating. It is given as 200 mg bid for 3 to 8 weeks; it yields a faster healing rate than placebo.

Client Education/Prevention

- A topical steroid should be used at first sign of tingling to abort the aphthous eruption.
- Topical anesthetics should be applied directly to a lesion that has dried.
- Nothing should be eaten within 1 hour of using anesthetic.
- A bland, soft diet should be followed during lesion eruptions.
- Intake of clear liquids should be increased.
- Lesions can recur.
- Avoid eating foods that seem to cause ulcers.
- Avoid touching areas of trauma in mouth with tongue.

Referral

- If a client, especially a child, becomes dehydrated, he or she may require hospitalization.
- Infants with multiple lesions should be referred to a pediatrician.

EVALUATION/FOLLOW-UP

- Children should be reevaluated within 24 to 48 hours, especially if multiple lesions are present, to ensure that client does not become dehydrated.
- Routine follow-up is not always indicated.

COMPLICATIONS

- Dehydration
- More serious illness not diagnosed

REFERENCES

Dello-Stritto, R. (2000). Dental problems. In D. Robinson, P. Kidd, K. Rogers (Eds.), *Primary care across the lifespan*, St. Louis: Mosby, 302-303.

McBride, D. (2000). Management of aphthous ulcers. *American Family Physician, 62*, 149-154, 160.

Verpilleux, M., Bastuji-Garin, S., Revuz, J. (1999). Comparative analysis of severe aphthosis and Behçet's disease: 104 cases. *Dermatology, 198*, 247-251.

Review Questions

1. Sylvio is complaining of fever, lumps on his neck, and painful vision along with mouth lesions. What should the NP consider in terms of diagnoses for Sylvio?

   a. Aphthous ulcers
   b. Reiter syndrome
   c. Herpes simplex
   d. Syphilis

2. Which of the following symptoms, provided by Sara, is typical of aphthous ulcers?

   a. "I have a funny pattern on my tongue."
   b. "I bit my cheek a couple days ago."
   c. "My mom has sores like this one."
   d. "My partner has a sore on his lip too."

3. During physical assessment, which finding is consistent with the diagnosis of aphthous ulcers?

   a. Small painless ulcer on lip
   b. Cervical lymphadenopathy
   c. Small ulcerated shallow lesion on inside of lip
   d. 20 mm ulcerated lesion on tongue

4. Aphthous ulcers must be differentiated from a more serious illness such as Behçet's disease. Compared with Behçet's disease, aphthous ulcers are associated with:

   a. Ulcers less than 10 mm
   b. Lesions on genitals

c. Uveitis
d. Lesions on hands

5. Which of the following drug choices is most appropriate for aphthous ulcers?
  a. Pain medication such as hydrocodone
  b. Nystatin swish and swallow
  c. Acyclovir five times a day
  d. Orabase tid

6. The NP provides instruction about pharmacologic treatment of aphthous ulcers. Which comment by the patient indicates a need for further instruction?
  a. "I should eat pudding and soft foods."
  b. "I should avoid drinking liquids when I have these ulcers."
  c. "I can take NSAIDs if my mouth is sore."
  d. "I can kiss my partner when I have these ulcers."

7. Which of the following is most helpful in terms of preventing aphthous ulcers?
  a. Brush teeth tid.
  b. Avoid foods that seem to increase ulcers.
  c. Wear dentures with adhesive.
  d. Use mouthwash on a daily basis.

8. Which of the following is most appropriate for the immuno-compromised client with mouth sores?
  a. Check CBC.
  b. Check HIV status.
  c. Check hepatitis B status.
  d. Perform mouth culture.

Answers and Rationales

1. *Answer:* **b** (analysis/diagnosis)
Rationale: Aphthous ulcers usually do not present with fever, adenopathy, or eye problems. This makes it more likely that Sylvio has an autoimmune disease such as Reiter's syn-

drome. Herpes simplex also does not cause the systemic side effects. Syphilis causes a painless ulcer in the primary stages (McBride, 2000).

2. *Answer:* **b** (assessment)
Rationale: Chemical or physical trauma can cause aphthous ulcers (McBride, 2000).

3. *Answer:* **c** (assessment)
Rationale: An aphthous ulcer is described as a shallow, painful ulcer on the buccal mucosa. A small, painless lesion should make you suspicious of syphilis. Aphthous ulcers generally are less than 10 mm and do not cause cervical lymphadenopathy (McBride, 2000).

4. *Answer:* **a** (analysis/diagnosis)
Rationale: Aphthous ulcers are typically less than 10 mm. Lesions on the genitals, a temperature, and uveitis are associated with autoimmune diseases such as Behçet's disease or Reiter's syndrome (McBride, 2000).

5. *Answer:* **d** (implementation/plan)
Rationale: Orabase provides a protective coating for the ulcer. Vicodin is not needed for the pain of aphthous ulcers. Nystatin is effective for candidiasis (thrush). Acyclovir is appropriate for herpes. (McBride, 2000).

6. *Answer:* **b** (evaluation)
Rationale: It is important to continue fluids when ulcers are present. Dehydration is a concern, so increased fluids should be stressed. All other answers are correct (McBride, 2000).

7. *Answer:* **b** (implementation/plan)
Rationale: for many people, specific foods seem to increase the frequency of ulcers. These foods should be avoided. No other answer provided helps decrease or prevent ulcers (McBride, 2000).

8. *Answer:* **b** (implementation/plan)
Rationale: those patients with large, and slow-to-heal ulcers should be evaluated for HIV (McBride, 2000).

APPENDICITIS *Denise Robinson*

OVERVIEW
Definition

Appendicitis is an inflammation of the appendix resulting from bacterial infection.

Incidence

- Develops in 1 of every 15 persons in the United States.
- Incidence rises after age 3 and peaks during late teens.
- Sixty-five percent of cases occur in people less than 30 years old.
- Males affected 1.5 times more frequently than women.
- Most common condition requiring emergency abdominal surgery in childhood.
- Diagnosis is difficult; perforation rates are 30% to 60%. Risk of perforation is greatest in 1- to 4-year-old age

group (70% to 75%) and lowest in adolescents (30% to 40%) (Hartmann, 1996).
- Cases occur more often in autumn and spring.
- The progression from onset of symptoms to perforation usually occurs over 36 to 48 hours.

Pathophysiology

Appendicitis arises from obstruction of the appendiceal lumen, usually by a fecalith, but also by foreign bodies such as seeds, barium, bones, wood, metal, or plastic. Obstruction prevents emptying of the intraluminal fluid into the cecum. The fluid accumulates and distends the appendix. The increased luminal pressure inhibits lymphatic and venous drainage. The congestion leads to thrombosis, necrosis, and perforation. Bacteria multiply and then invade the appendiceal wall. Common pathogens include *Escherichia coli, Bacteroides, enterococcus,* and *pseudomonas.*

Factors Increasing Susceptibility
- Dietary factors (fatty diet) increases susceptibility.
- Medications such as erythromycin, theophylline, and amoxicillin with clavulanate increase susceptibility.
- Suspect appendicitis in any patient with nonspecific complaints who is taking corticosteroids.
- Sexual activity increases susceptibility.
- Consumption of contaminated food increases susceptibility.
- Dysfunctional coping methods increase susceptibility.
- Stressful situations increase susceptibility.

ASSESSMENT: SUBJECTIVE/HISTORY
History of Present Illness
- Determine the time of onset and the duration of the pain.
- Describe the character of the pain.
- Ask whether the patient has nausea, vomiting, or diarrhea.
- Ask whether fever has been present.
- Determine whether there has been a history of trauma.
- Ask about the last BM and the passing of flatus.
- Ask about the patient's interest in eating.
- Ask about activities, such as running, and jumping (versus lying still).
- Ask about the patients typical diet and what he or she has eaten in the past 24 hours.

Symptoms
- *Classic triad: abdominal pain, vomiting, and fever*
- Abdominal tenderness
  - Right-sided abdominal pain is present.
  - Pain not always dull at first; intense and persistent later on.
  - Migration of pain from the umbilical area to right lower quadrant in 50% to 65% of patients only.
  - After age 2, symptoms of appendicitis become more typical.
  - In child, right-sided tenderness should never be considered insignificant no matter how mild.
  - Elderly patients have few or no prodromal symptoms.
  - Nausea is common.
  - Emesis almost always follows the onset of pain.
  - Children may be systematically ill with vomiting rather than presenting with abdominal pain and tenderness.
  - Ten percent to forty percent of clients have no loss of appetite (anorexia).

Past Medical History
- Ask about intestinal problems: diverticulitis, constipation, IBS.
- Ask about previous abdominal surgeries.

Medications
Ask whether the patient is taking erythromycin, theophylline, or amoxicillin with clavulanate.

Family History
Ask whether other family members have had appendicitis.

Psychosocial History
- Ask about tobacco dependence.
- Ask about alcohol ingestion.

ASSESSMENT: OBJECTIVE/PHYSICAL EXAMINATION
Physical Examination
Problem oriented, with particular attention to the following:
- Check vital signs. Is low grade fever present?
- Assess heart and lungs.
- Assess abdomen. Check bowel sounds; guarding; distention; tenderness; masses; and inability to jump, walk, and cough without pain. McBurney's sign should be evaluated last during the examination.
- Assess rectal area. Note tenderness on the right.
- Perform pelvic examination in women who are sexually active.
- In pregnant patients the appendix is displaced to a higher position with pain and tenderness outside the classic position.

In very young children, note the following:
- The abdomen commonly is distended and the child appears to be in a toxic state. The child is usually lethargic, with irritability and vomiting.
- In acute appendicitis, the child is likely to exhibit guarding and to lie on the left side with legs drawn up to reduce tension on the rectus muscle.
- Be alert to shock caused by dehydration or sepsis or both.

See Table 3-7 for special maneuvers.

Diagnostic Procedures
Perform the following diagnostic procedures primarily to rule out other conditions such as UTI, Henoch-Schönlein purpura, and others:
- WBC count (may have a shift to the left)
- U/A
- Pregnancy test
- Flat and upright radiographs of abdomen
- Fecal occult blood testing
- Amylase, lipase, alkaline phosphatase levels
- Ultrasound or CT of abdomen
- In pelvic examination, chlamydia, gonorrhea, and other STDs checks

TABLE **3-7** Special Maneuvers for Physical Examination

SIGN	ORGAN	PHYSICAL FINDINGS	MEANING
Murphy's	Gallbladder	Temporary inspiratory arrest with palpation of right subcostal margin	Cholecystitis, cholelithiasis
Iliopsoas	Psoas abscess	Psoas muscle pain with active hip flexion or passive extension	Peritoneal irritation
Rebound tenderness	Peritoneal irritation	Increased pain on release of deep palpation	Appendicitis
Obturator	Obturator muscle	Pain with internal/external rotation of flexed thigh	Peritoneal irritation
Punch tenderness	Liver, spleen, or adjacent structures	Tenderness with firm palpation to lower costal margin	Hepatitis, splenic injury
CVA tenderness	Kidney	Tenderness over costal vertebral angle	Pyelonephritis

Adapted from Burkhardt C: Guidelines for the rapid assessment of abdominal pain indicative of acute surgical abdomen, *Nurse Pract* 17(6):43–46, 1992. *CVA*, Costovertebral angle.

DIAGNOSIS

Think of appendicitis in every child, regardless of age, who has GI or other abdominal complaints. Differential diagnosis includes the following:

- Pneumonia
- Gynecologic problems, such as PID
- Gastroenteritis
- Gallbladder problems
- Crohn's disease
- UTI
- Irritable bowel disease

THERAPEUTIC PLAN

Nonpharmacologic Treatment

Whenever appendicitis is suspected, a prompt surgical consult is important.

Pharmacologic Treatment

Broad spectrum antibiotics are given before surgery.

Referral

- Seek early consultation for a child with a GI or abdominal complaint when the child appears to have a toxic condition.
- Obtain an obstetric consultation for a pregnant woman with right-sided abdominal pain, especially in the second or third trimesters.

Prevention

Increase dietary fiber. It lessens the risk of obstruction by decreasing the viscosity of the feces, reducing bowel transit time, and subsequently diminishing the likelihood that a fecalith will form.

EVALUATION/FOLLOW-UP

Serial evaluations are important to evaluate the abdomen if the history and physical do not clearly indicate appendicitis.

COMPLICATIONS

- Complications occur in 25% to 30% of children with appendicitis, especially those with perforation.
- Complications primarily infectious.
- Intestinal obstruction also may occur after surgery.

REFERENCES

Acosta R., Goldman H., Crain E.F. (2001). Computed tomography with rectal contrast in children with suspected appendicitis. English *Academy of Emergency Medicine, 8*(5), pp. 446-447.

Burkhardt C. (1992). Guidelines for the rapid assessment of abdominal pain indicative of acute surgical abdomen. *Nurse Practitioner 17*(6):43-46.

Finelli, L. (1991). Evaluation of the child with acute abdominal pain. *Journal of Pediatric Health Care, 5*(5), 251-256.

Hartman, G. (1996). Acute appendicitis. In W. Nelson (Ed). *Nelson Textbook of Pediatrics,* (15th ed., pp. 1109-1111). Philadelphia: Saunders.

Rice, P. (1996, April). Abdominal pain: Predicting who will need an operation. *Emergency Medicine,* 14-25.

Robinson, D. (2000). Appendicitis. In D. Robinson, P. Kidd, K. Rogers (Eds.), *Primary care across the lifespan,* (pp. 85-88). St. Louis: Mosby.

Stone, R. (1996). Primary care diagnosis of acute abdominal pain. *Nurse Practitioner, 21*(12), 19-40.

Review Questions

1. Colt is a 5-year-old boy. He is complaining of abdominal pain of a few hours duration. Which of the following historical data is consistent with a diagnosis of appendicitis?

    a. Vomiting followed by diarrhea
    b. Pain preceding emesis and fever
    c. Weight loss and prolonged symptoms
    d. Distended, hypoactive bowel sounds

2. During the physical examination, which action by Colt is typical of appendicitis?

    a. Jumping down from the examining table
    b. Vomiting when his abdomen is touched

A

c. Walking tentatively with a slight limp
d. Eating chicken noodle soup because he is hungry

3. Which of the following special maneuvers is appropriate when examining Colt for appendicitis?

a. McMurray test
b. Rebound tenderness
c. Drawer test
d. Palpation of the abdomen

4. Appendicitis must be differentiated from infectious enteritis. Compared against appendicitis, infectious enteritis is associated with which of the following?

a. Vomiting followed by crampy pain
b. Hypoactive bowel sounds
c. Anorexia
d. Hematuria

5. The NP provides instruction on how to observe 7-year-old Sally at home relative to her abdominal pain. Which of the following indicates that her mother needs further instruction?

a. "Sally can have pizza for lunch if she is hungry."
b. "If Sally has to walk bent over she should return to the hospital."
c. "Sally may have vomiting."
d. "If the pain moves from her right side to all over her abdomen, I will call."

6. Which of the following activities may help prevent the development of appendicitis?

a. Adequate exercise
b. Six to eight glasses of water per day
c. Regular bowel movements
d. High-fiber diet

7. Which of the following has the greatest priority at this time with regard to appendicitis?

a. Obtain surgical consult as soon as possible if appendicitis is suspected.
b. Watchful waiting and frequent abdominal examinations are appropriate.
c. The use of a laxative or enema helps if the client has abdominal pain.
d. Diagnostic procedures are more helpful in diagnosing appendicitis than the history and examination.

8. Jill is 6 months pregnant. She is complaining of abdominal pain and vomiting. Which of the following actions should be implemented immediately?

a. Have her lay on her left side and increase fluids.
b. Give appropriate antiemetic medication.
c. Call for obstetrical consult.
d. Begin nonstress testing.

Answers and Rationales

1. **Answer: b** (assessment)
   Rationale: In appendicitis, the pain usually precedes the emesis and fever (Hartman, 1996).

2. **Answer: c** (assessment)
   Rationale: Children with pain from appendicitis typically walk slightly bent over, and slowly; they may have a limp (Hartman, 1996).

3. **Answer: b** (assessment)
   Rationale: Checking for rebound tenderness is the appropriate special maneuver for appendicitis. The McMurray test demonstrates meniscal injury. The drawer test is specific for anterior cruciate ligament injury, and palpation of the abdomen is not a specific maneuver (Hartman, 1996).

4. **Answer: a** (analysis/diagnosis)
   Rationale: In appendicitis, the pain usually precedes vomiting. In infectious enteritis, vomiting occurs first, followed by crampy pain (Hartman, 1996).

5. **Answer: a** (evaluation)
   Rationale: During the time that a child is being watched at home for a potential appendicitis, it is important to give only clear liquids and light foods. A pizza will only aggravate symptoms if it is gastroenteritis (Robinson, 2000).

6. **Answer: d** (implementation/plan)
   Rationale: A high-fiber diet seems to decrease the occurrence of appendicitis. In countries where the fiber intake is higher, the incidence of appendicitis is less (Hartman, 1996).

7. **Answer: a** (implementation/plan)
   Rationale: If an appendicitis is suspected based on history and physical data, a surgical consult should be obtained without delay (Robinson, 2000).

8. **Answer: c** (implementation/plan)
   Rationale: If a pregnant woman complains of abdominal pain, especially in the second or third trimester, an obstetrical consult should be obtained immediately (Robinson, 2000).

3. Leukotriene modifiers are not indicated for children younger than 12 years. Close monitoring is critical, especially until control of symptoms has been achieved.
   - Asthma diaries should be kept, with symptom severity criteria for medication adjustments by parents (similar to the red/yellow/green stoplight categories used in diaries with PEFR measures).
   - Requires more frequent follow-up, especially during an exacerbation (days versus weeks).
4. Refer to specialist at step 3 (moderate, persistent); consider referral at step 2 level of care.

EVALUATION/FOLLOW-UP

- Initial follow-up depends on severity of exacerbation (1 day to 3 weeks).
- Schedule regular follow-up at 1- to 6-month intervals.
- Successful therapy is based on the following parameters:
  - Prevention of symptoms such as cough
  - Maintenance of nearly normal pulmonary function
  - Maintenance of regular activities
  - Prevention of exacerbations (no hospitalizations or visits to ED)
- At each visit, the following information should be determined: PEFR, triggers that affect asthma, correct medications are prescribed and client is taking them correctly; also discuss an action plan with every client (Schulte, O'Hea, Darling, 2001).
- Children should be monitored closely for growth; latest research reveals that inhaled corticosteroids do not stunt growth.

COMPLICATIONS

- Airway remodeling
- Serious to life-threatening airway obstruction
- Limitations on daily activities because of breathing problems

REFERENCES

Arvin, A.M., Behrman, R.E., Kliegman, R.M., & Nelson, W.E. (Eds.). (1996). *Nelson textbook of pediatrics* (15th ed.). Philadelphia: W.B. Saunders.

Boyton, R.W., Dunn, E.S., & Stephens, G.R., (Eds.). (1994). *Ambulatory pediatric care* (2nd ed.). Philadelphia: J. B. Lippincott.

Gross, K., & Ponte, C. (1998, July). New strategies in the medical management of asthma. *American Family Physician*. Retrieved July 13, 2002, from http://www.aafp.org/afp/980700ap/gross.html.

Kemp, J.P., & Kemp, J.A. (2001). Management of asthma in children. *American Family Physician, 63*, 1341-1348, 1353-1354.

Mellins, R. Evans, D., Clark, N., Zimmerman, B., & Wiesemann, S. (2000). Developing and communicating a long-term treatment plan for asthma. *American Family Physician, 61*, 2419-2428, 2433-2434.

Milgrom, H., Bender, B., Ackerson, L., Bowry, P., Smith, B., & Rand, C. (1996). Noncompliance and treatment failure in children with asthma. *Journal of Allergy and Clinical Immunology, 98*, 1051-1057.

National Asthma Education and Prevention Program. (1995). *Nurses: Partners in asthma care.* Bethesda, MD: National Heart, Lung and Blood Institute.

National Asthma Education and Prevention Program. (1997). *Expert panel report 2: Guidelines for the diagnosis and management of asthma.* Bethesda, MD: National Heart, Lung and Blood Institute.

Plaut, T.F. (1996). *One-minute asthma* (3rd ed.). Amherst, MA: Pedipress.

Satterly, C. (2000). Asthma. In D. Robinson, P. Kidd, K. Rogers (Eds.) *Primary care across the lifespan.* St. Louis: Mosby, 96-101.

Schulte, B., O'Hea, E., & Darling, P. (2001, May). Putting clinical guidelines into practice, *Family Practice Management.* Retrieved July 13, 2002, from www.aafp.org.fpm/20010500/45putt. html.

Stoloff, S., Janson, S. (1997, July). Providing asthma education in primary care. *American Family Physician.* Retrieved July 13, 2002, from http://www.aafp.org/afp/ap/asthma.html.

Suissa, S., Dennis, R., Ernst, P., Sheehy, O., & Wood-Dauphinee, S. (1997). Effectiveness of the leukotriene receptor antagonist Zafirlukast for mild to moderate asthma. *Annals of Internal Medicine, 126*, 177-183.

Warner, J., Naspitz C. (1998). Third international pediatric consensus statement on the management of childhood asthma. *Pediatric Pulmonology, 25*, 1-17.

Wise, R.A., & Liu, M.C. (1995). Obstructive airway diseases: Asthma and chronic pulmonary obstructive disease. In L. Barker, J. Burton, & P. Zieve (Eds.), *Principles of ambulatory medicine* (4th ed.). Baltimore: Williams & Wilkins.

Review Questions

1. A 3-year-old girl comes in with a history of cough that "will not go away." What associated history supports a diagnosis of asthma?
   - **a.** Smokers in the home
   - **b.** Recurrent skin problems since infancy
   - **c.** Older brother with seasonal allergies
   - **d.** Chronic otitis media during the first 2 years of life

2. A 5-year-old comes in with respiratory difficulty, respiratory rate (RR) of 48 breaths/min, mild intercostal retractions, and generalized wheezing. What further objective data supports a diagnosis of asthma?
   - **a.** Wheezing improves after treatment with albuterol in normal saline solution per nebulizer.
   - **b.** PEFR is 75% after treatment with albuterol in normal saline per nebulizer.
   - **c.** Associated signs of concurrent URI are present.
   - **d.** Barrel appearance of chest and clubbing of fingers are noted.

3. May has been using a steroid inhaler. She complains that it makes her voice hoarse. What suggestions can the NP give to May to decrease the occurrence of these side effects?
   - **a.** Stop taking the inhaler.
   - **b.** Use a spacer when taking the medication.

   c. Use cough drops.
   d. Decrease the dosage from qid to bid.

4. Appropriate management for a 6-month-old with generalized wheezing and moderate respiratory distress includes:
   a. Referral for hospitalization
   b. In-office nebulization treatment with 0.25 ml albuterol in 2 ml normal saline
   c. Education regarding PEFR monitoring
   d. Respiratory follow-up in 1 to 2 weeks

5. A 7-year-old with moderate persistent asthma uses an asthma diary to monitor the effectiveness of medications and the status of the disease. Which of the following tools or techniques could be used in this process to serve as an indicator for treatment change?
   a. PEFR
   b. RR
   c. Tissue perfusion
   d. Frequency and duration of cough

6. A 34-year-old female athlete is diagnosed with asthma. Sports activities tend to aggravate her condition, but she is able to participate successfully with additional medications. Daily control medication (nedocromil [Tilade] MDI) and supplements with quick-relief medication (albuterol [Proventil] MDI) before sports activity are included in current management. According to this level of therapy, this case of asthma is classified as:
   a. Mild intermittent
   b. Severe persistent
   c. Moderate persistent
   d. Mild persistent

7. Of the medications used for ongoing asthma management, which displays fewer side effects?
   a. Albuterol
   b. Cromolyn (Intal)
   c. Theophylline
   d. Beclomethasone nasal spray

8. A 19-year-old male comes in for asthma follow-up. After many years of ED visits for acute attacks, the client expresses new interest in achieving control as he gets ready to go away to college. Current management involves daily PEFR monitoring and two long-term control medications. Evidence of effective treatment with this plan includes which of the following?
   a. No more than three "yellow" PEFR readings per week
   b. Only one ED visit since initiation of the new treatment plan
   c. Consistent PEFR measures at 90% or better; no ED visits in 3 months
   d. Daily use of beta-agonist inhaler in addition to long-term medications

Answers and Rationales

1. *Answer:* **b** (assessment)
   Rationale: Atopy is the strongest predisposing factor associated with the development of asthma. Irritants and illnesses can serve as triggers for allergy attacks. A family history of allergies is not as much a support as are the symptoms of the child herself (National Asthma Education and Prevention Program, 1997).

2. *Answer:* **a** (assessment)
   Rationale: Reversible airway obstruction supports the diagnosis of asthma. PEFR of 75% demonstrates a lack of response or incomplete response to beta-agonist (albuterol). A concurrent URI might serve as a trigger but is not diagnostic. The barrel chest and clubbing of fingers demonstrate a chronic hypoxic state, more indicative of chronic lung disease such as cystic fibrosis or bronchopulmonary dysplasia (National Asthma Education and Prevention Program, 1997).

3. *Answer:* **b** (evaluation)
   Rationale: Using a spacer causes less deposition of the droplets in the mouth that cause the dysphonia. Stopping the medication or decreasing the dose is not an option unless the asthma is under control. A cough drop is not a satisfactory way to address the problem (Gross & Ponte, 1998).

4. *Answer:* **b** (implementation/plan)
   Rationale: A trial of short-acting beta-agonist is indicated for children younger than 5 years with wheezing and may be diagnostic (National Asthma Education and Prevention Program, 1997).

5. *Answer:* **a** (implementation/plan)
   Rationale: PEFR is used as an indicator of lung function. It provides an objective measure that can be used for assessment against a predicted value or personal best record (Plaut, 1996).

6. *Answer:* **d** (analysis/diagnosis)
   Rationale: According to the newest guidelines, this case of asthma is classified as mild persistent. This woman uses one antiinflammatory agent and inhaled beta-agonists for quick relief related to physical exercise (National Asthma Education and Prevention Program, 1997).

7. *Answer:* **b** (evaluation)
   Rationale: Cromolyn (Intal) is known for having virtually no side effects (Wise & Liu, 1995).

8. *Answer:* **c** (evaluation)
   Rationale: Successful therapy for asthma is determined according to prevention of troublesome symptoms, maintenance of nearly normal pulmonary function, prevention of exacerbations, and subsequent visits to the ED (National Asthma Education and Prevention Program, 1997; Wise & Liu, 1995).

ATTENTION DEFICIT/HYPERACTIVITY DISORDER   *Denise Robinson*

A

OVERVIEW
Definition
Attention-deficit/hyperactivity disorder (ADHD) is the current term applied to specific developmental disorders of both children and adults that are characterized by deficits in sustained attention, impulse control, and the regulation of activity level to situational demands. ADHD has had a variety of labels including hyperkinetic disorder of childhood, minimal brain dysfunction, and attention deficit disorder (with or without hyperactivity).

Incidence
- ADHD is one of the most common disorders of childhood, affecting 3% to 5% of children in the United States. It is the most common neurobehavioral disorder of childhood in the US (Herrerias, Perrin, Stein, 2001).
- ADHD is much more frequent in males than in females in the United States. The fourth edition of the Diagnostic and Statistical Manual of Mental Disorders (DSM-IV) states that the male-to-female ratio ranges from 4:1 to 9:1 depending on the setting (e.g., general population or clinics).
- It is estimated that one child in every classroom in the United States needs help for the disorder.

Pathophysiology
There are many different theories about the cause of ADHD. There may be a biologic basis such as imbalance in brain chemistry, especially in neurotransmitters such as dopamine, norepinephrine, and serotonin. ADHD has a genetic component; 30% to 40% of children diagnosed with ADHD have relatives with similar difficulties.

Studies of parent-child interactions of hyperactive children compared with normal children show the parents of the hyperactive child to be more likely to give commands to their children, more negative toward the child, and less likely to respond to the social initiatives of the child toward them. Hyperactive children compared with normal children are shown by these studies to be less compliant, more negative, and less able to sustain compliance to parental commands.

There is no scientific proof to render the following toxins responsible for the development of ADHD:
- Food additives
- Food dyes
- Preservatives
- Salicylates
- Refined sugar
- Florescent lighting

Factors Increasing Susceptibility
Higher rates of psychopathology are demonstrated among the biologic relatives of children with ADHD versus normal children. The heritability for the traits of ADHD is 30% to 50%. Between 20% and 32% of parents and siblings of children with ADHD also have the disorder. Susceptibility to ADHD is increased with the following:
- Prenatal and postnatal exposure to lead
- Cigarette smoking during pregnancy
- Alcohol consumption during pregnancy
- Drug abuse during pregnancy
- Poor maternal prenatal nutrition
- Brain injuries during and after birth
- Infections
- Possible side effects of sedatives or anticonvulsants

ASSESSMENT: SUBJECTIVE/HISTORY
History of Present Illness/Developmental Factors
- Ask about the onset of symptoms. ADHD onset is usually identified before the patient is 7 years old, with duration of symptoms lasting longer than 6 months.
- Determine the client's prenatal history, perinatal history, postnatal period and infancy history, and developmental milestones.
- Children with ADHD demonstrate the following characteristic behaviors during developmental stages:

  Infancy: Sleep problems, crying, feeding problems
  Preschool: Gross motor activity (running, etc.) rather than small muscle activities (coloring, etc.)
  School: Restlessness, inattention, impulsiveness
  Adolescence: Rebelliousness, antisocial behaviors

- Questions to ask include the following:
  How is your child doing in school?
  Are there any problems with learning that you or the teacher have seen?
  Are you concerned with behavior problems in school, at home, or when your child is playing with friends? (Herrerias, Perrin, Stein, 2001).

Symptoms
- Uninhibited behavior demonstrated by lack of ability to regulate behavior by awareness of rules and consequences
- Inability to sustain attention: easily bored with repetitive tasks, loss of concentration during lengthy tasks, and failure to complete tasks or activities without supervision

- Impaired impulse control: inability to stop and think about consequences before acting, interrupting conversations, not able to wait one's turn, needing immediate rewards rather than being able to wait for a long-term reward
- Excessive movements: typically "on the move," fidgeting, restlessness, cannot sit still, "bouncing off the walls"

Past Medical History

- Ask questions relevant to risk factors.
- Are there chronic health problems (e.g., asthma, diabetes, heart condition)?
- Is there a history of injury events?

Medication History

Has the child ever taken or is the child currently taking any of the following?
  - Methylphenidate (Ritalin)
  - Dextroamphetamine (Dexedrine)
  - Pemoline (Cylert)
  - Tranquilizers
  - Anticonvulsants
  - Antihistamines
  - Other prescription drugs

Family History

Identify parents or siblings with ADHD or similar symptoms.

Psychosocial History

- Ask about relationships with siblings and friends.
- Ask about physical and sexual abuse.
- Ask questions about involvement with the police and custody issues.
- Observe interaction between child and parent.
  - Parents of children with ADHD are more likely to be negative toward the child and less likely to respond to the social initiatives of the child toward them.
  - Children who are hyperactive are more negative, less compliant, and less able to sustain compliance to parental commands.
- Ask about school history
  - Inquire about the child's entire school history, including preschool and day care.
  - Ask about school changes and why.
  - Ask about attitude toward school, academic performance, relationship with teacher, best and worst subjects, and any modifications that have taken place.
  - Ask whether the child is receiving any special program or support services at the school.
- Ask about peer relationships
  - Ask about friends at school and in the neighborhood.

- What activities do the children normally engage in?
- Ask the ages of friends.
- Ask about drug/alcohol abuse and sexual activity.

ASSESSMENT: OBJECTIVE/PHYSICAL EXAMINATION

Physical Examination

- Conduct a full physical examination, including a thorough neurologic examination and hearing and vision testing.
- Determine if the child has any developmental difficulties such as problems with motor skills, motor coordination, memory, remembering sequences, listening and speaking, and recognizing and reproducing pictures and symbols.

Behavioral Assessment

- Obtain information about the child's behavior in a variety of settings: school, play, at home, organized sports, youth organizations, and after school programs.
- Use the DSM-IV criteria to make the diagnosis.
- Use any of the available "checklists" or behavior rating scales to have teachers and others who observe the child's behavior assess the child's behavior in different environments such as those developed by Connors and Taylor.

Diagnostic Procedures

There are currently no laboratory tests available to assist in the diagnosis of ADHD.

DIAGNOSIS

As many as one-third of children have one or more coexisting conditions. The differential diagnosis includes the following:

- Oppositional defiant disorder (ODD) has a 35% prevalence with ADHD.
  - Characteristic behavior is negativistic, hostile, defiant, lasting at least 6 months. These children demonstrate persistent stubbornness, resistance to directions, and unwillingness to compromise or negotiate with peers or adults.
- Conduct disorder (CD) has a 26% prevalence with ADHD.
  - Characteristic behavior includes a repetitive and persistent pattern of violating the rights of others or major age appropriate societal norms. They are quick to initiate aggressive behavior toward others as well as react aggressively toward others.
- GAD has a 26% prevalence with ADHD.
  - Behavior is characterized by excessive anxiety and worry that occurs on more days than not and lasts for at least 6 months. Children demonstrate restlessness, feeling keyed up or irritability.

- Depressive disorder has an 18% prevalence with ADHD.
- Learning disabilities are present in 12% to 60% of clients with ADHD.
  - Child's demonstrated achievement on standardized tests in reading, math, or written expression is substantially below the expected scores for age, schooling, and intelligence. These children demonstrate demoralization, low self esteem and poor social skills.
- Mental retardation is sometimes associated with ADHD.
  - Child demonstrates significantly subaverage general intellectual functioning accompanied by limited adaptive functioning.
- Understimulating environment is associated with ADHD.
- Developmentally inappropriate behaviors in active children are frequently seen.
- Comorbidity frequently occurs (ADHD and ODD, ADHD and CD, ADHD and depression, and ADHD and anxiety disorders).

DSM-IV Criteria

1. Either (a) or (b):
   a. Six (or more) of the following symptoms of inattention have persisted for at least 6 months to a degree that is maladaptive and inconsistent with developmental level:
   - Fails to give close attention to details or makes careless mistakes in schoolwork, work, or other activities.
   - Has difficulty sustaining attention in tasks or play activities.
   - Does not seem to listen when spoken to directly.
   - Does not follow through on instructions and fails to finish schoolwork, chores, or duties in the workplace (not as a result of oppositional behavior or failure to understand instructions).
   - Has difficulty organizing tasks and activities.
   - Avoids, dislikes, or is reluctant to engage in tasks that require sustained mental effort (such as schoolwork or homework).
   - Loses things necessary for tasks or activities (e.g., toys, school assignments, pencils, books, or tools).
   - Is easily distracted by extraneous stimuli.
   - Is forgetful in daily activities.
   b. Six (or more) of the following symptoms of hyperactivity-impulsivity have persisted for at least 6 months to a degree that is maladaptive and inconsistent with developmental level:
   - Fidgets with hands or feet or squirms in seat.
   - Leaves seat in classroom or in other situations in which remaining seated is expected.
   - Runs about or climbs excessively in situations in which it is inappropriate (in adolescents or adults

may be limited to subjective feelings of restlessness).
   - Has difficulty playing or engaging in leisure activities quietly.
   - Is "on the go" or often acts as if "driven by a motor."
   - Talks excessively.
   - Blurts out answers before questions have been completed.
   - Has difficulty awaiting turn.
   - Interrupts or intrudes on others (e.g., butts into conversations or games).
2. Some hyperactive-impulsive or inattentive symptoms that caused impairment were present before age 7 years.
3. Some impairment from the symptoms is present in two or more settings (e.g., at school [or work] and at home).
4. There must be clear evidence of clinically significant impairment in social, academic, or occupational functioning.
5. The symptoms do not occur exclusively during the course of a pervasive developmental disorder, schizophrenia, or other psychotic disorder and are not better accounted for by another mental disorder (e.g., mood disorder, anxiety disorder, dissociative disorder, or personality disorder) (APA, 1994).

THERAPEUTIC PLAN

- The best approach is via a multidisciplinary team.
- A consistent primary provider is essential.
- The nurse practitioner may serve as the case manager.

Pharmacologic Treatment

CNS stimulants are very effective for the management of symptoms, primarily attention span and impulse control. Changes in other behaviors are most likely the result of the improvement in attention span and impulse control. School performance also shows improvement as a result of medication. These are class 2 controlled substances, and include the following:
- Methylphenidate (Ritalin) (77% positive response)
  - Dosage 5 to 20 mg (0.3 to 0.7 mg/kg)
  - Bid dose given early morning and midday
  - Tid dose given early morning, midday, after school
  - Maximum dose not to exceed 60 mg/day
- Methylphenidate (Ritalin-SR) (1 dose/day; effect lasts 8 hours)
- Dextroamphetamine (Dexedrine) (74% positive response)
  - Dosage 2.5 to 10 mg bid or tid
  - Dosage intervals as for methylphenidate
- Dextroamphetamine (Dexedrine Spansules) (1 dose/day)

A

Nonpharmacologic Treatment

- Training the parents in the use of techniques for dealing with the child's behavior is one of the best therapeutic approaches when done properly. Behavior management skills help the parents reduce negative behaviors and promote positive behaviors.
- Parents need guidance on modifying the environment rather than the child. The child with ADHD functions best in a highly structured environment with clear rules/limits and consequences.
- Parents benefit from counseling in the areas of acceptance of ADHD and the potential for grief reaction.
- Psychotherapy may be needed to help some children with ADHD cope with the anxiety, depression, and self-esteem issues they are experiencing.
- Family therapy is helpful to improve communication within the family and help siblings deal with their concerns.
- Social skills training and peer relationship training may be beneficial to children with ADHD because they demonstrate problems in social situations and are at high risk for peer rejection.
- Some parents have found that a reduction in the use of artificial additives and the intake of simple sugars may help some children.

School Intervention

- Provide education on ADHD to teacher and staff.
- Provide training in classroom management of ADHD to teacher.
- Work with the teacher to develop educational approaches.

Client Education/Prevention

- Provide parent education on ADHD, including a review of symptoms, course, and what is known about the causative factors.
- There are no measures to prevent ADHD. A healthy prenatal course (avoiding lead, alcohol, cigarette smoking, drug abuse, and malnutrition) may decrease the incidence of ADHD.

EVALUATION/FOLLOW-UP

- Referral and/or consultation may be necessary.
- The family should be involved in the development of the treatment plan.
- A multidisciplinary approach is most successful.
- Treatment of ADHD is long term.
  - Adjustments in medications must be made as the child grows.
  - The interaction and plan developed with the child and the family changes as the child and family changes.
  - It was previously thought that children "outgrow" ADHD. Now it is more widely accepted that ADHD has an inborn biologic basis and that parents and children can learn how to cope with the behavioral difficulties rather than cure them. Of children diagnosed with ADHD, 50% to 80% carry the core symptoms into adulthood.

REFERENCES

American Psychiatric Association (1994). *Diagnostic and statistical manual of mental disorders (DSM-IV)* (4th ed.). Washington, DC: Author.

Barkley, R.A. (1991). *Attention-deficit hyperactivity disorder: A clinical workbook.* New York: Guilford Press.

Barkley, R.A. (1990). *Attention-deficit hyperactivity disorder: A handbook for diagnosis and treatment.* New York: Guilford Press.

Biederman, J., et al. (1996a). A prospective 4-year follow-up study of attention-deficit hyperactivity and related disorders. *Archives of General Psychiatry, 53* (5), 437-446.

Biederman, J., et al. (1996b). Is childhood oppositional defiant disorder a precursor to adolescent conduct disorder? Findings from a four-year follow-up study of children with ADHD. *Journal of the American Academy of Child and Adolescent Psychiatry, 35*(9), 1193-1204.

Biederman, J., et al. (1996c). Predictors of persistence and remission of ADHD into adolescence: Results from a four-year prospective follow-up study. *Journal of the American Academy of Child and Adolescent Psychiatry, 35*(3), 343-351.

Burns, C., & Shelton, K. (1996). Cognitive-perceptual patterns. In C. Burns, N. Barber, M. Brady, & A. Dunn (Eds.), *Pediatric primary care: A handbook for nurse practitioners.* Philadelphia: W. B. Saunders.

Dahl, R.E. (1996). The impact of inadequate sleep on children's daytime cognitive function. *Seminars in Pediatric Neurology, 3*(1), 44-50.

Herrerias, C., Perrin, J., Stein, M. (2001). The child with ADHD: using the AAP clinical practice guideline. *American Family Physician, 63,* 1803-1810, 1811-1812. Retrieved July 14, 2002, from http://www.aafp.org/afp/20010501/1803.html

Heidt, B. (2000). ADHD in D. Robinson, P. Kidd, K. Rogers (Eds). *Primary Care Across the Lifespan* (pp. 111-117). St. Louis: Mosby.

Javorsky, J. (1996). An examination of youth with attention-deficit/hyperactivity disorder and language learning disabilities: A clinical study. *Journal of Learning Disabilities, 29*(3), 247-258.

Lobar, S., Waecheter, M., Oher, L., Phillips, S. (1999). Parents', physicians', and nurse practitioners' perceptions of behaviors associated with attention deficit hyperactivity disorder. *Journal of the American Academy of Nurse Practitioners 11*(6): 237-242.

MacDonald, V.M., & Achenback, T.M. (1996). Attention problems versus conduct problems as six-year predictors of problem scores in a national sample. *Journal of the American Academy of Child and Adolescent Psychiatry 35*(9), 1237-1246.

Murphy, K.R., & Barkley, R.A. (1996). Parents of children with attention-deficit/hyperactivity disorder: Psychologic and attentional impairment. *American Journal of Orthopsychiatry 66*(1), 93-102.

Taylor, E., Chadwick, O., Heptenstall, E., Danckaerts, M. (1996). Hyperactivity and conduct problems as risk factors for adolescent development. *Journal of the American Academy of Child and Adolescent Psychiatry 35*(9), 1213-1226.

Review Questions

1. Which of the following symptoms best describes the child with ADHD, inattentive type?

    a. Makes careless mistakes in schoolwork, does not seem to listen when spoken to directly, has difficulty sustaining attention.

    b. Has difficulty organizing tasks, fidgets with hands, has difficulty waiting turn.

    c. Makes careless mistakes in schoolwork, has difficulty waiting turn, talks excessively.

    d. Interrupts others, talks excessively, does not seem to listen when spoken to directly.

2. Researchers have linked the development of ADHD to which of the following factors?

    a. Refined sugar, drug abuse during pregnancy, brain injuries after birth

    b. Food additives, fluorescent lighting, cigarette smoking during pregnancy

    c. Food additives, prenatal exposure to lead, poor maternal nutrition

    d. Cigarette smoking during pregnancy, prenatal exposure to lead, poor maternal nutrition

3. ADHD must be differentiated from ODD. Compared with ADHD, ODD is associated with:

    a. Fidgeting and squirming

    b. Persistent stubbornness, negativistic, hostile behavior

    c. Excessive anxiety and worry

    d. Aggressive behavior toward others

4. The physical examination of a child with ADHD most likely reveals which of the following abnormalities?

    a. Eye problems

    b. Gait problems

    c. Heart murmur

    d. None

5. Which of the following historical data is consistent with the diagnosis of ADHD?

    a. Brother has schizophrenia.

    b. Dad is impulsive and has changed jobs many times.

    c. Grandmother has diabetes.

    d. Mother has hyperthyroidism.

6. The parents of a 9-year-old boy with ADHD report that his behavior has improved at school, but they see no change in his behavior at home. The parents should be encouraged to:

    a. See a therapist who can teach them behavior management skills.

    b. Double check with the school to make sure he is taking his midday dose of methylphenidate (Ritalin) as prescribed.

    c. Do away with any rules or limits they set at home; he is not able to follow rules all day.

    d. Enroll the child in a social skills training program to improve his behavior in social situations.

7. The NP provides instruction about ADHD and appropriate nonpharmacologic management. Which comment by the parent indicates a need for further instruction?

    a. "Having clear rules and consequences makes sense to me."

    b. "We will enroll Kyle in behavior management classes."

    c. "I will have to be consistent with how I treat Kyle."

    d. "I will need to point out all of Kyle's negative behaviors to be an effective parent."

8. Which of the following is *not* a realistic goal for an ADHD treatment plan?

    a. Use a structured environment.

    b. Have child act like "all other kids."

    c. Have child placed in a class that uses specific ADHD techniques.

    d. On standardized test, score in top 10% of class.

Answer and Rationales

1. *Answer:* **a** (analysis/diagnosis)

    Rationale: Fidgeting, not waiting turn, talking excessively, and interrupting others are hyperactive behaviors. This question is asked for inattentive behaviors (American Psychiatric Association, 1994).

2. *Answer:* **d** (assessment)

    Rationale: There is no research to back up the theories about refined sugar, food additives, and fluorescent lighting being causes of ADHD (Barkley, 1990).

3. *Answer:* **b** (analysis/diagnosis)

    Rationale: ODD is described as being persistently stubborn, negative, and hostile. Answer *a* describes hyperactivity, answer *c* describes GAD, and *d* describes conduct disorder (Heidt, 2000).

4. *Answer:* **d** (assessment)

    Rationale: A thorough physical examination is necessary to rule out a developmental disorder, visual deficiencies, impaired hearing, and neurologic deficits. In most cases, no physical abnormalities are found (Barkley, 1990).

5. *Answer:* **b** (assessment)

    Rationale: In 30% to 40% of children, there is a family history of someone else with ADHD. Schizophrenia, diabetes, and hyperthyroid have no bearing on the incidence of ADHD (Heidt, 2000).

6. *Answer:* **a** (implementation/plan)

    Rationale: Many children demonstrate this phenomenon because the school often is a more structured environment than the home. When the parents and child begin to work with a therapist on behavior management skills, the behavior at home will improve (Barkley, 1990).

7. *Answer:* **d** (evaluation)

    Rationale: The parent does not need to point out all negative behaviors of the child to be effective. It is difficult to point out the positive behaviors of an ADHD child, because most behaviors are negative. Clear rules, consistency, and behavior management classes are all helpful tools to address ADHD (Barkley, 1990).

8. *Answer:* d (evaluation)
   Rationale: Aiming for a structured, clear environment is a realistic family goal. Having the child act like all the other kids,

and having ADHD-specific classroom techniques are helpful for an ADHD child. Having the child strive to score in the top 10% of the class on standardized tests may not be realistic (Barkley, 1990).

BEHAVIOR PROBLEMS (CHILDREN) *Pamela Kidd*

OVERVIEW
Definition

- Child's behavior is perceived by supervising adult to deviate from acceptable norms. They may be specific to a situation or person.
- Common behavior problems include temper tantrums, hitting, kicking, biting, noncompliance, back talk, fighting, arguing, yelling, refusing to go to bed.

Incidence

- Most children display one or more problematic behaviors during the first years of life through adolescence.
- Incidence is highest during preschool years—90% of mothers report at least mild concern.
- It is often undiagnosed (i.e., not addressed during health care encounters).

Pathophysiology

Unclear and irregular enforcement of parental expectations for behavior is the primary cause.

Factors Increasing Susceptibility
- Temperament of child and parenting skills contribute.
- Research has demonstrated associations with maternal smoking, increased family stress, increased family size, illness in family, socioeconomic status, and maternal marital status.

Protective Factors
- Positive functioning family
- Good parenting skills

ASSESSMENT: SUBJECTIVE/HISTORY
Symptoms

Obtain a description of misbehavior(s), parent response, and the effectiveness of that response. Consider the following:
- Age and sex appropriateness
- Persistence
- Life circumstance and precipitating events
- Setting/situation specificity
- Extent of disturbance
- Type, severity, and frequency of symptoms
- Change in behavior

Past Medical History

- Chronic illness of child
- Attention-deficit/hyperactivity disorder (ADHD)
- Anxiety disorder or depressive disorder in parent
- Alcohol abuse in parent

Medication History

- Any medication use that may suggest the previously listed conditions (under past medical history)
- Over-the-counter (OTC) use of upper- respiratory infection (URI)/allergy agents that could cause hyperactivity.

Family History

- Birth order
- Family composition
- Family dynamics
- Discipline techniques
- Illness
- Developmental milestones
- Family history of behavior problems

Dietary History

- Sugar intake of child
- Caffeine intake of child
- Recall of child's diet during the past 24 hours

ASSESSMENT: OBJECTIVE/PHYSICAL EXAMINATION
Physical Examination

- Complete physical examination (rule out illness or other physical cause for behavior change)
- Focus on the following areas:
  - General: observation of parent/child interaction, child's response to direction and correction, child's affect and behavior during play
  - Neurologic: neurodevelopmental screen, vision and hearing screen

Diagnostic Procedures
Behavior Rating Scale
- Select scale according to age and complaint.
- Scales may be completed by supervising adults other than parents (e.g., teachers).

- It is helpful to differentiate the psychologically disturbed child.

DIAGNOSIS
Common (Minor) Behavior Problem

Differential Diagnoses
- Normal behavior of childhood
- Major behavior problem
- Psychologic disturbance
- Learning disorder
- Ineffective parenting
- Dysfunctional parenting
- Child abuse

THERAPEUTIC PLAN
Nonpharmacologic Treatment
- Establish relationship with family.
- Acknowledge difficulty of developmental issues.
- Initiate behavior management system as appropriate.
- Refer for parenting classes, parent support groups, and/or social services as needed.
- Maintain open communication and support during process of implementing behavior management system—it may take weeks to notice consistent change.

Pharmacologic Treatment
- Short-term use of antidepressants or antianxiety agents may be indicated for parents.
- Child may need stimulants for ADHD (refer to ADHD section for specific information).

Client Education
- Developmental stages
  - Determine expected behaviors according to developmental level.

- Parents discuss and agree early in child's life what constitutes misbehavior (i.e., "cute" to some is "misbehaving" to others).
- Discuss appropriate parenting strategies, including a system for behavior modification, including the following:
  - Clear expectations
  - Consequences (punishment) for misbehavior (Table 3-10)
  - Positive reinforcement of appropriate behavior
- Reinforce consistency as key to a successful system (Box 3-8):
  - Between parents and all caretakers
  - Applicable across circumstances
- Identify parents as role models. (Encourage a consciousness for own behavior in all situations.)

Referral
- May need to refer to pediatrician and/or child psychologist for some hyperactivity and learning disorders.
- Consult with physician regarding aggressive or self-destructive behaviors.
- Report any suspected cases of child abuse to appropriate authorities.
- Refer complicated (multiple types) and/or major behavior problems (persistent, inappropriate for age/sex, increasing severity or frequency of symptoms) for evaluation by physician and possible psychiatric evaluation.

Prevention
Most minor behavior problems can be prevented if parents have good parenting skills. Parents should be enrolled in parenting classes during pregnancy with child age-appropriate follow-up courses as needed.

TABLE **3-10** Comparison of Mild Punishment

METHOD	DESCRIPTION	APPLICABLE AGES
Distraction	Removal from situation by providing alternative site for attention (e.g., provide another toy if one is in dispute)	Infants and toddlers
Time out	Interrupt disruptive or aggressive behavior by immediate isolation at onset; few words; boring place; timed for a minute per year of age	2-12 years
Scolding/disapproval	Naming misbehavior (stern voice) and expressing dissatisfaction	All ages
Natural consequences	Result occurs without intervention from parent and allowed only if it does not jeopardize safety (e.g., if play too roughly with cat, then may get scratched)	All ages
Logical consequences	Punishment determined by parent and logically connected to misbehavior (e.g., if ride bike without helmet, then no bike riding for 1 week)	3 years to adolescence
Behavioral penalty	Loss of privileges for misbehavior that has no clear consequence (e.g., if refuse to do chores, then "grounded" for the weekend)	5 years to adolescence

From Robinson, D., Kidd, P., Rogers, K. M. (2000). *Primary Care Across the Life Span.* St. Louis: Mosby.

Box 3-8 Guidelines for Using Punishment

Use sparingly
Use mild punishment (avoid physical punishment)
Punish quickly after misbehavior

Punish only if in control of self
Provide brief reason for punishment

EVALUATION/FOLLOW-UP

- Follow-up by phone in 1-2 weeks (encourage parent to call sooner with questions/difficulties with implementing behavior management)
- Schedule a return visit in 4-6 weeks.
  - Repeat neurodevelopmental screen if any developmental lags/deficits.
  - If misbehavior still unmanaged after 4 weeks, repeat neurodevelopmental screen.
- Consider 6-month interval between well-child visits until stability maintained.

COMPLICATIONS

- Child delinquency (socially inappropriate behavior)
- Child abuse

REFERENCES

Behrman, R. E., Kliegman, R. M., & Jenson, H. B., (Eds.). (2000). *Nelson textbook of pediatrics* (16th ed.). Philadelphia: W. B. Saunders.

Clark, L. (1985). *SOS! Help for parents.* Bowling Green, KY: Parents Press.

Coleman, W. L. (1997). Family-focused pediatrics: Solution-oriented techniques for behavior problems. *Contemporary Pediatrics, 14*(7), 121-134.

Herman-Staab, B. (1994). Screening, management and appropriate referral for pediatric behavior problems. *Nurse Practitioner, 19*(7), 40-49.

Satterly, C. (2000). Behavior problems: child. In D. Robinson, P. Kidd, & K. M. Rogers (Eds.), *Primary care across the lifespan* St. Louis: Mosby.

Schmitt, B. D. (1993). Time-out: Intervention of choice for the irrational years. *Contemporary Pediatrics, 10,* 64-71.

Schmitt, B. D. (1987). Seven deadly sins of childhood: Advising parents about difficult developmental phases. *Child Abuse & Neglect, 11,* 421-432.

Review Questions

1. Which of the following punishment strategies is most appropriate for a child age 18 months?
   - a. Distraction
   - b. Time out
   - c. Logical consequences
   - d. Behavioral penalty

2. Which of the following comments by the parent indicates understanding of the use of punishment?
   - a. "Wait to punish until the child has time to think about the behavior."
   - b. "Combine physical punishment with time out."
   - c. "Punish only if you are in control of yourself."
   - d. "Punish frequently so child will understand behavior is negative."

3. Ms. Smith brings in Molly (age 2) and complains of temper tantrums. To help determine if these temper tantrums constitute a behavior problem, the nurse practitioner (NP) should:
   - a. Conduct a developmental assessment of Molly.
   - b. Determine if Molly is holding her breath during the tantrum.
   - c. Have the parent explain what she means by temper tantrum.
   - d. Determine Molly's birth order.

4. A 10-year-old boy continues to dress in his dead sister's clothes and wet the bed. The NP decides to refer the client to a child psychiatrist and pediatrician for evaluation. Which of the following statements serves as appropriate rationale for this decision?
   - a. The behavior is not socially acceptable.
   - b. The behavior is not age- or gender-appropriate.
   - c. The behavior prevents him from sleeping over with friends.
   - d. The behavior may indicate a urinary tract infection (UTI).

5. Which of the following is a prevention strategy for child behavior problems?
   - a. Enroll the child in military school.
   - b. Allow the child limited choices in his or her environment.
   - c. Enroll the parents in parenting classes.
   - d. Encourage the parents to ignore disruptive behavior.

Answers and Rationales

1. **Answer: a** (implementation/plan)
   Rationale: Distraction (removal from the situation) is appropriate for infants and toddlers. Time out should not be used until age 2, when there is understanding that bad behavior brings a negative reaction. Logical consequence involves connecting the consequence (punishment) directly to the behavior and requires higher cognitive skills (age 3 and older). Behavioral penalty results in loss of privileges and requires the highest level of cognitive skills (age 5 and older).

2. **Answer: c** (evaluation)
   Rationale: Physical punishment should be avoided. Punishment should be used sparingly. To be effective punishment

must take place quickly after the misbehavior. Punishing when the parent is out of control may lead to abuse.

3. *Answer:* **c** (assessment)

Rationale: A developmental assessment is helpful in judging what is appropriate behavior for Molly. However, until the NP understands what the parent has identified as abnormal behavior (called a temper tantrum), it is not possible to determine if the displayed behavior is developmentally appropriate. Birth order may explain attention-seeking behavior, but until "temper tantrum" is defined the NP does not know if Molly is gaining attention through this behavior. Breath holding does not in itself make the behavior any more or less appropriate.

4. *Answer:* **b** (implementation/plan)

Rationale: The behavior is not age- or gender-appropriate; whether it is socially acceptable involves a better understanding of the social norms. There is not enough information to assume that the child is not sleeping over with friends. The NP should be able to assess and treat a UTI.

5. *Answer:* **c** (implementation/plan)

Rationale: Usually a child is enrolled in military school after behavior problems have surfaced. Parenting classes allow parents to define misbehavior and to act consistently in their parenting strategies when it occurs. Limited choices may cause rebellion or misbehavior. There is not enough information to understand what is meant by this option. Ignoring disruptive behavior may reinforce the behavior.

BELL'S PALSY *Pamela Kidd*

OVERVIEW
Definition

Bell's palsy is an acute idiopathic unilateral paralysis of the facial muscles innervated by the seventh cranial nerve.

Incidence

- Bell's palsy is the most common of all facial neuropathies, accounting for 60% to 80% of all cases.
- Affects all age groups, with frequency increasing with age.
- Women are more often affected before age 50; men are more often affected after 50.
- Encompasses all races.
- Occurs seasonally and is more common in winter.
- Higher-risk groups include women who are pregnant and people who have diabetes mellitus, hypothyroidism, hypertension, or a family history of Bell's palsy.
- May be an early manifestation of human immunodeficiency virus infection.

Pathophysiology

Inflammation of the seventh cranial nerve causes edema, which produces compression and entrapment, resulting in ischemia and degeneration of the nerve. The cause is unknown.

A theory of a viral cause (herpes viruses) most frequently is implicated in some studies. Other causal theories include autoimmune processes and inflammatory diseases such as sarcoidosis and Lyme disease.

Factors Increasing Susceptibility. Some viral or autoimmune diseases are implicated (see the previous section).

Protective Factors. None noted.

ASSESSMENT: SUBJECTIVE/HISTORY
Symptoms

- The onset of unilateral facial paralysis is sudden, usually occurring during a period of a few hours, with progression during 1 to 3 days.
- The individual may wake up and notice the problem.
- Associated symptoms include pain in or behind the ear.
- Mild transient tinnitus, slightly decreased hearing on affected side, and low-grade fever are possible at the onset.
- Other reported symptoms are taste disorder, hypersensitivity to sound, and drooling.

Past Medical History

- Current pregnancy
- Diabetes mellitus
- Hypothyroidism
- Hypertension
- Trauma
- Infection
- Risk factors for heart disease or stroke
- A URI preceding the paralysis (approximately 75% of clients)

Medication History

Note if client is already taking steroids or acyclovir.

Family History

Inquire about family members with Bell's palsy.

Dietary History

Not relevant.

ASSESSMENT: OBJECTIVE/PHYSICAL EXAMINATION

Physical Examination

- Observe general appearance for facial asymmetry with loss of voluntary and involuntary movement in both the upper and lower portions of the face. The forehead is smooth, the nasolabial fold is flattened, and the eyelid on the affected side does not close.
- Inspect for zosteriform lesions behind the ear or in the ear canal; also inspect for expanding target lesions, erythema chronicum migrans, Lyme disease, and neurofibroma.
- Look in the ear for cholesteatoma (pressure on the facial nerve) and otitis media (invasive infection).
- Observe the nose and jaw for trauma; palpate jaw for tenderness.
- Check the neck for lymphadenopathy.
- Auscultate the lungs for adventitious sounds (sarcoidosis).
- Perform a neurologic examination with assessment of cranial nerves; corneal reflex may be decreased.

Diagnostic Procedures

- No diagnostic procedures are required unless the diagnosis is uncertain.
- In severe cases, an electromyogram (EMG) obtained at least 72 hours after the onset of symptoms, and preferably within 7 to 10 days from onset, is indicated if there is no sign of improvement. The EMG helps predict the final prognosis.
- If there is no significant recovery in 6 months, a computed tomography (CT) scan or magnetic resonance imaging (MRI) is indicated to rule out other causes.
- If the onset of symptoms is in summer and the client lives in an area with endemic Lyme disease, consider serology testing.

DIAGNOSIS

The differential diagnosis includes the following:

- Surgery: history of middle ear or mastoid surgery
- Neoplasms: tumors, neurofibroma, cholesteatoma (put pressure on or invade the facial nerve)
- Blunt trauma: fracture of temporal bone
- Infections of the ear, parotid, mastoid, or facial nerve
- Lyme disease
- Infiltrations from sarcoidosis (can produce facial weakness)
- Guillain-Barré syndrome
- Hemiparesis

THERAPEUTIC PLAN

Nonpharmacologic Treatment

- Because approximately 60% of cases recover without treatment, some internists and neurologists do not treat with any medication.
- Surgical decompression of the nerve sometimes is used for recurrent facial palsy, although results may vary (Stennert & Sittel, 1997).
- Electric stimulation can lead to irreversible facial contractures and should be used cautiously, if at all.
- Safer alternatives are massage and facial exercises, which may be helpful during the recuperative phase.

Pharmacologic Treatment

The following is a list of treatment options with prednisone (after physician consultation):

- Prednisone 1 mg/kg PO for 5 to 6 days, with tapering dose during a period of 7 to 10 days, best started within 72 hours of onset of symptoms
- Prednisone 60 mg PO for 3 days, then tapering by 10 mg/day
- Prednisone 60 mg PO for 5 days; if improved during this period, taper for 10 more days. If not improved in the first 5 days, continue 60 mg for another 5 days, then taper for 10 more days.
- For children, prednisone 2 mg/kg for 1 week, then 1 mg/kg for another week.
- There is some evidence that prednisone plus acyclovir 400 mg 5 times a day for 10 days is more effective than prednisone alone (Bauer & Coker, 1996).
- In some cases, Bell's palsy may not be treated aggressively enough, and defective healing may occur. A poor prognosis is associated with advanced age, hyperacusis, and severe initial pain (Aminoff, 2001). This urges more aggressive treatment with antiinflammatory intravenous therapy.

Client Education

Advise the client to use artificial tears bid to prevent drying of the cornea; client may need to tape eyelid shut at night. Instruct the client to report eye pain or visual problems.

Discuss symptoms that might be expected, such as altered taste, hypersensitive hearing, decreased tearing, and saliva production. Defective regeneration of damaged nerves can lead to "crocodile tears" or lacrimation when eating.

The prognosis generally is considered favorable, but with varying rates of complete recovery ranging from 60% to 90%. Symptoms usually resolve within 3 to 4 weeks.

Referral

- Refer to a neurologist for severe cases or if in doubt about diagnosis.
- Bell's palsy with acute otitis media may infer an invasive process; refer immediately to physician/neurologist.
- Refer to an ophthalmologist in the case of corneal abrasion.

Prevention

Not currently preventable.

EVALUATION/FOLLOW-UP

Follow-up in 3 to 4 days and again in 2 to 4 weeks.

COMPLICATIONS

Usually none.

REFERENCES

Aminoff, M. J. (2001). Nervous system. In L. Tierney, S. McPhee, & M. Papadakis (Eds.), *Current medical diagnosis and treatment.* New York: McGraw Hill.

Bailey, E. (2000). Bell's palsy. In D. Robinson, P. Kidd, & K.M. Rogers (Eds.), *Primary care across the lifespan.* St. Louis: Mosby.

Bauer, C. A., & Coker, N. J. (1996, June). Update on facial nerve disorders. *Otolaryngologic Clinics of North America, 29*(3), 445-455.

Billue, J. A. (1997). Bell's palsy: An update on idiopathic facial paralysis. *Nurse Practitioner, 22,* 88-105.

Hughes, G. B. (1998). Acute peripheral facial paralysis. In R. Rakel, (Ed.), *Conn's current therapy.* Philadelphia: W. B. Saunders.

Pruitt, A. A. (1995). Management of Bell's palsy. In A. H. Goroll, L. A. May, A. G. Mulley (Eds.), *Primary care medicine* (3rd ed.). Philadelphia: J. B. Lippincott.

Stennert, E., & Sittel, C. (1997). Acute peripheral paralysis. In R. Rakel (Ed.), *Conn's current therapy.* Philadelphia: W. B. Saunders.

Review Questions

1. The incidence of Bell's palsy increases in which season of the year?
- **a.** Spring
- **b.** Summer
- **c.** Fall
- **d.** Winter

2. Bell's palsy is more common in:
- **a.** Children
- **b.** Adolescents
- **c.** Men older than 50
- **d.** Women older than 50

3. If the facial paralysis of Bell's palsy has not improved in 2 weeks, the diagnostic test sometimes used to predict outcome is:
- **a.** CT of the head
- **b.** MRI
- **c.** EMG
- **d.** Lumbar puncture

4. Improvement of the symptoms of Bell's palsy generally can be expected by:
- **a.** 1 week
- **b.** 4 weeks
- **c.** 3 months
- **d.** 6 months

5. The differential diagnosis considered in making the diagnosis of Bell's palsy might include all the following *except*:
- **a.** Lyme disease
- **b.** Trauma
- **c.** Epilepsy
- **d.** Tumor

Answers and Rationales

1. *Answer:* **d** (assessment)
Rationale: Bell's palsy is slightly more common in winter.

2. *Answer:* **c** (assessment)
Rationale: Bell's palsy increases in frequency with increasing age, but after the age of 50 men more often are affected.

3. *Answer:* **c** (implementation/plan)
Rationale: EMG testing of facial muscles after 72 hours can determine the degree of nerve degeneration, which helps predict the outcome.

4. *Answer:* **b** (evaluation)
Rationale: Client education regarding the expected time frame for improvement in the majority is usually 4 weeks, although more severe cases may take 3 to 6 months.

5. *Answer:* **c** (analysis/diagnosis)
Rationale: Lyme disease, trauma, and tumor are considerations in the differential diagnosis of facial palsy. Epilepsy does not cause symptoms of facial nerve paralysis.

B

BENIGN PROSTATIC HYPERTROPHY   *Pamela Kidd*

OVERVIEW
Definition

Benign prostatic hypertrophy (BPH) is a noncancerous enlargement of the prostate gland. This enlargement decreases the force/caliber of urinary stream and produces nocturia, sensation of incomplete emptying, hesitancy, frequency, urgency, and high postvoid residual (PVR).

Incidence

BPH affects one in every four men by age 80 in the United States. Symptomatology is reported in nearly half of men 50 to 64 years old in the general population.

Pathophysiology

The causes of BPH are not fully understood. The disorder is associated with two factors: male sex and increasing age. The cause of age-related hyperplasia is unknown, although it is thought to be related to androgenic changes at the cellular level. The earliest changes of BPH occur in the periurethral glands, with nodular hyperplasia. As these nodules grow and coalesce during a period of years, true prostatic tissue is compressed outward. As the gland enlarges, urethral resistance to urine flow increases and muscular hypertrophy of the bladder ensues.

Factors Increasing Susceptibility. Advancing age

Protective Factors. Young age.

ASSESSMENT: SUBJECTIVE/HISTORY
Symptoms

- Decreased force and caliber of urinary stream
- Nocturia (most frequent reason for seeking care [Pfeiffer & Giacomarra, 1999])
- Feeling of incomplete emptying
- Hesitancy
- Dribbling from penis
  Burning is not normal and may indicate infection, calculi, or cancer. The severity of symptoms does not correlate with the size of prostate gland.

Past Medical History

- Family history for prostatic disease(s)
- Medication history
- Delayed sexual drive
- Early cessation of sexuality
- Smoking

Medication History

Inquire about use of decongestants, antidepressants, or antihypertensives.

Family History

Not useful.

Dietary History

Inquire about amount and timing of fluid and caffeine intake. Too much fluid and/or caffeine, as well as drinking fluids late into the evening, may produce nocturia.

ASSESSMENT: OBJECTIVE/PHYSICAL EXAMINATION
Physical Examination

Given the wide variety of signs and symptoms in clients with BPH, a complete physical examination may be necessary.
- *Abdominal:* Check for distended bladder and abdominal pain.
- *Musculoskeletal:* Check for pain in back with range of motion or palpation.
- *Genital/rectal:* Perform an examination of the external genitalia. Assess for prostate tenderness, enlargement, or nodules. Determine if neurologic problems are causing the presenting symptoms.

Diagnostic Procedures

- First line procedure is a digital rectal examination (DRE).
- Second line procedure is a urinalysis.
- Third line procedure is a PVR/urinalysis by catheterization. A postvoid urine residual of more than100 mL suggests BPH or other obstruction and need for urinalysis. The American Urological Association index is an important aspect of the initial examination. Mild symptoms are scored between 0 and 7, moderate are rated between 8 and 19 (symptoms controlled with medications), and severe is between 20 and 35.

DIAGNOSIS

The differential diagnoses includes the following:
- Chronic nonbacterial prostatitis
- Prostatodynia
- Sexually transmitted disease
- Urethral stricture
- Acquired or congenital bladder neck contracture
- Chronic urethritis

THERAPEUTIC PLAN
Nonpharmacologic Treatment

Nonpharmacologic treatment for BPH can include herbal therapy, saw palmetto at 80 mg bid for 8 weeks, vitamin B_6 500 to 1000 mg qd, or zinc 50 to 100 mg qd. If zinc is taken for more than 1 month, copper at 1 to 2 mg/day

TABLE **3-11** Drug Treatment for BPH

DRUG	DOSE	COMMENTS
Finasteride (Proscar) (5-alpha reductase inhibitor)	5 mg qd PO	Shrinks prostate. Requires up to 6 months to be effective.
Prazosin (Minipress)	1 mg bid or tid up to 20 mg qd PO	Monitor for hypotension. Relaxes smooth muscle of urethra. Requires 2-3 month trial.
Doxazosin mesylate (Cardura)	1 mg hs PO, may increase to 8 mg	Monitor for hypotension. Relaxes smooth muscle of urethra. Requires 2-3 month trial.
Terazosin HCL (Hytrin) (alpha-1 blocker)	1 mg hs po, may increase to 10 mg	Monitor for hypotension. Relaxes smooth muscle of urethra. Requires 2-3 month trial.

should be added because zinc depletes the body's stores of copper.

The client may prefer a surgical or minimally invasive option (e.g., balloon dilation, laser prostatectomy, electrovaporization of the prostate, transurethral needle ablation). Transurethral resection of the prostate is still the gold-standard treatment for severe symptoms.

Pharmacologic Treatment

Pharmacologic treatment for BPH includes consideration of antiandrogens (finasteride) and alpha-adrenergic antagonists (prazosin, doxazosin, terazosin) given at bedtime to minimize side effects. Titrating the medications up to the desired/effective dose may be accomplished during a 3- to 4-week period. Before the dose is increased, blood pressure and the presence of orthostatic changes should be monitored (Table 3-11).

Client Education

- Possibly enhance voiding with obstruction by sitting when voiding.
- Avoid drinking fluids after 7 P.M.
- Take time to void properly.
- Reduce caffeine in diet (essential).
- Reduce consumption of alcoholic beverages.
- Avoid excess salt and diuretics (e.g., cucumbers).
- Comply with medication regimen (essential).
- Avoid OTC cold remedies that contain decongestants.

Referral

Refer men with BPH to a urologist if symptoms persist after 6 months of treatment with finasteride or after 2 to 3 months of treatment with other drugs. Refer immediately a client with abnormal DRE, hematuria, or PVR of 300 mL or greater.

Prevention

Maintenance of sexual activity.

EVALUATION/FOLLOW-UP

Indications for urologic investigation include treatment failures with appropriate medications, chronic/relapsing cases of bacterial prostatitis, BPH, or suspected prostate cancer.

COMPLICATIONS

- Renal failure
- Cystitis

REFERENCES

Birchfield, P. (2000). Prostate problems. In D. Robinson, P. Kidd, & K.M. Rogers (Eds.). *Primary care across the lifespan*. St. Louis: Mosby

Fugh-Berman, A. (1996, January). A better way to shrink an enlarged prostate. *Health Confidential*, 10.

Gorroll, A. H., May, L. A., & Mulley, A. G. (1995). *Primary care medicine: Office evaluation and management of the adult patient* (3rd ed.). Philadelphia: J. B. Lippincott.

Peters, S. (1997, April). For men only: An overview of three top health concerns. *ADVANCE for Nurse Practitioners, 5*(4), 53-57.

Pfeiffer, G. M. & Giacomarra, M. (1999). BPH: A review of diagnostic and treatment options. *ADVANCE for Nurse Practitioners. 7*(4), 31-36.

Tierney, L. M., McPhee, S. J., & Papadakis, M. A. (2001). *Current medical diagnosis and treatment* (40th ed.). New York: McGraw Hill.

U.S. Department of Health and Human Services (1994). *Benign prostatic hypertrophy: Diagnosis and treatment* (AHCPR Publication No. 94-0583). Rockville, MD: U.S. Department of Health and Human Services.

Zippe, C. D. (1996). Benign prostatic hyperplasia: An approach for the internist. *Cleveland Clinic Journal of Medicine, 63*(4), 226-236.

Review Questions

1. Alpha-adrenergic antagonists, used in the treatment of BPH, may be titrated to the desired dose during a period of:

    a. 5 to 6 weeks
    b. 1 to 2 weeks
    c. 1 to 2 months
    d. 3 to 4 weeks

2. Which symptoms would *not* cause the NP to consider a diagnosis of BPH?

    a. Frequency of urination
    b. Burning on urination
    c. Nocturia
    d. Decrease force of urine stream

B

3. What data support the diagnosis of BPH?

  a. Fever
  b. Pyuria
  c. Post void residual (PVR) urine of more than 100 mL
  d. Symptom score on the American Urological Association index of 2

4. Which of the following statements serve as appropriate rationale for the decision to refer a client with BPH to a urologist?

  a. Orthostatic changes with pharmacologic treatment
  b. No improvement in symptoms after 1 month
  c. PVR urine of 350 mL
  d. A client with American Urological Association Index score of 5

5. Which of the following questions should be asked by the NP in the dietary assessment of a client with a diagnosis of BPH?

  a. "Are you following a low-fat diet?"
  b. "When is the last time you drink something before bed?"
  c. "How much fiber do you eat each day?"
  d. "Do you drink a glass of orange juice each day?"

6. Which of the following remarks by the client with BPH indicates that teaching has been effective?

  a. "I will refrain from sex."
  b. "I will make position changes slowly."
  c. "I will urinate standing up."
  d. "I will not use antihistamines, but I will use decongestants for a cold."

7. Finasteride differs from other medications used in the treatment of BPH by its action of:

  a. Smooth muscle relaxation
  b. Dilating the urethra
  c. Reducing pelvic pressure
  d. Shrinking the prostate

Answers and Rationales

1. Answer: d (implementation/plan)
  Rationale: Because of the orthostatic side effects and the older age of the men being treated, the medications should be started at a low dose and titrated upward to reach the desirable dose.

2. Answer: b (assessment)
  Rationale: Burning is indicative of infection, calculi, or cancer.

3. Answer: c (analysis/diagnosis)
  Rationale: Fever and pyuria are associated with infection. A symptom score between 0 and 7 indicates mild symptoms and may not be indicative of a true problem. PVR indicates BPH or some other form of obstruction.

4. Answer: c (implementation/plan)
  Rationale: A PVR of 350 indicates major obstruction and the need for evaluation by a urologist. Most medications used to treat BPH cause hypotension side effects. The NP can adjust dose to decrease effects. These medications also require 2 to 3 months of use before symptoms may improve. A score of 15 on the American Urological Association index indicates moderate symptoms and that BPH should be able to be controlled with medications.

5. Answer: b (assessment)
  Rationale: Nocturia is the most common symptom associated with BPH. Drinking fluid in the evening may worsen nocturia.

6. Answer: b (evaluation)
  Rationale: BPH is not a contraindication for sexual activity. Urinating while sitting may enhance voiding. Decongestants also produce peripheral vasoconstriction and make voiding more difficult. Side effects of most BPH medications are relaxation of smooth muscle and hypotension.

7. Answer: d (analysis/diagnosis)
  Rationale: Finasteride shrinks the prostate and requires up to 6 months to see effects. Other classes of drugs used to treat BPH are smooth muscle relaxers.

BLEPHARITIS *Pamela Kidd*

OVERVIEW
Definition

Blepharitis is inflammation of the eyelid margin, resulting in redness, scaling and crusting.

Incidence

Blepharitis is more common in fair-skinned people. There is equal incidence in males and females. The nonulcerative form is associated with rosacea and seborrhea.

Pathophysiology

The nonulcerative form is considered a chronic condition with acute flare-ups. The exact mechanism is unknown, but it is related to increased skin shedding. The ulcerative form is produced by staphylococcal infection.

Factors Increasing Susceptibility
- Presence of rosacea or seborrhea
- Contact lens use

TABLE **3-12** Pharmacologic Treatment for Ulcerative Form

AGENT	DOSE	COMMENTS
Erythromycin ophthalmic ointment 0.5%	Apply to lid margin 4-6 times qd	May cause local irritation
Sulfacetamide ointment	Apply to lid margin 4-6 times qd	May cause local irritation

Protective Factors. Good handwashing to prevent spreading of staphylococcal infection.

ASSESSMENT: SUBJECTIVE/HISTORY
Symptoms

Assess duration of symptoms and previous episodes, use of contact lens and eye cosmetics, and any change in vision or tearing of eye. Common symptoms are irritation, burning, and itching of eyes with occasional tearing.

Past Medical History

Rosacea and seborrhea are indicative of blepharitis.

Medication History

Inquire about use of eye drops (OTC or prescribed). Check expiration date and if used by others.

Family History

Not applicable.

Dietary History

Not applicable.

ASSESSMENT: OBJECTIVE/PHYSICAL EXAMINATION
Physical Examination

Check visual acuity. If ulcerative form, there will be shedding of skin at eyelid margins. If skin is removed, there may be slight bleeding and shallow ulcer formation. Conjunctivitis may be present. In nonulcerative form, there will be greasy, removable scales on lid margins and eyelashes.

Diagnostic Procedures

Take a culture of lid margin if there is no improvement in 1 month.

DIAGNOSIS

The most common differential diagnoses are:
- Hordeolum: superficial lid infection resulting from staphylococcal infection of sebaceous, apocrine, or meibomian gland. Internal is on the conjunctival side of lid.
- Chalazion: tender, mildly inflamed mass on the lid
- Lice infestation: white or black specks attached to eyelashes

THERAPEUTIC PLAN
Nonpharmacologic Treatment

Use baby shampoo diluted 50% with water. Scrub eyelid with cotton ball soaked in the solution. Rinse with water. Afterward, apply hot compresses to closed lids for up to 10 minutes.

Pharmacologic Treatment

See Table 3-12.

Client Education

- No eye cosmetics or contact lens use during flare-ups.
- Clean eyelashes well after cosmetic use.

Referral

- Refer to ophthalmologist if no improvement.
- Refer to dermatologist for severe rosacea or seborrhea cases and for biopsy.

Prevention

Practice good hand and eye hygiene.

EVALUATION/FOLLOW-UP

Biopsy after 1 month if no improvement; it may be an unusual presentation of basal or squamous cell carcinoma.

COMPLICATIONS

- Scarring of eyelid margin
- Corneal infection

REFERENCES

Johnsen, D. A. (2000). Blepharitis. In D. Robinson, P. Kidd, & K. M. Rogers (Eds.), *Primary care across the lifespan*. St. Louis: Mosby.

Review Questions

1. A client presents with redness, scaling, and crusting of the right eye. Which of the following historical data would support a diagnosis of blepharitis?
   - a. Client is African American.
   - b. Client uses saline eye drops without relief.
   - c. Client has seborrhea.
   - d. Client wears eyeglasses.

2. In preventing blepharitis the NP should instruct a client to:
   - a. Wear sunglasses.

b. Avoid eye cosmetics.

c. Wear extended wear contact lens.

d. Use erythromycin ointment prophylactically.

3. Blepharitis must be differentiated from internal hordeolum. Compared with blepharitis, internal hordeolum is associated with:

a. Change in vision

b. Lesion on conjunctival side of lid

c. Affecting one eye

d. Presence of pain

4. Which of the following drug choices is the most appropriate for the ulcerative form of blepharitis?

a. Erythromycin orally

b. Erythromycin ophthalmic ointment

c. TMX-SMP (Bactrim) orally

d. Saline eye drops

Answers and Rationales

1. *Answer:* **c** (assessment)
   Rationale: Both rosacea and seborrhea are associated with nonulcerative blepharitis. It is more common in fair-skinned people who wear contact lenses.

2. *Answer:* **b** (implementation/plan)
   Rationale: Poor hygiene contributes to blepharitis. Use of eye cosmetics increases susceptibility. Contact lens wearing also increases susceptibility. There is no difference between daily and extended wear in relation to blepharitis. Antibiotic ointment is used to treat the ulcerative form of blepharitis. There are no data that support its use to prevent reoccurrence.

3. *Answer:* **b** (analysis/diagnosis)
   Rationale: Internal hordeolum is an inflammation of the internal meibomian gland. It is located on the conjunctival surface. Either blepharitis or hordeolum can affect both eyes, but usually only one is affected at a time. Blepharitis is inflammation of the edges of the eyelids, with the presence of greasy, removable scales on the eyelashes. Pain rarely is present in either condition. Neither condition produces a change in vision.

4. *Answer:* **b** (implementation/plan)
   Rationale: Systemic antibiotics are not indicated. Saline eye drops will not prevent corneal infection.

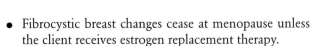

BREAST MASSES   *Cheryl Pope Kish*

OVERVIEW

Definition

A breast lump is a three-dimensional, dominant, palpable lump or area of thickening distinct from the surrounding breast tissue and generally asymmetric in comparison with the other breast.

Incidence

Four of five masses are benign, but malignancy always must be ruled out. According to the American Cancer Society (ACS), a woman has a 1:8 lifetime risk for breast cancer and a 1:28 lifetime risk for dying of breast cancer.

Pathophysiology

The most common benign breast masses—fibrocystic breast changes and fibroadenoma—represent a normal glandular response to fluctuating levels of estrogen.

Fibrocystic Breast Changes

- Not really pathologic, fibrocystic changes are a change in breast tissue associated with fluid-filled cysts within glandular structure.
- To some extent, fibrocystic changes are experienced by almost all women of reproductive age.
- Breast lumps are cyclic in nature. Areas of thickness, nodularity, or cystic masses may be palpable and tender 7 to 14 days before menses.

- Fibrocystic breast changes cease at menopause unless the client receives estrogen replacement therapy.
- Masses are multiple, round or lobular, soft and rubbery to thick, well circumscribed, and mobile, with no nipple retraction. Client can have tender, palpable axillary nodes.
- Fine, granular tissue or gross lumpiness can be palpated. Masses most often are found in the upper outer quadrant. Local edema or overall enlargement may be present, with symmetric findings in both breasts.

Fibroadenoma

- Fibroadenoma is the most common benign breast tumor.
- It is an abnormal growth of fibrous and ductal tissue under hormonal influence.
- It is not cyclic, with a 10% to 20% recurrence rate.
- Surgery provides definitive diagnosis and cure.
- Fibroadenoma is not associated with increased risk of breast cancer.
- A mass is single, nontender, soft or firm, freely moveable, and round or lobular in shape, with clear margins. It may cause premenstrual tenderness.
- Common age is 20 to 40 years; the condition is rare after menopause.
- Excessively large fibroadenoma (cystosarcoma phyllodes) grows rapidly and may stretch the skin to the

point of ulceration. It is a benign condition treated by wide local incision.

Intraductal Papilloma
- This is a small, wartlike growth in the lining of mammary duct, usually near the nipple.
- This is the most common cause of nipple discharge and is usually bloody or serous and spontaneous.
- Palpable mass occurs in approximately half of cases.
- Condition occurs commonly in women 45 to 55 years and increases after menopause.

Fat Necrosis
- The onset of mass, usually palpated superficially, is in direct response to trauma; half the cases are not remembered by the woman.
- It resolves slowly.
- There is no increase in cancer risk.
- It has been found that ecchymosis is possible, it is painless, it is a somewhat fixed mass, and nipple retraction is common.
- It is common in overweight women with large breasts or after breast surgery.
- It occurs at any age.
- It generally resolves with time.

Duct Ectasia
- Duct ectasia is the result of dilation of subareolar ducts, with fibrosis and inflammation behind the nipple. It is sometimes called periductal mastitis.
- The areola may be reddened.
- There is no increase in cancer risk.
- It causes burning pain exacerbated by cold, itching nipple, and nipple discharge (thin and watery in young women and thick, sticky, and pasty in older women; it may be dark green and arises from multiple duct openings); nipple retraction is possible.
- It is common in women 45 to 55 years old.
- It is treated with antibiotics.

Breast Cancer
- Breast cancer is the second leading cause of cancer death in women (first is lung cancer).
- Malignant cells invade breast tissue, with malignant potential for spread.
- Findings suggestive of malignancy are as follows: Mass is often single, irregular, or stellate; fixed, not clearly distinct from surrounding tissue; firm to rock hard; or unilateral. Nipple retraction and bloody discharge are common. There is a prominent vascular pattern on affected breast and peau d'orange (thick skin resembling orange peel) because of blocked lymphatic drainage.
- Pain may or may not be present.

- Common ages of occurrence are 30 to 80 years; prevalence significantly increases after menopause.
- Breast cancer is more than 100 times more common in women than men.
- Paget's disease: This type of breast cancer affects the epidermis of the nipple or areola. Its presenting symptoms include an eczema-like rash with excoriation and scaling.

Factors Increasing Susceptibility. Of women who get breast cancer, 85% have one of the following risk factors:
- Age older than 50 years
- Personal history of breast cancer
- Family history, first-degree relatives with breast cancer
- History of fibrocystic disease with epithelial hyperplasia diagnosed by at least one biopsy.
- Early menarche (younger than 12 years) and late menopause (older than 55 years)
- Nulliparity
- Age older than 30 years at first pregnancy
- Exposure to ionizing radiation
- Prolonged hormone replacement with unopposed estrogen
- Excessive alcohol use
- Exposure to toxic substances
- Smoking
- Increased fat in diet
- Obesity
- Diethylstilbestrol (DES) exposure
- Ashkenazi Jewish heritage (increased probability of inherited breast cancer gene)

Protective Factors. Breast feeding and early first pregnancy provide some protection against certain breast masses and breast cancer.

ASSESSMENT: SUBJECTIVE/HISTORY
A breast mass most likely is discovered by the client. The following subjective data should be elicited from the client with a breast mass:
- Location and description of mass
- When discovered
- What changes, if any, in mass since discovery
- Relationship to menstrual cycle
- Any changes in skin over area of mass
- Any trauma to breast
- Change in breast
- Previous mass (if yes, elicit details)
- Last menstrual period
- Menstrual and obstetric history, age at menarche
- Last breast self-examination (BSE), last clinical examination, last mammogram or breast ultrasound

- Evidence of risk factors for breast cancer
- Hormone replacement therapy

Symptoms

- Pain or tenderness: If present, describe when, where, how much on a 0- to 10-point scale, what makes it better, and what exacerbates it.
- Nipple discharge: If present, describe duration, color, and characteristics of fluid and whether it occurs spontaneously or is elicited. Note whether it arises from one or multiple duct openings from the nipple.
- Palpable, tender axillary lymph nodes, supraclavicular nodes.

Past Medical History

- Previous breast mass: Provide details about diagnosis and treatment
- Previous breast, ovary, colorectal or other cancer
- Trauma to breast

Medication History

Ask about use of the following medications:

- Oral contraceptives
- Medications associated with nipple discharge:
  - Tricyclic antidepressants
  - Diuretics
  - Phenothiazines
  - Steroids
  - Phenytoin
  - Digitalis
  - Reserpine
  - Methyldopa
- Medications with significant levels of methylxanthines, which exacerbate fibrocystic disease, are thought to increase mastalgia:
  - Aspirin plus caffeine (Anacin)
  - Aspirin, caffeine, and cinnamedrine (Midol)
  - Caffeine plus ergotamine tartrate (Cafergot)
  - Aspirin
  - Butalbital (Fiorinal)
  - Chlorpheniramine maleate plus phenylephrine hydrochloride, with or without aspirin (Dristan)
  - Theophylline
  - Aspirin plus oxycodone hydrochloride (Percodan)
  - Cimetidine, associated with gynecomastia

Family History

Ask about family history of breast, ovarian, and colorectal cancer; such history is especially significant in first-degree maternal relatives or men. Ask about other cancers.

Psychosocial History

Ask about OTC, prescription, and recreational drug use. Ask about smoking, caffeine use, and alcohol use. Determine client's feelings of uncertainty and anxiety and responses of her partner and family to the news of her finding the breast lump. The NP must appreciate that few findings are more alarming to a woman and her partner than a breast mass because the potential for malignancy always exists. Many fear the consequences of a cancer diagnosis and the possibility of pain, debilitating illness, disfiguring surgery, and death.

Dietary History

Ask about methylxanthines (coffee, tea, cola, chocolate) in diet because restricting these, although not research proven, seems to help relieve some cyclic breast pain. For the same reason, ask about caffeine use, vegetable consumption (especially those with carotene), and dietary sodium use. Ask about the amounts of beef and fat in the client's diet; excesses are believed to increase susceptibility to cancer.

ASSESSMENT: OBJECTIVE/PHYSICAL EXAMINATION
Physical Examination

A problem-oriented physical examination should be conducted with particular attention to the following:

- General appearance and examination of the breasts
- Axilla
- Supraclavicular lymph nodes
- With client sitting on examination table with arms at sides, observe uncovered breasts for symmetry, contour, and change in vascular pattern. Note discoloration or peau d'orange skin, retraction of nipple, crusting of areola and nipple, and local edema. Repeat observation with arms over head and with arms pressing against hips.
- With client supine, inspect breasts and skin. Begin palpation on opposite side from identified mass. Palpate entire breast, including tail of Spence, for masses. Palpate for axillary, supraclavicular, and infraclavicular lymphadenopathy. Massage entire breast toward nipple to attempt to elicit nipple discharge. If client has breast implants, check for location, extent of healing, symmetry, and presence of bulging.
- In a client with pendulous breasts, examine sitting up and leaning forward. Support breast with inferior hand and use other hand to palpate. Note the following:
  - Location, with distance of mass from nipple in centimeters
  - Size
  - Shape: oval, spherical, lobular, indistinct, stellate, irregular
  - Consistency: soft, firm, rubbery, hard
  - Mobility: freely movable versus fixed on chest wall

- Solitary versus multiple
- Nipple retraction
- Dimpling
- Discharge (suspicious discharge is bloody, serous, or serosanguineous; unilateral, especially if from one duct; and occurring with a mass)
  - Tenderness
- Men may have breast masses, too. Examination procedure is the same as in women.
- In the prepubertal male, breast enlargement is normal, usually with bilateral enlargement. Recheck in 6 months. If the client is embarrassed or distressed, refer him to a surgeon.

Diagnostic Procedures

Mammography is used in women older than 35 years to locate suspicious lesions. Masses can be localized to less than 1 cm, which is the smallest clinically detectable mass, increasing the survival potential and decreasing the necessity for extensive surgery. Mammography cannot distinguish benign from malignant disease; normal results occur in the presence of breast cancer in 10% of clients. Radiation dose approximates that received during a day in the sun. The ACS recommends that mammography should be done for the following:

- Women ages 30 and older—with suspected problem
- Women ages 40 and older—annually
- Women with first-degree relative with premenopausal breast cancer—schedule first mammogram 5 to 10 years before the age of the relative at diagnosis
- Men with breast mass—any age

Breast Ultrasonography
- Often is more effective for women younger than 35 years who have denser breast tissue.
- Differentiates cystic from solid masses.
- Exposes the client to less radiation.

Fine-Needle Aspiration. Fine-needle aspiration (FNA) is aspiration of fluid from a cystic mass with sterile technique, with or without local anesthesia, followed by cytologic analysis by a pathologist. (Note: Pap smear of breast fluid yields inconclusive results.)

Genetic Studies. BRCA-1 (long arm of chromosome 17) and BRCA-2 (chromosome 13) are gene mutations associated with an increased risk of breast cancer in those who inherit an abnormal gene. Routine screening is not recommended.

DIAGNOSIS

Differential diagnoses includes the following:
- Fibrocystic breast disease
- Mammary duct ectasia
- Fat necrosis
- Carcinoma
- Intraductal papilloma
- Paget's disease
- Mastitis
- Normal premenstrual breast tissue
- Costal cartilage disorder (Tietze's syndrome)
- Fibroadenoma

THERAPEUTIC PLAN
Pharmacologic Treatment
- Oral contraceptives daily or medroxyprogesterone acetate (Provera) days 15 to 25 of cycle may be used for cyclic pain.
- For fibrocystic disease, Vitamin E daily, evening primrose oil, and vitamin B_6 (pyridoxine) have received anecdotal support.
- As a last resort in cases of severe mastalgia, the following drugs may be used (consultation with physician is advised): danazol (Danocrine—only drug approved by Food and Drug Administration for fibrocystic disease), tamoxifen, and bromocriptine (Parlodel). All have significant side effects. A pregnancy test is advised because of teratogenicity.

Client Education
- Monthly BSE with ACS standards, reinforcing at each follow-up visit as necessary.
- With fibrocystic disease:
  - Restriction of caffeine, alcohol, and methylxanthines may lessen pain.
  - Decrease alcohol use to less than 3 drinks a week.
  - Increase consumption of vegetables, especially those with carotene.
  - Decrease sodium intake 10 days before menses.
  - Do not smoke.
  - Decrease weight if obese.
  - Wear support bra, day and night.
  - Avoid trauma.
  - Take mild analgesics.
  - Use warm compresses.
  - Eat a low-fat, high-fiber diet.
- Advise client regarding ways to alter lifestyle to decrease risk of breast cancer.

Referral
- Mass suspicious for cancer
- Cystic mass persisting after aspiration or 1 week past next menses
- Palpable lymph nodes
- Solid mass
- Woman who is difficult to examine completely because of breast size, density, or scarring
- Woman who is persistently worried about breast cancer despite negative workup

Prevention

Breast masses are not preventable in all cases.

EVALUATION/FOLLOW-UP

Ideal time for clinical breast examination is 7 to 9 days after menses. If office examination is performed during premenstrual phase and a mass is found, advise the client to return in 2 to 3 weeks for a recheck.

For a soft, mobile mass or thickness with suspicion of fibrocystic changes in low-risk clients, consider reexamination the week after next menses terminates. Refer if mass persists on reexamination.

Plan for follow-up of cystic mass:

- Do FNA. If cyst resolves, observe for 6 weeks. If it recurs, refer to surgeon.
- Do FNA. If cyst persists, obtain fluid for cytologic testing and refer to surgeon.

Treatment for breast cancer usually involves surgery, with or without breast reconstruction. Systemic treatment generally follows. This involves adjuvant therapy with radiation, chemotherapy, hormonal therapy, or immune system stimulants.

Survivors of breast cancer should continue monthly BSE and have a yearly mammogram and clinical examination with evaluation for a new breast cancer or metastasis every 3 to 6 months initially. Special attention is paid to the increased risk of bowel, endometrial, and ovarian cancer in this population.

COMPLICATIONS

A great concern of virtually all NPs caring for women is that a cancerous breast mass will be misdiagnosed. Careful adherence to clinical standards of practice and recommendations for screening as well as careful follow-up of women at risk minimize the potential of this complication.

REFERENCES

Alderman, E. M. (2001). Breast problems in the adolescent. *Patient Care, 34*(16), 56-80.

Appling, S. E. (1998). Prevention, early detection, and treatment of breast cancer: A collaborative approach. *Lippincott's Primary Care Practice, 2*(2), 111-118.

Berry, J. A. (2001). Breast pain: All that hurts is not cancer. *American Journal for Nurse Practitioners, 5*(4), 9-18.

Bowman, M. A., Braly, P. S., Johnson, S., & Mikuta, J. J. (1996). Who are you screening for cancer and when? *Patient Care, 30*, 54-87.

Bush, T. L., Cummings, S. R., & Hudis, C. A. (2000). Breast cancer prevention: Are we making progress? *Contemporary OB/GYN, 45*(4), 38-42, 45-52.

Cornell, S. (1999). Not just for women: Breast cancer affects men, too. *ADVANCE for Nurse Practitioners, 7*(6), 57-58.

Dains, J.E., Baumann, L.C., & Scheibel, P. (1998). *Advanced health assessment and clinical diagnosis in primary care.* St. Louis: Mosby.

Dixon, J. M. (1999). Managing breast pain. *The Practitioner, 243*(6), 484-491.

Fiorica, J. V., Schorr, S. J., & Sickles, E. A. (1997). Benign breast disorders—First rule out cancer. *Patient Care, 31*, 140-154.

Hindle, W. H. & Gonzalez, S. (2001). Breast disease: What to do when it's not cancer. *Women's Health in Primary Care, 4*(1), 21-24.

Johnson, C. (1999). Benign breast disease. *Nurse Practitioner Forum, 10*(3), 137-144.

Morrison, C. (1998). The significance of nipple discharge: Diagnosis and treatment regimes. *Lippincott's Primary Care Practice, 2*(2), 129-140.

Zieglfeld, C. R. (1998). Differential diagnosis of a breast mass. *Lippincott's Primary Care Practice, 2*(2), 121-128.

Review Questions

1. Which factor in a woman's history is considered positive protection against breast cancer?

- **a.** She has breast fed four children.
- **b.** She experienced menarche at age 10 years.
- **c.** She drank alcohol excessively for years but quit recently.
- **d.** Her mother and grandmother had early menopause.

2. Which objective finding is not usually associated with breast cancer?

- **a.** Rubbery, well-circumscribed, tender lesion
- **b.** Eczema-like scaling on one areola and nipple
- **c.** Peau d'orange dimpling of skin over breast
- **d.** Unilateral deviated and retracted nipple

3. The examination of a 27-year-old woman reveals an irregular, unilateral, stony-hard mass that is poorly defined, with spontaneous bloody discharge from a retracted nipple. What diagnosis is most appropriate?

- **a.** Fibroadenoma
- **b.** Paget's disease
- **c.** Breast cancer
- **d.** Intraductal papilloma

4. For which client should ultrasonography be ordered to evaluate a breast mass?

- **a.** 27-year-old Gail
- **b.** 39-year-old Merry
- **c.** 51-year-old Anna
- **d.** 68-year-old Thelma

5. Ms. Stelly, 20 years old, comes in for an annual examination. Her next menstrual period is due to start in 3 days. The family NP notes multiple cystic areas bilaterally, and the client's breasts are extremely tender. What follow-up is most appropriate?

- **a.** Client should return for recheck 7 to 10 days after her period ends.
- **b.** No follow-up is necessary because she is problem free.
- **c.** Ultrasonography of breasts should be performed within 24 hours.
- **d.** Client should return for recheck in 1 month.

6. A breast biopsy is considered mandatory with which of the following findings?

- **a.** Straw-colored fluid aspirated with FNA

b. Nonpalpable lesion found on mammogram
c. Ecchymotic area on the breast of a woman injured in a fall
d. Production of milky discharge after sexual stimulation of the breasts

7. Ms. Strauss, age 26 years, is a new client who comes in for a preemployment physical examination. History reveals that her mother had breast cancer diagnosed at age 38 years. In addition to a clinical examination and monthly BSE, this client should be advised to have a baseline mammogram when?

a. At 28 to 33 years of age
b. At 40 to 45 years of age
c. Within the next 6 months
d. Anytime before her 50th birthday

Answers and Rationales

1. ***Answer:*** **a** (assessment)
Rationale: Breast feeding appears to impart a protective effect against breast cancer (Bush, Cummings, & Hudis, 2000).

2. ***Answer:*** **a** (assessment)
Rationale: Peau d'orange and nipple retraction are common features of breast cancer; the cancer of Paget's disease reveals nipple and areola scaling, erythema, and erosion similar to eczema (Dains, Baumann, & Scheibel, 1998).

3. ***Answer:*** **c** (analysis/diagnosis)
Rationale: Cancerous masses are usually unilateral, hard, and rough edged. Nipple retraction and bloody discharge are common manifestations (Fiorica, Schorr, & Sickles, 1997).

4. ***Answer:*** **a** (implementation/plan)
Rationale: Ultrasonography is more effective for evaluating the dense breasts of the woman younger than 35 years (Fiorica, Schorr, & Sickles, 1997).

5. ***Answer:*** **a** (evaluation)
Rationale: Clinical breast examination is best performed a week or so after the onset of menses, when the breast is least congested (Fiorica, Schorr, & Sickles, 1997).

6. ***Answer:*** **b** (implementation/plan)
Rationale: Mammography identifies masses less than 1 cm smaller than when they are clinically palpable (Fiorica, Schorr, & Sickles, 1997).

7. ***Answer:*** **a** (evaluation)
Rationale: If a first-degree relative developed breast cancer, start screening the client when she is 5 to 10 years younger than that relative was at diagnosis (Bowman, Braly, Johnson, & Mikuta, 1996).

BRONCHIOLITIS   *Denise Robinson*

OVERVIEW
Definition

Bronchiolitis is a virally induced acute bronchiolar inflammation that is associated with signs and symptoms of airway obstruction.

Incidence

- It is the most common lower respiratory infection in infants.
- It occurs in a seasonal pattern, with highest incidence in the winter in temperate climates and during the rainy season in warmer countries.
- Of infants, 21% have lower respiratory tract disease.
- Of infants, 6 to 10:1000 require admission to the hospital for bronchiolitis.
- The peak rate of admission occurs in infants aged 2 to 6 months.
- Infants of Native-American or Inuit race tend to have a more complicated course.
- The mortality rate for bronchiolitis is less than 1% in those children without risk factors (Tang & Wang, 2001).

Pathophysiology

The organisms responsible for bronchiolitis are transmitted by respiratory secretions and droplet contamination.

Inflammation, excess mucus secretion, and epithelial hyperplasia and necrosis contribute to narrowing and blockage of the small airways of the bronchioles. The resultant obstruction contributes to increased airway resistance, air trapping, and respiratory compromise. The smaller bronchioles in infants exacerbate these processes and account for the higher mortality and morbidity in this group.

Respiratory syncytial virus (RSV) is responsible for bronchiolitis in approximately 70% of cases. This figure reaches 80% to 100% in the winter months. In early spring, parainfluenza virus type 3 also is responsible.

ASSESSMENT: SUBJECTIVE/HISTORY
History of Present Illness

- Ask about onset, fever, and prodromal and associated symptoms.
- Ask about recent exposures to persons with respiratory illness.
- Determine immunization status.
- Ask about feeding and sleeping difficulties and the infant's general behavior.

Symptoms

- Fever: low grade or absent
- Prodrome of mild rhinitis and cough for 1 to 2 days
- Rhinitis

- Tachypnea
- Expiratory wheezing (abrupt onset)
- Cough
- Rales
- Use of accessory muscles
- Apnea
- Retractions
- Nasal flaring

Aggravating Factors

Disease severity is related to the following:
- Size of the infant
- Congenital heart disease
- Chronic lung disease
- Premature birth
- Hypoxia
- Age younger than 6 weeks

Past Medical History

Assess for the following:
- Allergies/atopy
- Immune disorders
- Prematurity
- Congenital heart disease
- Possible foreign body aspiration

Family History

- Ask about allergies, asthma, and immune disorders.
- Ask about similar illness or viral illness in family members within the week preceding the illness.

Psychosocial History

Ask about smokers in the house—infants whose caregivers smoke are more likely to develop bronchiolitis.

ASSESSMENT: OBJECTIVE/PHYSICAL EXAMINATION

Physical Examination

- Obtain vital signs, which include low grade or absent fever and increased respiratory rate (RR) and heart rate.
- Observe general appearance; may be toxic with diminished sensorium and mild to moderate signs of respiratory distress and cyanosis.
- Observe the parent feeding the infant; monitor for feeding difficulties.
- Note skin pallor or mottling, delayed capillary refill, decreased skin turgor, and dryness of lips and mouth (may indicate dehydration).
- Observe head, eyes, ears, nose, and throat (HEENT) for possible concomitant infections (conjunctivitis, otitis media) and nasal flaring.
- Auscultate lungs for increased respiratory effort; shallow, rapid breathing (paradoxical or "see-saw" respira-

tions require immediate referral); grunting; prolonged expiration; hyperresonance; and diminished breath sounds with scattered rales and symmetric expiratory wheeze.
- Check heart for tachycardia.
- Examine abdomen—may be able to palpate liver and spleen because of hyperinflation of lungs.

Diagnostic Procedures

- Complete blood cell (CBC) count is not usually needed. White blood cell count usually is normal or slightly elevated.
- Chest radiograph is not usually needed. If taken, it shows hyperinflation, increased bronchovesicular markings, and mild interstitial infiltration.
- RSV culture is not usually done; it is positive if present.

DIAGNOSIS

Diagnosis is based on abrupt onset of wheezing and difficulty breathing. Physical examination findings that support hyperinflation corroborate the diagnosis.

Differential diagnoses include the following:
- Asthma
- Bronchitis
- Foreign body aspiration
- Gastroesophageal reflux disease
- Pneumonia
- Tuberculosis
- Viral croup

THERAPEUTIC PLAN

Nonpharmacologic Treatment

Fluid intake is important to prevent dehydration and to facilitate loosening and clearing of secretions.

Pharmacologic Treatment

- Antibiotics are given only if there is evidence of secondary infection.
- Aerosolized bronchodilators may provide transient improvement of the airway obstruction (Tang & Wang, 2001).
- There is conflicting evidence on the effects of corticosteroids in children with bronchiolitis.
- There is no evidence that ribavirin or immunoglobulins are effective in reducing mortality in children with bronchiolitis.

Client Education

- Parents need to be taught the signs of respiratory distress.
- Teaching caregivers how to use the bulb syringe to clear secretions or how to administer percussion and postural drainage may be helpful.

Prevention

Prophylactic RSV immunoglobulin or monoclonal antibody given to high-risk children (premature infants, bronchopulmonary dysplasia) on a monthly basis reduces hospital admissions and admission to intensive care (Tang & Wang, 2001).

Referral

- Hospitalization and mechanical ventilation are needed for 1% to 2% of infants with bronchiolitis. Medical consultation is warranted if the infant is in respiratory distress or has a RR greater than 60 breaths/min; has apnea; or is less than 3 months of age or less than 6 months of age with a history of prematurity or bronchopulmonary dysplasia or with congenital heart disease. In addition, if the child feeds with difficulty or shows signs of dehydration, the child should be referred.
- The child should be referred if there has been no resolution in 3 weeks or if bronchiolitis recurs (other pathology may be present).

EVALUATION/FOLLOW-UP

- Follow-up with a telephone call within 24 hours and daily thereafter until the symptoms of respiratory distress have abated.
- Schedule a return visit in 48 hours if there is minimal or no improvement with supportive therapy.
- Schedule a return visit in 1 week if symptoms are still present.

COMPLICATIONS

The prognosis for bronchiolitis is good, and most infants fully recover within 2 weeks. However, a number of these will experience recurrent episodes of wheezing and coughing for 3 to 5 years following the initial diagnosis. Very rarely the illness is so severe that permanent airway damage occurs.

REFERENCES

Niemer, L. (2000). Brochiolitis. In D. Robinson, P. Kidd, & K. Rogers (Eds.), *Primary care across the lifespan.* St.Louis: Mosby.

Orenstein, D. (1996). Bronchiolitis. In W. Nelson, R. Behrman, R. Kliegman, A. Arvin (Eds.). *Nelson textbook of pediatrics.* (15th Ed). Philadelphia: Saunders, 1211-1213.

Schuh, S., Coates, A., Binnie, R., Allin, T., Goia, C., Corey, M., et al. (2001). Efficacy of oral dexamethasone in outpatients with acute bronchiolitis. *Academic Emergency Medicine, 8*(5), 417.

Sharland, M., Bedford-Russell, A. (2001). Preventing respiratory syncytial virus bronchiolitis. *British Medical Journal, 322*(7278), 62-63.

Shay, D. K., Holman, R. C., Roosevelt, G. E., Clarke, M. J., Anderson, L. J. (2001). Bronchiolitis-associated mortality and estimates of respiratory syncytial virus-associated deaths among US children, 1979-1997. *Journal of Infectious Diseases, 183,* 16-22.

Tang, N., & Wang, E. (2001). Bronchiolitis. In S. Barton (Ed). *Clinical evidence* (pp 214-222). London: British Medical Journal Publishing Group.

Review Questions

1. A 6-month-old infant comes to your office with a 3-day history of worsening respiratory symptoms. The condition began as "a cold," but the infant now is "breathing so fast he can hardly eat or sleep." There is an intermittent, nonproductive cough, paroxysmal at times. On examination, respiratory rate is 64 breaths/min, and there are marked intercostal retractions and generalized wheezing. The parents are worried because the father has asthma. On the basis of these data, what is the most likely diagnosis?

    a. Asthma
    b. Pneumonia
    c. Bronchopulmonary dysplasia
    d. Bronchiolitis

2. A 3-month-old boy comes into the office with tachypnea with wheezing and rales. What associated history supports a diagnosis of bronchiolitis?

    a. Smokers in the home
    b. Older brother with seasonal allergies
    c. Recurrent skin problems since birth
    d. Otitis media 1 week ago

3. A 6-month-old boy comes in with respiratory difficulty, RR of 48 breaths/min, intercostal retractions, and generalized wheezing. What further objective data supports a diagnosis of bronchiolitis?

    a. Wheezing improved after treatment with albuterol in normal saline solution per nebulizer.
    b. Peak expiratory flow rate (PEFR) was 75% after treatment with albuterol.
    c. Barrel appearance of chest and clubbing of fingers are noted.
    d. Liver and spleen are palpable below the liver margin.

4. Appropriate management for a 6-month-old with bronchiolitis (generalized wheezing and respiratory distress, RR of 62 breaths/min) is which of the following?

    a. Referral for hospitalization
    b. In-office nebulization with albuterol
    c. Education regarding PEFR monitoring
    d. Respiratory follow-up in 2 weeks

5. The most likely differential diagnosis for bronchiolitis is which of the following?

    a. Pneumonia
    b. Asthma
    c. Foreign body aspiration
    d. Bronchitis

Answers and Rationales

1. *Answer:* d (analysis/diagnosis)
    Rationale: Bronchiolitis is at the top of the list of differential diagnoses for a 6-month-old with wheezing. Assuming that this

is the first episode of wheezing, a diagnosis of asthma is premature, even with his family history of a father with asthma. The progression of URI symptoms to respiratory distress signs and symptoms is typical of bronchiolitis (Orenstein, 1996).

2. *Answer:* a (assessment)
   Rationale: Smokers in the home make the infant much more susceptible to bronchiolitis. Infants that stay home with a heavy smoker are more likely to get sick than are their day care counterparts (Orenstein, 1996).

3. *Answer:* d (assessment)
   Rationale: The liver and spleen may be depressed because of hyperinflation of the lungs, with the result of being palpable below the liver (Orenstein, 1996).

4. *Answer:* a (implementation/plan)
   Rationale: Any child in severe respiratory distress with a RR greater than 60 breaths/min should be referred for hospitalization (Niemer, 2000).

5. *Answer:* b (implementation/plan)
   Rationale: The most likely differential diagnosis for bronchiolitis is asthma (Orenstein, 1996).

BRONCHITIS: ACUTE BRONCHITIS AND ACUTE EXACERBATIONS OF CHRONIC BRONCHITIS *Pamela Kidd*

OVERVIEW
Definition

Acute bronchitis has been defined as a transient infectious inflammatory condition of the trachea, bronchi, and bronchioles characterized by a cough. It is usually a diagnosis of exclusion. In conjunction with chronic obstructive pulmonary disease (COPD), acute exacerbations of chronic bronchitis (AECB) is defined as more frequent coughing, increased purulence or volume of sputum, and worsened dyspnea (Niederman, 2001).

Incidence

- Commonly affects all ages.
- In outpatients older than age 18, 7 million episodes per year occur.
- In AECB, there is an average of three exacerbations annually.

Pathophysiology

Smoking, environmental stimuli, and infection damage the mucociliary system. Loss of ciliated epithelium leads to impaired mucociliary clearance, allowing bacteria to multiply. A host inflammatory response is stimulated, resulting in release of neutrophils and toxins from the bacteria (free oxygen radicals). Airway damage results from damaged epithelium and mucus production.

Common Pathogens. Viral pathogens are the most common:
- Cold virus
- Influenza
- Adenovirus
- *Mycoplasma pneumoniae*

Secondary bacterial pathogens include the following:
- *Chlamydia pneumoniae*
- *Moraxella catarrhalis*
- *Streptococcus pneumoniae*
- *Haemophilus influenzae*

Factors Increasing Susceptibility
- Smoking
- Occupational exposures to bronchial irritants such as dust or toxic fumes
- Environmental tobacco smoke (ETS) exposure
- Environmental allergies
- Hypertrophied tonsils and adenoids in children
- Immunosuppression
- Chronic sinusitis
- COPD

Protective Factors. Competent immune system is a protective factor.

ASSESSMENT: SUBJECTIVE/HISTORY
Symptoms
- Productive cough is usually the hallmark symptom. Determine the following:
  - How long has cough been present?
  - Is cough productive or nonproductive?
  - Is cough mucoid (clear, white) or purulent (yellow, green)?
  - Was cough preceded by upper respiratory symptoms? If so, for how long?
  - Do others in the household have similar symptoms?
- Other symptoms include the following:
  - Substernal chest discomfort/burning
  - Dyspnea
  - Wheezing
  - Fatigue
  - Decreased appetite
  - Hemoptysis

- Fever
- Chills

Past Medical History

- Asthma/COPD
- Congestive heart failure (CHF)
- Chronic sinusitis
- Environmental allergies

Medication History

Note name, dosage, and amount of recently used medications:

- Antihistamines
- Decongestants
- Antibiotics
- Cough syrups
- Inhaled medications

Family History

- Asthma
- Cystic fibrosis
- Allergies

Dietary History

Ask about amount and type of liquids being consumed.

ASSESSMENT: OBJECTIVE/PHYSICAL EXAMINATION

Physical Examination

- Note general appearance, energy level, hydration status, and vital signs.
- Examine HEENT—look for signs of sinusitis/rhinitis/otitis, lymphadenopathy, jugular venous distention.
- Listen to heart; note any irregular rhythm, murmurs, rubs, gallops.
- Listen to lungs—may find scattered wheezes and rhonchi; should not have any focal areas of crackles, wheezes, or rhonchi (more indicative of pneumonia).
- Examine abdomen; there should be no hepatomegaly.
- Examine extremities; no edema should be present.

Diagnostic Procedures

- Diagnostic procedures are usually not necessary.
- Indications for CBC/chest radiograph examination include the following:
  - Children, adults, or older adults with any coexisting illnesses that could potentiate the seriousness of a pneumonia compared with a healthy client (e.g., cancer, diabetes, coronary artery disease, COPD, immunosuppression)
  - Symptoms persistent for longer than 2 weeks
  - Unclear clinical picture (e.g., possible CHF)
- Sputum Gram's stains generally are not helpful.

DIAGNOSIS

Differential diagnosis includes the following:

- Pneumonia
- Pertussis (particularly in children younger than 6 months or never immunized)
- Tuberculosis
- Asthma
- CHF
- Postnasal drainage from chronic sinusitis or allergic rhinitis
- Influenza

The diagnosis of acute bronchitis is acceptable after necessary diagnostic testing and the previously listed conditions have been suspected and ruled out on the basis of history and physical examination.

THERAPEUTIC PLAN

Nonpharmacologic Treatment

- Rest
- Fluids
- Humidification of heat or room where sleeping

Pharmacologic Treatment

Pharmacologic treatment used to be based on determining whether the cause was viral or bacterial. It now is believed that there may be some component of bacterial colonization in each episode. Use of antibiotics:

- Reduces duration of symptoms
- Avoids hospitalization frequently
- Allows earlier return to work
- Prevents progression to pneumonia and progressive airway damage (slows inflammatory cycle) (Niederman, 2001)

Children

- Erythromycin 30 to 50 mg/kg/day in divided doses every 6 hours
- Amoxicillin 20 to 40 mg/kg/day in divided doses every 8 hours

Adults/Older Adults

- Erythromycin 250 to 500 mg qid for 10 days
- Trimethoprim-sulfamethoxazole (TMP/SMX) bid for 10 days
- Doxycycline 100 mg bid for 10 days
- Amoxicillin 500 mg tid for 10 days
- Macrolides (azithromycin), tetracycline, quinolones (ciprofloxacin), and TMP/SMX good penetration into the sputum and bronchial mucosa
- Cough suppressants
  - Dextromethorphan
  - Codeine (mostly for nighttime use)
  - Acetaminophen

- Bronchodilators to decrease the cough and symptoms of dyspnea/chest tightness
  - Children 2 to 6 years: Albuterol syrup 0.1 mg/kg tid
  - Children older than 6 years to adult: Albuterol metered dose inhaler 2 puffs every 6 hours prn wheezing/chest tightness
- Prednisone taper for children and adults with underlying chronic respiratory disease and significant dyspnea

Client Education

Instruct client to return immediately if any of the following occur:
- Increase in fever
- Increase in dyspnea
- Dehydration and decreased voiding
- Worsening cardiovascular state

Referral

- Consider referral to allergy specialist if atopy/asthma is suspected.
- Consider referral to pulmonologist if COPD is suspected or if unable to manage symptoms.

Prevention

- Limit exposure to ETS.
- Do not smoke.

EVALUATION/FOLLOW-UP

- For client with coexisting illnesses, schedule return visit in 7 to 14 days to assess status.
- For client without coexisting illnesses, educate to return if no improvement after 7 to 14 days.
- Client who returns with complaints of continued dry, hacking cough, following acute bronchitis may represent temporary reactive airway disease and should be treated with bronchodilators as necessary for up to 1 month. If symptoms persist after 1 month, consider another cause for the cough.
- For client with more than two episodes per year, ascertain that bronchitis is the correct diagnosis instead of asthma. Bronchial provocation testing can aid in the diagnosis of asthma.

REFERENCES

Cropp, A. J. (1997). Acute bronchitis. In M. R. Dambro (Ed.), *Griffith's 5-minute clinical consult* (pp. 154-155). Baltimore: William & Wilkins.

Davis, A. L., Hahn, D. L., Niederman, M. S., & O'Connell, E. J. (1996, January 15). Acute bronchitis in adults and children. *Patient Care, 1,* 102-124.

Hoole, A. J., Pickard, C. G., Ouimette, R. M., Lohr, J. A., & Greenberg, R. A. (1995). *Patient care guidelines for nurse practitioners.* Philadelphia: J. B. Lippincott.

Leiner, S. (1997). Acute bronchitis in adults: Commonly diagnosed but poorly defined. *Nurse Practitioner, 22,* 104-114.

Mainous, A. G., III, Zoorob, R. J., & Hueston, W. J. (1996). Current management of acute bronchitis in ambulatory care. *Archives of Family Medicine, 5,* 79-85.

Niederman. M. S. (2001). Antibiotic therapy of acute exacerbations of chronic bronchitis. *Supplement to the Clinical Advisor, September,* 11-16.

Review Questions

1. Which of the following symptoms are suggestive of bronchitis?
- **a.** Sudden onset of fever, purulent sputum, shortness of breath
- **b.** Fever, cough, substernal chest pain following URI
- **c.** Rhinitis, headache
- **d.** Pharyngitis, nasal congestion

2. Which physical finding is most suggestive of bronchitis?
- **a.** Unilateral wheezing or rhonchi
- **b.** Scattered wheezing or rhonchi
- **c.** Unilateral decreased breath sounds
- **d.** Inspiratory crackles

3. A 46-year-old client complains of rhinitis and head congestion, followed by white productive cough and wheezing. Which diagnosis is *least* likely?
- **a.** Bacterial pneumonia
- **b.** Acute bronchitis
- **c.** Influenza
- **d.** Environmental allergy

4. A prednisone taper might be indicated for which client?
- **a.** A long-distance runner who has a scheduled competition and needs a speedy recovery
- **b.** A client with COPD and significant dyspnea
- **c.** A 24-year-old smoker
- **d.** A 48-year-old farmer

5. A 10-year-old boy is sent home with a diagnosis of viral bronchitis. Symptomatic treatment is prescribed. The mother calls 48 hours later and states that her son is now having purulent, productive cough, has a temperature of 103°F and chills, and is not eating. What plan is most appropriate?
- **a.** Call in a prescription of amoxicillin.
- **b.** Ask the client to return for a chest radiograph examination to rule out pneumonia.
- **c.** Encourage the mother to continue giving acetaminophen.
- **d.** Reassure the mother that symptoms will subside within 24 hours.

6. A 65-year-old client with a history of diabetes, coronary heart disease, and CHF has been diagnosed with bronchitis. What follow-up is appropriate?
- **a.** Inform the client to return if symptoms do not improve.
- **b.** Schedule a CBC and chest radiograph examination in 1 week.
- **c.** Schedule an office visit within 7 to 14 days.
- **d.** Advise the client to keep the regular 3-month checkup.

7. When suspecting bronchitis, in which client should the NP obtain a chest radiograph?
   a. Symptoms have been present for 7 days.
   b. Fever is present.
   c. Client is taking immunosuppressive drugs for a kidney transplant.
   d. Client has scattered wheezes and crackles.

8. A client has had four episodes of bronchitis this year. The next course of action for this client should be which of the following?
   a. Chest radiograph
   b. Workup for asthma
   c. Influenza vaccine
   d. Prophylactic antibiotics

Answers and Rationales

1. *Answer:* **b** (assessment)
Rationale: Fever, cough, and substernal chest burning following URI suggest bronchitis. Fever, purulent sputum, and shortness of breath are more indicative of pneumonia.

2. *Answer:* **b** (assessment)
Rationale: Focal findings such as unilateral wheezes, crackles, and unilateral decreased breath sounds may suggest foreign body, atelectasis, or pneumonia.

3. *Answer:* **a** (analysis/diagnosis)
Rationale: Bacterial pneumonia is least likely because clients usually have high fevers, crackles, and purulent sputum.

4. *Answer:* **b** (implementation/plan)
Rationale: Clients with preexisting lung disease may need systemic corticosteroids to help decrease bronchial hyperreactivity.

5. *Answer:* **b** (implementation/plan)
Rationale: A client who is not improving should return for a chest radiograph examination. Although pneumonia is suspected, there may be another underlying illness present. An on-site examination provides data (e.g., SaO_2, PEFR values) that helps determine if the client should be treated as an outpatient.

6. *Answer:* **c** (evaluation)
Rationale: Clients with coexisting illnesses should be evaluated for resolution of bronchitis symptoms. A CBC and chest radiograph in a week should not be obtained unless the symptoms have changed to suggest pneumonia.

7. *Answer:* **c** (implementation/plan)
Rationale: B and D are typical symptoms suggesting bronchitis. Usually pneumonia is not suspected until symptoms have been present for 2 weeks. Any client who is immunosuppressed could have severe complications from an undetected pneumonia. Thus a chest film should be obtained because symptoms may not appear as severe.

8. *Answer:* **b** (implementation/plan)
Rationale: Asthma frequently can present similar to bronchitis. Bronchial provocation testing can aid in diagnosis. A chest radiograph will not add any information. The flu vaccine will not decrease the number of episodes of bronchitis. Prophylactic antibiotics may create resistance and decrease their future effectiveness.

BURNS *Pamela Kidd*

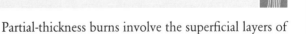

OVERVIEW
Definition

Burns are tissue injuries caused by heat, chemicals, electricity, or irradiation. The depth of the burn is a result of the intensity of the heat and the duration of the exposure.

Incidence

- More than 1.25 million people are burned each year (Brigham & McLoughlin, 1996).
- Burns are the leading cause of death in children; all ages are affected.
- Male and female prevalences are equal.

Pathophysiology

Burns occur as a result of excessive heat energy transferred to the skin, causing cellular protein coagulation and destruction of enzyme systems. Chemicals, electricity, and thermal energy can produce burns.

Partial-thickness burns involve the superficial layers of the epidermis.

- Superficial (first-degree): Erythema is present, skin blanches with pressure, and skin may be tender. Devitalization of superficial layers of epidermis and congestion of intradermal vessels occurs.
- Superficial partial thickness (second-degree): Erythema is present with blisters, and skin is extremely tender. There is coagulation of varying depths of epidermis, vesicles are present, and skin appendages are intact. Area blanches with pressure.
- Deep partial thickness (second-degree): Skin is pale to waxy white. It involves deep layers of dermis. Blisters are present but contain very little fluid. There is decreased pinprick sensation on pain assessment.
- Full thickness burn (third-degree): There is destruction of all skin elements, with destruction of subdermal plexus. With a third degree burn, the skin is tough and

leathery and may be black or white. Skin is not tender, and there is necrosis of all skin elements.

Causes of Burns

- Open flame and hot liquids are the most common causes of burns.
- Burns from caustic chemicals may show little damage for the first few days.
- Electricity may cause significant damage, with little damage seen on the surface.
- Topical medications (e.g., acne medications) may cause chemical burns in clients with sensitive skin.
- Excess sun exposure also is a common cause of burns.

Factors Increasing Susceptibility

- Hot-water heaters set too high (higher than 120° F)
- Workplace exposure to chemicals, electricity, or irradiation
- Thinner skin in young children and older adults
- Carelessness with cigarettes
- Inadequate or faulty wiring
- Use of alcohol or drugs
- Wearing flammable clothing

Protective Factors

- Flame-retardant clothing
- Working smoke detector
- Staying indoors during lightning and electrical storms
- Using personal protective equipment with chemical use

ASSESSMENT: SUBJECTIVE/HISTORY

Symptoms

Before obtaining a history, be sure that the burning process has stopped. If not, flush affected areas with tepid water. Remove all nonadhering clothing and jewelry in the area. Determine the following:

- Exposure to cause
- Possible smoke exposure
- Type of burning agent
- Previous treatment
- Use of alcohol or drugs
- Concurrent trauma

Most Common Symptoms

- Pain
- Redness of skin
- Blisters

Associated Symptoms

- Shortness of breath from smoke inhalation
- Palpitations from electrical burn
- Nausea and vomiting
- Chills
- Headache

Past Medical History

Ask about previous skin damage or burns.

Medication History

Determine whether client is taking any medications regularly.

Family History

Family history is not applicable.

Dietary History

Ask about time last meal was eaten in case client is transferred to emergency services or burn center and requires surgical debridement. Aspiration with potential pulmonary involvement from smoke inhalation may be needed.

ASSESSMENT: OBJECTIVE/PHYSICAL EXAMINATION

Physical Examination

A problem-oriented physical examination should be conducted, with particular attention to vital signs, weight, and general appearance.

- Determine extent of burn with respect to body surface area (BSA); use "rule of nines."
  - Each upper extremity, 9%
  - Each lower extremity, 18% for adults and 14% for children
  - Anterior trunk, 18% for adult, 36% for children and infants
  - Posterior trunk, 18% for adult, 36% for children and infants
  - Head and neck, 10% for adults, 14% for children, 18% for infants
  - For patchy areas, use palm (1%) to measure extent of burns
- Perform ear, nose, throat, and chest evaluation to rule out possible smoke inhalation.
- Do cardiovascular check for electrical burns.
- Check for circulation and neurologic status distal to burn.

Diagnostic Procedures

Procedures used are determined by the extent of the burn. Extensive laboratory tests may be necessary for serious burns. Perform an electrocardiogram with an electrical burn. Do a chest radiograph, and check arterial blood gases and carboxyhemoglobin level with possible smoke inhalation.

DIAGNOSIS

Differential diagnosis includes scalded skin syndrome and abuse.

THERAPEUTIC PLAN
Nonpharmacologic Treatment
- Remove all rings to avoid tourniquet effect.
- Flush chemical burn copiously with water.
- Do *not* apply ice to site.
- For initial care of first- and second-degree burns, gently cleanse with a mild detergent (such as Ivory) and rinse with warm water, then debride any broken blisters or dead skin. Blisters that are intact can be left alone. The burned areas should be covered with a thin layer of silver sulfadiazine cream and a fluffy dressing that absorbs drainage.

Pharmacologic Treatment
- Administer tetanus prophylaxis.
- Prophylactic antibiotics are not usually needed unless the client has a history of valvular heart disease.
- For pain relief give aspirin or ibuprofen every 4 hours.

Client Education
- To care for a burn at home, cleanse off old cream bid, dry well, and reapply cream and then dressing. Keep dressings clean and dry.
- Use sunscreens to avoid future burns.
- Identify risk of skin changes in future; monitor skin of burned area carefully.
- Decrease temperature of hot water heater to less than 120° F.
- Store household chemicals in a safe place, away from children.
- Do not smoke in bed.

Referral
All clients with second-degree burns over more than 10% BSA or with any third-degree burn should be hospitalized. Clients with any of the following burns also should be hospitalized:
- Any second-degree burns of hands, feet, or perineum
- Electrical burns or lightning strike
- Inhalation burns
- Chemical burns
- Circumferential burns

Prevention
- Practice fire safety drill at home.
- Ensure ladders are available inside for homes with more than one story.
- Have a working smoke detector.

EVALUATION/FOLLOW-UP
- First-degree burns: There should be complete resolution in 3 to 6 days without scarring.
- Second-degree burns: Epithelialization should occur in 10 to 14 days; deep second-degree burns may require skin grafts.
- Third-degree: Skin grafting is required.
- Follow-up initially in 48 hours and closely thereafter to make sure that healing is taking place.
- Consider child or elder abuse if burns are seen in a "dripping" pattern or there are cigarette or iron burns.

COMPLICATIONS
- Infection
- Scarring

REFERENCES
Brigham, P. A., & McLoughlin, E. (1996). Burn incidence and medical care in the United States: Estimates, trends, and data sources. *Journal of Burn Care Rehab, 17*(2), 95.

Dershewitz, R. A. (1993). *Ambulatory pediatric care* (2nd ed.). Philadelphia: J.B. Lippincott.

Fultz, J. (2001). Acute burn injury. In P. Kidd, K. Wagner (Eds.) *High acuity nursing* (pp. 805-829). Upper Saddle River, NJ: Prentice Hall.

Fultz, J., & Messer, M. (2000). Burns. In P. Kidd, P. Sturt, & J. Fultz (Eds.), *Mosby's emergency nursing reference* (pp. 180-214). St. Louis: Mosby.

Griffith, H., & Dambro, M. (1997). *The 5-minute clinical consult.* Philadelphia: Lea & Febiger.

Review Questions

1. A client is seen with a tender 10 × 2 × 2-cm region on the left lower arm that is red with blisters. The client sustained this injury from boiling water when a pot spilled. The NP diagnoses this as which of the following?
- **a.** Superficial burn
- **b.** Partial-thickness burn
- **c.** Full-thickness burn
- **d.** First-degree burn

2. When providing anticipatory guidance regarding burns, the NP should do which of the following?
- **a.** Discuss the temperature setting of water heaters with the family of an infant.
- **b.** Plan a fire escape route for the family.
- **c.** Demonstrate how to use a fire extinguisher.
- **d.** Discuss stop, drop, and roll.

3. All the following should be assessed when caring for a client with burns *except* which of the following?
- **a.** Treatment at home
- **b.** What caused the burn
- **c.** Family history
- **d.** Where the burn occurred

4. Which of the following systems should be examined in a client who was burned superficially when putting out a kitchen fire?
- **a.** HEENT
- **b.** Chest
- **c.** Abdomen
- **d.** Extremities

5. Education for a client treated for a partial-thickness burn should include which of the following?

    a. The future use of sunscreen on the area

    b. The need to return for tetanus immunization within 1 week

    c. Application of ice to decrease pain

    d. Explaining the proper way to debride blisters

6. A person is treated for a partial-thickness, second-degree burn. This client should be evaluated in 10 to 14 days for which of the following?

    a. Need for skin grafting

    b. Pain control

    c. Swelling

    d. Allergy to the silver sulfadiazine cream

7. A mother brings her daughter in with a scald burn to the feet and buttocks. There are fluid-filled blisters and erythematous areas to the region. A possible diagnosis for this child is which of the following?

    a. Full-thickness burn

    b. Neglect

    c. Child abuse

    d. Deep partial-thickness burn

8. Which of the following actions supports primary prevention of burns?

    a. Use of a fire extinguisher

    b. No smoking in bed

    c. Installation of a smoke detector

    d. Creating a planned escape route

Answers and Rationales

1. *Answer:* **b** (analysis/diagnosis)

    Rationale: A partial-thickness (second-degree) burn involves varying levels of epidermis and vesicles. Full-thickness burns destroy subdermal layers. A first-degree burn is one type of partial thickness burn, but there are no blisters (Fultz & Messer, 2000).

2. *Answer:* **a** (implementation/plan)

    Rationale: Although performance of all these actions would be nice, the NP does not have the time to perform them all in a

visit. The demonstration and discussion of how to extinguish a fire or how to perform in a fire should be left to fire professionals.

3. *Answer:* **c** (assessment)

    Rationale: Treatment at home, if incorrect, may have prolonged the burning process. Different agents produce different burning patterns, and severity may not be as readily apparent immediately after the event. A burn received from a fire in an enclosed area may also involve smoke inhalation. Family history is not relevant (Fultz & Messer, 2000).

4. *Answer:* **b** (assessment)

    Rationale: There is not enough information to determine where on the body the client was burned. However, a kitchen often is an enclosed area, and smoke inhalation may have occurred (Fultz & Messer, 2000).

5. *Answer:* **a** (implementation/plan)

    Rationale: A burned area is more susceptible to injury from thermal energy in the future. Tetanus prophylaxis must be administered within 72 hours. Ice is not used because vasoconstriction may further injure the area. Blisters should remain intact until they break on their own (Fultz & Messer, 2000).

6. *Answer:* **a** (evaluation)

    Rationale: Skin grafting may be necessary for second-degree burns. It takes 10 to 14 days for epithelialization to occur and an evaluation regarding grafting to be made. Pain and swelling are worse during the first 48 hours after the burn. Evidence of allergy to the cream occurs quickly after the first application (Fultz & Messer, 2000).

7. *Answer:* **c** (analysis/diagnosis)

    Rationale: This burn has a dipping pattern that is not created by a fall in a bathtub or a spill. A full-thickness burn involves destruction of all skin elements. A deep partial-thickness burn is characterized by pale, waxy, white skin.

8. *Answer:* **b** (implementation/plan)

    Rationale: The other actions will help if a fire occurs. Only not smoking in bed helps to prevent a fire from occurring.

CARPAL TUNNEL SYNDROME *Denise Robinson*

OVERVIEW
Definition

Carpal tunnel syndrome (CTS) is a neuropathy caused by compression of the median nerve at the wrist. Classic symptoms include tingling, numbness, burning, or pain in at least two of the first, second, or third fingers. CTS is associated with occupations or hobbies that involve frequent repetitive motion of the wrist. It is the most common entrapment neuropathy.

Incidence

- CTS is a common wrist–hand disorder.
- CTS occurs 3 to 5 times more in women than in men, peaking at age 45 to 54 years.
- The highest frequency is in the age group of 30 to 60 years old, with an age-adjusted incidence of 49 in 100,000 for men and 149 in 100,000 in women.
- Hormones and fluid retention may play a role in the higher incidence in women.

- Its incidence is increasing in industry with repetitive forceful flexion/extension, vibration, or awkward positioning of the wrist without sufficient rest.
- Pregnancy: There is an increased incidence of CTS in pregnancy, typically in the third trimester. Most cases resolve after childbirth.
- Childhood: CTS is not typically found in children.
- Statistics: The National Institute for Occupational Safety and Health (1989) estimates there are 20 million workers at risk for CTS; 23,000 new cases are reported every year; and 100,000 CTS release surgeries are performed annually. Treatment is expensive—surgery costs from $25,000 to $30,000.

Pathophysiology

The median nerve is compressed easily as it runs through the carpal tunnel of the wrist. The tunnel is made of carpal bones on the dorsal side and the transverse carpal ligament (flexor retinaculum) on the ventral (volar) side. The median nerve lies in this 2- to 3-cm tunnel along with the nine flexor tendons of the fingers. Any swelling, trauma, or systemic metabolic process can affect the tunnel and cause compression on the median nerve with accompanying symptoms. Frequent wrist flexion/extension causes increased friction of tendons against the carpal bones or ligaments with inflammation and swelling. The median nerve supplies sensory fibers to the thumb, second and third fingers, and radial side of the fourth finger. Pressure on the nerve produces symptoms of tingling, numbness, and pain. CTS resulting from repetitive factors can take weeks to years to develop with intermittent symptoms.

Factors Increasing Susceptibility. Causes of CTS are complex and multicausal; not everyone with exposure develops CTS. The following are the three categories of causes:

- Occupation/hobbies: Those most likely to develop carpal tunnel syndrome are computer keyboard typists, checkout clerks, meat cutters, seamstresses, hairdressers, those who use vibrating tools, musicians, mail handlers/sorters, domestics, cooks, bowlers, knitters, and gardeners.
- Trauma: Fractures, dislocations, a blow to the wrist, and structural defects are common causes. Anything that causes a decrease in the size of the carpal tunnel may produce symptoms.
- Metabolic/pregnancy: An increased incidence of CTS is associated with diabetes, rheumatoid arthritis, gout, hypothyroidism, obesity, very rapid weight loss, shorter height, recent menopause, birth control pill use, degenerative joint disease, and congenital defects of the wrist. CTS frequently is seen in pregnancy.

ASSESSMENT: SUBJECTIVE/HISTORY
History of Present Illness

- Do symptoms wake the client at night?
- What aggravates the symptoms?
- What impact do symptoms have on life activities?
- Are there problems with sensation, weakness, or fine motor tasks?
- Is there discomfort while driving a car?
- Are the symptoms intermittent or continuous?
- Are symptoms getting worse?

Symptoms

- Numbness, tingling, and pain to thumb and second, third, and fourth fingers of affected hand
- Most often wakes the person at night
- Onset insidious
- Sometimes intermittent for months

Associated Symptoms

- Wrist, forearm, and shoulder pain
- Chronic/late stages: thenar (muscle pad of thumb) wasting, weakness of hand with decreased grip strength, and decreased sensitivity of fingers

Past Medical History
Occupational/Hobbies

- What is the past job/work history and extensive current job description?
- Does the client perform repetitive forceful work, undergo vibration, or use small tools or a keyboard?
- What is the length of rest periods and breaks?
- What are the typical postures and motions?
- Does discomfort decrease when away from work or on vacations?
- What are the client's hobbies? How often does the client participate in hobbies?
- What is the type of discomfort?
- Does the client have any coworkers with similar symptoms?

Trauma and Metabolic/Pregnancy

- Diabetes (most commonly associated risk factor)
- Thyroid disease
- Any similar past problems during prior pregnancies
- Arthritis
- Use of oral contraceptive pills (OCPs)
- Medications/hormones
- Cancer
- Trauma

Medications

- Determine current medications and their impact on fluid retention.

C

- Determine which medication has been tried, whether there has been a trial of nonsteroidal antiinflammatory drugs (NSAIDs), and the results.

Family History

There is some indication of familial association with familial thickening of transverse carpal ligament.

ASSESSMENT: OBJECTIVE/PHYSICAL EXAMINATION

Physical Examination

- Always do a comparative evaluation.
- *Skin:* Examine dry skin of affected area.
- *Musculoskeletal:* Palpate affected area, grip strength, and active and passive range of motion (ROM). Look for thenar wasting and changes to skin.
- Palpate carpal bones and ligament to localize pain.
- Check pulses.
- *Cardiovascular:* Check pulses.
- *Neurologic:* Perform two-point discrimination, 6-mm distance along fingertips. Normal is able to discriminate at 6-mm or less (questionable reliability and is a late symptom).
- *Sensation:* Sensory signs within the median nerve are first evident and most pronounced in the fingertips.
- Perform the following specific maneuvers:
  - *Tinel's sign:* Tap at the volar surface of wrist. A positive result is reproduced symptoms or tingling into the median nerve distribution (50% accuracy) (Figure 3-1).
  - *Phalen's maneuver:* This maneuver has the greatest sensitivity. Flex wrists maximally and hold 60 seconds. A positive result is reproduced symptoms (Figure 3-2).
  - *Carpal compression:* Compress the median nerve with thumbs for 30 seconds. A positive result is reproduced symptoms. Preliminary results show more sensitivity and specificity than Tinel's or Phalen's sign.

Diagnostic Procedures

The following examinations may be considered. Diagnosis can be made based on history and physical examination with further studies used as confirmation.

- Quantitative grip and pinch studies: loss of strength; considered first-line test
- *Laboratory work:* Indicated by history of or suspected metabolic disorder; complete blood count (CBC); and thyroid, glucose, renal, uric acid, erythrocyte sedimentation rate, and rheumatoid factor evaluations
- *Nerve conduction tests:* Electromyogram/nerve conduction studies to show abnormality in time/velocity of nerve conduction and aids to verify clinical

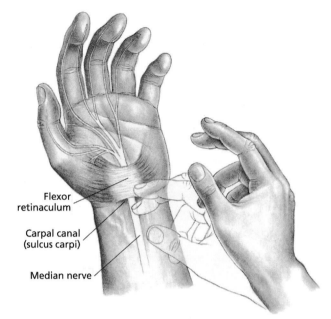

FIGURE **3-1**   Elicitation of Tinel's sign. (From Seidel, H. M., Ball, J. W., Dains, J. E., & Benedict, G. W. (1999). *Mosby's guide to physical examination* (4th ed.). St. Louis: Mosby).

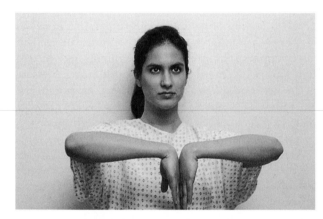

FIGURE **3-2**   Phalen's test for carpal tunnel syndrome. (From Thompson, J. M. & Wilson, S. F. [1996]. *Health assessment for nursing practice*. St. Louis: Mosby).

diagnosis; used as standard to confirm diagnosis; considered first-line test
- *Radiographic:* Used to assess trauma, fracture, tumor, structural defect; perform magnetic resonance imaging (MRI) and computed tomography (CT) for detailed studies

DIAGNOSIS

The differential diagnosis includes the following:

- Cervical radiculopathy (pressure on the nerve root as it exits the cervical spine)
- Thoracic outlet syndrome (pressure of vascular or neurogenic compression at neck/shoulder)
- de Quervain's disease (tenosynovitis of the thumb)

- Primal median nerve compression (median nerve compression higher in the arm)
- Guyon's canal (ulnar nerve compression)

THERAPEUTIC PLAN
Nonpharmacologic Treatment

Conservative treatment is 50% to 75% effective if started early, in the absence of thenar wasting, severe pain, or weakness.

- Limit activities/work that stress wrist. Client may need specific work restrictions.
- Apply cock-up splint to affected wrist with wrist in slight extension. Have client wear it at night to prevent hyperflexion in sleep. It also can be used during the day, if activity is restricted. Recent research results indicate that wearing a splint all the time improves symptoms and functional status in those clients with CTS.
- Apply cold to wrist to decrease inflammation.
- Client may consider physical therapy in conjunction with treatments listed previously, bioconductive therapy, and interference currents.
- Treat concurrent conditions (e.g., diabetes mellitus, thyroid disorders).
- If client is pregnant, she should avoid repetitive activities. Splinting is most effective, and cold should be applied to the wrist. Educate that CTS usually abates after delivery.

Pharmacologic Treatment

- Take NSAIDs with food daily for 4 to 8 weeks (e.g., ibuprofen 600 mg tid for 6 to 8 weeks). There have been conflicting reports of efficacy, although it may help in nonspecific tenosynovitis.
- Oral corticosteroids provide short-term relief of symptoms versus placebo, diuretics, and NSAIDs (Marshall, 2001).

Invasive Treatment

- Refer to an orthopedic hand specialist for invasive treatments after noninvasive measures fail.
- Steroid injection into the carpal tunnel may provide temporary relief, but there is an associated risk of infection, damage to nerve, and scarring.
- Surgical intervention is required to treat continued pain, thenar wasting, and progressive weakness.
  - Surgery is highly successful, with 90% to 95% improvement of symptoms (if not chronic disease).
  - The transverse carpal ligament is incised; this opens the tunnel and releases the pressure.
  - There are two procedures: an open procedure with ability to visualize and explore the tunnel, and an endoscopic procedure, which has less visualization but faster recovery.

- Postoperative care consists of splinting for 1 week or more, continued job restriction, and removal of sutures in 10 to 14 days.

Client Education/Prevention

- Prevention is the key. Modification of environment for proper joint alignment at the worksite is essential. Advise the client to seek ergonomic assessment of work tasks and tools. This strategy is important, especially in high-risk jobs. Conditioning exercises for hands and wrists with mild stretching and strengthening may help prevent CTS in nonsymptomatic clients.
- CTS takes a long time to heal following the treatment regimen. Healing may take months. If activities are not modified, symptoms will return.
- Wear a splint at night. Recent research results indicate that wearing a splint all the time improves symptoms and functional status in those clients with CTS."
- Wear the splint if there is no interference with activities during workday.
- Cases of CTS during pregnancy usually resolve without treatment. If symptoms continue after delivery and the client is not nursing, consider initiation of NSAIDs and referral.

Referral

If no improvement occurs after 1 to 2 months of conservative treatment, refer to orthopedic hand specialist for surgical evaluation.

EVALUATION/FOLLOW-UP

- Schedule initial follow-up in 2 to 4 weeks for noninvasive treatment. Assess for decrease in symptoms, grip and pinch strength, and thenar wasting (deterioration sign).
- Expect a decrease in symptoms 2 weeks after complaint, noninvasive treatment, and avoidance of cause. If CTS is work related, specific restrictions of job may be required (e.g., typing no more than 20 minutes every 2 hours). Work closely with an occupational health nurse at worksite if needed.
- If caught early, symptoms usually resolve following surgical intervention. If the client returns to the same activity postoperatively without modification and correct joint positioning, symptoms may recur.

COMPLICATIONS

Possible complications include pain, decreased ability to work, thenar wasting, decreased ROM of involved fingers, and loss of sensation.

REFERENCES

Dammer, S. J., Veering, M. M., Vermeulen, M. (1999). Injection with methylprednisolone proximal to the carpal tunnel:

randomised double blind trial. *British Medical Journal, 319,* 884-886.

Fox, H. (2000). Carpal tunnel syndrome. In D. Robinson, P. Kidd, K. Rogers (Eds.), *Primary care across the lifespan* (pp. 167-172). St. Louis: Mosby.

Lax, M., Grant, W., Manetti, F., & Klein, R. (1998, September). Recognizing occupational disease—taking an effective occupational history. *American Family Physician.* Retrieved May 24, 2002 from http://www.aafp.org/afp/980915ap/lax.html.

Marshall, S. (2001). Carpal tunnel syndrome. In S. Barton (Ed.), *Clinical Evidence, 5,* 717-728.

Miller, B. K. (1993). Carpal tunnel syndrome: A frequently misdiagnosed common hand problem. *Nurse Practitioner, 18*(12), 52-56.

National Institute of Occupational Safety and Health (1989, March). *Carpal tunnel syndrome selected references* (DHHS Publication No. 1992-648-179/ 60023). Cincinnati: U.S. Department of Health and Human Services.

Walker, W. C., Metzler, M., Cifu, D. X., & Swartz, Z. (2000). Neutral wrist splinting in carpal tunnel syndrome: a comparison of night-only versus full-time wear instructions. *Archives of Physical Medicine Rehabilitation, 81,* 424-429.

Review Questions

1. Which is *not* a common risk factor for CTS?
   a. Repetitive, forceful flexion, and/or extension wrist
   b. Metabolic disease such as diabetes and thyroid disorders
   c. Trauma to wrist
   d. Parkinsonism

2. Which best describes Phalen's maneuver?
   a. Perform ROM test for wrist.
   b. Tap on median nerve.
   c. Flex wrist maximally for 60 seconds and evaluate for symptoms.
   d. Compress median nerve with thumbs.

3. Which is not a diagnostic test used to assess for CTS?
   a. Grip and pinch test
   b. Phalen's maneuver, Tinel's sign
   c. Two-point discrimination
   d. Abduction of the shoulder

4. Preventive teaching is effective if clients recall all the following except:
   a. Keep joints in neutral positions at work.
   b. Increased speed and force of movements helps decrease symptoms.
   c. Rest breaks for recovery time are helpful to prevent CTS.
   d. Preventive mild conditioning exercises may be helpful for asymptomatic people in high-risk jobs.

5. Bridgett, an occupational health nurse practitioner, has responsibility for worksite management of CTS at the diamond processing plant where she works. Which of the following is the first strategy she must use in implementing this program?
   a. Splints for high-risk workers
   b. Easy access to ice machines for ice therapy
   c. Preventive teaching
   d. Prophylactic NSAIDs for workers at risk

6. Which of these occupations/hobbies are at least risk for CTS?
   a. Checkout clerks, seamstresses, typists
   b. Swimmers, opera singers, salesman
   c. Bowlers, knitters, musicians
   d. Meat cutters, jackhammer users, hairdressers

7. Which of the following results is not consistent with the physical findings of CTS?
   a. Numbness and tingling in the fourth and fifth fingers of the involved hand
   b. Numbness and tingling in the first, second, and third fingers of the involved hand
   c. Pain and discomfort in the forearm of the involved hand/wrist
   d. Thenar wasting

8. The nurse practitioner (NP) has finished teaching Stacy, who has CTS. She has been prescribed a neutral wrist splint. Which of the following statements indicates a need for further instruction?
   a. "I should wear my splint all night long."
   b. "I only need to wear my splint when I have pain."
   c. "Wearing the splint both day and night will be the most helpful for my symptoms."
   d. "I should wear the splint only when I am working."

Answers and Rationales

1. *Answer:* **d** (assessment)
   Rationale: Parkinsonism is not a risk factor for CTS. Prior trauma, metabolic disorders, and forceful repetitive motions are risk factors (Fox, 2000).

2. *Answer:* **c** (assessment)
   Rationale: The Phalen's maneuver is to maximally flex wrists for 60 seconds (Fox, 2000).

3. *Answer:* **d** (analysis/diagnosis)
   Rationale: Phalen's maneuver, Tinel's sign, grip and pinch test, and two-point discrimination are diagnostic maneuvers for CTS. Abduction of the shoulder is not a typical diagnostic maneuver for CTS (Fox, 2000).

4. *Answer:* **b** (evaluation)
   Rationale: Neutral positions, conditioning, and rest/recovery time for joints may help prevent CTS. Forceful repetitive movements increase the risk for CTS (Fox, 2000).

5. *Answer:* **c** (implementation/plan)
   Rationale: Prevention of CTS is the key, especially in large at-risk populations. Prevention is accomplished through workplace-wide programs and teaching, which include neutral joint positioning, rotation of jobs, rest periods, and knowledge of high-risk movements (Lax, 1998, & Fox, 2000).

6. Answer: b (assessment)
Rationale: Occupations/hobbies with repetitive forceful motions are risks for CTS. It is not a known problem in swimmers (National Institute of Occupational Safety and Health, 1989).

7. Answer: a (assessment)
Rationale: The median nerves provides sensory fibers to the thumb, second, third, and radial side of the fourth finger. It

does not provide sensation for the ulnar side of the fourth finger or the fifth finger (Fox, 2000).

8. Answer: b (evaluation)
Rationale: The wrist splint is the most effective if worn at all times, both night and day (Walker, 2000). It should not be worn only when there is pain. The median nerve can be compressed with few symptoms.

CATARACTS   *Pamela Kidd*

OVERVIEW
Definition

A cataract is an opacification of the crystalline lens of the eye. Cataracts usually lead to functional impairment caused by visual disturbances.

Incidence

- Cataracts are the leading cause of preventable blindness in adults in the United States.
- Incidence increases with age, with an incidence of approximately 50% in persons older than 75 years.
- Senile cataracts are typically bilateral, but progression may vary between eyes.
- Cataracts rarely occur in the pediatric population; cataracts that do occur in this population are a result of congenital factors.
- Congenital cataracts: In infants cataracts may occur as a result of inheritance of an autosomal dominant gene for cataracts. Many infants with Down syndrome may have congenital cataracts. Infants also may acquire cataracts as a consequence of prematurity. Intrauterine factors, such as maternal malnutrition, infection (cytomegalovirus or rubella), metabolic disease (diabetes), or medication ingestion (steroids), may lead to congenital cataract development.
- Traumatic cataracts: Factors such as eye injury, recurrent exposure to ultraviolet rays, foreign bodies (FBs), or scratches to the crystalline lens may hasten or cause cataracts.
- Secondary cataracts: A variety of eye disorders, including retinal dystrophy or detachment, atrophy of the iris, glaucoma, neoplasia, and ischemia, may lead to cataract formation. Medications, including steroids and radiation, also may lead to cataracts.
- Metabolic cataracts: Diseases leading to cataracts include diabetes mellitus, Wilson's disease, and hypoparathyroidism.

Pathophysiology

The lens is posterior to the iris and is suspended from the ciliary body. It is normally a transparent structure with an elastic capsule. The lens is avascular and acellular and lacks innervation. Transparency of the lens depends on active

metabolism of the epithelium. If the epithelium becomes traumatized, this may result in opacity of the lens. Density of the lens fibers increases with age, and chemical changes in protein of the lens occur. Both of these factors contribute to cataract formation. Cataracts may be either nuclear (central) or cortical (peripheral sunflower shape). Nuclear cataracts are most common, especially in older adults.

Factors Increasing Susceptibility
- Eye trauma increases risk.
- Eye disease increases risk.
- Diabetes increases risk.
- Aging increases risk.
- Cigarette smoking increases risk.
- Recreational or occupational exposure to ultraviolet B rays may predispose persons toward cataract development. Persons at risk include those who are frequently outdoors in the sun or in areas of high reflection, such as snow, beaches, or water.

Protective Factors. Routine eye examination to detect cataract formation early before a visual disability exists is considered protective.

ASSESSMENT: SUBJECTIVE/HISTORY
Symptoms

The most common symptom of cataract development is the gradual worsening of vision. Some clients report a constant fog over their eyes and rings or halos around lights and objects. Many clients note glare, especially affecting vision in bright-light situations. In clients with cataracts, vision appears more blue and yellow and distance vision becomes impaired. The location of the cataract determines the extent of visual loss. Persons with central opacities report improved vision in low light as a result of pupillary dilation, leading to a larger portion of the lens being available for viewing. Pain typically does not occur with this disorder. Part of the subjective evaluation should include an assessment of the degree of lifestyle impairment as a result of this condition and social isolation because of visual difficulties.

Past Medical History

Assess for history of long-term steroid use, as in clients receiving immunosuppressive therapy for transplants, or frequent steroid use, as in conditions with chronic inflammation. There may be a history of a former eye injury or recurrent eye trauma. Systemic disease, particularly diabetes, may predispose the client toward cataract development. A history of Wilson's disease or hypothyroidism also may lead to cataracts.

Medication History

Ask about use of steroids or radiation therapy.

Family History

With congenital cataracts, ask about family history of cataracts.

Dietary History

Not relevant.

ASSESSMENT: OBJECTIVE/PHYSICAL EXAMINATION
Physical Examination

Nuclear Cataract
- Absence of red reflex in children
- Gray-white opacity of the lens on direct lighted visual examination
- Black against the red reflex on ophthalmoscopic examination (use positive diopters to help visualize lens)

Peripheral Cortical Cataract
- Spokelike shadows that point inward
- As with nuclear cataract—gray-white on lighted examination and black against red per ophthalmoscope
  In both types of cataracts, no redness of the eye is present.

Diagnostic Procedures
- Visual acuity with Snellen chart
- Slit-lamp examination (most helpful to assist with diagnosis)

DIAGNOSIS

Differential diagnosis may include the following:
- Macular degeneration: This disease may result in loss of central vision in older adults. Onset is gradual, with distorted vision sometimes reported. Clients report no improvement of vision despite use of corrective lens. Macular degeneration is accompanied by characteristic physical findings, including neovascularization of the eye, exudates, drusen, and holes in the macula. These findings are visible on funduscopic examination of the macula.
- Retinal detachment: This results in a sudden impairment of vision in one eye, with a description of symptoms being "a curtain dropping over the eye" and loss of a portion of the visual fields. These findings often are preceded by symptoms such as flashing lights and "floaters." Retinal detachment may result from a blow to the head or eye trauma. The detached retina can be seen by ophthalmoscopy.
- Glaucoma (chronic wide-angle): Glaucoma is caused by increased intraocular pressure. It results in loss of peripheral vision, eventually leading to "tunnel vision." Measurement of intraocular pressure may lead to a diagnosis of glaucoma.
- Presbyopia, myopia: Worsening changes in the shape of the eye may result in visual distortions. This generally affects bilateral vision; the visual fields are not affected and may be improved by corrective lens adjustment.

THERAPEUTIC PLAN
Nonpharmacologic Treatment

The standard means of adaptation for the visually impaired should be pursued. Magnification, modification of spectacles, large print, and tactile cues may allow clients to delay or forgo surgery altogether.

Surgical Procedures

Surgery usually is done on an outpatient basis. The most common surgical procedure is extracapsular extraction of the opaque lens. Intracapsular extraction removes the lens through a small incision. In phacoemulsification (ultrasonic), the lens is broken up by vibration and removed extracapsularly, generally avoiding the need for sutures. Surgery also usually involves reimplantation of the intraocular lens. Aphakic glasses and contact lenses have been used in the past to restore vision but are rarely used today.

Preoperative Evaluation. Evaluation should address stabilization of chronic disease, including hypertension and diabetes; availability of a caregiver after the operation; and an understanding of client expectations of surgery. Anticoagulants are not generally stopped because their benefit in preventing possible surgical complications outweighs the risks of bleeding during this minimally invasive surgery.

Postoperative Complications. Primary care providers should be aware of signs and symptoms of postoperative complications, including altered lens adjustment, red eye or discharge indicating inflammation or infection, and delayed opacification of the posterior capsule (sometimes referred to as "after-cataracts"). Retinal detachment, macular edema, and glaucoma also may occur; screening for these conditions is therefore part of postoperative evaluation.

If surgery is delayed or avoided, continued assessment of the client's functional capacity as related to visual impairment should be assessed. Clients should be advised to wear sunglasses to protect against further cataract development from ultraviolet B radiation.

Pharmacologic Treatment

Mydriatics (e.g., atropine) occasionally are used to improve vision.

Client Education

The decision to pursue surgery is a highly individual decision because surgery is not without risk. However, if surgery is indicated, lens extraction improves visual acuity in 95% of cases.

- Discussion of the probability of surgical correction as a means of improving vision includes ruling out other possible causes for visual impairment. Evaluation of the effects of visual impairment on activities of daily living (ADLs) should contribute to the decision of whether to pursue surgical correction.
- The primary care provider should be aware of restrictions after cataract surgery, including the following:
  - An eye shield should be worn at night and glasses should be worn during the day to protect the eye.
  - Client should avoid bending, stooping, or heavy lifting for 3 to 4 weeks after surgery.
  - Client should not shower or wash hair for 2 weeks after the surgery.
  - Strenuous or excessive physical activity should be avoided for 4 weeks after surgery.
  - Client should not fly before full healing; this may increase intraocular pressure.

Referral

Ophthalmologic evaluation is indicated to help the client determine options for therapy. Visual acuity change can help determine when referral is necessary.

Prevention

Not smoking may help delay or lessen cataract formation.

EVALUATION/FOLLOW-UP

- If surgery is undertaken, the client is followed up primarily by ophthalmology.
- Postoperative cataract formation can recur, necessitating laser surgery.

COMPLICATIONS

Blindness may occur.

REFERENCES

Barker, R. (1995). *Principles of ambulatory medicine.* Baltimore: Williams & Wilkins.

Javitt, J. C. (1995). Cataract surgery in one eye or both. *Ophthalmology, 102,* 1583.

King, P. (2001). Cataracts. In D. Robinson, P. Kidd, & K. Rogers. (Eds.), *Primary care across the lifespan.* St. Louis: Mosby

Riordan-Eva, P. (2001). Eye. In L. Tierney, S. McPhee, & M. Papadakis. (Eds.), *Current medical diagnosis and treatment.* New York: McGraw Hill.

Schein, O. D. (1995). Predictors of outcome in patient who underwent cataract surgery. *Ophthalmology, 102,* 817.

Review Questions

1. You are working in a senior citizen center screening for sensory impairments affecting ADLs. Which of the following history information could indicate increased risk for visual impairment?

    a. Daily use of oxygen
    b. Alcohol or tobacco abuse
    c. Reading in low-light conditions
    d. Infrequent sun exposure

2. You are examining a 67-year-old woman for routine health screening. You are having difficulty visualizing the fundus of the eye. Which of the following is the most helpful in allowing you to conduct the funduscopic examination?

    a. Encourage the client to look directly at the light of the ophthalmoscope.
    b. Instill miotic drops to improve visualization of the optical field.
    c. Examine from an angle to the eye, shifting to positive diopters as you visualize the lens.
    d. Have the client lie flat and examine the eye from above.

3. The NP has been monitoring an 88-year-old man for cataracts for several years. In determining the appropriateness of referral for surgery, which of the following factors would be the most important to consider?

    a. Underlying pathology related to the age of the client
    b. Effect of visual defect on ADLs
    c. Whether the client still is driving
    d. Ability of the client to perform self-care

4. You are discussing surgical options with an 82-year-old woman who has acquired bilateral cataracts. Which of the following is correct information about surgery for cataracts?

    a. Bilateral cataract removal provides optimal postoperative progress.
    b. After the operation, clients typically are fitted for special aphakic lenses.
    c. Air travel plans may need to be delayed until full recovery occurs.
    d. Intraocular removal is the most commonly performed procedure for cataracts.

5. After the operation, the client experiencing cataract removal should expect which of the following?

    a. Rapid improvement (within 1 to 2 weeks) in central vision after lens implantation
    b. Need for continuing eyedrop use to prevent recurrence
    c. Some nausea and possible vomiting related to anesthesia
    d. A 1- to 2-day hospitalization for optimal recovery

C

6. The NP is seeing a 4-week-old infant who was born at 38 weeks' gestation. The infant's mother consults the NP about normal growth and development. She says she does not know what to expect in growth and development of a normal infant because her other child was several weeks premature and developed slowly. Which of the following points in a history given by the mother would lead the NP to be concerned about possible visual problems?

    a. History of cataract development in the preterm sibling
    b. Family history of visual astigmatism
    c. Infant's failure to track mother when she walks across the room
    d. Maternal exposure to cytomegalovirus

7. While examining a 58-year-old client with diabetes for retinopathy, the NP notes some cloudiness of the lens. Which of the following techniques is most helpful in determining whether a cataract is present?

    a. Additional visualization with the aid of a slit lamp
    b. Fluorescein stain to determine degree of opacity
    c. Measurement of eye pressure by tonometry
    d. Determination of visual acuity on a Jaeger chart

8. The NP is caring for an 80-year-old grandmother who has cataracts. Which of the following is true in planning for the care of this client related to her cataracts?

    a. Use of cholinergic eyedrops may help delay the necessity of surgery.
    b. The cataract needs to develop fully (ripen) before surgery is an option.
    c. Care for this woman will need to be managed by an ophthalmologist.
    d. Appropriate time for surgery may be guided by visual acuity measurement.

Answers and Rationales

1. Answer: b (assessment)
Rationale: Alcohol or tobacco abuse has been correlated with increased risk of cataracts.

2. Answer: c (assessment)
Rationale: Positive diopters are helpful in looking at visual lenses whose shapes have changed in response to cataracts.

3. Answer: b (analysis/diagnosis)
Rationale: Quality of life related to degree of sensory deprivation from visual defects is an important consideration in determining whether surgery is indicated.

4. Answer: c (implementation/plan)
Rationale: Flying before full healing has taken place may result in increased intraocular pressure and may disrupt surgical healing.

5. Answer: a (evaluation)
Rationale: Little adjustment is required for the intraocular implant to improve vision.

6. Answer: d (assessment)
Rationale: Maternal infection may result in congenital cataracts. The infant is too young to be able to track the mother. Family history is not a factor.

7. Answer: a (assessment)
Rationale: The slit lamp will be of most benefit in allowing the examiner to view the extent of the opacity of the lens.

8. Answer: d (implementation/plan)
Rationale: Visual acuity measurements will help evaluate the degree of visual impairment and show when surgery is indicated.

CELLULITIS   *Pamela Kidd*

OVERVIEW
Definition

Cellulitis is an acute, diffuse, inflammatory infection of the dermis and subcutaneous tissue.

Incidence

Incidence is not known.

Pathophysiology

- Cellulitis usually is caused by group A streptococcus.
- It also can be caused by non-group A streptococci, *Staphylococcus aureus*, *Haemophilus influenzae* type B, or *Campylobacter fetus*.
- Other causes include *Pseudomonas aeruginosa*, which may be present in puncture wounds. *Pasteurella multocida* may be present with bite wounds.
- Cellulitis often is precipitated by a break in the integrity of the skin from trauma, burns, bites, and puncture wounds. It also may result from scratches, insect bites, and stings.
- Tinea pedis with fissures has been implicated as a potential portal of entry in some cases.

Factors Increasing Susceptibility

Failure to wear shoes or failure to wear proper-fitting shoes increases risk.

Protective Factors
- Insect repellent
- Intact immune system

ASSESSMENT: SUBJECTIVE/HISTORY
Symptoms

- Inquire as to the presence and duration of erythema, warmth, edema, and pain.
- Inquire about portal of entry and whether an injury or break in the skin occurred.
- Investigate associated symptoms of fever, chills, or malaise.

Past Medical History

- History of recurrent cellulitis
- Saphenous venectomy for coronary artery bypass grafting (resulting in decreased circulation)
- Diabetes
- Peripheral vascular disease (PVD)

Medication History

Noncontributory.

Family History

Noncontributory.

Dietary History

Noncontributory.

ASSESSMENT: OBJECTIVE/PHYSICAL EXAMINATION
Physical Examination

- Warm, tender, erythematous plaques present.
- Lesions not well demarcated or elevated.
- May have purulent or serous drainage or superficial blisters.
- May have break in the integrity of the skin or portal of entry.
- Regional adenopathy or lymphadenitis with red streaking along lymphatics may be present.

- Concurrent pathology of the extremities as with PVD:
  - Edema
  - Decreased hair
  - Varicose veins
  - Dermatitis
  - Discoloration
  - Cool to touch
  - Ulcers
  - Pain
  - Decreased sensation
  - Absent or diminished pulses
  - Increased capillary refill

Orbital cellulitis causes proptosis, orbital pain, and restricted eye movement as well as erythema and edema of the eyelid and conjunctiva.

Diagnostic Procedures

- Children with cellulitis, fever, and an elevated white blood count (WBC) are at greater risk for bacteremia, and blood cultures should be considered.
- Osteomyelitis is a potential complication in some cases. The diagnosis is established by isolating *S. aureus* from the blood (culture) or bone of any client with signs and symptoms of focal bone infection.
- See Table 3-13 for common diagnostic tests.

DIAGNOSIS

See Table 3-14.

THERAPEUTIC PLAN
Nonpharmacologic Treatment

Cellulitis requires administration of antibiotics. Nonpharmacologic treatment is not helpful.

Pharmacologic Treatment

The first dose of oral antibiotic can be increased to achieve rapid high blood levels (Berger, 2001).

- Antibiotic of choice is penicillin for uncomplicated cellulitus.

TABLE **3-13** Diagnostic Testing

TEST	PURPOSE	INTERPRETATION
Wound culture	Culture and sensitivity	Aids in selection of antimicrobial treatment.
Complete blood count	Evaluate systemic response	Leukocytosis with left shift is consistent with a bacterial infection.
Doppler ultrasound of affected extremity	R/O DVT	Hypoperfusion appears in DVT, hyperperfusion in cellulitis.
Blood culture	R/O bacteremia	Cellulitis in an ill-appearing client with fever and an elevated white count means client is at risk for bacteremia.
X-ray film of site	R/O osteomyelitis	May present under the skin.

R/O, Rule out.

TABLE **3-14**   Common Differential Diagnoses

DIAGNOSIS	SYMPTOMS
Erysipelas	A distinct form of superficial cellulitis that usually occurs on the cheek. It is caused by B-hemolytic streptococci. It is an edematous, spreading, well-circumscribed, hot, painful, erythematous lesion with possible vesicular or bulla formation and there is systemic involvement of fever, chills and adenitis.
Necrotizing fascilitis	Resembles cellulitis. Caused by group A beta-hemolytic streptococci. Spreads rapidly; is associated with severe pain and marked systemic toxicity. As the infection progresses, involved skin loses normal sensation secondary to destruction of nerves.
Venous stasis dermatitis	Caused by venous insufficiency of the lower extremities and presents as edema, dermatitis with pruritis, hyperpigmentation, and skin breakdown. Ulcers may develop.
Thrombophlebitis	A partial or complete occlusion of the vein by a thrombus with secondary inflammation in the wall of the vein. Can present as calf pain, swelling, or erythema, with a palpable chord.
Gout	Involves erythema, pain, and swelling over a septic joint.

- Amoxicillin oral suspension 125mg/5mL or 250mg/ 5mL OR tablets 250mg or 500 mg
  - Children 20 to 40 mg/kg/day in divided doses every 8 hours for 10 days
  - Adults 250 to 500 mg PO every 8 hours for 10 days
- Pen Vee K oral suspension 125mg/5 mL or 250 mg/5 mL OR tablets 250 mg or 500 mg
  - Children 30 to 60mg/kg/day in divided doses every 6 hours for 10 days
  - Adults 250 to 500 mg PO every 6 hours for 10 days
- For clients allergic or intolerant to penicillin consider one of the following:
  - Cephalexin 50 mg/kg/day in 2 divided doses for 10 days for children. 250 mg to 500 mg PO every 6 to 12 hours for 10 days for adults.
  - Erythromycin ethylsuccinate 30 to 50 mg/kg/day in 3 divided doses for 10 days for children. 400 mg PO every 6 hours for 10 days for adults.
  - Azithromycin 500 mg PO on first day then 250 mg PO for 4 days for adults.

Cellulitis with an Associated Puncture Wound
- Consider treatment with ciprofloxacin 500 to 750 mg PO every 12 hours for 7 to 10 days for adults with a puncture wound, especially of the foot, for coverage of *Pseudomonas aeruginosa*.
- Consider a tetanus-diphtheria (Td) booster depending on the wound and the client's immunization status.

Erysipelas of the Face in an Adult
- Caused by group A beta-hemolytic streptococci.
- Trauma or a surgical wound may precipitate erysipelas, but most cases are without a portal of entry.
- Differs from cellulitis in that lymphatic involvement in the form of streaking may be present, lesions can be elevated with more definite borders, and the color becomes dark fiery red with vesicles appearing at the advancing border.

- Pain can be moderate to severe.
- Associated systemic symptoms of nausea, vomiting, fever, chills, and malaise are common.
- Treatment is the same for streptococcal cellulitis.

Orbital versus Periorbital Cellulitis
- Periorbital cellulitis is more common than orbital cellulitis.
- Infection is limited to the eyelid and presents with edema and erythema of the lid and conjunctiva.
- Sinusitis, upper respiratory infections (URIs), and trauma are the most common predisposing factors.
- Staphylococci and streptococci are the most common pathogens in adults.
- *Haemophilus influenzae* is the most common pathogen in children.
- Aggressive treatment is indicated to prevent progression to orbital cellulitis or spreading to the brain. Physician consultation is warranted.
- Immediate consultation and hospitalization is indicated.

Cellulitis Postsaphenous Venectomy for Coronary Artery Bypass Grafting
- Fever, erythema, and swelling may present for months to years after stripping of the veins in the legs or arms for coronary bypass surgery.
- It is caused by group C, G, or B beta-hemolytic streptococci.
- Concurrent tinea pedis may permit portal of entry of bacteria.

Immediate hospitalization should be considered in any client with the following emergent conditions:

- Extensive cellulitis with systemic involvement
- Diminished pulses in a cool, swollen, infected extremity
- Presence of cutaneous necrosis, periorbital and/or orbital cellulitis because of the proximity to the brain, or immunocompromised client or client with diabetes

Client Education

- Inform the client about fever care.
- Inform the client about proper wound care.
- Instruct client to return if no improvement in 24 to 48 hours.
- Stress that hospitalization may be necessary.
- Encourage smoking cessation (if applicable) if PVD is a concurrent problem.

Referral

- Consult with a physician about any client with decreased responsiveness, extremely elevated WBC, or PVD or who is immunocompromised.
- If osteomyelitis is evident on radiograph or bone scan, refer client to an orthopedic surgeon for surgical debridement to prevent further complications.

Prevention

- Properly cleanse all wounds to help prevent cellulitis.
- Wear shoes and protective gear during activities to protect skin integrity.

EVALUATION/FOLLOW-UP

- Reevaluate the client in 24 to 48 hours if no improvement; if drainage from the wound or systemic symptoms develop; or if the client has PVD, has diabetes, has had recent surgery, or is immunocompromised.
- Recheck at end of antibiotic course with improvement to ensure resolution.

COMPLICATIONS

- Septic shock
- Amputation

Complications associated with periorbital cellulitis include sinusitis, abscess formation, sinus thrombosis, visual disturbance, limited movement, diplopia, blindness, and meningitis.

REFERENCES

Berger, T. (2001). Skin, hair, and nails. In L. Tierney, S. McPhee, & M. Papadakis (Eds.), *Current Medical Diagnosis and Treatment.* New York: McGraw Hill.

Bisno, A. (1996). Streptococcal infections of the skin and soft tissue. *New England Journal of Medicine, 334*(4), 240-245.

Rogers, K. (2000). Cellulitis. In D. Robinson, P. Kidd, & K. Rogers (Eds.), *Primary care across the lifespan.* St. Louis: Mosby.

Review Questions

1. Mrs. Jones, a 50-year-old white female, comes to your clinic with a history of warmth, redness, and tenderness of the dorsum of her left foot for 3 days. Which of the following subjective data is *least* helpful in making a diagnosis?

    a. History of trauma to the affected extremity

    b. History of chronic dependent edema related to venous stasis

    c. Recent initiation of a walking program to promote weight loss

    d. History of fever and chills at home

2. Which of the following past medical problems should influence your decision when treating cellulitis?

    a. Hypertension

    b. Coronary artery disease (CAD)

    c. Obesity

    d. Diabetes

3. Which of the following objective signs are most indicative of cellulitis?

    a. Cool, erythematous, shiny, hairless extremity with diminished pulses

    b. Scattered, erythematous rings with clearing centers

    c. Clearly demarcated, raised, erythematous area of face

    d. Area of poorly differentiated, diffuse redness that is warm and tender to touch

4. Which of the following laboratory tests is most helpful in diagnosing cellulitis?

    a. Prothrombin time and international normalization ratio

    b. CBC count with differential

    c. Radiograph of affected area

    d. Uric acid

5. Which of the following is least likely to be the causal organism in cellulitis?

    a. Staphylococcus

    b. *Escherichia coli*

    c. *P. aeriginosa*

    d. Group A streptococci

6. If your client has no drug allergies, which of the following antibiotics is most appropriate in treating a wound from a cat bite?

    a. Erythromycin

    b. Penicillin

    c. Dicloxacillin

    d. Ciprofloxacin

Answers and Rationales

1. *Answer:* **c** (analysis/diagnosis)

    Rationale: Trauma can be associated with cellulitis if a break in skin integrity has occurred. Decreased circulation to an extremity from any cause contributes to infection once a break in skin integrity occurs. Fever and chills frequently are associated with cellulitis.

2. *Answer:* **d** (implementation/plan)

    Rationale: Although obesity, hypertension, and CAD may delay healing, their risks of complications are less than with diabetes, in which both increased blood sugar and decreased circulation may be present.

3. *Answer:* **d** (assessment)

    Rationale: Because cellulitis involves the subcutaneous tissue, it is less demarcated. The infection produces vasodilation and warmth.

C

4. *Answer:* **b** (analysis/diagnosis)
   Rationale: Of the tests listed, the CBC would be most helpful because the WBC count will be elevated. A radiograph will show in advanced cellulitis the presence of osteomyelitis, but it will not help diagnosis cellulitis.

5. *Answer:* **b** (analysis/diagnosis)
   Rationale: Staphylococci or streptococci frequently are associated with skin infections. *E. coli* most often is associated with internal organs.

6. *Answer:* **d** (implementation/plan)
   Rationale: A cat bite produces a puncture wound. This is a more penetrating wound, with greater consequences if not adequately treated. It requires a stronger, broad-spectrum, less frequently used antibiotic for treatment.

CHEST PAIN/ACUTE MYOCARDIAL INFARCTION *Pamela Kidd*

OVERVIEW
Definition
Chest pain is most closely associated with cardiac or pulmonary events. Acute myocardial infarction (AMI) is death of cardiac tissue resulting from occlusion of a coronary artery.

Incidence
CAD remains one of the most common causes of chest pain and death in our society, accounting for approximately 50% of all deaths. In 35- to 65-year-olds, CAD accounts for approximately 33% of deaths.

Pathophysiology
Acute coronary syndrome accounts for three different conditions: angina (chest pain resulting from cardiac ischemia), non-Q wave myocardial infarction (MI), and Q wave MI. These conditions begin with rupture of an atheromatous plaque in a coronary or epicardial artery. The ruptured plaque activates platelets and fibrin resulting in clot formation (ischemia and injury). Spontaneous fibrinoloysis determines how well the clot is dissolved or if full occlusion occurs (infarction).

   Factors Increasing Susceptibility. The most predictive risk factors for CAD include hypertension, smoking, and hyperlipidemia. Other factors that may play a part are obesity, sedentary lifestyle, psychosocial factors (e.g., stress), and heavy alcohol consumption.

   Protective Factors
- Estrogen
- Elevated high-density lipoprotein (HDL) levels

ASSESSMENT: SUBJECTIVE/HISTORY
Symptoms
Onset, duration, intensity, aggravating and alleviating factors, location, and quality are critical components to differentiate chest pain. These can help distinguish the cause of the pain. If a client reports diaphoresis, radiation down the left arm or into the jaw, shortness of breath, midsternal pain with exercise, or shortness of breath with exercise, consider the pain to be cardiac in nature until proved otherwise. Pain with inspiration indicates a pleuritic component. Assess smoking history and stress levels.

Past Medical History
- Hypertension
- Diabetes
- Hyperlipidemia
- Cardiovascular or peripheral vascular disease
- Gout
- Angina
- Previous or recent deep venous thrombosis (DVT)
- Cancer (from hypercoagulability)
- Chronic obstructive pulmonary disease (COPD)
- Previous spontaneous pneumothorax
- Previous or recent surgery (particularly orthopedic or trauma), recent delivery (possible pulmonary embolism [PE])
- Gastroesophageal reflux disease (GERD; may be associated with chest pain)

Medication History
- Ask about use of antihypertensive or vasoactive medications and use of OCPs.
- Be sure to include all over-the-counter (OTC) medications the client may have taken in the past 2 weeks.

Family History
- Determine presence of unmodifiable factors, such as advanced age, genetic predisposition, male gender, race (particularly black and Asian), and presence of diabetes mellitus type 1.
- Ask about history of cardiovascular disease.
- Ask about history of pulmonary disease.
- Ask about history of hypercoagulability or blood dyscrasias.

Dietary History
- Ask about increased or excessive intake of fats.
- Ask about excessive alcohol intake.

ASSESSMENT: OBJECTIVE/PHYSICAL EXAMINATION

Physical Examination

- Check general appearance for obvious pallor or diaphoresis.
- Take vital signs; check hydration status and look for orthostatic changes.
- Examine neck. Listen to carotid arteries for bruits and check for diminished or absent carotid pulsations.
- Determine cardiovascular status. Listen for irregular rhythms, S_3 or S_4 (indicative of left ventricular dysfunction) murmurs, or artificial heart valves. Check extremities for possible signs of DVT.
- Check pulmonary status for adventitious diminished or absent breath sounds.

Diagnostic Procedures

Special Tests

- Perform an electrocardiogram (ECG). Nonspecific ST-segment and T-wave changes have a low risk of AMI (but higher risk of unstable angina) (Brady, Perron, & Ghaemmaghami, 2001)
- In cases of left-sided heart failure, ST-segment and T-wave changes may "normally" be present. Depend more on serum markers (see Note).
    - AMI: ST-segment elevation greater than or equal to 1 mm in two contiguous leads
    - Presence of new-onset left bundle branch block
    - Q wave longer than 0.04 seconds and longer than 25% of R-wave amplitude (AHA, 1997)
- Stress testing (graded exercise test [GXT]). Consider doing a thallium or technetium Tc-99m sestamibi (Cardiolite) GXT if the client has bundle-branch block. Consider doing a dipyridamole thallium stress test if the client is unable to walk on the treadmill.

Laboratory Tests

- Obtain CBC.
- Obtain comprehensive metabolic profile (with lipid assay).
- Cardiac troponin I (cTnI) and cardiac troponin T (cTnT) if MI must be ruled out (found almost exclusively in cardiac tissue so more specific for AMI; elevates in cardiac ischemia; autoimmune disease may also falsely elevate these enzymes).
- Myoglobin is a sensitive and early marker of myocardial damage within 1 to 2 hours of onset, but because it also is found in skeletal muscle, other conditions (e.g., trauma) may elevate the myoglobin level.
- CK and CK-MB are elevated 2 to 24 hours post ischemia.

NOTE: *Trends with increasing elevation are more diagnostic than any single value of any marker. Serum markers become very important in non–Q-wave MI where ECG changes may not be present or readily apparent.*

Radiologic Tests

- Take a chest radiograph.
- Consider ventilation perfusion (V/Q) scan if pulmonary embolus is suspected; consult with physician before performing V/Q scan.

DIAGNOSIS

Differential diagnosis includes the following:

- Angina (chest pain lasts less than 15 minutes and is relieved with rest)
- MI
- Endocarditis
- Pericarditis
- Pulmonary embolus
- Pneumonia
- Pleurisy (pain on inspiration and with cough)
- Pneumothorax
- Hemothorax if related trauma
- GERD (clients sometimes have difficulty distinguishing between cardiac and epigastric pain)
- Chest wall pain (point tenderness on examination)

THERAPEUTIC PLAN

Nonpharmacologic Treatment

The therapeutic plan depends on the selected diagnosis. Acute life-threatening or potentially life-threatening problems should be referred to a physician, or at least a consultation should be obtained.

A non–life-threatening condition may require further workup during the next several days but may not require hospitalization. For example, clients with chest pain that they are not feeling at present but have had several times recently can be worked up for CAD as outpatients. However, if there is a strong indication that the pain is cardiac in nature, the client should be sent home with nitroglycerin tablets and a careful explanation of how and when to use them (1 tablet sublingually (SL) q5 minutes up to a total of 3 tablets).

If all cardiac workup results are negative and pain persists, begin a gastrointestinal (GI) workup for GERD or gastritis (refer to GERD section).

Pharmacologic Treatment

- If cardiac origin is suspected, inhibit platelet aggregation with aspirin 81 mg daily. Enteric-coated aspirin is best in the older adult.
- For MI, prescribe nitroglycerin sublingual and aspirin 325 mg PO, initiate intravenous line if available, and administer morphine sulfate intravenously for pain. Beta blockers (metoprolol, atenolol) can be given if no congestive heart failure (CHF) is present; client may receive thrombolytic therapy at emergency care center.

C

Client Education

Instruct the patient to stop smoking (if applicable), eat a healthy diet, and exercise regularly.

Referral

- For MI, immediately refer to a cardiologist with phone consultation and arrange emergency transportation.
- For DVT/PE, refer to an internal medicine/pulmonology/vascular service.
- For GERD, refer to a gastrologist.
- For COPD, refer to a pulmonologist.

Prevention

Eating a low-fat diet and getting regular exercise may help prevent this disease.

EVALUATION/FOLLOW-UP

Schedule a return visit for 1 to 2 weeks, depending on the diagnosis. If indicated, a GXT should be scheduled as soon as possible. Have the client document symptoms and notify health care provider about any new symptoms or change in the symptoms.

COMPLICATIONS

Some sources of chest pain resolve spontaneously without treatment (e.g., chest wall pain related to cold or local minor injury). Other causes of chest pain (e.g., AMI, bleeding, or GI ulcer) can lead to death if untreated.

REFERENCES

American Heart Association. (1997). *Textbook of advanced cardiac life support.* Dallas: American Heart Association.

Brady, W., Perron, A., & Ghaemmaghami, C. (2001). Acute MI: Could the ECG and the serum markers be masking the diagnosis? *Consultant, 41*(9), 1225-1228, 1229, 1235-1237, 1241.

Kidd, P., & Switzer, M. (2001). Acute cardiac dysfunction and electrocardiographic monitoring. In P. Kidd, & K. Wagner (Eds.), *High acuity nursing* (3rd ed.). Upper Saddle River, NJ: Prentice Hall.

Larsen, L. (2001). Chest pain. In D. Robinson, P. Kidd, & K. Rogers (Eds.), *Primary care across the lifespan.* St. Louis: Mosby.

Review Questions

1. Chest pain that lasts for less than 15 minutes and is relieved with rest is considered to be which of the following?
   a. COPD
   b. PE
   c. Angina
   d. MI

2. The presence of an S_3 heart sound in the presence of chest pain may be indicative of which of the following?
   a. Pneumonia
   b. Pericarditis
   c. Pulmonary embolus
   d. MI

3. All the following symptoms are associated with chest pain and are likely to represent CAD *except* which of the following?
   a. Jaw pain
   b. Shortness of breath
   c. Diaphoresis
   d. Pain with inspiration

4. Chest pain that is reproducible with palpation of the chest is most likely which of the following?
   a. MI
   b. Chest wall pain
   c. Pneumonia
   d. Angina

5. Which of the following can be worked up on an outpatient basis?
   a. Pulmonary embolus
   b. MI
   c. Angina
   d. Pneumothorax

6. How should clients sent home with SL nitroglycerin be taught to take this medication?
   a. 1 tablet SL q5 minutes to a total of 3 tablets
   b. 1 tablet SL q2 minutes to a total of 6 tablets
   c. 1 tablet SL q10 minutes to a total of 5 tablets
   d. 1 tablet only; if no relief, call ambulance

7. The NP obtained an ECG for a client with chest pain. Which of the following would indicate an AMI?
   a. S-T segment depression
   b. T-wave changes
   c. Longation of Q wave (longer than 0.04 seconds) and greater than 25% of R-wave amplitude
   d. Presence of premature ventricular contractions

8. When examining the laboratory work of a client with chest pain, the NP notices that the cardiac troponin I marker is elevated. The NP should do which of the following?
   a. Assess for the presence of autoimmune disease.
   b. Order myoglobin level.
   c. Order CPK panel.
   d. Repeat the ECG.

Answers and Rationales

1. *Answer:* c (analysis/diagnosis)
   Rationale: Angina is myocardial ischemia relieved by rest and, by definition, lasts less than 15 minutes.

2. *Answer:* d (assessment)
   Rationale: Because the injured myocardium is not functioning normally and part of the left ventricle can become dyskinetic, the S_3 indicates left ventricular function.

3. *Answer:* d (assessment)
   Rationale: Pain with inspiration indicates a pleuritic component; this indicates a lung problem rather than cardiac problem.

4. **Answer: b** (assessment)
   Rationale: Chest wall pain is the inflammation of the joint between the rib, sternum, and cartilage located between the rib and the sternum.

5. **Answer: c** (implementation/plan)
   Rationale: Although angina may be a precursor of MI, it can be worked up on an outpatient basis unless it is unstable and the client is experiencing ischemic changes on the ECG.

6. **Answer: a** (implementation/plan)
   Rationale: If pain relief has not been achieved with this regimen, the pain may be indicative of more extensive myocardial ischemia and possible MI.

7. **Answer: c** (analysis/diagnosis)
   Rationale: AMI is diagnosed by ST-segment elevation greater than 1mm in two contiguous leads, presence of a new left bundle branch block, and/or elongation of Q wave (longer than 0.04 seconds) and greater than 25% of R-wave amplitude (AHA, 1997).

8. **Answer: a** (analysis/diagnosis)
   Rationale: Cardiac Troponin I (cTnI) will elevate in autoimmune disorders. Therefore, before assuming the client had an AMI, the NP should assess if the result is most likely due to cardiac ischemia. Myoglobin also will elevate in cardiac ischemia but will elevate in other musculoskeletal conditions. A repeat ECG may not be necessary or helpful. If the client did not have an autoimmune disease, the cTnI could indicate cardiac ischemia without needing the CPK panel.

CHILD ABUSE *Denise Robinson*

OVERVIEW
Definition

Child abuse is a nonaccidental injury as a result of commission or omission on the part of a parent, guardian, spouse, or caretaker. Harm also may result because of neglect or inattention to physical, emotional, medical, and financial needs in a dependent situation.

Types of Abuse
- Physical abuse is inflicted injuries that are often a result of hitting, beating, shaking, or burning; may be unusual for age of victim or incompatible with history.
- Sexual abuse is assault, incest, or exploitation for the sexual gratification of an adult caregiver; also forced sexual activity without the consent of the sexual partner. Child sexual abuse is defined as engaging a child in sexual activity that the child cannot comprehend, for which the child is developmentally unprepared and cannot give informed consent (because of young age), or that violates societal taboos. It may include exhibitionism, fondling, genital viewing, oral–genital contact, insertion of objects, vaginal or rectal penetration, and pornography (Leder, Knight, & Emans, 2001). Sexual assault is defined as any sexual act performed by one person on another without that person's consent. The victim may not have the capacity to give consent because of age, mental or physical impairment, or the use of drugs or alcohol (Emans, 1998).
- Nontouching offenses include verbal sexual stimulation, exhibitionism, and invasions of privacy.
- Touching offenses are fondling, masturbation, intercourse, sodomy, anal penetration, and oral–genital contact.
- Emotional and psychologic abuse is an attack on the person's sense of self and social competence; it is concurrent with other forms of abuse. Types include ignoring, rejecting, isolating, terrorizing, corrupting, assaulting verbally, and overpressuring.
- Financial abuse is the exploitation of resources through misrepresentation, coercion, or theft.
- Neglect is the failure of the responsible person to provide adequate food, clothing, shelter, or medical care.

Incidence

Numbers are known to be underreported/underrecognized in the United States. The following are some statistics:
- In 1999, 826,000 victims of maltreatment were reported in the United State (DHHS, 2001).
- Regarding adolescent sexual assault, approximately 700,000 females report being raped; 61% are younger than 18 years of age. Male victims report about 5% of reported sexual assault cases.
- Each year, approximately 1% of children experience some form of sexual abuse.
- In 70% to 90% of cases, the victim knows the perpetrator; 50% of cases involve a relative (Leder, Knight, & Emans, 2001).

Pathophysiology
- Often physical abuse is explained as an accident, but it is more likely the result of a stressful situation and a caretaker or partner with poor decision-making and/or coping skills.
- Families under chronic strain from financial and health problems are particularly at risk.
- Isolation or lack of social support may contribute.
- Strong association of history of psychopathology or substance abuse by the abuser contributes.
- Vulnerable or powerless people, such as children, tend to be victims of abuse.

ASSESSMENT: SUBJECTIVE/HISTORY

If possible, take the history from the parents and child separately. Record the date and time of visit, sources of any information, and the date and time of the alleged abuse or assault. Focus your questions on what happened and, specifically, on whether genital, rectal, or oral contact occurred. Use developmentally appropriate language. Avoid leading the client. Clues that may indicate possible abuse include the following:

- Multiple health care providers or multiple emergency department visits
- Conflicting stories about how injuries occurred
- Information unknowingly revealed in the context of other questions (e.g., NP: "What was her last medicine for this condition?" Parent: "I did not get that prescription filled. I thought she was better.")
- Caretaker affect inappropriate for situation (e.g., laughter, anger, lack of concern)
- History of sleep disturbances, appetite changes, withdrawn behavior, aggressive behavior/violent outbursts, suicide attempts, regression
- Behavioral indicators of possible sexual abuse, such as temper tantrums, aggressive behavior, poor school performance, delinquent behavior, knowledge and use of sexual terms, excessive masturbation or sex play, suspicion of adults, depression, guilt, sleep disturbances (sexual acting out is the most specific indicator of possible sexual abuse)
- In adolescents, frequent requests for pain medication, frequent visits for somatic complaints, GI disturbances, chronic pain of unclear origin, suicidal behavior, and substance abuse

Appropriate questions include the following (Leder, Knight, & Emans, 2001):

- Do you know why you are here today?
- Can you tell me what happened?
- What happened next?
- Where did this happen?
- Where was everyone else?
- Has anybody told you to keep it a secret?
- Have you been hurt lately?

If there has not been any disclosure of abuse, the following questions may be helpful. Define for the client what body parts are private—use the terms of "good touch" and "bad touch" as reference.

- What would you do if someone gave you a bad touch?
- Who could you tell?
- Have you ever had to tell anyone you had a bad touch?
- Has anyone ever given you a bad touch?

With adolescent clients, ask about menstrual and contraceptive history, as well as any history of consensual sexual activity. Do not judge based on response of child; some are teary and upset, whereas others are more controlled. Younger children may not even understand what happened. With those clients who are reluctant to talk, a trained forensic examiner may be needed.

ASSESSMENT: OBJECTIVE/PHYSICAL EXAMINATION

If the event has taken place in the last 72 hours, refer the child to an emergency department for collection of forensic evidence. If rape has occurred, consider referral to a rape crisis team.

Explain each part of the examination, including the genital examination, and offer the family an opportunity to ask questions before the examination. Drawings or models may be helpful. Letting the child set the pace of the examination (i.e., having some control) and informing them that the NP will stop at any point if asked is important. In many cases physical findings may not be present because of the high elasticity of the tissue in the genital area.

Physical Examination

A complete physical examination is warranted with particular focus on the following areas:

- Determine general responsiveness/affect, hygiene, nutritional status, appropriateness of dress, presence of unattended physical problems.
- Examine head, eyes, ears, nose, and throat (HEENT) for head trauma, patchy hair loss, pupils.
- Perform funduscopic examination; check for retinal hemorrhage, hemorrhage of sclerae, bleeding from ears or nose, and blood behind tympanic membrane.
- Examine skin for bruises in different stages of healing; burns; physical marks of an object (e.g., looped cord, belt buckle); restraint marks on extremities, neck, or mouth; and human bite marks.
- Examine abdomen for tenderness, organomegaly, and bruising.
- Examine the musculoskeletal system for tenderness or swelling of joints and signs of spiral fractures or dislocations.
- Perform a neurologic examination for mental status; in children, do a neurodevelopmental screening.
- Examine genitalia for genital, urethral, vaginal, or anal bruising or bleeding; swollen, red vulva or perineum; and presence of foreign body in genital area. Using Muram's system or Adam's system to help detail genital findings may be helpful (Adams, 2001; Muram, 1988). Abnormalities of the hymen are most likely to be found between the 3 o'clock and 9 o'clock positions.
  - Place child in frog-leg position. In a prepubertal female, assess external genitalia (be sure to be

aware of anatomy of prepubertal female child). *Do not use a speculum* for internal examination. Use an otoscope or handheld lens with a bright light source. A trusted caregiver can stand close or hold hands with the child to reassure them. Look for signs of trauma and lesions suspicious for sexually transmitted disease (STDs).

- In an adolescent female, perform the same examination described for a prepubertal female, plus a speculum examination for adolescents who have reached menarche, had vaginal penetration, and can tolerate a speculum. For a sexually active adolescent a Pederson speculum is appropriate. The absence of physical findings is common in adolescent females.

- For male clients of any age, carefully examine the penis, scrotum, and anus for signs of injury such as bruises, lacerations, abrasions, or other lesions. Most male victims of sexual assault have a normal examination because some physical contact may not leave physical findings (e.g., fondling or oral–genital contact).

Diagnostic Procedures

- Growth measures are plotted on appropriate growth charts.
  - Determine height and weight (also head circumference of clients 2 years and younger).
  - Accurate/thorough descriptions of findings (photographs helpful); significant negatives are required.
- A flattening weight curve only may indicate early signs of neglect or nonorganic failure to thrive (FTT), whereas flattening of curves in all growth parameters is indicative of a more serious condition.
- Use other procedures such as radiographs and laboratory tests as indicated by subjective and objective data.
  - Do a set prep using KOH and saline; look for WBCs, clue cells, or trichomonad, and cytologic abnormalities caused by human papillomavirus.
  - Take cultures for gonorrhea and chlamydia from vaginal swabs or urine samples. The risk of acquiring chlamydia during sexual assault is estimated between 4% to 17% (Leder, Knight, & Emans, 2001). Nonculture results are not admissible in most states.
  - Examine a sample of any penile discharge for WBCs and trichomonads. The Centers for Disease Control and Prevention (CDC) estimates the rate of syphilis infection as a result of sexual assault to be 0.5% to 3%. The risk of acquiring human immunodeficiency virus (HIV) was found to be 0.25 in 1000 in one study (Geliert, 1994).
  - STDs are more common in adolescents as a result of the physiologic changes of the genital tract that occur during puberty and the higher likelihood of vaginal penetration during the assault (Emans, 1998).

- Sperm is a definitive finding of sexual abuse or assault (Muram, 1988).

DIAGNOSIS

The differential diagnosis includes the following:
- Unintentional injury
- Normal skin variations (e.g., mongolian spots)
- Organic FTT
- Blood dyscrasias (e.g., leukemia)
- Osteogenesis imperfecta
- Cultural practices (e.g., Asian practice of cupping)

THERAPEUTIC PLAN
Nonpharmacologic Treatment

Clear and complete documentation is vitally important; the more detailed the documentation, the more you will remember about the case when it is prosecuted. If the examinations are normal, say so. If not, use diagrams to describe the type and location of abnormal or unusual genital findings or physical abuse lesions. Verbatim questions and answers provide the most information and protection.

- Report any suspected abuse to the appropriate social service agency.

NOTE: *NPs are considered mandated reporters and are required by law to report suspected cases of abuse. NPs incur some form of legal immunity (varies by state) if they make a good faith report, but they also are subject to criminal charges if they fail to report a case of suspected abuse.*

- Treat or refer identified medical conditions.
- Ensure that the victim does not return to the hostile environment in the case of life-threatening situations (rare).
- Initiate team approach including medical, social services, and law enforcement members as appropriate.
- Reassure child concerning sexual abuse/assault that it is not his or her fault and that he or she is not in trouble. Recognize the bravery it took to tell the truth about what happened. Also emphasize that abuse does not render them sterile—in the future they will be able to have children. Same-sex abuse may cause the client to question their sexual orientation; counseling may be needed to address this concern.
- Refer to mental health support; as many as 80% of adolescent rape victims experience posttraumatic stress disorder. Provide information about counseling to clients and families.

Pharmacologic Treatment

- Treat for STDs if suspected based on the examination.
- Treat prophylactically for STDs if follow-up of the client is uncertain.

- Treat for STDs if parent or client requests it.
- Treat for STDs if the client is an adolescent who has been assaulted within the past 72 hours.
- Begin the hepatitis B series vaccination if the client has not been immunized.
- Discuss with HIV experts the merit of HIV postexposure prophylaxis.
- The risk of conception following rape is 2% to 6%. Female adolescent victims should be offered emergency contraception. Perform a urine or serum human chorionic gonadotropin level test to detect an existing pregnancy.

Client Education/Prevention

- Client education is most appropriate as a preventive measure.
- Incorporate screenings into practice that identify families at risk.
- Explain behavioral expectations by developmental level.
- Discuss parenting strategies for specific behaviors.
- Address further knowledge deficits regarding child behavior and parenting as identified.
- Parents need time away from their children to cool down or lessen stress.

EVALUATION/FOLLOW-UP

- Do a same-day phone follow-up if client is returning to same environment.
- Confirm social services investigation once a report is made (within 24 hours).
- Monitor progress of case until resolution.

COMPLICATIONS

- Death or severe physical, psychologic, or mental disorders secondary to abuse
- Continuation of abuse cycle in next generation
- Negative attitudes toward child or pregnancy may contribute to later abuse

REFERENCES

Adams, J. (2001). Evolution of a classification scale: medical evaluation of suspected child sexual abuse. *Child Maltreatment* 6(1), 31.

Arvin, A. M., Behrman, R. E., Kliegman, R. M., & Nelson, W. E. (1996). *Nelson textbook of pediatrics* (15th ed.). Philadelphia: W. B. Saunders.

Emans, S. (1998). Sexual abuse. In S. Emans, M. Laufer, & D. Goldsem (Eds.), *Pediatric and adolescent gynecology* (4th ed., pp. 751-794). Philadelphia: Lippincott-Raven.

Geliert, G. (1994). Pediatric acquired immunodeficiency syndrome testing as a barrier to recognizing the role of child sexual abuse (editorial). *Archives in Pediatric Adolescent Medicine, 148*, 766.

HHS News. (2001). HHS reports new child abuse & neglect studies. DHHS, April 2, 2001. Retrieved July 13, 2002, from http://www.hhs.gov/news/press/2001pres/20010402.html

Leder, M., Knight, J., & Emans, S. (2001). Sexual abuse: management strategies and legal issues. *Contemporary Pediatrics, 18*(5), 77-92.

Leder, M., Knight, J., & Emans, S. (2001a). Sexual abuse: when to suspect it, how to assess for it. *Contemporary Pediatrics, 18*(5), 59-74.

Lahoti, S., McClain, N., Girardet, R., McNeese, M., & Cheung, K. (2001). Evaluating the child for sexual abuse. *American Family Physician.* Retrieved May 25, 2002, from http://www.aafp.org/afp/20010301/883.html.

Mayer, B., & Burns, P. (2000). Differential diagnosis of abuse injuries in infants and young children. *Nurse Practitioner, 25*(10), 15-18, 21, 25-26.

Monteleone, J. A. (1994). *Recognition of child abuse for the mandated reporter.* St. Louis: Green-Warren Medical Publishing.

Muram, D. (1988). Classification of genital findings in prepubertal girls who are victims of sexual abuse. *Adolescent Pediatric Gynecology, 1*, 151.

Palmer, S., Brown, R., Rae-Grant, N., & Loughlin, M. (2001). Survivors of childhood abuse: their reported experiences with professional help. *Social Work 46*(2), 136-145.

Pulido, M. (2001). Pregnancy: a time to break the cycle of family violence. *Health & Social Work 26*(2), 120-124.

Robinson, D., Kidd, P, & Rogers, K. (2000). *Primary care across the lifespan.* St. Louis: Mosby.

Schmitt, B. D. (1987). Seven deadly sins of childhood: Advising parents about difficult developmental phases. *Child Abuse & Neglect, 11*, 421-432.

Toomey, S., & Bernstein, H. (2001). Child abuse and neglect: prevention and intervention. *Current Opinions in Pediatrics, 13*(2), 211-215.

Review Questions

1. Which aspect of an episodic history for a 12-year-old female is most suggestive of sexual abuse?

   a. Sleep disturbances
   b. Poor school functioning
   c. Thumb sucking
   d. Sexual acting out

2. The NP suspects abuse after completing a history and physical examination. Which finding most likely raised the red flag?

   a. Purulent nasal discharge with postnasal drainage
   b. Flat affect
   c. Multiple bruises on extremities and face ranging in color from purple to brown
   d. A 3-cm scar in the right lower quadrant of the abdomen

3. Which type of fracture is most often the result of abuse?

   a. Spiral
   b. Compound
   c. Simple
   d. Avulsion

4. The best intervention for the NP trying to prevent child abuse is to do which of the following?

    a. Refer the child for attention-deficit/hyperactivity disorder (ADHD) testing.
    b. Encourage parents to have time away from their children.
    c. Educate parents regarding appropriate developmental expectations.
    d. Screen families for child abuse potential.

5. If an STD is suspected based on the physical examination for sexual abuse, the most appropriate diagnostic testing is which of the following?

    a. DNA probe
    b. Wet prep
    c. Gonorrhea and chlamydia culture
    d. Urinary analysis (U/A)

6. Appropriate questions to elicit information about potential sexual abuse include which of the following?

    a. "How could you let someone touch you like that?"
    b. "Can you tell me why you are here today?"
    c. "What do you know about sexual rights and wrongs?"
    d. "Why didn't you yell for help when it happened?"

7. A 4-year-old boy comes to the clinic for a behavior problem. The mother reports problems at day care with sexual play and recent use of slang words for genital parts. The mother explains, "I don't know where he heard it. We don't use those words at home." The physical examination is normal. Although more data would be helpful, the first consideration for diagnosis is:

    a. Physical abuse
    b. Emotional abuse
    c. Behavior problem
    d. Sexual abuse

8. A child was placed in foster care 6 weeks ago after being physically abused. He visits the clinic today for a preschool physical examination. The child is withdrawn with minimal verbalization. The physical examination is significant for an erythematous loop-shaped mark on his back. The foster parents deny knowledge of the mark. Evaluation of management of this child for physical abuse includes which of the following?

    a. Physical marks are likely a result of abuse before foster care placement.
    b. Further investigation is needed to evaluate the situation.
    c. Physical abuse is still occurring; call the case worker immediately.
    d. Referral is needed to another foster care placement.

Answers and Rationales

1. *Answer:* **d** (assessment)
    Rationale: Sexual activity is the most significant behavior suggesting sexual abuse. The other behaviors might suggest sexual abuse, but they are not specific and also can be suggestive of other problems (Lahoti, McClain, Girardet, et al., 2001).

2. *Answer:* **c** (assessment)
    Rationale: Bruises in different stages of healing indicate multiple episodes of trauma over time, a key indicator of abuse (Monteleone, 1994).

3. *Answer:* **a** (analysis/diagnosis)
    Rationale: Spiral fractures, associated with a twisting motion, are the most common type of fracture associated with abuse (Lynch, 1997; Monteleone, 1994).

4. *Answer:* **c** (implementation/plan)
    Rationale: Parenting is difficult. Developmental issues such as colic and toilet training have high associations with abuse. All children are at risk during certain time periods. For this reason, proper education regarding developmental expectations is likely to prevent more cases of abuse (Schmitt, 1987). Referral for ADHD evaluation, respite for parents, and screening families for child abuse potential also may be helpful, but they are not the best of the actions offered for the NP.

5. *Answer:* **c** (analysis/diagnosis)
    Rationale: Cultures need to be done for gonorrhea and chlamydia because in most states nonculture results are not admissible in court. A nonculture method needs to have a culture done if the result is positive. U/A and wet prep may be done as part of the diagnostic tests for abuse, but they do not diagnose sexual abuse (Lahoti, McClain, Girardet, et al., 2001).

6. *Answer:* **b** (assessment)
    Rationale: Answers a and d are judgmental and should not be used to find out about sexual abuse. Answer c is too high level for most children. The best answer is b, a nonjudgmental way to start off the conversation (Leder, Knight, and Emans, 2001).

7. *Answer:* **d** (assessment)
    Rationale: Behavioral signs of sexual abuse in children include knowledge and use of sexual terms, excessive sexual play, and excessive masturbation (Lahoti, McClain, Girardet, et al., 2001).

8. *Answer:* **c** (analysis/diagnosis)
    Rationale: A loop mark (red, indicating a more recent infliction) is indicative of abuse. Abuse does occur in foster home placements. Reporting of this case is warranted (Monteleone, 1994).

c

CHLAMYDIA TRACHOMATIS   *Cheryl Pope Kish*

OVERVIEW
Definition

Chlamydia is an STD caused by the bacterium *Chlamydia trachomatis*. It is transmitted primarily by sexual contact, but it may be acquired by newborns as they are delivered through the cervix of an infected mother.

Incidence

- *C. trachomatis* is the most common STD in the United States.
- More than 10% of sexually active teens are infected with chlamydia. In college students, there is a 5% occurrence. Greatest incidence occurs in people ages 15 to 21 years old.
- Transmission to the infant occurs in 70% of women with untreated chlamydial infection during pregnancy.
- Frequently found concurrently with gonorrhea.
- Occurs more frequently in African-American and Hispanic populations and in lower socioeconomic groups.
- Symptoms do not occur in 1 in 4 infected men and 3 in 4 infected women.

Pathophysiology

C. trachomatis, the causative organism, is an obligate intracellular parasite bacterium that has some viral properties. It develops within the inclusion bodies in cytoplasm of host cells–primarily infecting the genital tract of women at the transformation zone of the endocervix and the urethra of men. Sexual contact that involves the anus exposes that mucous membrane to infection in both men and women. Maternal–newborn transmission occurs when birth takes place through an infected cervix.

Factors Increasing Susceptibility
- Sexual promiscuity, multiple sexual partners
- Early first sexual contact
- Use of nonbarrier contraception
- Concurrent gonorrhea or other STD
- New sexual partner within previous 2 months
- Use of OCPs (induces cervical eversion or ectopy, thereby exposing more susceptible squamocolumnar cells)

ASSESSMENT: SUBJECTIVE/HISTORY
History of Present Illness

Determine symptoms and their relationship to menstrual cycle and sexual activity. Note description, onset, duration, course, aggravating or relieving factors, and associated symptoms. Realize that many clients are infected but are asymptomatic.

Symptoms

- Endocervicitis: mucopurulent cervical discharge, post-coital or intermenstrual spotting or bleeding
- Urethral syndrome/urethritis: urinary frequency, dysuria, urethral itch lasting longer than 7 to 10 days; with involvement of epididymis: unilateral testicular pain, tenderness, and swelling
- Endometritis/salpingitis: intermenstrual spotting or bleeding, menorrhagia, dyspareunia, dysmenorrhea, abdominal or pelvic pain, fever/chills, malaise, nausea and vomiting
- Bartholinitis: localized tenderness and pain in area of Bartholin's gland, difficulty sitting and walking, and dyspareunia
- Proctitis: irritation of rectum, pain, hematochezia, tenesmus, mucus discharge, constipation, pain with defecation
- Perihepatitis (Fitz-Hugh Curtis syndrome): severe right upper quadrant pleuritic pain 6 days before or 14 days after lower abdominal pain, fever, nausea, and vomiting
- Reiter's syndrome (primarily in men): arthritis; non-specific rheumatoid complaints; skin, mouth, and nail lesions; conjunctivitis

Past Medical History

Ask about previous STDs and treatment. Determine if client has a chronic illness that might complicate management.

Medication History

Ask about oral contraception use.

Family History

Not applicable.

Psychosocial History

Conduct a sensitive assessment of sexual behaviors that increase risk. Determine number of partners, sexual practices, sexual relations with a new partner within the preceding 2 months, and age at first sexual contact. Ask about use of barrier contraception. Ask about date of last sexual contact.

ASSESSMENT: OBJECTIVE/PHYSICAL EXAMINATION
Physical Examination

- In men check for urethral discharge. Have client "milk" down the penile shaft to elicit discharge if present. Check the anus if sexual practice includes anal contact. Palpate for inguinal nodes. Assess for epidydimitis.

- In women check for guarding and rebound tenderness in abdomen. Examine perineum for excoriation, lesions, and ulcerations. Insert speculum and assess cervix for friability. Look for any mucopurulent discharge; if present, collect specimen. Perform bimanual examination to demonstrate cervical motion tenderness (Chandelier's sign) and uterine and adnexal tenderness or fullness.
- Assess vital signs in both men and women.

Diagnostic Procedures

Wet preparation may show increased WBC count and decreased normal vaginal flora. There are multiple laboratory tests available; sensitivities and specificities vary. Culture is the gold standard. To obtain a culture, a brush or swab should be inserted 1 to 2 cm and rotated for 30 seconds.

Because of high concurrence with gonorrhea, consider culture for gonorrhea at the same time. (DNA probes enable both tests from the same sample). Consider testing for syphilis, hepatitis B, and HIV if history indicates. Polymerase chain reaction and ligase chain reaction tests are available on first voided urine specimens; these cannot be used as test of cure.

Differential diagnosis includes gonorrhea, appendicitis, and urinary tract infection (UTI) in clients of both genders. In men, also consider urethritis, epididymitis, and proctitis. In women, consider cervicitis, Bartholinitis, endometritis, and pelvic inflammatory disease (PID). Infants born to affected women should be monitored for conjunctivitis and pneumonia related to *C. trachomatis*.

DIAGNOSIS

Diagnosis is difficult in women because 50% to 70% of infected women are asymptomatic. For that reason, screening programs are appropriate in high-risk populations, such as sexually active adolescents and young women with new or multiple sexual partners.

THERAPEUTIC PLAN

Pharmacologic Treatment

Goals of treatment are (1) prevention of infection of sexual partner or fetus and (2) minimization of sequelae. The following treatment options are recommended by the CDC:

- Doxycycline 100 mg PO bid for 7 days or azithromycin 1 g PO in a single dose; neither requires test of cure.
- Ofloxacin 300 mg PO bid for 7 days or erythromycin base 500 mg PO bid for 7 days or erythromycin ethylsuccinate (EES) 800 mg bid for 7 days or sulfisoxazole 500 mg PO bid for 10 days or tetracycline 500 mg bid for 7 days; all require a test of cure 3 to 4 weeks after treatment.

Pregnant or Lactating Clients. Erythromycin or amoxicillin is recommended; however, a test of cure 1 month after completion of therapy is necessary. Azithromycin (pregnancy category B) 1 g PO in a single dose may be used. A test of cure is appropriate 1 month after treatment.

Neonates. Erythromycin 50 mg/kg/day is 80% effective in 4 divided doses for 10 to 14 days. Follow-up to determine resolution.

Protection of public health requires that sexual partners be treated, including any partner within the preceding 60 days, regardless of symptoms. In most states chlamydia is a reportable disease.

Client Education/ Prevention

- Emphasize the importance of treating those sexual partners who have been contacts within 20 days of symptoms or 60 days if asymptomatic.
- Teach client to practice safe sexual behavior to decrease transmission of STDs, including barrier protection (latex condoms, latex dental dams for oral–genital and oral–anal contact).
- Inform client about possible sequelae of untreated chlamydia, including infertility.
- Teach client to use a backup method of contraception for remainder of cycle if on OCPs during antibiotic treatment.
- Instruct client to complete the full course of prescribed treatment so that the organism does not become dormant and cause reinfection.
- Client should not have sexual intercourse until treatment is completed in both partners.
- Doxycycline causes photosensitivity. Client should protect skin from sunlight.
- Tetracycline should be taken 1 hour before or 2 hours after meals, dairy products, antacids, or mineral-containing products for maximal efficacy.
- Inform client of the importance of test of cure after less effective medications are used.

Referral

Refer to treatment clients who are nonresponsive or experience complications beyond the scope of practice of the NP.

EVALUATION/FOLLOW-UP

- Clients do not need to be retested for chlamydia after completing treatment with doxycycline or azithromycin unless symptoms persist or reinfection is suspected. Repeat Pap smear if it was abnormal before treatment.
- Evidence of chlamydia in children requires evaluation for sexual abuse.

COMPLICATIONS

Women are disproportionately burdened with complications of chlamydial infection and should be followed closely. The most common complications in women include PID, which can lead to infertility or ectopic pregnancy related to tubal scarring; cervicitis; postpartum endometritis; and higher incidences of spontaneous abortion and stillbirth when chlamydia is present during pregnancy. In men, the predominant complications are Reiter's syndrome and epididymitis.

Nearly two thirds of newborns of infected mothers contract chlamydia; newborns should be followed at 5 to 14 days after birth for conjunctivitis and at 2 to 12 weeks after birth for pneumonia.

REFERENCES

Cash, J. C., & Glass, C. A. (2000). *Family practice guidelines.* Philadelphia: Lippincott.

Ferreira, N. (1997). Sexually transmitted *chlamydia trachomatis. Nurse Practitioner Forum, 8*(2), 70-76.

Gerrig, J. N. (1998). Preventing and recognizing STDs in the adolescent. *Lippincott Primary Care Practice, 2*(3), 312-314.

Hawkins, J. W., Roberto-Nichols, D. M., & Stanley-Haney, J. L. (1997). *Protocols for nurse practitioners in gynecologic settings.* New York: Tiresias Press.

Rawlins, S. (2001). Nonviral sexually transmitted infections. *Journal of Obstetric, Gynecologic, and Neonatal Nursing, 30*(3), 324-331.

Robinson, D., Kidd, P., & Rogers, K. (2000). *Primary care across the lifespan.* St. Louis: Mosby.

Shaffa, S. D. (1998). Vaginitis and sexually transmitted diseases. In E. Q. Youngkin, & M. S. Davis. *Women's health care: a primary care clinical guide.* (2nd ed., pp. 265-300). Stamford, CT: Appleton & Lange.

Smith, M. A. & Shimp, L. A. (2000). *20 common problems in women's health care.* New York: McGraw-Hill.

Star, W. L., Lommel, L. L., & Shannon, M. T. (1995). *Women's primary health care: protocols for practice.* Washington, DC: American Nurses Publishing.

Trotto, N. E. (1999). STDs: Are you up to date? *Patient Care, May 30,* 74-76, 81, 85-103.

Review Questions

1. Beth, age 20, presents to the university health service for an annual examination and Pap test. She desires birth control pills. She is sexually active and has had a total of two partners; she and her current partner have been together for 6 weeks. She discloses that he had numerous partners in the past but their relationship is mutually monogamous. Which findings in Beth's history place her at risk for *C. trachomatis* infection?

    a. Menarche at age 12
    b. Use of tetracycline for acne
    c. Sexual partner with history of promiscuity
    d. Strong family history of diabetes mellitus

2. In providing education about risk factors for chlamydial infection, the NP should be certain to list which of the following?

    a. First sexual contact after age 25
    b. Use of oral contraception
    c. White or Asian ancestry
    d. Lesbianism

3. The NP performs a vaginal examination and notes cervical friability and a mucopurulent discharge from the cervical os. She decides to collect a specimen for wet mount and culture. Which procedure is most appropriate for obtaining a culture to diagnose chlamydia?

    a. Remove excess secretions from cervix; insert swab into endocervix and rotate 30 seconds; place swab in appropriate medium; transport.
    b. Use Ayr spatula to scrape cells from os; spread cells evenly on glass slide; label for lab.
    c. Collect sample of discharge from cervical os; mix with drop of saline on glass slide; view under microscope at 40 × power to note intracellular parasite.
    d. Collect specimen as for Pap smear, but label "Chlamydia culture prior to Pap."

4. The NP views the wet prep under the microscope. The clinical finding consistent with chlamydial infection is which of the following?

    a. Motile flagellate organisms
    b. Numerous clue cells
    c. WBCs
    d. Budding yeast

5. Which finding on vaginal examination is consistent with a diagnosis of pelvic inflammation associated with chlamydia?

    a. Frothy green malodorous discharge
    b. Cervical motion tenderness
    c. Strawberry markings on a pale cervix
    d. Irregular contour of uterus

6. Mr. Lyles presents with complaints of frequent urination, burning, and a cloudy penile discharge. History and physical examination are consistent with chlamydia, and the NP is considering appropriate treatment. Which drug is most appropriate?

    a. Ampicillin 500 mg PO bid × 7 days
    b. EES 800 mg PO bid × 7 days
    c. Tetracycline 500 mg PO × 14 days
    d. Doxycycline 100 mg PO bid × 7 days

7. Mr. Lyles asks if there is some way to treat him more quickly. He hates taking pills and says, " I sure want to feel better, but I can't promise I'll take all that medicine." Which drug treatment meets Mr. Lyles's request and is effective for treating chlamydia?

    a. Procaine penicillin 1.2 million units IM in a single dose
    b. Ceftriaxone (Rocephin) 125 mg IM in a single dose
    c. Cefixime (Suprax) 400 mg PO in a single dose
    d. Azithromycin 1 gram PO in a single dose

8. In which of the following situations will a test of cure not be needed following treatment of chlamydia?

    a. Client was treated with doxycycline 100 mg bid × 7 days.
    b. Sexual partner did not receive full treatment.

c. Client received full course of treatment with erythromycin base.
d. Client reports inconsistent dosing of prescribed medication.

9. Brice is a 7-year-old boy who is brought in by his grandmother because he is "burning when he passes his water" and has milky drainage from his penis. Brice denies sexual contact, but the grandmother is concerned. Which action by the NP is most appropriate in this situation?
   a. Treat him presumptively for chlamydia.
   b. Reassure the grandmother and treat for UTI.
   c. Perform physical examination and obtain culture for chlamydia.
   d. Perform examination to rule out pyelonephritis.

10. The NP provides comprehensive client education for a woman with chlamydia. Which comment by the client suggests a need for further teaching?
   a. "I will need to tell all my sexual partners that they need to be treated."
   b. "While on doxycycline, I'll be sensitive to sunlight."
   c. "I should abstain from intercourse until both my partner and I complete treatment."
   d. "This kind of infection is not preventable except through sexual abstinence."

Answers and Rationales

1. Answer: c (assessment)
   Rationale: History of multiple partners or a partner with a history of multiple partners increases one's risk of chlamydia (Ferriera, 1997).

2. Answer: b. (implementation/plan)
   Rationale: OCP use increases the risk for chlamydia because they cause cervical eversion, thereby increasing cell susceptibility at the transformation zone (Ferriera, 1997).

3. Answer: a (implementation/plan)
   Rationale: The appropriate procedure for collecting a culture for chlamydia includes wiping away excess secretions, inserting the swab into the endocervical os and rotating 30 seconds, placing into medium, and transporting to lab (Shaffa, 1998).

4. Answer: c (analysis/diagnosis)
   Rationale: The wet mount in a client with chlamydia reveals less normal vaginal flora and the presence of WBCs, usually at least 8 per high-powered field (Ferriera, 1997).

5. Answer: b (assessment)
   Rationale: Cervical motion tenderness, also known as Chandelier's sign, is consistent with chlamydia (Cash & Glass, 2000).

6. Answer: d (implementation/plan)
   Rationale: Doxycycline 100 mg PO bid for 7 days is an effective treatment; it does not require a test of cure (Robinson, Kidd, & Rogers, 2000).

7. Answer: d (evaluation)
   Rationale: Azithromycin 1 g PO as a single dose is an effective treatment for chlamydia (Cash & Glass, 2000).

8. Answer: a (plan/implementation)
   Rationale: Doxycycline or azithromycin do not require tests of cure (Ferriera, 1997).

9. Answer: c (implementation/plan)
   Rationale: Assessment for chlamydial infection is appropriate despite denial of sexual contact (Robinson, Kidd, & Rogers, 2000).

10. Answer: d (evaluation)
   Rationale: Options a, b, and c are appropriate comments. Sexually responsible behavior that includes latex condoms as protective barriers offer protection against chlamydia (Cash & Glass, 2000).

CHRONIC OBSTRUCTIVE PULMONARY DISEASE *Pamela Kidd*

OVERVIEW
Definition
COPD, also referred to as *chronic airflow limitation,* is a disease of progressive airflow limitation that may be accompanied by airway hyperreactivity, and this hyperreactivity may be partially reversible. Most clients with COPD have components of bronchitis, emphysema, and sometimes asthma.

Chronic Bronchitis. The definition of chronic bronchitis is based on clinical criteria (a chronic productive cough for 3 consecutive months in 2 successive years). Chronic mucus hypersecretion by itself with chronic cough does not necessarily result in significant airway obstruction. When the hypersecretion leads to chronic obstructive bronchitis, rapid deterioration of pulmonary function results.

Emphysema. Based on morphologic features, emphysema is defined as the irreversible dilation and destruction of alveolar ducts and air spaces distal to the terminal bronchiole. This results in air trapping.

Incidence
- Sixteen million persons in the United States are affected by COPD.
- COPD is the fifth leading cause of death in the United States.
- Men are affected more than women.

- Mortality rates are higher among whites than among other ethnic groups.

Pathophysiology

- There is a 20- to 40-year preclinical period when the client is asymptomatic, but lung damage accumulates and function declines.
- Forced expiratory volume (FEV):
  - Mild forced expiratory volume in 1 second (FEV_1)/forced volume capacity (FVC) is >70%, FEV_1 ≥80% predicted for size.
  - Moderate stage has two phases. Phase 1 is with or without chronic symptoms of cough and shortness of breath, FEV_1 <50% to 80%, FEV_1/FVC <70%. Phase 2 is 30% ≤FEV_1 <50%.
  - Severe stage involves chronic oxygen therapy, FEV_1 <30% or <50%, plus signs of respiratory and heart failure (NHLBI, 2001).
  - A genetic factor is congenital homozygous alpha1-antitrypsin deficiency.

Factors Increasing Susceptibility. Cigarette smoking, recurrent infections, allergies, exposure to irritants, and tendency for bronchoconstriction to nonspecific airway stimuli all increase a person's susceptibility to COPD (Chesnutt & Prendergast, 2001).

Protective Factors. Having a nonsmoking household and work/school environment seems to protect against COPD.

ASSESSMENT: SUBJECTIVE/HISTORY
Symptoms

- Cough (time of day; onset, duration, and productivity; type, character, and amount of sputum)
- Wheezing
- Hemoptysis
- Dyspnea (onset, duration, and degree)
- Lost/gained weight
- Emphysema symptoms of progressive dyspnea/dyspnea on exertion, mild hypoxia, cough with clear sputum, muscle wasting, weight loss
- Chronic bronchitis symptoms of intermittent dyspnea, severe productive cough of mucopurulent sputum, obesity, cyanosis

Current History

- Smoking habits (past and present)
- Overall quality of life; ability to perform ADLs
- Exposure to passive smoking, past and present
- Foods
- Daily fluid intake
- Exercise
- Sexual activity
- Exposure to irritants or noxious materials, past and present

Past Medical History

Ask about allergies, previous respiratory diagnosis and recurrent pulmonary disease, hypertension, obesity, CHF, peptic ulcer disease, cor pulmonale, and morning headache.

Medication History

Ask about current prescription medications and OTC medications.

Family History

- Inquire about indications for alpha-antiprotease (AAT) deficiency (familial emphysema).
- Ask about environmental tobacco smoke exposure.

Dietary History

Not relevant.

ASSESSMENT: OBJECTIVE/PHYSICAL EXAMINATION
Physical Examination

- Check height, weight, and vital signs. Note respirations (tachypnea), pulse (tachycardia), blood pressure (pulsus paradoxus), and general appearance (cachexia, diaphoresis).
- Examine HEENT. Note pursed-lip breathing, mucous membrane, or perioral cyanosis.
- Check neck for jugular venous distention.
- Examine chest for increased anteroposterior diameter, retractions, and accessory muscle use; expect to hear expiratory wheezes; if crackles present, suspect accompanying heart failure.
  - Emphysema: barrel chest, hyperresonance, diminished breath sound
  - Chronic bronchitis: wheezes, rhonchi
- Listen to heart for right ventricular heave, S_3 gallop or premature atrial complexes, and atrial fibrillation if cor pulmonale is present.
- Palpate abdomen for organomegaly and liver engorgement (cor pulmonale).
- Check extremities for peripheral edema and pulses, cyanosis, and clubbing.
- Perform a neurologic examination for mental status (note somnolence and confusion).

Diagnostic Procedures

- Test clients with a positive family history of emphysema and clients who are younger than age 45 for 1-protease inhibitor deficiency.
- Perform spirometry at least once in every smoker at age 40 and in all clients who wheeze, cough, or have shortness of breath. Check for FEV greater than or less than 3 seconds, decreased vital capacity and expiratory flow rates in COPD, and increased respiratory volume and total lung capacity in emphysema.

- Obtain CBC (polycythemia in advanced stages of chronic bronchitis).
- Obtain a chemistry profile.
- Perform an ECG (advanced COPD, right atrial hypertrophy).
- Obtain a chest x-ray examination (check for hyperinflation and diaphragm flattening).
- Arterial blood gases (ABGs) (if FEV_1 is <1 L) indicate hypoxemia, respiratory alkalosis (early), acidosis (late), and hypoxia.
- For mild-to-moderate disease, perform all tests within normal limits except spirometry.
- For severe disease, obtain CBC (erythrocytosis).

DIAGNOSIS

Differential diagnosis includes the following:
- Cardiac causes
  - CHF
  - Infarction
  - Arrhythmia
- Pulmonary causes
  - Acute bronchitis
  - Pulmonary embolus
  - Lung cancer
  - Pneumothorax
  - Atelectasis
- Other causes
  - Deconditioning
  - Obesity
  - Psychogenic factors
  - Anemia
  - GERD
  - Postnasal drip
  - Chronic aspiration
  - Tuberculosis
  - Aspiration
  - Anaphylaxis
  - Epiglottitis

THERAPEUTIC PLAN

Treatment focuses on alleviating symptoms associated with chronic bronchitis or emphysema; therefore clients with both bronchitis and emphysema components may benefit from all proposed strategies.

Goals are the following (Goolsby, 2001):
- Prevent disease progression.
- Relieve symptoms.
- Improve exercise tolerance.
- Improve health status.
- Prevent and treat complications.
- Prevent and treat exacerbations.
- Reduce mortality.

Nonpharmacologic Treatment

- Goal is the prevention of progression of disease, improvement of symptoms, control of infection.

- NP functions as care coordinator.
- Encourage client to stop smoking.
- Educate client to prevent infection:
  - Smoking cessation and reduction in exposures to airway irritants
  - Avoidance of foods that increase bronchospasm and sputum (alcohol, spicy foods, dairy products)
  - Avoidance of extremes in temperature (wear a mask when exposure is unavoidable)
  - Home humidification and ingestion of 2 to 3 L of water per day for sputum liquefaction
  - Reduction of airflow obstruction
- Begin pulmonary rehabilitation program (pursed-lip breathing and diaphragmatic exercises).
- Encourage client to exercise to increase tolerance at a lower oxygen consumption rate.
- Educate client in upper extremity training to lessen diaphragmatic work.

Pharmacologic Treatment
Prevention of Infection
- Yearly influenza vaccine
- Pneumococcal vaccine polyvalent (Pneumovax) every 6 to 10 years

Stop Smoking. Try a nicotine transdermal patch or buproprion.

Treatment of Chronic Bronchitis
- Mild COPD: short acting bronchodilator when needed
- Moderate COPD: regular treatment with one or more bronchodilators (usually those listed as follows)
  - Anticholinergic: ipratropium (Atrovent) metered dose inhaler (MDI) (2 to 4 inhalations q6h) plus
  - Inhaled beta₂-selective agonist (albuterol [Ventolin] or metaproterenol [Alupent]) MDI) plus
  - Inhaled corticosteroid (beclomethasone, triamicinolone, or flunicolide) MDI (use only for corticosteroid responsive clients, determine response by trying oral steroids first with baseline and follow-up spirometry to determine improvement)
- Severe COPD: all of the medications listed previously plus extended-release theophylline (improves respiratory muscle performance and oxyhemoglobin saturation during sleep) plus
  - Extended-release oral albuterol plus
  - Oral corticosteroid (taper) plus home oxygen therapy
- Avoid sedatives, antihistamines, and beta blockers.

NOTE: *Sedatives can be used in cases of intractable dyspnea for very anxious clients.*

- Infection control (acute exacerbation): *S. pneumoniae, H. influenzae, Moraxella pneumoniae,* and *M. catarrhalis* are the most common infection-causing organisms.
- Trimethoprim-sulfamethoxazole (Bactrim DS) 1 tablet PO bid

- Erythromycin 250 mg qid or azithromycin (Zithromax) (if compliance with frequent medication dosing is a problem)
- Amoxicillin 250 to 500 mg PO tid

To treat a cough that is combined with a difficulty in clearing secretions, use mucolytic agents such as benzonatate (Tessalon) or guaifenesin.

Oxygen Therapy and Safety Issues

- Low (1-3 L/min) flow (or what concentration it takes to maintain PaO_2 greater than 55 mm Hg) has been shown to improve survival in clients with COPD. Oxygen must be used at least 15 hours per day.
- Use home oxygen when PaO_2 is less than 55 mm Hg or oxygen saturation is less than 88% at rest breathing room air while awake. (Do not use oxygen within 6 feet of open flame.)

Client Education

Instruct the client regarding the following:
- The need for a fire extinguisher and smoke alarms (with home oxygen use)
- Coughing (deep breath, then cough)
- Effects of COPD on lung function, breathing techniques, and coping skills
  - Educate family members.
  - Educate clients on the use of an MDI.
  - Counsel clients about advance directives, wishes concerning intubation and resuscitation, living will, and power of attorney.
  - Review signs and symptoms of respiratory infections.
  - Factors that contribute to upper respiratory tract infections

Signs and Symptoms

- Increased cough and sputum
- Thick/odorous sputum
- Change of sputum color
- Increased shortness of breath, fatigue, chest congestion, fever/chills

Referral

- Refer for multidisciplinary pulmonary rehabilitation.
- For AAT deficiency, refer to an endocrinologist.
- For cor pulmonale, refer to a pulmonologist.
- If oxygen is needed, refer to a pulmonologist.

Prevention

Not smoking cigarettes will help prevent COPD.

EVALUATION/FOLLOW-UP

- For acute attacks, phone contact within 24 to 48 hours must be made.

- If the client is taking theophylline, measure drug levels 1 to 2 weeks after initiation of therapy. (Desired level is 10 to 20 ng/dL.)
- Schedule follow-up visits every 3 to 6 months for stable chronic disease.
- Stress importance of early recognition of respiratory infection or distress.

COMPLICATIONS

- Pneumonia
- Pulmonary hypertension/cor pulmonale
- Chronic respiratory failure/death
- Spontaneous pneumothorax

REFERENCES

Boyars, M. C. (1997, June). COPD: A step-care approach when FEV$_1$ is deteriorating. *Consultant*, 1673-1687.

Celli, R., Costentino, A., Fiel, S., & Petty, T. (1997, January). COPD: Step by step through the workup. *Patient Care*, 20-52.

Chesnutt, M. & Prendergast, T. (2001). Lung. In L. Tierney, S. McPhee, & M. Papadakis. (Eds.), *Current medical diagnosis and treatment*. New York: McGraw-Hill.

Davis, A., Hahn, D., Niederman, M., & O'Connell, E. (1996, January). When chronic bronchitis turns acute. *Patient Care*, 124-127.

Goolsby, M. (2001). Chronic obstructive pulmonary disease. *Journal of the American Academy of Nurse Practitioners, 13*(8), 348-353.

National Heart, Lung, and Blood Institute. (2001). *Global initiative for chronic obstructive pulmonary disease: global strategy for the diagnosis, management, and prevention of COPD: NHLBI/WHO workshop report*. Bethesda, MD: United States Department of Health and Human Services, Public Health Services, National Institutes of Health, National Heart, Lung, and Blood Institute.

Witta, K. (1997). COPD in the elderly. *Advance for Nurse Practitioners, July*, 18-27, 72.

Review Questions

1. Which of the following is *not* a risk factor for COPD?
   a. Age
   b. Inhaled irritant and noxious agents
   c. Heredity
   d. Edema

2. Diagnostic testing for a client with COPD would include all *except* which of the following?
   a. Stress test
   b. Chest x-ray examination
   c. O_2 saturation
   d. Pulmonary function tests

3. A 56-year-old man complains of having a morning cough for the past 5 years that has increased during the last 2 days. He has smoked cigarettes for 30 years and has noticed wheezing lately. He also has experienced dyspnea for several months. What is the most likely diagnosis?
  a. COPD
  b. Lung cancer
  c. GERD
  d. Asthma

4. Pharmacologic interventions for a client with COPD include all *except* which of the following?
  a. Steroids
  b. Bronchodilators
  c. Sedatives
  d. Mucolytics

5. Theophylline was prescribed for Mrs. Crawford at her last office visit. She should have drug levels drawn at which of the following times?
  a. 2 weeks
  b. Never
  c. Every 3 to 6 months
  d. Yearly

6. The NP should prescribe home oxygen for a COPD client when which of the following occurs?
  a. Cor pulmonale is present.
  b. Oxygen saturation is less than 88% at rest.
  c. PaO_2 is less than 60 mm Hg.
  d. Client has shortness of breath doing ADLs.

7. Which of the following statements indicate the client with COPD understands his treatment plan?
  a. Avoid dairy products.
  b. Avoid humidification of home.
  c. Limit water intake to 1 L per day.
  d. Use salmeterol (Serevent) inhaler as rescue inhaler.

8. A client with COPD asks about pulmonary rehabilitation. What should the NP say to the client?
  a. "It is helpful in strengthening upper extremities to lessen diaphragmatic work."
  b. "It has not shown any benefit."
  c. "Exercise requires increased oxygen consumption and this is not helpful in COPD."
  d. "It does not help relieve dyspnea."

Answers and Rationales

1. *Answer:* d (assessment)
Rationale: A nonsmoking adult has a yearly decline of 15 to 30 mL in FEV_1. Cigarette smoking and urban/industrial pollution, first-degree relatives with COPD and an AAT deficiency, and airway hyperreactivity are risk factors for COPD.

2. *Answer:* a (implementation/plan)
Rationale: Spirometry assesses the risk of pulmonary disease in high-risk populations. Chest x-ray examination can confirm the diagnosis with hyperinflation and diaphragm flattening. O_2 saturation reading can indicate hypoxemia.

3. *Answer:* a (analysis/diagnosis)
Rationale: Nighttime cough might suggest asthma or GERD. With a history of a morning cough, significant smoking, and an age of 56 years or older, the most likely diagnosis is COPD.

4. *Answer:* c (implementation/plan)
Rationale: Avoid sedatives, antihistamines, and beta blockers in COPD because of diminished respiratory drive and bronchoconstriction side effect.

5. *Answer:* a (evaluation)
Rationale: To prevent caffeinelike side effects, theophylline should be started in low dosages and gradually increased to a maintenance level. It is important to monitor the client's serum level 1 to 2 weeks after initiation of the medication, dosage change, or switching brands.

6. *Answer:* b. (implementation/plan)
Rationale: PaO_2 should be below 55 mm Hg before prescribing home oxygen. In COPD, clients may become short of breath on activity even in less severe stages. Cor pulmonale may or may not be present with low oxygen saturations.

7. *Answer:* a (evaluation)
Rationale: Dairy products should be avoided because they increase bronchospasm. Humidification is needed to help with expectoration. Water intake should be increased up to 3 L per day to help expectoration. Salmeterol is a long-acting bronchodilator that does not take effect for at least 30 to 60 minutes and should not be used as a rescue inhaler.

8. *Answer:* a (implementation/plan)
Rationale: Pulmonary rehabilitation has been proved to increase tolerance to a lower oxygen consumption rate and to lessen diaphragmatic work through use of the upper extremities.

CLEFT LIP AND PALATE *Denise Robinson*

OVERVIEW
Definition
Cleft lip (CL) or cleft palate (CP) is the incomplete closure of the lip, the palate, or both at birth.

Incidence
- CL incidence: 1 in 600 births (with or without CP)
  - More common in males.
  - Genetic factors important.
- CP incidence: 1 in 1000 births
  - More common in females.
  - Highest incidence in Asians (1.61 in 1000 births) and whites (0.9 in 1000 births) and lowest among blacks (0.31 in 1000 births) (Sujansky, Stewart, & Manchester, 1999).
  - Associated with other congenital malformations, especially in those with cleft palate alone.

Pathophysiology
CL and CP are closely related embryologically, functionally, and genetically (Johnsen, 1996). CL results from hypoplasia of the mesenchymal layer, resulting in a failure of the medial nasal and maxillary processes to join. CP appears to represent failure of the palatal shelves to approximate or fuse (Johnsen, 1996).

ASSESSMENT: SUBJECTIVE/HISTORY
Symptoms
A CL may vary from a small notch in the vermilion border to a complete separation extending into the floor of the nose. Clefts may be unilateral (more often on the left). A CP can involve only the soft palate or it can involve both the soft and hard palates.

Past Medical History
Not applicable.

Medication History
Not applicable.

Psychosocial History
Not applicable.

Family History
- Ask about the incidence of CL/CP in the family
- Ask about history of alcohol ingestion during pregnancy, maternal seizures, and anticonvulsant usage during pregnancy.

ASSESSMENT: OBJECTIVE/PHYSICAL EXAMINATION
Physical Examination
- The examination should focus on the ear, nose, and throat system, although the examination should be complete because of the possibility of other congenital defects.
- Examine the HEENT system to determine the extent of the cleft.
- Look for other indicators of congenital problems (e.g., low-slung ears, prominent occiput).
- Examine the cardiovascular system; be alert to the possibility of congenital heart disease in affected infants.

Diagnostic Procedures
Perform diagnostic procedures as needed based on the extent of the disorder.

DIAGNOSIS
Determine if the CL/CP is an isolated occurrence or part of a syndrome. Some syndromes that typically have CL or CP include the following (Sujansky, Stewart, & Manchester, 1999):
- Trisomies 13 and 18 (CL/CP)
- Wolf-Hirschhorn (CL/CP)
- Shprintzen's (CP)
- Van der Woude's (CL/CP or CP)
- Treacher Collins (CP)
- Stickler (CP)

THERAPEUTIC PLAN
Nonpharmacologic Treatment
- Most immediate problem is feeding. The infant will be fitted with a plastic obturator to help in control of fluids.
- Soft artificial nipples with large openings are beneficial to infants with CP.
- Infants with isolated CL can be breastfed.
- Surgical closure is the treatment of choice for CL; it usually is performed by the time the child is 2 months old if the child is gaining weight and free of infection.
- The timing of surgical repair of CP is individualized based on the extent of the size, shape, and degree of the deformity. It usually is done before 1 year of age to enhance normal speech development.
- The control of secretions is most important because of the risk of choking.

Pharmacologic Treatment
Not applicable.

Client Education

- It is important after surgery to keep the infant's hands and toys away from the suture line. The child's elbows will be restrained.
- The child will be fed with a medicine dropper with a fluid or semifluid diet for 3 weeks.
- The parents should know that follow-up will be very important to assess for dental, speech, and hearing problems.
- The parents also should be advised on the need for genetic counseling; genetic counseling should include both parents, and a complete family history is needed.
- If the mother is considering having more children, supplementation with folic acid and a multivitamin may decrease the risk of neural tube defects and other congenital malformations (Hernandez-Diaz, Werler, Walker & Mitchell 2000).

Referral

Refer clients to a CL/CP multidisciplinary clinic.

EVALUATION/FOLLOW-UP

- The child needs frequent follow-up related to potential ear infection and hearing loss.
- Dental follow-up will be needed because the child usually requires orthodontic correction.
- Speech therapy may be needed even after closure of the palate.
- Ideally, care is given through a multidisciplinary CP clinic.

COMPLICATIONS

The main problems associated with treatment failure are ear, hearing, dental, and speech problems.

REFERENCES

Hernandez-Diaz S., Werler, M. M., Walker, A. M., & Mitchell, A. A. (2000). Folic acid antagonists during pregnancy and the risk of birth defects. *New England Journal of Medicine, 343,* 1608-1614.

Johnsen, D. (1996). The oral cavity. In W. Nelson, R. Behrman, R. Kliegman, & A. Arvin (Eds.), *Nelson textbook of pediatrics* (15th ed., pp. 1041-1042). Philadelphia: Saunders.

Sujansky, E., Stewart, J., & Manchester, D. (1999). Genetics and dysmorphology. In W. Hay, A. Hayward, M. Levin, & J. Sondheimer (Eds.), *Current pediatric diagnosis and treatment* (14th ed., pp. 881-916). Stamford, CT: Appleton & Lange.

Uhrich, K. & Mackin, A. (2001). Cleft lip and palate: what nurses can do to educate and reassure parents. *American Journal of Nursing, 101*(3), 24AA-BB, 24EE, 24GG.

Review Questions

1. An infant is born with a cleft lip and palate. What associated prenatal history supports a diagnosis of CL and CP?
   a. Maternal ingestion of alcohol
   b. Anxious mother during pregnancy
   c. Smokers in the home
   d. Taking prenatal vitamins during pregnancy

2. A child has a CL and CP. When conducting the physical examination of the newborn, the NP needs to pay particular attention to what aspect of the examination?
   a. Vital signs, general appearance
   b. Cardiovascular examination
   c. Abdominal examination
   d. Neurologic examination

3. Ways in which CL and CP might be avoided during pregnancy include all but which of the following?
   a. Folic acid supplementation
   b. Avoidance of anticonvulsant drugs
   c. Multivitamin supplementation
   d. Limited alcohol intake

4. The most important need of the infant with CL/CP immediately after birth is:
   a. Feeding
   b. Control of secretions
   c. Warmth
   d. Security

5. Follow-up after CL/CP surgery should focus on which of the following:
   a. Speech therapy
   b. Musculoskeletal needs
   c. Visual screening
   d. Smelling ability

Answers and Rationales

1. *Answer:* a (assessment)
   Rationale: One identified factor that may contribute to the development of CL/CP is maternal ingestion of alcohol. A safe amount has not been identified (Sujansky, Stewart, & Manchester, 1999).

2. *Answer:* b (assessment)
   Rationale: It is important to rule out other congenital defects if the infant has CL/CP. Cardiovascular defects are the most common (Sujansky, Stewart, & Manchester, 1999).

3. *Answer:* d (analysis/diagnosis)
   Rationale: Alcohol should be avoided during pregnancy. Although in most cases large amounts of alcohol ingestion may be related to the development of CL/CP, the minimum safe amount of alcohol ingestion is not known (Sujansky, Stewart, & Manchester, 1999).

4. *Answer:* b (analysis/diagnosis)
   Rationale: The issue of feeding is important with infants after birth, but the control of secretions is even more important because of the hazard of choking (Johnsen, 1996).

5. *Answer:* a (evaluation)
   Rationale: Speech therapy is needed after CL/CP surgery. Other areas that must be assessed and followed are hearing and dental care. (Sujansky, Stewart, & Manchester, 1999).

COLIC *Denise Robinson*

OVERVIEW
Definition

Infant colic is a poorly defined syndrome of paroxysmal infant crying that occurs in an infant who is 3 months of age or younger, who cries more than 3 hours a day, and who cries in this manner 3 or more days per week. Colicky babies are described as normal babies who are highly stimulated by the environment (Stein, 2001). Symptoms usually present at around 1 to 2 weeks and persist until approximately 3 months of age. The condition is self-limiting.

Incidence

- Colic occurs in 13% of the population.
- Colic occurs in equal rates in males and females.

Pathophysiology

Infant colic has no specifically known cause, but it is thought to have component physiologic, psychologic, and social factors. Physiologically there may be a predisposition for this syndrome because it is known to occur in family members. Psychologically it is thought that the infants' temperament may play a part, especially those infants described as difficult and those described as having a low sensory threshold. Socially, the infant with colic tends to have caregivers who demonstrate anxiety and frustration at dealing with excessive crying behavior.

Factors Increasing Susceptibility

- Infants on a cow's milk-based formula (10% to 15% of colicky infants have immunoglobulin E–mediated hypersensitivity)
- Infants who are poor feeders and never seem satisfied
- Infants with neurologic deficits
- Infants affected by prenatal drug abuse
- A genetic predisposition, such as a family history of parents or siblings with similar symptoms as an infant
- Difficult temperament in the infant
- Anxious/nervous caregivers

Protective Factors

- Infants with easy temperament
- Caregivers who are easy in their own temperament characteristics and who are not stressed by the crying

ASSESSMENT: SUBJECTIVE/HISTORY
History of Present Illness

- Ask about onset of symptoms and timing of the crying.
- Determine the frequency of the crying.
- Ask about stool patterns and frequency and consistency of bowel movements.

- Determine feeding patterns–how formula is mixed (if not breastfed), how long feedings last, and how much is taken by the baby.
- Determine comfort measures taken by the family and any tactics that do not work.
- Determine who is the caretaker when the episodes occur.

Symptoms

- Crying excessively and inconsolably
- Drawing up of knees
- Making hands into fists
- Demanding frequent feeding
- Having excess gas

Past Medical History

- Thoroughly analyze the labor, delivery, and postpartum period.
- Identify medications taken by the mother prenatally, natally, and presently.

Family History

Determine if any other siblings or family members had colic.

ASSESSMENT: OBJECTIVE/PHYSICAL EXAMINATION
Physical Examination

- Determine vital signs and rate of growth: measure temperature, pulse, respirations, weight, length, and head circumference.
- Plot the growth parameters on growth grids to see the trends.
- Examine general systems, assessing overall appearance, hydration, skin integrity, and any special features that you note about the overall appearance.
- Examine HEENT, checking the mouth for intact palate.
- Examine the abdomen, assessing for bowel sounds, masses, and hepatosplenomegaly.
- Because of the complaint of excessive crying, assess carefully for any bruises or abrasions that could indicate abuse.
- Watch the interaction of the parent and the child.
- If possible, watch the baby being fed.

Diagnostic Procedures

- No diagnostic procedures are indicated. Excessive testing tends to reinforce the parent's belief that the baby has a physical problem that can be treated medically.
- Test for immune globulin subclass profile if immune deficiency is suspected.

DIAGNOSIS

The differential diagnoses for colic include the following:
- Diaper dermatitis
- Otitis media
- Meningitis
- Gastroenteritis
- Child abuse/injury

THERAPEUTIC PLAN
Nonpharmacologic Treatment

- Decrease environmental stimulation during feedings or stressful crying periods.
- Dietary changes are not indicated if diarrhea or vomiting are not present and all physical findings are within normal limits for age. Lucessen, Assendelft, Gubbels, van Eijk, and Douwes (2000) found that in a double-blind trial of hydrolyzed whey formula, a 63-minute decrease in crying time was observed in the experimental group.
- Hold the baby prone, moving back and forth.
- If the colic continues, other treatments can be tried:
  - Elimination of cow's milk products in mother's diet if breastfeeding
  - Formula supplementation to relieve the mother at night

Pharmacologic Treatment

Try simethicone (Mylicon) drops for excessive gas.

Client Education

- Reassure the parents that the condition is self-limiting.
- Comfort measures include the following:
  - Swaddling
  - Holding close during feedings
  - Rubbing the tummy
  - Burping frequently
  - Feeding smaller quantities more frequently
  - Increasing the amount of time the infant is carried
  - Trying sleeping with or in close proximity to the infant
- Other methods to help with a crying bout include the following (Keeler, 2001):
  - Car rides
  - Vacuuming while carrying the infant or near the infant in an infant seat
  - Placement of an infant seat (well-monitored) on a noisy clothes dryer
  - Gentle bouncing/rocking
  - Walking outdoors
  - Any safe activity that uses rhythmic noise and movement (Keeler, 2001)
- Sometimes nothing can be done to stop the crying and the infant just needs to cry for an hour or so.
- Support caregivers by encouraging them to have someone come in and help care for infant when crying occurs.

- Colic may increase stress or cause marital discord. Reassure caregivers that colic is frustrating.
- There is a risk for child abuse/loss of control by parents if crying continues for more than 2 hours.

Referral

None indicated.

EVALUATION/FOLLOW-UP

- Encourage the family to call with a report in 1 to 2 weeks.
- Reassess at each office visit.

REFERENCES

Garrison, M. & Christakis, D. (2001). Early childhood: colic, child development and poisoning prevention. A systematic review of treatments for infant colic. *Pediatrics, 106,* 184-190.

Jan, M. & Al-Buhairi, A. (2001). Is infantile colic a migraine related phenomenon? *Clinical Pediatrics, 40,* 295-297.

Keeler, S. (2001). UNH research sheds light on colicky infants. *Nursing News, 25*(1), 16.

Lucassen, P. L., Assendelft, W. J., Gubbels, J. W., van Eijk, J. T., & Douwes, A. C. (2000). Infantile colic: crying time reduction with a whey hydrolysate: a double blind randomized, placebo controlled trial. *Pediatrics, 106*(6), 1349-1354.

Stein, M. (2001). Beyond infant colic. *Pediatrics, 107*(4), 813-821.

Zickler, C. (2000). Colic. In D. Robinson, P. Kidd, & K. Rogers (Eds.), *Primary care across the lifespan.* (pp. 220-228). St. Louis: Mosby.

Review Questions

1. A mother complains that her 8-week-old son is always crying, especially in the evening. What associated history supports a diagnosis of colic?
- **a.** Smokers in the home
- **b.** Family history of colic
- **c.** Recurrent skin problems in the family
- **d.** Older brother with seasonal allergies

2. The parents bring in their 10-week-old infant. He appears well hydrated, with no wheezing or other problems. What further objective data supports a diagnosis of colic?
- **a.** Abdomen soft with bowel sounds in all four quadrants
- **b.** Painful mass in epigastric area
- **c.** Hard, infrequent bowel movements
- **d.** Anal fissure

3. Appropriate management for a child with colic is which of the following?
- **a.** Antispasmodic and anticholinergic drops (Levsin)
- **b.** Stool softener
- **c.** Simethicone for gas
- **d.** Reassurance for parents that colic is self-limiting

4. After the NP teaches the parents of a child with colic, which of the following indicates that more teaching is needed?
- **a.** "I should not drink cow's milk."

b. "Steve's formula should be more concentrated because he gets so upset."

c. "Prone position with rocking back and forth is an option."

d. "Sitting the child on top of a clothes dryer might help him to quiet down."

5. Knowing that constant crying can be very frustrating for parents, what is the NP's initial recommendation?

a. Take the child on frequent walks in a stroller.

b. Switch to hydrolized whey formula.

c. Use a swaddling technique to wrap the child.

d. Have help when caring for the child, especially during the crying periods.

6. Mary, the NP, notices a swelling on the back of Amy's head (an 8-week-old infant). Her mother stated that Amy cries all the time and is difficult to get to sleep. The swelling raises Mary's suspicions about which of the following?

a. Leukemia

b. Head injury

c. Child abuse

d. Revenge of a sibling

Answers and Rationales

1. *Answer:* **b** (assessment)
Rationale: Colic tends to run in the family (Zickler, 2000).

2. *Answer:* **a** (assessment)
Rationale: The examination for a child with colic tends to be normal. The painful mass in the epigastric area may be significant for pyloric stenosis. An anal fissure could cause crying, as could constipation (Zickler, 2000).

3. *Answer:* **d** (implementation/plan)
Rationale: Most research clinical trials have not demonstrated any clearcut intervention that works for infants with colic (Garrison & Christakis, 2001); reassurance to the parents that nothing is wrong with their child is important.

4. *Answer:* **b** (evaluation)
Rationale: There do not need to be any changes to the concentration of the infant's formula. Sometimes a change from cow formula to soy formula is helpful (Zickler, 2000).

5. *Answer:* **d** (implementation/plan)
Rationale: When a child has colic and is crying for excessive periods, the risk of child abuse increases. It is important for the parents to have help during these periods (Zickler, 2000).

6. *Answer:* **c** (analysis/diagnosis)
Rationale: When a child has colic and is crying for prolonged periods, the NP needs to be alert to the signs/symptoms of child abuse (Zickler, 2000).

COMMON COLD/UPPER RESPIRATORY INFECTION *Pamela Kidd*

OVERVIEW
Definition

A cold, or a URI, is a mild, self-limited viral syndrome involving the upper respiratory tract that lasts 5 to 14 days. It is characterized by mildness of systemic findings (Baum, 1999).

Incidence

The most common acute illness in the industrialized world, a cold is highly contagious. It is a common cause for seeking medical attention and for absences from work and school. The number of colds per year tends to decrease with age, as shown in the following:

- Infants and preschool children: 4 to 8 per year
- School-age children: 2 to 6 per year
- Adults: 2 to 4 per year
- In households with children, adults tend to have higher rates, with the mother having more than the father.

Pathophysiology

The source of the common cold is viral.

Transmission

- Direct physical contact: nasal mucosa to hand to another person's hand to eyes or nasal membranes
- Large and small droplets produced by cough or sneeze

Common Pathogens

The most common pathogens include the following:

- Rhinoviruses: fall, mid-spring to summer
- Coronaviruses: winter

Other common pathogens include the following:

- Parainfluenza: fall, spring
- Respiratory syncytial virus (RSV): winter to early spring
- Influenza: winter

The most common pathogens in infants include the following:

- RSV
- Rhinovirus

Factors Increasing Susceptibility

- Exposure to others with URI

- Poor handwashing
- Sharing of toys among children
- Day care or school attendance
- Children in the home
- Smoking or exposure to environmental tobacco smoke

Protective Factors
- Breastfed infant
- Child cared for at home (not in day care situation)

ASSESSMENT: SUBJECTIVE/HISTORY
Symptoms

Symptoms lasting from 24 to 78 hours include:
- Dry, scratchy throat
- Clear nasal discharge
- Malaise
- Sneezing
- Loss of taste and smell
- Low-grade fever (less than 102° F)
- Redness and inflammation of nasal and pharyngeal membranes

Symptoms lasting 4 to 7 days include the following:
- Cough
- Hoarseness
- Thickening of nasal drainage
- In neonates, minimal respiratory signs and symptoms; nonspecific signs, including poor feeding and lethargy; severe signs include unexpected apnea episode
- In infants, anorexia, vomiting, and diarrhea
- In children, filling of eustachian tubes, causing obstruction and ear pain
- In smokers, more severe symptoms with same outcome

Past Medical History
Uusually noncontributory.

Medication History
Not helpful.

Family History
Ask about any family member with symptoms of a URI.

Dietary History
Not helpful.

ASSESSMENT: OBJECTIVE/PHYSICAL EXAMINATION
Physical Examination

A problem-oriented examination should be performed with special emphasis on the following:
- Tympanic membranes
- Mucous membranes
- Lymph nodes
- Breath sounds

Infants and Children
- Look for signs and symptoms of dehydration.
- Red flags include signs of upper airway obstruction (stridor, drooling, choking, inability to swallow; rule out epiglottis, peritonsillar abscess, retropharyngeal abscess); signs of lower airway obstruction (retractions, grunting, cyanosis, wheezing, tachypnea; rule out pneumonia, asthma, aspiration); severe headache (rule out meningitis, sinusitis, encephalitis, subarachnoid hemorrhage), and petechial or purpuric rash (rule out meningitis).

Diagnostic Procedures
- Sputum culture is done if copious amount of sputum are present; consider acid-fast bacilli (AFB) if tuberculosis is in the differential diagnosis.
- CBC is measured if temperature is elevated.
- Radiographs of sinus are taken if increased nasal congestion with sinus tenderness is present.
- It is difficult and unnecessary to identify the causative virus for management of the common cold.

DIAGNOSIS
Differential diagnoses may include the following:
- Pharyngitis
- Influenza
- Allergic rhinitis
- Lactose intolerance (leads to URI symptoms in infants)

THERAPEUTIC PLAN
Nonpharmacologic Treatment
- Bed rest is not necessary for a more rapid recovery.
- Steam or cool mist liquefies nasal secretions.
- Studies have shown that chicken soup helps to clear nasal secretions.
- Voice rest helps to decrease inflammation of vocal cords, which decreases hoarseness.

Pharmacologic Treatment
Stress that OTC medications may provide comfort but do not shorten the course of the URI.

Aspirin, Ibuprofen, or Acetaminophen
- Relieve body aches and fever.
- Aspirin and acetaminophen have been shown to excrete the virus more quickly from the mucous membranes.
- Aspirin products are not recommended in children younger than age 16.
- Acetaminophen (Tylenol) is the only recommended medication in pregnancy.

Antihistamines
- Chlorpheniramine (4 mg qd or bid)
  - Action: reduces sneezing, nasal mucous production
  - Side effects: drowsiness

- Can be used in controlled hypertension (blood pressure less than 140/90 mm Hg) (Baum, 1999)
- Diphenhydramine (Benadryl)
  - Action: does not differ from placebo effect
  - Side effects: drowsiness
- Triprolidine (Actifed)
  - Action: does not differ from placebo effect
  - Side effects: none
- Astemizole (Hismanal)
  - Action: treats seasonal allergic rhinitis
  - Side effects: weight gain

Decongestants

- Pseudoephedrine/phenylephrine spray or oral preparations
  - Action: congestion, sneezing reduction
  - Side effects: tachycardia, palpitations, elevated diastolic blood pressure, fatigue, dizziness, bladder outlet obstruction
- Pseudoephedrine 60 mg qid (can be used in controlled hypertension [blood pressure less than 140/90 mm Hg])
- Oxymetazoline spray (Dristan, Afrin) (can be used for 3 days only in uncontrolled hypertension [blood pressure higher than 140/90 mm Hg]) (Baum, 1999)
  - Action: improves nasal symptoms
  - Side effects: rebound nasal congestion

Expectorants

- Guaifenesin (400 mg q6h) can be used in controlled or uncontrolled hypertension
  - Action: thins sputum, does not reduce cough
  - Side effects: none

Anticholinergics

- Ipratropium spray (Atrovent aerosol) (Atrovent 2 puffs tid, or saline spray prn can be used in uncontrolled hypertension) (Baum, 1999)
  - Action: reduces sneezing and nasal discharge
  - Side effects: dry throat

Combinations

- Decongestant–antihistamine
  - Action: decreases congestion, postnasal drip, rhinorrhea
  - Side effects: dry mouth, nervousness, insomnia

Steroids

- Steroids (Medrol Dose Pack)
  - Action: reduces inflammation (e.g., vocal cords)
  - Side effects: weight gain, mood alteration

Client Education

- Avoid touching nasal or eye membranes.
- Wash hands after sneezing, coughing, or blowing nose.
- Throw tissues away.
- Cover nose and mouth during sneeze or cough.
- Avoid crowds.
- Do not use nasal preparations for longer than 5 days to avoid rebound congestion.
- Clean toothbrushes or purchase new ones.
- Clean pillow linens.
- Use well-dried pillows (viruses may remain in humid droplets).

Parents

- Do not share toys among children.
- Visitors should wash their hands before handling infant or child.

Referral

Symptoms of upper or lower airway obstruction, severe headache, and purpura/petechial rash should be examined by a physician and, depending on the severity of symptoms, emergency care should be sought.

Infants with apnea episodes should be admitted for observation and evaluation and treatment of RSV. In children and older adults, hospitalization may be required if pneumonia develops.

Prevention

Good handwashing helps prevent the common cold.

EVALUATION/FOLLOW-UP

Return if the following occur:

- Worsening of symptoms
- Increase in fever (higher than 102° F)
- Difficulty breathing, wheezing
- Color change of nasal drainage or sputum

Follow-Up Criteria

- In infants, follow up if fever is higher than 100.5° F. Take temperature rectally if younger than age 3 months.
  - Decreased responsiveness
  - Do not feed well
- In children, follow up if fever is higher than 101° F and persists for 3 or more days.
  - New symptoms develop after 3 to 5 days
  - Lethargic
  - Dyspnea
  - No improvement after 7 to 10 days
- In adults, follow up if symptoms are worse after 3 to 5 days.
  - No improvement after 14 days (Goolsby, 2001)

COMPLICATIONS

- In newborns through age 3 years, otitis media is associated 29% of the time.
- Of the infants who have died of sudden infant death syndrome (SIDS), 90% had cold symptoms reported before death.

● In adults and children, exacerbation of obstructive sleep apnea, disturbed sleep patterns, and bronchospasms are possible.

Refer to *Infants and Children*, p. 135, for more differential diagnoses.

REFERENCES

Baum, T. (1999). Upper respiratory symptoms in elderly patients. *ADVANCE for Nurse Practitioners, 7*(6), 44-48, 75.

Berman, S. & Schmitt, B. D. (1995). Ear, nose, and throat. In W. W. Han, J. R. Groothuis, A. R. Hayward, & M. J. Levin. *Current pediatric diagnosis and treatment* (12th ed., pp. 482-483). Norwalk, CT: Appleton & Lange.

Goolsby, M. J. (2001). Viral upper respiratory infections. *Journal of the American Academy of Nurse Practitioners, 13*(2), 50-54.

Koster, F. T. & Barker, L. R. (1995). Respiratory tract infections. In L. R. Barker, J. R. Burton, & P. D. Zieve (1995). *Principles of ambulatory medicine* (4th ed.). Baltimore: Williams &Wilkins.

Review Questions

1. A mother of a 7-year-old child is worried that her child has too many colds each year. The NP should reassure her by saying which of the following?

   a. It is probably allergies.
   b. It will get worse before it gets better; the number of colds increases during adolescence.
   c. The child should have between 2 to 6 colds a year.
   d. Give the child a flu shot each fall.

2. A mother asks how she can help prevent her child from experiencing a cold. The NP suggests which of the following?

   a. Avoid fans.
   b. Dress warmly.
   c. Avoid tobacco smoke.
   d. Wipe child's hands with rubbing alcohol.

3. Which of the following signs or symptoms may indicate a cold in a neonate?

   a. Tugging at ears
   b. Poor feeding
   c. More wet diapers
   d. Decrease of stool

4. A mother believes that the use of diphenhydramine (Benadryl) cured her 6-year-old son's cold. What should the NP say?

   a. Aspirin is the preferred agent because it causes excretion of the virus more quickly.
   b. OTC medications shorten the course of a cold.
   c. Benadryl reduces nasal congestion.
   d. OTC medications provide comfort only.

5. Which of the following statements is evidence of effective teaching of a client with a URI?

   a. "I will only use my Dristan nasal spray for 1 week."
   b. "I will get a new toothbrush."
   c. "I will avoid touching my ears."
   d. "I will smoke outside only."

Answers and Rationales

1. *Answer:* c (implementation/plan)
   Rationale: Allergies are not to be taken lightly and produce concern in parents. The number of colds decreases with age. A flu shot prevents influenza and is not recommended in children unless they are immunocompromised or living with a high-risk individual with a greater likelihood of experiencing a negative outcome postflu.

2. *Answer:* c (implementation/plan)
   Rationale: Avoiding fans and dressing warmly are not supported with research findings as ways to prevent a cold. Handwashing does prevent colds, but alcohol is a drying agent and could produce irritation. Exposure to environmental tobacco smoke does increase cold susceptibility.

3. *Answer:* b (assessment)
   Rationale: Ear pain occurs from pressure in the eustachian tubes. These are not well developed in the neonate. A change in bladder and bowel habits is not associated with colds. Poor feeding may indicate nasal congestion and drainage, which are associated with colds.

4. *Answer:* d (implementation/plan)
   Rationale: OTC medications do not shorten the course of the URI, but they do provide comfort. Aspirin does promote excretion of the virus from the mucous membranes, but it should not be used in a child younger than 16 years of age. Benadryl is an antihistamine, not a decongestant.

5. *Answer:* b (evaluation)
   Rationale: Nasal decongestant sprays should not be used for more than 5 days to avoid rebound congestion. Toothbrushes should be cleaned or discarded to prevent reinfection. Smoking increases susceptibility for a URI regardless of where one smokes. One should avoid touching the nose or eyes.

CONGENITAL HEART DEFECTS *Denise Robinson*

OVERVIEW
Definition

A congenital heart defect (CHD) is a cardiac lesion present in neonates.

Incidence

Approximately 8 in 1000 of all neonates are born with a congenital heart defect. This includes lesions diagnosed later in life.

Types

Acyanotic Heart Defects. Congenital heart defects in which no deoxygenated or poorly oxygenated blood enters the systemic circulation are acyanotic. Types include the following:

- Left-to-right shunting through abnormal opening:
  - Patent ductus arteriosis (PDA)
  - Atrial septal defect (ASD)
  - Ventricular septal defect (VSD)
- Obstructive lesions that restrict ventricular outflow:
  - Aortic valvular lesions
  - Pulmonary artery stenosis
  - Coarctation of the aorta

Cyanotic Heart Defects. Congenital heart defects in which deoxygenated blood enters the systemic circulation are cyanotic. Types include the following:

- Right-to-left-shunting:
  - Tetralogy of Fallot
  - Tricuspid atresia
  - Transposition of great arteries (TGA)
  - Truncus arteriosus
  - Hypoplastic left heart syndrome
  - Total anomalous pulmonary venous communication

Risk Factors

- Fetal and maternal infection during the first trimester (especially rubella) (increased risk of PDA)
- Maternal alcoholism
- Maternal use of other drugs with teratogenic effects (indomethacin)
- Maternal age older than 40 years
- Maternal dietary deficiencies
- Maternal insulin-dependent diabetes
- Residence at high altitudes (PDA)
- Other congenital defects with abnormalities of other system and those with abnormal karyotypes
- History of heart disease in a first-degree relative

NOTE: *All children with congenital heart lesions should be followed closely by cardiology or cardiothoracic specialists.*

Information is provided to review the lesions, presenting symptoms, and diagnostic findings. Treatment options are discussed briefly as a point of interest; it is not necessary to be familiar with specifics of diagnostics or treatment because most NPs are not primary caregivers of these clients.

Acyanotic Lesions—Patent Ductus Arteriosus

OVERVIEW
Definition

PDA is the persistent patency of the fetal structure bridging the pulmonary artery and the descending aorta. Two types of shunting are possible. One is left-to-right shunting, in which CHF is possible, depending on the size of the PDA. The other is right-to-left shunting, in which oxygenation is a problem.

Incidence

In term infants the ductus arteriosus usually closes at birth. PDA accounts for between 2% and 5% of symptomatic cardiac diseases seen in the first 28 days. Premature infants of less than 34 weeks' gestational age have a significantly higher incidence of PDA in conjunction with respiratory distress syndrome.

Pathophysiology

Factors that influence ductal patency include the following:
- Muscle mass
- Low oxygen tension (living at high altitudes)
- Low pH
- Acetylcholine
- Prostaglandin E_2
- Catecholamines
- Bradykinin
- Exposure to rubella during first trimester

ASSESSMENT: SUBJECTIVE/HISTORY
History of Present Illness

- Difficulty in feeding is common.
- Tachypnea, sweating, and subcostal retraction may occur.
- Feeding takes longer than 30 minutes.

ASSESSMENT: OBJECTIVE/PHYSICAL EXAMINATION
Physical Examination

A physical examination should be conducted, with particular attention to the following:

- Take blood pressure.
- Determine pulse pressure.
- Obtain vital signs.
- Determine weight.
- Observe general appearance.
- Assess respiratory and cardiac status.
- Assess circulatory status. Bounding pulses with wide pulse pressure, hyperactive precordium, enlarged heart, and pulmonary edema can all be signs of decompensation.
- Assess cardiac status. A continuous "machinery" grade I to IV/VI murmur also may be audible at the upper left sternal border or left intraclavicular area, S_3, rales.
- If the murmur is heard within the first 24 hours, the risk of CHD is 1 in 12, and PDA is usually the underlying defect.
- Assess urinary status. Decreased urinary output may be seen.
- Assess extremities for femoral and brachial pulses.

Diagnostic Procedures

- ECG with Doppler detects the structural defect.
- Chest radiograph findings depend on the direction of flow across the PDA and on the degree of the shunt.
- ECG findings may be normal or reveal left ventricular hypertrophy in small to moderate PDAs.
- Obtain pulse oximetry measure.
- Perform MRI.

DIAGNOSIS

Differential diagnoses include the following:
- Noncardiogenic pulmonary edema
- Respiratory distress syndrome
- ASD
- VSD

THERAPEUTIC PLAN

- Client may be free of symptoms and in hemodynamically stable condition with a small PDA; this requires no immediate intervention.
- Client should be monitored closely for any respiratory or hemodynamic instability.
- In clients with symptoms and hemodynamic instability, surgical ligation is the treatment of choice.

Acyanotic Lesions—Atrial Septal Defects

OVERVIEW
Definition

An ASD is an opening between the two atria that permits the shunting or mixing of blood. The overall rate of spontaneous closure of the secundum type of atrial defect is 87% in the first 4 years of life. Most children with ASD remain asymptomatic.

Incidence

ASD occurs in approximately 10% of clients with CHD. It is twice as common in females as in males.

Pathophysiology

There is no pressure differential between the right and left sides of the heart during the first month of life as a result of relatively elevated pulmonary artery pressures. As the right-sided pressures begin to fall, more blood is shunted along the path of least resistance from both atria into the right ventricle and pulmonary vessels. This creates an increased volume load on the right ventricle. Excessive flow passes through the pulmonic valve, creating a relative pulmonic stenosis with a concomitant murmur. It also leads to right-sided heart failure. In addition, over time this may lead to pulmonary hypertension as a result of high blood flow through the pulmonary arteries.

ASSESSMENT: SUBJECTIVE/HISTORY

Client may have no symptoms or may demonstrate varying degrees of right-sided heart failure. Older children are seen with fatigue, shortness of breath, and poor growth and development.

ASSESSMENT: OBJECTIVE/PHYSICAL EXAMINATION
Physical Examination

A physical examination should be conducted with particular attention to general appearance and cardiac status. Note the following:
- Observe general appearance. Note FTT and cyanosis with pulmonary hypertension only.
- Assess cardiac status. Arterial pulses are normal and equal; the heart is hyperactive, with heave best felt at left lower sternal border; S_2 is widely split and fixed at pulmonic area, with no thrills; a grade I to III/VI systolic ejection murmur (SEM) is heard best at the left sternal border.

Diagnostic Procedures

- ECG shows right axis deviation, right ventricular hypertrophy, and right atrial enlargement.
- Chest radiograph demonstrates cardiac enlargement, with the main pulmonary artery dilated.
- ECG shows paradoxic motion of the ventricular septal wall and a dilated right ventricular cavity.
- Cardiac catheterization reveals a significant increase in oxygen saturation at the atrial level. Pulmonary pressures are normal or elevated.

THERAPEUTIC PLAN

Surgery is recommended for clients with a ratio of pulmonary to systemic blood flow greater than 2:1. Elective surgery is performed in clients between ages 2 and 4 years. Early surgery is recommended for infants with CHF or critical pulmonary hypertension.

Acyanotic Lesions—Ventricular Septal Defects

OVERVIEW
Definition

A VSD is an opening between the two ventricles permitting the shunting or mixing of blood. Defects may occur in the membranous, muscular, or apical portions of the ventricular septum.

Incidence

VSD is the most common form of congenital cardiac heart defect, representing 20% to 25% overall. From 30% to 50% of all VSDs close spontaneously. From 60% to 70% of small defects also close.

Pathophysiology

There is only a slight pressure difference between the right and left ventricles during the first month of life as a result of relatively elevated pulmonary artery pressures. Therefore there is little flow across the VSD and only a slight murmur is heard. As the right-sided pressures begin to fall, more blood is shunted along the path of least resistance from the left ventricle into the right ventricle and pulmonary vessels. As the pressure gradient increases, turbulence of circulation between the two ventricles increases and creates a louder murmur. It also creates an increased volume load on the right ventricle and left atrium. This leads to biventricular failure or right-sided heart failure. In addition, in time this may lead to pulmonary hypertension as a result of high blood flow through the pulmonary arteries.

ASSESSMENT: SUBJECTIVE/HISTORY
Symptoms

- Acyanosis
- Frequent respiratory infections during infancy or early childhood
- Dyspnea
- Exercise or feeding intolerance
- Edema
- Abdominal distention
- Fatigue

Past Medical History

Ask about frequent respiratory infections, as noted previously.

Dietary History

Inquire about feeding intolerance and high salt intake if edema is present.

ASSESSMENT: OBJECTIVE/PHYSICAL EXAMINATION
Physical Examination

A problem-oriented physical examination should be conducted with particular attention to vital signs and weight, general appearance, respiratory status, and cardiac status.

- Assess general status. Many children demonstrate FTT, with slow growth and poor weight gain. Some even may demonstrate developmental delay. This is predominantly caused by CHF, which develops between 1 and 4 months.
- Assess respiratory status. Signs of respiratory distress include grunting, flaring, retracting, and increased respiratory rate. Inspiratory rales and expiratory wheezing may occur.
- Assess cardiac status. The degree of symptoms varies depending on the size of the shunt.
  - Small left-to-right shunts (grade II or III pansystolic murmur, left sternal border)
  - Moderate left-to-right shunts (grade III to IV/VI harsh, pansystolic murmur, lower left sternal border at fourth intracostal space; no heaves, lifts or thrills)

Diagnostic Procedures

- ECG is normal in most cases.
- Chest radiograph also may vary according to the size of the shunt.
- ECG identifies VSDs larger than 4 mm only.
- Angiography shows normal to increased left atrial pressures.
- Pulmonary vascular resistance varies from normal to markedly increased.

DIAGNOSIS

Differential diagnoses may include the following:
- ASD
- Tetralogy of Fallot (the acyanotic type, "pink tet")
- PDA

THERAPEUTIC PLAN

If the client does not respond to selective therapy, has growth failure, or has increasing pulmonary hypertension, surgery is indicated. Age at elective surgery ranges from younger than age 2 to age 5 years. Postoperative complications include conduction defects, such as right bundle branch block.

Acyanotic Lesions—Obstructive Lesions: Coarctation

OVERVIEW
Definition

Coarctation is a constricture of the aorta most commonly (98%) surrounding the insertion site of the ductus arteriosus into the descending thoracic aorta.

Incidence

Coarctation occurs in 0.2 per 1000 live births, with a male predominance of almost 2 to 1. As the eighth most common defect among all age groups, it is seen frequently in infancy when collateral circulation is poor.

Pathophysiology

Left ventricular outflow tract obstruction occurs with development of left ventricular hypertrophy and eventually CHF.

Factors Increasing Susceptibility. One parent with coarctation increases susceptibility.

Other Associated Defects
- Bicuspid aortic valve
- VSD
- PDA
- TGA
- Hypoplastic left ventricle

ASSESSMENT: SUBJECTIVE/HISTORY

Most common symptoms include the following:
- Dyspnea
- Tachypnea
- Irritability
- Feeding difficulties
- Tachycardia
- FTT
- Cool lower extremities with decreased pulses
- Ashen color
- Cyanosis

These symptoms are typically not present until 2 weeks of age. Circulatory shock, as demonstrated by oliguria, anuria, or any of the symptoms listed previously, may not appear until 2 to 6 weeks of age. Relatively symptom-free children may report leg pains only.

ASSESSMENT: OBJECTIVE/PHYSICAL EXAMINATION

Physical Examination

Attention should focus on four-extremity blood pressure, vital signs, weight, and general appearance. Classic clinical signs of coarctation are a higher blood pressure in the arms than in the legs and pulses that are bounding in the arms but decreased in the legs—typically, upper extremity blood pressure higher than that of lower extremities by more than 10 mm Hg.
- *Respiratory:* pulmonary rales
- *Circulatory:* mild periorbital edema, dorsum hand and feet edema
- *Cardiac:* SEM most common at left sternal border; frequent hypertension from poor renal perfusion
- *Hepatic:* hepatosplenomegaly
- *Renal:* oliguria or anuria

Diagnostic Procedures
- ECG reveals left ventricular hypertrophy for mild cases and right axis deviation with right ventricular hypertrophy in more severe forms.
- Chest radiograph shows normal or enlarged heart.
- Two-dimensional (2-D) echocardiography shows shelf-like narrowing of descending aorta.
- Cardiac catheterization measures an increased pressure gradient or pressure drop across the coarctation.

DIAGNOSIS

Differential diagnoses include the following:
- Hypoplastic left heart syndrome
- CHF

THERAPEUTIC PLAN

The plan of care depends on whether a client has symptoms. Observe for increasing symptoms. In some cases balloon angioplasty may be necessary. The surgical options of choice include resection of the coarctated segment with an end-to-end anastomosis.

Cyanotic Congenital Heart Defects

When pulmonary disorders are the cause of cyanosis, administration of O_2 increases saturation to at least 95%. In clients with cyanotic CHD, oxygen saturation increases only to 80% to 85%.

Cyanotic Congenital Heart Defects— Transposition of the Great Arteries

OVERVIEW
Definition

TGA is defined as a switch of the origin of the great arteries from their normal ventricular origins so that the aorta originates from the right ventricle and the pulmonary artery arises from the left ventricle.

Incidence

Prevalence is 2 in 10,000 live births, representing the second most common defect in the first year of life.

Pathophysiology

The aorta and pulmonary arteries are transposed, so that the two circulations are separate and parallel rather than in sequence. The infant with transposition depends on the opening of the ductus arteriosus; this allows the mixing of the blood for the survival of the infant.

Associated Factors
- Male (3 to 1)
- Normal to slightly increased birthweight
- No maternal or fetal distress

Associated Defects

- VSD
- Tricuspid regurgitation
- Pulmonic stenosis

ASSESSMENT: OBJECTIVE/PHYSICAL EXAMINATION

Physical Examination

- Assess general status. Infant is normal or large at birth; however, a growth and developmental delay is seen if the condition remains undetected.
- Assess circulatory status. Baseline cyanosis increases with crying and has little or no response to increased inspired oxygen. Clubbing of the digits is seen.
- Assess cardiac status. The S_2 is single and loud. When auscultating, no murmur is audible if ventricular septum is intact. CHF may be present.

Diagnostic Procedures

- Chest radiograph indicates right axis deviation and right ventricular hypertrophy, "egg on a string" appearance.
- Electrolytes indicate hypoglycemia, hypocalcemia, and acidosis.

DIAGNOSIS

Differential diagnoses includes the following:
- Truncus arteriosus
- Hypoplastic right ventricle syndrome
- Hypoplastic left ventricle syndrome
- Double-outlet right ventricle
- Double-outlet left ventricle

THERAPEUTIC PLAN

Before surgical intervention, temporizing measures include infusion of prostaglandin E_1, to maintain patency of the ductus arteriosus, and treatment of CHF. The treatment is the arterial switch operation, in which the aorta and pulmonary artery are divided and reattached to their proper positions. The survival rate after the switch procedure is 82%.

Cyanotic Congenital Heart Defects—Tetralogy of Fallot

OVERVIEW

Definition

Tetralogy of Fallot is a congenital heart disease consisting of four different abnormalities, including pulmonary stenosis or atresia (outflow tract obstruction), large VSD, right ventricular hypertrophy, and overriding or dextroposition of aorta.

Incidence

Tetralogy of Fallot accounts for 10% to 15% of all congenital heart disease, representing the most prevalent form of heart disease beyond infancy. Incidence is the same for males and females.

Pathophysiology

Severe right ventricular outflow tract obstruction coupled with a large VSD results in a right-to-left shunt at the ventricular level, with subsequent desaturation of arterial blood. The size of the shunt determines the degree of desaturation and amount of cyanosis. The greater the obstruction, the larger the VSD; the lower the systemic vascular resistance, the greater the right-to-left shunt noted. Therefore right ventricular pressure cannot surpass left ventricular pressure, but they may be equal.

Associated Defects

- Right-sided aortic arch, 25%
- ASD, 15%

ASSESSMENT: SUBJECTIVE/HISTORY

Most common symptoms include the following:
- Dyspnea is experienced on exertion.
- Cyanosis is present, especially during vagal maneuvers.
- Tet spells occur, causing hyperpnea, irritability, cyanosis, and decreased murmur intensity.
- Squatting decreases venous systemic return by trapping blood in the legs, breaking the overloading hypoxia cycle

ASSESSMENT: OBJECTIVE/PHYSICAL EXAMINATION

Physical Examination

A physical examination should be conducted with particular attention to vital signs, weight, general appearance, and the following:
- Assess respiratory status. Client may have hypoxic spells, peaking at 2 to 4 months. These begin with rapid and deep respirations, followed by irritability with crying.
- Cyanosis and heart murmur intensity decrease. An intense spell can lead to limpness, seizures, cerebrovascular accident (CVA), or even death. Death during a cyanotic spell is extremely rare.
- Assess cardiac status. Look for a thrill at lower left sternal border, aortic ejection click, normal S_1, loud and single S_2, III to V/VI SEM at middle to upper left sternal border.

Diagnostic Procedures

- CBC shows polycythemia, iron-deficiency anemia with normal hematocrit, and coagulopathies.

- ECG shows right axis displacement and right ventricular hypertrophy. Rhythm disturbances occasionally occur.
- Chest radiograph shows decreased pulmonary vascular markings. Heart size is normal overall, but CHF may be present in acyanotic clients. The classic finding of a boot-shaped heart is due to a normal heart size with significant right ventricular hypertrophy and upturning of the apex of the heart. Right aortic arch may be present in 25% of clients.
- A 2-D echocardiography reveals a large PDA and overriding of the aorta. Doppler studies confirm antegrade pulmonary flow or continuous or diastolic pulmonary flow. A VSD also is seen.

DIAGNOSIS

Differential diagnoses include the following:

- Severe valvular pulmonic stenosis with intact ventricular septum
- Truncus arteriosus with decreased pulmonary flow
- Double-outlet right ventricle
- TGA with subpulmonic stenosis, VSD, and tricuspid atresia

THERAPEUTIC PLAN

- Diagnose and treat iron-deficiency anemia because clients are predisposed toward CVAs.
- Prescribe prophylactic treatment for subacute bacterial endocarditis.

Palliative Treatment

- Detect and treat hypoxic spells.
- Propanol decreases heart rate and may increase stroke volume.
- Prostaglandin E_1 is indicated for severe cyanosis and ductal dependence in infancy.
- Atrial septostomy is performed by means of cardiac catheterization.
- Surgical procedure is shunt insertion to allow flow to bypass the obstructive lesion to the lungs.

Definitive Treatment

Closure of VSD with removal of ventricular outflow obstruction frequently results in rhythm disturbances.

Cyanotic Congenital Heart Defects—Truncus Arteriosus

OVERVIEW
Definition

Truncus arteriosus is a condition in which the arterial trunk arises out of both ventricles in fetal life and later divides into the aorta and the pulmonary artery with the development of the bulbar septum.

Incidence

Truncus arteriosus accounts for less than 1% of all cases of CHD. Occurrence is 3 in 100,000 live births, with frequency more in females than in males.

Pathophysiology

Associated defects include the following:

- Large VSD
- Right aortic arch in 50% of cases
- DiGeorge syndrome should be considered in any infant with this defect.

ASSESSMENT: OBJECTIVE/PHYSICAL EXAMINATION
Physical Examination

A physical examination should be conducted with particular attention to vital signs, weight, general appearance, and the following:

- Assess circulatory status. Variable degrees of cyanosis may be present after birth.
- Assess respiratory status. Signs of CHF may develop within several weeks.
- Assess cardiac status. A harsh grade II to IV/VI systolic murmur, similar to VSD, that can go into diastole may be present at the upper left sternal border. An apical diastolic rumble with or without gallop may be present if pulmonary blood flow is large. A constant ejection click, bounding pulses, and wide pulse pressure may be present.

Diagnostic Procedures

- ABGs show mild desaturation, with little improvement with hyperoxia.
- ECG shows electrographic signs of CHF in 70% of cases.
- Chest radiograph shows cardiomegaly (biventricular and left atrial enlargement), narrow mediastinum, and increased pulmonary blood flow. Right aortic arch is present 50% of the time.
- A 2-D echocardiography reveals large PDA right under truncal valve.

DIAGNOSIS

Differential diagnoses include the following:

- TGA
- Hypoplastic right ventricle syndrome
- Hypoplastic left ventricle syndrome
- Double-outlet right ventricle
- Double-outlet left ventricle

THERAPEUTIC PLAN

Diuretics and digoxin are required to decrease pulmonary congestion. Cardiac catheterization demonstrates the abnormal anatomy as well as the hemodynamics and pressures. It can determine the size and branching pattern of the main pulmonary artery. An aortogram rules out truncal insufficiency and major stenosis in pulmonary arteries.

Early surgical repair is the treatment of choice. Most infants die of CHF between ages 6 and 12 months unless surgery is performed.

General Care Strategies for Congenital Heart Defects

When caring for a client with a CHD in either the preoperative or postoperative period, some simple principles should be followed to ensure optimized care. The three major areas of concern are worsened CHF, increased shunt, and inadequate surgical correction. These can be followed up easily with careful histories and physical examinations. Parents also should be alerted to these same signs so that they can seek the earliest possible care to correct the problem. If an infant is experiencing a hypoxic spell, place the infant over the shoulder in the knee-chest position.

ASSESSMENT: SUBJECTIVE/HISTORY

The history should concentrate on the following:
- Respiratory status
  - Shortness of breath
  - Dyspnea
  - Inability to feed
  - Cyanosis (at rest or exacerbating factors)
  - Cough
  - Retractions
  - Grunting
  - Flaring
- Cardiovascular status
  - Sweating
  - Cyanosis
  - Pallor
  - Increased facial ruddiness
  - Increasing head size
  - Limb discrepancies
  - Mottling
  - Increasing edema
- Abdominal status
  - Increased abdominal girth
  - Vomiting
  - Constipation
  - Diarrhea
- Renal status: decreased wet diapers or decreased urination
- Neurologic status
  - Lethargy
  - Irritability
  - Seizures
  - Disorientation
  - Developmental delay (inability to achieve milestones)

Family History

Determine if any first-degree relatives have heart disease.

ASSESSMENT: OBJECTIVE/PHYSICAL EXAMINATION
Physical Examination

The physical examination should concentrate on the following:
- Vital signs/general status
  - FTT/poor weight and height gain (acyanotic lesions tend to jeopardize weight gain, whereas cyanotic lesions affect both height and weight)
  - Tachypnea
  - Tachycardia
  - Hypotension
  - Hypertension
- Respiratory status
  - Shortness of breath
  - Dyspnea
  - Cyanosis (at rest or exacerbating factors)
  - Cough
  - Retractions
  - Grunting
  - Flaring
  - Inspiratory rales
  - Wheezing
- Cardiovascular status
  - Murmur changes
  - Decreased pulses
  - Decreased capillary refill
  - Sweating
  - Cyanosis
  - Pallor
  - Increased facial ruddiness
  - Increasing head size
  - Limb discrepancies, mottling, and edema
- Abdominal status: hepatosplenomegaly (a cardinal sign of right heart failure)
- Neurologic status
  - Lethargy
  - Irritability
  - Seizures
  - Disorientation
  - Developmental delay (inability to achieve milestones)
- Extremities: clubbing of fingers and toes, edema

THERAPEUTIC PLAN

Adequate nutrition is extremely important for infants with CHD. If the child is not able to gain weight, supplementation with a high caloric, nocturnal enteral feeding or continuous 24-hour feeding is indicated. A caloric intake of 140 to 200 calories/kg/day in addition to the regular amount of calories are needed to induce catchup growth. In most clients, growth is caught up within 6-12 months after surgery.

- Routine childhood immunizations should be scheduled.
- More frequent evaluations are needed if CHF is present.
- These children should receive the measles-mumps-rubella and varicella vaccines at age 12 months.
- Influenza should be given yearly beginning at age 6 months.
- Pneumococcal 7-valent conjugate vaccine (Prevnar) should be given according to schedule.
- Children should receive prophylaxis against bacterial endocarditis when undergoing certain procedures, according to the American Heart Association recommendations.
- Assess activity on an individual basis. Graded exercise testing should be done before athletic endeavors. Children with severe forms of CHD, aortic stenosis, and coarctation of the aorta with residual hypertension are at risk for sudden death during exercise. In the absence of pulmonary hypertension, ASD, VSD and PDA are usually asymptomatic.

EVALUATION/FOLLOW-UP

During follow-up appointments, the client always must be evaluated for recurrence of symptoms.

REFERENCES

Bernstein, D. (1996). The transitional circulation. In W. Nelson, R. Behrman, R. Kliegman, & A. Arvin (Eds.), *Nelson textbook of pediatrics* (15th ed., pp. 1283-1335). Philadelphia: Saunders.

Korones, S. & Bada-Ellzey, H. (1993). *Neonatal decision making.* St. Louis: Mosby.

Saenz, R., Beebe, D. & Triplett, L. (1999). Caring for infants with congenital heart disease and their families. *American Family Physician.* Retrieved May 28, 2002, from http://www.aafp.org/afp/990401ap/1857.html.

Suddaby, E. (2001). Contemporary thinking for congenital heart disease. *Pediatric Nursing, 27*(3), 233-238, 270.

Wolfe, R., Boucek, M., Schaffer, M., & Wiggins, J. (1999). Cardiovascular diseases. In W. Hay, A. Hayward, M. Levin, & J. Sondheimer (Eds.), *Current pediatric diagnosis and treatment* (14th ed., pp. 465-527). Stamford, CT: Appleton & Lange.

Review Questions

1. All the following are signs of CHF in an infant except:
   a. Sweating during feedings
   b. Tachycardia
   c. FTT
   d. Cyanosis

2. At birth an infant is noted to be cyanotic with respiratory distress. The test most specific for detection of congenital heart disease is which of the following?
   a. Physical examination for a heart murmur
   b. Chest radiograph
   c. Echocardiography
   d. ABG analysis

3. Steve is 4-year-old who had a CHD with successful surgery. You are seeing him in the office with complaints of a swollen tooth and abscess. He is scheduled for a dental appointment in 2 days. You order penicillin (Pen Vee K) for him as prophylaxis for which of the following?
   a. Otitis media
   b. Sinusitis
   c. Bacterial endocarditis
   d. Appendicitis

4. A 5-year-old boy is seen for his preschool physical examination and is noted to have cool lower extremities with weak pulses and hypertension (blood pressure 164/92 mm Hg). Initial tests to examine for possible coarctation of the aorta include all the following except:
   a. Four-extremity blood pressures
   b. ECG
   c. Chest radiograph
   d. GXT

5. In evaluation of TGA, the classic chest radiograph reveals which of the following?
   a. A figure of 3
   b. A snowman in a snowstorm
   c. A boot
   d. An egg on a string

6. A child (with cyanotic CHD) presents in your office with tachypnea. You are not sure whether it is pulmonary or cardiac in origin. When you apply oxygen to the child, the oxygen saturation increases to within a normal range. This indicates that the problem is most likely which of the following?
   a. Pulmonary in origin
   b. Cardiac in origin
   c. Diaphragmatic in origin
   d. Neurologic in origin

7. Physical findings consistent with a clinically significant ASD include all the following except:
   a. Hypertension
   b. A murmur consistent with pulmonic stenosis
   c. FTT
   d. Normal pulses

8. Which of the following CHDs is considered cyanotic?
   a. ASD
   b. VSD
   c. Transposition of the great vessels
   d. PDA

Answers and Rationales

1. **Answer: d** (assessment)
   Rationale: Although it can be associated with CHF, cyanosis is a sign of shunting of blood from the right to the left side of the heart without oxygenation in the lungs. Signs of CHF in an infant include tachycardia, tachypnea, FTT, sweating, oliguria, edema, lethargy, respiratory distress, pallor, coughing,

seizures, developmental delay, and hepatosplenomegaly (Saenz, Beebe, & Triplett, 1999).

2. *Answer:* **c** (analysis/diagnosis)

Rationale: Heart murmurs are very common in the neonatal period and either may represent congenital heart lesions or may be simple benign flow murmurs. This is an extremely nonspecific test. Although chest radiograph and ABGs can assist in the assessment of cyanosis and dyspnea, they fail to distinguish between pulmonary and cardiac primary lesions (Saenz, Beebe, & Triplett, 1999). ECG can be used to visualize the heart and to examine blood flow and to estimate pressures within the chambers and overall ventricular function. Therefore this is the most specific of the examinations listed and is superseded only by the highly invasive procedures of cardiac catheterization and direct observation of the heart for true specificity.

3. *Answer:* **c** (evaluation)

Rationale: Children who have had surgery for CHD should receive prophylaxis for bacterial endocarditis before procedures (Saenz, Beebe, & Triplett, 1999).

4. *Answer:* **d** (analysis/diagnosis)

Rationale: Coarctation of the aorta essentially can be diagnosed with simple tests that can be performed in the office, such as four-extremity blood pressures to examine for significant blood pressure discrepancies between the upper and lower extremities. ECG and chest radiograph add evidence of left-sided heart failure with this obstructive lesion. GXT is not appropriate unless there is evidence of myocardial ischemia (Saenz, Beebe, & Triplett, 1999).

5. *Answer:* **d** (analysis/diagnosis)

Rationale: Although chest radiograph frequently does not demonstrate clearcut findings, it does demonstrate many

features of the classic picture. A figure of 3 is seen with coarctation of the aorta as the stricture narrows the aorta at a single fixed location. The snowman in the snowstorm represents the extreme heart failure and pulmonary edema seen in total anomalous pulmonary venous return. The boot is the right ventricular hypertrophy and lack of pulmonary blood flow in tetralogy of Fallot. The egg on the string in TGA represents significant CHF with a narrowed mediastinum as a result of alignment of the great vessels in the midline.

6. *Answer:* **a** (analysis/diagnosis)

Rationale: When oxygen is applied to a child with cyanotic CHD, the saturation only goes to approximately 80% to 85%. In this case the saturation goes to within normal limits, so it must be pulmonic in origin (Saenz, Beebe, & Triplett, 1999).

7. *Answer:* **a** (assessment)

Rationale: Initially, ASDs can go undetected until pulmonic pressures decrease. As right ventricular overload occurs, the client has increased flow across the pulmonic valve and a murmur of relative stenosis. Left ventricular output remains within normal limits until extremely late in the disease process. Therefore pulses and blood pressure remain normal. As ventricular failure progresses, clients fail to thrive as they expend increased energy to maintain normal metabolism (Wolfe, Boucek, Schaffer, et al., 1999).

8. *Answer:* **c** (analysis/diagnosis)

Rationale: Transposition of the great vessels is considered a cyanotic heart defect. The others are all acyanotic (Saenz, Beebe, & Triplett, 1999).

CONGESTIVE HEART FAILURE   *Pamela Kidd*

OVERVIEW
Definition

Congestive heart failure occurs when the heart is unable to maintain an output adequate to meet the metabolic demands of the body.

Incidence

- In the United States, 2 million people have CHF.
- Each year 400,000 new cases are diagnosed.
- The 6-year mortality rate is 80% for men and 65% for women.
- CHF is the most common inpatient diagnosis.

Pathophysiology

Symptoms occur as a result of organ hypoperfusion and inadequate tissue oxygen delivery caused by a decreased

cardiac output and decreased cardiac reserve and pulmonary and venous congestion.

Systolic dysfunction (ejection fraction less than 40%, depressed contraction of myocardium [Fletcher & Thomas, 2001]) is associated with AMI.

- Inotropic abnormalities
- Decreased systolic emptying

Pathology of diastolic dysfunction (impaired filling caused by loss of myocardium elasticity associated with hypertension) is related to compensatory mechanisms.

- Left ventricular dilatation and hypertrophy
- Increase in systemic vascular resistance related to activation of the sympathetic nervous system and an increase in catecholamines
- Activation of the renin-angiotensin system

The primary cause of CHF during the first 3 years of life is congenital heart disease.

Factors Increasing Susceptibility
- Fluid overload/increased salt intake in clients with coronary artery disease (CAD)/hypertension
- Lack of adherence to medications

Protective Factors. Getting regular exercise, eating a low-fat diet, and not smoking all protect against CHF.

ASSESSMENT: SUBJECTIVE/HISTORY
Symptoms

- Dyspnea on exertion
- Orthopnea with paroxysmal nocturnal dyspnea (PND)
- Edema
- Decreased exercise capacity
- Dry, hacky cough
- Fatigue
- Recent weight gain
- Bloating or abdominal fullness
- Change in mental status (mainly in older adults)

Children
- Feeding difficulties
- FTT

Past Medical History

- CAD
- COPD
- Renal disease
- Diabetes
- Hypertension
- Previous MI
- Valvular disease
- Anemia (severe)
- Thyroid disease
- Cardiomyopathy
- Arrhythmias
- Pregnancy
- Congenital heart disease

Medication History

Medications (e.g., beta blockers, calcium-channel blockers, or NSAIDs) can induce CHF through decreased heart rate and increased fluid retention, respectively.

Family History

Ask about a history of CAD, HPT, or diabetes mellitus.

Dietary History

- Inquire about a recent increase in the use of sodium.
- Ask about increased consumption of fluids in clients with previous decompensated heart failure and known left ventricular dysfunction.
- Ask about fat content of diet.

ASSESSMENT: OBJECTIVE/PHYSICAL EXAMINATION
Physical Examination

A problem-oriented examination should be performed with attention to the following areas:
- Assess vital signs, weight, and general appearance.
  - Client may be hypotensive, normotensive, or hypertensive.
  - Pulse rate may be tachycardic.
  - Weight may be increased (it is important to assess the time span in which the weight gain occurred).
- Assess neck. Jugular venous distention may be present.
- Assess chest for the following:
  - Basilar crackles (rales) that do not clear with cough
  - Wheezes
  - Cough
  - Respiratory distress in children
- Assess cardiac status for the following:
  - S_3 gallop
  - Laterally displaced point of maximal impulse
  - Murmur
- Assess abdomen for the following:
  - Hepatomegaly
  - Hepatojugular reflex
- Assess extremities for peripheral edema.
- The most specific diagnostic physical findings in a client with symptoms include S_3 and ventricular gallop for ventricular overload/systolic dysfunction. S_4, atrial gallop, and pulsus alternans (alternating weaker and stronger pulses in peripheral arteries) are most characteristic of diastolic dysfunction (Shamsham & Mitchell, 2000).

Diagnostic Procedures

- Perform chest x-ray examination to check for cardiomegaly, pulmonary venous congestion (butterfly pattern), and Kerley B lines (horizontal lines representing dilated and thickened interlobar septa).
- Perform ECG to check for ischemia, arrhythmias, conduction abnormalities, and left ventricular hypertrophy.
- Obtain CBC to check for anemia.
- Obtain electrolytes levels.
- Obtain serum creatinine.
- Perform thyroid function tests. Thyroxine and thyroid-stimulating hormone should be checked in all clients 65 years old and older who have heart failure with no obvious cause.
- Check serum albumin level. There may be an increase in extravascular volume as a result of hypoalbuminemia.

- Perform U/A to check for presence of proteinuria and red blood cells.
- Perform ECG or radionuclide ventriculography to measure left ventricular ejection fraction.

DIAGNOSIS

New York Heart Association (NYHA) functional class (I through IV) for heart failure is as follows:
- Class I: No dyspnea with exertion
- Class II: Dyspnea with maximal exertion
- Class III: Dyspnea with minimal exertion
- Class IV: Dyspnea at rest

Differential diagnoses include pulmonary disease, pneumonia, MI, arrhythmias, cirrhosis, and nephrotic syndrome.

THERAPEUTIC PLAN

The goal is to improve the quality of life; treatment is aimed at controlling the underlying cause and symptoms.

Nonpharmacologic Treatment

- Dietary restrictions include a 2 g sodium diet, fluid restriction if appropriate, and a decrease in ethanol consumption.
- Restrict fluids to 1.5 to 2 L/day
- Encourage regular exercise and activity to improve functional capacity; begin cardiac rehabilitation program *for clients with stable heart failure* (Simon-Weinstein, 1999). Rehabilitation has shown improved quality of life, functional status, and exercise tolerance without prolongation of life.
- Cardiac transplantation may be an option for some clients.

Pharmacologic Treatment

- Angiotensin-converting enzyme (ACE) inhibitors decrease mortality and prolong survival in clients with CHF. They should be prescribed for all clients with systolic dysfunction unless contraindicated.
  - Contraindications include intolerance or side effects, potassium level higher than 5.5 mEq, or signs and symptoms of hypotension.
  - Starting doses may need to be adjusted in the older adult.
  - Benefits usually are seen within 90 days of initiation.
  - Most common ACE inhibitors are captopril 6.25 to 25.0 mg tid, enalapril 2.5 mg qd/bid, and fosinopril 5 to 10mg qd.
  - Angiotensin receptor blockers should be used by only those clients who cannot tolerate ACE inhibitors because of side effects (e.g., cough).
- Diuretics can be used in clients with CHF.

- Do not use as monotherapy. Start with thiazides (12.5 to 25 mg qd) in clients with normal renal function. Progress to loop diuretics if necessary. Diuretics decrease preload, dyspnea on exertion, orthopnea with PND, and edema.
- Increased doses may be needed in clients with renal failure, and decreased doses may be necessary in older adults.
- When using in conjunction with ACE inhibitors, dose low.
- Use loop diuretics when a rapid response is needed (acute presentation of CHF).

⚕CAUTION: *Overdiuresis may lead to renal insufficiency or hypotension.*

- Complications of diuretic use include electrolyte imbalances and carbohydrate intolerances. Check electrolytes and renal chemistries within 2 weeks of starting therapy.
- Digoxin increases the force of ventricular contraction in clients with left ventricular systolic dysfunction. It should be used in conjunction with diuretics and ACE inhibitors in clients with severe heart failure, preferably of systolic dysfunction type.
- Aspirin should be used with CHF secondary to CAD.
- Beta blockers should be used with caution because they can increase dyspnea and edema. Carvedilol (3.125 to 6.25 mg bid) is preferred because it improves renal function in CHF. However, it is contraindicated in clients with asthma.

Client Education

Client and family education includes explanation of the diagnosis, prognosis, and symptoms of worsening heart failure and resultant interventions.
- Avoid highly processed foods, canned foods, and luncheon meats because of high salt content.
- Obtain and record daily weights. A weight gain of 2 to 4 pounds in a 2- to 3-day period should be reported.
- Stop smoking.
- Include rationale for importance of compliance with medication regimen and the side effects. Avoid use of OTC NSAIDS.
- Seek care if unable to perform ADLs without increased fatigue.

Referral

- Refer clients to a physician in cases of new-onset heart failure or heart failure refractory to conventional therapy.
- Refer children.
- Refer client to a physician if CHF is refractory to intervention.

Prevention

- Low-fat diet
- Regular exercise

EVALUATION/FOLLOW-UP

- Return to clinic as necessary until CHF is compensated.
- Once compensated, routine follow-up is every 1 to 3 months.

COMPLICATIONS

- Cardiogenic shock
- Dysrhythmias

REFERENCES

Aronow, W. (1997). Treatment of congestive heart failure in older persons. *Journal of the American Geriatric Society, 45*, 1252-1258.

Fletcher, L. & Thomas, D. (2001). Congestive heart failure: Understanding the pathophysiology and management. *Journal of the American Academy of Nurse Practitioners, 13*(6), 249-257.

Konstam, M. & Dracup, K. (1994). *Heart failure: Evaluation and care of patients with left ventricular systolic dysfunction.* Clinical Practice Guideline No. 11. AHCPR Publication 94. Rockville, MD: Agency for Health Care Policy and Research, Public Health Service, U.S. Department of Health and Human Services.

Shamsham, F. & Mitchell, J. (2000). Essentials of the diagnosis of heart failure. *American Family Physician, 61*(5), 1319-1328.

Simon-Weinstein, M. (1999). Cardiac rehabilitation: nonpharmacologic treatment for congestive heart failure. *Journal of the American Academy of Nurse Practitioners, 11*(7), 293-296.

Review Questions

1. Which of the following is *not* a compensatory mechanism of CHF?
   a. Progressive left ventricular dilatation and hypertrophy
   b. Activation of the sympathetic nervous system
   c. Activation of the renin-angiotensin system
   d. Decrease in systemic vascular resistance

2. Which of the following is *not* considered a precipitating risk factor for CHF?
   a. Hypertension
   b. CAD
   c. Severe anemia
   d. Family history

3. A 68-year-old man with known systolic dysfunction seeks treatment with increasing dyspnea and signs of recurrent heart failure. Which of the following medications may be contributing to these symptoms?
   a. Aspirin, 325 mg/day
   b. Digoxin, 0.125 mg/day
   c. Lisinopril, 10 mg/day
   d. Metoprolol, 50 mg bid

4. Which of the following diagnostic tests is indicated for evaluation of left ventricular ejection fraction?
   a. Echocardiogram
   b. ECG
   c. Chest radiograph
   d. GXT

5. A 52-year-old woman with known CHF reports dyspnea with minimal exertion (walking from room to room). In what NYHA functional class is she?
   a. Functional class I
   b. Functional class II
   c. Functional class III
   d. Functional class IV

6. Which of the following drugs have been proved to decrease mortality and increase survival in persons with CHF?
   a. Diuretics
   b. Digoxin
   c. ACE inhibitors
   d. Nitrates

7. Which of the following is *not* a contraindication to use of an ACE inhibitor?
   a. Hypotension
   b. Serum potassium level less than or equal to 5.5 mEq
   c. History of intolerance or reaction to ACE inhibitors
   d. Renal insufficiency

8. Which of the following remarks made by the client indicates a need for further teaching?
   a. "I should avoid canned soup."
   b. "I should report a weight gain of 2 pounds in a week."
   c. "I may walk each day."
   d. "I may drink two glasses of water a day."

Answers and Rationales

1. *Answer:* d (analysis/diagnosis)
   Rationale: There is an increase in systemic vascular resistance as a result of activation of the sympathetic nervous system and an increase in catecholamines.

2. *Answer:* d (assessment)
   Rationale: Although family history is considered a risk factor for CAD, it is not a precipitating risk factor for CHF. There is an underlying pathophysiologic cause for development of CHF. Anemia and CAD can produce CHF as a compensatory mechanism for inadequate oxygenation of the myocardium. Hypertension increases afterload and results in ventricular hypertrophy from trying to eject blood into the aorta against a high pressure.

3. *Answer:* d (assessment)
   Rationale: Negative inotropic agents such as beta-blockers, verapamil, diltiazem, and class IA and IC antiarrhythmics can cause a decompensation in CHF. NSAIDs also can contribute to CHF.

4. *Answer:* a (assessment)
   Rationale: ECG or radionuclide ventriculography can be used to measure left ventricular ejection fraction. GXT

measures functional capacity but does not provide a definitive measure of left ventricular function unless it is used with ECG or radionuclide ventriculography.

5. *Answer:* **c** (analysis/diagnosis)
Rationale: Class I, no limitation in activity; class II, dyspnea with normal to maximal physical activity; class III, dyspnea with minimal activity; class IV, dyspnea at rest.

6. *Answer:* **c** (implementation/plan)
Rationale: ACE inhibitors have been shown to reduce mortality and increase functional status in persons with CHF. None of the other drugs listed have been shown to decrease mortality.

7. *Answer:* **d** (implementation/plan)
Rationale: ACE inhibitors can be used with caution in clients with elevated creatinine (levels less than 3 mEq) but require close monitoring with follow-up basic metabolic profile. ACE inhibitors should not be instituted in clients with elevated serum potassium and the presence of hypotension.

8. *Answer:* **c** (evaluation)
Rationale: Processed and canned foods have a higher sodium content and should be avoided. Fluid restrictions still allow 1.5 to 2 L/day. Regular exercise has improved functional capacity in CHF. A weight gain of 2 to 4 pounds within a 3-day period should be reported.

CONJUCTIVITIS   *Denise Robinson*

OVERVIEW
Definition

Conjunctivitis is an inflammation of the conjunctiva. Ophthalmia neonatorum is a type of conjunctivitis that occurs in the first month of life.

Incidence

A common infection in children, conjunctivitis is less common in the adult population. Children are at increased risk as a result of physical contact with large groups of other children, inadequate handwashing, and increased incidences of URIs and acute otitis media.

Several studies have concluded that bacteria is the most frequent cause of conjunctivitis. The next most frequent cause is viruses.

Pathophysiology

The conjunctiva is a thin, transparent mucous membrane covering the globe of the eye and inner surface of the eyelids. Irritants, including bacteria, viruses, chemicals, allergens, and FBs, can result in inflammation of this tissue. Incubation for bacterial conjunctivitis is 2 to 3 days; for viral conjunctivitis it is 5 to 14 days.

Factors Increasing Susceptibility
- Poor handwashing
- Exposure to someone with conjunctivitis
- Exposure to impetigo
- Presence of URI
- Presence of allergens
- Lack of tears or moisture in eye
- Pathogenesis
  Bacterial Causes
- *Streptococcus pneumoniae* (10% of cases in children)
- *Haemophilus influenzae:* often concurrent with acute otitis media (40% to 50% of cases in children)
- *Moraxella catarrhalis*
- Staphylococcus aureus *(most common in adults*
- Pneumococcus
- Proteus
- *Neisseria gonorrhoeae* (hyperacute bacterial conjunctivitis)
- *Chlamydia trachomatis*
  Viral Causes
- Adenovirus (most common)
- Enterovirus
- Coxsackievirus
- Herpes simplex: complications, optic neuritis
  Ophthalmia Neonatorum
- *Neisseria gonorrhoeae:* complications, destruction and/or perforation of the cornea
- *Chlamydia trachomatis* (leading cause of ophthalmia neonatorum): complications, conjunctival scarring
- Herpes simplex: complications, cataracts, keratitis, optic neuritis
- Other listed bacteria
- Antibiotics: primarily silver nitrate and erythromycin
  Allergic/Vernal Causes
- Irritant chemicals
- Medications, antibiotics: gentamicin, neomycin, tobramycin atropine, eyedrop preservatives

Protective Factors. Tears continually wash the eye, inhibiting colonization and diluting and flushing irritants. Tears do not develop in infants until approximately 1 month of age.

ASSESSMENT: SUBJECTIVE/HISTORY
History of Present Illness
- Photophobia
- Itching of eyes
- Burning of eyes
- Discharge from eyes
- Eyelids stick together
- Visual changes

Associated Symptoms

URI, fever, ear pain, acute otitis media, and throat pain may be associated.

Past Medical History

- Ask about history of previous ear infection, eye diseases, recent illness, concurrent illness, allergies, recent herpes simplex infection, exposure to someone with conjunctivitis, exposure to someone with impetigo, use of contact lenses, history of an STD in self or partner(s), and recent eye trauma. Also ask about dry eyes (with collagen vascular disease).
- Ask mothers of infants about treatment for STD during pregnancy.

Medication History

- Ask about recent use of antibiotics or any eye preparations.
- If corneal abrasion or trauma is suspected, inquire about tetanus immunity status.
- Diuretics or antidepression drugs may cause dry eyes.

Family History

Ask about family history of eye diseases or atopic diseases (allergic rhinitis, asthma, or eczema).

ASSESSMENT: OBJECTIVE/PHYSICAL EXAMINATION
Physical Examination

Use a problem-oriented approach to the physical examination.

- Check vital signs, including temperature, heart rate, respiratory rate, and blood pressure in everyone older than age 3 years.
- Assess skin for color and character, and check for lesions of herpes simplex.
- Assess heart sounds and record.
- Assess breath sounds and record.
- Assess ears, nose, and throat. Look for concurrent URI and acute otitis media.
- Assess eyes. Determine visual activity in school-age and older clients. Assess visual fields, extraocular movements, and pupillary functions. Examine sclera and conjunctiva for inflammation, edema, and discharge. Examine cornea for clarity and ulceration. Examine eyelid margins. Perform funduscopic examination on all clients, although this may not be possible for infants and small children.
- Assess lymphatics. Focus on head and neck. Enlarged preauricular nodes often are present in viral and chlamydial conjunctivitis.

Diagnostic Procedures

- Culture and Gram stain are not usually necessary, unless infection is recurring or resistant to routine treatment.
- Cultures always should be done on infants younger than 1 month of age. Cultures of the eye and nasopharynx should be done concurrently. Culture should be done for *Chlamydia trachomatis, Neisseria gonorrhoeae,* and bacteria. If a child has gonococcal or chlamydial ophthalmia neonatorum, both parents need to be screened for gonococcal and chlamydial infection (Baker, 1996).
- Perform fluorescein stain with examination under cobalt-blue light source for corneal abrasion or trauma. Epithelial abrasion is brilliant green; deeper injuries are darker.

DIAGNOSIS

Differential diagnoses may include the following:

- Bacterial conjunctivitis presents with mucopurulent discharge; eyes matted on wakening; itching of the affected eye; mild pain; injection of conjunctival vessels; unilateral involvement that often becomes bilateral after 48 hours; and, less frequently, mild photophobia.
- In *Chlamydia trachomatis* discharge is thinner, more mucoid. Photophobia is pronounced. Not self-limited; can persist for months.
- Ophthalmia neonatorium presentation is 24 to 48 hours after birth, with dramatic symptoms, including erythremic, edematous conjunctiva and profuse purulent discharge, usually bilateral.
- Assess for viral conjunctivitis. Ask about watery discharge, eyes matted on wakening, presence of URI, and bilateral eye involvement.
- Allergic conjunctivitis presents with mild to moderate inflammation of conjunctiva, severe itching, marked burning, rhinorrhea, watery drainage, and bilateral involvement. Presentation is seasonal. Conjunctiva of the eyelids may have cobblestone appearance; symptoms often are reported as more severe than clinical presentation.
- Chemical conjunctivitis presentation is within the first 24 hours of life. It is usually related to instillation of silver nitrate and, to a lesser extent, erythromycin, both used as chlamydial and gonococcal prophylaxis. There is mild injection and mucopurulent discharge. The condition is self-limited, usually resolving in 24 to 48 hours.
- In other chemical causes, ask about watery discharge, injected conjunctiva, photophobia, marked burning, and history of exposure to irritant.
- In case of corneal abrasion or trauma, ask about watery discharge (usually unilateral), photophobia of infected eye, and exposure to trauma or FB.
- Assess for iritis.
- Assess for glaucoma.
- Herpes simplex conjunctivitis: presentation is 48 hours to 14 days after birth; with marked inflammation, mucoid drainage, and herpetic vesicles; look for possible presence of fever blister, vesicles on eyelids (Table 3-15).

TABLE **3-15** Comparison of Different Types of Conjunctivitis

TYPE	DISCHARGE	CONJUNCTIVA	UNILATERAL VS. BILATERAL ITCHING	PAIN/PHOTOPHOBIA/ BLURRED VISION
Bacterial	Purulent/mucopurulent	Mildly injected to markedly inflamed	Unilateral initially	Not usually a feature of typical conjunctival inflammatory process; consider more serious disease process: uveitis, keratitis, acute glaucoma, or orbital celulitis; blurred vision is rarely associated with conjunctivitis
Viral	Serous or mildly mucopurulent	Hyperemic	Unilateral initially	
Allergic	Watery or stringy mucoid	Edematous or moderately inflamed	Itching bilateral	
Chemical	Serous	Inflamed and edematous	Depends on exposure	

From Robinson, D., Kidd, P., & Rogers, P. M. (2000). *Primary care across the lifespan.* St. Louis; Mosby.

THERAPEUTIC PLAN
Pharmacologic Treatment

Bacterial Conjunctivitis
- Administer sulfacetamide sodium 10%. Apply 0.5- to 1-cm ribbon of ointment in conjunctival sac qid for 7 days or 10% solution 2 gtts every 2 to 3 hours while client is awake. This medicine is effective, well tolerated, and inexpensive.
- Administer bacitracin or polymyxin. Apply 0.5 to 1 cm ointment in conjunctival sac qid for 7 days.
- Alternative treatments include tobramycin ointment or solution and erythromycin ointment or solution. Gentamicin and neomycin preparations are options for use but have higher incidence of allergic reaction (Merenstein, Kaplan, & Rosenberg, 1994).
- If concurrent acute otitis media is present in a child, the child can be treated with systemic antibiotic therapy. It is best to use a beta-lactamase resistant drug, such as amoxicillin (Augmentin). You do not need to use topical antibiotics concurrently (Robinson, 2000). Trimethoprim/sulfamethoxazole (Bactrim) should not be given to children younger than 2 months.

Ophthalmia Neonatorum
- For gonococcal conjunctivitis, administer ceftriaxone 50 mg/kg IM as single dose. If organism is sensitive to penicillin, give aqueous penicillin G 100,000 u/kg/day (Baker, 1996).
- The infant may need frequent eye irrigation with sterile normal saline solution to clear discharge.
- For *Chlamydia trachomatis*, administer erythromycin suspension 30-40 mg/kg/day PO in 3 divided doses.

Allergic Conjunctivitis
- Administer systemic antihistamines:
  - For children, administer diphenhydramine 5 mg/kg/day for 4 days in 4 divided doses. Be alert for drowsiness.
  - For adults, administer diphenhydramine 25 to 50 mg tid for 4 days.

- For children older than 4 years and adults, administer cromolyn sodium ophthalmic solution 4%. When administering 1 to 2 gtts 4 to 6 times per day or when the client is older than 3 years, you can use olopatadine (Patanol), a mast cell stabilizer and antihistamine. Give 1-2 drops bid.
- Do not prescribe ophthalmic steroids for clients of any age. They are associated with increased incidence of cataracts and glaucoma.

Nonpharmacologic Treatment
Comfort Measures
- Provide wet compresses, cool or warm per client's preference. Use cotton balls.
- Children may need distraction to keep from rubbing eyes.

Infection Control
- Encourage good handwashing with client and family.
- Client should keep hands away from face and eyes.
- Client's face cloths and towels should be kept separate from others. These linens should be used one time only, then washed.
- Monitor other family members, especially siblings, for symptoms of conjunctivitis.
- Client should refrain from wearing contact lenses for 24 hours.
- Clean contact lenses and storage case with appropriate disinfectant.
- Children should stay home from school or day care until inflammation and discharge are gone, 24 to 48 hours after treatment begins.

Client Education
Medication Administration
- Clean eye before any medication administration.
- To apply or instill, gently separate eyelids, pulling lower lid down toward the center of the eye. Place the drops or a thin line of ointment in pocket that is formed (Boynton, Dunn, & Stephens, 1998).

- Infection should respond to treatment in 2 to 3 days. Client or parent should call after 48 hours if response to medication is poor. Instruct client or parent to call if symptoms worsen or vision decreases.

Referral

- Infants younger than 1 month
- All ages in the case of any of the following:
  - Corneal ulcer
  - Extensive corneal defect
  - Corneal inflammation
  - Suspected gonococcal infection
  - Suspected herpes simplex infection
  - Any irregularities in pupil size or reaction
  - No improvement after 48 hours of treatment
  - Client reports any of the following: moderate to severe pain, severe photophobia, or decreased visual acuity

Prevention

Conjunctivitis can be avoided through good handwashing.

EVALUATION/FOLLOW-UP

Bacterial Infection

- No follow-up is necessary if client responds to treatment.
- Practitioner may want to follow up with severe cases.

Viral Infection

Follow-up is done for persistent symptoms.

Allergic Conjunctivitis

Follow-up is done for persistent symptoms. Referral to allergist or ophthalmologist may be necessary.

Corneal Abrasion or Trauma

Follow-up is done as needed.

Ophthalmia Neonatorum

Follow-up is done as advised by referred physician.

COMPLICATIONS

- Blindness
- Changes in visual acuity

REFERENCES

Baker, R. C. (1996). *Handbook of pediatric primary care.* Boston: Little, Brown.

Barker, L. R., Burton, J., & Zieve, P. (1995). *Principles of ambulatory medicine.* Baltimore: Williams & Wilkins.

Boynton, R. W., Dunn, E. S., & Stephens, G. R. (1998). *Manual of ambulatory pediatrics* (5th ed.). Philadelphia: J.B. Lippincott.

Eisenbaum, A. (1999). Eye. In W. Hay, A. Hayward, M. Levin, & J. Sondheimer (Eds.), *Current pediatric diagnosis and treatment* (14th ed.). Stamford, CT: Appleton & Lange:

Hara, J. (1996). The red eye: diagnosis and treatment. *American Family Physician, 54*(8), 2423-2430.

Merenstein, G. B., Kaplan, D. W., & Rosenberg, A. A. (1994). *Handbook of pediatrics.* Norwalk, CT: Appleton & Lange.

Morrow, G., & Abbott, R. (1998). Conjunctivitis. *American Family Physician, 57*(4), 735-746.

Nelson, L. (1996). Disorders of the eye. In W. Nelson, R. Behrman, R. Kliegman, & A. Arvin (Eds.), *Nelson textbook of pediatrics* (15th ed., pp. 1779-1782). Philadelphia: Saunders.

Pellerano, R. A., Bishop, V., & Silber, T. J. (1994). Gonococcal conjunctivitis in adolescents. Recognition and management. *Clinical Pediatrics, 33*(2), 114-116.

Robinson, D. (2000). Conjunctivitis. In D. Robinson, P. Kidd, & K. Rogers (Eds.), *Primary care across the lifespan.* (pp. 257-263). St Louis: Mosby.

Ruppert, S. D. (1996). Differential diagnosis of pediatric conjunctivitis. *Nurse Practitioner, 21*(7), 12-26.

Uphold, C. R. & Graham, M. V. (1994). *Clinical guidelines in family practice.* Gainesville, FL: Barmarrae Books.

Weiss, A. (1994). Acute conjunctivitis in childhood. *Current Problems in Pediatrics, 24*(1), 4-11.

Weiss, A., Brinser, J. H., & Nazar-Stewart, V. (1993). Acute conjunctivitis in childhood. *Journal of Pediatrics, 24*(1), 10-14.

Review Questions

1. You are taking a history for a 2-week-old infant. The mother has reported an infection in the right eye. In your history, it is important to ascertain which of the following?

   a. Mother's history of STD or STD treatment during pregnancy

   b. Day of life when onset of symptoms occurred

   c. Description of drainage

   d. All of the above

2. Which of the following symptoms is not usually identified by a client with a corneal abrasion?

   a. Photophobia

   b. Mild to moderate pain

   c. Mucopurulent discharge

   d. Hyperemia

3. You diagnose your client, a 2-year-old girl, with acute otitis media and bacterial conjunctivitis. The pathogen is unknown. Your treatment choice is which of the following?

   a. Sulfacetamide sodium 10% ophthalmic ointment

   b. Bactrim suspension

   c. Amoxicillin suspension and sodium sulfacetamide ophthalmic solution 10%

   d. Augmentin suspension

4. The NP provides instruction about eye drops to a mother of a child with conjunctivitis. Which comment by the mother indicates a need for further instruction?

   a. "I'm going to give these eye drops every 4 hours."

   b. "I should clean the eye before I put in the eye drops."

   c. "I can use my other son's eye drops—he had conjunctivitis a couple months ago."

   d. "I should not touch the dropper to his eye."

5. Your client, a 22-year-old man, has a diagnosis of chlamydial conjunctivitis. Which of the following symptoms are consistent with this diagnosis?
   a. Photophobia
   b. Profuse purulent discharge
   c. Condition present for 2 months
   d. Enlarged tender preauricular nodes

6. All the following statements are true regarding follow-up for bacterial conjunctivitis except:
   a. Usually no follow-up is necessary.
   b. Practitioner may want to follow up severe cases.
   c. Follow-up is necessary if symptoms persist after 48 hours of treatment.
   d. All cases of bacterial conjunctivitis require a follow-up visit.

7. Which statement is true regarding diagnostic cultures in conjunctivitis?
   a. All cases of suspected bacterial conjunctivitis require culture and sensitivities.
   b. Culture and sensitivity testing are necessary when conjunctivitis is recurring or resistant to routine treatment.
   c. All infants younger than 3 months should have culture testing, Gram stain, and cultures for chlamydia and gonorrhea.
   d. All teenagers should have culture testing for bacteria, chlamydia, and gonorrhea.

8. Which of the following problems of clients should be referred to an ophthalmologist?
   a. Corneal abrasion
   b. Allergic conjunctivitis
   c. Suspected gonococcal infection
   d. 10-week-old client

Answers and Rationales

1. *Answer:* **d** (assessment)
   Rationale: The infection possibly is due to the STD gonorrhea, chlamydia, trachomatis, or herpes simplex. Obtaining a history of STDs, onset of symptoms, and description of drainage helps narrow the practitioner's differential diagnosis (Baker, 1996).

2. *Answer:* **c** (assessment)
   Rationale: Photophobia, mild to moderate pain, and hyperemia are all associated with corneal abrasion. Mucopurulent drainage is associated with bacterial conjunctivitis (Ruppert, 1996).

3. *Answer:* **d** (implementation/plan)
   Rationale: A beta-lactamase resistant systemic antibiotic is the drug of choice. Augmentin is an appropriate treatment (Robinson, 2000).

4. *Answer:* **c** (evaluation)
   Rationale: The mother should not use a medication prescribed for someone else. She would be giving the eye drops every 4 hours, cleaning the eye before administration of the eye drops, and not touching the dropper to the eye (Robinson, 2000).

5. *Answer:* **a** (analysis/diagnosis)
   Rationale: Profuse purulent discharge is associated with gonococcal conjunctivitis. The discharge seen in chlamydial conjunctivitis is thin and mucoid. The hallmark of chlamydial conjunctivitis is photophobia (Pellerano, Bishop, & Silber, 1994).

6. *Answer:* **d** (evaluation)
   Rationale: Usually no follow-up is necessary for bacterial conjunctivitis. Follow-up is needed when symptoms persist or client is unresponsive to treatment (Uphold & Graham, 1994).

7. *Answer:* **b** (analysis/diagnosis)
   Rationale: Culture and sensitivity testing should be done when the conjunctivitis is recurring or resistant to treatment, with all infants younger than 1 month, and in suspected cases of gonorrhea or chlamydial conjunctivitis (Baker, 1996; Ruppert, 1996).

8. *Answer:* **c** (implementation/plan)
   Rationale: A 10-week-old with new-onset conjunctivitis can be treated by a practitioner, as can a client with a corneal abrasion and allergic conjunctivitis. Gonococcal conjunctivitis should be referred (Morrow & Abbott, 1998).

CONSTIPATION *Pamela Kidd*

OVERVIEW
Definition

Constipation is defined as a decrease in the frequency, size, or liquid content of stool. The term refers more to the consistency of stool than to the frequency of stools. Constipated stools are small, hard, and dry.

Incidence

- Constipation is common among children, adolescents, and older adults.
- Accounts for 2.5 million health care visits annually and 4% of all pediatric visits.

Pathophysiology

Distention of the bowel wall from stool passing into the rectum stimulates mass peristalsis, producing the defecation reflex. The urge to defecate can be voluntarily controlled through tightening of the external sphincter. When this occurs, stool remains in the rectum and produces relaxation and cessation of the defecation reflex. Liquid content continually is reabsorbed, producing hard, dry stool that is difficult and painful to pass. Most constipation is functional, with no organic cause.

Factors Increasing Susceptibility
- Sedentary lifestyle

- Voluntarily ignoring the urge to defecate because of lack of privacy or painful anal fissures or hemorrhoids

Protective Factors
- Daily exercise
- Adequate fluid intake
- "Home"-cooked meals (less dependence on fast/convenience foods)

ASSESSMENT: SUBJECTIVE/HISTORY
Symptoms

The history should include client's definition of constipation, usual bowel pattern including recent changes, dietary recall, activity level, and current or recent use of medications (including laxatives).

NOTE: *Many people, especially the elderly, consider one bowel movement a day to be "normal." In fact, one bowel movement a week may be normal. "Normal" means the bowel movement is passed without pain or bloating (Peters, 1997).*

Symptoms of constipation are the following:
- Children: nausea, vomiting, excessive urination, blood in stools, soiling of underclothes, behavioral problems
- Adults: abdominal pain, blood in stools, weight loss, depression, diarrhea
- Decrease in the number of stools from normal stooling patterns
  - Breastfed babies may stool after every feeding.
  - Bottle-fed babies stool less often.
  - Neonates stool more often than four times per day.
  - Four-month-olds produce two stools per day.
  - Four-year-olds through adults generally produce one stool per day. Stool size increases with age.
- Hard, dry, small stools
- Straining required to push stool out (normal during neonatal period)
- Pain with defecation

Past Medical History
- Organic causes include Hirschsprung's disease, strictures, anal–rectal stenosis, and volvulus.
- Neuromuscular defects include spinal cord lesions.
- Metabolic causes include hypokalemia, dehydration, and hypothyroidism.
- Anorexia nervosa also causes constipation.

Medication History
- Narcotics
- Psychoactive drugs
- Antidepressants
- Iron supplements
- Nasal decongestants
- Antihistamines
- Diuretics

Family History
Noncontributory.

Dietary History
- Low fiber in the diet
- Low fluid intake

ASSESSMENT: OBJECTIVE/PHYSICAL EXAMINATION
Physical Examination

Abdominal Examination
- The abdomen is distended with a palpable mass in the midline or lower left quadrant.
- Auscultate bowel and percuss for dullness over fecal mass.

Rectal Examination. Check for fissures, hemorrhoids, irritation, fecal impaction, and sphincter tone.

NOTE: *Clients with functional constipation usually have normal sphincter tone and large rectal vaults.*

Diagnostic Procedures

A radiographic examination of the abdomen is sometimes helpful to estimate the amount of stool retained. In adults, three separate stools should be obtained for occult blood testing. Barium enema or endoscopy may be needed to look for diverticulitis and Crohn's disease.

DIAGNOSIS
Differential diagnoses include the following:
- Toilet-training resistance
- Normal straining in infancy–soft stools
- Hirschsprung's disease–constipation from birth, rectal ampulla empty
- Encopresis
- Partial bowel obstruction
- Irritable bowel syndrome
- Rectal fissures or hemorrhoids
- Hypothyroidism

THERAPEUTIC PLAN
Nonpharmacologic Treatment

Infant
- At 0 to 4 months, discontinue solids and increase water and fruit juice in the diet.
- At 4 to 12 months, introduce fruits and nonstarchy vegetables into diet. Encourage an occasional juice or water bottle. Avoid rice cereal.

Child (1 to 12 Years)
- If significant constipation is seen on initial examination, give one or more pediatric Fleet enemas to evacuate the bowel.

- Retrain bowels; have the child sit on the toilet for 20 minutes after meals. Educate child and parents on gastrocolic reflex.
- Encourage dietary changes, increasing fiber, fluids, vegetables, and fruit.
- If a toddler is not completely potty-trained, put the child back in diapers and remove all pressure related to toileting.

Adult

- Increase fluid intake to 1.5 to 2 L daily (6 to 8 glasses/day).
- Increase fiber (25 to 35 g/day [Peters, 1997]) in the diet, and add fresh fruits and vegetables, bran cereals, and whole-grain breads.
- Increase daily exercise.
- Retrain bowel habits; client should sit on the toilet for 15 minutes after meals. Client should not ignore the urge to defecate.

Elderly. Encourage use of "natural" laxative: mix together 2 cups applesauce, 2 cups unprocessed bran, and 1 cup 100% prune juice; take 1 oz of mixture per day (Shuler, Huebscher, & Hallock, 2001).

Pharmacologic Treatment

Child

- Use stool softeners only if other measures fail.
  - Docusate sodium (Colace), 5 mg/kg/day
  - Maltsupex:
    - For ages 4 to 12 months, it may be necessary to use Maltsupex, 1 to 2 teaspoons tid.
    - For ages 1 to 5 years, administer 1 teaspoon bid; may increase to 2 tablespoons bid.
    - For ages 5 to 15 years, administer 2 teaspoons bid; may increase to 2 tablespoons bid.
- Reduce daily dose once stools are soft.
- Continue for 2 to 3 months until regular bowel habits are established.

Adult

- Stool softeners/emollient laxative are for short-term use only. These include Docusate sodium (Colace), 50 to 300 mg/day and docusate calcium (Doxidan), 240 mg/day.
- Fiber additives are the safest laxative. These include polycarbophil (Fibercon), methylcellulose (Citrucel), or psyllium (Effersylium). Begin with 1 tablespoon daily and increase as needed to 3 tablespoons daily. Must be accompanied by plenty of fluids; may be used long term
- Saline laxatives (milk of magnesia, Maalox) should not be used in clients with renal failure due to possible hypermagnesia and hypocalcemia.

Client Education

- Instruct the client to avoid chronic laxative use.
- The client can substitute flavored gelatin for fluids to maintain adequate fluid intake.

Referral

Refer the following clients to a gastroenterologist:

- Any child who has a poor response to therapy or who exhibits emotional problems
- Adults older than 50 with constipation representing a change from their usual pattern
- Any client who has hemoccult-positive stools

Prevention

- Attending to urge to defecate
- Eating a well-balanced diet with adequate fiber and fluid intake
- Exercising daily

EVALUATION/FOLLOW-UP

Schedule follow-up visits every 2 weeks until normal bowel function resumes.

COMPLICATIONS

- Impaction
- Fecal incontinence
- Bowel obstruction
- Obstipation (dilated colon/rupture)

REFERENCES

Arvin, A. M., Behrman, R. E., Kliegman, R. M., & Nelson, W. E. (Eds.), (1996). *Nelson textbook of pediatrics* (15th ed.). Philadelphia: W. B. Saunders.

Gordy, C. (2000). Constipation. In D. Robinson, P. Kidd, & K. Rogers (Eds.) *Primary care across the lifespan.* St. Louis: Mosby.

Groothuis, J. R., Hay, W. W., Hayward, A. R., & Levin, M. J. (Eds.), (1995). *Current pediatric diagnosis and treatment* (12th ed.). Norwalk, CT: Appleton & Lange.

McCargar, L. J., Hotson, B. L., & Nozza, A. (1995). Fibre and nutrient intakes of chronic care elderly patients. *Journal of Nutrition for the Elderly, 15*(1), 13-31.

Peters, S. (1997). Constipation: Assessment and treatment in elderly patients. *ADVANCE for Nurse Practitioners, 5*(8), 45-46, 49-50.

Shuler, P., Huebscher, R., & Hallock, J. (2001). Providing wholistic health care for the elderly: Utilization of the Shuler Nurse Practitioner practice model. *Journal of the American Academy of Nurse Practitioners, 13*(7), 297-303

Review Questions

1. While taking the history of a 30-year-old woman, the NP learns that the client has a bowel movement every third day. What should the NP do?

a. Prescribe a bulk-forming agent such as polycarbophil (Fibercon).

b. Instruct the client to take a laxative if she fails to have a bowel movement by bedtime.

c. Take a detailed dietary history, looking especially for high-fiber foods.

d. Ask the client whether this represents a change from her usual pattern before assessing further.

2. The NP needs to consult the physician for which of the following cases?

a. An 8-month-old infant with a 24-hour history of diarrhea and mild dehydration

b. An 8-year-old with a familial tendency toward constipation who reports having a bowel movement once a week

c. A 55-year-old woman who reports a bowel history of stools qod

d. A 60-year-old man who reports constipation after having previously been regular

3. During the physical examination of an elderly client with a history of chronic constipation, the NP expects to find all the following *except:*

a. Occult blood in the stool

b. Hemorrhoids or rectal irritation

c. Hard, impacted stool in the rectal vault

d. Mild abdominal tenderness, with a fecal mass palpable in the left lower quadrant

4. An NP is trying to assess if a bowel movement was normal for a client. What should the NP ask?

a. "What color was the stool?"

b. "Was it passed without pain or bloating?"

c. "Was it formed?"

d. "Did you feel you emptied completely?"

5. When advising a mother how to adapt the diet of an infant who has experienced constipation, the NP should suggest which of the following?

a. Avoiding wheat cereal

b. Encouraging the child to drink cow's milk

c. Using jello water

d. Avoiding rice cereal

6. In helping an older client establish regular bowel habits, the NP suggests which of the following?

a. Increasing fluid to 1L/day

b. Sitting on the toilet for 1 hour after meals

c. Increasing fiber to 35 g/day

d. Avoiding beef

7. Which of the following laxatives are considered the safest to prescribe?

a. Emollients

b. Fiber additives

c. Saline laxatives

d. Stool softeners

Answers and Rationales

1. *Answer:* d (assessment)

Rationale: Bowel habits are unique to individuals. A daily bowel movement may not be normal for everyone. The NP first should determine whether the pattern is a problem for this individual before attempting to treat. A dietary history and perhaps a bulk-forming agent would be appropriate if it is determined that constipation exists. Regular laxative use always should be discouraged.

2. *Answer:* d (implementation/plan)

Rationale: A physician should be consulted for any adult older than 50 years of age with constipation that represents a change from his or her usual pattern. Both the 8-month-old and the 8-year-old could be managed by the NP. The 55-year-old is continuing in an established pattern considered normal.

3. *Answer:* a (assessment)

Rationale: Older clients with chronic constipation often have fecal impaction. Rectal irritation and hemorrhoids frequently accompany constipation as a result of straining to pass large, hard stools. The presence of occult blood in any client's stool is an indication of a more serious problem and warrants a consultation.

4. *Answer:* b. (assessment)

Rationale: A normal bowel movement is considered the passing of stool without pain or bloating (Peters, 1997). Color can be determined by diet and may vary considerably. A movement may be normal and the client still may not feel completely emptied if the client had to rush or has eaten more solid food lately. A normal bowel movement may not be solidly formed.

5. *Answer:* d (implementation/plan)

Rationale: Rice, not wheat, cereal is constipating. Cow's milk should never be introduced during the first 12 months of life. Jello water is used to treat diarrhea.

6. *Answer:* c (implementation/plan)

Rationale: Beef is needed to promote iron intake in the elderly and should not be avoided unless personal preference. Fluids should be increased to 1.5 L/day up to 2 L/day. The gastrocolic reflex occurs within 15 to 20 minutes after meals. Fiber should be increased to 35 g/day.

7. *Answer:* b (implementation/plan)

Rationale: Stool softeners and emollients should be used only for the short term. Saline laxatives can produce hypermagnesia and hypocalcemia, particularly in the client who also has some degree of renal failure. Fiber additives are the safest.

c

COUGH *Denise Robinson*

OVERVIEW
Definition

Cough can be acute or chronic. Acute cough generally is defined as being one that is present for less than 3 weeks. Chronic cough is one that has lasted longer than 3 weeks. Chronic cough is a physiologic reflex to protect the airways by clearing secretions and foreign particles.

Incidence

- Cough is the fifth most common symptom seen in outpatient clinics, resulting in 30 million visits annually.
- Persistent cough is reported in 14% to 23% of nonsmokers.
- In smokers who smoke half a pack of cigarettes per day, 25% report a cough.
- In smokers who smoke two packs per day, 50% report a chronic cough.

Pathophysiology

The cough reflex has five components:

1. Cough receptors
2. Afferent nerves (vagus, trigeminal, glossopharyngeal, and phrenic)
3. A cough center located in the medulla and separate from the respiratory center
4. Efferent nerves (vagus, phrenic, intercostal, lumbar, trigeminal, facial, and hypoglossal)
5. Effector organs (diaphragm, intercostal, and abdominal muscles; muscles of the larynx, trachea, and bronchi; and upper airway and accessory respiratory muscles) (Corrao, 1996)

An effective cough has three components:

1. Rapid inhalation of a large volume of air, followed by closure of the glottis
2. Elevation of intrathoracic pressures caused by the contraction of abdominal and thoracic muscles
3. With increased pressure, a sudden opening of the glottis that expels the trapped air, thus producing the cough

ASSESSMENT: SUBJECTIVE/HISTORY
History of Present Illness

- How long has the cough been present? Was the onset sudden or insidious?
- Is it productive or nonproductive?
- If productive, is it clear, mucoid, or purulent?
- Is it harsh, barking, or coarse?
- Was it preceded by upper or lower respiratory tract infection symptoms, allergy exposure, or a choking/feeding episode?
- Is it present during the day, night, or both?
- Is there associated shortness of breath or wheezing with the cough?
- Are there any other precipitating factors?
- With a child (1 to 3 years old), is there a possibility of exposure to small items (i.e., suspect a foreign body ingestion).

Symptoms

Cough usually is accompanied by other symptoms, which can help lead to the diagnosis, which may be one of the following:

- Dyspnea on exertion or orthopnea (consider CHF)
- Bloody sputum, weight loss (consider tuberculosis or lung cancer)
- Substernal burning, indigestion, regurgitation of digested material, hoarseness, choking, bitter taste in mouth (consider GERD)
- Paroxysmal dry, hacking cough made worse by cold air, cardiovascular exercise, laughing, or allergy exposure (consider asthma)
- Tickle in throat, sensation of secretions in throat, frequent clearing of throat (consider a postnasal drainage syndrome)
- Cough that disappears with sleep and worsens when attention is drawn to it (consider psychogenic cough [a very rare cause])
- Children with recurrent URIs, poor weight gain, fatty stools (consider cystic fibrosis [CF])
- High fever, dyspnea, productive purulent cough (consider pneumonia)
- Acute onset with upper respiratory tract symptoms (consider bronchitis)
- Dry cough after acute bronchitis (consider hyperreactive airways)

Past Medical History

- Asthma
- COPD
- CHF
- GERD
- Postnasal drainage syndromes
  - Allergic rhinitis
  - Acute sinusitis
  - Chronic sinusitis
  - Vasomotor rhinitis
  - Primary nasal polyposis
  - Psychiatric illnesses

Medication History

- Recent ACE inhibitor therapy (may cause cough)
- Frequent use of antacids
- Cough syrups

Family History

- CF
- Asthma/COPD
- Allergies

Psychosocial History

- Tuberculosis exposure
- Smoker/smoke exposure
- Occupational/environmental irritants

Dietary History

- Food allergies
- Eating late at night or lying down after meals

ASSESSMENT: OBJECTIVE/PHYSICAL EXAMINATION

Physical Examination

- Observe general appearance: comfort level, use of accessory muscles, spontaneous coughing, dyspnea, and cyanosis.
- Examine HEENT for signs of sinusitis, postnasal drainage, boggy nasal membranes, cobblestone appearance of pharyngeal mucosa, lymphadenopathy, jugular venous distention, and position of trachea.
- Examine heart for murmurs, rubs, gallops, S_3, and S_4.
- Listen to lungs for any wheezes, rhonchi, crackles, anteroposterior diameter, or decreased breath sounds.
- Palpate abdomen for any organomegaly or epigastric tenderness.
- Examine extremities for edema and digital clubbing.

Diagnostic Procedures

The following procedures should be used based on the suspected diagnosis:

- Chest x-ray examination (pneumonia, CHF, tuberculosis, unexplained cough)
- Pulmonary function tests (COPD; often normal results even with diagnosis of asthma)
- Peak expiratory flow
- Sputum for AFB (tuberculosis)
- Barium swallow (GERD)
- 24-hour esophageal probe (GERD)
- Nasal smear (postnasal drainage syndromes)
- Sweat test (CF)
- Purified protein derivative (PPD) (tuberculosis)
- Bronchial provocation test (asthma)
- Pertussis culture

In children, bronchoscopy is the most helpful test (Lawler, 1998).

DIAGNOSIS

The most common causes of an acute cough are upper and lower respiratory tract infections. Other causes include FB aspiration (especially in children) and allergy or irritant exposure.

The most common differential diagnoses of chronic cough in nonsmokers are postnasal drainage, asthma, and GERD. Other diagnoses include recurrent viral infections, CF, tuberculosis, pneumoconiosis, carcinoma, CHF, psychogenic cough, ACE inhibitor-induced cough, environmental allergies, bronchiectasis, pertussis, and chronic bronchitis.

Keep in mind that cough can be the sole manifestation of asthma and GERD.

THERAPEUTIC PLAN

General measures for acute cough include the following:

- Smoking cessation
- Avoiding environmental irritants
- Air humidification
- Cough suppressants (should only be used temporarily for acute cough syndromes and should be limited to nighttime usage to provide adequate rest)
- Inhaled beta-agonist (if wheezing present with lower respiratory tract infection)
- Antibiotics rarely are needed for cough in children

Treatment for chronic cough depends on the suspected diagnosis. Appropriate empiric treatment should be started if there is enough evidence from the client's history and physical examination to suggest one of the five most common causes of chronic cough: GERD, asthma, postinfectious bronchial inflammation, chronic bronchitis, or postnasal drainage.

If the history and physical examination do not suggest a cause for cough, the client should be treated first for postnasal drip, followed by asthma and GERD (Philp, 1997). In children, the most common cause of chronic cough depends on age.

- 0 to 18 months: cough variant asthma or aberrant innominate artery, congenital causes
- 18 months to 6 years: cough variant asthma, sinusitis
- 6 to 16 years: cough variant asthma and psychogenic cough

Client Education

- Teach the importance of smoking cessation.
- Identify and treat allergies.
- Encourage the use of preventive gear for occupational exposures.

Referral

If coughing continues, consider referral for a bronchoscopy or to a pulmonologist for further workup. If chronic cough is being treated empirically for GERD, asthma, or postnasal drainage and there is no improvement within 4 to 6 weeks, consult with or refer to a collaborating physician or pulmonologist.

EVALUATION/FOLLOW-UP

Acute cough syndromes should improve within 3 weeks as the underlying illness resolves. If cough persists for longer than 3 to 4 weeks, begin workup for chronic cough.

COMPLICATIONS

- Continued smoking
- Lung cancer or COPD

REFERENCES

Collins, R. D. (1995). *Algorithmic diagnosis of symptoms and signs.* New York: Igaku-Shoin.

Corrao, W. M. (1996). Chronic persistent cough: Diagnosis and treatment update. *Pediatric Annals, 25*(3), 162-168.

Dowell, S., Schwartz, B., & Phillips, W. (1998). Appropriate use of antibiotics for URIs in children: Part II. Cough, pharyngitis, and the common cold. *American Family Physician.* Retrieved May 29, 2002, from http://www.aafp.org/afp/981015ap/dowell.html.

Lawler, W. (1998). An office approach to the diagnosis of chronic cough. *American Family Physician.* Retrieved May 29, 2002, from http://www.aafp.org/afp/981200ap/lawler.html.

Newman, K. B. & Milgrom, A. C. (1995). Chronic cough: A step-by-step diagnostic workup. *Consultant, October,* 1535-1542.

Philp, E. (1997). Chronic cough. *American Family Physician, 56*(5), 1395-1404.

Robinson, D. (2000). Cough. In D. Robinson, P. Kidd, & K. Rogers. *Primary care across the lifespan.* (pp. 277-282). St. Louis: Mosby.

Scott, P., Clark, J., & Miser, W. (1997). Pertussis: an update on primary prevention and outbreak control. *American Family Physician, 56*(4), 915-923.

Smith, P. L., Britt, E. J., & Terry, P. B. (1995). Common pulmonary problems: Cough, hemoptysis, dyspnea, chest pain and the abnormal chest x-ray. In L. R. Barker, J. R. Barton, & P. D. Zieve (Eds.), *Principles of ambulatory medicine* (4th ed., pp. 633-649). Baltimore: Williams & Wilkins.

Uphold, C. & Graham, M. (1994). *Clinical guidelines in adult health.* Gainesville, FL: Barmarrae Books.

Review Questions

1. Which of the following medications may cause a cough?
   a. ACE inhibitors
   b. Dextromethorphan
   c. Sulfonylureas
   d. Ibuprofen

2. Which initial test is most appropriate for a client with a cough if the history and physical examination have failed to lead the examiner to a diagnosis?
   a. PPD
   b. Pulmonary function test
   c. Sweat test
   d. Chest radiograph

3. Which test is most appropriate in the diagnosis of asthma?
   a. Bronchial provocation test
   b. Nasal smear
   c. Sputum for AFB
   d. Sweat test

4. The most common differential diagnosis for chronic cough includes all except which of the following?
   a. Postnasal drainage
   b. CHF
   c. GERD
   d. Asthma

5. General measures for cough include all except which of the following?
   a. Smoking cessation
   b. Vitamin and mineral supplementation
   c. Air humidification
   d. Avoidance of environmental irritants

6. When is it most appropriate to use cough suppressants?
   a. When the client has coronary artery disease.
   b. When sleep/rest patterns are disrupted significantly.
   c. When the client's family members are disturbed by the cough.
   d. When chronic cough of unknown cause is present.

7. When chronic cough is treated empirically for GERD, asthma, or postnasal drainage, the client should be referred at what time?
   a. No improvement within 6 months
   b. No improvement within 4 to 6 weeks
   c. No improvement within 2 weeks
   d. No improvement within 1 year

8. John, a 45-year-old, complains of a chronic cough. Which of the following historical data is consistent with a diagnosis of chronic cough?
   a. "I work as an accountant."
   b. "I take metoprolol (Lopressor) for my HTN."
   c. "I just had strep throat."
   d. "I smoke two packs of cigarettes a day."

Answers and Rationales

1. **Answer: a** (assessment)
   Rationale: ACE inhibitor therapy causes coughing in about 5% to 20% of persons who are treated with these medications (Newman & Milgrom, 1995).

2. **Answer: d** (analysis/diagnosis)
   Rationale: If no cause can be identified, a chest radiograph should be obtained (Newman & Milgrom, 1995).

3. **Answer: a** (analysis/diagnosis)
   Rationale: If a client has a positive bronchial provocation test and responds to a bronchodilator, the diagnosis of asthma is more certain (Corrao, 1996).

4. *Answer:* **b** (analysis/diagnosis)
   Rationale: Corrao (1996) describes several studies that show the three most common causes of chronic cough to be postnasal drainage, GERD, and asthma.

5. *Answer:* **b** (implementation/plan)
   Rationale: Smoking cessation, air humidification, and avoiding environmental irritants are more likely to decrease airway irritability (Smith, Britt, & Terry, 1995).

6. *Answer:* **b** (implementation/plan)
   Rationale: There are few situations in which cough suppressants are necessary; their use should be for the purpose of allowing clients to sleep and to avoid posttussive syncope or stress incontinence (Smith, Britt, & Terry, 1995).

7. *Answer:* **b** (evaluation)
   Rationale: After trying empiric treatment for 4 to 6 weeks and the client has shown no improvement, more testing is warranted (Newman & Milgrom, 1995). Further testing includes 24-hour monitoring with an intraesophageal pH probe, fiberoptic laryngoscopy, and fiberoptic bronchoscopy.

8. *Answer:* **d** (assessment)
   Rationale: Of clients who smoke, 50% also have a chronic cough.

CROUP *Denise Robinson*

OVERVIEW
Definition
Croup is an acute viral inflammatory disease of the subglottic mucosa. It usually is proceeded by a viral URI.

Incidence
- Croup is at least 10 times more common than epiglottitis.
- Croup is most common in the fall and winter months, peaking between October and December.
- Croup is the most common cause of stridor in young children.
- Croup rarely occurs in infants younger than 1 month or in school-age children.
- The age group that most commonly suffers from croup is 6 months to 6 years; incidence declines with age.
- Boys are at higher risk than girls, with a ratio of 3 to 2.
- Croup is generally self-limited.
- Fewer than 2% are admitted to the hospital, and 0.5% to 1.5% require intubation (Osmond & Evans, 2001).

Pathophysiology
Viruses that cause the inflammation of the larynx include the following:

- Parainfluenza virus, type 1 (most common)
- Parainfluenza virus, type 3
- RSV
- Adenoviruses
- Rubeola
- Influenza

ASSESSMENT: SUBJECTIVE/HISTORY
History of Present Illness
- Ask about eating and past behavior (sleeping, playing).
- Ask about URI symptoms.

Most Common Symptoms
- Low-grade fever
- Rhinorrhea
- Barking cough, especially during the night

Associated Symptoms
- URI symptoms
- Hoarse voice
- Inspiratory and/or expiratory stridor

   Symptoms are aggravated by agitation and crying.

Past Medical History
- Recent viral infections
- Exposures
- Allergies/atopy
- Medications
- Immunization status

Family History
Inquire about any recent illness.

Psychosocial History
- School or day care exposure
- Smoking
- Profession (possible exposure to inhaled irritants such as paints, chemicals, dust particles, and smoke)

Dietary History
Ask about decreased oral intake.

ASSESSMENT: OBJECTIVE/PHYSICAL EXAMINATION
⚕**CAUTION:** *Ensure that the airway is not compromised before proceeding with any physical examination.*

Physical Examination
⚕**CAUTION:** *Have emergency life-support equipment available.*

   A problem-oriented physical examination should be conducted with particular attention to the following:

- Airway compromise
- Vital signs
- General appearance
- Respiratory status (nasal flaring, retractions, prolonged and labored expiratory phase, bilaterally diminished breath sounds, rhonchi, and scattered crackles)
- Ears
- Nose
- Lymph nodes

Diagnostic Procedures

°**CAUTION:** *Diagnostic procedures should not be attempted until the airway is secured.*

- Lateral neck radiograph
  - Croup: normal epiglottis, with narrowing of the subepiglottic area, steeping sign

DIAGNOSIS

Differential diagnoses may include the following:
- FB
- Traumatic obstruction
- Neoplasm
- Angioneurotic edema
- Laryngitis
- RSV
- Bacterial tracheitis
- Inhalation injury
- Epiglottitis

THERAPEUTIC PLAN

Pharmacologic Treatment

Croup without Stridor at Rest. Prescribe acetaminophen or ibuprofen to control fever.

Croup with Stridor at Rest
- Prescribe racemic epinephrine 2.25% solution by nebulizer every 2 hours while stridor continues at rest. (Lasts approximately 4 hours; watch for rebound effect.)
  - Weight less than 20 kg: 0.25 ml in 2.25 mL saline solution
  - Weight between 20 and 40 kg: 0.50 ml in 2.25 mL saline solution
  - Weight more than 40 kg: 0.75 ml in 2.25 mL saline solution
- Administer dexamethasone (Decadron) 0.6 mg/kg/dose IV, IM, or PO for 1 to 4 doses every 6 to 12 hours. (Use in handheld nebulized treatments has the same results.) Inhaled steroids also are effective.
- Administration of oxygen requires admission to intensive care unit; the client should be hospitalized

for observation if recurrent epinephrine administration is required or if respiratory distress persists.

Nonpharmacologic Treatment
- Oral fluids to maintain hydration
- Cool-mist humidifiers

Client Education
- Keep room humidified with cool mist.
- Keep fever under control.
- Encourage child to intake oral fluids.
- If stridor begins, take child outside into the cool air for 5 minutes; if it does not resolve, then take child to emergency center.

Referral
- Epiglottitis
- Croup with stridor at rest
- Dehydration or inability to drink fluids
- Inability to control fever
- Inability to maintain airway

Prevention

None.

EVALUATION/FOLLOW-UP
- Recurrent croup episodes
- No improvement in 4 to 5 days
- Increase in stridor
- Stops drinking
- Inability to control fever
- New symptom development

Children who have wheezing along with croup may be at risk for airway or lung abnormalities that predispose them to more persistent subsequent wheezing.

COMPLICATIONS
- Intubation with potential laryngeal damage
- Subsequent airway or lung abnormalities

REFERENCES

Ausejo, M., Saenz, A., Pham, B., Kellner, J. D., Johnson, D. W., Moher, D., Klassen, T. P. (1999). The effectiveness of glucocorticoids in treating croup: Meta-analysis. *British Medical Journal, 319,* 595-600.

Castro-Rodriguez, J., Holberg, C., Morgan, W., Wright, A., Halonen, M., Taussig, L. M., Martinez, F. D. (2001). Relation of two different subtypes of croup before age three to wheezing, atopy and pulmonary function testing during a childhood: A prospective study. *Pediatrics, 107*(3), 512-518.

Dello-Stritto, R. (2000). URI. In D. Robinson, P. Kidd, & K. Rogers. *Primary care across the lifespan.* (pp. 1131-1134). St. Louis: Mosby.

Larson, G., Accurso, F., Deterding, R., Halbower, A., & White, C. (1999). Croup. In W. Hay, A. Hayward, M. Levin, & J. Sondheimer (Eds.), *Current pediatric diagnosis and treatment* (14th ed.). Stamford, CT: Appleton & Lange:

Leung, A. & Cho, H. (1999). Diagnosis of stridor in children. *American Family Physician, 60*, 2289-2296.

Miller, J., Eastburn, L, & Fregeau, D. (1999). An update on selected pediatric respiratory infections. *Modern Medicine, 67*(12), 57-66.

Orenstein, D. (1996). Croup. In W. Nelson, R. Behrman, R. Kliegman, & A. Arvin (Eds.), *Nelson textbook of pediatrics* (15th ed., pp. 1667-1680). Philadelphia: Saunders.

Osmond, M., & Evans, D. (2001). Croup. In S. Barton (Ed). *Clinical Evidence*, Vol. 5, 236-245.

Rittichier, K., & Ledwith, C. (2000). Outpatient treatment of moderate croup with dexamethasone: Intramuscular versus oral dosing. *Pediatrics, 106*(6), 1344.

Review Questions

1. C.W., 2 years old, has a sudden onset of stridor. There is no history of a viral illness, fever, or vomiting. The child's mother states that C.W. was well this morning. What would be of highest suspicion on your differential diagnosis?

- **a.** Croup
- **b.** Epiglottitis
- **c.** Neoplastic tumor
- **d.** FB aspiration

2. Croup most commonly is caused by which of the following?

- **a.** *Staphylococcus aureus*
- **b.** *Streptococcus* group A
- **c.** RSV
- **d.** Parainfluenza

3. Which of the following symptoms are indicative of croup?

- **a.** Cough, mild fever, sore throat
- **b.** Barking cough, fever, URI symptoms
- **c.** Rapid onset of fever, drooling, toxic-looking appearance
- **d.** Stridor

4. Once Sara's airway is stabilized, she is sent for a lateral neck radiograph. Which of the following is characteristic for croup?

- **a.** Thumbprint sign
- **b.** Steeple sign
- **c.** White out sign
- **d.** Tracheal narrowing

5. Which of the following has *not* been shown to be effective in treating croup?

- **a.** Racemic epinephrine
- **b.** Antibiotics
- **c.** Inhaled steroids
- **d.** Oral corticosteroids

6. David is a 5-year old boy with a sore throat, fever, and barking cough. Which of the following historical data is consistent with a diagnosis of croup?

- **a.** Members of the family are sick with a viral illness.
- **b.** No one else in the family is sick.
- **c.** His mother has asthma.
- **d.** His father has COPD.

7. What is the best means of preventing croup?

- **a.** Prevnar immunization
- **b.** Hemophilias influenza B immunization
- **c.** Careful handwashing
- **d.** Use of antipyretics and other cough/cold products

8. Croup must be differentiated from epiglottitis. Compared to epiglottitis, croup is associated with which of the following?

- **a.** Drooling
- **b.** High fever
- **c.** Toxic-looking client
- **d.** Barking cough

Answers and Rationales

1. *Answer:* d (analysis/diagnosis)
   Rationale: This child has no other clinical symptoms that suggest croup or epiglottitis, such as fever. Neoplastic tumor is not associated with a sudden onset of stridor. Two-year-old children often place objects into their mouths; therefore they are at greater risk for accidental aspiration of FBs. In any child with a sudden onset of stridor, FB aspiration always should be considered (Leung & Cho, 1999).

2. *Answer:* d (analysis/diagnosis)
   Rationale: Croup is a viral illness, caused by parainfluenza in most cases (Larsen, Accurso, Deterding, Halbower, & White, 1999).

3. *Answer:* b (assessment)
   Rationale: The hallmark of croup is a barking cough. A rapid onset of fever with toxic-looking child is the hallmark of epiglottitis (Larsen et al., 1999).

4. *Answer:* b (analysis/diagnosis)
   Rationale: The steeple sign is characteristic of croup on a lateral neck radiograph. A thumbprint is characteristic of epiglottitis (Orenstein, 1996).

5. *Answer:* b (implementation/plan)
   Rationale: Epinephrine and steroids (inhaled or oral) are effective treatment for croup. Because croup is a viral illness, antibiotics are not effective (Ausejo, Saenz, & Pham, 1999).

6. *Answer:* a (assessment)
   Rationale: In most cases, family members have a viral illness when the client has croup (Orenstein, 1996).

7. *Answer:* c (implementation/plan)
   Rationale: Because croup is a viral illness, there is no true way to prevent the illness. Good handwashing is the most effective means of prevention.

8. *Answer:* d (analysis/diagnosis)
   Rationale: Drooling and toxicity are hallmarks of epiglottitis. Barking cough is the hallmark of croup (Miller, Eastburn, & Fregeau, 1999).

CUSHING'S DISEASE   *Pamela Kidd*

OVERVIEW
Definition

Cushing's disease is a result of extended glucocorticoid excess (hypercortisolism).

Incidence

- Occurs in 2 to 4 persons per million per year.
- More common in women age 20 to 50.
- Rare in children.

Pathophysiology

The adrenal gland regulates the following:

- Controls the body's adjustment to an upright position.
- Permits accommodation to intermittent rather than a constant intake of food.
- Influences immune reactivity, blood cell formation, cerebral function, protein synthesis, and many other body processes.
  Cortisol regulates the following:
- Is the principal glucocorticoid excreted by the adrenal gland.
- Influences appetite and well-being.
- Maintains blood sugar concentrations by promoting hepatic glucogenesis.
- Indirectly affects heart rate and pumping force by controlling synthesis of epinephrine in the adrenal medulla.
- Is critical in the physiologic response to stress and illness.

Hypercortisolism, or Cushing's disease, is a result of pathology of the pituitary gland or the adrenal cortex.

- Most cases of Cushing's disease are due to hypersecretion of the adrenocorticotropic hormone (ACTH) from the pituitary gland with resultant bilateral adrenal hyperplasia. It is five times more frequent in women (Fitzgerald, 2001).
- Almost all cases are due to pituitary microadenomas. A smaller number are due to adrenal adenomas or carcinoma.
- Nonpituitary neoplasms (e.g., small-cell lung cancer) may produce ectopic ACTH.
- An iatrogenic cause of Cushing's disease is long-term corticotropic or glucocorticoid use. This is the most common cause in children.

Factors Increasing Susceptibility
- Female gender
- Neoplasm

Protective Factors. Male gender.

ASSESSMENT: SUBJECTIVE/HISTORY
Symptoms

- Weight gain
- Increased deposition of fat in upper body resulting in classic moon face, buffalo hump, and truncal obesity
- Plethora or beefy red discoloration of the face
- Muscle wasting as evidenced by thin extremities
- Muscle weakness
- Fatigue
- Hypokalemia
- Skin changes including telangiectasia over the face
- Atrophy and thinning of the skin with easy or spontaneous bruising
- Ecchymoses
- Acne
- Hyperpigmentation
- Poor wound healing
- Hypertension and diabetes mellitus

Associated Symptoms

- Development of purplish abdominal striae
- Menstrual irregularities including amenorrhea and oligomenorrhea
- Hirsutism and slight balding in women
- Impotence and decreased libido
- Bone mineral loss producing osteoporosis and back pain
- Crush fractures of the vertebrae
- Hip or wrist fractures may occur after minimal trauma
- Lability of mood, depression, insomnia, anxiety, mania, and/or psychoses

Past Medical History

- Hypertension
- Diabetes
- Osteoporosis
- Amenorrhea
- Medical conditions that utilize glucocorticoids including but not limited to:
  - Rheumatoid arthritis
  - Asthma
  - COPD
  - Lymphoma
  - Skin disorders
  - Allergic disorders

Medication History

Glucocorticoids

Family History

- Autoimmune disorders
- Hypertension
- Diabetes

Dietary History

- Weight gain
- Increased appetite

ASSESSMENT: OBJECTIVE/PHYSICAL EXAMINATION

Physical Examination

A complete physical examination should be performed with particular attention to the following:

- Vital signs (blood pressure)
- Weight (weight gain)
- Body habitus (increased subcutaneous fat in the upper body: moonface, buffalo hump, truncal obesity)
- Cardiovascular (edema)
- Musculoskeletal (muscle wasting, muscle weakness)
- Skin (telangiectasia over the face, atrophy and thinning with bruising, ecchymoses, purplish abdominal striae)
- Hair (thinning, coarse, hirsutism)

Laboratory precision of the testing listed in Table 3-16 is imperative.

- If ACTH is normal or high, CT or MRI of the pituitary is indicated to rule out the presence of a tumor. If ACTH is suppressed, evaluation should focus on the adrenals.
- Additional testing should include a comprehensive metabolic panel to identify hypokalemia, hypernatremia, or hyperglycemia.

DIAGNOSIS

- Alcoholism
- Anorexia nervosa
- Obesity
- Diabetes mellitus
- Hypertension
- Depression

THERAPEUTIC PLAN

Nonpharmacologic Treatment

- If the screening and diagnostic testing is equivocal and clinical features strongly suggest Cushing's disease, referral to an internist or endocrinologist is indicated to confirm the presence of hypercortisolism and establish a plan of care.
- The internist or endocrinologist establishes an ACTH–dependent from a non-ACTH–dependent source of the hypercortisolism.
- The primary treatment for Cushing's disease in adults secondary to pituitary ACTH excess is transsphenoidal microadenomectomy. The cure rate is as high as 90%, with a recurrence rate between 5% and 20%.
- External irradiation, not adenomectomy, is the treatment of choice in children.
- Bilateral adrenalectomy also has been used for years in the treatment of adults, but it has significant operative mortality and morbidity. All clients experience adrenal insufficiency after an adrenalectomy and risk the development of an enlarging pituitary adenoma accompanied by hyperpigmentation known as Nelson's syndrome.

Pharmacologic Treatment

See Table 3-17.

TABLE **3-16** Screening and Diagnostic Testing

TEST	PURPOSE	INTERPRETATION
Dexamethasone suppression test Dexamethasone 1mg is given PO at 11:00 PM, then plasma cortisol level is drawn at 8:00 AM	Screening test to exclude the diagnosis of Cushing's disease. It is used when the diagnosis seems unlikely or the presentation is vague. It results in more false positives than does the urinary free cortisol test.	Normal: <5 µg/dL If value >5 µg/dL a workup for Cushing's disease is indicated. Results can be affected by obesity, acute stress, agitated depression, and alcoholism.
24-hour urinary excretion of cortisol (free cortisol)	Screening test used when the diagnosis of Cushing's disease seems likely. The urinary cortisol is more widely used. Using both urinary and plasma tests are at times advisable.	Normal <120 µg Minimal elevations of plasma cortisol result in marked elevations in urinary cortisol. Not affected by obesity.
Dexamethasone 0.5 mg PO every 6 hours for 2 days	This test is more definitive and is used if the screening tests are positive.	A 24-hour urinary 17-OHS level <3.5mg on the second day or a plasma cortisol level <5 µg/dL on the third day rules out Cushing's disease.

TABLE **3-17** Drug Therapy

DRUG	COMMENT
Mitotane 9-10 g PO qd	An inhibitor of adrenal synthesis and is used alone or in combination with pituitary irradiation. Causes vomiting.
Aminoglutethimide (Cytadren) 250 mg PO qid at 6-hr intervals not to exceed 2 g/day	Usually used as an interim measure until surgery
Ketoconazole (Nizoral)	High doses used for Cushing's disease. NOT U.S. FOOD AND DRUG ADMINISTRATION APPROVED.

Client Education

- Development of signs and symptoms
- Diagnosis
- Treatment
- Medication
- Complications including symptoms of adrenal insufficiency after treatment
- Emotional support to improve body image and self-esteem

Referral

Consultation with an internist or endocrinologist is indicated for evaluation and treatment.

Prevention

Monitor administration of glucocorticoids in clients. Taper dose when possible.

EVALUATION/FOLLOW-UP

Schedule follow-up appointments every 3 months to monitor blood pressure, electrolytes, and symptoms of adrenal insufficiency. Signs and symptoms of adrenal insufficiency include the following:
- Weakness
- Anorexia
- Weight loss
- Hypotension
- Hypovolemia
- Hyperpigmentation concentrated over palmar and other body creases, over pressure points, and around the areolas of the nipples
- Hyperkalemia
- Hyponatremia
- Hypoglycemia
- BUN elevations

COMPLICATIONS

- Death
- Hypertension
- Diabetes
- Compression fractures
- Psychosis

REFERENCES

Davis-Martin, S. (1996). Disorders of the adrenal glands. *Journal of the American Academy of Nurse Practitioners, 8,* 323-326.

Fitzgerald, P. (2001). Endocrinology. In L. Tierney, S. McPhee, & M. Papadakis (Eds.), *Current medical diagnosis and treatment.* New York: Mc-Graw Hill.

Gumowski, J., & Loughran, M. (1996). Diseases of the adrenal gland. *Nursing Clinics of North America, 31,* 747-768.

Loriaux, T. (1996). Endocrine assessment: Red flags for those on the front lines. *Nursing Clinics of North America, 31,* 695-712.

Price, S., & Wilson, L. (1997). *Pathophysiology: clinical concepts of disease processes.* St. Louis: Mosby.

Rogers, K. (2001). Cushing's disease. In D. Robinson, P. Kidd, & K. Rogers. (Eds.), *Primary care across the lifespan.* St. Louis: Mosby.

Rusterholtz, A. (1996). Interpretation of diagnostic laboratory tests in selected endocrine disorders. *Nursing Clinics of North America, 31,* 715-724.

Review Questions

1. Adults or children with Cushing's disease typically complain of which of the following?

    a. Mood swings, weight gain, muscle weakness
    b. Menstrual irregularities, mood swings, muscle weakness
    c. Weight gain, muscle weakness, fatigue
    d. Fatigue, mood swings, weight gain

2. Children usually develop Cushing's disease because of which of the following?

    a. Pituitary microadenoma
    b. Adrenal tumor
    c. Long-term glucocorticoid administration
    d. Adrenal pathology

3. Ms. Jones is a 45-year-old woman seen by the NP. She is concerned about weight gain, fatigue, and edema of her lower extremities. What systems should be checked during physical examination to aid in the diagnosis of Cushing's disease?

    a. Cardiovascular, musculoskeletal, skin
    b. Respiratory, skin, musculoskeletal
    c. Cardiovascular, skin, ophthalmic
    d. Cardiovascular, musculoskeletal, abdominal

4. A person with Cushing's disease has which of the following chemistry values?

    a. Hyponatremia, hypokalemia, hyperglycemia
    b. Hyponatremia, hyperkalemia, hyperglycemia
    c. Hypernatremia, hypokalemia, hyperglycemia
    d. Hypernatremia, hyperkalemia, hyperglycemia

5. An education plan for a client with Cushing's disease includes all the following *except:*
   a. Medication, diagnosis, treatment
   b. Development of symptoms of adrenal insufficiency
   c. Injection of hydrocortisone
   d. Emotional support to improve body image

Answers and Rationales

1. Answer: c (assessment)
   Rationale: The most common presenting symptoms for Cushing's disease are weight gain, muscle weakness, and fatigue. The symptoms are the result of the excessive glucocorticoid effect.

2. Answer: c (analysis/diagnosis)
   Rationale: Children usually develop Cushing's disease after long-term therapy with glucocorticoids causing hypercortisolism.

3. Answer: a (assessment)
   Rationale: The systems with the most noted change from Cushing's syndrome are cardiovascular, musculoskeletal, and skin. The changes include hypertension, edema, increased subcutaneous fat, muscle weakness, and telangiectasia.

4. Answer: c (analysis/diagnosis)
   Rationale: Because of the elevation of glucocorticoids, sodium and glucose usually increase. Potassium is lost.

5. Answer: c (implementation/plan)
   Rationale: Hydrocortisone is used in adrenal insufficiency. If a client develops adrenal insufficiency after treatment, then instruct the client regarding injection of hydrocortisone.

CYSTIC FIBROSIS *Denise Robinson*

OVERVIEW
Definition
CF is a multisystem disorder characterized by cough, maldigestion, and excessive sodium chloride excretion in sweat and saliva.

Incidence
- Has an autosomal recessive inheritance.
- The CF gene is located on chromosome 7.
- Most common genetic disorder of the white population.
- Occurs in approximately 1 in 3000 white live births and 1 in 17,000 black live births in the United States.
- It is a chronic progressive disease with a life expectancy of 30 to 35 years.
- Usually presents before age 1 (70%).
- Presentation of milder forms often do not occur until childhood and, rarely, adulthood.

Pathophysiology
Respiratory Tract. Defective chloride ion transport in respiratory epithelial cells leads to cellular dehydration, causing bronchial secretions to become viscous and difficult to clear. In addition, pH-sensitive enzymes function abnormally, producing epithelial cell composition abnormalities that result in glycoprotein secretions on cell surfaces that adhere to *Pseudomonas* and *Staphylococcus aureus,* increasing the individual's susceptibility to infection.
Digestive Tract. Increased viscosity of mucous gland secretions obstruct pancreatic ducts, resulting in pancreatic fibrosis. Pancreatic enzymes are unable to reach the duodenum, and the digestion and absorption of nutrients is impaired. Intrahepatic bile ducts become blocked with viscous secretions, leading to biliary cirrhosis. The disease may first appear as prolonged neonatal jaundice; however, the condition usually occurs over a more prolonged period.
Reproductive System. Cervical glands become distended with mucus, and the cervical canal is filled with copious amounts of mucus. Endocervicitis develops in many teenagers and young women. In males the epididymis, vas deferens, and seminal vesicles become occluded.

ASSESSMENT: SUBJECTIVE/HISTORY
Newborn
- Family history of CF
- Meconium ileus (failure to pass meconium within first 48 hours) (17% of infants with CF)

Infant
- Chronic cough
- Recurrent URI
- FTT (50% of clients with CF present with FTT and respiratory compromise)
- Chronic diarrhea
- Abdominal distention
- Persistent vomiting, especially with cough
- Salty taste when kissed

Child
- Frequent bulky and foul-smelling stools that float
- Rectal prolapse
- Wheezing
- Recurrent upper and lower respiratory tract infections
- Poor weight gain
- Exercise intolerance

Adolescent/Adult (Rarely Diagnosed this Late)

- Delayed puberty
- Pansinusitis
- COPD

ASSESSMENT: OBJECTIVE/PHYSICAL EXAMINATION

Physical Examination

Newborn
- Prolonged jaundice
- Intestinal atresia
- Meconium ileus
- Abdominal distention

Infant
- Recurrent bronchiolitis
- Persistent infiltrates
- Atelectasis
- Chronic cough
- FTT
- Chronic diarrhea and abdominal distention
- Persistent vomiting (with cough)
- Use of accessory muscles to breathe

Child
- Hyperinflation
- Infiltrates
- Rales
- Rhonchi
- Wheezes
- Digital clubbing
- Barrel chest
- Rectal prolapse
- Nasal polyps
- Steatorrhea

Adolescent/Adult
- Delayed puberty
- Growth failure
- Portal hypertension
- Sterility in males
- Nasal polyps
- Persistent sinusitis
- COPD

Diagnostic Procedures

- Perform sweat test. Quantitative pilocarpine iontophoretic test is done. Sweat chloride values of 60 mEq/L generally are considered diagnostic for CF. Results of 40 mEq/L are considered normal.
- Obtain chest x-ray examination. Early changes include hyperinflation and increased peribronchial markings. Later findings include infiltrates, bronchial thickening, bronchiectasis (tram lines, parallel bronchial markings), and patchy atelectasis.

- Obtain sputum culture. Findings are positive for bacteria.
- Perform pulmonary function tests. Not reliable until age 6 years. Findings include decreased midmaximal flow rate and increased residual volume and residual capacity.
- Elevated serum glucose levels, elevated serum amylase levels, and vitamin deficiency may be found on blood chemistry profiles.

DIAGNOSIS

Differential diagnoses include the following:

- Infant: bronchiolitis, *Chlamydia pneumonitis*, gastroesophageal reflux with aspiration, celiac disease, immune deficiency syndromes, and GI allergies
- Child: asthma, upper and lower respiratory tract allergies, tuberculosis
- Adolescent/adult: asthma, upper and lower respiratory tract allergies or infections, acquired immunodeficiency syndrome, tuberculosis

THERAPEUTIC PLAN

NOTE: *The family NP or pediatric NP may participate in the therapeutic plan as a member of the pulmonary center team. Pulmonary care of these children always should be managed by the pulmonary specialty team, not by the family/pediatric care provider. The community NP role is to serve as a case finder for CF, maintaining a suspicion for children with symptoms of CF, and initiating a workup.*

Nonpharmacologic Treatment

- Refer to pediatric or adult pulmonary disease specialist for long-term management.
- Goals are to prevent bronchial obstruction and respiratory infection, optimize nutrition, and promote a positive psychosocial climate to allow the client to live as normal a life as possible.
- Ensure client receives regular, vigorous chest physiotherapy (percussion and postural drainage, vibratory vest).
- Monitor sputum for pathogens.
- Give infants predigested formula (Pregestimil or Portagen).
- Client should eat high-calorie foods of choice in multiple small meals throughout the day.

Pharmacologic Treatment

- Bronchodilators by MDI (controversial; reserve for those with response to bronchodilation)
- Antiinflammatory agents such as corticosteroids: prednisone (0.1 to 0.2 mg/kg/day) on qod schedule
- Nutritional supplements: fat-soluble vitamins A, D, and E; pancreatic enzyme capsules with every meal and snack; high-protein, high-calorie diet

- Dornase alfa (recombinant DNase) by nebulizer to break down extracellular DNA in sputum; decreases viscosity of secretions and subsequent respiratory infections; 2.5 mg/nebulizer
- Antibiotics: inhaled antibiotics (tobramycin) to suppress pseudomonas to reduce hospitalizations, improve lung function, and lead to fewer days requiring antibiotics for treatment of pseudomonas
- Other antibiotics include chloramphenicol for use against *Staphylococcus* or *H. influenzae.*

Client Education

- Encourage client to follow the routine health maintenance plan carefully. Stress the importance of immunizations (including influenza and pneumonia vaccines).
- If the client's weight is not routinely followed by a nutritionist, monthly weight checks are required.
- Psychosocial help may be required in dealing with chronic illness. Counsel adolescents regarding sexual maturation, potential reproductive problems (males are usually sterile, and females have difficulty becoming pregnant because of thick cervical mucus), and increased risk for STDs.
- Teach clients to recognize the early signs of respiratory infection and the steps to take when symptoms are noted.
- Stress the importance of administering pancreatic enzymes with every meal and snack.

Referral

- All children with CF should be referred to an accredited cystic fibrosis center. These centers provide financial assistance and educational and psychologic support.
- Refer to the Cystic Fibrosis Foundation.
- Refer for genetic counseling.
- Refer for treatment of atelectasis, persistent or severe hemoptysis, or acute respiratory failure. Evaluate unexplained or persistent GI symptoms carefully (increased risk for digestive tract malignancy).
- Refer to nutritionist for poor weight gain.
- Refer adolescent to psychologist for counseling regarding sexual maturation and potential reproductive problems.

EVALUATION/FOLLOW-UP

Respiratory infections must be treated vigorously. Hospitalize for acute exacerbations. Follow growth and development closely, especially weight gain. Children with CF usually remain at or below the 5th percentile, but they should not be permitted to lose weight or fail to gain weight for extended periods. Seasonal immunizations are essential.

COMPLICATIONS

- Pneumonia
- FTT
- Death

REFERENCES

Arvin, A. M., Behrman, R. E., Kliegman, R. M., & Nelson, W. E. (Eds.), (1996). *Nelson textbook of pediatrics* (15th ed.). Philadelphia: W. B. Saunders.

Bindler, R. M. & Howry, L. B. (1997). *Pediatric drugs and nursing implications* (2nd ed.). Norwalk, CT: Appleton & Lange.

Duffield, R. A. (1996). Cystic fibrosis and the gastrointestinal tract. *Journal of Pediatric Health Care, 10*(2), 51-57.

Kidd, P. (2000). Cystic fibrosis. In D. Robinson, P. Kidd, & K. Rogers. (Eds.), *Primary care across the lifespan.* (pp. 288-291). St. Louis: Mosby.

Larson, G., Accurso, F., Deterding, R., Halbower, A., & White, C. (1999). In W. Hay, A. Hayward, M. Levin, & J. Sondheimer (Eds.), *Current pediatric diagnosis and treatment* (14th ed., pp. 436-438). Stamford, CT: Appleton & Lange.

Neglia, J. P., FitzSimmons, S. C., Maisonneuve, P., Schoni, M. H., Schoni-Affolter, F., Corey M, Lowenfels, A. B. (1995). The risk of cancer among patients with cystic fibrosis. Cystic fibrosis and cancer study group. *New England Journal of Medicine, 332,* 494-499.

Orenstein, D. (1996).Cystic fibrosis. In W. Nelson, R. Behrman, R. Kliegman, & A. Arvin (Eds.), *Nelson textbook of pediatrics* (15th ed., pp. 1239-1250). Philadelphia: Saunders.

Stern, R. (1997). The diagnosis of cystic fibrosis. *New England Journal of Medicine, 336,* 487-491.

White, K. R., Munro, C. L., & Pickler, R. H. (1997). Therapeutic implications of recent advances in cystic fibrosis. *The American Journal of Maternal Child Nursing, 20*(6), 304-308.

Wilmott, R. W. & Fiedler, M. A. (1994). Recent advances in the treatment of cystic fibrosis. *Pediatric Clinics of North America, 41,* 431-451.

Review Questions

1. Which of the following symptoms are least suggestive of CF?

  a. Three episodes of bronchiolitis and one episode of pneumonia in the past 8 months
  b. A history of meconium ileus
  c. Abdominal distention with a history of constipation
  d. Failure to gain weight with a steady decline on the growth chart

2. Which of the following findings is considered diagnostic of CF?

  a. Sweat test result of 40 mEq/L
  b. Wheezes and crackles bilaterally on chest auscultation
  c. Digital clubbing and use of accessory muscles with respiration
  d. Sweat test result of 70 mEq/L

3. A 14-year-old girl comes into the clinic because she is concerned about not having started her period. In looking over her records, the family NP notes that the client is below the 5th percentile for height and weight and has a history of recurrent respiratory infections. The differential diagnosis for this client includes all of the following except:

    a. CF
    b. Asthma
    c. Pneumonia
    d. Turner's syndrome

4. An 18-year-old female with CF comes to the clinic with midepigastric pain and recurrent nausea. This is her second visit with the same complaints. The most appropriate action by the family NP is which of the following?

    a. Obtain a careful history and complete physical examination including an upper GI tract x-ray examination.
    b. Ask the client to keep a dietary record for the next week and return to the clinic for follow-up.
    c. Question the client regarding compliance with her nutritional supplements.
    d. Reassure the client that these problems go along with CF and help her identify which foods seem to "upset" her stomach.

5. After a diagnosis of CF has been established, appropriate management by the family NP includes which of the following?

    a. Start a short course of corticosteroids.
    b. Begin antibiotics for any current infection, and refer the client for long-term treatment by a pulmonary specialist.
    c. Admit the client to the hospital for further evaluation and development of a long-term treatment plan.
    d. Teach the client and parents how to use the nebulizer to administer dornase alfa at home.

6. The family NP knows that teaching regarding pancrelipase administration has been effective when the client's mother makes which of the following statements?

    a. "I'll make sure he takes his pancrelipase every time he eats."
    b. "I'll make a schedule so that I can be sure he gets his pancrelipase 4 times every day."
    c. "It embarrasses him to take medicine at school, so I'll make sure he gets in all his doses at home."
    d. "I'll make sure he takes his pancrelipase as soon as he wakes up in the morning so that he will be covered for the day."

7. Danielle is a 4-year-old child who is reported to have wheezing and poor weight gain. Which of the following historical data is consistent with a diagnosis of CF?

    a. She has frequent diarrhea with foul-smelling stools.
    b. She is able to play with her friends when they run.
    c. Her mother has asthma.
    d. She plays on a small-fry soccer team.

8. Which of the following findings on the physical examination is consistent with the diagnosis of CF?

    a. Allergic shiner
    b. Erythema of tympanic membrane
    c. Enlarged abdomen, stool palpated in colon
    d. Hyperinflation of lungs

Answers and Rationales

1. *Answer:* **c** (assessment)
Rationale: Recurrent respiratory infections, meconium ileus, and poor weight gain are consistent with the diagnosis of CF. Diarrhea is consistent with the diagnosis of CF, whereas constipation is not (Larsen, Accurso, Deterding, et al., 1999)

2. *Answer:* **d** (analysis/diagnosis)
Rationale: The diagnosis of CF is based on a quantitative sweat test result of 60 mEq/L (Arvin, Behrman, Kliegman, & Nelson, 1996). Answers b and c may be found on physical examination in a child with CF, but they are not diagnostic.

3. *Answer:* **c** (analysis/diagnosis)
Rationale: Recurrent respiratory infections and poor weight gain can indicate both asthma and CF. Short stature and delayed puberty are consistent with a diagnosis of Turner's syndrome. A diagnosis of pneumonia is not logical in the absence of current respiratory symptoms (Larsen, Accurso, Deterding, et al., 1999).

4. *Answer:* **a** (evaluation)
Rationale: Unexplained or persistent GI symptoms must be evaluated carefully because of the increased risk of digestive tract tumors in individuals with CF (Neglia, FitzSimmons, Maisonneuve, et al., 1995).

5. *Answer:* **b** (implementation/plan)
Rationale: Although the family NP can function as a valuable member of the treatment team, all clients with CF should be referred to a CF treatment center where a team approach can be used (Duffield, 1996).

6. *Answer:* **a** (evaluation)
Rationale: Creon is a pancreatic enzyme replacement that must be taken with all food to aid in the digestion of fats, starches, and proteins (Bindler & Howry, 1997).

7. *Answer:* **a** (assessment)
Rationale: A child with CF usually has exercise intolerance and therefore would not be running with friends or on a soccer team. The child with CF has bulky and foul-smelling stools that float (Kidd, 2000).

8. *Answer:* **d** (assessment)
Rationale: The chest would be hyperinflated on examination in a person with CF (Kidd, 2000).

DELIRIUM *Pamela Kidd*

OVERVIEW
Definition

Delirium is an acute confusional state. A potentially reversible syndrome of acquired cognitive impairment of attention, alertness, and perception, it develops over hours to days and exhibits fluctuations in cognitive function. Hallucinations and visual illusions are common. Delirium is usually caused by a general medical condition such as infection, metabolic disturbance, or pharmacologic toxicity. Drug toxicity is the most common cause of delirium in the elderly.

Incidence

The exact incidence of delirium is not known. Up to 80% of elderly clients with terminal illness experience delirium near death (Breitbart et al., 1997).

Pathophysiology

The pathophysiology of delirium directly relates to the precipitating cause, usually hypoxia, impaired perfusion, impaired metabolism, or neural structural defect.

Factors Increasing Susceptibility
- Chronic illness
- Poor nutrition and hydration
- Impaired immunocompetence

Protective Factors
- Correct management of chronic illness through primary care provider
- No functional decline, ability to fix meals

ASSESSMENT: SUBJECTIVE/HISTORY
Symptoms

Ask about the presence of impaired vision or hearing, illness, dehydration, constipation, depression, fatigue, and infection. Determine pattern, if any, to behaviors. Lack of pattern is more indicative of delirium and not dementia. In dementia, the client usually has difficulty with multitask events (e.g., meal, shower).

Past Medical History

Chronic illness with possible systemic exacerbation.

Medication History

Medications commonly causing delirium are anticholinergic agents, antipsychotic agents, antidepressants, digoxin, H_2 blockers, and antihypertensive agents. Encourage patient to bring all medications, including over-the-counter (OTC), herbal, and prescription, to each visit.

Family History

Alzheimer's in family history.

Dietary History

Dietary history is applicable only in that a nutritious diet contributes to a positive immune system and lack of anemia.

ASSESSMENT: OBJECTIVE/PHYSICAL EXAMINATION
Physical Examination

- Perform complete examination to identify any source of infection or illness.
- Observe for evidence of decreased attention span, alterations in level of consciousness, and perceptual disturbances. Conduct baseline mental status and depression measures.

Diagnostic Procedures

- Urinalysis (U/A) with culture and sensitivity screening
- Chest radiograph if warranted by examination
- Complete blood count (CBC) with differential
- Folate
- Vitamin B_{12}
- Rapid plasma reagin (RPR)
- Comprehensive metabolic profile
- Thyroid-stimulating hormone level

DIAGNOSIS

The most common differential diagnoses related to delirium are depression, drug and alcohol toxicity, normal pressure hydrocephalus, metabolic changes, hepatic disease, hyponatremia, calcium disorders, vitamin B_{12} deficiency, thyroid disease, and hypoglycemia.

THERAPEUTIC PLAN
Nonpharmacologic Treatment

Clients with delirium often require hospitalization for stabilization depending on severity of symptoms and precipitating cause. Until the cause of the delirium is removed, the behaviors are treated in the same manner as that for dementia. Treatment options follow:
- Provide assistance during meals to encourage intake.
- Increase lighting; use contrasting colors.
- Create a routine.
- Give simple, step-by-step instructions; may need to model action.
- Praise generously.
- Be aware of caregiver's tone and voice; client will respond directly in same manner.

Pharmacologic Treatment

Agitation can be treated using neuroleptics, anxiolytics, anticonvulsants, selegiline, and trazodone.

Client Education

Once confusion has been corrected, explain to the client the source of the problem and ascertain why the problem occurred (e.g., did not understand how to take medication). Develop a plan jointly with the client to prevent recurrence.

Referral

Refer to specialist as indicated by diagnosis (e.g., endocrinologist for thyroid condition or diabetes, metabolic problem).

Prevention

Adherence to treatment plan for underlying condition that precipitated the delirium

EVALUATION/FOLLOW-UP

Depends on condition diagnosed as precipitating cause of delirium. Refer to appropriate chapter for the specific condition (e.g., hypothyroidism).

COMPLICATIONS

Death caused by underlying pathological condition.

REFERENCES

Breitbart, W., Rosenfeld, B., Roth, A., Smith, M., J., Cohen, K., Passik, S. (1997). The Memorial Delirium Assessment Scale. *Journal of Pain Symptom Management, 13,* 128.

Kidd, P., & Kitchen, D. (2001). Nursing care of the acutely ill elderly patient. In P. Kidd & K. Wagner (Eds.), *High acuity nursing* (3rd ed.). Stamford, CT: Appleton & Lange.

Review Questions

1. Which of the following statements best describes delirium?
   a. It is a gradual onset of cognitive impairment.
   b. It is a nonreversible condition.
   c. Clients have most difficulty with activities of daily living (ADLs).
   d. It is an acute onset of symptoms that are potentially reversible.

2. In trying to ascertain the source of a client's cognitive impairment, the nurse practitioner (NP) should assess which of the following as a priority?
   a. Client's diet
   b. Family history
   c. Medication history
   d. Home environment

3. Which of the following assessment data would best help the NP make a diagnosis of delirium?
   a. Client has difficulty taking a shower.
   b. There is a pattern of cognitive deterioration present.

   c. The client has experienced hallucinations.
   d. The client has a history of diabetes.

4. Which of the following diagnostic tests would be *least* helpful in diagnosing delirium?
   a. U/A
   b. CBC with differential
   c. Chest radiograph
   d. Cardiac enzyme panel

5. Which of the following specialists is often consulted in treating a client with delirium?
   a. Cardiologist
   b. Pulmonologist
   c. Endocrinologist
   d. Gastroenterologist

Answers and Rationales

1. *Answer:* d (analysis/diagnosis)
   Rationale: Dementia is gradual onset and nonreversible. Cognitive impairment occurs first in both delirium and dementia, followed by difficulty completing ADLs.

2. *Answer:* c (assessment)
   Rationale: Drug toxicity is the most common cause of delirium. Diet will not provide essential information. Family history is relevant in ruling out Alzheimer's disease but is not a priority. Home environment will help determine how to cope with the condition/symptoms but not necessarily provide clues to the cause.

3. *Answer:* c (analysis/diagnosis)
   Rationale: In dementia there is difficulty performing multitask activities (e.g., showering, eating/cooking). There is a lack of a pattern of decline in delirium, and there is great fluctuation. Diabetes may be present as a co-morbidity with either condition, although an uncontrolled blood sugar or associated infection may precipitate delirium. Hallucinations and visual illusions are common in delirium.

4. *Answer:* d (analysis/diagnosis)
   Rationale: Infection is a common cause of delirium. The CBC, U/A, and CXR help identify common sites of or provide information about infection. Cardiac enzymes are not helpful because myocardial infarction is not usually associated with delirium.

5. *Answer:* c (implementation/plan)
   Rationale: Metabolic problems (e.g., diabetes, thyroid disorders) are common causes of delirium. Pneumonia, if present, usually can be treated by the NP. Gastrointestinal and cardiac events are not associated with delirium as often.

DEMENTIA *Pamela Kidd*

OVERVIEW
Definition

Dementia is an acquired syndrome that deteriorates intellectual abilities sufficient to erode daily life in an alert person. Impairment occurs in short- and long-term memory, abstract thinking, judgment, and personality change severe enough to interfere with social activities and relationships with others.

Incidence

Two thirds of all dementias are Alzheimer's disease (AD). Fifteen percent are vascular in origin. The remaining 15% are mixed AD and vascular disease in origin (D'Epiro, 1998).

Pathophysiology

Vascular dementias account for 15% of dementias and are associated with hypertension and cardiovascular disease. The clinical course is stepwise and variable. Focal motor and sensory signs, except fluent aphasia and apraxia, suggest vascular dementia.

A positive diagnosis of *dementia associated with Diffuse Lewy Bodies (DLB)* requires a finding of dementia and at least one of three core symptoms: detailed visual hallucinations, parkinsonian signs, and alterations in alertness or attention. Parkinsonian rigidity and bradykinesia accompanying the onset of dementia suggest DLB. (Parkinsonian signs, especially pill rolling tremor in years predating cognitive decline, usually are indicative of Parkinson's disease, not DLB.)

Pick's disease is a rare brain condition of unknown cause. Atrophy occurs in a relatively circumscribed area of the brain, usually the frontal and temporal regions. Occurs in the age range of 40 to 60 and rarely in old age.

Creutzfeldt-Jacob disease may be caused by a slow-acting virus. Once expressed, it is progressive and fatal, with death usually occurring in 2 years. It is found in middle-aged women and men, and produces ataxia, muscle spasms, seizures, incontinence, psychotic behavior, and visual symptoms. Electroencephalogram (EEG) of clients with Creutzfeldt-Jacob disease shows a characteristic pattern.

Factors Increasing Susceptibility
- Vascular insufficiency
- Small vessel disease
- Nutritional deficiencies
- Hypoglycemia
- Head trauma

Protective Factors
- Proper and adequate nutrition
- Use of helmets and seat belts

ASSESSMENT: SUBJECTIVE/HISTORY

NOTE: *Always speak to both client and another family member/friend separately.*

Symptoms

Increased difficulty with any of the following:
- Learning and retaining new information
- Handling complex tasks
- Reasoning ability
- Spatial ability and orientation
- Language
- Behavior (Costa et al., 1996)

In dementia, the client usually has difficulty with multitask events (e.g., meal, shower). Common behaviors include anger, agitation, insomnia, paranoia, delusions, wandering, screaming, repetitive actions and speech, inappropriate sexual behavior, hoarding, verbal or physical assault, and difficulty eating (Bryant, 1998).

Past Medical History

Assess for chronic illness that may be exacerbating and producing symptoms.

Medication History

Several medication classes can cause or worsen cognitive impairment. Some of the most common are antiarrhythmics, antibiotics, anticholinergics, anticonvulsants, antiemetics, antihypertensives, histamine receptor antagonists, narcotics, and sedatives.

Family History

Family history of AD suggests need to consider AD-type dementia.

Dietary History

Assess 24-hour diet recall to rule out metabolic cause of cognitive impairment (delirium).

ASSESSMENT: OBJECTIVE/PHYSICAL EXAMINATION
Physical Examination

The goal is to assess severity of impairment and to rule out treatable, reversible causes of symptoms (delirium). For example, mild cognitive impairment involves some loss of memory skills, but general cognitive functioning is intact and there is ability to perform ADLs (Petersen et al., 2001).

Diagnostic Procedures

- Noncontrast computed tomography (CT) scan or magnetic resonance imaging (MRI) to rule out central nervous system (CNS) disorder

- CBC with differential to rule out anemia and infection
- Electrolytes to rule out metabolic disorder
- Glucose to rule out diabetes
- Blood urea nitrogen /creatinine levels to affirm kidney function
- Folate level and Vitamin B_{12} level to rule out pernicious anemia
- Thyroid function tests to rule out hypothyroidism

DIAGNOSIS

Rule out infections, CNS disorders, and systemic conditions (e.g., hypothyroid, anemia, neurosyphilis, human immunodeficiency virus [HIV]).

THERAPEUTIC PLAN
Nonpharmacologic Treatment

The NP can help the family/caregiver respond to behavior problems defined as recurrent deviant actions that do not conform to social norms (Bryant, 1998). Have family keep a 1-week behavioral log to describe events associated with the behavior and what was related to a stop in the behavior.

- Remove clutter and keep a small, simple environment.
- Increase lighting; use contrasting colors.
- Create a daily routine.
- Give simple, step-by-step instructions; may need to model action.
- Praise generously.
- Be aware of caregiver's tone and voice; client will respond directly in same manner.
- Identify one behavior at a time to modify.

Pharmacologic Treatment

Agitation can be treated using neuroleptics, anxiolytics, anticonvulsants, selegiline, and trazodone.

Client Education

In this case, the caregiver benefits from education rather than the client. Refer to the nonpharmacologic treatment section.

Referral

Initiate antiagitation therapy in consultation with the neurologist, geriatrician, or psychiatrist.

Prevention

Prevention of cardiovascular disease and hypertension through proper diet and exercise reduces vascular dementias.

EVALUATION/FOLLOW-UP

Schedule patient surveillance and health maintenance visits every 3 to 6 months or more often as needed for problems.

COMPLICATIONS

- Institutionalization of client because of antisocial behavior
- Death from inadequate nourishment

REFERENCES

Bryant, H. (1998). Dementia in the primary care setting. *ADVANCE for Nurse Practitioners, 6*(7), 29-33.

Costa, P. T., et al. (1996, November). *Recognition and initial assessment of Alzheimer's disease and related dementias: Clinical Practice Guideline No. 19.* Rockville, MD: U.S. Department of Health and Human Services, Public Health Service, Agency for Health Care Policy and Research, ACHPR Publication # 97-0702.

D'Epiro, N. W. (1998). Alzheimer's disease: Current progress, future promise. *Patient Care Nurse Practitioner, 1*(3), 22-24, 26-32, 35.

Petersen, R. C., et al. (2001). Practice parameter: early detection of dementia: mild cognitive impairment (an evidence-based review). *Neurology, 56,* 1133-1142.

Review Questions

1. Which of the following behaviors suggest the diagnosis of dementia?
  - **a.** Getting lost
  - **b.** Forgetting the name of a person
  - **c.** Slurred speech
  - **d.** Personality change

2. In assessment of a client suspected of having dementia, the NP should assess if the client has difficulty in which of the following?
  - **a.** Getting dressed
  - **b.** Walking down stairs
  - **c.** Reading the newspaper
  - **d.** Balancing the checkbook

3. Which event presents the most difficulty for a client with dementia?
  - **a.** Making the bed
  - **b.** Folding clothes
  - **c.** Washing dishes
  - **d.** Taking a shower

4. Which of the following medications should the NP avoid in the demented client?
  - **a.** Disopyramide (Norpace)
  - **b.** Glipizide (Glucotrol)
  - **c.** Salmeterol (Serevent) inhaler
  - **d.** Tenormin (Atenolol)

5. Which action should the NP instruct the family of a client with dementia to perform?
  - **a.** Keep the area around the client cluttered with familiar items.
  - **b.** Use dim lighting to decrease agitation.
  - **c.** Do not show the client how to do a task, but let the client initiate the activity.
  - **d.** Use contrasting colors in the house.

Answers and Rationales

1. *Answer:* **d** (analysis/diagnosis)
   Rationale: In dementia, impaired judgment and personality change occur. Getting lost and forgetting the name of a person can happen to anybody and may not indicate short-term memory impairment. Slurred speech is associated with brain attack/stroke.

2. *Answer:* **d** (assessment)
   Rationale: Difficulty getting dressed or walking may be associated with arthritis or a mobility problem. Reading the newspaper may be related to a visual problem. Inability to balance the checkbook is a sign of a problem with reasoning ability and complex cognitive tasks (indications of dementia).

3. *Answer:* **d** (analysis/diagnosis)
   Rationale: Multitask events cause the most difficulty in dementia. The other activities described are single actions.

4. *Answer:* **a** (implementation/plan)
   Rationale: Antiarrhythmics can cause or worsen dementia.

5. *Answer:* **d** (implementation/plan)
   Rationale: Contrasting colors are effective in helping the client engage with his or her environment and find items. Lighting should be bright. Role modeling a task may help the client. Removing clutter and keeping a simple environment is best.

DENTAL PROBLEMS (GINGIVITIS, ACUTE NECROTIZING ULCERATIVE GINGIVITIS, APHTHOUS ULCERS, TOOTH FRACTURE)
Denise Robinson and Pamela Kidd

OVERVIEW
Definition

Gingivitis is the inflammation of the gingiva caused by tooth-borne bacteria (plaque) build-up, which initiates lymphocyte proliferation and the activation of cytokines. This results in the destruction of the periodontal ligament and the alveolar bone, the supporting structures of the teeth.

Acute necrotizing ulcerative gingivitis (ANUG) (trench mouth, Vincent's infection) is a bacterial infection of the gingival tissue. It usually begins between the teeth and spreads in a lateral direction. It may lead to tooth and bone loss.

Aphthous ulcers (canker sores) are superficial ulcerations of the mucous membranes of the mouth and lips. They are further defined as the following:

- *Occasional aphthae*: Occasional aphthae are single lesions that occur in intervals of months or years. They usually heal without complications.
- *Acute multiple aphthae*: Acute multiple aphthae are associated with gastrointestinal disorders. An acute episode may last for weeks. The lesions develop sequentially at different sites in the mouth.
- *Chronic recurrent aphthae*: Chronic recurrent aphthae are one or more lesions that are always present for years.

A tooth fracture is a fracture of the tooth caused by blunt trauma to the tooth. Anterior teeth fractures (Figure 3-3) are classified as the following:

- *Ellis I:* Fracture of the enamel, resulting in a rough edge to the tooth
- *Ellis II:* Fracture that penetrates the dentin; leads to exposure of the pulp
- *Ellis III:* Full-thickness fracture of the tooth; involves the enamel, dentin, and pulp; pink tissue or blood is seen in the fracture
- *Avulsed:* Tooth removed from the socket; may have bone involvement

Incidence
Gingivitis

- Pandemic; occurs in 90% of the population
- Occurs in up to 50% of children; increases in severity with age
- May lead to tooth and bone loss if untreated

ANUG (Trench Mouth, Vincent's Infection)

- Most common in adolescents and young adults who are usually under physical or psychological stress
- First described by the early Romans
- During World War I, this inflammation was referred to as trench mouth

Aphthous Ulcers (Canker Sores)

- Approximately 20% to 50% of adults; females more than males
- Familial tendencies
- More common during the winter and spring months

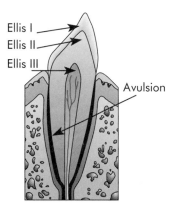

FIGURE **3-3** Ellis classification of tooth fractures.

Pathophysiology

Gingivitis. Gingivitis is an increased bacterial plaque build-up with an acute inflammatory response at the junctional epithelium (the attachment of the gingiva to the enamel surface of the tooth). Common pathogens are gram-positive filamentous rods; actinomyces is most common.

ANUG. It is believed that all of the following pathogens are present:

- Fusospirochetal complex: *Fusobacterium fusiforme*
- Forms:
  - Vibrios
  - Streptococci
  - Diplococci
  - Filamentous
- Spirochete: *Borrelia vincentii*

Aphthous Ulcers. Aphthous ulcers (canker sores) were once thought to be herpes simplex virus (HSV), but the actual cause is not known.

Factors Increasing Susceptibility

Gingivitis. Systemic factors include the following:

- Drugs may cause hyperplasia:
  - Phenytoin (Dilantin)
  - Calcium channel blockers
  - Cyclosporine
- Pregnancy leads to exaggerated inflammatory response, especially in the third trimester
- Vitamin C deficiency
- Diabetes mellitus

Local factors include the following:

- Food impaction
- Trauma
- Smoking
- Mouth breathing, which leads to drying of the gingiva

ANUG

- Stress: physical and psychological
- Systemic diseases

Aphthous Ulcers. None.

Tooth Fracture. Contact sports.

Protective Factors

Gingivitis and ANUG

- Good oral hygiene
- Good nutrition

Aphthous Ulcers

- Good oral hygiene
- Avoidance of oral exposure to others with same

Tooth Fracture

- Use of safety equipment, such as mouth guards

ASSESSMENT: SUBJECTIVE/HISTORY

Symptoms

Gingivitis

Early:

- Bleeding gums after brushing or flossing
- "Bad breath"
- Red gums
- Painless gum swelling

Late:

- Sensitivity to sweets and hot and cold
- Dull, throbbing pain after eating and when awakening

ANUG. Most common symptoms include the following:

- Sudden onset of acute gingival pain
- Bleeding gums with minimal stimulation
- "Bad" taste: foul, metallic
- Breath odor
- Increased salivation
- Fever
- Malaise
- Loss of appetite

Aphthous Ulcers

- Burning sensation 1 to 48 hours before eruption of ulcer
- Pain
- Swelling
- Redness

Tooth Fracture

- Tooth pain
- Bleeding gum line
- Swelling to gum line
- Paraesthesia
- Jaw pain
- Difficulty opening or closing mouth

Past Medical History

Gingivitis

- Mouth breather
- Dental hygiene habits
- Treatment for malocclusion
- Poor dental restorations: poorly done or deteriorated
- Diabetes
- Pregnancy
- Last menstrual period (LMP)
- HIV exposure
- Access to dental care: last dental exam or pattern for dental exams
- Smoking history

ANUG
- Recent emotional or physical stressors
- Diabetes
- HIV
- Dental hygiene habits: date of last dental exam

Aphthous Ulcers
- Allergies to chocolate, nuts, tomatoes
- Autoimmune disease
- Recent trauma
- Drugs: possible reaction
- Stressors: physical or emotional

Tooth Fracture
- Recent mouth trauma
- Dental work: caps, dentures, partials, and others
- Tetanus status, especially if laceration is noted to lips, tongue, or gums
- Allergies to medications
- Chronic diseases such as diabetes and HIV
- LMP
- Last dental hygiene exam

Medication History
Gingivitis
- Antibiotics
- Oral contraceptives
- Dilantin
- Corticosteroids: oral and inhaled
- Insulin
- Chemotherapy

ANUG
- Corticosteroids: oral or inhaled
- Chemotherapy agents
- Immunosuppressive therapy

Aphthous Ulcers
- Antibiotics
- Corticosteroids, especially inhaled

Tooth Fracture
- Aspirin products: increased bleeding tendencies
- Corticosteroids, especially inhaled: associated with gum disease, which increases the risk of tooth loss to trauma

Family History
Gingivitis
- Diabetes
- Periodontal disease

ANUG
- Others in household with same
- Diabetes
- HIV

Aphthous Ulcers
- History of the same
- Autoimmune diseases

Tooth Fracture. Noncontributory.

Dietary History
- *Gingivitis:* poor nutritional intake
- *ANUG:* poor nutritional status, especially the lack of Vitamin C; recent decrease in oral intake related to pain in mouth
- *Apthous ulcers:* recent decrease in oral intake because of pain
- *Tooth fracture:* noncontributory

ASSESSMENT: OBJECTIVE/PHYSICAL EXAMINATION
Physical Examination

Gingivitis. A problem-oriented examination should be conducted with particular attention to the following:
- *General appearance:* Does the patient look healthy or ill?
- *Gingiva:* Note the presence of inflammation and redness surrounding the neck of the tooth, erosion, presence of plaque, hyperplasia, or recession of gums.

ANUG. A problem-oriented examination should be conducted with particular attention to:
- *General appearance:* Does the client look ill?
- *Hydration status:* May become dehydrated related to decreased oral intake because of pain.
- *Gingiva:* Classic triad is the following:
  - Intense pain
  - "Punched-out" interdental papillae, covered with a white pseudomembrane
  - Foul mouth odor
- *Vital signs:* Fever, tachycardia may be present.
- *Neck:* Lymphadenopathy may be present.

Aphthous Ulcers. A problem-oriented examination should be conducted with particular attention to the following:
- *General appearance:* Does the patient look ill?
- *Hydration status:* May become dehydrated because of decreased oral intake
- Oral membrane characteristic lesions include the following:
  - Located on buccal or labial mucosa, pharynx, or lateral tongue
  - One or more
  - Small—less than 10 mm
  - Superficial, shallow, and oval
  - Light yellow to grey fibrinoid center
  - Red ridges

Tooth Fracture. A problem-oriented examination should be conducted with particular attention to the following:

- Perform neurologic examination to rule out possible head injury from trauma.
- Evaluate oral cavity for possible laceration to tongue or gum line, and evaluate for pieces of broken tooth.
- Examine the cervical spine to ensure no injury to cervical spine as a result of trauma to the mouth.
- Assess airway to ensure tooth fragments have not been aspirated or block airway.
- Assess for loose teeth.
- Assess for instability of maxillary bone.

Diagnostic Procedures

- *Gingivitis:* No tests are indicated.
- *ANUG:* Obtain CBC if elevated fever and lymphadenopathy are present.
  - Electrolytes if dehydrated.
  - Consider blood cultures if high fever is present to rule out systemic infection.
- *Aphthous ulcers:* Perform an incisional biopsy of the lesion if unsure of the cause of the lesion, or if the lesions become larger or change color, which is inconsistent with previous aphthous ulcers.
- *Tooth fracture:* Obtain facial, cervical spine, and mandibular radiographs as indicated to rule out fractures of the bones. Obtain a chest radiograph to rule out aspiration of missing tooth fragments.

DIAGNOSIS
Differential Diagnoses for Gingivitis and ANUG

- Dental abscess: local and not generalized
- Periodontitis: involves decay of tooth
- Stomatitis: associated with superficial ulcer formation, not located on gingiva
- Drug reaction: should be linked to medication in history

Aphthous Ulcers

- HSV
- Drug allergies
- Behçet's syndrome
- Inflammatory bowel disease
- Squamous cell carcinoma

Tooth Fracture

- Fracture of mandible
- Le Fort fractures
- Malocclusion injuries
- Closed head injury
- Newly erupting tooth
- Dental infection

THERAPEUTIC PLAN (Table 3-18)
Nonpharmacologic Treatment

Gingivitis and ANUG

- Removal of plaque and other irritants
- Warm saline and water rinses 2 to 3 times a day

TABLE **3-18** Therapeutic Plan for Dental Problems

INFECTION	ORGANISM	PRESENTATION	MEDICATIONS	OTHER TREATMENTS
Gingivitis	Gram-positive filamentous rods	Bleeding gums Red gums Sensitivity to sweet, hot, and cold	None	Tooth plaque removal by dentist Warm saline and water rinses 2-3 times per day
Acute Necrotizing Ulcerative Gingivitis	Fusospirochetal complexes and spirochetes	Classic triad: Intense pain "Punch-out" interdental papillar covered with white pseudomembranes Foul mouth odor Fever, tachycardia	Penicillin V (B), or Erythromycin (B), or Topical anesthetics Chlorhexidine gluconate 0.12% (B)	Increase vitamin C intake Regular dental hygienist care
Apthous Ulcer (Canker Sore)	Herpes simplex virus unknown	Burning sensation 1-48 hours before eruption, pain, swelling, redness, small oval lesion <10 mm	Topical corticosteroids: Amlexanox (Apthasol) 5% paste qid Triamanolone acetonide 0.1% (C), or Fluocinonide ointment 0.05% (C)	Mouth rinse: Benadryl/Maalox (B) Viscous lidocaine (B) Tetracycline (D) Chloraseptic (B)

Aphthous Ulcers. None.

Tooth Fracture
- Apply ice to affected area.
- Apply pressure dressing to bleeding socket.
- Place dislodged tooth in saline.

Pharmacologic Treatment
Gingivitis
- Rinse mouth with antibacterial mouthwash.

ANUG
- Provide penicillin V 250 to 500 mg every 6 hours for 10 days (children 25-50 mg/kg/24 hours in 4 divided doses).
- Provide erythromycin 250 mg every 6 hours for 10 days (children 30-40 mg/kg/day in 4 divided doses).
- Rinse mouth with chlorhexidine gluconate 0.12% and warm water.
- Apply topical anesthetic.
- Use cotton pellets soaked in 3% hydrogen peroxide to debride lesions 3 to 4 times a day.

Aphthous Ulcers
- Amlexanox (Apthasol): Apply 5% paste to area qid.
- Topical corticosteroids are the following:
  - Triamcinolone acetonide, 0.1%, or
  - Fluocinonide ointment 0.05% in an adhesive base (Orbase Plain) to lesions 3 times a day
- Mouth coating: Use a mixture of pseudoephedrine (Benadryl) suspension (5mg/ml) and calcium carbonate (Maalox or Mylanta) in equal parts.
- Mouth rinse: Use viscous lidocaine (Xylocaine) 15 ml swished in mouth every 4 hours for clients more than 12 years of age; 3-5 ml for children 5 to 12 years of age.

Tooth Fracture
- Narcotic pain medications if no head injury
- Nonnarcotic if head injury is suspected

Client Education
Gingivitis and ANUG. The client should do the following:
- Get regular dental and hygienist check-ups.
- Improve diet nutrition, especially Vitamin C.
- Stop smoking.

Aphthous Ulcers
- Use of topical corticosteroid at first sign of tingling may abort the aphthae eruption.
- Topical anesthetics should be applied directly to a lesion that has been dried.
- Do not eat within 1 hour of using anesthetic.
- Eat a bland, soft diet during lesion eruptions.
- Push clear liquids.

- Lesions can recur.
- Provide tetracycline 250 mg capsule opened and the powder mixed in 30-50 ml of water, 3 to 4 times a day for 5 to 7 days.
  - Tetracycline tends to abort the lesions and prevent secondary infections.
  - Tetracycline should not be used during pregnancy.
- Provide Chloraseptic mouthwash every 2 hours for children more than 6 years of age.

Tooth Fracture
- Use proper safety equipment (correctly fitted mouth guard) during contact sports.
- Close follow-up by dentist is essential.
- Eat soft diet until injury is resolved.
- Maintain good oral hygiene.

Referral
- *Gingivitis:* These patients must be referred to the dentist for treatment and further education. This usually results in the return of healthy gingiva.
- *ANUG:* If patient appears ill (i.e., fever, dehydrated, or experiencing severe pain), the patient should be admitted for intravenous (IV) antibiotic and rehydration. Must be seen by a dentist immediately for definitive care.
- *Aphthous ulcers:* If client, especially a child, becomes dehydrated, he or she may require hospitalization. Infants with multiple lesions should be referred to a pediatrician.
- *Tooth fracture:* All tooth fractures must receive follow-up with a dentist.
  - **Ellis I:** Needs referral to a dentist within 24 hours to have crown filed to remove rough edges.
  - **Ellis II:** Needs urgent referral to dentist within 24 hours to have crown placed to prevent bacterial contamination of the pulp.
  - **Ellis III:** Needs urgent referral to an oral surgeon for probable tooth extraction or root canal.
  - **Avulsion:** Needs emergent referral to an oral surgeon within 2 hours for possible tooth reimplantation and root canal.

Prevention
Gingivitis and ANUG
- Brush and floss teeth between each meal.
- Schedule dental hygiene visits every 6 months

Aphthous Ulcers. None.

Tooth Fracture
- Wear protective mouth equipment during contact sporting activity.
- Provide environment safe from falls.

EVALUATION/FOLLOW-UP
Gingivitis

- Close follow-up by the dentist and oral hygienist is essential for continued healthy gingiva. Visiting the oral hygienist every 6 months is recommended.
- During pregnancy, visiting the oral hygienist every 3 months is recommended.
- Children should have the first dental exam between the ages of 12 and 18 months.

ANUG

- Must be followed closely by the dentist for continued care. (This usually requires 2 to 4 visits until healthy gingiva is restored.)
- Nutritional status must be monitored.

Aphthous Ulcers

- Children should be reevaluated within 24 to 48 hours, especially if multiple lesions are present, to ensure that the patient does not become dehydrated.
- Routine follow-up is not always indicated.

Tooth Fracture

Close follow-up by an oral surgeon or dentist is essential.

COMPLICATIONS

Loss of teeth.

Gingivitis, ANUG

- Periodontal disease
- Septicemia

Aphthous Ulcers

- Dehydration
- Weight loss

REFERENCES

Dambro, M. R., Griffth, J., & Cann, C. (1997). *Griffith's 5-minute clinical consult* (pp. 163-165, 424-425). Baltimore: Williams and Wilkins.

Dello-Stritto, R. (2000). Dental problems. In D. Robinson, P. Kidd, & K. Rogers (Eds.), *Primary care across the lifespan.* St. Louis: Mosby.

Parshall, M. (2000). Ear, nose, throat, facial, and dental conditions. In P. Kidd, P. Sturt, & J. Fultz (Eds.), *Emergency nursing reference* (2nd ed.). St. Louis: Mosby.

Rund, D. A. (1996). Facial and oral trauma. In D. A. Rund (Ed.), *Essentials of emergency medicine* (2nd ed., pp. 231-242). Mosby, St. Louis.

Review Questions

1. A client with acute gingivitis asks the NP, "What is the most common cause of gingivitis?" Which of the following would the NP reply?

    a. "No one really knows the exact cause of gingivitis, but good dental care is important for its prevention."
    b. "Gingivitis is caused by both *Fusobacterium fusiforme* and *Borrelia vincentii*."
    c. "Gingivitis is caused by plaque bacteria that builds up below the gum line."
    d. "Gingivitis is caused by the trauma related to a hard-bristled toothbrush."

Situation: P.D. is a 15-year-old boy who states that he fell from his bicycle, striking his face on the ground. He is reporting severe tooth pain. During the evaluation, the NP notes that P.D. has fractures of his eighth and ninth teeth (upper central incisors). On further evaluation, the NP notes pink tissue within the teeth, and the fracture appears to have penetrated the enamel and dentin. (Applies to questions 2 to 4.)

2. On the basis of the Ellis classification for fractures of the anterior teeth, these fractures should be classified as which of the following?

    a. Ellis I fracture
    b. Ellis II fracture
    c. Ellis III fracture
    d. Ellis IV fracture

3. P.D. states that he is not sure where the remainder of the tooth is. During the evaluation of his mouth, the NP does not see teeth fragments. The next step in the evaluation of this client should include which of the following?

    a. Chest radiograph
    b. CBC and U/A
    c. Skull series
    d. No indication for radiologic or laboratory analysis

4. The referral for this client would be which of the following?

    a. Client needs an emergency referral to an oral surgeon within 2 hours for a possible reimplantation of the tooth.
    b. Client needs an urgent referral to an oral surgeon for possible tooth extraction or root canal.
    c. Client needs an urgent referral to a dentist within 24 hours for crown placement and reduction of the risk of bacterial contamination.
    d. Client needs a referral to the dentist to have the crown of the tooth filed to remove the rough edges.

Situation: A child presents with mouth sores. (Applies to questions 5 to 7.)

5. In obtaining the history, the NP notes that the child has a history of asthma, dental caries, and is allergic to chocolate. The mother smokes in the home. The child is not performing well at school. Which information is important to note in relation to the chief complaint?

    a. History of asthma
    b. Allergy to chocolate
    c. School performance
    d. Dental caries

6. Which of the following mouth rinses should be recommended to the mother?

    a. Benadryl and antacid
    b. Saline
    c. Listerine
    d. Viscous xylocaine

7. Effective education of the mother is indicated by which of the following statements?
  a. "I should be most concerned about infection."
  b. "I should take my child to the dentist for follow-up within one week."
  c. "I will make sure my child drinks plenty of fluids."
  d. "I will take my child's temperature every 3 to 4 hours."

Answers and Rationales

1. *Answer:* **c** (analysis/diagnosis)
  Rationale: Gingivitis is caused by the build-up of plaque at the dentogingival junction. The bacteria, if not removed by brushing, will proliferate and lead to this inflammatory process. Answer b: ANUG is caused by these microorganisms.

2. *Answer:* **c** (analysis/diagnosis)
  Rationale: This is an Ellis III fracture. An Ellis I fracture is a fracture of the enamel, resulting in a rough edge to the tooth. An Ellis II fracture is a fracture that penetrates the dentin, which leads to exposure of the pulp. An Ellis III fracture is a full-thickness fracture of the tooth; it involves the enamel, dentin, and pulp. Pink tissue or blood is seen in the fracture. An avulsion fracture is a tooth removed from the socket; it may have bone involvement. There is no such classification as an Ellis IV fracture.

3. *Answer:* **a** (implementation/plan)
  Rationale: It is essential to account for missing tooth fragments. If you are unable to account for the missing fragments, a chest radiograph is indicated to rule out possible aspiration of the tooth fragments. There is no indication for the remainder of the studies, unless you suspect kidney injury or skull fracture in this bicycle crash.

4. *Answer:* **b** (implementation/plan)
  Rationale: This is the correct referral for an Ellis III fracture. Answer a: An avulsion of the tooth. Answer c: Ellis II fracture. Answer d: Ellis I fracture.

5. *Answer:* **a** (assessment)
  Rationale: A history of asthma should alert the NP to assess medications and use of inhalers. Corticosteroid use is frequently associated with apthous ulcers. School performance is not related to the chief complaint. Allergies to chocolate, nuts, and tomatoes are associated with apthous ulcers. Dental caries are not associated with apthous ulcers.

6. *Answer:* **d** (implementation/plan)
  Rationale: Benadryl and antacids are used as a mouth coating, not rinse. Listerine and saline would burn and irritate the mucosa. Viscous xylocaine would provide local anesthesia.

7. *Answer:* **c** (evaluation)
  Rationale: Infection is rarely a complication of apthous ulcers. Fever is not associated with apthous ulcers. Follow-up is not necessary with a dentist. A major concern is dehydration resulting from pain.

DEPRESSION   *Pamela Kidd, Cheryl Pope Kish, and Denise Robinson*

OVERVIEW
Definition

Depression is a disturbance in mood or affect. Depressive disorders are classified as the following:

- *Major depressive disorder* is characterized by two or more episodes of a depressed mood or loss of interest lasting at least 2 weeks.
- *Dysthymia* is defined as symptoms of depression that are less intense but of longer duration (2 years or more) with impaired functioning.
- *Adjustment disorder depression* is defined as the onset of depression symptoms in response to an identifiable event within the preceding 3 months. This does not include posttraumatic stress disorder.
- *Postpartum depression, or "baby blues,"* is a type of adjustment disorder that occurs during the first few days to weeks after childbirth, and is self-limited. Postpartum blues are believed to be caused by sudden changes in estrogen, progesterone, and prolactin levels after childbirth. Major depression may also occur postpartum.

Incidence

- Depression is twice as common in women as in men.
- It is believed that 8% to 12% of men and 18% to 25% of women suffer a major depression in their lifetime.
- At any given time, 10 to 14 million Americans are suffering from some form of a mood disorder.
- Depression is the most common reason for seeking mental health treatment. It accounts for 75% of the hospitalized psychiatric clients and 6% to 8% of all outpatients in a primary care setting.
- There is an increased incidence of depression in older adults who are living in long-term facilities.
- Depression is more common in young women and tends to decrease with age; however, the incidence increases in women older than 50 with hypothyroidism.
- In men, the incidence tends to increase with age.
- Older adults are at a high risk for depression because of the multiple losses and health problems that frequently occur at this stage of life.
- No significant relationship has been found between race and mood disorders.
- Incidence increases once a person has experienced a depressive episode (50% after the first, 70% to 80% after the second).

- Suicide is a risk for all clients with a mood disorder. It is the eighth leading cause of death in the United States across all age groups, and the third leading cause of death for adolescents and young adults. Suicide is also a leading cause of preventable death for adults older than 60.
- Depression affects 2% of prepubertal children and 5% to 8% of adolescents.
- The incidence of postpartum depression is 8% to 26%; recurrence in subsequent pregnancy is common. As many as 80% of new mothers experience postpartum "blues."

Pathophysiology

Various theories have been formulated to explain the cause and dynamics of mood disorders. It is believed that these disorders are a syndrome with common features and a variety of causative factors. The most common theoretical perspectives are the following:

- *Biochemical/neurobiologic:* There is a functional deficiency of the neurotransmitters serotonin, dopamine, norepinephrine, and acetylcholine, with a probable genetic component.
- *Psychodynamic:* This theory focuses on perceived loss and the unresolved grieving that occurred in the early child-parent relationship. The unresolved grieving is accompanied by repressed anger, resulting in anger turned against the self.
- *Cognitive:* Schemas direct the way people experience others and themselves. Those who are depressed ignore the positive and focus on the negative messages, thus contributing to a view of self as unworthy, incompetent, and unlovable. When this occurs, cognitive distortions result.

Factors Increasing Susceptibility
- Marital status: single and divorced persons
- Seasonal: increase in spring and fall
- Previous episode: prior episodes of depression increase chance of another episode
- Age: less than 40
- Postpartum state
- Physical illness
- Inadequate social support
- Substance abuse
- Ineffective psychosocial functioning

Risk Factors For Suicide
- White race
- Physical illness
- Substance abuse
- Male
- Increasing age
- Living alone

- Previous suicide attempts
- Less education
- Relationship conflict
- Family or other suicide
- Loss of income/employment
- Impaired impulse control

ASSESSMENT: SUBJECTIVE/HISTORY

The clinical interview is the most effective method for detecting depression.

History of Present Illness
- Determine the level of depression and severity of symptoms.
- Identify when the symptoms began, as well as aggravating and relieving factors.
- In postpartum woman, identify abnormal bonding behaviors and evidence that the woman may harm her infant.

Past Medical History
- Obtain a complete personal history of panic attacks, depression, and suicide attempts.
- Obtain a history of cerebral vascular accident, myocardial infarction, or other chronic debilitating illness.

Medication History
- Reserpine
- Oral contraceptive pills
- Steroids
- Amphetamine/cocaine withdrawal

Family History
- Ask about family history of depression/suicide attempts and mental illness.
- If the history indicates previous depressive episodes, ask about treatment obtained.

Psychosocial History
- Discuss the client's support systems and coping techniques.
- Determine whether there is substance abuse. Illegal or legal drug use and alcohol can complicate or cause depression. It is essential that the clinician obtain a complete list of all substances used by the client.
- Ascertain the client's perceived losses and current stressors.
- Suicide risk must be critically assessed. Specific and clear questions should be asked by the NP regarding the following:
  - Suicidal thoughts and history of past suicide attempts
  - Presence of a plan for suicide
  - Access to a means of suicide

TABLE **3-19** Lethality Assessment Scale

DANGER TO SELF	INDICATORS
No predictable risk of immediate suicide	No notion of suicide, no history of attempts, satisfactory social support network, close contact with significant others
Low risk of immediate suicide	Person has considered suicide with low lethal method, no history of attempts or recent serious loss, has satisfactory support network, no alcohol problems, basically wants to live
Moderate risk of immediate suicide	Has considered suicide with high lethal method but no specific plan or threats or has plan with low lethality, history of low lethal attempts; has tumultuous family history and reliance on benzodiazepines for stress relief; is weighing the odds between life and death
High risk of immediate suicide	Has current high lethal plan, obtainable means, history of previous attempts, has a close friend but is unable to communicate with him or her; has a drinking problem; is depressed, wants to die
Very high risk of immediate suicide	Has current high lethal plan with available means, history of high lethal suicide attempts, is cut off from resources; is depressed and uses alcohol to excess, and is threatened with a serious loss, such as unemployment or divorce or failure in school

From Hoff, L. A. (1995). *People in crisis* (4th ed.). San Francisco: Jossey Bass.

D

- The more specific and structured the plan, the greater the risk for suicide (Table 3-19)

Symptoms

Symptoms most often associated with depression include the following:

- Feelings of sadness, guilt, low self-esteem
- Pessimistic thoughts
- Suicidal thoughts, gestures, attempts
- Tearfulness, anxiety, irritability
- Anhedonia (loss of interest or pleasure in activities that were previously enjoyed)
- Sleep disturbances
- Changes in appetite, with either weight gain or loss
- Decreased libido
- Impaired cognitive reasoning (all-or-nothing thinking, jumping to conclusions, mental filtering, personalization, and "should" statements)
- Physiologic symptoms include the following:
  - Fatigue
  - Headache
  - Chest pain
  - Alteration in bowel and bladder function
  - Amenorrhea
  - Nausea and vomiting
  - Psychomotor agitation or retardation

Children
- Loss of appetite
- Fatigue
- Conduct problems
- Aggression: temper tantrums, other behavioral problems

- Anhedonia
- Fear of separation from caregiver or fear of caregiver
- Failure to achieve developmental tasks
- Low self-esteem, guilt
- Somatic complaints: stomachache, headaches

Adolescents
- Isolation
- Self-destructive behavior
- Sexual promiscuity
- Antisocial behavior
- Negative thinking
- Weight change
- Anhedonia
- Substance abuse

Older Adults. Many of the physical symptoms of depression, such as fatigue, anorexia, and bowel and bladder problems, are often attributed to "old age." Older adults may also manifest symptoms that must be differentiated from those of dementia. These symptoms may include the following:
- Disorientation
- Impaired memory
- Inability to concentrate
- Anhedonia

Postpartum Women. Appetite change, sleep disturbances, fatigue, and decreased libido are associated with normal adjustment to parenting and the presence of a newborn in a home. These temporary changes must be differentiated from a serious depression.

Depression is manifested by impaired responses in the four following areas:

1. *Emotional:* sadness, worthlessness, apathy, guilt and anger, suicidal ideation or gestures
2. *Behavioral:* anhedonia, poor hygiene, psychomotor retardation
3. *Cognitive:* impaired concentration, obsessive thoughts, indecisiveness
4. *Physical:* fatigue, appetite, sleep, constipation

ASSESSMENT: OBJECTIVE/PHYSICAL EXAMINATION
Physical Examination

The physical examination should be thorough, with particular attention given to the following:

- *General appearance:* poor eye contact, tearful, downcast, inattentive to appearance
- *Speech:* little or no spontaneous speech, monosyllabic, long pauses, slow, low, monotone
- *Mental status:* memory, affect, judgment, cognitive abilities, thought content, preschool and school-aged children appear sad
- Thyroid enlargement
- Neurologic status

Diagnostic Procedures

Currently there are no conclusive diagnostic physical examination findings or laboratory tests for depression; however, certain abnormal results have been noted in a few tests. These abnormal results include the following:

- Abnormal sleep EEGs are seen in about 50% of all outpatients with depression.
- The dexamethasone suppression test is sometimes employed to help establish a diagnosis of depression.
- Thyroid function studies are often done to rule out hypothyroid disorder.
- Many clinicians use various rating scale instruments designed to measure the client's mood to aid in the diagnosis of depression.
- Use postpartum depression checklist such as the Edinburgh Postnatal Depression Scale to facilitate diagnosis after childbirth.
- In children, perform a CBC to rule out anemia, obtain a lytes level to rule out electrolyte or renal problems, and perform an EEG to rule out seizure disorder.

DIAGNOSIS

- Conduct a clinical interview for signs/symptoms of depression.
- Investigate the possibility of substance abuse.
- Conduct a medical review of systems to identify a medical disorder.

- Identify the presence of another concurrent psychiatric disorder.
- Exclude alternative causes.
- The differential diagnoses include the following:
  - Organic mood disorder
  - Schizophrenia
  - Grief
  - Delirium
  - Dementia
  - Substance abuse
  - Endocrine disorders
  - Liver failure
  - Chronic fatigue
  - Renal failure

THERAPEUTIC PLAN
Nonpharmacologic Treatment

- The initial and primary goal of nonpharmacologic treatment is to provide for the safety of the client. Determine the lethality of the client's suicidal ideation/plan. Remember that suicide is most likely when a client is going into or emerging from depression.
- Avoid excessive cheerfulness, which might diminish the significance of the client's feelings.
- Establish a no-suicide contract with the client.
- Assist the client in contacting immediate support systems. If the client is clearly suicidal and unwilling to contract not to harm self, immediate hospitalization must be considered.
- Exercise appears to be beneficial. Initially, a 10-minute walk is suggested.
- Psychotherapy is recommended to treat depression, either alone or in combination with medication. Individual and group therapy are both effective modalities.
- Electroconvulsive therapy is recommended to treat the most severe forms of psychotic depression that are not responsive to other forms of therapy.

Pharmacologic Treatment

Antidepressants are effective in the treatment of all types of depression ranging from dysthymia to severe depression. Appropriate agents include the tricyclic antidepressants, monoamine oxidase inhibitors (MAOIs), and the selective serotonin reuptake inhibitors (SSRIs). The choice of medication is based on consideration of the following factors:

- Client history of previous treatment and response; family response to antidepressants
- Type of depression
- Side effects of the medication
- Other medications the client may be taking
  - In general, doses for children and elderly should be half of normal starting dose

- Discontinuation syndrome occurs when medications stopped abruptly; taper medications if stopped
- Whether postpartum client is breastfeeding when prescribing antidepressants

SSRIs

- Begin fluoxetine or paroxetine 20 mg qd. This can be increased in 1 week to 40 mg qd.
- The side effect profile of SSRIs includes headache, dry mouth, sexual dysfunctioning, sleepiness, restlessness, and insomnia. These side effects generally improve over time.
- Decreased libido may continue; patients should be asked specifically about their sexual desire.
- SSRIs are the best choice if suicide is a concern.

Tricyclic Antidepressants

- Have potential for overdose.
- Need to do an electrocardiogram (ECG) before starting medications because a cardiotoxic effect can occur in children, especially with overdose.
- Examples include amitriptyline (Elavil) and nortriptyline (Pamelor). Anticholinergic side effects include dry mouth, constipation, blurred vision, urinary retention, orthostatic hypotension, and sleepiness.

MAO Inhibitors. MAOIs are reserved for treatment when other medications have failed. In general, NPs do not prescribe MAOIs.

Client Education

- Most antidepressant medications take 4 to 6 weeks before any significant results are obtained, although benefits may be seen in as little as 2 weeks.
- Inform the client and family of medication side effects, with special emphasis on those effects that must be reported. Include dietary and activity restrictions related to the medication.
- Instruct the client and family when to seek professional help. Teach the client and family to report increasing signs of depression or suicidal thoughts.
- Advise the family of a postpartum client that the woman should not be left alone with the infant when exhibiting symptoms of delusions, hallucinations, or the illogical thought patterns of psychotic depression.
- Remind the woman's partner that postpartum depression is likely to recur in subsequent pregnancies.
- Reinforce effective coping behaviors, nutrition, exercise, rest, and socialization.
- It is important for the family to make the patient feel as though she is a valued and important member of the family.

Referral

- Referral to a mental health specialist for counseling should be seriously considered.
- Any patient who is difficult to diagnose and treat should be referred. These patients include the following:
  - Very young patients: infants, toddlers
  - Those with significant co-morbidities
  - Bipolar disorder
- Immediate consultation is needed for anyone who is actively suicidal.
- Immediate consultation is needed for the woman whose newborn is at risk.

Prevention

Unknown

EVALUATION/FOLLOW-UP

- Clients who are depressed and receiving antidepressant medications should return weekly for evaluation. If improvement is seen after 5 to 6 weeks, the follow-up can be decreased to two times a month, then monthly, and so on.
- Counseling combined with antidepressant therapy is critical to obtaining the most improvement.
- Each successive episode of depression suggests that psychosocial events have little or no role in the disorder as the disorder becomes more firmly established.
- The most common reasons for continuing depression are prescribing too low a dose of antidepressants, not treating the depression long enough, or an underlying substance abuse or medical condition.
- Maintain the client on medication for at least 4 to 9 months for the first episode of depression, 1 to 2 years for the second episode, and lifelong for three or more episodes.
- Treat clients indefinitely who are more than 40 years old and have had two or more episodes, or those who are more than 50 years old and have had one episode.
- Relapse rate is 50% during the first 6 to 18 months.
- Improvement is seen when the client accomplishes the following:
  - Verbalizes and demonstrates compliance with treatment plan.
  - Experiences no suicidal thoughts and does not have a suicide plan.
  - Verbalizes positive feelings about the future.
  - Demonstrates resolution of presenting symptoms.

COMPLICATIONS

- Continued depression
- Suicide
- In postpartum women, harm to infant

- Problems with mothering; occurs when the postpartum client experiences depression; children of such women experience cognitive and social problems in development, are more likely to have frequent illnesses during childhood

REFERENCES

American Psychiatric Association (APA). (1994). *Diagnostic and statistical manual of mental disorders* (DSM-IV) (4th ed.). Washington, DC: APA.

Beck, C. T. (1998). A checklist to identify women at risk for developing postpartum depression. *Journal of Obstetric, Gynecologic, and Neonatal Nursing, 27*(1), 39-46.

Beck, C. T. (1999). Postpartum depression: Stopping the thief that steals motherhood. *AWHONN Lifelines, 3*(4), 41-44.

Flowers, M. E. (1997). Recognition and psychopharmacologic treatment of geriatric depression. *Journal of the American Psychiatric Nurses Association, 3*(2), 32-39.

Kish, C. P. (in press). The postpartum family at risk. In S. Olds, M. London, & P. Ladewig (Eds.), *Maternal newborn nursing: A family and community-based approach* (7th ed.). Upper Saddle River, NJ: Prentice Hall.

The Harvard Mental Health Letter. (1994, December). Update on mood disorders. Part 1, 1-4.

The Harvard Mental Health Letter. (1995, January). Update on Mood Disorders. Part 2, 1-4.

The Harvard Mental Health Letter. (1996, November). Suicide. Part 1, 1-4.

Robinson, D. (2000). Depression. In D. Robinson, P. Kidd, & K. Rogers (Eds.), *Primary care across the lifespan* (pp. 307-320). St. Louis: Mosby.

Rush, A., et al. (1993, April). *Depression in primary care*: Volumes 1 and 2, Clinical practice guidelines, No. 5. Rockville, MD: U.S. Department of Health and Human Services, Public Health Service, Agency for Health Care Policy and Research, AHCPR Publication No. 93-0550.

Sung, S., & Kirchner, J. (2000). Depression in children and adolescents. *American Family Physician, 62,* 2297-2308, 2311-2312.

Wilson, H., & Kneisl, C. (1996). *Psychiatric nursing* (5th ed., pp. 324-359, 793-802). Menlo Park, CA: Addison-Wesley.

Review Questions

1. Which of the following patients is more at risk for suicide?
- **a.** Sam, who has a close relationship with his wife
- **b.** Sue, who has no history of suicide attempts in the past
- **c.** Terry, who is dependent on alcohol
- **d.** John, who recently changed jobs

2. Which of the following symptoms are representative of depression in a child?
- **a.** Chest pain
- **b.** Stomach ache
- **c.** Alteration in bowel and bladder function
- **d.** Impaired memory

3. A client complains of severe anticholinergic side effects following 4 weeks of treatment on a tricyclic antidepressant (imipramine [Tofranil]). Which of the following drugs has a lower side effect profile in terms of anticholinergic symptoms?
- **a.** SSRI (sertraline [Zoloft])
- **b.** Tricyclic (nortriptyline [Pamelor])
- **c.** MAOI (phenelzine [Nardil])
- **d.** Antianxiety/sedative (alprazolam [Xanax])

4. A client with severe clinical depression who has been treated for 3 weeks is starting to show signs of improvement. During this recovery period, which of the following applies to the client?
- **a.** The client is no longer at risk for suicide.
- **b.** The client is at a greater risk for suicide than when severely depressed.
- **c.** The client is less of a risk for suicide than when severely depressed.
- **d.** The client will always be at a high risk for suicide.

5. A middle-aged married couple comes to the clinic. During the interview assessment, the wife verbalizes concern about her husband's major mood swings and not knowing what to expect from him. What information should the NP elicit first?
- **a.** Family history of mental illness
- **b.** Information about their sexual relationship
- **c.** Information about any stresses or losses that have occurred within the past year
- **d.** More detailed information about the symptoms and what impact they have on the couple's daily life

6. Subjective symptoms of clinical depression include all the following, *except*:
- **a.** Grandiosity
- **b.** A sense of worthlessness
- **c.** Fatigue
- **d.** Anhedonia

7. Which of the following interventions is not appropriate in treating a client with clinical depression?
- **a.** Convey unconditional acceptance and respect.
- **b.** Assist in the identification of real achievements to promote self-esteem.
- **c.** Consistently maintain a very cheerful attitude when interacting with the client.
- **d.** Keep all commitments to build trust.

8. What should the NP teach the family of a client with clinical depression?
- **a.** It is important that the client feel a sense of being a useful and valued member of the family.
- **b.** The family should hide any negative feelings from the client.
- **c.** The family needs family therapy to prevent a relapse in the client.
- **d.** Depression will be a constant problem throughout the client's life.

Answers and Rationales

1. *Answer:* **c** (assessment)
  Rationale: The person who is dependent on alcohol is more likely to run a high risk of immediate suicide (Robinson, 2000).

2. *Answer:* **b** (assessment)
   Rationale: Children are more likely to have somatic symptoms, which conveys their inner turmoil (Sung & Kirchner, 2000).

3. *Answer:* **a** (evaluation)
   Rationale: SSRIs are thought to have less anticholinergic effects than the tricyclic drugs (Wilson & Kneisl, 1996).

4. *Answer:* **b** (evaluation)
   Rationale: Individuals are at a greater risk for suicide when going into or emerging from depression (Harvard Mental Health Letter, 1996, November).

5. *Answer:* **d** (analysis/diagnosis)
   Rationale: Although all the information may be essential, the NP first needs accurate information about the symptoms to complete a comprehensive assessment (Wilson & Kneisl, 1996).

6. *Answer:* **a** (assessment)
   Rationale: Grandiosity implies feelings of self-importance, which is more characteristic in mania (Wilson & Kneisl, 1996).

7. *Answer:* **c** (implementation/plan)
   Rationale: Excessive cheerfulness can diminish the significance of the depressed person's feelings (Wilson & Kneisl, 1996).

8. *Answer*: **a** (implementation/plan)
   Rationale: A major emotional symptom seen in depression is a sense of worthlessness (American Psychiatric Association, 1994).

DERMATITIS *Pamela Kidd*

OVERVIEW
Definition
Contact dermatitis is an eruption of the skin related to contact with an irritating substance or allergen. Secondary bacterial infection can occur, increasing inflammation.

Incidence
Dermatitis occurs in all ages and both genders. No ethnic predisposition exists.

Pathophysiology
An epidermal reaction is caused by sensitized T lymphocytes after contact with an antigen or irritating substance. If produced by an antigen, it is considered a type IV delayed hypersensitivity reaction that takes several hours to manifest.

Factors Increasing Susceptibility
- Jewelry
- Cosmetics
- Travel
- Nickel
- Rubber, latex
- Plants
- Detergents

Protective Factors. Avoid known antigens.

ASSESSMENT: SUBJECTIVE/HISTORY
Symptoms
- Rash 10 to 12 hours after exposure
- Pruritus
- Edema and erythema
- Stinging, burning, and pain
- Fever

- Ask about hiking, grass cutting, new clothes, perfume, detergent, food, occupation, and exposures.

Past Medical History
History of previous allergen exposure followed by pruritic rash.

Medication History
Recent use of antimicrobial, topical antihistamine, or anesthetic.

Family History
Usually not significant.

Dietary History
Usually not significant.

ASSESSMENT: OBJECTIVE/PHYSICAL EXAMINATION
Physical Examination
- Undress patient and check entire body for lesions.
- *Skin:* Erythematous macules, papules, and vesicles. May have bullae with drainage. Secondary lesions with crusting, excoriation, and lichenification may be present. Lesions are on exposed parts and have bizarre distribution patterns. Swelling may be present.
- Location of the rash helps provide clues to the offending antigen, which may include any of the following:
  - *Generalized:* airborne (paint, ragweed), bath oil, soap, powder, topical medications
  - *Scalp:* hair dyes, sprays, shampoos, hair preparations
  - *Forehead:* hat bands
  - *Eyelids:* cosmetics
  - *Earlobes:* nickel in earrings
  - *Face:* cosmetics

- *Perioral:* lipstick, toothpaste, mouthwash
- *Neck:* perfumes
- *Hands:* soap, nickel, lotion, chemicals
- *Arms:* wristbands; soap; poison ivy or other plant; chemicals; new, unwashed clothing
- *Axilla:* deodorants
- *Trunk:* new, unwashed clothing; nickel or rubber in clothing (belts, bra straps)
- *Anogenital:* menstrual pads, contraceptives (condoms, foams, gels), plant/poison ivy (camping in a location without restroom facilities)
- *Feet:* powders, shoes, athlete's foot medicine

Diagnostic Procedures

- May be none necessary.
- Gram's stain and culture rules out impetigo.
- Scraping rules out scabies.
- KOH prep test rules out tinea.
- Patch test helps client learn what to avoid in the future. The patch test cannot be performed during acute episode (Berger, 2001).

DIAGNOSIS

- *Tinea:* linked with heat and humidity; rash is more round; usually affects face, neck, and arms
- *Impetigo:* classically occurs in children; history of siblings, other family member with similar lesions increases probability of impetigo; poor hygiene may be evident
- *Irritant form of contact dermatitis:* scaling and erythema (Berger, 2001)
- *Allergic form of contact dermatitis:* weepy and crusted lesions (Berger, 2001)

THERAPEUTIC PLAN
Nonpharmacologic Treatment

- Administer cool, moist compresses or tub bath with colloidal oatmeals.
- Apply calamine lotion to affected area.
- Bandage areas with wet dressings several times a day.

Pharmacologic Treatment

See Table 3-20.

NOTE: *For more information about prescribing topical corticosteroids, please refer to the eczema and atopic dermatitis section.*

- Antihistamine of choice may be used for itching and to decrease edema.
- Antibiotics may be used for secondary infection.

Client Education

- Avoid irritant/antigen if known.
- Remove allergen promptly with prolonged washing with water or isopropyl alcohol soon after exposure.

Referral

- Refer to dermatologist for patch testing.
- Consult with dermatologist if no improvement.

Prevention

- Wear personal protective equipment at work to prevent exposure or change work activity.
- Use barrier cream (e.g., Ivy Shield, Vioform) before exposure to allergen.

EVALUATION/FOLLOW-UP

See client until symptoms subside (usually 2 to 3 weeks).

COMPLICATIONS

- Skin infection
- Scarring

REFERENCES

Berger, T. (2001). Skin, hair, & nails. In L. Tierney, S. McPhee, & M. Papadakis (Eds.), *Current medical diagnosis and treatment* (40th ed.). New York: McGraw-Hill.

Berger, T., Goldstein, S., & Odom, R. (1998). Skin and appendages. In L. Tierney, S. McPhee, & M. Papadakis (Eds.), *Current medical diagnosis and treatment* (36th ed.). Stamford, CT: Appleton & Lange.

TABLE **3-20** Pharmacologic Treatment for Contact Dermatitis

DRUG	DOSE	COMMENT
Topical corticosteroids	Mid-potency (Fluocinonide gel 0.05% bid or tid, Triamcinolone 0.1%) to high-potency (amcinonide 0.1%, desoximetasone 0.25%) corticosteroids	Use for localized involvement only and *never* on the face or in body folds. Taper number of applications per day.
Prednisone	60 mg for 4-7 days 40 mg for 4-7 days 20 mg for 4-7 days	Key is to use enough for effectiveness and taper slowly to prevent rebound. Medrol dosepack will not achieve desired effect and prevent rebound (Berger, 2001).

Boynton, R., Dunn, E., & Stephens, G. (1998). *Manual of ambulatory pediatrics* (4th ed.). Philadelphia: Lippincott.

Kidd, P. (2000). Contact dermatitis. In D. Robinson, P. Kidd, & K. Rogers (Eds.), *Primary care across the lifespan*. St. Louis: Mosby.

Pierce, N. (1995). Bacterial infections of the skin. In L. Barker, J. Burton, & P. Zieve (Eds.), *Principles of ambulatory medicine* (4th ed.). Baltimore: Williams & Wilkins.

Review Questions

1. Which of the following actions promotes primary prevention of contact dermatitis?

   a. Wear personal protective equipment at work.
   b. Use Ivy Shield cream before exposure.
   c. Wash with water after exposure.
   d. Take diphenhydramine (Benadryl) before exposure.

2. Which of the following diagnostic tests should the NP perform when he or she suspects contact dermatitis?

   a. None
   b. KOH prep test
   c. Gram's stain and culture
   d. Microscopic scraping of lesion

3. Which of the following findings should cause the NP to consider a diagnosis of contact dermatitis?

   a. Rash
   b. Pruritus
   c. Erythema
   d. Papules

4. In the assessment of a client with suspected contact dermatitis, the NP should do which of the following?

   a. Check behind the ears of the client.
   b. Assess the popliteal regions.
   c. Completely undress the client and assess the total body.
   d. Check the conjunctiva.

5. Which of the following should the NP prescribe for a client with contact dermatitis of the face caused by cosmetic use?

   a. Fluocinonide gel
   b. Triamcinolone cream
   c. Medrol dosepack
   d. Prednisone 60 mg for 5 days, 40 mg for 5 days, 20 mg for 5 days

Answers and Rationales

1. *Answer:* a (implementation/plan)
   Rationale: Personal protective equipment (e.g., clothes) prevents exposure to potential allergens. The other three options are meant to prevent reaction postexposure. They are secondary preventive efforts.

2. *Answer:* a (analysis/diagnosis)
   Rationale: No diagnostic test is necessary. KOH rules out tinea. Microscopic scraping rules out scabies. Gram's stain and culture rules out impetigo.

3. *Answer:* b (analysis/diagnosis)
   Rationale: A key finding in contact dermatitis is pruritus. The other signs may be present in multiple dermatologic disorders.

4. *Answer:* c (assessment)
   Rationale: Because contact dermatitis is a result of contact with an allergen, it is important to completely undress the client to assess the body for lesions. In contact dermatitis, a linear pattern is present, and the location helps to identify the agent. Popliteal regions are often involved with eczema. Behind the ears and the conjunctiva are not associated with contact dermatitis.

5. *Answer:* d (implementation/plan)
   Rationale: Steroids may be used to treat severe cases of contact dermatitis. A medrol dosepack produces rebound effect and may not produce the desired effect (Berger, 2001). Steroid cream is never used on the face.

DEVELOPMENTAL DELAYS AND DISABILITIES   *Denise Robinson*

OVERVIEW

Definition

Developmental delays and disabilities constitute a spectrum characterized by deficits in cognitive, social, and emotional functioning. Competence is defined by comparing performance levels of an individual child with norms accumulated from observation and testing of children of the same age (Goldson, 1999). Inability to use meaningful words other than "dada," "mama," "bye-bye," and "hello" by 18 months and the inability to speak in short sentences by 24 months are considered developmental delays. Mental retardation is the most common cause of speech delay, accounting for 50% of cases.

Incidence

Approximately 2% to 3% of the general population is considered mentally retarded. About 10% of the mentally retarded are identified as such during infancy and early childhood; most fall into the moderate to profound group (intelligence quotient [IQ] lower than 50). Most have clear-cut evidence of brain damage, genetic disorder, or other pathologic condition. Mental retardation is more common in males than females. Those children who are profoundly retarded (IQ lower than 30) usually require continuous care; these are the severely deformed, nonambulatory, and minimally communicative individuals.

The remaining 90% of the mentally retarded fall into the mildly retarded range (IQ 50 to 69). Most are not identified before going to school and most commonly come from families characterized by low intelligence and low socioeconomic status. The following are common characteristics:

- Approximately 6% are considered borderline intelligence.
- Approximately 6% to 7% of the population shows clumsiness, awkwardness, choreiform movements, or generally poor coordination but with no signs of systemic disease. Many of these children show learning disabilities.
- In 30% to 40% of children with mental retardation, the cause of the retardation cannot be determined, even after extensive investigation.

Prevalence of selected developmental disabilities:

- Cerebral palsy: 2 per 1000
- Visual impairment: 0.3 to 0.6 per 1000
- Hearing impairment: 0.8 to 2 per 1000
- Learning disability: 75 per 1000
- Attention deficit hyperactivity disorder: 150 per 1000
- Behavioral disorders: 6% to 13% (Needlman, 1996)

Pathophysiology

Causes of developmental delays include the following possibilities:

- *Genetic:* inborn errors of metabolism and chromosome disorders
- *Intrauterine:* congenital infections, placental-fetal malfunction, complications of pregnancy
- *Perinatal:* prematurity, postmaturity, metabolic disorders
- *Postnatal:* endocrinopathies, metabolic disorders, trauma, infections, poisoning, maltreatment
- *Cultural–familial:* low family intelligence, environmental deprivation

These disorders include but are not limited to cerebral palsy, mental retardation, blindness and deafness, central processing disorders, and pervasive developmental delay such as autism, Asperger's syndrome, Down syndrome, fragile X syndrome, or childhood schizophrenia.

ASSESSMENT: SUBJECTIVE/HISTORY

Information obtained in a developmental evaluation should be based on the following:

- Child's level of cognitive and social functioning
- Data that assist in making an etiologic diagnosis
- Data relevant to developing a plan of care

These objectives are best obtained using a multidisciplinary team. Developmental disabilities usually are seen as a result of the child's failure to meet developmental milestones or age-related expectations. Other disabilities may be seen as being related to failure to establish feeding or poor interaction with caregivers. Gross motor failures, such as failure to sit, predominate after 9 months, whereas language delay becomes the major reason for referral between 21 and 30 months (Dershewitz, 1999). If there is concern, an assessment should be performed.

History

History taking includes the following areas:

- *Family history:* Obtain information regarding CNS disorders, mental retardation, epilepsy, evidence of school problems, and specific learning disabilities in other family members. Details of mother's pregnancy history, including stillbirths, deaths, and other problems may be helpful.
- *Prenatal history:* Obtain information about use of drugs, radiographs taken during pregnancy.
- *Perinatal history:* Obtain information about neonatal infections, asphyxia, elevated bilirubin levels, and difficulty during labor.
- *Past medical history:* Obtain information about CNS insult or injuries, failure to thrive, chronic illnesses, hospitalizations, or abuse.
- *Current functioning/developmental history:* Determine the age at which various milestones were achieved, especially those pertaining to speech and language.
- Obtain information about behavioral functioning.
- Obtain information about educational and learning history.
  - *Preschool:* Determine what the child has learned in an informal setting. If in formal setting, obtain information about relationships with other children and teachers. Gather information from teachers who can report on child's performance and behavior in the classroom.
  - *School age:* Determine grade placement, whether special education evaluations have been performed and the results, whether grades have been repeated, and standardized test scores. Gather information about how instruction is being provided, whether the method is appropriate for the child's learning needs, and whether the content is aligned with the child's experience.
- *Psychosocial history:* Gather information about family problems and parental characteristics; assess the family's abilities to promote cognitive abilities, and social development, including parents' language and cultural background, the quality of verbal interaction, disciplinary practices, and the ability to set standards. Also include any investigation for neglect, family instability, marital discord, a hostile attitude toward the child, signs of maladjustment (e.g., alcohol abuse, chronic unemployment, criminal or psychiatric problems), and general unrest within the family. The most complete way to provide details about the home environment is to include a home observation for measurement of the environment (HOME) assessment. This instrument is used to identify families that are unlikely to support development in their children. The home screening questionnaire (HSQ) is a shorter version of the HOME assessment that can be done and scored in the office. Neither scale is

helpful when evaluating middle or upper socioeconomic families.

- Children of hostile, rejecting authoritarian parents tend to be the most severely affected. Parents who are too lax, provide too little nurturance, are too harsh in punishment, or fail to supervise their children tend to have children with aggressive behavior problems that persist into adolescence and adulthood.
- *Environmental exposures:* Determine exposures to lead, alcohol, and others.
- *Emotional and social behavior:* Use scales to record teacher and parent ratings of general behavior. Scales are available to evaluate children as young as 2 (e.g., the Child Behavior Checklist). Scales that rate for hyperactivity and attention deficit also are helpful to complete.
- *Evaluation of family and social resources:* Determine the type, extent, and cost of educational and counseling services available to the child, and the family's ability to carry through with treatment plans; these are important to know soon in the process. Sixty percent of families with learning disabilities have clear-cut social and emotional problems.
- *Evaluation of intelligence:* Intelligence tests measure general knowledge, reasoning, judgment, and analytic skills that are expected to develop through experiences encountered in the process of growing up (Goldson, 1999).

ASSESSMENT: OBJECTIVE/PHYSICAL EXAMINATION
Physical Examination

A comprehensive physical examination is performed, with particular attention to the following:
- Assess growth parameters and head circumference.
- Assess for dysmorphism.
- Assess pigmentary abnormalities.
- Assess physical anomalies: abnormal palmar crease, syndactyly, unruly hair, malformed ears, skin tags, and facial abnormalities.
- Perform an expanded neurologic examination.
- Assess neurologic soft signs: clumsiness, right–left confusion, disordered temporal orientation, overflow phenomenon, choreiform movements, and finger agnosia. These signs may be associated with school learning and behavior problems, although children without developmental delays may also have them
- Perform a sensory evaluation to assess visual and auditory problems. In infants and young children, sensory deficits may be confused with developmental delays.
- Evaluate the four milestones, which follow:
  1. Gross motor milestone: independent locomotion

2. Language milestones (best predictor of later cognition); includes the following:
   - Reception
   - Expression
   - Visual language
3. Fine motor and problem-solving milestones (these form the basis for most infant intelligence scales); includes the following:
   - Hand function
   - Problem solving
   - Visual–motor abilities
4. Personal social abilities: mastery of child over environment; feeding, dressing, hygiene

Diagnostic Procedures

No specific lab tests are indicated. Screen at birth for the following:
- Screening requirements for phenylketonuria, hypothyroidism, and other metabolic disorders vary from state to state.
- Iron deficiency and lead toxicity are easily done.
- EEG and neuroimaging might be appropriate if there is a clinical suspicion of seizure or encephalopathy, microcephaly, or rapidly expanding head circumference.
- Perform chromosomal and molecular biologic testing for fragile X, the most common inherited cause for mental retardation.

DIAGNOSIS

- It can be difficult to distinguish behavior disorders from developmental delays, particularly in disadvantaged children because they often have delays in both social and cognitive abilities and combinations of developmental delays and behavior problems.
- Three components appear to be very important for school learning and behavior: attention, memory, and the coordination of these processes.
- Diagnosis includes the following three levels of developmental delay:
  1. *Delay:* This is the most common type, usually less than 75% normal rate of development. Infants and toddlers with 25% deficit in development are eligible for early intervention services.
  2. *Dissociation:* This is a state in which one phase of development is out of synchrony with others.
  3. *Deviance:* This nonsequential development is most commonly seen in processing disorders, for example, in a child who walks without crawling (Dershewitz, 1999).
- Disorders with IQ achievement discrepancy are areas in which achievement is below IQ in selected areas and the disorder is not caused by a sensory impairment. Other areas are at the level of expectancy. Specific learning disorders may occur in any area of academic achievement, but the most common involve the following:

- Reading (dyslexia)
- Arithmetic (dyscalculia)
- Writing (dysgraphia)
- Children with minimal brain dysfunction are those who fail to learn despite conventional instruction, adequate familial opportunity, and adequate intelligence. This is thought to represent an idiopathic or genetic syndrome. A family history usually shows affected family members, especially among males. Physical examination is normal. Behavior problems may be present. Intelligence tests reveal average intelligence.
- Disorders without IQ discrepancy include disorders in which IQ and achievement are equal, but at low-normal to below-normal levels.
- Children who are slow learners tend to have IQs in the 80s. The following is a breakdown of children who are slow learners:
  - Neurologic dysfunction: 11%
  - Questionable neurologic findings: 25%
  - Clumsiness in copying geometric figures: 60%
  - Language delay: 40%
- Clumsiness, motor impersistence, and right–left confusion are twice as common in slow learners than children with learning disorders.
- History reveals developmental delay, especially in language area.
- A family history of school problems may be present.
- In mental retardation, IQ and achievement are 2 standard deviations below average. The following is a breakdown of mental retardation:
  - Educable: IQ usually 50 to 70
  - Trainable: IQ usually below 50
- Sensory deficits are common in this group of children, as are motor handicaps, speech and language delays, seizure disorders, and behavior problems. Signs of significant developmental delay are evident by the age of 2.

Therapeutic Plan

- Developmental disorders are complex cases because they often require inpatient or residential placement for stabilization and medication management. Self-help skills are delayed, and normal socialization skills may be absent. The disorders are chronic, placing a strain on normal family resources. Family dysfunction is common (Pearson, 1995).
- The earlier the diagnosis, the better for the child because the older the child is at the time of the diagnosis, the less likelihood there is of reversing the retardation even if a reversible cause is present.
- Schools have the responsibility for providing educational services for children from 3 to 21 years of age in the least restrictive, most normalized environment possible in which the child can reasonably receive educational benefit. They must be served through the local school system.

Client/Family Education

- Tactful discussion about the child's needs, including social support, infant education programs, and physical therapy
- Counseling to help the whole family adapt to the impact of a developmentally delayed child

Prevention

The only significant approach to treatment is through prevention. These efforts include the following:
- Screening for early detection of inborn errors in metabolism before damage can occur to the CNS
- Preventive programs for children at risk for familial–cultural retardation
- Head Start preschool

EVALUATION/FOLLOW-UP

All clients who may have a developmental delay or disability should be quickly referred to a professional or center (preferably multispecialty) who can conduct a thorough examination and follow through with the needed treatment plan. A center for developmental disabilities is usually part of a children's hospital medical center. Management is directed toward the support and impact on the family.

REFERENCES

Derschewitz, R. (1999). *Ambulatory pediatric care* (3rd ed.). Philadelphia: Lippincott.

Goldson, E. (1999). Developmental disorders and behavioral problems. In W. Hay, A. R. Hayward, M. Levin, & J. M. Sondheimer (Eds.), *Current pediatric diagnosis and treatment* (14th ed., pp. 77-101). Stamford, CT: Appleton & Lange.

Leung, A., & Kao, C. (1999, June). Evaluation and management of the child with speech delay. *American Family Physician*. Retrieved July 16, 2001, from www.aafp.org/aft/990600ap/3121.html.

Needlman, R. (1996). Growth and development. In W. Nelson, et al. (Eds.), *Nelson textbook of pediatrics* (15th ed., pp. 67-72). Philadelphia: W. B. Saunders.

Pearson, G. (1995). Pervasive developmental disorders. In B. Johnson (Ed.), *Child, adolescent, and family psychiatric nursing*. Philadelphia: J. B. Lippincott.

Saenz, R. (1999, January). Primary care of infants and young children with Down syndrome. *American Family Physician*. Retrieved July 16, 2001, from www.aafp.org/afp/990115ap/381.html.

Review Questions

1. Maggie is a 12-month-old infant who is unable to sit without assistance. The NP should do which of the following?
   a. Suspect abuse.
   b. Encourage the family to stimulate Maggie more.
   c. Refer Maggie for investigation of developmental delay.
   d. Recheck Maggie in 1 month to assess progress.

2. To appropriately refer a client with a developmental disability, the NP must first assess all the following, *except* which of the following?

    a. Gross motor function
    b. Language use
    c. Social abilities
    d. Abdominal circumference

3. Deshawn is a child with a developmental delay. Which of the following historical data is consistent with a diagnosis of developmental disorder?

    a. Deshawn was an early walker.
    b. His brothers and sisters all have made A's in school.
    c. He has attended Head Start since the age of 3.
    d. His mother smoked marijuana during the pregnancy.

4. Which of the following objective information gleaned from the physical examination is consistent with a diagnosis of developmental delay?

    a. 75th percentile for height and weight
    b. 5th percentile for head circumference
    c. Red reflex present; extra occular movement (EOM); pupils equal, round, reactive to light, and accomodating (PERRLA)
    d. S_1 and S_2 within normal limits, no murmurs, rubs or gallops

5. Learning disability must be differentiated from mental retardation. Compared to mental retardation, learning disabilities are associated with which of the following?

    a. Achievement below IQ in selected areas
    b. IQ below 50
    c. IQ below 70
    d. Achievement and IQ equal

6. Which of the following diagnostic tests are first line in cases of developmental delays?

    a. Lead level
    b. CBC
    c. MRI
    d. Basic metabolic panel

7. Which of the following is the best way to treat developmental delays and mental retardation?

    a. Prevention of the syndrome from occurring
    b. Early screening
    c. Thorough history and physical at each well-child examination
    d. Special diet

8. The NP provides instruction regarding developmental delays to the mother of a 9-year-old child. Which comment by the mother indicates a need for further instruction?

    a. "Delicia will be able to attend the local school."
    b. "Delicia will need special help with speech and language development."

    c. "The whole family will be in counseling."
    d. "Treatment of her problem will return her to normal."

Answers and Rationales

1. ***Answer: c*** (implementation/plan)
    Rationale: Gross motor failures are the major reason for referral in infants and toddlers. At 12 months, Maggie needs to be sitting alone and standing, at least with assistance. Earlier intervention carries better outcomes (Pearson, 1995).

2. ***Answer: d*** (assessment)
    Rationale: Height and weight should be recorded for every client and the growth charts examined for trending. Abdominal circumference is not needed for the assessment (Goldson, 1999). Baseline language, fine motor, gross motor, and social skills must be assessed.

3. ***Answer: d*** (assessment)
    Rationale: In the history-taking evaluation for a developmental delay, it is important to determine things that may have influenced the development of problems. In this case, the mother smoking marijuana on a regular basis could have contributed to the development of problems (Goldson, 1999).

4. ***Answer: b*** (assessment)
    Rationale: A persistent head circumference in the 5% range or below is consistent with microcephaly and is cause for concern (Leung & Kao, 1999).

5. ***Answer: a*** (analysis/diagnosis)
    Rationale: The hallmark of learning disabilities is the incongruence between IQ and achievement. Mental retardation demonstrates equal IQ and achievement. An IQ lower than 80 is considered mental retardation (Goldson, 1999).

6. ***Answer: a*** (analysis/diagnosis)
    Rationale: A first-line test is lead screening. It is fairly noninvasive, and a high lead level can contribute to a developmental delay (Needlman, 1996).

7. ***Answer: a*** (implementation/plan)
    Rationale: Prevention is the only means to address or treat developmental disorders and mental retardation (Goldson, 1999).

8. ***Answer: d*** (evaluation)
    Rationale: In most cases, once the developmental disorder or mental retardation is diagnosed, it is unlikely that any treatment can address or reverse the cause (Needlman, 1996).

DEVELOPMENTAL DYSPLASIA OF THE HIP *Denise Robinson*

OVERVIEW
Definition

Developmental dysplasia of the hip (DDH) is displacement of the femoral head in respect to normal orientation with the acetabulum. Dislocation refers to hips that completely move out of the socket. It also includes hips that are poorly developed and hips that are abnormal after the newborn period. Subluxation describes hips that have movement within the joint. The movement feels like "popping out" or a "click."

Incidence

- One to two for every 1000 births in children of European origin; rare in blacks
- More common in cultures that practice swaddling or use infant cradle boards
- Occurs in girls more often than boys
- Unilateral dislocation twice as frequent as bilateral
- Unknown genetic link; association of first-born females with positive family history of affected first-degree relatives

Pathophysiology

In utero, the acetabulum starts as a flat surface, which later cups around the head of the femur. This process is completed during the first months of extrauterine life. DDH is the failure of this normal cup to form around the head of the femur.

Factors Increasing Susceptibility. Congenital dislocation can be divided into two types: idiopathic and teratogenic.
Idiopathic
- More frequent and often related to family history; can range from subluxed to dislocated and reducible or dislocated and irreducible
- Abnormal intrauterine positioning
- Relaxing effect of hormones acting on soft tissue during pregnancy
- History of breech presentation; exhibits generalized increased ligamentous laxity
Teratogenic
- More severe form of the disorder
- Associated congenital anomalies common in infants; significant association with clubfoot deformities and neuromuscular conditions; approximately 30% to 50% of infants with hip abnormality have other risk factors

Common Pathogens. There are no known infectious etiologic factors.

ASSESSMENT: SUBJECTIVE/HISTORY
Symptoms

Infants
- Legs held in adduction and external rotation
- Asymmetry of skinfolds of thighs and buttocks; not true of bilateral dislocation
- Limited abduction
- Irritability on leg motion

Children
- Gait disturbance
- Inability to crawl
- Hip or medial knee pain
- Low activity level

Past Medical History

Infants
- Birth order
- Family history: 20% of children treated for DDH have a family history of the disorder
- Abnormal intrauterine positions
- Congenital deformities
- Muscle disorder
- Progress of ambulation

Children
- Abnormal gait
- Uneven length of legs
- Difficult diapering

Psychosocial History

This information is noncontributory.

Dietary History

This information is noncontributory.

ASSESSMENT: OBJECTIVE/PHYSICAL EXAMINATION
Physical Examination

Infants
- Conduct a problem-oriented examination, with particular attention to height and general appearance.
- *Skin:* Assess for asymmetry of skinfolds of thighs and buttocks.
- *Lower extremities:* Do a complete examination of the legs and hips. Perform the Barlow's test and Ortolani's sign. These maneuvers cannot be performed on a crying, fussy newborn whose muscle activity may inhibit the movement of an unstable hip.

- *Ortolani's sign:* Place the infant in the supine position with the pelvis on a flat surface; abduct and externally rotate the hip with the middle finger of the examiner over the greater trochanter. A palpable "clunk" confirms reduction of the dislocated hips. The clunk is less pronounced in those infants with a poorly developed acetabulum. This is less common after the newborn period (Figure 3-4).
- *Barlow's test:* Place the infant in the supine position with pelvis flat. Adduct and internally rotate the hips. A palpable "clunk" confirms the hip dislocation.
- *Allis' sign:* Position child supine with knees fully adducted and held together. The test is positive if one femur is shorter than the other (Figure 3-5).

Children

- Assess gait status for limping, swayback, toe walking, lurch gait, or delay of ambulation.
- Skin: Assess for excessive thigh or buttocks folds.
- Limited abduction is the predominant sign as the hip becomes fixed in the dislocated position. Limitation of hip abduction is the best indicator in the older infant. In the neonate, each thigh should abduct to almost 90 degrees; abduction less than 60 to 70 degrees indicates abnormality.
- Galeazzi sign: Place the child in the supine position with the knees fully adducted and held together. If one femur is shorter than the other, the result is positive.

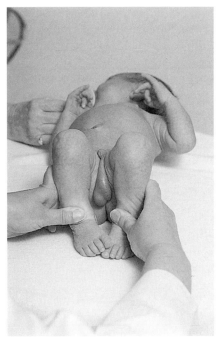

D

FIGURE **3-5** Examination for the Allis sign: unequal upper leg length indicates a positive sign. This is also known as Galeazzi sign. (From Seidel, H. M., et al. 1999. *Mosby's guide to physical examination*, 4th ed. St. Louis: Mosby.)

Diagnostic Procedures

Based on documented positive hip "click" or "clunk," the following radiographic studies should be performed. Also consider testing if the infant has no signs of DDH, but there is a history of DDH in a parent or sibling.

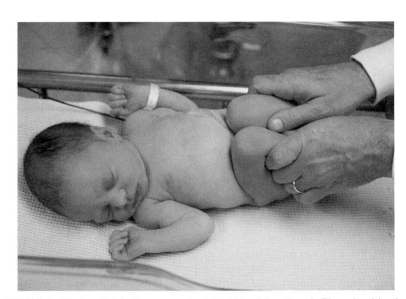

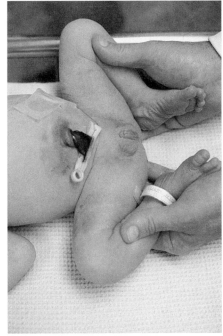

FIGURE **3-4** Barlow-Ortolani maneuver to detect hip dislocation. A, Phase I, adduction. B, Phase II, abduction. (From Seidel, H. M., et al. 1999. *Mosby's guide to physical examination*, 4th ed. St. Louis: Mosby.)

- *Ultrasound:* Confirms real-time dislocation of the femoral head in an immature, unossified anatomy. This is best done at 4 to 6 weeks because, by this time, immature hips have stabilized.
- *X-ray examination:* This is best done after 4 months of age. Before this time, the femoral nucleus is not ossified. Obtain the following views:
  - "Frog-legged" view
  - Upright anteroposterior view; hips internally rotated
- *Hip arthrography:* Inject radiopaque dye into hip joint; this may require sedation.
- Obtain a CT/MRI.

DIAGNOSIS

The differential diagnoses includes the following:
- Spina bifida
- Arthrogryposis
- Lumbosacral agenesis
- Neonatal Marfan syndrome
- Fetal hydantoin syndrome
- Larsen's syndrome
- Septic hip
- Proximal femoral epiphyseal separation
- Coxa vara

THERAPEUTIC PLAN

- Always refer the child to a pediatric orthopedic surgeon for evaluation.
- Therapy depends on the age of the child at the time of diagnosis and the age of the abnormality on clinical examination. The following breaks down therapy by age:
  - *Age 0 to 6 months:* A Pavlik harness permits a relaxed motion of the hip while maintaining a flexed and abducted position for natural development of joint space, until the capsule tightens in approximately 6 weeks. The primary complication of the harness is avascular necrosis of the femoral head (1% to 5% incidence). Most cases of avascular necrosis are related to the improper application of the harness.
  - *Age 6 months to 2 years:* Consider closed reduction versus open reduction, spica cast, or preliminary traction.
- The prognosis is excellent if treated early. Failure to diagnose early can result in more extensive management and a less favorable outcome.

Client Education

- Despite traditional use of double and triple diapering, no clinical evidence supports the benefit of these treatments. These therapies are not recommended because the adductor muscles of the thigh usually overpower saturated diapers and abduction is not maintained.

- The Pavlik harness should stay in place during all sleeping and waking hours, with the exception of bathing.
- Harness straps should be adjusted by a medical professional only.
- Parents may apply skin moisturizer in areas of strap erosions.
- The use of a Pavlik harness requires the special attention of all family members who change diapers. Extra time for changing diapers is needed.
- Spica casts affect family life to a greater degree than Pavlik harnesses. The child must be carried everywhere, and diaper care may be difficult. Special attention must be paid to the neurovascular status of the lower extremities and to possible breaks in the skin at the edges of the case.
- The cast is changed every 4 to 6 weeks to allow for the child's growth.

EVALUATION/FOLLOW-UP

- Even though spontaneous reduction of the hip may occur in 6 weeks, it is recommended that the Pavlik harness be worn for several months, until the hips are stable.
- The spica cast should be changed every 6 weeks to allow for the child's growth. The cast should not be used for more than 6 months.

COMPLICATIONS

- Complications if DDH is untreated include no stable reduction, avascular necrosis of the femoral head, and decreased range of movement.
- Without therapy, DDH results in permanent degenerative changes of the hip that eventually lead to arthritis.

REFERENCES

Aronsson, D., Goldberg, M. J., Kling, T. F. Jr, & Roy D. R. (1994). Developmental dysplasia of the hip. *Pediatrics, 94*(2), 201-208.

Conrad, A. (2000). Developmental dysplasia of the hip. In D. Robinson, P. Kidd, & K. Rogers (Eds.), *Primary care across the lifespan* (pp. 327-332). St. Louis: Mosby.

Donaldson, J., & Feinstein, K. (1997). Imaging of developmental dysplasia of the hip. *Pediatric Clinics of North America, 44*(3), 591-614.

French, L., & Dietz, F. (1999). Screening for developmental dysplasia of the hip. *American Family Physician, 60*, 177-188.

Swartz, M. W. (1997). *The 5-minute pediatric consult.* Baltimore: Williams & Wilkins.

Zitelli, B., & Davis, H. (1994). *Atlas of pediatric physical diagnosis* (2nd ed.). London: Mosby-Wolfe.

Review Questions

1. Besides Ortolani's maneuver, what is another physical examination technique to test for DDH?

a. Pavlik
b. Phalen
c. Galeazzi
d. Iliopsoas

2. Signs associated with DDH in an infant include all *except* which of the following?

a. Asymmetric or extra skinfolds of the thigh
b. Legs adducted and externally rotated
c. Hip "clunk"
d. Full or unlimited abduction

3. All of the following diagnostic procedures can be useful in diagnosing DDH, *except:*

a. Radiographs
b. Ultrasound
c. Arthrography
d. Rheumatoid factor with antinuclear antibodies (ANA)

4. A 4-year-old girl visiting from Mexico has a 2-year history of a progressively increasing limp. She is diagnosed with DDH. Her prognosis for correction will likely be which of the following?

a. Excellent
b. Complicated management and less favorable outcome
c. Unknown
d. No correction possible

5. Whom does DDH affect more often?

a. Girls more often than boys
b. Boys more often than girls
c. Both boys and girls equally
d. Boys later in life than girls

6. The best time to do the physical examination for DDH for a newborn is when the child is which of the following?

a. Fussy
b. Feeding
c. Crying
d. Quietly awake

7. For a hip that is dislocatable and relocatable, a reliable form of fixation such as a Pavlik harness is used. Which of the following is true about the Pavlik harness?

a. It should be removed only for each diaper change.
b. It should be removed only for bathing.
c. It should be removed as desired.
d. It should never be removed.

8. At his first well-child visit, a 14-day-old infant is noted to have a positive result from a Barlow's test but negative results from Galeazzi sign and Ortolani's sign. Appropriate management would include which of the following?

a. Reassure the mother that this may be a variant of normal and reexamine the hip at 2 months of age.
b. Obtain anteroposterior and frog-legged radiograph views of the pelvis to confirm the diagnosis.
c. Obtain a hip ultrasound to confirm the diagnosis.
d. Immediately place the child in a Pavlik harness.

Answers and Rationales

1. *Answer:* c (assessment)
Rationale: Galeazzi is a test for DDH, Parlik is the harness, phalen is for carpal tunnel, and PSOAS is for peritoneal irritation (French & Dietz, 1999).

2. *Answer:* d (assessment)
Rationale: In the neonate, each thigh should abduct to almost 90 degrees; abduction less than 60 to 70 degrees indicates abnormality (Behrman & Vaughan, 1997).

3. *Answer:* d (analysis/diagnosis)
Rationale: No laboratory tests are helpful in diagnosing DDH (Conrad, 2000).

4. *Answer:* b (evaluation)
Rationale: If DDH is diagnosed early, the prognosis is uniformly excellent (Zitelli & Davis, 1994).

5. *Answer:* a (analysis/diagnosis)
Rationale: Girls are more commonly affected than boys (Conrad, 2000).

6. *Answer:* d (assessment)
Rationale: A crying infant's hip is nearly impossible to examine accurately (Swartz, 1997).

7. *Answer:* b (implementation/plan)
Rationale: The harness should not be removed with each diaper change. It should be removed only with bathing (Conrad, 2000).

8. *Answer:* c (implementation/plan)
Rationale: By 14 days of age, normal ligamentous laxity should be resolved; however, the diagnosis of DDH should still be confirmed before instituting prolonged therapy because Pavlik harness placement can cause necrosis of the femoral head. The femoral head is not calcified, and its relationship to the acetabulum cannot be seen on x-ray examination; however, these same structures are easily visualized on ultrasound, and the motion of the femoral head over the acetabulum can be confirmed. This has the added advantage of not subjecting the infant to unnecessary radiation. Delay of diagnosis and treatment by 2 months may provide a less favorable outcome (French & Dietz, 1999).

DIABETES MELLITUS *Pamela Kidd*

OVERVIEW
Definition

Diabetes mellitus is a disease in which glucose is not metabolized correctly because of either inadequate insulin levels or poor utilization of insulin.

Incidence

- There are approximately 10 million people with diabetes in the United States.
- Of these, 80% to 90% have non–insulin-dependent diabetes mellitus (type 2 diabetes), and 10% to 20% have insulin-dependent diabetes mellitus (type 1 diabetes).

Pathophysiology

- In type 1 diabetes, the pancreas ceases to produce insulin. The beta-cells of the pancreas are slowly destroyed. Type 1 diabetes is an autoimmune disorder with a genetic predisposition. Type 1 diabetes usually occurs before age 40.
- In type 2 diabetes, there is a defect in the insulin receptors. The pancreas continues to produce insulin, but the body is not able to use the available insulin. Type 2 diabetes usually occurs after the age of 40.
- Syndrome X consists of obesity, glucose intolerance, dyslipidemia, and hypertension (Gavin & Peters, 1999). Insulin resistance predisposes to hyperglycemia, which leads to hyperinsulinemia. Hyperinsulinemia may or may not correct the hyperglycemia, but it does increase very low-density lipoprotein (VLDL) production by the liver, leading to hyperlipidemia. Increased VLDL causes the kidney to retain sodium, producing hypertension (Barbrey, 1999).

Factors Increasing Susceptibility
- Smoking
- Alcohol
- African, Asian, Native American, Hispanic, Pacific Islander

Protective Factors. Exercise.

ASSESSMENT: SUBJECTIVE/HISTORY
Symptoms

Most Common Symptoms
- In adults with type 2 diabetes, the most common symptoms are polyuria, polydipsia, and polyphagia.
- In children and young adults with type 1 diabetes, the most common symptoms are rapid onset of polydipsia, polyuria, weight loss, polyphagia, and fatigue.

Associated Symptoms
- In adults with type 2 diabetes, paresthesia, dysesthesias, blurred vision, vaginal candidiasis, or fungal skin infections may occur.

- In type 1 diabetes, in addition to the symptoms just mentioned, abdominal pain, nausea, vomiting, or fruity breath may occur.

Past Medical History
- Hypertension
- Hypoglycemia
- Retinopathy
- Obesity
- Gestational diabetes

Medication History
- Recent use of steroids or diuretics may raise blood glucose levels.
- Use of beta-blockers may raise blood glucose levels, although this is debatable.

Family History
- Diabetes
- Hyperlipidemia
- Hypertension

Dietary History
- Weight gain or loss
- 24-hour diet recall
- Polyphagia and polydipsia

ASSESSMENT: OBJECTIVE/PHYSICAL EXAMINATION
Physical Examination

A complete physical examination should be performed, with particular attention to the following:

- Vital signs (hypertension, tachycardia, or tachypnea)
- Weight (gain or loss)
- Ophthalmic (funduscopic examination: check for retinopathy)
- Oral (mouth and dental: attention to teeth and gums)
- Cardiovascular (bruits, pulses, or edema)
- Thyroid (palpable or nonpalpable)
- Abdomen (hepatomegaly, bruits)
- Skin (infections, integrity)
- Feet (integrity, callus, infection, or deformity)
- Neurologic (sensation): use monofilament to check sensation (push filament into the skin until filament bends at 10 g of force) at plantar aspect of foot on the first, third, and fifth toes, middle toe joint, fifth toe joint, arch, and heel; clients who cannot feel 75% of these points have significant neuropathy, higher risk for lower extremity amputation later (Caballero, Habershaw, & Pinzur, 2000)

Diagnostic Procedures

Glycosylated hemoglobin or hemoglobin A_1C: The glycosylated hemoglobin test or the hemoglobin A_1C (Hgb A_1C) test can give the average glucose value for the past 3 months. For the Hgb A_1C test, the normal value for a person with diabetes is approximately 7% to get an average of 150 mg/dL. The glycosylated hemoglobin should be maintained at approximately 8% to get an average glucose of 150 mg/dL. The latest guidelines from the American Association of Clinical Endocrinologists recommend a target Hgb A_1C level of 6.5%, whereas the American Diabetic Association suggests a 7% goal. The Hgb A_1C test can further validate the diagnosis.

Other Laboratory Data
- Fasting lipid profile
- Liver profile, if client is taking lipid-lowering agent
- Serum creatinine in adults; in children only if proteinuria exists
- U/A: glucose, ketones, protein, sediment
- Urinary microalbuminuria (overnight specimen) on diagnosis with type 2 diabetes or after 5 years diagnosis in type 1 diabetes
- Thyroid function tests, when indicated by history and examination
- ECG, in adults only
- Cardiac stress testing if indicated

DIAGNOSIS
Diagnostic Laboratory Data

Plasma Glucose. In adults, the diagnosis is based on the following:
- Classic symptoms of diabetes, polyuria, polydipsia, polyphagia, and weight loss, and a "casual" (without regard to time of last meal) plasma glucose level of 200 mg/dL or higher; or
- Fasting (no caloric intake for the preceding 8 hours) plasma glucose level of 126 mg/dL or higher; or
- A plasma glucose level of 200 mg/dL or higher at the 2-hour mark of an oral glucose tolerance test (Expert committee on Diagnosis and Classification of DM, 1997)

In children, the diagnosis is based on the following:
- Classic symptoms of diabetes, polyuria, polydipsia, polyphagia, and weight loss and a plasma glucose level of 200 mg/dL or higher; or
- Fasting plasma glucose level of 140 mg/dL or higher and two oral glucose tolerance tests demonstrate a 2 hour postprandial glucose and one other value 200 mg/dL or higher (of the three values obtained)

The differential diagnoses includes the following:
- Cushing's disease
- Transient hyperglycemia
- Acromegaly
- Pheochromocytoma
- Diabetes insipidus

THERAPEUTIC PLAN
Treatment goals for diabetes are the following:
- Preprandial plasma glucose level of 80 to 120 mg/dL
- Bedtime plasma glucose level of 100 to 140 mg/dL
- Glycosylated hemoglobin A_1C level less than 7%

Nonpharmacologic Treatment
Type 1 Diabetes Mellitus
- *Nutrition:* Many nutrition plans are available. The easiest plan for most people is to avoid concentrated sugar with 50% to 60% carbohydrate, 30% fat, and 10% to 20% protein (i.e., food guide pyramid). Client should eat three meals per day with an optional bedtime snack.
- *Exercise:* Exercise is recommended for 30 to 45 minutes per day, 3 to 4 days per week. Check blood glucose level before exercise. If blood glucose level is less than 60 mg/dL, eat protein. If blood glucose level is 250 mg/dL or higher, avoid exercise (may actually raise blood glucose).
- *Home glucose level monitoring:* Home glucose monitoring is recommended four times a day (before meals and at bedtime) at least 3 to 4 days per week, or more if blood glucose level is elevated or during illness.

Type 2 Diabetes Mellitus
- *Nutrition:* The guidelines are similar to type 1 diabetes, except weight loss is focal. More restriction of calories through fat intake reduction is necessary.
- *Syndrome X:* High-fiber, high-complex carbohydrate, low-fat, calorie-restricted diet is recommended.
- Regular aerobic exercise (30 to 45 minutes at least 5 times per week) is recommended.

Pharmacologic Treatment
Type 1 Diabetes Mellitus
- *Insulin:* Total daily insulin requirement is 0.5 U/kg/day. One third of the dose is short onset (1 to 3 hours; regular type) and remaining two thirds of the dose is long to intermediate type (4 to 8 hours onset; NPH, L, U types). Combination types are 50/50 or 70NPH/30R. Adjustment of insulin dose is based on glucose level monitoring results (see Table 3-21).

Type 2 Diabetes Mellitus
- *Oral agents:* If blood glucose is less than 250 mg/dL, the exercise and nutrition guidelines for type 1 diabetes are sufficient. If blood glucose is 250 mg/dL or higher, an oral agent must be started. The following are the current oral medications used to treat Type 2 diabetes:

TABLE **3-21**   Adjustment of Insulin Based on Glucose Monitoring Results

HOME GLUCOSE MONITORING RESULTS	REGULAR INSULIN DOSE
Fasting glucose >140	Increase evening or supper intermediate insulin
Prelunch glucose >140	Add or increase regular insulin at breakfast
Presupper glucose >140	Increase morning intermediate insulin
Bedtime glucose >140	Add or increase regular insulin at supper
Fasting glucose <75	Add snack at bedtime or decrease intermediate insulin at bedtime or supper
Glucose <75 after exercise	Snack before exercise or decrease previous dose of regular insulin

From Robinson, D., Kidd, P., & Rogers, K. M. (2000). *Primary care across the lifespan.* St. Louis: Mosby.

- Sulfonylureas (second generation)
- Glimepiride (Amaryl) 1-, 2-, 4-mg tablets; maximum dose 8 mg/day
- Glyburide (Diabeta) 1.25-, 2.5-, 5-, 10-mg tablets; maximum dose 20 mg/day
- Glyburide (Glynase) 0.75-, 1.5-, 3-, 6-mg tablets; maximum dose 12 mg/day
- Glipizide (Glucotrol) 5-, 10-mg tablets; maximum dose 20 mg bid
- Glipizide (Glucotrol-XL) 5-, 10-mg tablets; maximum dose 20 mg/day
- Biguanides: Metformin (Glucophage) 500-mg tablets; maximum dose 2.5 g tid
- Alpha-glucosidase inhibitors: acarbose (Precose) 50-, 100-mg tablets; maximum dose 100 mg tid
- Glitazones (insulin-resistance reducers; not for first-line therapy)
- Rosiglitazone (Avandia) 4-8 mg/day
- Pioglitazone (Actos) 15-45 mg/day
- *Insulin:* Can use any form used in type 1 diabetes; however, insulin lispro is especially good for avoiding postprandial hyperglycemia often seen in type 2 diabetes. Glargine (long-acting, used once daily) does not peak and reduces the risk of hypoglycemia (Colwell, Gerich, Seley, & Struebing, 2000).
- Metabolic syndrome *(syndrome X):* Glipizide increases insulin secretion in direct response to diet and avoids hyperinsulinemia and lipid involvement.

Client Education

Include the family in the education process. It takes several visits to complete the education plan. Goals should be set based on priority for most-needed items. The first visit should include the basics for survival (e.g., medications, signs and symptoms of low blood glucose). At the second visit, assess the knowledge base and determine the next level. Some people may not be able to afford home glucose monitoring. Education is based on each individual, and should take the following factors into account:

- Pathophysiology of diabetes
- Home glucose monitoring with diary completion
- Foot care
- Medication
- Insulin administration
- Nutrition

- Complications of diabetes: retinopathy, neuropathy, nephropathy, and cardiovascular disorders
- Signs and symptoms of hypoglycemia and hyperglycemia and treatment
- Sick days (e.g., fluids, insulin, medicine, monitoring during illness)
- Exercise plan
- Diabetes identification bracelet

Referral

- A person age 10 or older diagnosed with type 1 diabetes should have an initial eye examination within 5 years of diagnosis and annually after the initial examination. Type 2 diabetics should have annual eye examinations.
- Consult with a physician for any newly diagnosed client with diabetes.
- Children with diabetes should be referred to a pediatric endocrinologist if possible.
- Refer to podiatrist for significant neuropathy.

Prevention and Detection

- *Type 2:* Maintain ideal body weight.
- Measure fasting blood glucose at 45 years of age. Repeat q3 years if result is less than 110 mg/dL. Repeat annually if result is greater than 110 but less than 126 mg/dL.
- Screen at younger age if following risk factors are present:
  - Blood pressure (BP) higher than 140/90 mm Hg
  - Diabetes in a first-degree relative
  - African, Asian, Native American, Hispanic, Pacific Islander race
  - Obese (body mass index 27 kg/m² or greater)
  - History of gestational diabetes or birth of baby larger than 9 lb
  - High-density lipoprotein (HDL) 35 mg/dL or less, triglyceride level 250 mg/dL or greater (Genuth, Palmer, & Zimmerman, 1999)

EVALUATION/FOLLOW-UP

After the initial diagnosis, visits should be scheduled every 1 to 2 weeks until blood glucose level is closer to 180 to 200 mg/dL. For clients starting insulin, visits may need to be every 1 to 2 days. Phone contact can supplement.

- *Type 1 diabetes:* Schedule visits q3 mo to monitor Hgb A_1C and assess diabetes control.
- *Type 2 diabetes:* Schedule visits q6 mo if condition is well controlled (Hgb A_1C less than 7%) and the client does not take insulin.
- Schedule visits q3 mo if the condition is poorly controlled (Hgb A_1C 9% or higher). For clients treated with insulin, follow the recommendations of type 1 diabetes (q3 mo).
- *Syndrome X:* Measure Hgb A_1C quarterly with goal of 7%; client should have a yearly eye examination.

COMPLICATIONS

- Retinopathy
- Neuropathy
- Nephropathy
- Cardiovascular disorders
- Hypertension

REFERENCES

American Diabetes Association. (1996a). Office guide to diagnosis and classification of diabetes mellitus and other categories of glucose intolerance. *Diabetes Care, 19* (Suppl. 4).

American Diabetes Association. (1996b). Nutrition recommendations and principles for people with diabetes mellitus. *Diabetes Care, 19* (Suppl. 16-19).

American Diabetes Association. (1996c). Standards of medical care for patients with diabetes mellitus. *Diabetes Care, 19* (Suppl. 8-15).

Baliga, S. B., & Fonseca, V. A. (1997). Recent advances in the treatment of type II diabetes mellitus. *American Family Physician, 55*(3), 817-824.

Barbrey, C. M. (1999). Managing cardiovascular risk in noninsulin dependent diabetes mellitus. *Journal of the American Academy of Nurse Practitioners, 11*(6), 261-265.

Barker, L. R., Burton, J. R., & Zieve, P. D. (1995). *Principles of ambulatory medicine.* Baltimore: Williams & Wilkins.

Bohannon, N. J. V., & Jack, D. B. (1995). Type II diabetes: How to use the new oral medications. *Geriatrics, 51,* 33-37.

Caballero, E., Habershaw, G., & Pinzur, M. (2000). Preventing amputation in patients with diabetes. *Patient Care for the Nurse Practitioner, 3*(5), 17-19, 23-24, 27-28, 31-32, 35-38.

Cefalu, W. T. (1996). Treatment of type II diabetes. *Postgraduate Medicine, 99*(3), 109-122.

Colwell, J., Gerich, J., Seley, J. J., & Struebing, P. (2000). At the front line of type 2 diabetes therapy. *Patient Care for the Nurse Practitioner,* December (Suppl.), 6-13.

Genuth, S., Palmer, J., & Zimmerman, B. (1999). New diagnostic criteria for diabetes. *Patient Care for the Nurse Practitioner,* February (Suppl.).

Hay, W., Hayward, A. R., Levin M., Sondheimer, J. M. (1997). *Current pediatric diagnosis and treatment.* Norwalk, CT: Appleton & Lange.

Hiss, R. G. (1996). Barriers to care in non–insulin-dependent diabetes mellitus. *Annals of Internal Medicine, 124,* 146-148.

Jaspan, J. B. (1995). Taking control of diabetes. *Hospital Practice, 30*(10), 55-62.

Report of the Expert Committee on the Diagnosis and Classification of Diabetes Mellitus. (1997). *Diabetes Care, 20*(7), 1183-1197.

Singh, I., & Marshall, M. C. (1995). Diabetes mellitus in the elderly. *Endocrinology and Metabolism Clinics of North America, 24*(2), 255-272.

Stolar, M. W. (1995). Clinical management of Type 2 diabetes patient. *Diabetes Care, 18*(5), 701-707.

Willis, J. (1995). Diabetes dietary management. *Nursing Times, 91*(49), 42-44.

Review Questions

1. An adult who develops type 2 diabetes is most likely to experience all the following symptoms, *except:*

    a. Polyuria

    b. Nausea

    c. Polydipsia

    d. Polyphagia

2. Mr. Jones has polyuria and polydipsia at his first visit to the NP. The NP suspects type 2 diabetes. Which of the following is *not* included in the physical examination?

    a. Ear, nose, and throat (ENT)

    b. Ophthalmic

    c. Neurologic

    d. Cardiovascular

3. To assess renal function in a client with type 1 diabetes, urinary microalbuminuria should be assessed at what time?

    a. On diagnosis

    b. 2 years after diagnosis

    c. 3 years after diagnosis

    d. 5 years after diagnosis

4. Mr. Bates is a 50-year-old man who visits the NP for evaluation. He has been experiencing fatigue, polyuria, polydipsia, and nocturia. Plasma glucose is 240 mg/dL. Which of the following would *not* be included in the differential diagnosis?

    a. Diabetes mellitus

    b. Cushing's syndrome

    c. Diabetes insipidus

    d. Pheochromocytoma

5. The NP completed an examination of a 15-year-old, 60-kg male with type 1 diabetes. After consulting with the physician, it is agreed to prescribe NPH and regular insulin, 0.5 U/kg/day. Two thirds of the total dose will be NPH, and one third will be regular (R) insulin. The total dose will be divided into two doses, before breakfast and supper. What is the correct dose?

    a. 10 U NPH + 5 U R bid

    b. 15 U NPH + 5 U R A.M.; 10 NPH + 5 R P.M.

    c. 15 U NPH + 5 U R bid

    d. 10 U R + 5 NPH bid

6. Which of the following is the easiest nutrition plan for a client with diabetes to follow?

    a. Carbohydrate counting

    b. Calorie counting

   c. Food guide pyramid
   d. Counting fat grams

7. Ms. King was seen by her NP for follow-up on type 2 diabetes. Her Hgb A_1C level was 9%. Her current treatment is glipizide (Glucotrol-XL) 10 mg/day. When should Ms. King's next appointment be scheduled?

   a. 6 months
   b. 3 months
   c. 2 weeks
   d. 1 month

8. What is the best explanation for the relationship between hyperglycemia and hyperlipidemia?

   a. Insulin resistance promotes lipid production.
   b. The liver uses the increased glucose to produce lipids.
   c. Increased insulin production corrects hyperglycemia and hinders lipid breakdown.
   d. Hyperinsulinemia increases VLDL production by the liver.

Answers and Rationales

1. *Answer:* **b** (assessment)
   Rationale: Nausea is typical in type 1 diabetes only.

2. *Answer:* **a** (assessment)
   Rationale: The ear is not associated with any specific changes in type 2 diabetes. The other systems provide pertinent data.

3. *Answer:* **d** (evaluation)
   Rationale: The American Diabetes Association (ADA) recommends screening for renal disease in type 1 diabetes 5 years after diagnosis. It usually takes 5 to 10 years for complications to develop in type 2 diabetes (ADA, 1996c).

4. *Answer:* **c** (analysis/diagnosis)
   Rationale: In diabetes insipidus, clients experience polyuria and polydipsia but lack hyperglycemia.

5. *Answer:* **a** (implementation/plan)
   Rationale: $0.5 \text{ U} \times 60 \text{ kg} = 30 \text{ U/day}$
2 doses/30 U/day = 15 U/dose
$15 \times 0.66 = 9.9 = 10 \text{ U NPH}$
$15 \times 0.33 = 4.95 = 5 \text{ U R}$
10 U NPH + 5 U R bid

6. *Answer:* **c** (implementation/plan)
   Rationale: The food pyramid is the easiest tool for people with diabetes to use.

7. *Answer:* **b** (evaluation)
   Rationale: The level of glycemic control is 9% for Ms. King. The medication can be increased to the maximum dose and the visit scheduled in 3 months (ADA, 1996c).

8. *Answer:* **a** (analysis/diagnosis)
   Rationale: Insulin resistance predisposes to hyperglycemia that leads to hyperinsulinemia. Hyperinsulinemia may or may not correct the hyperglycemia, but it does increase VLDL production.

DIAPER RASH   *Denise Robinson*

OVERVIEW
Definition

Diaper dermatitis is a skin irritation located in the perineal area, usually caused by diapers.

Incidence

- Exact incidence is unknown.
- Present from 2 weeks of life until child is toilet trained.
- The young and the old are more likely to be colonized.

Pathophysiology

Dermatitis results from prolonged contact of urine and feces with skin, leading to skin irritation. In 80% of cases if the dermatitis lasts more than 3 days, the area is colonized with *Candida* even before the characteristic lesions are seen. Some cases may be caused by *Candida* and passed to the child from the mother through a maternal vaginal candidiasis at birth. The rash is usually caused by the yeast *Candida albicans*, and less often by other *Candida*. *Candida albicans* is an oval yeast. More than 100 species of the genus have been identified. Candida albicans and other species often colonize the gastrointestinal (GI) tract of humans. Colonization may occur during birth, infancy, or later in life. Fecal colonization is present in about 40% to 67% of people (Fitzpatrick, 2001).

Factors Increasing Susceptibility
- Tightly applied diapers
- Use of rubber pants or plastic pants over diaper
- Diarrheal stools
- Immune or chronic debilitation
- Diabetes mellitus
- Systemic and topical glucocorticoids

Protective Factors. Frequent diaper changing.

ASSESSMENT: SUBJECTIVE/HISTORY
History of Present Illness

- Rash in diaper area
- Irritability
- Cries when voiding

Past Medical History

Prior episodes of rash (suggests neglect, carelessness).

Medication History

- Use of neomycin ointment (can cause allergic dermatitis in infants)
- Recent antibiotic use suggests candidal infection

Family History

Maternal vaginal candidiasis.

Psychosocial History

- History of abuse or neglect
- Cultural differences in hygiene
- Parents' low education level

Associated Symptoms

- Eczema or other skin lesions present
- Oral thrush

ASSESSMENT: OBJECTIVE/PHYSICAL EXAMINATION

Physical Examination

- Observe head, ears, eyes, nose, throat (HEENT), particularly mouth and throat, for white patches on tongue and buccal mucosa.
- Examine genitalia. Erythema, papules or vesicles, ulcerations may be present.
- Skin may have a burned, scalded, or shiny appearance if caused by contact with irritant. Skin folds are spared. If rash is caused by *Candida*, it is intensely red and inguinal folds are involved. There are confluent erythema and satellite lesions beyond the main area of the eruption. If bullae or yellow crusts are present, suspect a secondary infection *(Staphylococcus aureus)*.

Diagnostic Procedures

- Culture to rule out Staphylococcus aureus
- KOH wet prep reveals yeast cells and pseudohyphae if *Candida*

DIAGNOSIS

Differential diagnoses include the following:
- Atopic dermatitis
- Impetigo
- Psoriasis
- Irritant dermatitis
- Seborrheic dermatitis

THERAPEUTIC PLAN

Nonpharmacologic Treatment

- Increase fluids.
- Provide cranberry juice if child is 1 year or older.
- Exclude other juices.

Pharmacologic Treatment

- Topical treatment:
  - Glucocorticoid preparation: judicious short-term use speeds resolution
  - Topical antifungal agents
  - Nystatin, azole, or imidazole cream to affected area bid or more often with diaper dermatitis
  - Oral antifungal agents
  - Nystatin: eliminate GI colonization; not absorbed from bowel; may be effective in recurrent diaper dermatitis

Client Education

- Avoid petroleum products because they trap moisture.
- Change diapers frequently.
- Cleanse diaper area with water at each diaper change; avoid commercial wipes because they contain alcohol.
- Change brand of diapers.
- Wash hands carefully.
- Let infant/child go without diapers as much as possible.
- Avoid talcum powder; it may produce aspiration pneumonia.

Referral

- If patient fails to respond in 1 week, case should be referred to dermatologist.
- If condition worsens, refer to collaborating physician. An immunodeficiency may be present.

Prevention

- Keep area dry.
- Washing with benzoyl peroxide may reduce *Candida* colonization.
- Powder with miconazole applied daily.

EVALUATION/FOLLOW-UP

Return in 48 hours for recheck or follow-up by phone.

COMPLICATIONS

Secondary bacterial infection possible.

REFERENCES

Brilliant, L. (2000). Perianal streptococcal dermatitis. *American Family Physician, 61,* 391-397.

Fitzpatrick, T., Wolff, K., Suurmond, D. (2001). *Color atlas and synopsis of clinical dermatology.* New York: McGraw-Hill.

Kidd, P. (2001). Diaper rash. In D. Robinson, P. Kidd, & K. Rogers (Eds.), *Primary care across the lifespan.* St. Louis: Mosby.

Morelli, J., & Weston, W. (1999). Skin. In W. Hay, A. R. Hayward, M. Levin, & J. M. Sondheimer (Eds.), *Current pediatric diagnosis and treatment* (14th ed., pp. 347-350). Stamford, CT: Appleton Lange.

D

Review Questions

1. Shaunté is a 10-month-old girl with a rash in her diaper area. Which of the following historical data are consistent with a diagnosis of diaper dermatitis?

   a. Recent trip to Alaska
   b. Liquid bowel movements 2 to 3 times a day
   c. Use of cloth diapers
   d. Recent change of formula

2. Which of the following symptoms is common in children with a diaper rash?

   a. Decreased appetite
   b. Crying when voiding
   c. Excessive sleep
   d. Tylenol helps the rash

3. During physical assessment, which finding is consistent with a diagnosis of diaper dermatitis?

   a. Bright red erythema, satellite lesions
   b. Bullous lesions with clear drainage
   c. Small papular lesions that cause intense itching
   d. Vesicular lesions with honey-colored discharge

4. Which of the following diagnoses must be considered a differential to diaper dermatitis?

   a. Scabies
   b. Impetigo
   c. Tinea corporis
   d. Eczema

5. Which of the following organisms is the most frequent cause of diaper dermatitis?

   a. *Staphylococcus aureus*
   b. *Streptococcus*
   c. *Candida albicans*
   d. Histoplasmosis

6. Which of the following drug choices is appropriate as a first-line treatment for diaper dermatitis?

   a. Griseofulvin PO
   b. Clotrimazole 1% (Lotrimin)
   c. Hydrocortisone 5%
   d. Neomycin ointment

7. The NP provides instruction to the mother concerning the treatment for diaper dermatitis. Which of the following comments indicates a need for further instruction?

   a. "I should not use baby wipes for diaper care."
   b. "I should change the diaper frequently."
   c. "I should switch from disposable diapers to cloth with plastic overpants."
   d. "Good handwashing is important."

8. If a child still has a diaper rash even after 2 weeks of treatment, which of the following is appropriate?

   a. Change from topical treatment to oral antifungal therapy.
   b. Obtain a culture from the diaper area.
   c. Increase hydrocortisone from 1% to 5%.
   d. Begin hot lamp treatments.

Answers and Rationales

1. *Answer:* **b** (assessment)
   Rationale: Diarrhea is a precipitating factor to the development of diaper dermatitis (Kidd, 2000).

2. *Answer:* **b** (assessment)
   Rationale: Chemical irritation occurs when a child urinates or defecates onto the erythematous areas, causing pain (Kidd, 2000).

3. *Answer:* **a** (assessment)
   Rationale: Characteristic lesions of diaper dermatitis caused by *Candida* are erythema, papular and pustular lesions, collarette-like scaling at the margins of the lesions, with satellite lesions on the thighs (Fitzpatrick, 2001).

4. *Answer:* **b** (analysis/diagnosis)
   Rationale: Impetigo caused by Staphylococcus needs to be considered as a differential for diaper dermatitis (Kidd, 2000).

5. *Answer:* **c** (analysis/diagnosis)
   Rationale: In more than 80% of children with diaper dermatitis lasting longer than 3 days, the causative agent is *Candida albicans* (Morelli & Weston, 1999).

6. *Answer:* **b** (implementation/plan)
   Rationale: Appropriate treatment for diaper dermatitis caused by *Candida albicans* is an antifungal topical preparation (Fitzpatrick, 2001).

7. *Answer:* **c** (evaluation)
   Rationale: Care of an infant with diaper dermatitis includes frequent diaper changes, using water rather than commercial baby wipes to clean the genital area, and good handwashing. Switching from disposable diapers to cloth diapers is helpful, but not if plastic pants are then applied over the cloth diaper. The same effect of heat and moisture occlusion is obtained as with disposable diapers (Kidd, 2000).

8. *Answer:* **b** (evaluation)
   Rationale: A diaper rash that has not improved in 2 weeks needs definitive treatment. A culture of the diaper area may indicate that *Staphylococcus* or *Streptococcus* is causing the symptoms. If the culture is negative, a referral to a dermatologist is appropriate (Brilliant, 2000).

DIARRHEA   *Denise Robinson*

OVERVIEW
Definition

Diarrhea is defined as an increase in the frequency and fluid content of stools.

Incidence

- Diarrhea accounts for approximately 20% of all pediatric office visits in the United States.
- It affects approximately 10% of all infants younger than 1 year in the United States.
- In the United States, each child has 7 to 15 episodes of diarrhea by age 5.
- Nine percent of all hospitalizations of children younger than age 5 are associated with diarrhea.
- Approximately 300 to 500 children die from diarrhea each year.
- Incidence varies with age, causative organism, geographic location, season, and host susceptibility.

Pathophysiology

Rotovirus is the most common cause of acute diarrhea among children, causing 25% of the cases (incubation 2 to 4 days). Other pathogens include Norwalk-like viruses, enteric adenoviruses, astroviruses, and caliciviruses. Bacterial pathogens include salmonella, shigella, yersinia, campylobacter, and certain strains of *Escherichia coli*. Parasitic causes include giardia, cryptosporidium, and *Entamoeba histolytica*.

Factors Increasing Susceptibility

- Poor handwashing increases susceptibility.
- Improper food handling increases susceptibility.
- Recent use of antibiotics increases susceptibility.
- Immunocompromised host increases susceptibility.
- Poor sanitation increases susceptibility.
- Recent travel increases susceptibility.
- *Acute diarrhea* increases susceptibility. Viral or bacterial toxins stimulate the active transport of electrolytes into the small intestines. The mucosal lining of the intestines becomes irritated, resulting in secretion of excess amounts of fluid and electrolytes from the cells.
- *Lactose intolerance* increases susceptibility. Inflammation of the intestinal mucosal cells decreases the ability to absorb nutrients, electrolytes, and water.
- *Overfeeding and some medications* increase susceptibility. With overfeeding or medications such as antibiotics, laxatives, and antacids excess fluid in the gut produces increased motility and rapid emptying.

Causes of Chronic Diarrhea

- Malabsorption
- Acquired immunodeficiency syndrome (AIDS)
- Hyperthyroidism
- Fecal impaction
- Functional bowel disease
- Congenital (e.g., short-gut syndrome, gastroschisis)

ASSESSMENT: SUBJECTIVE/HISTORY

- Possible elevated temperature
- Anorexia
- Lethargy
- Sudden or gradual increase in number and liquidity of stools
- Crampy abdominal pain

In addition, ask about the following:

- Onset
- Description of stools
- Frequency of stools
- Usual pattern of elimination
- Associated symptoms, such as vomiting or localized abdominal pain
- Current or recent drugs
- Exposure to others with diarrhea
- Detailed dietary history, including introduction of new foods
- Recent travel
- Psychologic upsets
- Treatments tried
- Urinary output

Family History

- Family history of inflammatory bowel disease
- Family history of bleeding disorder
- Other family members with diarrhea or bloody diarrhea

ASSESSMENT: OBJECTIVE/PHYSICAL EXAMINATION
Physical Examination

- Weight, orthostatic vital signs (drop in arterial BP of at least 30 systolic and 20 diastolic indicates orthostatic hypotension)
- Signs and symptoms of dehydration (see Table 3-22):
  - Mucous membranes
  - Skin turgor
  - Urinary output
  - Fontanel
  - Tears
  - Heart rate
  - Level of consciousness
  - Temperature elevation may be related to dehydration or infection.
- Abdominal examination:

TABLE **3-22** Signs and Symptoms of Dehydration

INDICATOR	MILD DEHYDRATION* (3%-5% DEFICIT)	MODERATE DEHYDRATION* (6%-9% DEFICIT)	SEVERE DEHYDRATION* (>10% DEFICIT)
Thirst	Increased	Increased	Severe
Mucous membranes	Slightly dry	Dry	Mottled or gray, very dry
Skin	Normal	Tenting, loss of skin turgor, pale (use abdominal or thoracic wall to check for tenting)	Prolonged skin tenting and skin retraction time (more than 2 seconds), color markedly decreased
Mental status	Normal, restless	Normal to listless, restless, irritable to touch or drowsy	Severe lethargy or altered consciousness
Capillary refill	2-3 seconds	3-4 seconds	Decreased >4 seconds
Fontanelle	Normal	Slightly decreased	Depressed
Tears	Decreased	Decreased	Absent
Eyes	Normal	Sunken	Deeply sunken
Urinary output	Slightly decreased	Decreased	No urine
Pulses	Normal	Slight increase	Tachycardia, cool and poorly perfused extremities**
Blood pressure	Normal	Normal	Low
Urinary specific gravity	>1.020	>1.020	No urine
Urine sodium	<20mEq/L	<20mEq/L	No urine

Adapted from Ford, D. (1999). Fluid, electrolyte, and acid-base disorders and therapy. In W. Hay, A. Hayward, M. Levin, & J. Sondheimer (Eds.), *Current pediatric diagnosis and treatment* (14th ed.). Stamford, CT: Appleton & Lange, 1113; V. Uphold, C. Uphold, & G. Uphold. (1999). *Clinical guidelines in family practice* (p. 527). Gainesville, FL: Barmarrae Press; and Centers for Disease Control and Prevention (CDC). (1992). The management of acute diarrhea in children: Oral rehydration, maintenance and nutritional therapy. *Morbidity and Mortality Weekly Report, 41,* October (No. RR-16): 1-20.
*Infants with acute diarrhea are more apt to dehydrate than older children because they have a higher body surface to weight ratio, have a higher metabolic rate, and depend on others for fluid.
** Rapid deep breathing, prolonged skin retraction, and decreased perfusion are more reliably predictive of dehydration than sunken fontanelle or absence of tears.

- Distention
- Hyperactive bowel sounds
- Diffuse tenderness
- Increased tympany to percussion
- Splenomegaly (bacterial)
- Other infections that can produce diarrhea and vomiting and therefore should be ruled out in examination:
  - Streptococcal pharyngitis
  - Pneumonia
  - Otitis media

Diagnostic Procedures

Diagnosis can usually be made by careful history alone. If any of the following conditions occur, lab testing may provide important diagnostic clues:
- Bloody diarrhea
- Weight loss
- Diarrhea leading to dehydration
- Fever
- Prolonged diarrhea (3 or more unformed stools per day, for several days)
- Neurologic involvement (paresthesias, motor weakness, cranial nerve palsies)
- Severe abdominal pain

- No tests if duration less than 48 hours
- Dehydration, especially in small children, check serum electrolytes
- Wet preparation for white blood cells (WBCs)
- Stool for ova and parasites (check if travel history given, immunocompromised, persistent diarrhea, unresponsive to antibiotic therapy)
- Stool culture for enteric pathogens (indicated if the patient is immunocompromised, febrile, has bloody diarrhea, severe abdominal pain, or if illness is severe or persistent)

DIAGNOSIS

Summary information for diagnosis of acute diarrhea is included in Table 3-23.

Acute Diarrhea

Differential diagnoses include the following:

- Diarrhea induced by food or drug sensitivities
- Starvation diarrhea
- Parenteral infections: urinary tract infection (UTI), upper respiratory infection (URI)
- Sepsis in neonates

TABLE **3-23** Acute Diarrhea

AGENT*	AGE AFFECTED	INCUBATION	SOURCE	SYMPTOMS	STOOL CHARACTERISTICS	TREATMENT
Viral	Any; infants/children, elderly, and immunocompromised most vulnerable	24-48 hr	Food, person-to-person	Nausea, vomiting, diarrhea, low-grade fever may precede diarrhea, URI, lasting 4-8 days	Large and liquid, variable odor, negative for blood, WBCs	Varies with age (see text)
Bacterial *Campylobacter*	Any; most common bacterial diarrhea in 1- to 5-year-olds	2-5 days	Raw and undercooked poultry, unpasteurized milk, contaminated water	Diarrhea, cramps, fever and vomiting, diarrhea may be bloody, lasts approximately 2-10 days	Bloody and watery, may be positive for blood and WBCs	Erythromycin for 5-7 days
Escheria coli	More common in children younger than 4	1-8 days	Undercooked beef, unpasteurized milk and juice, raw fruits and vegetables, salad dressing, and contaminated water	Severe diarrhea that is often bloody, abdominal pain, vomiting; usually little or no fever is present, lasts 5-10 days	Green, slimy, foul-smelling, positive for WBCs	Same as shigella
*Salmonella**	Any	1-3 days	Contaminated eggs, poultry, unpasteurized milk or juice, cheese, contaminated raw fruits and vegetables	Diarrhea, fever, abdominal pain, vomiting, lasts 4-7 days	Loose, slimy, and green with rotten egg odor, positive for WBCs and blood	Ampicillin
Shigella	Any; peaks 2-10 years	24-48 hours	Food or water contaminated with fecal matter, usually person-to-person spread, fecal-oral transmission; ready-made foods touched by food workers, raw vegetables, egg salad	Abdominal cramps, fever, and diarrhea; stool may contain blood and mucus, lasts 4-7 days	Watery, yellow-green, mucus and bloody, no change in odor; positive for blood and WBCs	Bactrim
Parasitic *Giardia*	Any; peaks at 4 years	1-4 weeks	Drinking water, other sources	Acute or chronic diarrhea, flatulence, bloating, lasts weeks	Pale, bulky, greasy with foul odor; negative for blood and WBCs; 30%-60% are positive for casts	Metronidazole

URI, Upper respiratory infection; *WBCs*, white blood cells.
*Foodborne diseases and conditions designated as notifiable in the U.S. (CDC, 2001b).

Chronic Diarrhea

Differential diagnoses include the following:

- Malabsorption (cystic fibrosis, lactose deficiency, celiac disease)
- Reye syndrome
- AIDS
- Inflammatory bowel disease
- Food allergies
- Metabolic disease
- Pseudomembranous colitis

THERAPEUTIC PLAN
Infants and Children

Diarrhea is usually self-limiting and requires no aggressive therapy. The family nurse practitioner (FNP) treatment plan should be based on careful assessment of the degree of dehydration. Treat as follows:

Diarrhea without Dehydration
- Continue breast milk, formula, or age-appropriate diet.
- Push oral fluids at a rate of 150 ml/kg/day.
- Follow each stool with 10 ml/kg electrolyte solution (Pedialyte or Infalyte).

Mild Dehydration
- Oral rehydration therapy (ORT) with a solution containing 75 to 90 mEq/L sodium. Give 40 to 50 ml/kg over 2 to 4 hours.
- Reassess hydration status every 2 to 4 hours.
- When dehydration is corrected, move to maintenance therapy.
- Maintenance therapy; resume breast milk, formula, or age-appropriate diet.
- Push oral fluids at a rate of 150 ml/kg/day.
- Follow each stool with a solution containing 40 to 60 mEq/L sodium (Pedialyte or Infalyte) at 10 ml/kg and follow each emesis with 2 ml/kg.

Moderate Dehydration
- Administer ORT at 100 ml/kg over 2 to 4 hours.
- Reassess hydration status every 2 to 4 hours.
- When dehydration is corrected, move to maintenance therapy.

Severe Dehydration. Consult physician and refer for hospitalization and IV rehydration.

Pharmacologic Treatment

Usually pharmacologic treatment is not indicated, and at times it may prolong the course. Pharmacotherapy may be used in severe cases to shorten the course, prevent complications, or decrease excretion of the causative agent (see Table 3-23).

Oral Rehydration Therapy
- Give children younger than 2 years $1/2$ cup ORT solution every hour.
- Give children older than 2 years one-half to 1 cup ORT solution every hour.
- If vomiting occurs, give 1 teaspoon ORT solution every 2 to 3 minutes until vomiting stops, and then continue ORT as previously indicated.
- Have parent notify the FNP if diarrhea is not improved in 24 hours, there is an increase in the frequency or amount of vomiting or diarrhea, or if blood appears in either the stool or the emesis.
- Avoid using antidiarrheal agents, including OTC preparations.

Adults
- For acute episodes, discontinue solids for 12 hours.
- Reintroduce food as soon as possible and advance as tolerated.
- Pharmacologic therapy is usually not indicated. It may be used in severe cases to shorten the course, prevent complications, or decrease excretion of the causative agent.
- Give kaolin-pectin (Kaopectate) 60 ml PO every 3 to 4 hours. Use is not to exceed 2 days.
- Give loperamide (Imodium) 4 mg PO initially, then 2 mg after each loose stool, to a maximum dose of 16 mg in 24 hours. Use is not to exceed 2 days.
- See Table 3-23 for treatment of bacterial infections.

Client Education
- Teach parents the signs and symptoms of dehydration:
  - Dry mouth
  - No tears
  - Less moisture in diaper
  - Lethargy
  - Weight loss
  - Irritability
  - Sunken fontanel
- Parents should keep ORT at home and use the solution when diarrhea first occurs in the child.
- Children and adults eating a regular diet should continue receiving a regular diet. Foods to be avoided include those that are high in simple sugars (they can exacerbate diarrhea by the osmotic effects). These foods include soft drinks, undiluted apple juice, Jell-O, and presweetened cereals. Foods high in fat may not be tolerated because of their tendency to delay gastric emptying.
- Remind parents not to use the "BRAT" (bananas, rice, cereal, applesauce, toast) diet for a prolonged time because it results in inadequate energy and protein content.

Prevention
- Practice food safety:
  - Clean and wash hands often.

- Separate; don't cross contaminate (raw meat, poultry, seafood, and eggs).
- Cook food to proper temperatures.
- Chill and refrigerate food properly.
- When traveling in developing countries or in any area where water supply is questionable, drink bottled water.

EVALUATION/FOLLOW-UP
Infants and Small Children

- Conduct telephone follow-up in 12 hours and then daily until diarrhea has subsided. Infants need daily weight checks.
- Instruct caregiver to call if fluids are refused or continually vomited.

Adults

- Return to clinic in 3 days if diarrhea has not resolved.

Referral

- Consult and/or refer in the following cases:
  - Infants younger than 3 months
  - Severe dehydration
  - Diarrhea persisting longer than 3 days in children and longer than 2 weeks in adults
  - Bloody diarrhea or emesis
- Depending on the cause of diarrhea, some clients may need to be reported to the local health department.

COMPLICATIONS
Death.

REFERENCES

Centers for Disease Control and Prevention (CDC). (1992). The management of acute diarrhea in children: Oral rehydration, maintenance and nutritional therapy. *Morbidity and Mortality Weekly Report, 41,* (No RR-16), 1-20.

Centers for Disease Control and Prevention (CDC). (2001a). Norwalk like viruses. *Morbidity and Mortality Weekly Report, 50* (RR09), 1-18.

Centers for Disease Control and Prevention (CDC). (2001b). Diagnosis and management of foodborne illness. *Morbidity and Mortality Weekly Report, 50* (RR02), 1-69.

Goepp, J. G., & Santosham, M. (1993). Oral rehydration therapy. In M. D. Oski & J. A. McMillan (Eds.), *Principles and practice of pediatrics updates*. Philadelphia: J. B. Lippincott.

Hay, W., Hayward, A., Levin, M., & Sondheimer, J. (1999). *Current pediatric diagnosis and treatment* (14th ed.). Norwalk, CT: Appleton & Lange.

McCargar, L. J., Hotson, B. L., & Nozza, A. (1995). Fibre and nutrient intakes of chronic care elderly patients. *Journal of Nutrition for the Elderly, 15*(1), 13-31.

Nelson, W. (1996). *Nelson textbook of pediatrics* (15th ed.). Philadelphia: W. B. Saunders.

Robinson, D., Kidd, P., & Rogers, K. (2000). *Primary care across the lifespan*. St. Louis: Mosby.

Rosenthal, M. (1997). Diarrhea organisms are becoming media stars. *Infectious Diseases in Children, 10*(1), 10-11.

Schreiber, D., et al. (2001). A clinical prediction rule to predict positive stool cultures in ED patients with acute diarrhea. *Academic Emergency Medicine, 8*(5), 478-479.

Straughn, A., & English, B. (1996). Oral rehydration therapy: A neglected treatment for pediatric diarrhea. *Maternal Child Nursing, 6*(5), 144-147.

Review Questions

1. A 3-year-old comes to the clinic with a 24-hour history of vomiting, diarrhea, fever (103° F), and severe abdominal tenderness. What should the NP do?
- **a.** Reassure the mother that this is gastroenteritis and it should be self-limiting.
- **b.** Conduct a complete dietary history and physical examination before making a diagnosis.
- **c.** Take a complete dietary history, looking especially for other family members who might have eaten the same contaminated foods.
- **d.** Send a stool culture for ova and parasites and for enteric pathogens.

2. A 6-year-old boy has had diarrhea for 1 day. What associated historical data is consistent with a diagnosis of viral diarrhea?
- **a.** "I have blood in my stools."
- **b.** "The stools have a terrible odor and float."
- **c.** "Steve's sister has diarrhea too."
- **d.** "Steve has lost 10 pounds."

3. The most common cause of diarrhea in children is which of the following?
- **a.** Rotavirus
- **b.** Campylobacter
- **c.** Shigella
- **d.** Norwalk virus

4. During the physical examination, which of the following findings is *not* consistent with viral diarrhea?
- **a.** Occult blood in the stool
- **b.** Moist mucous membranes, slight tenderness of the abdomen
- **c.** Hyperactive bowel sounds
- **d.** Mild abdominal tenderness

5. The FNP has prescribed ORT for a 14-month-old with mild dehydration. The mother asks what she should do if the child vomits the solution. What instructions should the FNP give?
- **a.** Hold the ORT solution until the child stops vomiting.
- **b.** Continue to give the ORT solution in small, frequent amounts (1 teaspoon every 1 to 2 minutes).
- **c.** Hold the ORT solution for 2 to 3 hours until the child's stomach has settled and then resume feeding.
- **d.** Continue to give the ORT solution as ordered.

6. Four hours after beginning ORT on an infant with moderate dehydration, the FNP phones to check the child's progress. The mother reports that he has vomited all the ORT solution and is continuing to have liquid stools. The FNP should do which of the following?

D

a. Ask the mother to continue ORT in the clinic under a controlled situation.
b. Ask the mother to observe the child for 1 hour and then attempt to restart ORT.
c. Change the ORT solution to juice or gelatin water.
d. Consult the physician about the need for parenteral fluid therapy and refer the child to the emergency department.

7. A man comes in complaining of diarrhea and a 10-pound weight loss in the past week. He has explosive diarrhea and gas, but no fever. He had been camping in a local campground and bathed in the nearby creek. This history is most consistent with which type of diarrhea?
a. Rotavirus
b. Shigella
c. Giardia
d. Salmonella

8. Which of the following sets of symptoms is most consistent with severe dehydration in a child?
a. Dry mucus membranes, decreased urinary output, increased heart rate
b. Decreased urinary output, abdominal distention
c. Very dry lips, very thirsty, increased heart rate, sunken orbits
d. Slightly dry lips, thick saliva

Answers and Rationales

1. **Answer: b** (assessment)
Rationale: Significant abdominal tenderness suggests a more serious problem than gastroenteritis. A thorough history and physical examination should always be conducted before making any diagnosis (CDC, 1992).

2. **Answer: c** (assessment)
Rationale: With viral diarrhea, there are often other family members at home with similar symptoms. Blood in the stools does not occur with viral illness, nor does a terrible odor with floating. Viral diarrhea generally does not produce a significant weight loss (Robinson, Kidd, Rogers, 2000).

3. **Answer: a** (analysis/diagnosis)
Rationale: The most common cause of diarrhea in children is the rotavirus (CDC, 1992).

4. **Answer: a** (assessment)
Rationale: Blood in the stool is not present with viral diarrhea (CDC, 1992).

5. **Answer: b** (implementation/plan)
Rationale: Giving the ORT in very small quantities will limit gastric distention while helping to correct dehydration and acidosis. Vomiting is generally triggered by gastric distention and acidosis. Both choices a and d would fail to give the child fluid and would contribute to increasing dehydration. Choice c would require large quantities of solution, which would lead to gastric distention and more vomiting (CDC, 1992).

6. **Answer: d** (evaluation)
Rationale: Children who continue with a negative fluid balance 4 hours into ORT should receive IV fluids (Goepp & Santosham, 1993). High-osmolar fluids, such as gelatin water and fruit juices, tend to draw water into the intestines and actually increase the number of stools (Straughn & English, 1996).

7. **Answer: c** (analysis/diagnosis)
Rationale: Giardia usually causes increased gas and bloating. Weight loss is common. It is caused by inadequate water treatment (CDC, 2001b).

8. **Answer: c** (analysis/diagnosis)
Rationale: A child with more than 10% loss by dehydration would have sunken orbits, severe thirst, and increased heart rate (CDC, 1992).

DIVERTICULAR DISEASE *Denise Robinson*

OVERVIEW
Definition
Diverticula are abnormal herniations of mucosa through the muscle layer of the colon wall. Asymptomatic diverticular disease is referred to as diverticulosis. Diverticulosis often is diagnosed serendipitously when searching for other diagnoses. Diverticulitis represents inflammation caused by infection.

Incidence
- Diverticular disease affects men and women equally.
- Although there is no known genetic pattern, it is present in 20% of the adult population older than 40 years, increasing progressively with age.
- It is estimated that 70% of those older than 70 years have diverticular disease.
- Diverticulitis occurs in 10% to 25% of those individuals with diverticulosis.
- Thirty-three percent of those treated for diverticulitis will likely have subsequent episodes.
- Two or three occurrences during 1 to 2 years is an indication to consider surgical removal of that portion of the bowel.
- It most commonly occurs in Europe and North America, where diets are typically low in fiber.

Pathophysiology
Diverticula most commonly occur in the sigmoid colon, where the colon is narrowest and the pressure is highest; however, diverticula can occur anywhere in the GI tract. The saclike outpouchings occur at a weak point in the colon, often where arteries penetrate the tunica muscularis.

Thickening, hypertrophy, and contraction of the muscles in the colon wall increase intraluminal pressure and the degree of the herniation. Trapped, undigested food and bacteria in the diverticular sacs can result in an infection.

Factors Increasing Susceptibility
- Age older than 40 years
- Low-residue diets reduce fecal bulk, reducing the diameter of the colon
- Previous episodes of diverticulitis

ASSESSMENT: SUBJECTIVE/HISTORY
History of Present Illness

Ask about the following:
- Duration of symptoms
- Location/and quality of discomfort
- What provides relief
- Bowel habits
- Nausea/vomiting
- Fever or chills
- Flatulence
- Rectal bleeding
- Diverticulosis
- Symptoms possibly vague or absent; fewer than 25% have symptoms
- Intermittent lower left quadrant abdominal pain, worse after eating; some relief after bowel movement or flatulence
- Constipation alternating with diarrhea

Diverticulitis. Symptoms vary; any of the following symptoms may be present:
- Pain localized to the left lower quadrant; usually sudden onset
- Fever and chills
- Poor appetite
- Nausea and vomiting
- Constipation or diarrhea
- Guarding, rebound tenderness
- Gas and flatulence
- Rectal bleeding

Past Medical History

Ask about previous episodes of diverticulitis or severe abdominal pain.

Medication History

Inquire about current medications, including laxative and oral corticosteroid use.

Psychosocial History

Not applicable.

Dietary History
- Ask about the amount of fiber in the diet.
- Ask about fluid intake.

ASSESSMENT: OBJECTIVE/PHYSICAL EXAMINATION
Physical Examination

A problem-oriented physical examination should include vital signs, height, and weight. Age and level of acuity may require a more comprehensive examination than an assessment of the abdomen and rectum.

Diverticulosis
- Abdomen may be distended and tympanic.
- Flatulence present.
- Rectal examination may reveal a palpable firm, tender mass in left lower quadrant.
- Melena present if diverticular bleed.
- Brisk rectal bleeding present.

Diverticulitis
- Rigid abdomen, or distended and tympanic present.
- Tender, firm, fixed palpable mass present in left iliac fossa.
- Bowel sounds depressed, or increased if obstruction.
- Rectum may be tender on examination; there may be a mass in the cul de sac.
- Melena present if diverticular bleed.
- Brisk rectal bleeding present.
- Check for guarding, perform iliopsoas muscle test, and assess obturator sign (abdominal pain in response to passive internal rotation of the right hip from 90-degree hip/knee flexion position).
- Elderly clients and those taking corticosteroids may present with mild symptoms only, no fever, no elevated WBC count and only vague complaints of abdominal pain.

Diagnostic Procedures
- Obtain CBC with differential (WBC count elevated with immature polymorphs in diverticulitis).
- Check hemoglobin—low if bleeding.
- Determine sedimentation rate—elevated in diverticulosis.
- Obtain the following imaging:
  - Abdominal flat-plate supine and upright radiographs are useful in peritonitis and perforation.
  - Barium enema is used to diagnose diverticulosis. It is controversial for diagnosing diverticulitis in the acute phase because it may cause rupture of the diverticula. Diagnostic accuracy of the barium enema in distinguishing between diverticular disease and cancer has been questioned.
  - Colonoscopy and flexible sigmoidoscopy are helpful in differentiating diverticulosis, ulcerative colitis, and cancer.
  - CT scan, although expensive, is an excellent alternative diagnostic procedure to the barium enema.

D

DIAGNOSIS

Differential diagnoses include the following:

- Irritable bowel syndrome
- Lactose intolerance
- Appendicitis
- Gastroenteritis
- Fecal impaction
- Ulcerative colitis, Crohn's disease
- Carcinoma
- Ectopic pregnancy
- UTI

THERAPEUTIC PLAN

Nonpharmacologic Treatment

A high-fiber diet is recommended to improve symptoms and slow the progression of the diverticular disease process. It is recommended that persons with diverticulosis take in 20 to 35 g of fiber per day (average U.S. intake is 15 to 20 g/day) (Box 3-9). Consider adding a fiber supplement such as Metamucil or Fiber Con.

For clients with diverticulitis, a clear liquid diet is prescribed, gradually increasing to soft foods as symptoms improve. Eventually these clients go to a high-fiber diet when they have fully recovered. Clients should increase their fluid intake to 10 8-ounce glasses per day.

Pharmacologic Treatment

Diverticulosis

- Manage pain with antispasmodic dicyclomine [Bentyl], 10 to 20 mg bid to qid with meals. Anticholinergics need to be used with caution (they may reduce the painful spasm, but they increase the risk of constipation).
- Manage constipation and diarrhea similarly to irritable bowel syndrome (IBS).
  - Loperamide (Imodium), 2 mg after each diarrheal stool, or diphenoxylate (Lomotil), 2.5 to 5 mg after each diarrheal stool

- Psyllium products, Metamucil 1 tablespoon bid or tid for constipation or Fiberall 1 to 2 wafers bid or tid with 8 ounces of water
- Antiflatulents, simethicone (Flatulex), 80 mg after meals and at bedtime

Diverticulitis. Treat only mild, nontoxic individuals in primary care (temperature less than 101°F, WBC level 13,000 to 15,000 cells/mm³).

- Administer metronidazole (Flagyl), 250 to 500 every 8 hours for 7 days, and amoxicillin, 500 mg combination every 8 hours, or ciprofloxacin, 500 mg bid (to cover enterococcal and Gram-negative aerobes).
- Client should respond within 3 days.
- Use mild analgesics (nonopiates) for pain.

Client Education

- Maintain adequate fluid intake (2000 mL/day).
- Good sources of fiber include bran, raw carrots, and fruit. Bran can cause bloating or flatulence, which resolves with continued use.
- Avoid foods with seeds or those that are indigestible, such as nuts, popcorn kernels, corn, cucumber seeds, tomato seeds, strawberry seeds, or caraway seeds on buns. These can block the neck of the diverticulum.
- Avoid laxatives, enemas, and opiates because they can lead to chronic constipation.
- *Signs and symptoms of complications* include severe abdominal pain, vomiting, temperature higher than 101°F, hard or firm abdomen, no bowel movements, and frank rectal bleeding.
- Discuss *stress management* methods; consider relaxation techniques. Participate in support groups if helpful to manage symptoms.
- There are no *activity* restrictions for diverticulosis. Restrict activity in diverticulitis, with bed rest during the acute phase.

Box 3-9 Food High in Fiber			
CEREALS	**GRAINS**	**FRUITS**	**VEGETABLES**
Branflakes, oatmeal, shredded wheat	Bran muffins, brown rice, whole-wheat bread	Artichokes, apples, blackberries, dates, figs, oranges, pears, prunes, raspberries, tomatoes	Beans (baked, black, kidney, lima, pinto), broccoli, brussels sprouts, carrots, chick peas, green peas, lentils, pumpkin, rutabaga, winter squash

From Robinson, D., Kidd, P., & Rogers, K. M. (2000). *Primary care across the lifespan.* St. Louis: Mosby.

- Develop and maintain a regular exercise program (walking and exercise increases peristalsis and decreases constipation).

Prevention

- High-fiber diet
- Exercise
- Adequate fluid intake

Referral

- Refer very ill older clients with a history of diverticulosis (older clients may not look toxic yet have an acute abdomen with no pain and no fever).
- Refer toxic clients with diverticulitis (septicemia, peritonitis).
- Refer if failure to resolve in 48 to 72 hours.
- Refer in cases of brisk rectal bleeding.
- If client's condition is worsening, consider hospitalization immediately if temperature is higher than 101° F, if there is a marked change in abdominal pain and continuous increase in WBCs, and if peritoneal signs develop.
- Two or more episodes of diverticulitis during a 1- to 2-year period may be an indication for surgery.

Consultation

Consultation is needed if there is no change in symptoms regardless of management regime.

EVALUATION/FOLLOW-UP
Diverticulosis

- Follow-up in 1 to 2 weeks, then every 3 months to 1 year, then annually as needed.
- Barium enema may be repeated every 3 to 5 years, followed by a colonoscopy if needed.

Diverticulitis

- Do telephone follow-up at 24 to 72 hours; if there is no progress or symptoms are worse, client should return to clinic for further evaluation.
- Follow-up in 10 days to 2 weeks if recovery has progressed as expected.
- Follow-up at 1- to 3-month intervals, expanding to annual check-ups based on symptoms.

COMPLICATIONS

- Abscess formation (bowel may rupture)
- Peritonitis
- Obstruction
- Bleeding
- Fistula development into bladder, gut, or vagina

REFERENCES

Bradshaw, L. (2000). Diverticulosis/diverticulitis. In D. Robinson, P. Kidd, & K. Rogers (Eds.), *Primary care across the lifespan* (pp. 366-371). St. Louis: Mosby.

Braunwald, E., & Fauci, A. (2001). *Harrison's principles of internal medicine* (15th ed.). New York: McGraw-Hill.

Goroll, A., May, L., & Mulley, A. (Eds.), (1995). *Primary care medicine: Office evaluation and management of the adult patient.* Philadelphia: J. B. Lippincott.

Hurst, J. W. (1996). *Medicine for the practicing physician.* Norwalk, CT: Appleton & Lange.

Lonergan, E. (Ed.). (1996). *Geriatrics: A clinical manual.* Norwalk, CT: Appleton & Lange.

Rakel, R. (Ed.). (1995). *Textbook of family practice* (5th ed.). Philadelphia: W. B. Saunders.

Review Questions

1. Which of the following is most indicative of diverticulosis?
   a. Generalized abdominal pain, better after eating
   b. Lower right quadrant abdominal pain, worse after eating
   c. Intermittent epigastric pain
   d. Intermittent lower left quadrant abdominal pain, worse after eating

2. B.B., a 58-year-old man reports to the clinic with a temperature of 100° F, bloating, and cramping abdominal pain throughout his entire abdomen for the preceding 2 days. He notes mild constipation and increasing nausea. He has a 5-year history of diverticulosis. He reports no surgeries. He ate popcorn 3 days ago. His WBC count is 15,000 cells/mm^3. On physical examination, you note generalized abdominal tenderness, no rebound tenderness, no rectal point tenderness, and a negative guaiac test result. On the basis of this history, what is the most likely diagnosis?
   a. Diverticulitis
   b. Gastroesophageal reflux disease (GERD)
   c. IBS
   d. Appendicitis

3. What is the best treatment for B.B., the subject of the previous question?
   a. Lifestyle changes and H$_2$ blockers
   b. Anticholinergic agents
   c. Hydrocodone bitartrate (Vicodin) for pain
   d. Antibiotics

4. Which of the following comments indicate a need for more teaching related to diverticulosis?
   a. "I should drink 8 to 10 glasses of water a day."
   b. "I should eat low-fiber foods to avoid an infection."
   c. "I should eat 25 g of fiber a day."
   d. "Exercise will help with my constipation."

5. Which of the following is most indicative of diverticulitis?

D

a. Nausea and vomiting, distended abdomen
b. Epigastric pain radiating upward
c. Pain improving with eating
d. Pain improving with bowel movement

6. Which of the following sets of findings is most common in persons with diverticulitis?

a. Elevated WBC count, fever, left lower quadrant abdominal pain
b. Elevated WBC count, fever, right lower quadrant abdominal pain
c. Rectal bleeding
d. Constipation

7. A 65-year-old female comes in complaining of vague abdominal symptoms, including lower left quadrant pain, especially after eating. Which of the following historical statements is consistent with a diagnosis of diverticulosis?

a. "I eat apples, tomatoes, and bran muffins every day."
b. "I eat cereal every morning and have fruits and vegetables often."
c. "I eat eggs and bacon for breakfast, fast food for lunch, and usually have pasta for dinner."
d. "I exercise every day and eat a healthy diet."

8. Abigail is an 80-year-old with diverticulosis. She has followed a high-fiber diet, and she exercises and drinks adequate water; however, her abdominal pain and constipation/diarrhea still continues. What is the appropriate action at this point?

a. Try Bentyl with meals and at bedtime.
b. Prescribe a H_1 blocker.
c. Increase the fiber she is eating.
d. Refer her to a GI specialist.

Answers and Rationales

1. *Answer:* **d** (assessment)
Rationale: Increased bulk and motility after eating result in pressure irritation of the diverticula, most commonly found in the sigmoid colon located on the left lower side of the abdomen. Right-sided pain is rarely worse after eating and is most often associated with appendicitis; intermittent epigastric pain is more likely gastric or cardiac in nature (Goroll, May, & Mulley, 1995; Hurst, 1996; Rakel, 1995).

2. *Answer:* **a** (analysis/diagnosis)
Rationale: The elevated temperature, elevated WBC count, abdominal tenderness, and history of diverticulosis are strongly indicative of a diagnosis of diverticulitis; however, appendicitis also needs to be a consideration because the client has had no surgeries. Although you would expect right-sided pain, presenting symptoms of disease processes are not always predictable. The client's history and physical findings do not support a diagnosis of GERD or IBS (Goroll, May, & Mulley, 1995; Hurst, 1996; Rakel, 1995).

3. *Answer:* **d** (implementation/plan)
Rationale: Antibiotics are an appropriate treatment for a person with diverticulitis. The client notes mild constipation, so constipating medications such as anticholinergic medications or Vicodin are avoided. Lifestyle changes may be relevant after this acute phase, but they and H_2 blockers are more appropriate therapy for a diagnosis of GERD or peptic ulcer disease (Goroll, May, & Mulley, 1995; Hurst, 1996; Rakel, 1995).

4. *Answer:* **b** (evaluation)
Rationale: Patients with diverticulosis need to eat a high-fiber diet to help prevent progression of the disease. A low-fiber diet is what contributed to the illness (Bradshaw, 2000).

5. *Answer:* **a** (assessment)
Rationale: The inflammatory process in the bowel often results in an alteration in motility, leading to abdominal distention, nausea, and vomiting. These symptoms may also be accompanied by abdominal pain. Epigastric pain radiating upward is often referred to as heartburn, common in GERD. Pain that improves with eating is associated with a duodenal ulcer. Pain improvement with bowel movements is noted among individuals with IBS. Such improvement may also occur with diverticulosis (Goroll, May, & Mulley, 1995; Hurst, 1996; Rakel, 1995).

6. *Answer:* **a** (analysis/diagnosis)
Rationale: Elevated WBC count and fever are signs of an infection and inflammation. The left-sided abdominal pain is common in diverticulitis (the sigmoid colon seems to be somewhat more vulnerable to the development of diverticula). Right-sided lower quadrant pain is more common in appendicitis. Rectal bleeding and constipation may be present regardless of any inflammatory process (Goroll, May, & Mulley, 1995; Hurst, 1996; Rakel, 1995).

7. *Answer:* **c** (assessment)
Rationale: Answer c describes a low-fiber diet. This is contributory to the development of diverticulosis (Bradshaw, 2000).

8. *Answer:* **d** (evaluation)
Rationale: A patient who makes the lifestyle changes by adding fiber, exercise, and fluids, and who has no improvement, should be referred (Bradshaw, 2000).

DYSMENORRHEA *Cheryl Pope Kish*

OVERVIEW

Definition

Dysmenorrhea refers to painful menstruation. Primary dysmenorrhea occurs with ovulatory menstrual cycles and in the absence of pelvic pathology. The painful menses of secondary dysmenorrhea is caused by either intrauterine or extrauterine pelvic pathology (endometriosis is the most common cause).

Incidence

- Primary dysmenorrhea is the most common medical problem in young women. Of all menstruating women, 70% have dysmenorrhea; 10% have symptoms severe enough to interfere with school, work, or other activities. Onset is usually at least 6 to 12 months after menarche, or when ovulatory cycles begin. Incidence increases and peaks in the late teens and early twenties, then gradually declines with age.
- Onset of secondary dysmenorrhea usually is after 25 to 30 years of age. Incidence gradually increases with age.

Pathophysiology

Primary dysmenorrhea is due to increased levels of prostaglandins in the uterine endometrium during the luteal phase of the menstrual cycle that are released as the lining is shed. Prostaglandin causes increased myometrial muscle tone, uterine contractions, ischemia, and sensitization of nerve endings. Because it causes smooth muscle contractions, prostaglandin is responsible for many of the associated symptoms as well.

The tendency to synthesize prostaglandin is hereditary, so daughters of mothers with primary dysmenorrhea are more likely to have primary dysmenorrhea. Women with anovulatory cycles do not have luteal increases in prostaglandins and thus do not have primary dysmenorrhea. Secondary dysmenorrhea is associated with pelvic pathology and is suggested by the following:

- Dysmenorrhea in first cycles after menarche (possibly related to congenital outlet obstruction)
- Symptoms beginning after age 25
- Onset after a history without previous menstrual pain (possibly related to ectopic pregnancy or threatened abortion)
- Abnormal physical examination indicative of pelvic abnormality
- Heavy menstrual flow or irregular cycles (possibly fibroids, polyps, adenomyosis)
- Dyspareunia

- Infertility (possibly pelvic inflammatory disease [PID] scarring, endometriosis)
- Failed response to nonsteroidal anti-inflammatory drugs (NSAIDs), oral contraceptive pills (OCPs), or both

For common causes of secondary dysmenorrhea, see Table 3-24.

Factors Increasing Susceptibility

- Earlier menarche
- Longer menstrual periods
- Nulliparity
- Obesity
- Smoking
- Alcohol consumption
- Stress

ASSESSMENT: SUBJECTIVE/HISTORY

- Obtain detailed menstrual history, including age at menarche and age at onset of symptoms, frequency and duration of menses, timing of symptoms in relation to onset of menstrual flow, associated symptoms, factors that alleviate symptoms, and factors that make symptoms worse.
- Determine last menstrual period (LMP).
- Ask about contraception.
- Ask about previous pregnancies.
- Determine if client is sexually active and if the pain is related to intercourse.
- Ask how she protects herself from sexually transmitted disease (STDs).
- Inquire about treatment of STDs in past.
- Does she have a new partner? A vaginal discharge?
- Determine date of last Pap smear.

TABLE **3-24** Common Causes of Secondary Dysmenorrhea

UTERINE CAUSES	EXTRAUTERINE CAUSES
Adenomyosis	Endometriosis
PID	Adhesions related to
Cervical stenosis and	inflammation and scarring
polyps	(PID)
IUD	Functional ovarian cysts
Fibroids	Benign or malignant tumors
Congenital malformations	in pelvis
Threatened abortion	Inflammatory bowel disease
	Ectopic pregnancy

D

Symptoms

Primary Dysmenorrhea

- Pain is crampy; spasmodic midline over lower abdominal and pelvis.
- Pain may radiate to the upper thighs, groin, or lower back.
- Symptoms usually begin several hours before or at the onset of menses and last 24 to 72 hours, at which time they begin to abate.
- Pain may be moderate to severe; some women have more severe pain than they experience during childbirth.

Associated symptoms may include nausea, vomiting, diarrhea, headache, fatigue, weakness, diaphoresis, flushing, anxiety, tension, depression, bloating with weight gain, and breast tenderness. Severe cases may have dizziness and fainting.

Secondary Dysmenorrhea

- Symptoms are more variable, depending on the cause.
- Pain may occur at any time during the menstrual cycle and tends to increase with age. Pain may occur at times other than during menstruation. There may be dyspareunia.
- Associated symptoms of secondary dysmenorrhea depend on the cause.

Past Medical History

Obtain a detailed menstrual and gynecologic history; also ask about hospitalizations, surgery and procedures, liver or renal disease, other chronic medical conditions, and allergies.

Medication History

Ask about any current prescription drugs, all OTC medications, contraceptive agents, and allergies. Query previous use of analgesics.

Family History

Look for positive family history for dysmenorrhea or other gynecologic problems.

Psychosocial History

Assess support systems, coping skills, and previous mechanisms for coping with pain.

Dietary History

Assess for diet high in refined sugar and salt, and for excessive caffeine. Obtain a complete nutritional history for the obese client.

ASSESSMENT: OBJECTIVE/PHYSICAL EXAMINATION

Physical Examination

A problem-oriented physical examination should be conducted, with particular attention to the following:

- Observe general appearance.
- Check vital signs.
- Determine weight.
- Assess abdomen for masses and tenderness.
- Perform pelvic examination. Inspect external genitalia and palpate for masses and tenderness. Perform speculum visualization of cervix and bimanual examination to assess for cervical motion tenderness, adnexal tenderness and abnormality, uterine tenderness, size, and contour. Note cervical erosion, stenosis, discharge, and intrauterine device (IUD) string.

Primary Dysmenorrhea. Physical examination is normal, although client may have some uterine and cervical tenderness if examined during symptoms. If evaluating for the first time, rule out pregnancy and pelvic infection.

Secondary Dysmenorrhea. Pelvic pathology may or may not be found on examination; additional tests are necessary to confirm diagnosis.

Diagnostic Procedures

- There are no diagnostic tests that confirm primary dysmenorrhea; diagnosis is made from clinical presentation and history.
- Tests for secondary dysmenorrhea are based on physical findings and symptoms and may include the following:
  - CBC, erythrocyte sedimentation rate (ESR) to rule out infection or inflammation
  - RPR to rule out syphilis
  - Cervical culture to rule out gonorrhea and chlamydia
  - Vaginal wet mount to rule out bacterial vaginosis, trichomoniasis, and candidiasis
  - Pap smear to rule out cervical cancer
  - Pregnancy test
  - Vaginal and pelvic ultrasonography to rule out pelvic pathology
  - Referral for additional tests, such as hysteroscopy, laparoscopy, or hysterosalpingogram if necessary to exclude other pathology and confirm diagnosis

DIAGNOSIS

Differential diagnoses include the following:

- Endometriosis
- PID
- Pregnancy complications (ectopic, spontaneous abortion)
- Uterine, ovarian, cervical congenital malformation, or other pathology
- Appendicitis
- Intestinal disease
- Renal or biliary colic

THERAPEUTIC PLAN

Primary Dysmenorrhea

Pharmacologic Treatment

- Prostaglandin synthetase inhibitors (NSAIDs) are effective in 75% to 90% of cases; try various agents for 6 months before considering treatment a failure.
- Three FDA-approved NSAIDs for primary dysmenorrhea are the following:
  - Ibuprofen (Motrin, Advil, other analogs)
  - Indomethacin (Indocin)
  - Naproxen sodium (Anaprox)
- Mefenamic acid (Ponstel), aspirin, and other NSAIDs are effective.
- Treat 2 to 3 days when symptoms are present.
- Assess for sensitivity before administration.
- Take with food or milk to lessen GI side effects.
- Contraindications include hypersensitivity, peptic ulcer disease, renal or hepatic disorder, asthma, anticoagulant therapy, bleeding disorder.
- Side effects include nausea, abdominal pain, indigestion, constipation, diarrhea, fluid retention, rash, tinnitus, GI bleeding; renal, hepatic, or CNS toxicity.
- OCPs are effective.
  - Combined estrogen-progesterone pill is drug of choice if client also desires contraception and has no contraindications. The daily use of medication to prevent symptoms 2 days per month is cumbersome and exposes the client to unnecessary side effects for a first-line therapy; therefore OCPs are usually limited to those who desire contraception as well as pain prevention. Norplant and DepoProvera are also effective to relieve dysmenorrhea.
  - Effective pain relief is obtained in 90% of cases. Mechanism of action is reduction of menstrual fluid volume and suppression of ovulation.
  - Because OCPs and NSAIDs work through different mechanisms of action, a combination of the two can be of value. For reasons that are not currently understood, approximately 10% of women fail to respond to treatment with NSAIDs or OCPs. Nonresponse is an indication to consider a secondary cause.
- Antiemetics are used if nausea and vomiting are major symptoms.
- Surgery is used rarely, in severe cases. Surgical procedures include presacral neurectomy, laser uterosacral nerve ablation (LUNA), and hysterectomy.

Nonpharmacologic Treatment

- Local heat, gentle abdominal massage, pelvic tilt, and stretching increase uterine blood flow and decrease muscle spasm.
- Transcutaneous electrical nerve stimulation stimulates release of endorphins.
- Regular aerobic exercise, three to four times per week for 20 to 30 minutes, suppresses prostaglandin release, increases endorphin release, promotes fitness and weight loss, and improves overall sense of well-being.
- Stress reduction and relaxation techniques are effective.
- Adjust diet. Decrease salt, caffeine, alcohol, and refined sugar; increase complex carbohydrates and foods that cause diuresis. Moderate amount of protein. If obese, lose weight.
- Stop smoking.
- Sexual activity can help. Sexual arousal and orgasm cause arteriolar vasodilation in uterus, decreasing ischemic pain.
- Pregnancy reduces the number of adrenergic nerves with only partial regeneration after delivery, resulting in decreased pain perception.

Secondary Dysmenorrhea

Treatment of secondary dysmenorrhea depends on the cause.

Client Education

Primary Dysmenorrhea

- Educate client about physiology of menstrual cycle and how it relates to pain.
- Inform client of nonpharmacologic measures for comfort.
- Teach about purpose, dosage, expected results, and potential side effects of medications.
- Teach warning signs associated with oral contraceptive use.
- Encourage client to keep record of menses, symptoms, and effects of medications.
- Encourage follow-up with health care provider.

Secondary Dysmenorrhea. Educational needs are determined by cause and treatment.

D

Prevention

Dysmenorrhea can rarely be prevented entirely but can be minimized with NSAIDs and OCPs.

Referral

- Refer to consultant if secondary dysmenorrhea is suspected.
- Refer client with primary dysmenorrhea to consultant for further evaluation if condition fails to improve on aforementioned treatment.

EVALUATION/FOLLOW-UP

Primary Dysmenorrhea

After initial evaluation, client should return at 2 months and at 4 months to evaluate therapy, then annually for Pap smear and pelvic examination. Client should return to clinic with new or worsening symptoms.

Secondary Dysmenorrhea

Follow-up with consultant as instructed or with health care provider when diagnosis and treatment are established.

COMPLICATIONS

Failure to treat primary dysmenorrhea can cause additional pain for the young woman that affects the quality of life and alters perceptions of menstruation as a normal physiologic process. Magnification of menstruation and negativity could occur as a result. Misdiagnosis or inappropriate treatment of secondary dysmenorrhea, depending on cause, could be life-threatening, depending on the cause.

REFERENCES

Cash, J. C., & Glass, C. A. (2000). *Family practice guidelines.* Philadelphia: Lippincott.

Coco, A. S. (1999). Primary dysmenorrhea. *American Family Physician, 60*(2), 489-495.

Hawkins, J., Roberto-Nichols, D., & Stanley-Haney, J. (1997). *Protocols for nurse practitioners in gynecologic settings* (6th ed.). New York: Tiresias Press.

Murphy, J. (1995). Dysmenorrhea. In W. Star, L. Lommel, & M. Shannon (Eds.), *Women's primary health care: Protocols for practice.* Washington, DC: American Nurses Publishing, 12/30-12/35.

Robinson, D., Kidd, P., & Rogers, K. M. (2000). *Primary care across the lifespan.* St. Louis: Mosby.

Smith, M. A., & Shimp, L. A. (2000). *20 common problems in women's health care.* New York: McGraw-Hill.

Uphold, C., & Graham, M. (1997). *Clinical guidelines in family practice* (3rd ed.). Gainesville, FL: Barmarrae Books.

Webb, T. (1996). Common menstrual disorders. *ADVANCE for Nurse Practitioners, 4*(1), 21-23.

Wolf, L.L., & Schumann, L. (1999). Dysmenorrhea. *Journal of American Academy of Nurse Practitioners, 11*(13), 125-132.

Review Questions

1. The cause of pain in primary dysmenorrhea is which of the following?
   a. Uterine muscle dysfunction
   b. Shedding of uterine lining
   c. Prostaglandin release and synthesis
   d. Endometriosis

2. Which of the following descriptions of symptoms is consistent with a diagnosis of primary dysmenorrhea?
   a. Spasmodic abdominal cramps and low back pain on days 1 through 3 of menses
   b. Pain intermittently throughout menstrual cycle
   c. Onset of menstrual pain at 38 years, increasing in severity
   d. Frequent dyspareunia

3. Which of the following drugs is most appropriate for Annie, a 16-year-old with primary dysmenorrhea?
   a. Naproxen sodium on a set schedule
   b. High-dose ibuprofen prn
   c. Tylenol on a set schedule
   d. Tylenol with codeine prn

4. Annie's mother, who accompanied her to the clinic, asks why a narcotic is not ordered because her daughter has such severe pain. How should the NP answer?
   a. Narcotics are given to teenagers only as a last resort because of the risk of psychologic dependence.
   b. NSAIDs decrease the level of prostaglandin, the chemical that causes the cramping.
   c. The consulting physician will be notified that a narcotic has been requested.
   d. The protocol for care demands a 3-month trial with NSAIDs before a narcotic can be considered.

5. Mary, 28 years old, seeks treatment. She has intermittent lower abdominal pain, dyspareunia, postcoital bleeding, and foul-smelling vaginal discharge. Of the following, the *least* likely diagnosis is:
   a. Primary dysmenorrhea
   b. Secondary dysmenorrhea
   c. Endometriosis
   d. PID

6. Mrs. Brown, 24 years old, has irregular, anovulatory menstrual cycles associated with intermittent abdominal pain. On the basis of this information, the most likely assessment is which of the following?
   a. Primary dysmenorrhea
   b. Endometriosis
   c. Secondary dysmenorrhea
   d. Uterine leiomyoma

7. Which of the following statements is *true* regarding the treatment of primary dysmenorrhea?

a. Oral contraceptives are the drug of choice when birth control is desired.

b. Mild narcotics often are necessary for the pain.

c. NSAIDs are completely safe and have no contraindications.

d. Medication is not necessary because the pain and symptoms are psychologic.

8. Jane, 29 years old, has just had primary dysmenorrhea diagnosed and has started on a regimen of NSAIDs. How often should she be evaluated?

a. As needed

b. Annually

c. In 2 months, then in 4 months

d. Weekly for 2 months

9. Betty, 35 years old, was referred to a consultant, and secondary dysmenorrhea was diagnosed. Her treatment and follow-up will:

a. Be determined by the cause of the secondary dysmenorrhea

b. Include a Pap smear every 6 months

c. Consist of low-dose narcotics

d. Include annual endometrial biopsy

10. Merritt, a 17-year-old, has primary dysmenorrhea. The NP provides education about dysmenorrhea and treatment measures. Which behavior by Merritt indicates that she has understood the instruction?

a. She tells her mother the menstrual pain will become increasingly worse until menopause.

b. She begins a strict low-fat diet and limits her intake of dairy products.

c. She places a heating pad on her lower abdomen during episodes of cramping.

d. She tells her friends she will not be able to have children because of her diagnosis.

Answers and Rationales

1. *Answer:* **c** (assessment)

Rationale: Prostaglandin release and synthesis occur during the luteal phase of the menstrual cycle. Prostaglandins stimulate uterine contractions, which results in menstrual cramps (Wolf & Schumann, 1999).

2. *Answer:* **a** (assessment)

Rationale: Primary dysmenorrhea commonly begins at or slightly before the menses and rarely lasts longer than 3 days (Robinson, Kidd, & Rogers, 2000).

3. *Answer:* **a** (implementation/plan)

Rationale: Naproxen sodium is an FDA-approved NSAID for treatment of dysmenorrhea. A scheduled dose is more

effective than prn dosing because NSAIDs not only minimize pain, they also prevent pain by inhibiting prostaglandin release (Wolf & Schumann, 1999).

4. *Answer:* **b** (implementation/plan)

Rationale: NSAIDs inhibit the synthesis and release of prostaglandin, which causes increased resting tone of the uterus, dysrhythmic uterine contractions, and vasoconstriction (Wolf & Schumann, 1999).

5. *Answer:* **a** (analysis/diagnosis)

Rationale: Primary dysmenorrhea is characterized by pain associated with ovulatory cycles, with the pain occurring just before or with the onset of menses and lasting for 2 to 3 days. Pain between menstrual periods, dyspareunia, postcoital bleeding, and foul-smelling vaginal discharge are not associated with primary dysmenorrhea (Webb, 1996).

6. *Answer:* **c** (analysis/diagnosis)

Rationale: Primary dysmenorrhea is associated with ovulatory cycles, with pain occurring just before or with the onset of menses. On the basis of the information provided, this client has secondary dysmenorrhea. Further diagnostic tests are necessary to establish the diagnosis of endometriosis or uterine leiomyoma (Cash & Glass, 2000).

7. *Answer:* **a** (implementation/plan)

Rationale: A combined estrogen and progesterone OCP is the drug treatment of choice for primary dysmenorrhea when birth control is also desired and there are no contraindications to taking OCPs. Narcotics are rarely indicated. Although NSAIDs are relatively safe, there are potential side effects and contraindications to their use, such as hypersensitivity, renal or liver disease, asthma, and peptic ulcer disease (Robinson, Kidd, & Rogers, 2000).

8. *Answer:* **b** (implementation/plan)

Rationale: As many as 90% of all primary dysmenorrhea cases are successfully treated with pharmacologic and nonpharmacologic approaches. Hysterectomy is indicated extremely rarely as a treatment for primary dysmenorrhea (Gerbie, 1994).

9. *Answer:* **c** (evaluation)

Rationale: Treatment should be evaluated at 2 months and then at 4 months to evaluate effectiveness and to assess for any problems. Other choices listed are inappropriate (Uphold & Graham 1997),

10. *Answer:* **c** (evaluation)

Rationale: Heat promotes comfort during episodes of cramping and is an appropriate action on the part of the client (Cash & Glass, 2000).

EATING DISORDERS   *Denise Robinson and Cheryl Pope Kish*

OVERVIEW
Definition

Anorexia nervosa (AN) is the intentional loss of weight and refusal to maintain a body weight at or above 85% of a normal weight for height and age. There are four criteria for diagnosis and according to the *Diagnostic and Statistical Manual of Mental Disorders* (DSM-IV):

1. Refusal to maintain body weight at or above minimally normal weight for age and height (body weight less than 85% of expected body weight)
2. Intense fear of gaining weight or becoming fat, even though underweight
3. Disturbance in the way in which one's body weight or shape is experienced, undue influence on body weight or shape on self-evaluation, or denial of the seriousness of the current low body weight
4. In postmenarcheal females, amenorrhea (i.e., the absence of at least three consecutive menstrual cycles)

There are two types of AN, according to the DSM-IV:
- *Restricting:* During the current episode of AN, the person has not regularly engaged in binge eating or purging behaviors (i.e., self-induced vomiting or the misuse of laxatives, diuretics, or enemas).
- *Binge-eating/purging:* During the current episode of AN, the person has regularly engaged in binge eating or purging behaviors (i.e., self-induced vomiting or the misuse of laxatives, diuretics, or enemas). Similar to bulimia nervosa (BN); body weight is the criteria for whether it is AN or BN. If clients are 15% below their natural body weight with bingeing and purging, they have AN.

BN is an eating disorder characterized by binge eating and inappropriate compensatory acts to prevent weight gain. Bulimia nervosa is characterized by recurrent episodes of binge eating and purging by use of vomiting, laxatives, or enemas. Binge eating disorder is defined as episodes of uncontrolled eating, without purging. The criteria and types of BN according to the DSM-IV are as follows:

1. A recurrent episode of binge eating is characterized by both of the following:
   - Eating in a discrete period of time (e.g., within any 2-hour period) an amount of food that is definitely larger than most people would eat during a similar period of time and under similar circumstances
   - A sense of lack of control over eating during an episode (e.g., a feeling that one cannot stop eating or control what or how much one is eating)
2. Recurrent inappropriate compensatory behaviors are used to prevent weight gain, such as self-induced vom-

iting; misuse of laxatives, diuretics, enemas, or other medications; fasting; or excessive exercise.
3. The binge eating and inappropriate compensatory behaviors both occur, on average, at least twice a week for 3 months.
4. Self-evaluation is unduly influenced by body and weight.
5. The disturbance does not occur exclusively during an episode of AN.

There are two types of BN, according to the DSM-IV:
- *Purging type*: During the current episode of BN, the person has regularly engaged in self-induced vomiting or misuse of laxatives, diuretics, or enemas.
- *Nonpurging type*: During the current episode of BN, the person has used other inappropriate compensatory behaviors, such as fasting or excessive exercise, but has not regularly engaged in self-induced vomiting or the misuse of laxatives, diuretics, or enemas.

It has been estimated that 75% to 94% of persons with BN use vomiting at least once per day.

Incidence

- Approximately 5% of adolescent and young women have an eating disorder.
- Only 1% of men have an eating disorder.
- Two percent of all adults in the United States are affected by a binge eating disorder.

Anorexia

- AN typically occurs in young, white, middle to upper middle class females (90% to 95%), an estimated 0.5% to 1% of the young female population in the United States; however, an increase of AN in all socioeconomic classes and other ethnic groups has been noted.
- There is a higher risk of AN if first-degree biologic relatives have an eating disorder.
- Age of onset of AN is concentrated between 12 and 25 years. Bimodal peak of AN is between 14 and 18 years.
- AN usually occurs after puberty begins and rarely occurs after 40 years of age.

Bulimia

- The incidence of BN is estimated at 1% to 3% of adolescent and young adult females in the United States.
- Age of onset of BN is usually late adolescent or early adult life. Binge eating usually begins after a diet.
- Most persons with BN are average weight, slightly underweight, or slightly overweight.
- One third to one half of cases have a history of being overweight.

General

- It is not unusual for persons with an eating disorder to slide from AN to BN and vice versa.
- An estimated 5% to 10% of persons with AN are male. An estimated 1 of 10 or 1% to 3% of persons with BN are male. An increased incidence of AN and BN are noted in the homosexual population.
- Persons involved in sports with emphasis on weight and shape, such as wrestling, gymnastics, swimming, and long-distance running, or persons involved in activities such as modeling or ballet are at higher risk for AN and BN. Eating disorder develops after participation in these sports and/or activities is initiated.
- Approximately 10% of all persons hospitalized with AN die. Death is related to complications associated with starvation or suicide. Mortality figures for persons with BN are unknown.

Pathophysiology

It is difficult to identify the cause of AN/BN because the disorders are multidetermined. Persons with AN/BN share many of the same characteristics/factors. These factors include individual, family, sociocultural, and biologic ones.

Individual Factors

- Weight disturbance as child/adolescent
- Low self-esteem
- Sense of ineffectiveness/lack of control/powerlessness
- Need for approval
- Perfectionism
- Fear of growing up
- Self-criticism
- Inability to identify or tolerate feelings
- Dependence
- High value placed on self-control and self-discipline
- For males, sexual identity issues
- Impulsivity in persons with BN
- Obsessive traits in persons with AN
- Difficulty developing a sense of "self"/problems with being able to separate from family and individuate

Family Factors

- Lack of conflict resolution
- Parental overprotectiveness
- Disengagement/enmeshment rigidity
- Unbearable rules
- No compromises
- Blurring of generational boundaries (the child acts as the parent)
- High parental expectations
- Overly concerned with appearance/achievement
- Affective and substance abuse disorders

Sociocultural Factors

- Pressure to be thin in society
- Mixed messages about women's worth in relation to their bodies–"appearance is your worth"
- Changing roles of women and role destabilization
- Prejudice against obesity/"fat phobias"
- Emphasis on achievement and perfection

Possible Biologic Factors

- AN may have a genetic predisposition, based on twin studies in which concordance rates were 50% for monozygotic twins versus 10% for dizygotic.
- Higher incidences of affective disorders in family members of the eating disordered person may indicate a genetic predisposition.

ASSESSMENT: SUBJECTIVE/HISTORY
History of Present Illness

- Ask about eating habits: "Are you satisfied with your eating patterns?" "Do you ever eat in secret?"
- Symptoms may be vague.

Symptoms

- Denial of any problems, especially in persons with AN
- Feelings of guilt or shame in persons with BN
- Body distortion (i.e., feel "too fat" although emaciated), intense fear of gaining weight
- Unusual eating rituals like cutting food into tiny pieces
- Strict exercise routines
- Dizziness
- Menstrual irregularities, amenorrhea
- Complaints of being cold
- Decreased energy/fatigue
- Complaints of increased sensitivity to heat, cold, acid substances in teeth/mouth
- Gastrointestinal (GI) disorders, including constipation, diarrhea, nausea, vomiting, bloating, and heartburn
- Social withdrawal, anhedonia
- See Table 3-25

Past Medical History

Include questions pertaining to the associated symptoms, as well as to the following:

- Substance abuse (especially in males and persons with BN)
- Use of ipecac (extremely dangerous, cardiotoxic), laxatives, diuretics, enemas, purging
- Swelling in extremities
- Seizures
- Activity level, especially exercise history (type, frequency, duration, compulsiveness), increased restlessness, changes in strength and endurance

E

TABLE **3-25** Common Symptoms of Eating Disorders

SYMPTOMS	ANOREXIA NERVOSA	BULIMIA NERVOSA	BINGE EATING DISORDER
Excessive weight loss in relatively short period	×		
Continuation of dieting although bone thin	×		
Dissatisfaction with appearance; belief that body is fat, even though severely underweight	×		
Loss of monthly menstrual periods	×	×	
Unusual interest in food and development of strange eating rituals	×	×	
Eating in secret	×	×	×
Obsession with exercise	×	×	
Serious depression	×	×	×
Binging—consumption of large amounts of food	×	×	
Vomiting or use of drugs to stimulate vomiting; bowel movements and urination		×	
Binging but no noticeable weight gain		×	
Disappearance into bathroom for long periods to induce vomiting		×	
Abuse of drugs or alcohol		×	×

From National Institutes of Health. Eating disorders. United States Department of Health and Human Services, National Institutes of Health Publication No 94-3477-1944.
Some individuals suffer from anorexia nervosa and bulimia nervosa and have symptoms of both disorders.

- Obesity-related diseases: gallbladder, diabetes, heart disease, hypertension (HTN)

Family History

- Parents' ages, careers, general health, relationship with client, attitudes toward food, physical appearance
- Age and sex of siblings and their relationships
- History of psychiatric illnesses in the family, especially incidence of eating disorders, substance abuse, affective disorders

Psychosocial History

- Involvement in activities and educational history
- Ways the client views self (especially looking for perfectionism and self-criticism and body distortions)
- Relationships outside family
- Physical and sexual abuse
- Mood fluctuations, inability to describe feelings, suicidal ideation, past psychiatric history and treatment
- Several co-existent psychiatric conditions—mood disorders, anxiety disorders, and personality disorders, along with substance-related disorders
- High co-morbidity of affective, obsessive, compulsive, anxiety, and personality disorders in persons with AN
- In persons with BN, possible co-morbidity of affective, anxiety, or personality disorders and substance abuse and impulsivity (e.g., promiscuity, shoplifting)

Dietary History

- Onset of weight loss
- Highest and lowest weights
- Fluctuations in weights

- Changes in appetite
- Typical pattern of eating
- Binge-purge episodes (75% of BN clients self-induce vomiting)
- Habits of hiding/throwing away food
- Preoccupation with food
- Unusual handling of food (e.g., cutting into small pieces)
- Guilt after eating

Sexual History

- Ask about development of secondary sexual characteristics, menstrual history, preparation for puberty, sexual orientation, attitudes toward sexual development/sexuality, and history of sexually transmitted diseases (STDs).
- Inquire about sexual activity.
  - Adolescents/young adults with AN report no to little sexual activity.
  - Older persons with AN usually report decreased sexual interests.
  - Persons with BN may report multiple partners and high-risk sexual activity.

ASSESSMENT: OBJECTIVE/PHYSICAL EXAMINATION

Physical Examination

Perform a problem-oriented physical examination with particular attention to the following:

- *Vital signs:* Assess for orthostatic hypotension, decreased temperature (may be decreased to 95° F [35° C] or below), bradycardia, and arrhythmias.

- *Weight/height:* Compare against expected weight charts.
- *General appearance:* Look for yellowing of skin (hypercarotenemia), jaundice (may be present in older persons with AN), lanugo hair, and parotid salivary gland tenderness (in 8% of clients with BN) and enlargement.
- *Skin:* Assess for dry skin, brittle nails, pruritus, loss of muscle, alopecia.
- *General hydration status:* Look for signs of dehydration secondary to purging or restricting.
- *Mouth and teeth:* Assess for discolored tooth enamel and excessive caries, halitosis, and sore oral and esophageal mucosa.
- *Extremities:* Look for acrocyanosis, pedal edema, and scarring on the dorsum of hands from self-induced vomiting.
- Note delayed development of secondary sexual characteristics in persons with AN.
- *Cardiovascular:* Assess for irregular heartbeat and bradycardia.
- *Neurologic/mental status:* Assess for alterations in state of consciousness related to starvation, suicidal thoughts and intentions, obsessions, compulsions, and anxieties and fears related to food, getting fat, and growing up.
- *Musculoskeletal:* Observe for loss of muscle mass and subcutaneous fat, muscle weakness, tetany, and decreased reflexes.
- *Anal:* Determine presence of bleeding or hemorrhoids.
- There may be a lack of physical signs and symptoms in persons with BN.

Diagnostic Procedures

Abnormalities in laboratory and diagnostic test results are related to the severity of the restricting or purging activities of the person with an eating disorder.

- *Renal/electrolytes:* Monitor for increased blood urea nitrogen (BUN), hypokalemia, hypochloremia, hypoglycemia, hyponatremia, hypomagnesemia, hypocalcemia.
- *SMA-12/60:* Hypercholesterolemia is possible.
- *Decreased phosphorus:* Monitor carefully when refeeding a person with AN to avoid "re-feeding syndrome" (edema in lower extremities and possible congestive heart failure).
- *CBC with differential:* Leukopenia and mild anemia are possible.
- *Thyroid function studies:* Thyroxine (T4) low-normal, triiodothyronine (T3) subclinical.
- *Liver function tests:* Abnormalities (elevations) possible in chronically starved or older persons with AN or in persons with significant substance abuse.

- *pH balance:* Monitor for possible signs of metabolic acidosis or metabolic alkalosis (related to hypochloremia and hypokalemia).
- *Urine/stool:* May show evidence of diuretic or laxative abuse (e.g., occult blood in stool).
- *Endocrine studies in persons with AN:* Female—look for decreased luteinizing hormone, follicle-stimulating hormone, and estrogen; males—look for decreased testosterone.
- *ECG:* Sinus bradycardia and rarely arrhythmias are possible.
- *Gynecologic:* Refer for examination as indicated for possible STDs.
- *Psychologic/psychiatric evaluation:* Refer for diagnostic evaluation.

DIAGNOSIS

The differential diagnoses for AN includes the following disorders because they may have significant weight loss and should be ruled out; however, none of these disorders includes the intense body distortions or the desire for weight loss that is present in persons with eating disorders:

- Thyroid disease
- Diabetes
- Acquired immune deficiency syndrome (AIDS)
- Inflammatory bowel disease
- Malignancy
- Major depressive disorder
- Schizophrenia

The differential diagnoses for BN includes the following:

- AN binge-eating/purging type
- Neurologic or medical conditions such as Kleine-Levin syndrome
- Major depression with atypical features
- Borderline personality disorder

THERAPEUTIC PLAN
Nonpharmacologic Treatment

- The severity of the orthostasis/cardiac and hydration status, including hypokalemia, determines if hospitalization is warranted. The stabilization of homeostasis is paramount before any psychiatric/psychologic treatment can occur.
- Suicidal tendency should also be assessed, and hospitalization should occur if the nurse practitioner (NP) believes that the client is at imminent risk.
- Cognitive-behavioral therapy alone or with other techniques has resulted in the most significant reductions of binge eating (McGilley & Pryor, 1998).
- Development of therapeutic rapport between caregivers and client and family is important.
- It is also important that an agreement be made between the primary health provider, the client and family, and the client's therapist about the manner in which vital

signs, weight, and pertinent laboratory data will be monitored. Within the agreement, the parameters for when hospitalization will occur, if necessary, should be set.

- A dietitian to assist with nutritional counseling and any medical specialist(s) needed to manage medical complications should also be members of the treatment team.
- The client needs ongoing medical as well as psychiatric/psychologic treatment.

Pharmacologic Treatment

Pharmacologic treatment should be initiated by a psychiatrist or advanced-practice psychiatric nurse, as follows:

- *Antidepressants:* It is estimated that at least 50% of persons with an eating disorder are depressed. Controversy exists regarding how effective antidepressants are in persons with AN because many show a decrease in depression once starvation has been addressed. However, it is estimated that 40% to 60% may benefit from antidepressants.
- *Selective serotonin reuptake inhibitors (SSRIs) (first-line choice):* Fluoxetine (Prozac) and other SSRIs are used because these medications do not cause orthostasis and have minimal effects on cardiac rhythms, unlike the tricyclic antidepressants imipramine, desipramine, and amitriptyline, which have been used but have significant cardiac effects.
- *Benzodiazepines:* Benzodiazepines are sometimes used in hospitalized clients for short intervals to decrease anxiety before meals.
- Other medications may be needed to address associated medical conditions related to the effects of eating disorders (e.g., potassium/phosphorus supplements, estrogen replacement for decreasing bone loss).

Client Education/Prevention

Discuss with client the following:

- Disease process and possible results
- Nutritionally sound diet
- Need for counseling
- Long-term commitment
- Keeping a food and exercise diary

Referral/Consultation

The treatment of eating disorders must be of a collaborative "team" nature. A referral for a psychiatric/psychologic evaluation must be made to assist with the diagnosis.

EVALUATION/FOLLOW-UP

Monitor client's weight weekly until stable, then monthly.

COMPLICATIONS

Binge Eating

- Gastric rupture (uncommon)
- Nausea
- Abdominal pain and distention
- Prolonged digestion
- Weight gain

Purging

- Dental erosion
- Enlarged salivary glands
- Esophageal/pharyngeal damage
- Upper GI tears
- Perforation of upper digestive tract, esophagus, and stomach
- Hypokalemia
- Seizures
- Cardiac arrhythmias

Approximately 50% of clients who undergo treatment for eating disorders stop the bingeing and purging. The remaining clients show some improvement, with a small number not responding at all to treatment.

REFERENCES

American Psychiatric Association. (1994). *Diagnostic and statistical manual of mental disorders* (DSM-IV) (4th ed.). Washington, DC: APA.

Eckert, E. D. (1985). Characteristics of anorexia nervosa. In *Anorexia and bulimia: Diagnosis and treatment.* Minneapolis: University of Minnesota Press.

Garfinkle, P. E., & Kennedy, S. H. (1992). Advances in diagnosis and treatment of anorexia nervosa and bulimia nervosa. *Canadian Journal of Psychiatry, 37,* 309-315.

Harper-Guiffre, J., & MacKenzie, K. R. (1992). *Group psychotherapy for eating disorders.* Washington, DC: American Psychiatric Press.

Hofland, S. L., & Dardis, P. O. (1992). Bulimia nervosa. Associated physical problems. *Journal of Psychosocial Nursing, 30*(2), 23-27.

Maxmen, J. S., & Ward, N. G. (1995). *Eating disorders: Essential psychopathology and its treatment* (2nd ed.). New York: W. W. Norton.

McGilley, B., & Pryor, T. (1998). Assessment and treatment of bulimia. *American Family Physician,* Retrieved July 19, 2002, from www.aafp.org/afp/980600ap/mcgilley.html.

Muscari, M. E. (1996). Primary care of adolescents with bulimia nervosa. *Journal of Pediatric Health Care, 10*(1), 17-25.

Wachsmuth, J. R., & Garfinkel, P. E. (1993). Treatment of anorexia nervosa in young adults. *Child and Adolescent Psychiatry Clinics of North America, 2,* 145-160.

Zerbe, K. J. (1996). Anorexia nervosa and bulimia nervosa. *Postgraduate Medicine, 99*(1), 161-169.

Review Questions

1. Lisa Evans, 21 years old, has a history of BN for the past 3 years. When obtaining a history, the NP could expect to find which of the following?

  a. A history of maternal depression and substance abuse in the paternal family
  b. A strong sense of self-esteem
  c. Several school failures
  d. No weight disturbances in childhood and adolescence

2. Ms. Evans describes a "binge" episode. The description will probably include which of the following?

  a. A feeling of being in control of the type and amount of food consumed
  b. The intake of an extra ice cream cone when out with friends
  c. Eating two 13-ounce bags of potato chips in less than 45 minutes
  d. Consuming two pieces of pizza and a salad for dinner

3. While talking with a mother and her 15-year-old daughter with AN, the NP may observe which of the following interactional patterns?

  a. Mother and daughter do not interact.
  b. Mother and daughter are openly hostile to each other.
  c. Mother and daughter sit close, and mother answers all the questions.
  d. Mother and daughter equally interact.

4. When considering a diagnosis of AN, the NP should consider which of the following differential diagnoses?

  a. Major depressive disorder with atypical features and thyroid disease
  b. Kleine-Levin syndrome and AIDS
  c. Diabetes and borderline personality disorder
  d. Malignancy and thyroid disease

5. Because of the complex medical and psychologic components of AN, treatment must include which of the following?

  a. Provide educational opportunities for clients and families to learn about AN.
  b. Develop a "team" approach with the health care professionals, client, and family members involved.
  c. Start antidepressant medications.
  d. Hospitalize the client.

6. Participation in which of the following activities could indicate improvement in a person with BN?

  a. Exercise group
  b. Drama club
  c. Substance abuse program
  d. Classes at a community college

7. While interviewing a 14-year-old suspected of being anorexic, the NP may observe which of the following psychiatric symptoms?

  a. Anxiety and irritability
  b. Delusions of grandeur
  c. Paranoia
  d. Hallucinations

8. Which laboratory result is not expected in AN, purging type?

  a. Hypokalemia
  b. Hyponatremia
  c. Decreased BUN
  d. Hypochloremia

Answers and Rationales

1. *Answer:* a (assessment)
  Rationale: It has been noted that there is a higher likelihood of affective disorders and substance abuse in families of persons with BN. Low self-esteem usually is present. Persons with BN tend to be perfectionists and "overachievers" and are not likely to have school failures. They often have histories of weight disturbances (Harper-Guiffre & MacKenzie, 1992).

2. *Answer:* c (assessment)
  Rationale: A "binge" is defined as eating a larger amount of food than most people would eat during a similar period of time and under similar circumstances. Options b and d do not meet this definition; there is a sense of loss of control over eating, not a sense of control (American Psychiatric Association, 1994).

3. *Answer:* c (assessment)
  Rationale: In families of anorexic persons, often there is enmeshment, in which the individuals of the family are "lost" and separation is not allowed to occur (Harper-Guiffre & MacKenzie, 1992).

4. *Answer:* b (analysis/diagnosis)
  Rationale: Because of the significant weight loss often associated with this disease process, one should consider Kleine-Levin syndrome and AIDS when assessing an individual. The other options include a differential diagnosis for BN (American Psychiatric Association, 1994).

5. *Answer:* b (implementation/plan)
  Rationale: The coordination of the treatment plan for AN is extremely important because of the serious and complex nature of the illness. A team approach in which the professional caregivers, family, and client work together is essential. The other options presented may or may not be part of the treatment plan (Wachsmuth & Garfinkel, 1993).

6. *Answer:* c (evaluation)
  Rationale: Because of the increased incidence of substance abuse in persons with BN, involvement in a substance abuse group could indicate improvement (Harper-Guiffre & MacKenzie, 1992).

7. *Answer:* a (assessment)
  Rationale: Irritability and anxiety are symptoms associated with depression, which anorexic persons often have as a comorbid diagnosis. The other symptoms are usually associated with thought disorders (Harper-Guiffre & MacKenzie, 1992).

8. *Answer:* c (analysis/diagnosis)
  Rationale: One can expect a decrease in potassium chloride, sodium, and chloride if the client is purging through diuretic and or laxative use/vomiting and an increase in BUN related to volume depletion may be present (Hofland & Dardis, 1992).

E

ECTOPIC PREGNANCY *Cheryl Pope Kish*

OVERVIEW
Definition

Ectopic pregnancy refers to the implantation of a fertilized ovum outside the uterine cavity. Although ectopic pregnancies may implant on the cervix, ovary, or within the abdominal cavity, the most common (95%) ectopic site is within a fallopian tube. None of these anatomic sites can sustain an advancing pregnancy; therefore the potential for a life-threatening tubal rupture with hemorrhage always exists. The most common time for the fallopian tube to rupture is between 8 and 12 weeks' gestation.

Incidence

Ectopic pregnancy occurs in 1 of 50 pregnancies in the United States and is a leading cause of maternal mortality. Worldwide incidence has increased, but the rate varies among different population groups. It is most common in non-white ethnic groups and in women aged 15 to 19 and those older than 35 years of age. The increase in rates of ectopic pregnancy is attributable to increases in certain risk factors but also to improved diagnostics.

Pathophysiology

Normally, the ovum is fertilized in the outer third of the fallopian tube and travels through the tube to the uterus, where it implants. Any factor that interferes with the normal function of the fallopian tube during this process increases the risk of ectopic pregnancy. Obstruction of the fallopian tube and impaired tubal motility are common mechanisms of cause.

Factors Increasing Susceptibility
- More than one half of women with ectopic pregnancy have no identifiable risk factor.
- Pelvic inflammatory disease (PID)
- Previous ectopic pregnancy
- Endometriosis
- Previous tubal surgery
- Uterotubal anomalies
- Intrauterine exposure to diethylstilbesterol (DES)
- Cigarette smoking
- Infertility and infertility treatment; induced superovulation; in vitro fertilization
- Multiple sexual partners
- Early age at first coitus
- Vaginal douching
- Past or current intrauterine device (IUD): indication that IUDs do not actually cause ectopic pregnancy; rather, are less effective in preventing ectopic pregnancy than intrauterine pregnancy
- Prior voluntary interruption of pregnancy
- Low-dose progestins or emergency contraception in recent history

ASSESSMENT: SUBJECTIVE/HISTORY
Common Symptoms

The classic symptom is some type of pelvic or abdominal pain, which may vary from dull aching to sharp colicky pain that is either diffuse or unilateral. Up to 90% of women experience pain. Often the pain is associated with spotting approximately 6 to 8 weeks after the last normal menstrual period. Less commonly, ectopic pregnancy presents with syncope, pain radiating to the shoulder (from blood accumulating under the diaphragm), and dizziness. With tubal rupture, the woman is likely to complain of acute pelvic pain associated with backache, dizziness, and syncope, related to blood loss. Because the woman is in the early part of a pregnancy, albeit an ectopic one, she often has the classic signs of early pregnancy as well: 1- to 2-month history of amenorrhea, fatigue, nausea and vomiting, and breast tenderness. Many women present with vague or mild symptoms, making diagnosis difficult. Ectopic pregnancy must be a differential diagnosis for any woman of child-bearing age who reports abdominal discomfort, whether mild or severe, especially associated with menstrual irregularity or scant dark brown spotting.

Past Medical History
- Identification of risk factors from the medical history raises the index of suspicion of ectopic pregnancy.
- Ask about previous pregnancies.
- Determine last menstrual period.

Medication History

Ask about the use of fertility drugs or low-dose progestins and emergency contraception.

Family History

Inquire about use of DES in the client's mother's pregnancy.

Psychosocial History
- Ask about the number of current and lifelong sexual partners and sexual behaviors that increase risk of STDs and PID.
- Ask about cigarette smoking and drug and alcohol use.
- Determine the existence of a support system.
- Assess for evidence of grief.

ASSESSMENT: OBJECTIVE/PHYSICAL EXAMINATION
Physical Examination

A problem-oriented physical examination should be performed, with a focus on the following areas:

- *Vital signs*: Hypotension and tachycardia may be evident with blood loss. Fever is not expected.

- Assess general appearance and evidence of acuity.
- *Skin color*: Pallor may be evident with blood loss.
- Perform abdominal examination.
  - Abdominal tenderness is present in 80% to 90% of cases. May be associated with rebound tenderness and guarding with a leaking or ruptured ectopic pregnancy.
  - Assess for Cullen's sign, a periumbilical bluish discoloration secondary to hemoperitoneum (if leaking or rupture has occurred, causing significant blood loss).
  - Assess uterine size, which may be normal size or only slightly enlarged.
- Perform pelvic examination.
  - Note blood at introitus, within vaginal cavity, or from cervical os on visualization with speculum.
  - Determine uterine size.
  - Expect cervical motion tenderness.
  - Note palpable adnexal mass and tenderness.
  - May note doughy sensation along posterior vaginal wall at cul de sac of Douglas secondary to accumulation of blood.

Diagnostic Procedures

Diagnostic testing ordered depends on the clinical status— stable versus emergent—of the woman presenting for care. *The woman who presents with the possibility of an ectopic pregnancy should be referred immediately to an emergency department or obstetrician/gynecologist or surgeon.* The following tests may be needed:

- Complete blood count (CBC) is important if woman is experiencing blood loss.
- Obtain blood type and Rh if woman is hemorrhaging and blood replacement is a possibility.
- Obtain a urine pregnancy test (99% sensitive and 99% specific for pregnancy and quicker results than beta-human chorionic gonadotropin (beta-hCG).
- The gold standard test is serum beta-hCG–B-hCG radioimmunoassay (usually requires 24 hours to obtain results). The small amount of trophoblastic tissue in an ectopic pregnancy produces a small amount of hCG without the doubling normally seen in an intrauterine pregnancy every 2 to 4 days.
- Serum progesterone level lower than 15 ng/mL raises the index of suspicion of an abnormal pregnancy but is not diagnostic as a single factor.
- Transvaginal ultrasound is preferred over abdominal ultrasound because the transvaginal ultrasound is more sensitive and has a lower discriminatory zone, allowing diagnosis to be made an average of 1 week earlier. The discriminatory zone is the level of serum B-hCG above which a gestational sac can be consistently visualized. With transvaginal ultrasound, this value is a level greater than 1500 IU /L, contrasted with abdominal ultrasound, which has a discriminatory zone value of 6500 IU/L. *An ectopic pregnancy should be expected if transvaginal ultrasonography shows no intrauterine gestational sac when the B-hCG level is higher than 1500 mIU/ml (1500 IU/L).*
- Culdocentesis can be performed by a consulting physician. It is performed rarely today, and its use is generally confined to situations in which ultrasound is not readily available. Presence of nonclotted blood is consistent with ruptured ectopic pregnancy; yellow or straw-colored fluid is consistent with ruptured ovarian cyst.
- Laparoscopy may be necessary to confirm ectopic pregnancy.

DIAGNOSIS

The following differential diagnoses should be considered with ectopic pregnancy:

- Normal intrauterine pregnancy with inaccurate gestational age dating
- Intrauterine pregnancy with corpus luteum cyst
- Ruptured corpus luteum cyst
- Threatened abortion
- PID
- Appendicitis
- Endometriosis
- Gestational trophoblastic disease
- Renal calculus

THERAPEUTIC PLAN
Nonpharmacologic Treatment

If the woman's condition is stable, expectant or pharmacologic management can be used. If her condition is deteriorating, surgical management is indicated, with prompt hemodynamic management to stabilize her. Laparoscopy may be necessary to remove the ectopic products of conception. Emergency laparotomy may be necessary when the woman is hemodynamically unstable because of tubal rupture. Salpingostomy is the preferred treatment; however, at times salpingectomy may be necessary.

Pharmacologic Treatment

Methotrexate, a folic acid antagonist that interferes with DNA synthesis and cell multiplication, is a fairly new medical treatment for ectopic pregnancy. The rapidly dividing cells of trophoblastic tissue are most vulnerable to the drug. The low dosages of methotrexate (Rheumatrex) required for ectopic pregnancy generally cause mild, self-limited reactions: nausea, vomiting, urinary frequency, and diarrhea. The potential for serious toxic effects on buccal and intestinal mucosa, bladder, bone marrow, and skin does exist. Criteria for use of the drug are as follows:

- Unruptured ectopic mass must be determined less than 3.5 cm in size.
- Woman must be hemodynamically stable.

E

- Ultrasound must indicate findings consistent with ectopic pregnancy.
- Woman must be willing to undergo follow-up with serial decline in B-hCG levels.

Single-dose regimens are common; a second single dose may be ordered. This therapy is so new that a standard protocol has not yet been developed. This therapy is prescribed and managed by a physician. Women taking methotrexate should be cautioned about photosensitivity.

Early ectopic pregnancies sometimes spontaneously resolve; therefore expectant management is sometimes possible. Careful follow-up is essential because complications may occur and include tubal rupture with hemorrhage and shock. Criteria for treating a woman with ectopic pregnancy expectantly include the following:

- Initial B-hCG level is less than 2000 IU and continues to decline.
- Woman is asymptomatic.
- Ultrasonography and/or laparoscopy reveal patent tube and no bleeding.
- Woman is compliant with serial testing required and with follow-up visits.

The woman followed expectantly needs guidance for recognizing and responding quickly in the event that an emergent situation arises.

Referral

All women with ectopic pregnancy must be referred to a physician for management; it is outside the scope of an NP. Expectant medical management for a stable client may be co-managed with a physician. Conservative management, whether watchful waiting or medication administration, is associated with less recurrence than surgical management.

Client Education

Clients should be educated about the condition, the inherent risks, and the management required. If they are candidates for and agree to expectant or medical management, women should be aware of the potential for sudden rupture with rapid blood loss and anticipate how they will respond to ensure timely treatment. They should not drive in case of dizziness or syncope; they should have a plan for immediate access to emergency care, should rupture occur.

Women who have one ectopic pregnancy are at risk for future ectopic pregnancy. If pregnancy is suspected, they should seek care promptly to enable evaluation for a recurrence.

Rh-negative women need to be educated about Rh incompatibility and the need for RhoGAM. Women should be informed about the follow-up required and the importance of preventing another pregnancy for at least 3 months. The woman who has had surgical treatment for ectopic pregnancy needs instructions specific to postoperative care.

Prevention

Some ectopic pregnancies are unavoidable; however, prevention of PID may eliminate some risk. Prevention of STDs is the primary strategy for decreasing PID risk.

EVALUATION/FOLLOW-UP

Women with ectopic pregnancy who are Rh negative and antibody screen (Du) negative should receive RhoGAM (RhDu) immune globulin as follows:

- MicroRhoGAM 50 µg IM: if gestational age is less than 13 weeks
- RhoGAM 300 µg IM: if gestational age is more than 13 weeks.

Approximately 50% of women experience grief related to the loss; others perceive pregnancy loss as an unfortunate event and are temporarily sad but do not experience an intense grief response. Careful attention to her words will reveal the woman's perceptions of loss. For example, she may refer to losing the pregnancy versus losing her baby. Anticipatory guidance related to the grief response is individualized accordingly. Emotional support is an essential element of care when women are grieving. Referral to a support group may be helpful.

Weekly blood tests for B-hCG are monitored until it is no longer detectable. Anticipatory guidance about contraception is extremely important because conception should be avoided for a minimum of 3 months following ectopic pregnancy to allow the implantation site to completely recover.

COMPLICATIONS

Ectopic pregnancy is a life-threatening condition because of hemorrhage, hypovolemic shock, or other related problems such as disseminated intravascular coagulation. This diagnosis accounts for 10% to 15% of all maternal deaths and is the most common reason women die in the first trimester of pregnancy. Early diagnosis and appropriate treatment are critical.

REFERENCES

Brown, K. (2000). *Management guidelines for women's health nurse practitioners.* Philadelphia: F. A. Davis.

Matteson, P. S. (2001). *Women's health during the childbearing years.* St. Louis: Mosby.

Meredith, P. V., & Horan, N. M. (2000). *Adult primary care.* Philadelphia: W. B. Saunders.

Shannon, M. T. (1999). Ectopic pregnancy. In W. L. Star, M. T. Shannon, L. L. Lommel, & Y.M. Gutierrez, *Ambulatory obstetrics* (3rd ed., pp. 367-378). San Francisco: UCSF Press.

Smith, R. P. (1997). *Gynecology in primary care.* Baltimore: Williams & Wilkins.

Tenore, J. L. (2000). Ectopic pregnancy. *American Family Physician*, February 15, 61(4), 1080–1088.

Youngkin, E. Q., & Davis, S. M. (1998). *Women's health: A primary care clinical guide.* Stamford, CT: Appleton & Lange.

Review Questions

1. Andrea is a 22-year-old who presents with left lower quadrant pain and scant brown vaginal spotting for 3 days; her pain is increasing steadily. Her period is overdue; she is uncertain if the spotting represents an unusual period. Which factor in Andrea's history does not indicate a risk for ectopic pregnancy?

    a. Nulliparity
    b. Multiple sexual partners
    c. Endometriosis
    d. Treatment for chlamydia

2. Which medication in Andrea's recent history has been associated with increased risk of ectopic pregnancy?

    a. Nitrofurantoin
    b. Progestin-only oral contraceptive pills (OCPs)
    c. Tegretol
    d. Nonsteroidal antiinflammatory drugs (NSAIDs)

3. Peggy presents with symptoms suggesting ectopic pregnancy. Which factor in her history raises the index of suspicion for a diagnosis of ectopic pregnancy?

    a. Induced superovulation for infertility
    b. Diagnosed rheumatoid arthritis
    c. Frequent vaginal yeast infections
    d. Irregular periods

4. Which of the following descriptions suggests ectopic pregnancy with tubal rupture?

    a. Stabbing pelvic pain, nausea, vaginal bleeding, and hematochezia
    b. CVA tenderness, colicky pain, HTN, and tachycardia
    c. Syncope, pelvic pain, spotting, and shoulder pain
    d. Right upper quadrant tenderness, vomiting, hypotension, and bradycardia

5. Which objective sign is associated with hemoperitoneum in ectopic pregnancy?

    a. Murphy's sign
    b. Apley's sign
    c. Lachman's sign
    d. Cullen's sign

6. Which of the following differential diagnoses is not typically considered when the clinician is attempting to rule out ectopic pregnancy?

    a. Appendicitis
    b. Urinary calculus
    c. Cholecystitis
    d. Threatened abortion

7. A review of B-hCG levels and transvaginal ultrasonography findings is helpful to diagnosing ectopic pregnancy. Which finding suggests ectopic pregnancy as a likely diagnosis?

    a. B-hCG less than 1500 IU/L with intrauterine fetal pole identifiable
    b. B-hCG less than 1500 IU/L and no intrauterine gestational sac visible
    c. B-hCG greater than 1500 IU/L and no intrauterine gestational sac visible
    d. B-hCG greater than 1500 IU/L with intrauterine gestation identifiable

8. In which case will methotrexate be justified as a treatment for ectopic pregnancy?

    a. Blood pressure (BP): 86/50, P: 120, Hgb: 6.8
    b. Unruptured ectopic mass 2.1 cm
    c. B-hCG levels 7200 IU/L
    d. Client uncertainty about risk of drug

9. In which woman is RhoGAM indicated following ectopic pregnancy?

    a. B-positive, Du-negative woman
    b. O-negative, Du-positive woman
    c. AB-negative, Du-negative woman
    d. A-positive, Du-negative woman

10. At her follow-up visit after successful treatment of ectopic pregnancy with methotrexate, Julie receives anticipatory guidance from the NP who co-managed her care. Which comment made by Julie indicates that she has understood the instructions?

    a. "The risk of another ectopic pregnancy is too great to justify another pregnancy."
    b. "I will need to have frequent ultrasound tests over the next 6 to 8 months."
    c. "Because I had this drug, weekly blood tests will be required for a year."
    d. "If I get pregnant again, I will need careful follow-up to rule out another ectopic."

Answers and Rationales

1. *Answer:* **a** (assessment)
    Rationale: Nulliparity is not considered a risk factor for ectopic pregnancy. Multiple partners, endometriosis, and a history of STDs are all risk factors (Tenore, 2000).

2. *Answer:* **b** (assessment)
    Rationale: Progestin-only oral contraceptives have been associated with some risk of ectopic pregnancy because of their tendency to slow transport of ovum from ovary to uterus (Star et al., 1999).

3. *Answer:* **a** (assessment)
    Rationale: Infertility treatment, including superovulation, imply increased risk of ectopic pregnancy (Tenore, 2000).

4. *Answer:* **c** (assessment)
    Rationale: Abdominal pain, syncope, shoulder pain, and vaginal spotting, especially 6 to 8 weeks after a missed period, are highly suggestive of a ruptured tubal pregnancy (Youngkin & Davis, 1998).

5. *Answer:* **d** (assessment)
    Rationale: Cullen's sign is bluish periumbilical discoloration associated with hemoperitoneum (Star et al., 1999).

6. **Answer: c** (analysis/diagnosis)
   Rationale: Cholecystectomy is not considered a typical differential diagnosis when evaluating ectopic pregnancy (Tenore, 2000).

7. **Answer: c** (analysis/diagnosis)
   Rationale: An intrauterine gestational sac confirming a normal intrauterine pregnancy is associated with a B-hCG level higher than 1500 IU/L. Absence of an intrauterine gestational sac with this level of B-hCG indicates an abnormal, perhaps ectopic pregnancy (Tenore, 2000).

8. **Answer: b** (implementation/plan)
   Rationale: Option a indicates a hemodynamically unstable client; option c does not indicate a diagnosis of ectopic preg-

nancy; and option d indicates an uninformed client. These are all reasons to exclude methotrexate as a treatment option. An unruptured ectopic mass smaller than 3.5 cm is an appropriate criterion (Tenore, 2000).

9. **Answer: c** (evaluation)
   Rationale: Rh-negative, Du-negative women receive RhoGAM following ectopic pregnancy (Star et al., 1999).

10. **Answer: d** (evaluation)
    Rationale: A woman with a history of one ectopic pregnancy is at risk for another, and if she became pregnant would need to have ectopic pregnancy ruled out. The risk of recurrence is less for women who are treated medically than for those treated surgically (Tenore, 2000).

ECZEMA/ATOPIC DERMATITIS   *Pamela Kidd*

OVERVIEW
Definition

Genetically determined chronic skin disorder with relapsing pattern

Incidence

- Occurs in 1.9% to 5% of the population.
- More common in children and more severe in males.
- Approximately 80% are detected before age 5 years.
- Affects 1 in 10 children.
- Up to 75% of cases resolve spontaneously by adolescence.

Pathophysiology

- Cause is not completely understood.
- Defects in cell-mediated immunity are present.
- Increased water loss from the epidermis reduces the pliability of the skin.
- Skin is at greater risk of penetration by environmental irritants (Nicol, 2000).
- Effects are worse in winter when humidity is low.

Factors Increasing Susceptibility
- Genetics
- Dust mites
- Pet dander
- Pollen

Protective Factors. Intact immune system.

ASSESSMENT: SUBJECTIVE/HISTORY
Symptoms

- Infantile stage occurs from 2 to 6 months of age, resolving by 3 years of age.
- Pruritus, redness and blisters on cheeks, forehead, scalp, and extensor aspects of arms and legs may be present.
- Childhood stage occurs from 4 to 10 years of age.

- Look for dry, scaly, rash on antecubital, popliteal regions, flexures of wrists, ankles, neck, buttock-thigh creases; less pruritic. Papules rather than exudation is common.
- Adolescent or adult stage appears on the face, neck, and body.
- Scaling skin with xerosis and lichenification is present.
- Older adult stage appears on the hands.
- Consider the stigma of having a visible skin disorder.
- Psychological stresses are triggers.
- Assess living conditions, especially exposure to dust mites.

Associated Symptoms
- Wheezing
- Runny nose
- Tearing of eyes

Past Medical History
- Of clients with atopic dermatitis, 50% also have hayfever and/or asthma (Nicol, 2000).
- Food allergies may also be present.
- Other skin disorders may exist.

Medication History

Ask client about new medication, particularly topical medicine to rule out contact dermatitis.

Family History (in First-Degree Relative)
- Hayfever
- Asthma
- Food allergies
- Other skin disorders, including atopic dermatitis

Dietary History

Most common food allergens are eggs, milk, wheat, soy, seafood, and nuts.

ASSESSMENT: OBJECTIVE/PHYSICAL EXAMINATION

Physical Examination

- Undress client and check entire body for lesions.
- Assess skin. As the condition progresses with aging, there is a change in the type of lesion.
  - Infants have more vesicles with exudation and scarring; extensor surfaces are involved.
  - Children have less exudate and crusting and more papular, well-circumscribed patches.
  - Adults have more scaling and lichenification of flexures.
- Acute flare-ups may be in the form of red patches that are weepy, shiny, or lichenified.
- Hypopigmentation occurs in dark-skinned persons.
- Assess hands. Palms may have hyperlinear, xerotic creases.
  - Facial pallor with infraorbital darkening
  - Fissures under the earlobes
- Severity of the disease can be scored using the Eczema Area and Severity Index (Rosen, 2001).

Diagnostic Procedures

- None are usually necessary.
- Serum immunoglobulin E (IgE) levels are elevated.
- Cultures of drainage may help in ruling out other causes.

DIAGNOSIS

Differential diagnoses include the following:
- Psoriasis is silvery scales on red plaques on knees, elbows, scalp. Separation of nail from nail bed is common (onycholysis).
- Contact dermatitis does not involve eczema's characteristic distribution or chronic course; usually linear pattern.
- Vesicles may occur at any age.

THERAPEUTIC PLAN

Nonpharmacologic Treatment

- Wear cotton gloves at bedtime to minimize scratching.
- Soak skin in water, then seal with emollient. Use emollient after each handwashing. Eucerin cream, Aquaphor, and Vanicream are effective moisturizers.
- If client does not respond to tacrolimus or corticosteroids, consider ultraviolet light therapy.

Pharmacologic Treatment

See Table 3-26.

NOTE: *Use water-miscible corticosteroid creams, not ointments. Can use in conjunction with warm wet wraps at night to increase penetration and decrease pruritus. To prevent maceration, use for 5 to 10 consecutive nights only.*

- Use mildest corticosteroids on face.
- Use moderate corticosteroids on other parts of body and change to mild potency as condition improves.
- Monitor use at each visit; have client bring tube in and check application format and amount.
- Tachyphylaxis may occur (progressive loss of effectiveness). To minimize tachyphylaxis, use for 10 days, then allow 4 treatment-free days.
- Herpes simplex infection may occur from improper use of corticosteroids; if so treat with acyclovir.
- Oral corticosteroids should be avoided because of steroid dependency caused by the relapsing nature of the disease that necessitates repeated use.
- Antihistamines can be used for pruritus but have limited value because pruritus appears to be due to factors other than histamine release. Sedatives may be necessary to promote sleep.

Client Education

- Avoid pets.
- Avoid dry environments.

TABLE **3-26**   Pharmacologic Treatment of Eczema/Atopic Dermatitis

DRUG	DOSE	COMMENT
Tacrolimus (Protopic)	0.03% ointment for children, 0.1% for adult; apply thin layer bid. Do not occlude or apply to wet skin. Not recommended for children younger than 2 years of age.	Allows reduction or elimination of corticosteroids. Inhibits T cell activation and thus cytokinin production. Side effects are local erythema.
Triamcinolone	1%; apply sparingly 2-4 times daily and rub in well.	Never use on face. Taper to avoid rebound flares. Use for short time in children.
Doxepin cream	5%; apply four times daily to lesions.	Treats pruritus.
Tar preparations (LCD)	5% in Aquaphor; apply to area.	Best for thickened, lichenified lesions when topical steroids are not helping.
Burrow solution	Apply 4-6 times a day for 10 minutes using wet compresses.	Best for acute, weeping lesions.
Salicylic acid solution	3-5%; apply to area.	Used more in chronic phase.

- Avoid exposure to dust mites (post carpet cleaning).
- Eliminate one food at a time to determine triggers.
- Teach to avoid anything that dries or irritates the skin (e.g., skin preparations with alcohol).
- Do not use bubble bath.
- Bathe minimally.
- Do not sit in tub for prolonged periods.
- Do not use washcloths or brushes.
- Use soap only on armpits, groin, and feet. Use mild soap (Neutrogena, Dove).
- Pat skin dry and apply emollient.
- Avoid scratchy material (wool).
- Avoid overheating because perspiration can trigger itching.
- Consider removing pet from the environment.

Referral/Consultation

- Refer to dermatologist if there is minimal or no response to basic management measures.
- Refer to dermatologist for skin testing (detects dust mite allergy).

Prevention

There is no known prevention of atopic dermatitis. The goal is to minimize flare-ups, as described in the Client Education section.

EVALUATION/FOLLOW-UP

- Frequently during flare-up; every 2 to 3 days
- No secondary infection of lesions
- Less primary lesions

COMPLICATIONS

- Skin infections (usually staphylococcus)
- Herpes simplex (eczema herpeticum)

REFERENCES

Berger, T., Goldstein, S., & Odom, R. (1998). Skin and appendages. In L. Tierney, S. McPhee, & M. Papadakis (Eds.), *Current medical diagnosis and treatment* (36th ed.). Stamford, CT: Appleton & Lange.

Boynton, R., Dunn, E., & Stephens, G. (1998). *Manual of ambulatory pediatrics* (4th ed.). Philadelphia: Lippincott.

Kolmer, H. L., Taketomi, E. A., Hazen, K. C., Hughs, E., Wilson, B. B., & Platts-Mills, T. A. (1996). Effect of combined antibacterial and antifungal treatment in severe atopic dermatitis. *Journal of Allergy and Clinical Immunology, 98*(3), 702-706.

Nicol, N. H. (2000). Managing atopic dermatitis in children and adults. *The Nurse Practitioner, 25*(4), 58-59, 63-64, 69-70, 73-74, 76.

Rosen, T. (2001). Update on atopic dermatitis. *Consultant, 41*(7), 1066-1067.

Roth, M., & Grant-Kels, J. (1996). Diagnostic criteria for atopic dermatitis. *The Lancet, 348,* 769-770.

Review Questions

1. A child has a diagnosis of eczema. Parent education should include which statement?
- **a.** "It is worse in the summer because of humidity."
- **b.** "It may disappear by adolescence."
- **c.** "It is worse in females."
- **d.** "It is associated with allergies."

2. Characteristics of an eczema rash are which of the following?
- **a.** Maculopapular without vesicles
- **b.** Nonpruritic
- **c.** Dry with acute papules or vesicles
- **d.** Occurring on the trunk

3. Medications used to treat eczema include all of the following, *except*:
- **a.** Antihistamines
- **b.** Acyclovir
- **c.** Corticosteroids
- **d.** Penicillin

4. When is it appropriate to refer a client with eczema to the dermatologist?
- **a.** With the occurrence of secondary infection
- **b.** No improvement with steroids
- **c.** When the client is allergic to steroids
- **d.** When scarring occurs

5. A differential diagnosis for eczema is which of the following?
- **a.** Scabies
- **b.** Contact dermatitis
- **c.** Varicella
- **d.** Tinea versicolor

Answers and Rationales

1. *Answer:* d (implementation/plan)
Rationale: Eczema is worse in the winter because of low humidity. It is more commonly seen in males. Infantile forms may disappear by the age of 5 years. It is associated with allergies.

2. *Answer:* c (assessment)
Rationale: Vesicles may be present. The condition is pruritic and occurs on flexural regions.

3. *Answer:* b (implementation/plan)
Rationale: No viral infections are associated with eczema.

4. *Answer:* b (evaluation)
Rationale: A client cannot be allergic to steroids. Glucocorticoids are naturally occurring substances in the body and cannot trigger an inflammatory response because they are not recognized as foreign. Scarring most likely necessitates referral to a plastic surgeon, but it is not common with eczema. Hypopigmentation or hyperpigmentation may occur. A person is referred for alternative treatment (e.g., ultraviolet) when steroids do not improve the condition. A primary care provider can treat secondary infection.

5. *Answer:* b (analysis/diagnosis)
   Rationale: Scabies involves burrows and a maculopapular rash. Varicella does not include dry, patchy areas. Tinea versicolor involves only changes in pigmentation.

EDEMA *Pamela Kidd*

OVERVIEW
Definition

Edema is an abnormal accumulation of fluid in the interstitial space. It can be localized or generalized.

Localized Edema

- Localized edema is produced by regional obstruction to venous flow, lymphatic flow, or both.
- Loss of vascular integrity occurs with urticaria and angioneurotic edema.
- Increase in tissue osmotic pressure may occur, for example from surgical trauma, such as edema of the arm after a radical mastectomy (occurs in 10% to 30% of clients).
- Increase in hydrostatic pressure results from increase in venous resistance.

Generalized Edema

- Generalized edema is soft-tissue swelling of most or all regions of the body. It indicates an increase in the interstitial fluid but also in the sodium content of the extracellular compartment and signifies potentially serious disease.
- Idiopathic edema occurs most commonly in young women. They need to be asked about the periodic or cyclic nature of the edema formation and any apparent relationship to the menstrual cycle.
- Orthostatic sodium retention (an abnormal capillary leak of protein resulting in a reduction in blood volume, most pronounced in the upright posture) may be present.
- Heat edema may be present.
- Altitude edema may be present.

Incidence

Sixteen percent of persons 65 years old have swelling of ankles and lower calves, with pitting to 1 cm depth or more in response to firm pressure from the examiner's finger.

Pathophysiology

Edema occurs when (1) the osmolality of the blood is not great enough to retain fluid within the vessel (albumin/protein loss); (2) there is retention of fluid, causing "spillover" into the interstitial space (renal failure, drug side effects); and (3) fluid through the vessel is blocked, causing increased hydrostatic pressure and "spillover of fluid" (e.g., thrombophlebitis, lymphatic obstruction).
   Edema that develops quickly excludes lymphedema and lipedema. Generalized edema involving the face or sacrum or associated with abdominal swelling or shortness of breath (SOB) suggests cardiac, renal, or hepatic disease.

Factors Increasing Susceptibility. Presence of chronic disease (see Past Medical History section).

Protective Factors. Adequate endocrine, renal, and cardiac function.

ASSESSMENT: SUBJECTIVE/HISTORY
History of Present Illness

- Distribution of edema (e.g., lower extremities versus more generalized)
- How quickly edema developed
- Associated trauma, SOB, or pain
- Urinary output
- Weight gain

Idiopathic Edema

- Unexplained weight gain
- Tightness of a ring
- Puffiness of the face
- Swollen extremities
- Enlarged abdominal girth
- Persistence of indentation of the skin after pressure

Generalized Edema

- Jaundice
- Dyspnea
- Orthopnea
- Cough
- Fatigue
- Weakness
- Abdominal distention
- Paroxysmal nocturnal dyspnea
- Anorexia
- Weight loss or gain

Past Medical History

- Renal disease (acute and chronic)
- Liver disease
- Cardiac and pulmonary disease (congestive heart failure [CHF] or CHF coexisting with chronic obstructive pulmonary disease [COPD]); edema is a late feature of heart failure
- Nutritional disease (insufficient protein or malnutrition)
- GI disease

E

- Trauma
- History of deep venous thrombosis
- Thrombophlebitis
- Venous insufficiency
- Ethanol abuse
- Coronary artery disease
- Renal disease
- Diabetes mellitus
- Systemic lupus erythematosus

Medication History

Any drugs that cause sodium retention (e.g., antihypertensives, corticosteroids, androgenic and anabolic steroids, estrogens, and NSAIDs) may aggravate or cause generalized edema. The following may exacerbate edema:

- Diuretic and laxative abuse
- NSAIDs
- Vasodilators
- Adrenal steroids
- Corticosteroids
- Estrogens
- Calcium agonist
- All of these drugs can contribute to the formation of edema through water and sodium retention and loss of protein.

Family History

A family history of chronic health problems should be elicited.

Psychosocial History

- Work history (how much time spent standing)
- Past or current substance abuse
- Smoking history
- Alcohol use history
- Support networks (who cooks and cleans)
- Exercise and recreational activities
- Inactivity (especially in the older adult)

Dietary History

- Carbohydrate loading
- Salt intake
- Protein intake
- Fluid intake

ASSESSMENT: OBJECTIVE/PHYSICAL EXAMINATION

Physical Examination

- *General appearance:* vital signs, weight (In pregnancy, more than 5-pound weight gain in 1 week with HTN and proteinuria is indicative of preeclampsia)
- *Head, ears, eyes, nose, and throat (HEENT):* jugular venous distention, carotid pulse
- *Cardiovascular:* cardiomegaly, displacement of point of maximal impulse, atrial fibrillation, S_3 gallop (left ventricular dilation), rubs

- *Chest:* breath sounds, crackles, wheeze, dullness to percussion, bibasilar rales
- *Abdomen:* hepatomegaly, ascites, splenomegaly
- *Extremities:*
  - Pitting or nonpitting edema with firm pressure of examiner's finger (NOTE: pitting edema occurs when accumulation of fluid exceeds what can be absorbed interstitially [Porth, 1998])
  - Varicose veins
  - Redness
  - Warmth
  - Mottled, brown discoloration of ankle skin (venous insufficiency)
  - Leg circumference
  - Tenderness
  - Homans' sign (dorsiflexion elicits pain in thrombosis)
  - Pulses
  - Cyanosis
  - Clubbing
  - Decreased hair on lower extremities

Diagnostic Procedures

- CBC may indicate anemia, infection, hemodilution.
- Urinalysis (U/A) may indicate infection or need for renal panel.
- Chest x-ray film may indicate pleural effusion and heart failure.
- Echocardiogram may reveal low ejection fraction, which indicates heart failure.
- Liver function test may reveal elevated enzymes, which may indicate cirrhosis, liver failure.
- Thyroid panel may reveal low thyroid hormone levels, which may indicate hypothyroidism.
- Thyroid-stimulating hormone (TSH)

DIAGNOSIS

- Localized edema of the face may characterize both local allergic reactions and anaphylaxis.
- Edema may be the first sign of a new health problem (e.g., chronic venous insufficiency).
- Edema that occurs in conjunction with chronic illness may signify exacerbation (e.g., peripheral edema with COPD may indicate right heart failure).
  Differential diagnoses includes the following:
- Venous or lymphatic obstruction
- Chronic venous insufficiency
- CHF
- Cirrhosis
- Renal disease
- Nephrotic syndrome
- Hypothyroidism
- Drug-associated edema
- Hypoalbuminemia (malnutrition, enteropathies)
- Anemia
- Angioedema

- *Rectal:* Check for sacral dimple, position of anus, anal wink, sphincter tone, rectal vault size, and presence or absence of stool in rectum. May reveal anal fissures, decreased tone, or hard-formed stool in rectal vault.
- Do neurologic screening examination.

Diagnostic Procedures

- Obtain an abdominal x-ray examination to rule out obstruction and look for fecal mass.
- Check for UTI with U/A.
- Flat plate of abdomen may be helpful in diagnostic process.
- Further testing using laboratory tests, barium enemas, rectal manometry, or biopsy is reserved for those who fail conservative therapy or whose history and physical examination suggest organic causes (Kuhn, et al., 1999).

DIAGNOSIS

The differential diagnoses include the following:

Retentive

- Functional constipation (95%)
- Organic (5%)
  - Hirschsprung's disease (usually do not pass large bowel movements and rarely soil)
  - Neuromuscular defect
  - Spinal cord lesion
  - Cerebral palsy
  - Anal stricture/fissure
  - Lead poisoning
  - Hypothyroidism
  - Drugs: codeine, antacids, others

Nonretentive

- Nonorganic (99%)
- Organic (1%)
  - Ulcerative colitis

THERAPEUTIC PLAN
Nonpharmacologic Treatment

- Initial treatment is retentive.
  - Relieve constipation and/or impaction.
  - Prescribe hypertonic phosphate enemas 3 ml/kg bid until return is free of solid stool.
  - Prescribe mineral oil 1 to 2 ml/kg bid until incontinence develops; reduce dose until child has two to three loose stools daily.
- Bowel retraining is necessary (6 to 12 months).
  - Taper laxatives as tolerated.
  - Prescribe stool softeners (docusate sodium [Colace] 5 mg/kg/day).
  - Have child sit on the toilet immediately after meals for 15 to 20 minutes at the same time every day.
  - Increase the child's intake of fiber, fruits, vegetables, and fluids.

- Increase exercise.
- Teach behavior modification: reward success, never punish failure.
- Nonretentive treatment as follows:
  - Keep toileting diary: determine when bowel movements occur and information that may be helpful in treatment.
  - Address toilet refusal behaviors.
  - Develop positive toilet sits to help overcome negative associations with bathroom.
  - Encourage fathers and male caretakers to sit during urination. Boys should be encouraged to sit while urinating until fully bowel trained.
- Dietary changes as necessary:
  - Recommend supplements such as flavored fiber drinks or bran sprinkles to increase the number of bowel movements and maximize daily toileting opportunities.
  - If having a soft daily bowel movement is a problem, use stool softeners or laxative such as Milk of Magnesia.
- Schedule prompted toilet sits.
  - Begin after child is not resistant to sitting on the toilet and is having normal bowel movements.
  - Schedule up to 5 per day for 3 to 5 minutes each.
  - Schedule 5 to 20 minutes after each meal.
  - Reward for successful implementation of toilet sits.
- Provide incentives for appropriate bowel movements and self-initiation.

Client Education

- Encourage parents to keep toileting diary.
- Discuss developmental issues related to toilet training.
- Have parents role model positive toileting practices.

Prevention

- Begin toileting when child is developmentally ready.
- Provide a nutritionally sound diet with adequate fiber, fruits, and vegetables.
- Do not punish the child for bowel movement accidents; treatment must be approached in a calm, relaxed manner.
- Explain the physiology of constipation to parents.

Referral

- Any child with suspected neurologic problems should be referred to a neurologist.
- Any child with suspected sexual abuse should be referred to social service, law enforcement, and mental health services.
- Refer for psychologic evaluation if child has poor response to treatment.
- Children's specialty hospitals may have units specifically designed to address and deal with all of the issues associated with encopresis.

E

EVALUATION/FOLLOW-UP
Retentive

- Follow up by telephone prn and in 1 week.
- Recheck every month until rectal vault is normal size.
- Taper stool softeners once regular elimination pattern is established.

Nonretentive

- If child withholds stool for 4 days, have parents call for appointment.
- Begin specific plan to address withholding.

COMPLICATIONS

- Megacolon
- Chronic constipation
- Anal fissure
- Impaction

REFERENCES

Boynton, R. W., Dunn, E. S., & Stephens, G. R. (Eds.). (1998). *Manual of ambulatory pediatrics* (4th ed.). Philadelphia: J. B. Lippincott.

Chaney, C. A. (1995). A collaborative protocol for encopresis management in school-aged children. *Journal of School Health, 65*(9), 360-364.

Dershewitz, R. A. (Ed.). (1993). *Ambulatory pediatric care* (2nd ed.). Philadelphia: J. B. Lippincott.

Gordy, C. (2000). Enuresis and encopresis. In D. Robinson, P. Kidd, & K. Rogers (Eds.), *Primary care across the lifespan* (pp. 410-412). St. Louis: Mosby.

Hay, W. W., Hayward, A. R., Levin, M., & Sondheimer, J. (1999). *Current pediatric diagnosis and treatment* (14th ed.). Norwalk, CT: Appleton & Lange.

Kuhn, B., Marcus, B., & Pitner, S. (1999). Treatment guidelines for primary nonretentive encopresis and stool toileting refusal. *American Family Physician*, April. Retrieved July 16, 2002, from www.aafp/org/afp/990415ap/2171.html.

Loening-Baucke, V. (1996a). Balloon defecation as a predictor of outcome in children with functional constipation and encopresis. *The Journal of Pediatrics, 128*(3), 336-340.

Loening-Baucke, V. (1996b). Encopresis and soiling. *Pediatric Clinics of North America, 43*(1), 279-299.

Nelson, W., Behrman, R. E., Kliegman, R. M., & Arvin, W. E. (Eds.). (1996). *Nelson textbook of pediatrics* (15th ed.). Philadelphia: W. B. Saunders.

Sprague, J. M., Lamb, W., & Homer, D. (1993). Encopresis: A study of treatment alternatives and historical and behavioral characteristics. *Nurse Practitioner, 18*(10), 52-63.

Review Questions

1. Seven-year-old Robert is brought to the clinic for his annual physical examination. When the family NP asks how things are going, Robert's mother flashes him an angry look and says, "Everything would be fine if I could just get him to stop pooping in his pants every afternoon." To evaluate this situation, the family NP needs to do which of the following?

   a. Ask about other behavioral problems.
   b. Ask for a complete description of Robert's stooling patterns.
   c. Ask about psychosocial upsets such as divorce or the birth of a sibling.
   d. Assist the mother in planning a program of behavior modification.

2. Robert's mother goes on to explain that one of the most frustrating components of his soiling is that "he tries to hide his underwear, and when I find it, he acts like he just doesn't care." Which of the following statements about encopresis helps the family NP explain this behavior?

   a. "Children with encopresis frequently have major psychosocial problems."
   b. "Boys with encopresis generally do not consider it a problem."
   c. "Since Robert only soils in the afternoon, he is probably just trying to get his mother's attention."
   d. "Hiding soiled clothing and acting indifferent are common coping strategies used by children with encopresis."

3. Before a diagnosis of encopresis is made, the family NP should consider all of the following, *except*:

   a. Hirschsprung's disease
   b. Lead poisoning
   c. Chronic diarrhea
   d. Iron-deficiency anemia

4. Sam, a 12-year-old who has been undergoing treatment for encopresis, returns to the clinic for his 1-month follow-up. He is currently taking 2 teaspoons of mineral oil bid and is having regular soft-to-loose stools. The family NP should do which of the following?

   a. Praise Sam for his success and continue current treatment.
   b. Increase the amount of mineral oil until stools are liquid.
   c. Discontinue all pharmacologic intervention and continue dietary therapy.
   d. Decrease and then discontinue the mineral oil, begin docusate sodium (Colace) 10 mg/kg/day, and continue a high-fiber diet.

5. Marvion has been diagnosed with encopresis. What associated history would support this diagnosis?

   a. He was 20 months old when he started toilet training.
   b. He has older siblings.
   c. His mother is a single parent.
   d. He likes fruits and vegetables.

6. A boy comes into the office with constipation and liquid stools. What further objective data supports a diagnosis of encopresis?

   a. Normal examination
   b. Hard stool in rectal vault
   c. Normal anal sphincter tone
   d. Neurologic system grossly intact

7. If a child has negative thoughts about using the toilet and bathroom for bowel movements, which of the following is the initial step in addressing this problem?

   a. Identify medical, developmental, or behavioral pathology.
   b. Encourage positive toilet sits.

c. Ensure well-formed, soft stools.
d. Schedule prompted toilet sits.

8. Once the child with encopresis has success in having a bowel movement in the toilet, what is the most appropriate next step?
a. Use strict consequences if "accidents" occur in the future.
b. Reward the child for his accomplishment.
c. End the toileting program.
d. Continue the mineral oil indefinitely.

Answers and Rationales

1. **Answer: b** (assessment)
Rationale: Soiling in the afternoon is suggestive of encopresis. Knowledge of stooling patterns either supports or rules out this diagnosis. The soiling involved with encopresis is involuntary and not a reflection of a behavioral problem or a psychosocial upset. It is inappropriate to develop a plan before conducting a complete assessment (Boynton, Dunn, & Stephens, 1998).

2. **Answer: d** (implementation/plan)
Rationale: Children who experience soiling are usually ashamed and embarrassed. Hiding soiled clothing and pretending indifference are common coping strategies (Chaney, 1995).

3. **Answer: d** (analysis/diagnosis)
Rationale: Hirschsprung's disease sometimes is characterized by chronic constipation. Lead poisoning also frequently produces constipation, abdominal pain, and anorexia. Soiling may occur with any case of diarrhea. Iron-deficiency anemia may be characterized by anorexia but usually does not produce soiling, constipation, or abdominal pain (Nelson, Behrman, Kliegman, & Arvin, 1996).

4. **Answer: d** (evaluation)
Rationale: Mineral oil therapy should be continued at 3 to 4 teaspoons bid until liquid stools develop. The dose should then be reduced to 1 to 2 ml/kg until soft stools occur bid. The client can then be treated with dietary therapy and stool softeners until regular bowel habits are well established. Mineral oil therapy is unpleasant, and clients usually will not comply for extended periods. Moving the client toward nonpharmacologic therapy should always be the goal (Boynton, Dunn, & Stephens, 1998).

5. **Answer: a** (assessment)
Rationale: Toilet training that starts before a child is physiologically and developmentally ready is likely to fail and may contribute to later continence problems (Kuhn et al., 1999).

6. **Answer: b** (assessment)
Rationale: A finding of hard stool in the rectal vault is common in children with encopresis, retentive type (Kuhn, et al., 1999).

7. **Answer: a** (implementation/plan)
Rationale: It is important to determine if there are any medical, developmental, or behavioral problems before beginning treatment for the toilet phobia. A complete history and physical, along with a toileting diary, should be done before starting any interventions (Kuhn, et al., 1999).

8. **Answer: b** (evaluation)
Rationale: Incentives and rewards for having a bowel movement in the toilet may decrease fecal withholding and the risk of constipation. It is important that rewards are age appropriate and given immediately after the desired behavior is displayed (Kuhn, et al., 1999).

ENDOMETRIOSIS   *Cheryl Pope Kish*

OVERVIEW
Definition
Endometriosis refers to the growth of endometrial tissue outside the uterine cavity. Although most aberrant endometrial implants are scattered through the pelvis, implants have been identified in the lungs and brain. The disease progresses under the repetitive influence of menstrual cycles. Adenomyosis refers to the condition of the endometrial lining invading the myometrium of the uterus.

Incidence
All racial, ethnic, and socioeconomic groups are affected by endometriosis; it affects 5% to 15% of women of reproductive age. Endometriosis typically affects women from their teens through early thirties; adenomyosis is more common in 40- to 50-year-old women.

Pathophysiology
The pathophysiology of endometriosis is not fully understood; it is likely multifactorial in nature. One popular theory of causation relates to retrograde menstrual flow through the fallopian tubes, with implantation of tissue in the pelvis. Another common theory is that coelomic cells lie dormant on the peritoneal surface until they are stimulated to become ectopic endometrium in situ. Adenomyosis grows during menses and bleeds into the myometrium.

Factors Increasing Susceptibility
- Increased exposure to menstruation
  - Increased flow
  - More frequent flow (shorter cycles)
  - Decreased parity
- Family history

Adenomyosis
- Previous cesarean childbirth
- Induced abortion
- Abnormal uterine bleeding
- Late menarche

ASSESSMENT: SUBJECTIVE/HISTORY

History of Present Illness

Ask about the onset of symptoms, duration, and factors that provide relief and those that make symptoms worse. Determine if there are associated symptoms. Quantify the pain with a 0 to 10 pain scale and ask for specific descriptions of the pain and how it relates to the menstrual cycle. Inquire about the relationship of symptoms with menarche, noting the age at which the client's periods began. Ask if there is any relationship between pain and voiding or defecating. Ask about dyspareunia. Ask about abnormal uterine bleeding and infertility.

NOTE: *One third of women with endometriosis are asymptomatic. In women who do experience symptoms, the degree of pain does not correlate directly with the extent of endometrial implants.*

Past Medical History

Complete an obstetrical history. Note number of pregnancies, outcomes, years it took to become pregnant, and any fertility methods used. Ask about gynecologic or other surgery and chronic diseases.

Medication History

Determine what, if any, medications are being used for pain. Identify current medications used. Inquire about current contraceptive method.

Family History

Ask if any first-degree female relatives have endometriosis (this factor increases a woman's risk 10-fold).

Psychosocial History

Inquire about use of alcohol, tobacco, and illicit drugs. Determine if coping mechanisms in place are working effectively and if situational support is in place.

Common Symptoms

- Dysmenorrhea (50% to 66%)
- Pelvic pain and dyspareunia (20% to 33%): Early in disease, pain is worse 1 to 2 days premenstrually; later in the disease, pain can be more chronic.
- Infertility (25% to 70%)
- Intermenstrual bleeding: midcycle spotting (12% to 14%)
- Dyschezia and rectal pain
- Low back pain
- Dysuria

ASSESSMENT: OBJECTIVE/PHYSICAL EXAMINATION

Physical Examination

Many symptomatic women have normal findings on physical examination. The focus of the physical examination is the pelvic examination; conducting the examination at the beginning of the menses increases the probability of finding diagnostic signs. Note these common clinical findings on pelvic examination: diffuse or focal pelvic tenderness; uterosacral nodularity and nodules along the cul de sac; retroversion of uterus; decreased uterine mobility; and adnexal masses (possible). With adenomyosis, expect an enlarged, boggy, tender uterus.

Diagnostic Tests

- Pelvic ultrasound is not diagnostic but is able to detect some degree of pelvic pathology when physical examination is compromised by pain.
- Magnetic resonance imaging (MRI) is diagnostic.
- Laparoscopy is considered the gold standard for diagnosis by enabling direct visualization of endometrial implants: classic brown "powder burn" lesions; reddish-blue lesions on pelvic viscera; endometrioma "chocolate cysts" on ovary.
- Pathology report after hysterectomy is often the only diagnosis for adenomyosis.
- CA 125 is increased in cases of endometriosis, pregnancy, infection, and cancer. Cannot be used as screening test. Has no clinical significance at present.

DIAGNOSIS

The following differential diagnoses should be considered:

- PID
- Pelvic adhesions
- Pregnancy
- Leiomyoma
- Ovarian cancer
- Irritable bowel syndrome
- Diverticulitis

THERAPEUTIC PLAN

At present, hysterectomy is considered the only definitive treatment for adenomyosis. Factors that should be considered before attempting treatment for endometriosis include client age, desire for fertility, severity of symptoms, and the extent and location of implants. Consultation with a gynecologist is appropriate in decision making about treatment; the goals of treatment are to (1) preserve fertility, if desired; (2) decrease signs and symptoms; and (3) simplify future surgical procedures or make them unnecessary. There are four treatment approaches to consider:

1. Expectant management is provided for young women with milder disease and a desire for pregnancy.
2. Conservative surgeries include ablation of implants with electrocautery or laser, lysis of adhesions, and assessment of tubal occlusion.
3. Medical treatment interrupts or decreases menstrual cycles; drugs do not improve adhesions or regress disease but do keep the symptoms from becoming worse.

4. Extensive surgery: Hysterectomy with bilateral salpin-gooophorectomy is often a final alternative for those in whom earlier treatment options have failed.

Pharmacologic Treatment

Pharmacologic management of endometriosis is typically prescribed in consultation with a physician or on referral. Pain relief with NSAIDs or other analgesics is an important component of client management. Other drugs are used to control symptoms and improve fertility:

- Danazol (Danocrine) is used to suppress menses for 6 to 9 months; produces a hyperandrogenic state and shrinks endometrial implants. Side effects are decreased breast size, weight gain, acne, and hirsutism.
- Medroxyprogesterone to suppress luteinizing hormone (LH) and follicle-stimulating hormone (FSH); can be given PO or IM.
- OCPs are combined estrogen/progesterone to cause atrophy of implants. Administered 6 to 12 months; continuous dosing without pill-free days.
- GnRH agonists creates a hypoestrogen state of pseudomenopause for 6 months; administer synarel (Nafarelin) nasal spray or leuprolide (Lupron) either subcutaneously daily for 6 months or as depot injection each month. Side effects are hot flashes, vaginal atrophy, and bone demineralization. Osteoporosis is a concern when these drugs are used for 6 months or longer.

Prevention

Prevention of endometriosis and adenomyosis is not possible.

Client Education

The NP will not manage endometriosis independently but may be involved in collaborative management to some extent. NPs may be involved in explanations of the disease process and therapies, support during the chronicity of the disease and recurrence when medical therapy is discontinued, and discussion of timing pregnancy because infertility is so common.

Referral

All women with this disorder are referred.

EVALUATION/FOLLOW-UP

Follow-up is determined by management strategy. Medical treatment is limited; implants do recur after the medication is discontinued.

COMPLICATIONS

- Pain that increases with each menstrual cycle disrupts life. The disorder improves with menopause.
- Other complications include infertility and the possibility of hysterectomy to remedy the disorder.

REFERENCES

Brown, K. M. (2000). *Management guidelines for women's health nurse practitioners*. Philadelphia: F. A. Davis.
Cash, J. C., & Glass, C. A. (2000). *Family practice guidelines*. Philadelphia: Lippincott.
Corwin, E. J. (1997). Endometriosis: Pathophysiology, diagnosis, and treatment. *The Nurse Practitioner, 22*(10), 35-57.
Meredith, P. V., & Horan, N. M. (2000). *Adult primary care*. Philadelphia: W. B. Saunders.
Newkirk, G. R. (1996). Endometriosis. In C. A. Johnson, B. E. Johnson, & J. L. Murray (Eds.), *Women's health care handbook* (pp. 319-322). Philadelphia: Hanley & Belfus.
Propst, A. M., & Loufer, M. R. (2000). Diagnosing and treating adolescent endometriosis. *Contemporary Nurse Practitioner, 4*(1), 11-18.
Robinson, D., Kidd, P., & Rogers, K. M. (2000). *Primary care across the lifespan*. St. Louis: Mosby.
Smith, M. A., & Shimp, L. A. (2000). *20 common problems in women's health care*. New York: McGraw-Hill.
Smith, R. P. (1997). *Gynecology in primary care*. Baltimore: Williams & Wilkins.
Tarney, C. M., & DeCherney, A. H. (1999). Update on endometriosis: Medical therapy, surgery, or both. *Women's Health in Primary Care, 2*(2), 126-138.
Tierney, L. M., McPhee, S. J., & Papadakis, M. A. (2001). *Current medical diagnosis and treatment*. New York: Lange Medical Books/McGraw-Hill.
Wellberg, C. (1999). Diagnosis and treatment of endometriosis. *American Family Physician, 60*, 1753-1768.

E

Review Questions

1. Which of the following factors is known to increase the risk of endometriosis?
   a. OCP use
   b. Multiparity
   c. Family history
   d. History of chlamydia

2. Which of the following pairs of clinical findings in a 26-year-old is consistent with a diagnosis of endometriosis?
   a. Pelvic pain and dyspareunia
   b. Amenorrhea and frequent diarrhea
   c. Vulvar edema and erythema
   d. Postcoital bleeding and frothy discharge

3. Which objective finding is commonly found in women with endometriosis?
   a. Severe cervical motion tenderness
   b. Inguinal lymphadenopathy
   c. Nodules along the cul de sac
   d. Cervical friability

4. Ellen, a new client, presents to the clinic with symptoms of upper respiratory infection (URI). She tells the NP that she is undergoing medical treatment for endometriosis in the hopes of being able to get pregnant. Ellen provides a list of all the medications she has taken in the last 6 months. Which drug from the list would have been used for endometriosis?
   a. Diflucan

b. Danazol
c. Tessalon
d. Nitrofurantoin

5. What diagnostic procedure is considered the gold standard for diagnosing endometriosis?
  a. Culdocentesis
  b. Transvaginal ultrasonography
  c. Hysterosalpingogram
  d. Laparoscopy

6. Miriam is a 32-year-old with a diagnosis of endometriosis. Which statement by Miriam indicates that she understands the disease process and management?
  a. "This is a sexually transmitted disease that might have been prevented with safer sexual behaviors."
  b. "I will likely have pain from this disorder until I experience menopause; then it should get better."
  c. "The most common cause of endometriosis is having an elective abortion in one's teen years."
  d. "I got endometriosis because my mother took DES while she was pregnant with me."

7. Anne asked the NP how the prescription for NSAIDs will help her endometriosis. The NP explains that NSAIDs work by which of the following?
  a. Shrinking the endometrial implants by at least 60%
  b. Blocking the production of prostaglandin, thereby decreasing painful periods
  c. Preventing the disease progression
  d. Reversing the disease progression

8. Susan has suffered with endometriosis for years. The NP's collaborative physician orders leuprolide (Lupron) for Susan. The NP provides comprehensive education about the drug. Which comment by Susan about the potential adverse effects of the drug shows that she has understood the information?
  a. "I can expect my breasts to become distended and tender."
  b. "I should get my blood pressure checked every few months because of the risk of hypertension."
  c. "This drug puts me at risk for loss of bone."
  d. "Most people experience some degree of stomach problems."

Answers and Rationales

1. Answer: c (assessment)
  Rationale: Women with a mother or sister with endometriosis have a 10-fold increase in risk because of that family history (Propst & Laufer, 2000).

2. Answer: a (assessment)
  Rationale: Pelvic pain and dyspareunia are classic symptoms of endometriosis (Tarney & De Cherney, 1999).

3. Answer: c (assessment)
  Rationale: Endometrial implants often contribute to nodules along the cul de sac and uterosacral space (Tarney & De Cherney, 1999).

4. Answer: b (implementation/plan)
  Rationale: Danocrine (Danazol) is a drug that is often used to medically manage endometriosis, with a goal of decreasing symptoms and improving fertility (Tarney & DeCherney, 1999).

5. Answer: d (analysis/diagnosis)
  Rationale: Laparoscopy is considered the gold standard procedure for diagnosing endometriosis because it requires direct visualization of the classic lesions for diagnosis (Brown, 2000).

6. Answer: b (evaluation)
  Rationale: Endometriosis is a disease that progresses under the influence of menstruation; at menopause the implants regress and symptoms improve or disappear (Tarney & DeCherney, 1999).

7. Answer: b (implementation/plan)
  Rationale: NSAIDs are used to treat endometriosis because of their ability to inhibit prostaglandin, thereby decreasing painful periods. They do not affect the course of the disease otherwise (Corwin, 1997).

8. Answer: c (evaluation)
  Rationale: The GnRH agonists, such as lupron, are antiestrogenic and cause osteoporosis. Breasts shrink, virilization occurs, and GI distress is uncommon, making these choices incorrect (Corwin, 1997).

ENURESIS   *Denise Robinson*

OVERVIEW
Definition

Involuntary voiding after the age when control should have been established (usually 5 years old) is called *enuresis*. It may be nocturnal (85%) or diurnal (15%). Enuresis is subdivided into two categories. In primary enuresis, bladder control has never been established. In secondary enuresis, there is loss of bladder control in a child who has been consistently dry for at least 6 months.

Incidence
- Approximately 5 to 7 million children in the United States have primary nocturnal enuresis.
- More common in boys than girls.
- There is a familial tendency.
- More common in large families and in the lower socioeconomic groups.
- Approximate incidence by age group is as follows:
  - 10% to 15% of 6-year-olds
  - 5% of 10-year-olds

- 3% of 12-year-olds
- 1% of 15-year-olds

Pathophysiology
Primary Enuresis

- Urinary control is a function of the central nervous system (CNS).
- Delayed maturation of that portion of the CNS that permits bladder control results in the child not sensing bladder fullness and therefore not awakening to void.
- Contributing factors include the following:
  - Immature bladder with small capacity
  - Arousal from non-rapid eye movement (REM) sleep
  - Psychologic or emotional problems (e.g., new sibling, divorce)
  - Neurologic deficit (neurogenic bladder, spinal cord lesion)
  - Urologic abnormalities (UTI, vesicoureteral reflex, bifurcated bladder, tumors)
  - Diabetes mellitus/diabetes insipidus
- Genetics appear to play a role; appears to be a major dominant gene on chromosome 13. No specific gene locus has yet been identified.

Secondary Enuresis

- Psychologic problems can cause secondary enuresis.
- UTIs: The presence of bacteria is irritating to the bladder mucosa, producing frequency, urgency, and dysuria.
- Sexual abuse may result in secondary enuresis.
- Diabetes mellitus/diabetes insipidus can cause secondary enuresis.

ASSESSMENT: SUBJECTIVE/HISTORY
History of Present Illness

- Determine onset, frequency, and time frame (at what time of night does the bed-wetting usually occur? Is it consistent?).
- Determine voiding patterns.
- Note fluid intake related to bedtime.
- Ask about method used by parents to correct the problem.
- Note the attitude of parents and the child regarding the enuresis, response to therapy tried.
- Determine any previous workup for the problem.
- Depending on the child, the family NP might choose to conduct a portion of the interview with the parents and child separated.

Symptoms

- Frequency, urgency, pain, or burning on urination
- Nocturnal seizures (bitten tongue or sore muscles on awakening)

Past Medical History

- UTI
- Congenital anomalies
- Toilet training methods (were parents demanding or punitive?)

Family History

- Enuresis in parents, especially in father (both parents of 77% of children currently with enuresis had enuresis themselves; one parent of 44% of children currently with enuresis had enuresis themselves; only 15% of children with enuresis have parents who did not have enuresis.)
- Diabetes

Psychosocial History

- Births
- Deaths
- Divorce
- Moves
- School problems

ASSESSMENT: OBJECTIVE/PHYSICAL EXAMINATION
Physical Examination

- Perform complete physical and neurologic examinations; findings from these examinations are usually within normal limits.
- Focus on constant dribbling, external anomalies of the genitalia, rectal sphincter tone, café au lait spots, abdominal masses, spinal bony defects, hairy tufts, masses, and gait. Also palpate/percuss for a distended bladder. Check for flank pain.
- Assess for chronic urinary tract disease; suspect disease if the client's height and weight are below the fifth percentile or if the client's average blood pressure is above the 95th percentile for age and sex.

Diagnostic Procedures

- U/A and a clean, voided culture are recommended. A culture is only recommended if the client has symptoms consistent with UTI.
- More invasive procedures (e.g., cystoscopy, ultrasound) are not indicated unless an abnormality is discovered on physical examination or the problem persists past age 6 years and all other diagnostic procedure results are negative.

DIAGNOSIS

This is a diagnosis of exclusion. All other causes of enuresis need to be ruled out. The differential diagnoses include the following:

- Normal developmental enuresis
- Toilet training resistance

- Altered parenting
- UTI or anatomic abnormalities
- Diabetes mellitus, diabetes insipidus (specific gravity less than 1.006)
- Seizure disorder
- Excessive fluid intake
- CNS deficit

NOTE: *In most cases, no organic pathologic condition can be found.*

THERAPEUTIC PLAN

- Involve the child in the treatment plan.
- The decision to treat or not to treat must be made jointly by the child and the parents.
- Treat only children who are 8 years old or older and who have a bladder capacity of 200 ml or greater (determined by measuring output after having the child wait to urinate as long as possible).
- Investigate and treat the cause of secondary enuresis.

Nonpharmacologic Treatment

- Motivational therapy results in approximately 70% improvement; try for 3 to 6 months, especially for younger children.
  - Reassure the parents and child.
  - Remove the guilt associated with bed-wetting.
  - Provide emotional support to the child.
  - Instruct the child on taking responsibility for his or her bedwetting; give the child a role in the treatment plan.
  - Provide positive reinforcement for dryness: Use a gold-star chart.
- Behavioral therapy is effective.
- Conditioned response therapy includes the following:
  - "Enuresis alarm" is worn at night and is triggered by moisture. A success rate up to 80% has been reported. The typical course is 4 months. The alarm must be worn until 21 consecutive nights of dryness are achieved. There is roughly a 25% relapse rate.
  - Parental involvement is important with alarms. Also may use diary and reward system to help reinforce behavior.
  - Requires a long-term commitment because results may not be evident for several months.
  - Use for 3 weeks of complete dryness; relapses are common if discontinued too soon.
- Bladder training exercises involve increasing fluid and having child hold off voiding as long as possible.

Pharmacologic Treatment

Usually reserved for children older than 7 years of age. These medications are stop-gap measures until children are able to wake on their own during the night to void.

- Imipramine (Tofranil) can be used. The initial dose is 15 to 25 mg PO hs, which may be increased to a maximum dose of 50 mg for children younger than 12 years and 75 mg for children older than 12 years. (This drug has an anticholinergic effect and may alter secretion of antidiuretic hormone [ADH].)
  - Prescribe a 6- to 8-week treatment, then taper the dose during a 4- to 6-week period.
  - Drug tolerance is common.
  - Watch for cardiac side effects (dysrhythmia, postural hypotension, anemia) and anticholinergic effects (dry mouth).
  - Overdose may be fatal; warn parents to keep medicine out of child's reach.
- Anticholinergic therapy involves the following:
  - Hyoscyamine (Levsin) and Oxybutynin (Ditropan) have a direct effect on smooth muscle control and reduce the bladder's ability to contract. Give 5 mg at bedtime.
  - Side effects include dry mouth, facial flushing, drowsiness, constipation, and dizziness. In the summer, elevated temperature can be a problem.
- Desmopressin acetate (DDAVP; synthetic analog of ADH): Use 20 to 40 mg intranasally with children age 6 years and older.
  - Treatment is expensive.
  - Effectiveness is controversial.
  - There is a high relapse rate.
  - Needs to be tapered because abrupt discontinuation causes a high rate of relapse.
  - Long-term therapy appears to be safe.
  - Helpful for short-term needs (e.g., sleepovers, camps).

Client Education

- Parents need to be actively involved in the treatment process.
- Do not shame, place guilt, or embarrass the child when accidents occur.
- Involve the child in the treatment plan.
- Be patient: treatment will take several months to work.

Prevention

- Begin toilet training when child is developmentally ready.
- Do not attempt toilet training or treatment plan when family stress is present, such as birth of sibling, divorce, or move.

Referral

- Refer for any anatomic abnormalities.
- Once a UTI has been ruled out, children with chronic enuresis should have a thorough urologic workup simultaneously with behavioral therapy.

EVALUATION/FOLLOW-UP
Primary Enuresis

- Contact by telephone in 2 weeks to check progress.
- Schedule a return visit in 1 month.
- Continue follow-up at 2- to 4-week intervals. Phone calls and office visits may alternate.

Secondary Enuresis

- Draft an individualized counseling contract.
- Schedule initial follow-up in 10 to 14 days.
- If medication is prescribed, the client should be seen monthly.
- If a UTI is diagnosed, follow up after antibiotics are completed.

COMPLICATIONS

- Family stress may result if treatment is not successful.
- In most cases enuresis is a self-limiting problem; as the child grows, the incidence of enuresis decreases.

REFERENCES

Boynton, R., Dunn, E., & Stephens, G. (1998). *Manual of ambulatory pediatrics* (4th ed.). Philadelphia: Lippincott.

Cendron, M. (1999). Primary nocturnal enuresis: current concepts. *American Family Physician*, March. Retrieved July 16, 2002, from www.aafp.org/afp.990301ap/1205.html.

Gordy, C. (2000). Enuresis. In D. Robinson, P. Kidd, & K. Rogers (Eds.), *Primary care across the lifespan*. St. Louis: Mosby, 420.

Son, S., & Kirchner, J. (2000). Depression in children and adolescents. *American Family Physician, 62*, 2297-2308, 2311-2312.

Review Questions

1. A mother brings in her 7-year-old son because he wets the bed at night. What associated historical datum is consistent with this diagnosis?

   a. Smokers in the home
   b. Recurrent skin problems since infancy
   c. Recent birth of brother
   d. Father had enuresis as child

2. Which of the following questions is most associated with an organic cause of enuresis and should be asked by the NP in the client/family assessment?

   a. "Describe the prenatal course of Marvion."
   b. "Does he have flank pain and decreased appetite?"
   c. "How much fluid does he drink in the evenings?"
   d. "Does he drink a lot of fruit juice?"

3. A 10-year-old boy has primary nocturnal enuresis. What further objective data supports this diagnosis?

   a. Liver and spleen palpable below the costal margin
   b. Bowel sounds positive, no abdominal tenderness

   c. Abdominal tenderness with guarding
   d. Hard stool in rectal vault

4. All of the following findings help the family NP rule out an organic cause for secondary enuresis, *except*:

   a. Urine specific gravity of 1.011
   b. No evidence of glycosuria and acetonuria from U/A
   c. Presence of protein and leukocytes in the urine
   d. No evidence of bacteria in the urine

5. The therapeutic plan of care for a 5-year-old diagnosed with enuresis who has a negative physical examination includes all of the following, *except*:

   a. Reassure the parents and wait for maturation.
   b. Refer for a renal ultrasound and a voiding cystogram.
   c. Suggest the use of exercises to increase bladder capacity.
   d. Suggest the use of a behavior modification program such as "gold stars" for dryness.

6. Jeremy is started on DDAVP for primary enuresis. Which comment from the mother indicates a need for further teaching?

   a. "Jeremy can take the medication when he goes to a friend's house to sleep over."
   b. "After Jeremy is dry for 3 weeks, I will stop the medication."
   c. "DDAVP has few side effects."
   d. "I will continue Jeremy's reward chart for no enuresis."

7. Josh is a 6-year-old who has enuresis. Which of the following is most appropriate to use as initial therapy for this problem?

   a. Motivational therapy
   b. Behavioral therapy
   c. Pharmacologic therapy
   d. Psychological counseling

8. Thomas is started on imipramine (Tofranil) for enuresis. Which of the following is very important to emphasize with his parents?

   a. "It causes a dry mouth."
   b. "It has a high potential for fatal overdose; keep it away from the children."
   c. "He can drink as much as he wants before bedtime."
   d. "Side effects include seizures and headaches."

Answers and Rationales

1. *Answer:* d (assessment)
   Rationale: With one parent with a history of enuresis, the incidence in children is 44%. This is especially true if the father has a similar problem (Cendron, 1999).

2. *Answer:* b (assessment)
   Rationale: Painful urination and flank pain are indicative of UTI and should be investigated further as a cause of the enuresis (Gordy, 2000).

3. *Answer:* b (assessment)
   Rationale: In most cases, no objective findings support the diagnosis of enuresis; it is a diagnosis by exclusion (Gordy, 2000).

E

4. Answer: c (analysis/diagnosis)

Rationale: A urine specific gravity higher than 1.006 rules out diabetes insipidus, absence of glycosuria and acetonuria rules out diabetes mellitus, and absence of bacteriuria rules out a UTI. The presence of protein and leukocytes in the urine might indicate glomerulonephritis or nephrotic syndrome (Boynton, Dunn, & Stephens, 1998).

5. Answer: b (implementation/plan)

Rationale: Most cases of primary enuresis have no organic cause. Extensive or invasive laboratory or radiologic examination should be avoided in the absence of physical findings. An estimated 10% to 15% of all 6-year-olds continue to be incontinent at night. At age 5 years, this is probably a normal variant; if the parents desire treatment, the least invasive methods should be tried first (Cendron, 1999).

6. Answer: b (evaluation)

Rationale: DDAVP should not be discontinued abruptly because it has a high relapse rate. It should be tapered gradually when discontinued (Cendron, 1999).

7. Answer: a (implementation/plan)

Rationale: Use of motivational therapy is a reasonable first-line approach for younger children (Cendron, 1999).

8. Answer: b (implementation/plan)

Rationale: Imipramine has been associated with accidental overdose of clients and siblings; it should be kept away from children (Cendron, 1999).

EPIDIDYMITIS   *Pamela Kidd*

OVERVIEW
Definition

Infectious process of the epididymis.

Incidence

Two different causes exist, with males younger than 40 most susceptible for sexually transmitted disease as the agent. Males 40 and older have associated UTI or prostatitis. Gram-negative rods are the causative agent.

Pathophysiology

The organism travels through the urethra to the ejaculatory duct, then down to the vas deferens to the epididymis.

Factors Increasing Susceptibility
- Unprotected sex
- Benign prostatic hypertrophy

Protective Factors
- Condoms
- Frequent sexual intercourse after age 40

ASSESSMENT: SUBJECTIVE/HISTORY
Symptoms
- Acute swelling of epididymis and groin
- Pain in the scrotal area, with possible radiation to flank
- Ask about recent history of sexual activity, heavy lifting, or trauma.
- Urethral discharge
- Dysuria
- Fever and chills

Past Medical History
- Sexually transmitted disease
- Mumps (may cause epididymitis)

Medication History

Anticholinergics.

Family History

Noncontributory.

Dietary History

Noncontributory.

ASSESSMENT: OBJECTIVE/PHYSICAL EXAMINATION
Physical Examination

Examine genitalia. Pain in the scrotum radiating along spermatic cord or to flank during palpation indicates epididymitis.

- Genitalia is extremely tender to touch.
- Erythema is present.
- Scrotum is swollen.
- Prostate may be tender.
- Urethral discharge present.
- Elevation of scrotum above symphysis pubis improves pain.

Diagnostic Procedures
- *Complete blood count (CBC):* leukocytosis and a left shift
- *Gram stain of urethral discharge:* Gram-negative diplococci (gonorrhea), WBC count (nongonococcal, probably chlamydia)
- Culture of urethral drainage
- *U/A:* pyuria, bacteria, hematuria; urine culture to demonstrate pathogen in non–sexually transmitted form
- Scrotal ultrasound to demonstrate hyperperfusion in epididymitis, hypoperfusion in testicular torsion

TABLE **3-27**   Differential Diagnoses

CONDITION	SIGNS	SYMPTOMS
Testicular tumor	Palpable mass Negative U/A Positive mass on ultrasound	No pain
Testicular torsion	Negative U/A and Gram stain Hypoperfusion on ultrasound	Prepubertal client Acute onset of symptoms
Epididymitis	Positive Gram stain Positive U/A Hyperperfusion on ultrasound	Gradual onset with symptoms worsening over time
UTI	Positive U/A Fever	Pain may radiate to flank Acute onset of pain

TABLE **3-28**   *Pharmacologic Treatments*

DRUG	DOSE	COMMENT
Ceftriaxone	250 mg as a single dose IM plus doxycycline	Treat sexual partner.
Doxycycline	100 mg PO q12h × 10-21 days	Treat sexual partner.
Azithromycin	1 g PO as single dose for nongonococcal urethritis Use 2 g PO single dose for gonococcal	WBC count present, elevated on smear; positive chlamydia culture; treat sexual partner.
Ciprofloxacin	250-500 mg PO q12h × 21-28 days	Use for non-sexually transmitted disease, gram-negative rods.
Ofloxacin	300 mg q12h × 10 days	Use for non–sexually transmitted disease, gram-negative rods.

Trimethoprim/
  sulfamethoxazole
  DS (Bactrim)
	160/800 mg PO q12h × 21-28 days	Use for non-sexually transmitted disease, gram-negative rods.

DIAGNOSIS

The most common differential diagnoses are testicular torsion and testicular mass. Table 3-27 illustrates the differences among these diagnoses.

THERAPEUTIC PLAN
Nonpharmacologic Treatment

- Elevation/support of testes relieves pain.
- Apply ice packs to scrotum to reduce swelling (be sure to tell client to use a barrier between the ice and skin).
- Take bed rest during the acute phase.

Pharmacologic Treatment

Use antibiotics for up to 21 days for the sexually transmitted variety and up to 28 days for the non–sexually transmitted variety (See Table 3-28). Pain medication may be ordered for acute phase.

Client Education

Use condoms and limit sexual partners.

Referral

Consider referral to a urologist for urinary tract evaluation in cases of Gram-negative rod infection.

EVALUATION/FOLLOW-UP

Repeat urethral culture (sexually transmitted variety) or U/A (non–sexually transmitted variety) after antibiotic course.

Complications

Delayed or inadequate treatment may decrease fertility or produce an abscess.

REFERENCES

Denman, S., & Murphy, P. (1995). Genitourinary infections. In L. Barker, J. Burton, & P. Zieve (Eds.), *Principles of ambulatory medicine* (4th ed.). Baltimore: Williams & Wilkins.

Kidd, P. (2000). Genitourinary conditions. In P. Kidd, P. Sturt, & J. Fultz (Eds.), *Mosby's emergency nursing reference*. St. Louis: Mosby.

Kidd, P. (2000). Epididymitis. In D. Robinson, P. Kidd, & K. Rogers (Eds.), *Primary care across the lifespan*. St. Louis: Mosby.

Stoller, M., Presti, J., & Carroll, P. (2001). Urology. In L. Tierney, S. McPhee, & M. Papadakis (Eds.), *Current medical diagnosis and treatment* (40th ed.). New York: McGraw-Hill.

E

Review Questions

1. In trying to discriminate the causative agent for epididymitis in a client, which of the following symptoms and signs are important?

  a. Urethral discharge
  b. Fever
  c. Pain in the scrotal area
  d. Acute swelling of the groin area

2. Which of the following co-morbidities are associated with epididymitis?

  a. Diabetes
  b. HTN
  c. Prostatitis
  d. Inguinal hernia

3. A scrotal ultrasound indicates which of the following in epididymitis?

  a. Hypoperfusion
  b. Lesion
  c. Hyperperfusion
  d. Presence of fluid

4. The common differential diagnoses to epididymitis are all of the following, *except:*

  a. Erectile dysfunction
  b. Testicular tumor
  c. Testicular torsion
  d. UTI

5. An NP prescribes antibiotics for treatment of epididymitis caused by Gram-negative rods. The treatment should include which of the following?

  a. Dosing for 21 to 28 days
  b. IM injection followed by PO therapy
  c. Antibiotics for the sexual partner(s)
  d. Use of probenecid

Answers and Rationales

1. *Answer:* **a** (assessment)
  Rationale: Both forms of epididymitis present with pain, swelling, and fever. Urethral discharge more commonly occurs when the condition is produced by a sexually transmitted disease.

2. *Answer:* **c** (assessment)
  Rationale: There are no systemic diseases associated with epididymitis. The presence of an inguinal hernia suggests a history of heavy lifting, and lifting may be associated with testicular torsion but not epididymitis. Prostatitis is associated with epididymitis produced by Gram-negative rods.

3. *Answer:* **c** (analysis/diagnosis)
  Rationale: A lesion suggests a testicular mass or cancer. Fluid indicates a hydrocele. Hypoperfusion occurs with testicular torsion caused by obstruction of blood flow. Infection and inflammation (as with epididymitis) produces hyperperfusion.

4. *Answer:* **a** (analysis/diagnosis)
  Rationale: Erectile dysfunction does not produce physical illness or pain.

5. *Answer:* **a** (implementation/plan)
  Rationale: Gram-negative rods are produced by non–sexually transmitted disease and may be caused by abnormal growth of existing flora. Treatment is with PO antibiotics. Probenecid is used as an adjunct in penicillin treatment. Penicillin is not a recommended treatment for epididymitis.

EPIGLOTTITIS *Denise Robinson*

OVERVIEW
Definition

Epiglottitis is a rapidly developing, life-threatening bacterial infection of the supraglottic area. A true medical emergency, it may or may not be preceded by a URI syndrome.

Incidence

- Epiglottitis is rare and generally occurs in children aged 2 to 6 years. Adult cases do occur and are most often seen between the second and fourth decade of life.
- Epiglottitis can occur at any time of the year and is most often seen in temperate climates.

Pathophysiology
Common Pathogens

- Haemophilus influenzae: The incidence is decreasing in children with the use of the Haemophilus influenzae vaccine, whereas the incidence is increasing in adults.
- High fever is associated with epiglottis.
- Drooling and difficulty swallowing are associated with epiglottis.
- In children, possible presenting symptoms include URI symptoms, sore throat, and voice change.
- In infants, possible nonclassic presentation includes URI symptoms, croupy cough, excoriated nares, and low-grade fever.

ASSESSMENT: SUBJECTIVE/HISTORY
Associated Symptoms

- Toxic-looking
- Muffled voice
- Dysphagia
- Inspiratory stridor
- Sitting position preferred

Past Medical History

- Recent viral infections
- Exposures
- Allergies
- Medication
- Immunization status

Family History

Inquire about any recent illness.

Psychosocial History

- School or day care exposure
- Smoking
- Profession (possible exposure to inhaled irritants such as paints, chemicals, dust particles, and smoke)

Dietary History

Ask about decreased oral intake.

ASSESSMENT: OBJECTIVE/PHYSICAL EXAMINATION

ⓕ**CAUTION:** *Ensure that the airway is not compromised before proceeding with any physical examination.*

Physical Examination

ⓕ**CAUTION:** *Have emergency life support equipment available.*

A problem-oriented physical examination should be conducted, with particular attention to the following:

- Airway compromise
- Vital signs
- General appearance
- Respiratory status
- Ears
- Nose
- Lymph nodes

Diagnostic Procedures

ⓕ**CAUTION:** *Diagnostic procedures should not be attempted until the airway is secured.*

- Lateral neck radiograph
  - Croup: normal epiglottis, with narrowing of the subepiglottic area
  - Epiglottitis: "thumbprint" sign consistent with inflammation of the epiglottis (children near C2-3; adults near C5-6)
- *CBC with differential:* WBC count 10,000 to 25,000 cells/mm^3 with elevated bands
- *Arterial blood gases (ABGs) and pulse oximetry:* results variable, depending on degree of respiratory distress
- Blood cultures

DIAGNOSIS

Differential diagnoses may include the following:

- Foreign body (FB)
- Traumatic obstruction
- Neoplasm
- Angioneurotic edema
- Laryngitis
- Respiratory syncytial virus (RSV)
- Bacterial tracheitis
- Inhalation injury

THERAPEUTIC PLAN
Pharmacologic Treatment

- Croup without stridor at rest: acetaminophen or ibuprofen to control fever
- Croup with stridor at rest:
  - Racemic epinephrine 2.25% solution by nebulizer every 2 hours while stridor continues at rest (lasts approximately 4 hours; watch for rebound effect)
  - less than 20 kg: 0.25 ml in 2.25 ml saline solution
  - 20 to 40 kg: 0.50 ml in 2.25 ml saline solution
  - more than 40 kg: 0.75 ml in 2.25 ml saline solution
  - Dexamethasone (Decadron): 0.6 mg/kg per dose IV, IM, or PO for 1 to 4 doses every 6 to 12 hours (handheld nebulized treatments has the same results)
  - Oxygen: requires intensive care unit admission.
- Epiglottitis: Refer/consult immediately.
  - Oxygen at 100% followed by intubation
  - Antibiotics via IV for at least 5 days then may switch to PO
  - Cefotaxime: 50 to 150 mg/kg/day divided every 6 to 8 hours
  - Ceftriaxone: 50 to 75 mg/kg/day divided every 12 hours
  - Cefuroxime: 100 mg/kg/day divided every 6 to 8 hours
- Epiglottitis: Explain need for intubation and procedures to family.

Referral

- Epiglottitis
- Croup with stridor at rest
- Dehydration or inability to drink fluids
- Inability to control fever
- Inability to maintain airway

EVALUATION/FOLLOW-UP

- Recurrent croup episodes
- If no improvement in 4 to 5 days
- Increase in stridor
- Stops drinking
- Inability to control fever
- New symptom development

E

REFERENCES

Bamberger, B. M., & Jackson, M. A. (1994). Upper respiratory tract infections: Pharyngitis, sinusitis, otitis media and epiglottitis. In M. S. Niederman, G. A. Sarosi, & J. Glassroth (Eds.), *Respiratory infections: A scientific basis for management* (pp. 77-87). Philadelphia: W. B. Saunders.

Barker, L. R., Burton, J. R., & Zieve, P. D. (1995). *Principles of ambulatory medicine* (4th ed.). Baltimore: Williams & Wilkins.

Barkin, R. M., & Rosen, R. (1994). Pulmonary disorders. In R. M. Barkin & R. Rosen (Eds.), *Emergency pediatrics: A guide to ambulatory care* (4th ed., pp. 712-720). St. Louis: Mosby.

Berman, S., & Schmitt, B. D. (1995). Ear, nose, and throat. In W. W. Han, J. R. Groothuis, A. R. Hayward, & M. J. Levin. *Current pediatric diagnosis and treatment* (12th ed., pp. 482-483). Norwalk, CT: Appleton & Lange.

Casmmassima, P. S., & Belanger, G. K. (1994). Ear, nose, and throat disorders. In R. M. Barkin & R. Rosen (Eds.), *Emergency pediatrics: A guide to ambulatory care* (4th ed., pp. 552-555). St. Louis: Mosby.

Hall, C. B., & McBride, J. T. (1994). Upper respiratory tract infections: The common cold, pharyngitis, croup, bacterial tracheitis and epiglottitis. In J. E. Pennington (Ed.), *Respiratory infections: Diagnosis and management* (3rd ed., pp. 101-119). New York: Raven Press.

Jacoby, D. B. (1995). Adult epiglottitis. *Journal of the American Academy of Nurse Practitioners, 7*(10), 511-512.

Komaroff, A. L. (1994). Disease of the respiratory tract: Pharyngitis, Coryza, and related infections in adults. In W. T. Branch (Ed.), *Office practice of medicine* (3rd ed., pp. 148-163). Philadelphia: W. B. Saunders.

Koster, F. T., & Barker, L. R. (1995). Respiratory tract infections. In L. R. Barker, J. R. Burton, & P. D. Zieve (Eds.), *Principles of ambulatory medicine* (4th ed). Baltimore: Williams &Wilkins.

Larson, G., Accurso, F., Deterding, R., Halbower, A., & White, C. (1999). In W. Hay, A. Hayward, M. Levin, & J. Sondheimer (Eds.), *Current pediatric diagnosis and treatment* (14th ed.). Stamford, CT: Appleton & Lange.

Orenstein, D. (1996). In W. Nelson, R. Behrman, R. Kliegman, & A. Arvin (Eds.), *Nelson textbook of pediatrics* (15th ed., pp. 1667-1680). Philadelphia: Saunders.

Paluzzi, R. G. (1995). Respiratory tract infections: Pharyngitis. In K. R. Epstein (Ed.), *Manual of office medicine* (pp. 562-567). Boston: Blackwell Science, 562-567.

Review Questions

1. Epiglottitis is most commonly caused by which of the following?

   a. *Staphylococcus aureus*
   b. *Streptococcus* group A
   c. *Haemophilus influenzae*
   d. RSV

2. Which of the following symptoms are more indicative of pharyngitis in an infant?

   a. Cough, fever of 101° F, and sore throat
   b. Cough, increased nasal secretions, and vomiting

   c. Rapid onset of fever (101°F), muffled voice, toxic-looking appearance
   d. Excoriated nares

3. Ms. White comes to your clinic with the complaint of sore throat. She denies fever, nausea, vomiting, or diarrhea. During the review of symptoms, Ms. White admits to an itchy vaginal discharge for several weeks. Which of the following diagnostic procedures should be performed?

   a. Throat culture on swab
   b. Throat culture applied to chocolate agar
   c. Throat culture placed in saline solution (wet mount)
   d. Throat culture placed in KOH

4. Which of the following clients would you suspect as having group A streptococcal pharyngitis?

   a. A 6-month-old with fever and barking cough
   b. An 8-year-old with fever and sore throat
   c. A 29-year-old mother of three with sore throat, low-grade fever, without exudate
   d. A 50-year-old man with complaint of sore throat

5. Which of the following clients should be referred to the ear, nose, and throat (ENT) clinic?

   a. Child with viral pharyngitis for the second time in 1 year
   b. Child with group A streptococcal pharyngitis for the fourth time in 1 year
   c. Adult woman with group A streptococcal pharyngitis for the first time in her life time
   d. Adult man with a sore throat, fever, rhinitis, and productive cough

Answers and Rationales

1. *Answers:* **c** (analysis/diagnosis)
   Rationale: The most common bacteria associated with epiglottitis is Haemophilus influenzae (Hall & McBride, 1994).

2. *Answer:* **d** (assessment)
   Rationale: Infants often have unusual presenting signs and symptoms for pharyngitis; one of the most common signs is excoriated nares. Answer c is associated with epiglottitis, which is rare in an infant. Answers a and b could be associated with the common cold and pharyngitis (Bamberger & Jackson, 1994).

3. *Answer:* **b** (analysis/diagnosis)
   Rationale: The female client who has a sore throat without symptoms consistent with a bacterial or a viral throat infection and also has a vaginal discharge should be evaluated for the presence of an STD. In this case, the client should be tested for *Neisseria gonorrhoeae* by application of a throat culture specimen to a chocolate agar. A culture swab is used for culture and sensitivity studies. Wet mount and KOH studies generally are not useful throat culture media (Koster & Barker, 1995).

4. *Answer:* **b** (analysis/diagnosis)
   Rationale: The age group that most commonly contracts group A streptococcal pharyngitis is 5 to 10 years. Answer a is

the most common presentation for croup. The 29-year-old woman does not have exudate, which suggests streptococcal pharyngitis. The 50-year-old man is not in the population age group consistent with streptococcal pharyngitis (Hall & McBride, 1994).

5. *Answer:* b (implementation/plan)

Rationale: Clients with recurrent group A streptococcal pharyngitis should have an ENT referral for possible tonsillectomy. The others do not need referral unless the present condition persists despite treatment (Berman & Schmitt, 1995).

EPISTAXIS   *Denise Robinson*

OVERVIEW
Definition

Epistaxis, or nosebleed, is a hemorrhage from the nose.

Incidence

- Epistaxis is the most common ENT emergency.
- Nosebleeds are rare in infancy, common in childhood, and decrease in adolescence.
- Incidence increases during winter.
- More common in morning, with a smaller peak in the afternoon (Manfredini, 2000).

Pathophysiology

Ninety-five percent of nosebleeds are caused by rupture of small vessels that overlie the anterior nasal septum; they are usually self-limiting. The most common cause of epistaxis is trauma and inflammation. Trauma includes nose picking, foreign bodies, and blunt trauma to the nose. Inflammation can be the result of rhinitis, sneezing, blowing the nose forcibly, dryness from air that is not well-humidified, and inhalant drugs and drug abuse.

- Five percent originate in the posterior cavity and can be life-threatening because they are more brisk. The condition is often accompanied by HTN, which is not thought to be the cause but is probably an anxiety reaction.
- Ninety percent of epistaxis in children are anterior nosebleeds that originate in the Kiesselbach's triangle of the anterior portion of the nares.

Cause

- Nasal trauma such as FB, forceful blowing, blunt trauma, or penetrating trauma (e.g., a finger)
- URI
- Irritants (over-the-counter [OTC] nose sprays, cocaine)
- Mucosal drying in low humidity
- Septal deviation
- Vascular abnormalities
- Children: usually FB
- Older adults: usually spontaneous from dry or thinned mucosa

ASSESSMENT: SUBJECTIVE/HISTORY
History of Present Illness

- Ask about time of onset (usually spontaneous onset or trauma), which nostril it started in, and whether blood ran out of the nose or down throat. (Anterior bleeding exits primarily from the anterior nares. Posterior bleeding presents with blood in mouth, nasopharynx, and nares.)
- Ask about bleeding in gums, urine, or stool.
- Ask about possible obstruction and FB.

Past Medical History

- Ask about previous epistaxis (if so, what controlled it?) or bleeding.
- Ask about concurrent sinus problems, URI, and allergies.
- Inquire about blood disorders, including anemia, leukemia, clotting abnormalities, thrombocytopenia, or platelet dysfunction.
- Inquire about liver disease.
- Look for presence of HTN.

Past Surgical History

Inquire about any previous ENT procedures.

Medication History

- Anticoagulants, including aspirin use and NSAIDs
- Nasal sprays

Psychosocial History

- Ask about smoking habit.
- Inquire about drug abuse/use, especially cocaine.

Family History

- Inquire about family history of blood or bleeding disorders, including familial hereditary telangiectasia.
- Frequently a family history of childhood nosebleeds is reported.

ASSESSMENT: OBJECTIVE/ PHYSICAL EXAMINATION
Physical Examination

Focused physical examination is appropriate.
- *General:* Look for signs of anxiety, fear, hypovolemia, shock.

E

- *Vital signs:* Include orthostatics and oxygen saturation.
- *HEENT:* Typical examination includes examination of anterior septum with nasal speculum. Client should be sitting upright with head in "sniffing" position, not with neck extension. Remove all clots and look for bleeding site, signs of septal erosion (cocaine), trauma, and color of mucosa. In children, the Kiesselbach's triangle reveals a red, raw surface with fresh clots or old crusts. Check posterior pharynx for signs of bloody drainage. Check buccal mucosa for bleeding. FB in the nose presents with unilateral, foul-smelling, purulent nasal drainage.
- *Children:* Look for FB.

Diagnostic Procedures

- CBC if bleeding is prolonged or if orthostatic vital signs changes are present.
- Coagulation studies if taking anticoagulants, prolonged bleeding, orthostatic changes.
- U/A and stool guaiac if history of bleeding.
- Type and cross-match packed red blood cells if necessary.

DIAGNOSIS

Differential diagnoses may include the following:

- Anterior epistaxis (primary versus secondary) may be present.
- Posterior epistaxis may be present.
- Clotting abnormality may be present.
- Septal perforation may be present.
- Children: usually secondary to trauma or FB.
- Older adults: Usually primary epistaxis is from dry mucosa, but it may indicate a vascular problem.

THERAPEUTIC PLAN

- Reassure client.
- Treat definitively.
- Anterior nosebleeds account for most nosebleeds and should respond to the application of pressure to the anterior nasal septum. Tilt the head slightly forward. Apply pressure for 10 to 15 minutes.
- Ice may be applied to the nose and lips or around the neck to promote vasoconstriction.
- If bleeding, try instilling 1 or 2 sprays of phenylephrine (Neo-Synephrine).
- If bleeding continues, topical 4% cocaine or cauterization (silver nitrate) is indicated.
- If bleeding persists, nostril must be packed with 1/2-inch iodoform gauze lubricated with petroleum jelly or bacitracin or with commercial nose packs. The packing should remain in place for 3 days.

Posterior Nosebleeds

These bleeds typically do not respond to cauterization and anterior packing. Posterior packing consists of passing a rubber catheter through the nose into the oropharynx and out of the mouth, where a sterile gauze pack is tied to the catheter. The catheter is then withdrawn through the nose, and the pack is positioned and secured. A Foley catheter may also be used through the nose and into the oropharynx. When it is inflated and under traction, it creates hemostasis and controls the bleeding. Posterior packing should remain in place for 3 to 5 days.

Antibiotics

If packing is used, place client on a short course of prophylactic antibiotics.

Client Education

- Avoid vigorous exercise and blowing nose for several days.
- Avoid hot or spicy foods and tobacco (may cause vasodilation).
- Avoid chronic use of nasal sprays; use petroleum jelly or bacitracin for dry mucosa.
- Children: Instruct parents to keep small objects out of reach. If children are old enough, instruct them not to put anything smaller than their elbow in their nose.

Prevention

A bedside humidifier, petroleum jelly applied to the inside of the nose, and the reduction of trauma from picking or blowing the nose will help reduce the incidence of episodic anterior nosebleeds.

Referral

- Return to clinic or emergency department if epistaxis recurs or signs of infection appear.
- If anterior packing is used, return to clinic in 2 to 4 days for removal.
- If posterior packing is used, return to clinic in 3 to 5 days for removal. Posterior bleeds may require hospitalization secondary to the risk of hemorrhage or hypoxemia from the nasal packing.
- Referral may be needed to remove an FB from the nose.
- Referral to an otolaryngologist is indicated in the case of a suspected intranasal tumor.
- If a blood disorder is found, referral to a hematologist is appropriate.

EVALUATION/FOLLOW-UP

- Reassess vital signs and check for hemostasis before dismissing.
- Any recurrence of epistaxis is an indication for ENT referral.

COMPLICATIONS

Shock if the bleeding cannot be controlled.

REFERENCES

Barbarito, C. (1999). Hypertension-induced epistaxis. *American Journal of Nursing, 98*(2), 48.

Jackler, R., & Kaplan, M. (1996). Ear, nose and throat. In L. Tierney, Jr., S. McPhee, & M. Papadakis (Eds.), *Current medical diagnosis and treatment* (pp. 198-199). Norwalk, CT: Appleton & Lange.

Manfredini, R., Portaluppi, F., Salmi, R., Martini, A., & Gallerani, M. (2000). Circadian variation in onset of epistaxis: Analysis of hospital admissions. *British Medical Journal, 321*(7269), 1112.

Roberts, J., & Hedges, J. (1998). *Clinical procedures in emergency medicine* (3rd ed.). Philadelphia: W. B. Saunders.

Robinson, D., Kidd, P., & Rogers, K. (2000). *Primary care across the lifespan.* St. Louis: Mosby.

Review Questions

1. The proper way to examine a client with epistaxis is with the client in which of the following positions?

   a. Sitting upright in the "sniffing" position
   b. With the neck fully extended
   c. Lying supine
   d. With one naris occluded, and then the opposite naris occluded

2. When assessing a client with epistaxis, the NP should ask about which of the following?

   a. Family history
   b. Medication history
   c. Immunizations
   d. Sexual history

3. When caring for a child with epistaxis, the NP should assess which of the following?

   a. Growth patterns
   b. Presence of an FB
   c. Blood pressure
   d. Signs of abuse

4. A client returns for a second episode of epistaxis in a week period. The NP should do all of the following, *except:*

   a. Refer the client to a specialist.
   b. Perform a hematocrit and hemoglobin test.
   c. Increase the dose of topical cocaine used.
   d. Repack the nose.

5. Evidence of effective client education for a client successfully treated for epistaxis is when the client states that he will do which of the following?

   a. Avoid cold beverages.
   b. Not play racquetball for 3 days.
   c. Use saline nose drops faithfully.
   d. Avoid caffeine.

6. A child is brought to the clinic with a nosebleed. Which of the following objective descriptions is consistent with an anterior nosebleed?

   a. Blood seen in oropharynx
   b. Red, raw Kiesselbach triangle
   c. Unilateral, foul-smelling nasal discharge
   d. Clear discharge from both nares

7. Preventive measures for epistaxis include all but which of the following?

   a. Use Neo-Synephrine nose drops on a daily basis to promote vasoconstriction.
   b. Use petroleum jelly to help moisturize the nose.
   c. Use a humidifier by the bedside.
   d. Stop nose picking.

8. A client comes into the emergency department complaining of a severe nosebleed. He has tried to apply pressure at home, but it has not worked. He complains of blood in his mouth and running down the back of his throat. This history is most consistent with which type of nosebleed?

   a. Anterior
   b. Posterior
   c. Middle turbinate
   d. Superior turbinate

Answers and Rationales

1. *Answer:* **a** (assessment)
   Rationale: Placing the client supine or with the neck fully extended can occlude the airway. Having one naris occluded while examining the other naris also diminishes air intake (Jackler & Kaplan, 1996).

2. *Answer:* **b** (assessment)
   Rationale: The use of aspirin or aspirin products increases the risk for epistaxis. The other information is less relevant (Jackler & Kaplan, 1996).

3. *Answer:* **b** (assessment)
   Rationale: Children usually experience epistaxis from nose picking, traumatic injury (e.g., fall), or placement of an FB. The abused child rarely has a nose injury. HTN may produce epistaxis in the adult (Jackler & Kaplan, 1996).

4. *Answer:* **c** (evaluation)
   Rationale: The client should be referred to an ENT specialist. A hemoglobin and hematocrit or CBC should be performed to determine blood loss. The nose may need to be repacked. The dose of cocaine used for vasoconstriction remains the same (Jackler & Kaplan, 1996).

5. *Answer:* **b** (evaluation)
   Rationale: Vigorous exercise should be avoided. Hot, spicy foods should be avoided. Nasal sprays should not be used. Caffeine is not significant (Jackler & Kaplan, 1996).

6. *Answer:* **b** (assessment)
   Rationale: In children, bleeding is usually from the Kiesselbach's triangle. It can be seen on examination as a red, raw area with clots present (Robinson, 2000).

7. *Answer:* **a** (analysis/diagnosis)
   Rationale: Using Neo-Synephrine nose drops does produce vasoconstriction but is not recommended for use in

E

preventing a nosebleed. It causes rebound congestion when used for more than 3 days. All other answers are helpful to prevent nosebleeds (Robinson, 2000).

8. **Answer: b** (analysis/diagnosis)
   Rationale: Posterior nosebleeds are more severe, unlikely to be stopped by constriction, and typically cause bleeding into the mouth, oropharynx, and nares. (Robinson, 2000).

ERECTILE DYSFUNCTION   *Pamela Kidd*

OVERVIEW
Definition

Erectile dysfunction (ED) is the inability to achieve and maintain an erection of the penis with sufficient rigidity (tumescence) to allow for sexual intercourse. It may be chronic, occasional, or situational.

Incidence

- Fifty-two percent of men between the ages of 40 and 70 experience ED (Moskowitz, 2000).
- Prevalence is related to decade of life (e.g., prevalence in 40 year olds is 40%).
- Erectile dysfunction can affect any male after puberty.
- Chronic erectile dysfunction can affect younger men as well as older men.
- Treatment can restore sexual function in approximately 95% of cases.
- Eighty-five percent of cases of chronic erectile dysfunction result from physical causes, although many cases have coinciding psychologic factors.

Pathophysiology

- Vascular problems: arteriosclerosis, HTN, coronary artery disease, peripheral arterial insufficiency, chronic renal insufficiency, or renal failure
- Endocrine disorders: diabetes mellitus (most frequent cause of organic origin [Doerfler, 1999]), thyroid disease, adrenal disorders, hyperprolactinemia, hypogonadism, and pituitary disorders
- Neurologic disorders: brain or spinal cord injuries, Alzheimer's disease, Parkinson's disease, multiple sclerosis, and epilepsy
- Psychologic disorders: affective, psychotic, and personality disorders
- Oncologic radiation treatments
- Prostate, bladder, rectum, and colon surgery
- Alcohol, cigarettes, illegal drugs, and substance abuse
- Penile deformities and prostate infections
- Congenital syndromes

Factors Increasing Susceptibility
- Chronic illness
- Delayed sexual maturity
- Use of medications to treat chronic illness

Protective Factors. Lifestyle (no alcohol, tobacco, or street drugs/cocaine, amphetamines, barbiturates, or opiates).

ASSESSMENT: SUBJECTIVE/HISTORY
History of Present Illness

- Inquire about onset and duration of symptoms, including libido, the ability to achieve and maintain an erection, orgasm, ejaculation, and satisfaction with sex life.
- Inquire about current sexual relationships and past sexual experiences and behaviors.
- Inquire about concurrent medical conditions, including endocrine disorders, vascular problems, neurologic problems, and psychiatric problems.
- Inquire about smoking, alcohol, and substance abuse.
- Try to differentiate psychogenic from organic cause:
  - Psychogenic: Can obtain an erection with masturbation, different partners, and/or erotic stimuli; presence of nocturnal or morning erections, complains of intermittent ED.
  - Organic: ED is persistent.

Past Medical History

- Inquire about past genitourinary surgeries.
- Inquire about prior pelvic trauma, bicycling, or horseback riding.
- Inquire about sexual development and secondary sex characteristics.

Medication History

Inquire about all current prescription and OTC medications. Many of these can cause erectile dysfunction. Beta-blockers are most often implicated (Doerfler, 1999). Cimetidine, digoxin, antidepressants, and diuretics may also produce ED (Moskowitz, 2000).

Family History

Not relevant.

Dietary History

Not relevant.

ASSESSMENT: OBJECTIVE/PHYSICAL EXAMINATION
Physical Examination

- Assess vital signs, including BP, to rule out hypotension, effects of medications.
- Assess body habitus and secondary sex characteristics to rule out pituitary tumor, hypogonadism.

- Assess for gynecomastia to rule out pituitary tumor.
- Assess abdomen and inguinal area for scars from past genitourinary surgeries to rule out hernia, pelvic/perineal trauma.
- Assess genitourinary–penis, scrotum, testes–to rule out hydrocele, Peyronie's disease.
- Assess prostate and anal sphincter tone to rule out sacral nerve impingement.
- Assess femoral and lower extremity pulses to rule out diabetic vasculopathy and atherosclerosis.
- Perform a neurologic examination of perianal sensation and lower extremities to rule out a problem with spinal cord/sacral reflex circuit.

Diagnostic Procedures

- High serum glucose may indicate diabetes.
- Abnormal lipid profile may indicate atherosclerosis.
- Low testosterone level may indicate hypogonadism.
- High TSH level may indicate hypothyroidism.
- If serum prolactin is increased, consider pituitary tumor.
- More invasive testing (e.g., penile doppler ultrasound, penile angiography) is not considered first-line treatment.

DIAGNOSIS

See Table 3-29. See pathophysiology section for the many causes of ED.

THERAPEUTIC PLAN

Nonpharmacologic Treatment

- Underlying medical conditions, such as diabetes, thyroid disease, coronary heart disease, or renal disease, should be treated.
- Sex therapy or psychotherapy may be indicated for ED of psychogenic origin or dysfunctional intimate relationships.
- Vacuum constrictive devices are appropriate for clients with venous disorders of the penis. The device draws the penis into an erect state by inducing a vacuum within a cylinder. Once an adequate erection is achieved, a constrictive rubber band is placed around the proximal end of the penis to prevent loss of erection. The cylinder is removed before intercourse.

Surgery

- Penile prostheses may be directly implanted into the corporal body of the penis. The protheses vary and may be rigid, malleable, hinged, or inflatable. Sensation, ejaculation, or orgasm generally is not altered. Penile implants are irreversible and are often considered a last resort.
- Clients with arterial disorders or venous occlusions may be candidates for vascular reconstruction.

Pharmacologic Treatment

- Consider substituting different medications for managing chronic illness (e.g., ACE inhibitor instead of beta-blocker for HTN).
- Androgen deficiency can be treated with testosterone injections 200 mg IM every 2 to 3 weeks.
- Sildenafil (Viagra) 50 mg PO 1 hour before sexual intercourse. May be taken 30 minutes to 4 hours before intercourse. Dose may be adjusted to the maximum dose of 100 mg per day or decreased to 25 mg per day. *Viagra is contraindicated in clients who take concurrent organic nitrates and should not be prescribed to any client who may have access to nitrates in any form, at any time, for any reason.* Success rate is 66%. Side effects are headache, flushing. If client is taking a cytochrome P-450 isoenzyme 3A4 inhibitor (see Appendix for a list of these drugs) (e.g., cimetidine, erythromycin, ketoconazole, mibefradil), use a smaller dosage because clearance of sildenafil is decreased.
- Intraurethral alprostadil (MUSE) penile suppository side effects are penile pain and hypotension. Inconsistent efficacy has been reported.
- Injection therapy consists of the direct injection of vasoactive substances into the penis. A tuberculin syringe is used, and the injection site is the base and lateral aspect of the penis. Complications include dizziness, hypotension, nausea, pain, fibrosis, infection, and priapism.

TABLE **3-29**   Differential Diagnoses of Male Sexual Dysfunction

Loss of libido	May indicate an androgen deficiency secondary to hypothalamic, pituitary, or testicular disease. Serum testosterone and gonadotropin levels should be assessed.
Loss of erections	May result from arterial, venous, neurogenic, or psychogenic causes. Can be secondary to many medications. Occasional impotence despite nocturnal or early morning erections indicates a probable psychogenic cause. A gradual loss of erections over time suggests an organic cause.
Loss of emission	Retrograde ejaculation may occur as a result of surgery, medications, or diabetes. May be secondary to an androgen deficiency.
Loss of orgasm	Usually psychogenic if libido and erection are intact.
Premature ejaculation	Usually anxiety related.

Client Education

- ED is not necessarily a part of aging.
- Spouses and/or sexual partners should be included in the treatment plan.
- Smoking and alcohol cessation should be recommended.
- Encourage couples to discuss sex, their likes and dislikes, show each other how they want to be touched, relax, and slow down to allow time for arousal.

Consultation/Referral

Consultation with a physician, psychiatrist, urologist, plastic surgeon, vascular surgeon, endocrinologist, or neurologist may be indicated depending on the cause of ED.

EVALUATION/FOLLOW-UP

Depends on cause, severity, and client motivation. Follow-up every 6 to 12 months is recommended once ED is treated (Padma-Nathan & Forrest, 2000).

COMPLICATIONS

- Infertility
- Social isolation and poor self-esteem
- Dysfunctional sexual/intimate relationships

REFERENCES

Albaugh, J. (1999). Erectile dysfunction: Newer treatment options don't reduce need for education, counseling. *ADVANCE for Nurse Practitioners, 7*(4), 43-44.

Doerfler, E. (1999). Male erectile dysfunction: A guide for clinical management. *Journal of the American Academy of Nurse Practitioners, 11*(3), 117-123.

Dunn, S. A. (1998). *Primary care consultant* (pp. 198-199). St. Louis: Mosby.

Gerchufsky, M. (1995). Impotence: The problem men don't talk about. *ADVANCE for Nurse Practitioners, 3*(3), 13-16.

Moskowitz, M. (2000). The challenges of diagnosing erectile dysfunction in the primary care setting. *Nurse Practitioner*, June (Suppl.), 1-3.

Padma-nathan, H., & Forrest, C. (2000). Diagnosis and treatment of erectile dysfunction: The process of care model. *Nurse Practitioner*, June (Suppl.), 4-10.

Rogers, K. (2001). Impotence. In D. Robinson, P. Kidd, & K. Rogers (Eds.), *Primary care across the lifespan*. St. Louis: Mosby.

Review Questions

1. A client presents with erectile dysfunction. Which of the following should the NP assess in attempting to determine an organic cause?

- **a.** History of diabetes mellitus
- **b.** Caffeine intake
- **c.** Repair of inguinal hernia
- **d.** OTC use of aspirin

2. Which of the following drugs may induce erectile dysfunction?

- **a.** Verapamil
- **b.** Glucophage (Metformin)
- **c.** Atenolol (Tenormin)
- **d.** Ergotamine

3. Which of the following indicates a psychogenic cause of erectile dysfunction?

- **a.** Gradual loss of erections over time
- **b.** Nocturnal emission
- **c.** Loss of libido
- **d.** Erection can be achieved with masturbation

4. Which of the following diagnostic tests should be used as first-line treatment to determine the cause of erectile dysfunction?

- **a.** Penile Doppler ultrasound study
- **b.** Penile angiography
- **c.** TSH level
- **d.** U/A

5. Which of the following statements indicates that the client understands how to manage premature ejaculations?

- **a.** "Take 7.5 mg buspirone orally as needed before intercourse."
- **b.** "Take 50 mg Sildenafil (Viagra) 1 hour before intercourse."
- **c.** "Use an alprostadil penile suppository before sexual activity."
- **d.** "Urinate before sexual activity."

6. Which of the following clients should *not* be prescribed Sildenafil for erectile dysfunction?

- **a.** Hypertensive client taking a beta-blocker
- **b.** Client with angina taking nitroglycerin prn
- **c.** Diabetic client taking Glucotrol
- **d.** Hypothyroid client taking Synthroid

Answers and Rationales

1. *Answer:* **a** (assessment)
Rationale: Diabetes is the most common cause of organic-related erectile dysfunction. Caffeine and aspirin intake or use is not related to erectile dysfunction. Prostate, bladder, rectum, and colon surgery are related, but not hernia repair.

2. *Answer:* **c** (assessment)
Rationale: Beta-blockers are most often associated with erectile dysfunction.

3. *Answer:* **d** (analysis/diagnosis)
Rationale: Gradual loss of erections over time is associated with an organic cause. Nocturnal erection but not emission may be associated with psychogenic ED. Obtaining an erection with stimulation is associated with a psychogenic cause. Libido is not affected in psychogenic-related erectile dysfunction.

4. *Answer:* **c** (analysis/diagnosis)
Rationale: Penile angiography and ultrasound are not first-line diagnostic tests. A U/A is not indicated. A TSH level may

indicate hypothyroidism, which is an organic cause of erectile dysfunction.

5. *Answer:* a (evaluation)

Rationale: Premature ejaculations are usually related to anxiety. Buspirone decreases anxiety. Urination is not related to premature ejaculations. Sildenafil and alprostadil are used to treat loss of erection, not premature ejaculation.

6. *Answer:* b (implementation/plan)

Rationale: Sildenafil is contraindicated in clients who take concurrent organic nitrates and should not be prescribed to any client who may have access to nitrates in any form, at any time, for any reason.

FAILURE TO THRIVE *Denise Robinson*

OVERVIEW

Definition

Failure to thrive (FTT) is defined as the client's weight consistently measuring below the third percentile on standardized growth charts, or a drop in weight across two major growth lines in 6 months or less. FTT is usually differentiated as organic or nonorganic. Organic failure refers to growth failure related to a physiological cause; nonorganic failure to thrive refers to an unexplained growth failure—often there is an alteration in the parent-child relationship, resulting in difficulties in feeding and absorption.

Incidence

- FTT occurs in children younger than 5 years of age; average age at diagnosis is 16 weeks.
- Approximately 5% to 10% of all low-birthweight children are identified as FTT.
- Approximately 3% to 5% of all pediatric hospitalizations are for evaluation of FTT.
- Approximately 70% of FTT cases have nonorganic causes (Box 3-12).

Pathophysiology

FTT occurs when caloric intake is not sufficient to meet the metabolic needs of the child. This lack of adequate nutrition often results in developmental delays, delayed growth, decreased immune response, cognitive delays, and academic failures.

Factors Increasing Susceptibility. Several parental stressors predispose a child to FTT. These stressors include the following:

- Poverty
- Little social support
- Depression or other mental health problems
- Low intelligence
- Substance abuse
- Immaturity
- Preterm or sick newborns or those with physical deformities
- Parents who have excessive concerns about the infant's fat intake or obesity
- Abnormal feeding practices

Protective Factors

- Parents with good parenting skills, good interpersonal skills with their infant, and low stress place their infants at low risk for FTT.
- Infants who are identified as being adaptable, who are full-term, responsive, easy to comfort, and who feed easily are at low risk for FTT.

ASSESSMENT: SUBJECTIVE/HISTORY

History of Present Illness

- Obtain history of child vomiting frequently, having a decreased appetite, having a poor suck reflex, having aversive behavior, or having other trouble with feeding.
- Elicit a thorough feeding history, including the following:
  - Type of formula/food; how mixed if concentrate
  - How often fed, how much taken
  - Problems with sucking, swallowing, regurgitation
  - If breastfed, problems with milk supply or fat content
- Review stool patterns.
- Ask about possible parasite exposure.

Box 3-12 Causes of Failure to Thrive

IMPROPER FEEDING (50%-90%)	OTHER CAUSES (10%-50%)
Economic: 10%-40%	Hypothyroidism
Education (lack of understanding of feeding techniques, adequate diet, etc.): 10%-40%	Cystic fibrosis
	Subdural hematoma
	Celiac disease
	Mental retardation, unspecified
Psychologic (poor parent-child interaction, emotional or maternal deprivation): 30%-40%	Brain tumors
	Chronic liver disease
	Congenital heart disease
Feeding intolerance: <5%	Ulcerative colitis

From Barnes, L: Failure to thrive. In Hoekelman R, editor: *Primary pediatric care*, ed 2, St Louis, 1997, Mosby.

F

Symptoms

- Aversive behaviors, particularly with respect to eating
- Poor suck reflex, turns away from bottle
- Spits up excessively
- Poor eye contact
- Difficult to cuddle
- Cries or whines frequently
- Difficult to comfort
- Associated symptoms: frequent diarrhea or vomiting

Past Medical History

- Child's birth weight, gestational age
- Prenatal history:
  - Tobacco/drug use by mother
  - Other toxin exposure
  - Presence of human immunodeficiency virus (HIV)
  - Labor/delivery
- Illnesses since birth
- Possible lead exposure
- Food allergies

Dietary History

Elicit 24-hour diet recall; 3- to 7-day recall is best.

Medication History

Maternal medication use or sedation during labor may contribute to FTT.

Family History

- Important to identify heights and weights of parents, grandparents, and siblings.
- Determine family history of malabsorption problems (cystic fibrosis, lactose intolerance, other inborn errors of metabolism).
- Determine childhood history of parents (parents who give a history of being poorly parented are at high risk of having FTT infants).

Psychosocial History

Assess parent/infant bonding. Determine if mother's illness, separation of infant from mother, financial stressors, or other factors that impair attachment behavior are present.

ASSESSMENT: OBJECTIVE/PHYSICAL EXAMINATION

Physical Examination

A complete physical examination should be done, with particular attention to the following:

- General appearance: Measure height/weight, head circumference; may see a gradually declining height/length (infants fall off the growth chart with respect to weight; height is near normal until late in the disease, and there is no significant change in head circumference).
- Head, eyes, ears, nose, and throat (HEENT): Assess for oral defects, thyroid enlargement, status of fontanelles.
- Cardiovascular (CV): Listen for murmurs.
- Gastrointestinal (GI): Note whether abdomen is protuberant.
- Musculoskeletal (MS): Assess for signs of wasting and other evidence of malnourishment (decreased fat pads in cheeks, buttocks waster, poor muscle tone).
- Neurologic: Assess hypotonia, gag and swallow reflexes, muscle strength, sensation, deep tendon reflexes.
- Observe parental/infant interaction.
- Perform Denver Developmental screening to help identify developmental delays.

It is also helpful to observe the feeding of the infant whenever possible (Table 3-30).

TABLE **3-30** Common Findings in Infants with Inorganic Failure to Thrive

AGE (MONTHS)	FINDINGS
0-6	Prematurity
	Neonatal illness or anomaly necessitating early separation
	Feeding difficulties
	Height and weight below third percentile for age
	Unresponsiveness and withdrawal
	Watchfulness, little smiling
	Delayed socialization and vocalization
	Irregular sleep patterns
	Developmental delays
6-12	Absence of stranger anxiety
	Rumination
	No displeasure at separation
	Apathy/passivity
	Delayed milestones, such as sitting and standing
	Muscular hypotonia
12-18	Indifference to caregivers
	Small physical size
	Delayed dentition
	Little vocalization
	Little eye contact
	Intense watchfulness
	Repetitive self-stimulation behavior (rocking, head banging)

Adapted from Silva, F., Needleman, R. (1993). Failure to thrive: Mystery, myth and method. *Contemporary Pediatrics* 10, 114-133.

Diagnostic Procedures

Before a diagnosis of nonorganic FTT is made, diagnostic testing is done to rule out possible organic causes for poor weight gain. Diagnostic tests include the following:

- Complete blood count (CBC)
- Lead level
- Sweat chloride screening
- Renal, liver panel, electrolytes
- Growth hormone
- Albumin
- Calcium phosphate, phosphatase
- Thyroid panel
- Stool samples
- Tuberculosis (TB), HIV

DIAGNOSIS

- Must differentiate physiologic versus nonorganic causes.
- Diagnosis is made based on poor progression on the growth chart (Table 3-31).

THERAPEUTIC PLAN

Pharmacologic Treatment

No drugs are indicated for FTT unless an underlying disease is found.

Nonpharmacologic Treatment

- Every effort should be made to enhance parent/child attachment.
- Parents must be followed closely in the home to observe feeding behaviors and parent-child interaction and to promote bonding.
- The child may need hospitalization to provide for nutritional needs.

Diet

- Increase caloric intake by calculating the amount of kcal/kg/day based on the age of the child. This can be done by dividing the average caloric requirement for age by the child's percentile of median weight for age.
  - 0 to 6 months: 108 kcal/kg/day
  - 6 to 12 months: 98 kcal/kg/day
  - 1 to 3 years: 102 kcal/kg/day

Client Education

- Teach feeding techniques:
  - How to feed without introducing extra air
  - How often to burp
  - Average daily number of ounces of formula needed
  - Types and amount of other food needed
  - Review of how to prepare formula
  - Multiple vitamin with iron
- Teach ways to comfort baby, expected normal baby behaviors, child nutrition, community resources available.
- FTT is a family condition with disruption in normal parent-child bonding; the impact on the family is significant.
- Direct efforts to alter feeding toward all caregivers.
- Ways to strengthen family unity may play a direct role in resolution of the FTT.
- Force feeding is not recommended.

Referral

- Refer to home health/social services if appropriate.
- Refer to Women, Infants, and Children (WIC) if appropriate.
- Refer to nutritionist.
- Child Protective Services may be appropriate if FTT is caused by maternal neglect.

TABLE **3-31**   Why Isn't This Baby Growing?

AGE AT ONSET	DIAGNOSTIC CONSIDERATIONS
IUGR, prematurity	Especially in symmetrical IUGR, consider prenatal infections, congenital syndromes, teratogenic exposures (anticonvulsants, alcohol)
Neonatal (0-3 mo)	Incorrect formula preparation; failed breastfeeding; neglect; poor feeding interactions; metabolic, chromosomal, or anatomic abnormality (less common); GERD; cystic fibrosis
3-6 mo	Underfeeding (possibly associated with poverty), improper formula preparation, milk protein intolerance, oral motor dysfunction, celiac disease, HIV infection, cystic fibrosis, congenital heart disease, GERD
7-12 mo	Autonomy struggles, overly fastidious parent, oral-motor dysfunction, delayed introduction of solids, intolerance of new foods
After 12 mo	Coercive feeding, highly distractible child, distracting environment, acquired illness, new psychosocial stressor (divorce, job loss, new sibling, death in the family)

Adapted from Silva F, Needleman R: Failure to thrive: mystery, myth and method, *Contemp Pediatr* 10:114, 1993; and Bauchner H: Children with special health needs. In Nelson W et al, editors: *Nelson textbook of pediatrics*, ed 15, Philadelphia, 1996, WB Saunders.
GERD, Gastroesophageal reflux disease; *HIV*, human immunodeficiency virus; *IUGR*, intrauterine growth retardation.

- Children with obvious signs of malnutrition or those unresponsive to efforts to increase growth should be evaluated in conjunction with a physician regarding the need for hospitalization.

Prevention

- Good infant-parent bonding is preventative.
- Parenting classes are preventative.

COMPLICATIONS

- Complications associated with treatment failure are possible.
- FTT in the first year of life is ominous.
- Most brain growth occurs in the first 6 months.
- Approximately one third of children with nonorganic FTT are developmentally delayed and have social/emotional problems.

EVALUATION/FOLLOW-UP

- Child with FTT must be followed frequently.
- Although early efforts may be successful, the parent may not be able to carry out these efforts over time.
- High rate of relapse occurs in FTT.
- Follow child weekly and then monthly for several months until child returns to a normal growth curve.

REFERENCES

Frank, D., Silva, M., & Needleman, R. (1993). Failure to thrive: mystery, myth and method. *Contemporary Pediatrics, 10,* 114-133.

Lobo, M., & Barnard, K. (1992). Failure to thrive: a parent-infant interaction perspective. *Journal of Pediatric Nursing, 7,* 251-260.

King, P. (2000). Failure to thrive. In D. Robinson, P. Kidd, & K. Rogers (Eds.), *Primary care across the lifespan.* St. Louis: Mosby, 427-434.

Review Questions

1. Which of the following children might be diagnosed with FTT?
- **a.** A 10-month-old premature infant at 10% on weight chart
- **b.** A 7-month-old with muscle hypotonia and passivity
- **c.** A 15-month-old who weighs 30 pounds
- **d.** A 2-year-old child with limited vocabulary

2. A mother brings her 6-month-old child to be seen. Which of the following historical data is consistent with a diagnosis of FTT?
- **a.** "Marvion is eating well."
- **b.** "Heavenly smiles and is happy."
- **c.** "Lakendra is watching me; she doesn't make sounds or smile."
- **d.** "Steven sits up and grabs at toys."

3. Which of the following are causes of FTT?
- **a.** Improper formula preparation
- **b.** Breastfeeding
- **c.** Divorce
- **d.** Poor parenting skills

4. If a child of 4 months develops FTT, what is the most likely cause?
- **a.** Overfeeding
- **b.** Decreased stimulation
- **c.** Underfeeding
- **d.** Decreased iron

5. To avoid FTT, which of the following recommendations is *not* appropriate to give to the parents regarding feeding?
- **a.** Offer finger foods.
- **b.** Force feeding increases intake.
- **c.** Limit junk foods.
- **d.** Eat with your child whenever possible.

6. Which of the following is the first change seen in FTT?
- **a.** Weight
- **b.** Height
- **c.** Head circumference
- **d.** Weight for height

7. Which of the following indices indicates FTT?
- **a.** Change of 1 percentage group (75th to 50th)
- **b.** Loss of 5 pounds
- **c.** Change of 2 percentage groups (75th to 25th)
- **d.** Mismatch of weight and height

8. Once an infant is diagnosed with FTT, how often should follow-up occur?
- **a.** Every 6 months
- **b.** Every 3 to 4 days
- **c.** Every year
- **d.** Every 2 months

Answers and Rationales

1. *Answer:* **b** (assessment)
Rationale: Symptoms of FTT include hypotonia and passivity (King, 2000).

2. *Answer:* **c** (assessment)
Rationale: Symptoms of FTT at 6 months include watchfulness, delayed socialization, and vocalization (Frank, Silva, & Needlman, 1993).

3. *Answer:* **a** (assessment)
Rationale: Improper formula preparation leads to FTT in 50% to 90% of cases. Although poor parenting skills can contribute to FTT, improper mixing of the formula leads to the physical symptoms of FTT (King, 2000).

4. *Answer:* **c** (analysis/diagnosis)
Rationale: The most likely cause of FTT in a child is when the parents do not offer enough food to meet the infant's increased nutritional needs (Frank, Silva, & Needlman, 1993).

5. *Answer:* **b** (implementation/plan)
Rationale: Force feeding, bribing, or cajoling to help the child eat will backfire and is not recommended to treat FTT (Frank, Silva, & Needlman, 1993).

6. *Answer:* **a** (analysis/diagnosis)
   Rationale: The first change seen in FTT is in weight; later height and head circumference may be affected if FTT continues (Frank, Silva, & Needlman, 1993).

7. *Answer:* **c** (analysis/diagnosis)
   Rationale: A change of 2 percentiles (e.g., from 50th to 10th) is indicative of FTT (Frank, Silva, & Needlman, 1993).

8. *Answer:* **b** (evaluation)
   Rationale: Follow-up should occur frequently to monitor the infant's weight closely. Initially follow-up should be every 3 to 4 days and then weekly until normal growth is established (Frank, Silva, & Needlman, 1993).

FATIGUE   *Cheryl Pope Kish*

OVERVIEW
Definition

Fatigue is a sensitive but nonspecific indicator of underlying medical or psychological problems or a physiologic response to overexertion or deficient rest and sleep. Fatigue can be classified as physiologic, acute, or chronic. *Physiologic fatigue* is that normal expected tiredness associated with exertion, inadequate rest, or poor nutritional status. *Acute fatigue* is a normal or expected tiredness that is intermittent in nature, lasting less than 6 months that is not responsive to bed rest. *Chronic fatigue* is unusual and extreme tiredness that has a cumulative effect and lasts longer than 6 months.

Incidence

- Fatigue is a common problem seen in primary care; as a chief complaint, it accounts for 1% to 7% of visits to primary care providers and is within the top 10 of chief complaints voiced in primary care.
- For chronic fatigue syndrome (CFS), the prevalence rate is 4 to 10 per 100,000 persons older than 18.
- CFS is more prevalent in women than men by 3:1; why the prevalence is greater for women is unknown.

ASSESSMENT: SUBJECTIVE/HISTORY
History of Present Illness

When the client presents with a complaint of fatigue, ask what they mean when they say "fatigued." Are they referring to physical fatigue consistent with overexertion, poor physical conditioning, sleep deficits, or mental fatigue associated with emotional stress? Determine when the fatigue is most noted and how it changes during the course of a day. Ask about the duration and inquire about how the fatigue is affecting their activities of daily living (ADLs) and work habits or their school performance, leisure activity, and relationships. (Functional fatigue is present on awakening and may actually improve during the course of the day. Fatigue that increases over the course of the day, without unusual activity, and abates with rest is more likely to be organic in cause.)

Review the health and lifestyle habits, including sleep and rest patterns that might contribute to fatigue. Ask about associated, aggravating, and ameliorating factors.

In women of childbearing age, determine the last menstrual period (LMP) and method of contraception. Fatigue may be among the first indicators of pregnancy. Ask about recent childbearing. Postpartum fatigue is common for at least 6 weeks after delivery, and often much longer. Inquire about the activity change or differences in play in children because this can be a manifestation of fatigue.

Determine if the client is experiencing the clinical manifestations of depression, has experienced losses, or shows evidence of low self-esteem. Assess for suicide ideation or intent.

An instrument for quantifying fatigue, such as the Piper Fatigue Scale, may be helpful in understanding the subjective findings. The Beck Depression Inventory is useful in assessing depression. Inquire about anxiety or persistent nervousness or life conflict that may be affecting rest and sleep.

Symptoms

Fatigue seldom presents as an isolated symptom; other subjective and objective features increase the index of suspicion of a cause of fatigue. Consequently, a complete and careful review of systems is necessary to determine if the client has symptoms of any of these diseases that cause fatigue (Box 3-13).

Past Medical History

Inquire about a history of anemia, rheumatic fever, mononucleosis, heart murmur or other problems, recurrent urinary tract infection (UTI), liver disease, substance abuse, depression, or anxiety. Determine if there been exposure to TB, hepatitis, or HIV. Has there been travel-related exposure to parasitic or endemic infections? Is there a history of sleep disorders? Has there been a recent weight gain or loss?

Medication History

Ask about both prescription and over-the-counter (OTC) drugs. Antihypertensive agents, drugs with anticholinergic effects, antidepressants, and antihistamine drugs may cause fatigue. Determine if the client is taking sedatives for sleep or has used any other medications to attempt self-treatment.

F

Box 3-13   Common Conditions Presenting with Complaints of Chronic Fatigue

PSYCHOLOGIC
Depression
Anxiety
Somatization disorder

ENDOCRINE
Hypothyroidism
Diabetes mellitus
Pituitary insufficiency
Hyperparathyroidism
Hypercalcemia
Addison's disease
Chronic kidney failure
Liver failure

HEMATOLOGIC
Anemia

NEOPLASTIC
Cancer (especially pancreatic cancer)

INFECTIOUS
Bacterial endocarditis
Tuberculosis
Mononucleosis
Hepatitis
Parasitic disease
HIV
Cytomegalovirus

CARDIOPULMONARY
Chronic congestive heart failure
Chronic obstructive pulmonary disease

CONNECTIVE TISSUE
Rheumatoid disease

OTHER DISEASE THAT AFFECTS NORMAL SLEEP
Sleep apnea
Esophageal reflux

Family History

A family history of chronic health problems should be elicited. Certain anemias (e.g., sickle cell anemia) and autoimmune diseases (e.g., lupus) have familial tendencies.

Psychosocial History

Psychosocial assessment provides helpful evidence for evaluating fatigue. Assess the following:

- Sleep patterns and bedtime routines; napping to have energy to make it through normal daily activities (suggests an organic cause of chronic fatigue)
- Occupation: work routines, requirements, schedule, shift work
- Past or current substance abuse
- Support networks
- Sexual behavior associated with risk
- Exercise patterns and leisure activities
- Usual coping skills
- Life changes within the current year, including significant losses

Dietary History

- Poor nutrition or inadequate protein intake can lead to muscular fatigue with activity.
- Evaluate a 24-hour dietary recall for both weekdays and weekends.

ASSESSMENT: OBJECTIVE/PHYSICAL EXAMINATION
Physical Examination

A complete physical examination is indicated for a chief complaint of fatigue to discover findings that provide a high suspicion of medical problems. A mental status assessment should be included.

Diagnostic Procedures

The physical examination focuses on localizing findings that support one differential over another because fatigue is associated with many possibilities. Appropriate first-level tests with a chief complaint of fatigue include CBC with differential, erythrocyte sedimentation rate (ESR), albumin, blood urea nitrogen (BUN) level, creatinine level, transaminase level, thyroid-stimulating hormone (TSH) or thyroxine level, urinalysis, serum or urine pregnancy test (if indicated), and blood glucose level. If lymphadenopathy coexists with fatigue, a heterophile test, HIV screen, and hepatitis profile should be added. A Lyme titer is appropriate, with exposure. Antinuclear antibody (ANA) and rheumatoid factor (RF) tests are appropriate with arthralgias. With abnormal results, a search for cause continues.

Clients at high risk should have syphilis, HIV, and TB tests, with exposure. If client is at geographic risk, a Lyme titer may be helpful.

Perform a mammogram, Pap smear, fecal occult blood test, and sigmoidoscopy if these tests have not been performed recently and are appropriate to the age of the client.

It is unnecessary to order a test for Epstein-Barr virus, which was once considered a causative agent for CFS; it is no longer considered a factor.

DIAGNOSIS

Differential diagnoses include the following:

- Anemia
- Thyroid dysfunction

- Adrenal gland dysfunction
- Heart or lung disease
- Liver disease
- Diabetes mellitus
- Tuberculosis
- Opportunistic infection
- Autoimmune disease (rheumatoid arthritis, systemic lupus erythematosus [SLE])
- Multiple sclerosis
- Myasthenia gravis
- CFS
- Infection (HIV, hepatitis, endocarditis)
- Cancer

Chronic Fatigue Syndrome

This is an idiopathic, nonprogressive illness associated with complaints of fatigue with a new or definite onset (not lifelong) that is not alleviated by rest and contributes to a substantial reduction in previous levels of occupational, educational, social, or personal activities. For many, this begins as a flulike syndrome but persists. A cause has not been determined, but recent studies indicate a neurally mediated hypotension as an associated factor. There are similarities between CFS and fibromyalgia; it has not been determined if this is an overlap in diagnostic criteria or a common pathology. For a diagnosis of CFS, four or more of the following symptoms must be present, all of which must have begun after the fatigue and been consecutively present for at least 6 months:

- Impaired memory or cognition
- Sore throat
- Tender cervical or axillary lymph nodes
- Muscle pain
- Multijoint pain
- New headaches
- Unrefreshing sleep
- Postexertional malaise

CFS is excluded as a diagnosis if depression predates the fatigue, other medical conditions explain the symptoms, or alcohol or other substance abuse has occurred within two years of the onset of chronic fatigue and in any time thereafter.

Objective examination often reveals trigger points that, when touched, cause radiating pain.

THERAPEUTIC PLAN

Fatigue has a vast number of potential causes. The client and significant others must be helped to understand that the workup may take one to two visits. The ultimate treatment plan will depend on the final diagnosis. The plan may involve referral to a different type of provider, such as a physician, psychologist, or sleep specialist.

For a diagnosis of CFS, a strong provider–client alliance is particularly beneficial, and the following elements are part of appropriate treatment:

- Reassure clients of the legitimacy of their signs and symptoms and discuss the syndrome. For most clients, there are initial troublesome symptoms, followed by improvement and a plateau stage. Most symptoms usually resolve within 12 to 18 months. With cognitive behavioral therapy, 75% of clients feel normal within 12 months.
- Recommend healthy behaviors that will optimize health and well-being for clients.
- Recommend a structured day and a specified bedtime that allows 6 to 8 hours of sleep (for adults). Discuss bedtime rituals and actions that promote sleep.
- Prescribe a graded aerobic exercise program with warmup and cool-down stages.
- Refer to the Chronic Fatigue and Immune Dysfunction Association of America for information, research findings, treatment suggestions, and support groups.
- Refer to a psychologist for cognitive behavioral therapy. Select a professional with expertise in this area of psychology.
- Refer to a support group if available.

Pharmacologic Treatment

No specific medications have been approved for CFS; however, several kinds of drugs may be valuable for symptom management. Nonsteroidal antiinflammatory drugs (NSAIDs) are often useful for myalgia, arthralgia, and headaches. Anxiolytics or medications for insomnia may be helpful. The tricyclic antidepressants (TCAs), in dosages less than those for treating depression, such as amitriptyline (Elavil) 10 to 25 mg at bedtime, improves the quality of sleep and reduces some other symptoms for many clients. Pharmacologic treatment for fatigue in general depends on identified cause.

Nonpharmacologic Treatment

Cause determines management in general. For CFS, the following treatments have been helpful:

- Program of gradually increasing activity. Clients have likely experienced an exacerbation of symptoms following exercise and are understandably hesitant. Advising activity in the form of a "prescription" might be beneficial for some: 5 to 10 minutes of activity followed by 5 minutes of rest in three to four cycles is helpful.
- Extra salt and water. For clients who experience orthostasis as part of the neurally mediated hypotension sometimes associated with CFS, this approach may be helpful.
- Cognitive behavioral therapy. This approach addresses ways in which negative beliefs about clients' illness and the expectations of self and others contribute to symptoms, and the way in which assumption of the sick role is affecting their health. Clients examine the role of stress on their health and mod-

F

ification of the lifestyle and self-expectations as a means for improvement.

Client Education

Summarize the work-up for fatigue and the rationale for each element. Explore the findings. Provide information appropriate to the final diagnosis. If the ultimate diagnosis is CFS, suggest the following:

- Eat a nutritious diet that includes eight glasses of water per day. Limit caffeine and alcohol.
- Quit smoking.
- Do not restrict salt intake unless there is concurrent hypertension.
- Have realistic expectations for daily activity. Get extra rest before a day that demands high activity levels. Do not stay in bed too long.
- Participate in a graded aerobic exercise program of walking, bicycling, or swimming 5 days per week for at least 12 weeks, starting with 5 minutes and building to 30 minutes by adding 1 to 2 minutes each week until the total is achieved. Do not exceed the exercise prescription, and if fatigue worsens, go back to the previous week's exercise prescription. (The nurse practitioner (NP) should appreciate that the concept of exercise as a prescription for fatigue is often difficult for clients to accept and may be accepted better when linked to research findings.)
- Use nighttime rituals and schedule at least 6 to 8 hours of sleep every night.
- The Social Security Administration (SSA) has produced a document related to disability status for persons with CFS, available at their Website. To qualify for benefits, the individual must have symptoms severe enough to keep him or her from working for 12 consecutive months and be physically or mentally incapable of doing any available job. Documentation to enable such disability benefits is extensive. (NPs cannot submit disability requests.)

EVALUATION/FOLLOW-UP

Clients should be referred to an appropriate physician specialist for further evaluation if a cause cannot be found for the fatigue or if the client's condition is deteriorating rapidly. Those clients with CFS should schedule a return visit for 2 to 3 weeks.

At times, it is helpful to suggest that the person bring a significant other to the next visit to obtain another's appraisal of how fatigue is affecting the person. It can also be helpful in follow-up for the client to keep a diary of symptoms and bring it to the next visit. Documentation should include the effects of fatigue on daily activities, sleep patterns, and diet. Fatigue should be rated on a standardized scale each day, such as the Pearson Byars Fatigue Feeling Checklist, Rhoton 10-point fatigue scale, Piper's fatigue scale, or a visual analog or 0-10 fatigue scale.

REFERENCES

Dunphy, L. M., & Winland-Brown, J. E. (2001). *Primary care: The art and science of advanced nursing practice.* Philadelphia: F. A. Davis.

Farrar, D., Locke, S., & Kantrowitz, F. (1995). Chronic fatigue syndrome 1: Etiology and pathogenesis. *Behavioral Medicine, 21,* 5-16.

Goroll, A. H., & Mulley, A. G. (1995). *Primary care medicine: Office evaluation and management of the adult patient.* Philadelphia: Lippincott Williams & Wilkins.

Kantrowitz, F., Farrar, D., & Locke, S. (1995). Chronic fatigue syndrome 2: Treatment and future research. *Behavioral Medicine, 21,* 17-24.

Robinson, D., Kidd, P., & Rogers, K. M. (2000). *Primary care across the lifespan.* St. Louis: Mosby.

Ruffin, M., & Cohen, M. (1994). Evaluation and management of fatigue. *American Family Physician, 50,* 625-632.

Saunders, C. S. (1998). New directions in chronic fatigue syndrome. *Patient Care Nurse Practitioner, 1*(7), 29-38.

Schumann, L., & Rodriquez, T. (2000). The challenge of evaluating fatigue. *Journal of American Academy of Nurse Practitioner, 12*(8), 329-338.

Seller, R. H. (2000). *Differential diagnosis of common complaints.* Philadelphia: W. B. Saunders.

Thiedke, C. C. (2000). Fibromyalgia and chronic fatigue syndrome. In C. C. Thiedke & J. A. Rosenfeld (Eds.), *Women's health* (pp. 145-146). Philadelphia: Lippincott Williams & Wilkins.

Review Questions

Mrs. Weems, a 43-year-old homemaker and mother of three school-age children, presents with complaints of "feeling tired all the time." She says, "I don't even have the energy or strength to brush my hair, and on days that my hair needs shampooing, I can't do that and shower; I must decide which is most important at the time." She also discusses the difficulty the fatigue is causing in her managing a busy home and active children.

1. Which comment from the history for Mrs. Weems suggests an organic cause for her fatigue?
   a. "I have to take a nap every day just to have enough energy to do basic cooking."
   b. "I had a tubal ligation after my last child."
   c. "My mother came last weekend to help me cook enough food to last several days."
   d. "I have been taking an over-the-counter vitamin with iron but it has not helped."

2. Which drug taken by Mrs. Weems on a routine basis may produce some level of fatigue?
   a. Advil
   b. Maalox
   c. Claritin
   d. Robitussin

3. Which of the following objective measures is definitely warranted if recent results are not available?

a. Visual acuity testing
b. Weber's test
c. Fecal occult blood test
d. Gallbladder ultrasound

4. Which diagnostic test is *not* considered a first-line test in determining a cause of chronic fatigue?

a. ESR
b. Electrocardiogram (ECG)
c. CBC with differential
d. TSH

5. If Mrs. Weems had a recent vacation to Mexico, which differential diagnosis should be considered in the workup because of its association with chronic fatigue?

a. Lyme disease
b. Hepatitis
c. Sprue
d. Shigella

6. The NP suspects CFS as a diagnosis based on the results of all the tests done thus far. Which factor is *not* consistent with the current case definition for that diagnosis?

a. Impaired concentration starting after the fatigue was noticed and lasting for 6 months
b. Muscle and joint pain that began after the fatigue and has lasted for 6 months
c. Postexertional malaise and nonrefreshing sleep for 6 months and noted after the onset of fatigue
d. Difficulty with swallowing and esophageal reflux lasting 6 months and noticed after the fatigue started

7. The NP diagnoses CFS and is deciding on an appropriate course of treatment. Which drug has a questionable place in treating CFS?

a. Hydrocortisone
b. Ibuprofen
c. Elavil
d. Multivitamin

8. On a follow-up visit 2 weeks after her diagnosis, Mrs. Weems tells the NP that a friend who had the same diagnosis of CSF several years ago wonders why an Epstein-Barr titer was not ordered. Which comment by the NP is most appropriate?

a. "In the past, the medical community believed that Epstein-Barr virus caused chronic fatigue, but more recent research has proved otherwise."
b. "That's a good idea. I'll order the test immediately."
c. "The Epstein-Barr titer is no longer available."
d. "I'll consult my collaborative physician and see if she believes an Epstein-Barr titer is warranted in your case."

9. The NP has explained the nature of CFS and the treatment plan thoroughly. Which comment by Mrs. Weems suggests that further teaching is warranted?

a. "I can expect to have this disorder for the rest of my life and to be totally disabled by my early sixties."

b. "I should follow the graded aerobic exercise plan carefully and increase by 1 to 2 minutes weekly to a maximum of 30 minutes 5 days each week."
c. "I understand that there is no specific medication for this problem, but ibuprofen may help with the aches and pains associated with it."
d. "My husband agrees that we should have you refer me to the psychologist for cognitive behavioral treatment."

10. Miss Tucker is a 50-year-old with CFS. She works on a production line at a local manufacturing company and asks the NP to do the workup for Social Security disability. Which action is most appropriate in responding to Miss Tucker's request?

a. Explain that NPs cannot legally conduct disability testing but that a referral to a physician for such evaluation will be made.
b. Schedule the physical examination and diagnostic testing immediately to secure disability benefits.
c. Explain that disability payments are not allowed for a diagnosis of CFS.
d. Advise Miss Tucker that she will not be eligible for Social Security disability benefits for another 10 years.

Answers and Rationales

1. *Answer:* a (analysis/diagnosis)
Rationale: Napping during the day to enable one to complete usual activities of daily living suggests an organic cause of fatigue (Gorroll & Mulley, 1995).

2. *Answer:* c (assessment)
Rationale: Antihistamines are a common cause of fatigue (Schumann & Rodriquez, 2000).

3. *Answer:* c (implementation/plan)
Rationale: Fecal occult blood testing is an appropriate option for this client who is older than 40 (Schumann & Rodriquez, 2000).

4. *Answer:* b (analysis/diagnosis)
Rationale: An ECG is not part of first-line diagnostic testing for CFS (Schumman & Rodriquez, 2000).

5. *Answer:* b (analysis/diagnosis)
Rationale: Hepatitis is an endemic disease in parts of Mexico and is highly likely to cause fatigue (Saunders, 1998).

6. *Answer:* d (assessment)
Rationale: Difficulty swallowing and esophageal reflux are not common causes of fatigue (Saunders, 1998).

7. *Answer:* a (implementation/plan)
Rationale: Cortisone is not warranted in the treatment of CFS (Saunders, 1998).

8. *Answer:* a (implementation/plan)
Rationale: Epstein-Barr virus, which was once considered a causative agent in CSF, is no longer considered such, and a titer is no longer warranted for diagnosis (Saunders, 1998).

F

9. *Answer:* **a** (evaluation)
Rationale: CFS is not a lifelong illness; it rarely lasts beyond 12 to 18 months (Saunders,1998).

10. *Answer:* **a** (implementation/plan)
Rationale: NPs cannot evaluate clients for Social Security disability benefits for any diagnosis. Referral is warranted (Saunders, 1998).

FEVER   *Denise Robinson*

OVERVIEW

Definition

Fever is a symptom and is a nonspecific response to an infectious or noninfectious disease process. There is a normal diurnal temperature variation, with the body temperature being lowest in the morning and highest in the late afternoon. Fever that arises when there is no obvious bacterial focus or characteristic viral infection is referred to as fever without source (FWS). Fever is defined as follows:

- Rectal or aural temperature higher than 100.4° F (38° C)
- Oral temperature higher than 99.5° F (37.5° C)
- Axillary temperature higher than 98.6° F (37° C)
- Fever of unknown origin: Fever with temperature higher than 100.9° F (38.3° C) for 3 weeks in which the diagnosis is not apparent after one week or more of studies
- Low fever: Oral reading of 99° to 100.4° F (38° C)
- Moderate fever: Oral reading of 100.5° to 104° F (38° to 40° C)
- High fever: Oral reading of 104° F (40° C)
- Fever higher than 108° F (42.2° C) (produces unconsciousness and brain damage if sustained)

Incidence

- Infection is the most common cause of fever in both adults and children.
- In general, children tend to have a greater febrile response than adults. Elderly persons, neonates, and those receiving medications such as NSAIDs or corticosteroids may have a less marked or absent febrile response even in the presence of bacteremia.
- Serious bacterial infection occurs in approximately 9% of well-appearing febrile infants and young children and includes UTI, bacteremia, enteritis, meningitis, and bone and joint infections.
- The risk of occult bacteremia is drastically reduced in those infants and children who have received two or more doses of Haemophilus influenzae b conjugate vaccine and two or more doses of pneumococcal conjugate vaccine.

Pathophysiology

- Body temperature is a set point regulated by the hypothalamus.
- Fever occurs when bacteria, viruses, or toxins are phagocytosed by leukocytes and cytokines are released.

Shivering increases heat production. Peripheral vasoconstriction prevents heat loss.
- Usually a viral organism initiates phagocytosis, but fevers can also be bacterial, rickettsial, fungal, or parasitic in origin.
- Hyperthermia is not mediated by cytokines and occurs when body metabolic heat production or environmental heat load exceeds normal heat loss capacity or when there is impaired heat loss. Heatstroke is an example.

ASSESSMENT: SUBJECTIVE/HISTORY

History of Present Illness

- Ask about onset, duration, and pattern of fever.
- Ask how the temperature was determined. Was a thermometer used or was the temperature determined by touch? If a thermometer was used, by what route?
- Ask about hydration status, including fluid intake, urination, vomiting, and diarrhea.
- Ask about level of discomfort.
- Ask about recent immunizations or new medications.
- Ask about last dose of antipyretic or other self-care measures.

Neonates. In infants less than 2 months old, ask about the following:
- Prematurity, maternal illness, including a primary herpes infection
- Maternal screenings, including B *Streptococcus*, premature rupture of membranes
- Prolonged nursery stay with antibiotic treatment
- Infant smile, which is a useful negative predictor of meningitis

Children

- Ask parent about the child's activity and whether child seems irritable, more drowsy, or not playing as usual.
- Inquire about previous episodes of febrile seizures, which affect approximately 4% of children.
- Children tend to have greater febrile responses than do adults. Teething does not cause fever with temperature higher than 101.1° F (38.4° C).
- Factors in history that influence the risk of serious bacterial infection in a febrile infant or young child include the following:
  - Current or recent antibiotics
  - Recent infectious contacts

- Recent infectious or unexplained illness
- Underlying medical problems
- Immunization status (especially Hib and conjugate pneumococcal vaccines)
- Birth history such as prematurity, prenatal antibiotics
- Fever history (measurement method, onset, duration)
- Social history (availability of telephone and car, distance from provider)

Symptoms

- Changes in activity
- Appetite
- Chills
- Headache
- Nasal congestion
- Earache
- Sore throat
- Cough
- Abdominal pain
- Vomiting
- Diarrhea
- Painful urination

Past Medical History

- Current medications
- Previous illnesses and diseases, particularly any cardiac or chronic debilitating disorders, especially immunosuppressive treatments or disorders
- Infections
- Trauma
- Surgery
- Diagnostic testing
- Use of anesthesia

Family History

Ask whether family members are ill or have traveled recently.

ASSESSMENT: OBJECTIVE/PHYSICAL EXAMINATION

Physical Examination

- Measure temperature. If the child is overdressed, remove the clothes and retake temperature in 15 minutes.
  - Rectal or aural temperature is 0.5° C higher than oral temperature.
  - Axillary temperature is 0.5° C lower than oral temperature.
  - Record rectal temperature in infant younger than 3 months.
- Measure vital signs, including respirations, pulse, and blood pressure.
- Observe the general appearance and mental alertness of both adults and children.
- Assess the quality of the cry of an infant.

- Assess skin for color rash, petechiae, purpura, dryness, turgor, capillary refill, redness, and warmth.
- Assess for nuchal rigidity.
- Assess anterior fontanelle of an infant.
- Assess for both upper and lower respiratory involvement.
- Assess for lymphadenopathy.
- Assess for swollen joints.

A complete examination may be indicated, depending on the presenting complaint and the age of the client, to find a localized infection such as otitis media, pharyngitis, sinusitis, meningitis, or pneumonia. See specific chapters for more information about individual diagnoses.

Diagnostic Procedures

Usually the history and physical examination uncover the source of the fever. Perform a complete history and physical examination for the following clients:

- Younger than 3 months
- Looking toxic
- Immunocompromised
- With underlying chronic disease
- With extremely elevated temperature

Consider ordering the following tests:

- *Urinalysis and culture:* Obtain by catheterization; bagged specimens are false-positive up to 85% of the time and should be avoided.
- Obtain CBC with differential, ESR, and blood cultures.
  - A white blood cell (WBC) count between $5000/mm^3$ and $15,000/mm^3$ has a negative predictive value as high as 97% in infants younger than 60 days. Check CBC in a child 61 days to 36 months if the fever is 102.2° F, and assess for risk of occult bacteremia. If WBC is less than $15,000/mm^3$, continue with appropriate follow-up.
  - A WBC count higher than $15,000/mm^3$ raises the risk of bacteremia fivefold (Bower & Powell, 2001).
- Obtain chest radiograph.
- Obtain cerebrospinal fluid for culture, cell count and differential, and chemistries.
- Obtain stool specimen for those children who have diarrhea of more than four stools a day with no associated vomiting. Salmonella is frequently overlooked.
- Physician consultation is indicated for any infant younger than 2 months. In most cases, hospitalization is necessary even if the source of the fever is identified because of the risks of dehydration, sepsis, meningitis, and pneumonia.

DIAGNOSIS

Infection is the most common cause of fever and may be viral, bacterial, rickettsial, fungal, or parasitic. Differential diagnoses include the following:

F

- Assess for autoimmune disease.
- Assess for malignant neoplastic disease.
- Assess for hematologic disease.
- Assess for cardiovascular disease.
- Assess for GI disease.
- Assess for endocrine disease.
- Drug reactions, including serum sickness, neuroleptic malignant syndrome, and malignant hyperthermia of anesthesia, are diseases that cause fever as a result of chemical agents. Central nervous system (CNS) disease interferes with the thermal regulatory process and is seen with fever.

Infants younger than 60 days with the following are at low risk for serious bacterial infection:

- Previously healthy, born at term, no antibiotics, no hyperbilirubinemia, no chronic or underlying illness, not hospitalized longer than the mother
- WBC count between 5000/mm³ and 15,000/mm³
- A spun urine sample shows fewer than 10 WBCs per high-power field
- If the infant has diarrhea, high-power analysis shows less than 5 leukocytes per field (Bower & Powell, 2001b)

THERAPEUTIC PLAN

Clients with fever who are disoriented or delirious, or who have meningismus, petechiae, or purpura, should be transported to the emergency department immediately by another responsible person or by ambulance.

Clients who are immunodeficient, have cardiac disease, or have another serious disease also need immediate evaluation because the heart rate increases approximately 10 beats per minute for every degree Fahrenheit. Respiration rate also increases.

The following children with fever need immediate evaluation (Hay, 1995):

- Younger than 2 months with temperature of 100.4° F
- With temperature higher than 104.2° F (40.1° C)
- Crying inconsolably or whimpering
- Crying when moved or touched
- Difficult to awaken
- With stiff neck
- With purple spots on the skin
- With difficulty breathing
- Drooling saliva and unable to swallow food or fluids
- With history of convulsion
- Looking or acting extremely sick

Children between 2 months and 2 years of age with fever can be treated on an outpatient basis in the presence of a localized, nonserious infection, as long as they are playful, drinking, and voiding and they do not appear toxic. Bacteremia is more likely in a child with a temperature higher than 105° F (40.6° C) and should be considered even if a localized infection is found.

Pharmacologic Treatment

Antipyretic Indications

- In fevers of 103° F (39.4° C), treat with antipyretics.
- In children with a history of febrile seizures, treat with antipyretics.
- In clients who have compensated cardiac disease or chronic debilitating disorders, who become dehydrated easily, or who are alcoholics, treat with antipyretics.
- In clients who are uncomfortable and cannot rest, treat with antipyretics.
- Considerations for not treating low to moderate fevers include the fact that antipyretics may mask the signs or symptoms of a serious disease and possibly confuse the clinical picture.

Medications

- Acetaminophen, PO or rectal every 4 to 6 hours, for adults and for children older than 2 months
- Ibuprofen, PO every 6 to 8 hours, for adults and for children older than 6 months
- Aspirin, PO every 4 to 6 hours, for adults only (increased risk of developing Reye syndrome in children)

Client Education

- Teach parents the proper method of assessing temperature. If child is younger than 3 months, use a rectal thermometer. Oral thermometers can be used for children older than 3 years.
- Avoid OTC medications that contain aspirin, such as Pepto-Bismol.
- Keep the child well hydrated by offering fluids every 15 to 30 minutes. Use oral rehydration solution in cases of vomiting. Consume extra fluids during a fever.
- Avoid overdressing when febrile.
- Avoid strenuous activity. Rest.
- Use lukewarm water sponge baths in the following cases:
  - Fever with temperature level higher than 106.2° F (41.2° C)
  - Clients with liver disease who cannot take acetaminophen
  - Clients with neurologic problems in which temperature regulation is impaired
- Alcohol is never used for sponging.
- Sponging should not cause the client to shiver.
- Adults should be taught when to administer antipyretics and the correct dose to avoid overdosing and underdosing. Pediatric formulations vary in their concentration. For example, elixir is 160 mg/mL, whereas drops are 80 mg/0.8 mL and chewable tablets are 80 mg each.

Consultation

Consider consultation with a physician or referral for the following:

- Any febrile infant less than 2 months of age
- Clients with underlying medical conditions in which fever may increase risk for complications

Prevention

- Increased temperature can be avoided by overdressing
- Adequate hydration

EVALUATION/FOLLOW-UP

Follow-up depends on age, diagnosis, clinical presentation, the reliability of the caregiver, and the level of support from friends and family.

- Recheck infants, young children, older adults, and clients with chronic conditions in 24 hours in person or by phone.
- Have the client return if fever persists for 2 to 3 days.

COMPLICATIONS

Death from bacteremia.

REFERENCES

Baraff, L. J., Bass, J. W., Fleisher, G. R., Klein, J. O., McCraken, G. H. Jr., Powell, K. R., & Schriger, D. L. (1993). Practice guideline for the management of infants and children 0 to 36 months of age with fever without source. Agency for Health Care Policy and Research. *Annals of Emergency Medicine, 22*(7), 198-210.

Bower, J., & Powell, K. (2001a). Unexplained fever in infants and young children: When is it serious? *Consultant, 41*(5), 653-656.

Bower, J., & Powell, K. (2001b). Unexplained fever in infants and young children: How to manage. *Consultant, 41*(5), 712-715.

Hay, W., Hayward, A., Levin, M., & Sondheimer, J. (1999). *Current pediatric diagnosis and treatment* (14th ed.). Norwalk, CT: Appleton & Lange.

Professional guide to signs and symptoms (2nd ed.). (1996). Springhouse, PA: Springhouse.

Robinson, D., Kidd, P., & Rogers, K. (2000). *Primary care across the lifespan*. St. Louis: Mosby.

Wells, N., King, J., Hedstrom, C., & Youngkins, J. (1995). Does tympanic temperature measure up? *American Journal of Maternal/Child Nursing, 20*(1), 95-100.

Review Questions

1. Which of the following symptoms associated with fever indicates a serious illness?
   a. Degree of the temperature
   b. Concurrent nasal congestion, cough
   c. Other family members with similar symptoms
   d. Change in behavior, such as irritability or lethargy

2. Which of the following measurements of temperature with a mercury thermometer is most reliable for a 2-year-old?
   a. Oral temperature, left in place for 2 minutes
   b. Rectal temperature, left in place for 2 minutes
   c. Axillary temperature, left in place for 2 minutes
   d. Ear temperature, left in place for 2 minutes

3. The most common cause of fever in both adults and children is which of the following?
   a. Bacterial infection, such as otitis and sinusitis
   b. Autoimmune illness, such as rheumatic fever and rheumatoid arthritis
   c. Viral illness, such as enteroviruses and adenoviruses
   d. Drug reaction

4. Children should be evaluated immediately in which of the following cases?
   a. Temperature is higher than 101° F.
   b. Child is sleeping more but is easily awakened.
   c. Child looks or acts sick.
   d. Child is drinking but not eating.

5. A child arrives in the office all bundled up in winter clothes. He has a temperature of 101° F. Before initiating any treatment for the fever, which of the following actions would be prudent?
   a. Retake the temperature after the child has been undressed for 15 minutes.
   b. Obtain blood cultures.
   c. Begin alcohol sponge bath.
   d. Give antipyretic so the child is more comfortable.

6. The medication of choice for moderate fever in children is which of following?
   a. Acetaminophen
   b. Aspirin
   c. Ibuprofen
   d. None

7. A 70-year-old man comes in to be seen because he does not feel well. Which of the following is a cause for concern?
   a. Temperature of 102° F
   b. Looking extremely sick
   c. Awake and alert, responds appropriately to questions
   d. WBC 8000/mm^3

8. Which of the following is a good indicator of the seriousness of fever in a young child?
   a. Activity
   b. Ability to feed
   c. Urination
   d. Skin temperature

Answers and Rationales

1. *Answer:* **d** (assessment)
   Rationale: The degree of the temperature does not correlate well with the severity of the illness. Clients with viral infections may have upper respiratory symptoms and may have household contacts with similar symptoms. CNS involvement

may show irritability, as with meningitis, and lethargy may be seen with bacteremia, both of which are serious (Hay, 1995).

2. *Answer:* b (assessment)

Rationale: With a mercury thermometer, rectal temperatures are most accurate. Oral temperatures are also reliable if done properly but are reserved for older children. Axillary temperatures are the least accurate, but they are better than no measurement. The thermometer must be left in place 2 minutes for a rectal temperature, 3 minutes for an oral temperature, and 5 to 6 minutes for an axillary temperature. A mercury thermometer is not placed in the ear (Robinson, Kidd, & Rogers, 2000).

3. *Answer:* c (analysis/diagnosis)

Rationale: Infection is the most common cause of fever in both adults and children. Most infections are viral in cause (Robinson, Kidd, & Rogers, 2000).

4. *Answer:* c (evaluation)

Rationale: Children should be evaluated immediately if the temperature is higher than 104° F, if the child is difficult to awaken, or if the child is not drinking or eating, the last because of the risk of dehydration (Hay, 1999). The behavior and appearance of the child are important determinants,

and a child who looks or acts ill should be seen immediately.

5. *Answer:* a (implementation/plan)

Rationale: Children are often overdressed when they have a fever. The most accurate way to determine the level of fever is to retake the temperature after the child has been undressed for 15 minutes (Bower & Powell, 2001a).

6. *Answer:* a (implementation/plan)

Rationale: Acetaminophen is the drug of choice for fever for adults and children older than 2 months. Ibuprofen is an alternative for adults and children older than 6 months. Aspirin can be used in adults, but not children, for the management of fever. At times, it is appropriate not to use antipyretics for low-grade fever (Robinson, Kidd, & Rogers, 2000).

7. *Answer:* b (assessment)

Rationale: Although the temperature may be an indicator for fever and serious illness, a more important clue is that the client looks sick (Robinson, Kidd, & Rogers, 2000).

8. *Answer:* b (assessment)

Rationale: Ability to feed is a good indicator of the seriousness of a child's illness (Robinson, Kidd, & Rogers, 2000).

FIBROMYALGIA *Cheryl Pope Kish*

OVERVIEW
Definition

Fibromyalgia syndrome (FMS) is a chronic, clinically defined pain syndrome characterized by diffuse pain and palpable tender points. According to The American College of Rheumatology, fibromyalgia includes both a 3-month history of widespread pain and the presence of tender points in soft tissue at 11 of 18 defined anatomic sites using a digital palpation force of 4 kg. Widespread pain involves pain perceived both above and below the waist and on both the right and left sides. This finding is often accompanied by generalized body aches, morning stiffness, fatigue, and nonrestful sleep.

Incidence

- Occurs in 2% to 5% of general population.
- Accounts for 5% to 10% of clients in internal medicine practices.
- Accounts for 4% to 20% of clients in rheumatology practices; is second only to those with rheumatoid arthritis
- Approximately 73% to 90% of those with fibromyalgia are women.
- Average age of clients with fibromyalgia is 40 to 60 years, with the peak incidence at age 45 to 55.
- Now considered twice as common as rheumatoid arthritis.

Pathophysiology

The cause of fibromyalgia has not been determined, and there is no clearly documented pathophysiologic cause; however, aberrations in CNS processing, altered cerebral blood flow, changes in neurotransmitters, a stresslike response, and alterations in growth hormone may account for much of the pain. The following additional organic features help to explain the disorder:

- Restorative delta-wave stage IV (non-REM) sleep is disrupted by nonrestorative alpha-wave sleep.
- Emotional stressors may alter CNS serotonin, a chemical mediator of deep sleep and pain perception. Changes in neurotransmitters alter perception so that nonnoxious stimuli are perceived as painful; this feature is known as *allodynia.*
- Pain and fatigue often result in inactivity, depression, and sleep difficulties, which contribute to more pain and fatigue, beginning a vicious cycle.

ASSESSMENT: SUBJECTIVE/HISTORY
Symptoms

- Widespread, persistent musculoskeletal pain is the central feature of the disorder. Most common areas of pain are the axial skeleton (especially cervical and low back), shoulder, and pelvic girdles. Pain on palpation occurs at 11 of 18 identifiable anatomic points; diagnosis depends on client's use of the word "pain" not just "tender." Two thirds report pain to palpation all over, not just at the tender points; this may be related to diminished pain threshold.

- Many clients do not realize that they are having problems sleeping because they are able to fall asleep but wake up fatigued. Ninety percent wake up tired and nonrefreshed.
- Fatigue is experienced by 55% to 100% of clients.
- Morning stiffness is experienced by 76% to 91% of clients.
- Depression is experienced by 26% of clients.
- The client experiences a subjective sensation of swollen joints.
- The client may experience headache (migraine or tension type).
- Symptoms similar to Raynaud's disease (pallor, cyanosis, and paresthesias) may be present.
- Irritable bowel or bladder symptoms, or both, may be present.
- The client may experience anxiety.

Aggravating Factors. Several factors have been associated with fibromyalgia; the NP should inquire about the following:

- Exposure to cold, humid weather
- Physical/mental fatigue
- Extremes of physical activity (too much or too little)
- Stress and mental fatigue
- Decreased tolerance to pollution, fumes, perfumes, loud noise, and bright light

Relieving Factors. Ask about factors that provide relief of symptoms. Moderate activity; warm, dry weather; and hot showers and baths are commonly reported as relieving factors.

Past Medical History

Depression is common in the history of those with fibromyalgia; 71% have a current or past history of depression. Fibromyalgia often complicates existing rheumatic disorder. If not well controlled, hypothyroidism may mimic fibromyalgia. Ask about previous history of CFS: both conditions have similar symptoms, except fibromyalgia causes more pain. In one third of cases, viral illness is a precedent; in another one third, trauma is a triggering event. Sometimes there is no obvious trigger.

Medication History

It is always appropriate to ask about medications, both current and past. Asking about previous pain relief from steroids or NSAIDs is particularly helpful because these drugs do not usually provide pain relief in fibromyalgia. Determine if the client is using drugs or alcohol to attempt to blunt symptoms.

Family History

It is not uncommon to see a family history of autoimmune disorders or depression in those with fibromyalgia. It has long been thought to "run in families"; recently a human leukocyte antigen (HLA) genetic marker has been identified in clients with fibromyalgia, but it is not used in clinical diagnosis at this time.

Psychosocial History

Because of the pain and fatigue of fibromyalgia, clients are often unable to perform ADLs, hold a job, or engage in enjoyable leisure activities. Moreover, relationships are often strained as a result. Determine how the illness has affected lifestyle and relationships, as well as how it has affected the client's self-perception and esteem.

ASSESSMENT: OBJECTIVE/PHYSICAL EXAMINATION

Physical Examination

Physical examination includes manual palpation of tender points employing a rolling motion with either the thumb or first two fingers (using 4 kg of pressure, approximately the force it takes to blanch a fingernail). According to the American College of Rheumatology 1990 Criteria for the Classification of Fibromyalgia (Multicenter Criteria Committee, 1990), pain must be elicited in 11 of 18 tender points to diagnose fibromyalgia. The defined anatomic points are both above and below the waist and on both sides of the body (see Figure 3-6).

- Occiput: bilateral, at the suboccipital muscle insertions
- Low cervical: bilateral, at the anterior aspects of the intertransverse spaces at C_5-C_7
- Trapezius: bilateral, at the midpoint of the upper border
- Supraspinatus: bilateral, at origins, above the scapula spine near the medial border
- Second rib: bilateral, at the second costochondral junctions, just lateral to the junctions on the upper surfaces
- Lateral epicondyle: bilateral, 2 cm distal to the epicondyles
- Gluteal: bilateral, in the upper outer quadrants of the buttocks in the anterior fold of muscle
- Greater trochanter: bilateral, posterior to the trochanteric prominence
- Knee: bilateral, at the medial fat pad proximal to the joint line

Tender points must be differentiated from trigger points. Pressure on trigger points causes radiating pain, which is associated with myofascial syndromes but not with fibromyalgia.

Physical examination results are otherwise negative. There should be no visible swelling or objective weakness unless it is caused by other concomitant illnesses.

F

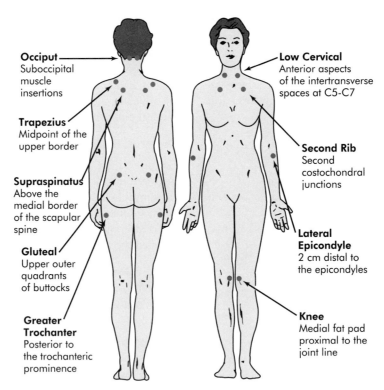

Occiput
Suboccipital
muscle
insertions

Trapezius
Midpoint of the
upper border

Supraspinatus
Above the
medial border
of the scapular
spine

Gluteal
Upper outer
quadrants
of buttocks

**Greater
Trochanter**
Posterior to
the trochanteric
prominence

Low Cervical
Anterior aspects
of the intertransverse
spaces at C5-C7

Second Rib
Second
costochondral
junctions

**Lateral
Epicondyle**
2 cm distal to
the epicondyles

Knee
Medial fat pad
proximal to the
joint line

FIGURE **3-6**   Location of specific tender points for diagnostic classification of fibromyalgia (From Phipps, W., Sands, J., & Maerek, J. 1999. *Medical-surgical nursing: concepts and clinical practice,* ed. 6. St. Louis: Mosby).

(This is despite subjective complaints of swelling and weakness.)

It is not uncommon to note hypermobility or laxity of the joints in clients with FMS; when asked, they often acknowledge being "double jointed."

Diagnostic Procedures

Fibromyalgia is a diagnosis of exclusion. All test results should be negative in the absence of concomitant disease. The initial workup includes CBC, ESR, chemistries, and TSH. If other causes are suspected, creatine phosphokinase (CPK), serum protein electrophoresis, ANA, and rheumatoid factor are ordered. X-ray examination is appropriate if pain is more localized. Unless the client is falling asleep in situations compromising safety (i.e., while driving), sleep studies are not justified.

DIAGNOSIS

The differential diagnoses include the following:
- Rheumatoid arthritis
- Metabolic myopathies
- Endocrine disorders (thyroid, parathyroid)
- Adrenal disorders (most commonly hypothyroidism)
- Polymyositis
- Polymyalgia rheumatica
- Osteoarthritis
- Metastatic cancer

- Myofascial pain syndrome
- Ankylosing spondylitis
- Depression/anxiety
- Disk herniation
- Connective tissue disease
- CFS

THERAPEUTIC PLAN
Pharmacologic Treatment

- Tricyclics help induce stage IV sleep and provide non-specific analgesia for chronic pain:
  - Cyclobenzaprine (Flexeril) 10 to 30 mg hs Use caution with clients with urinary retention or closed-angle glaucoma. May have additive toxicity with TCAs.
  - Amitriptyline (Elavil) 10 to 50 mg hs Contraindicated in pregnancy and lactation, narrow-angle glaucoma and with monoamine oxidase inhibitors (MAOIs). Has anticholinergic side effects; use with caution in urinary retention, hyperthyroidism, hepatic, or renal impairment.
- NSAIDs and corticosteroids are not usually helpful. Narcotics are not advised.
- Selective serotonin reuptake inhibitors (SSRIs): Fluoxetine (Prozac) 20 to 40 mg is effective, especially if there is a depressive component. Contraindicated with MAOIs; use caution in cases of hepatic impairment or seizure disorders.

Nonpharmacologic Treatment

- Offer reassurance. Give a name to the symptoms. Validate that this is a recognized organic syndrome that is very real and not "all in the head." Reinforce that it is not a progressive or crippling disease.
- Relate symptoms to modifiable factors (stress, sleep, exercise) to give clients a sense of control over their body and symptoms. Emphasize that the ultimate goal is to reduce pain and enable functional improvement; elimination of pain is not a realistic option for most. Acknowledge that this is a time-consuming and frustrating illness but support will be provided.
- Low-impact aerobic exercise for at least 30 minutes three times per week is essential to overall management. Stretching, range-of-motion, and aquatic exercises are also effective.
- Moist heat (e.g., heating pads, warm showers or baths, whirlpools) applied to painful areas may be comforting.
- Refer to support groups, therapeutic biofeedback programs, relaxation therapy, yoga, tai chi, and hypnotherapy as appropriate.
- Transcutaneous electrical nerve stimulation may be helpful.
- Cognitive behavior therapy can be helpful because common beliefs about symptoms contribute to perpetuation of symptoms. This therapy encourages examination and challenge of negative beliefs. Encourage clients to look at how they have assumed a sick role and how that may be affecting their improvement. Also examine how stress affects symptoms and clients' need for support during stressful times.
- Contact the Arthritis Foundation and Fibromyalgia Network for client education booklets. Education is empowering and decreases the sense of helplessness experienced by many clients. Education also helps shift the person's perception from one of helplessness, frustration, and anger to more positive feelings of hope and self-efficacy.
- Encourage stress reduction, including job modification as needed.
- Encourage self-paced activities with frequent rest periods. Avoiding daytime naps may enhance nighttime sleep. Encourage bedtime rituals. Activity is increased gradually, and client is advised not to "overdo it."
- Explore with individual ways to prioritize life activities to enable pleasurable leisure events as well as required activities. This may involve reappraisal of standards for housework and a change in self-criticism when activities take longer than in the past. It is helpful for these clients to experience a sense of accomplishment.

Prevention

Because the origin of FMS is unknown, prevention is impossible at this time.

EVALUATION/FOLLOW-UP

Because there are no diagnostic tests for fibromyalgia, evaluation must be based on the client's subjective feeling of decreased pain, fatigue, and stiffness.

- Follow monthly at first until some improvement in symptoms is noticed. Then decrease the frequency of visits as symptoms warrant.
- Consult with a physician about additional testing if there is any reason to suspect other disorders.

COMPLICATIONS

Untreated FMS results in functional disability, pain, and fatigue and the inherent lower quality of life these symptoms bring to suffering individuals.

REFERENCES

Alarcon, G. S. (1999). Fibromyalgia: Dispelling diagnostic and treatment myths. *Women's Health in Primary Care, 2*(10), 775-784.

Barbour, C. (2000). Use of complementary and alternative treatments by individuals with fibromyalgia syndrome. *Journal of the American Academy of Nurse Practitioners, 12*(8), 311-316.

Clark, S., & Odell, L. (2000). Fibromyalgia syndrome: Common, real, and treatable. *Clinician Reviews, 10*(5), 57-59, 63-64, 69-76, 81-83.

Cunningham, M. D. (1996). Becoming familiar with fibromyalgia. *Orthopedic Nursing, 15*(2), 33-36.

Dunphey, L. M., & Winland-Brown, J. E. (2001). *Primary care: The art and science of advanced practice nursing.* Philadelphia: F. A. Davis.

Geel, S. E. (1994). The fibromyalgia syndrome: Musculoskeletal pathophysiology. *Seminars in Arthritis and Rheumatism, 23,* 347-353.

Harmon, C. E. (1996). Fibromyalgia: Treatments worth trying. *Internal Medicine, 17*(1), 64-75.

Johnson, S. P. (1997). Fluoxetine and amitriptyline in the treatment of fibromyalgia. *Journal of Family Practice, 44*(2), 128-130.

Jones, K. D., & Burckhardt, C. S. (1997). A multidisciplinary approach to treating fibromyalgia syndrome. *American Journal for Nurse Practitioners, 1*(4), 7-14.

Kennedy, M., & Felson, D. T. (1996). A prospective long-term study of fibromyalgia syndrome. *Arthritis and Rheumatism, 39,* 682-685.

Martin, L., Nutting, A., MacIntosh, B. R., Edworthy, S. M., Butterwick, D., & Cook, J. (1996). An exercise program in the treatment of fibromyalgia. *Journal of Rheumatology, 23,* 1050-1053.

Multicenter Criteria Committee. (1990). The American College of Rheumatology 1990 Criteria for the Classification of Fibromyalgia. *Arthritis and Rheumatism, 33,* 160-172.

Thiedke, C. C. (2000). Fibromyalgia and chronic fatigue syndrome. In C. C. Thiedke & J. A. Rosenfeld, *Women's health.* Philadelphia: Lippincott Williams & Wilkins, 145-156.

Unger, J. (1996). Fibromyalgia. *Journal of the American Academy of Nurse Practitioners, 8*(1), 27-29.

F

White, K. P., & Harth, M. (1996). An analytical review of 24 controlled clinical trials for fibromyalgia syndrome (FMS). *Pain, 64,* 211-219.

Wilke, W. S. (1995). Treatment of "resistant" fibromyalgia. *Rheumatic Disease Clinics of North America, 21,* 247-257.

Review Questions

1. Carly Newsome, a 37-year-old teacher, presents with complaints of fatigue, pain, and stiff joints of 3 weeks' duration. Which of the following historical data are consistent with a diagnosis of fibromyalgia?

 a. Her husband is an Air Force captain recently deployed overseas for 2 years.
 b. She has two children, ages 7 and 10.
 c. She uses Depo-Provera for contraception.
 d. Her hobby is designing with stained glass.

2. Which of the following symptom descriptions provided by Mrs. Newsome, in addition to pain and fatigue, is typical of FMS?

 a. "I have frequent hot flashes; when others around me are cool, I'm turning on the fan."
 b. "Even though I get 8 hours of sleep every night, I rarely feel rested when I awaken."
 c. "I have noticed recently that my urine has a stronger odor and is darker in color."
 d. "Ibuprofen has made my pain tolerable."

3. During the physical assessment, which comment made by Mrs. Newsome in response to the palpation of the 18 defined anatomic areas is consistent with a diagnosis of FMS?

 a. "When you touch that spot on my knee, the pain radiates down my leg to my toes."
 b. "That area you touched on my shoulder was really tender."
 c. "Ouch. It hurts when you push on that spot on my arm."
 d. "The pressure you're putting on those spots feels good."

4. Which of the following diagnostic tests are first line in cases of FMS?

 a. CBC, ESR, thyroid profile, and blood chemistry
 b. RF, ANA, uric acid, and creatinine
 c. Bone scan, EMG, arthritis profile, and x-ray examination of the spine
 d. MRI, muscle biopsy, LSE profile, and growth hormone assay

5. Fibromyalgia must be differentiated from CFS. Compared with CFS, fibromyalgia is associated with which of the following?

 a. More severe fatigue because of disruptions of stage IV sleep
 b. Higher levels of depression as indicated by Beck Depression Inventory scores
 c. Greater functional disability
 d. More severe and widespread pain

6. What is the primary difference between tender points and trigger points as an objective finding in physical examination?

 a. The amount of pressure required to elicit them is different.
 b. Palpation of trigger points causes radiation of pain; palpating tender points does not.
 c. Tender points cause radiating pain, whereas trigger points do not.
 d. Eliciting trigger points requires use of the reflex hammer; evaluating tender points does not.

7. Which of the following drug choices is the most appropriate for FMS?

 a. Naproxen (Naprosyn) 500 mg PO bid
 b. Demerol 25 mg PO q4h for severe pain
 c. Amitriptyline (Elavil) 50 mg PO hs
 d. Ibuprofen 200 mg PO q6h

8. The NP provides instruction about FMS and appropriate nonpharmacologic management. Which comment by the client indicates a need for further instruction?

 a. "I'm going to walk 20 minutes several times a week."
 b. "A warm bath or shower before bedtime may be helpful."
 c. "Imaging, relaxation breathing, or yoga might be helpful in managing my illness."
 d. "I can expect to become progressively worse over time, maybe even crippled from this disease."

9. Which of the following comments by a client with FMS indicates attainment of a realistic goal of treatment?

 a. "My pain and fatigue are better; I am able to manage my home with some help from my husband and to work part-time."
 b. "Mercifully, my pain is completely gone."
 c. "Thanks to treatment, I can realize my dream of cross-country skiing."
 d. "Now that my treatment regimen is completed, I sleep soundly every night."

10. The NP initiates treatment for a client with FMS and provides comprehensive instruction. How soon should a follow-up visit be scheduled?

 a. 3 to 4 days
 b. 1 week
 c. 1 month
 d. 3 months

Answers and Rationales

1. *Answer:* **a** (analysis/diagnosis)
 Rationale: Stressful events precipitate FMS in one third of cases (Alarcon, 1999).

2. *Answer:* **b** (assessment)
 Rationale: Nonrestorative sleep is a classic feature of FMS (Clark & Odell, 2000).

3. *Answer:* **c** (assessment)
 Rationale: A diagnostic criterion is that clients respond to tender point palpation by describing pain, not tenderness (Alarcon, 1999).

4. *Answer:* a (analysis/diagnosis)
   Rationale: FMS is a diagnosis of exclusion, but first-line diagnostic tests (i.e., CBC, ESR, thyroid profile, and blood chemistry) help rule out the most common competing differential diagnoses (Clark & Odell, 2000).

5. *Answer:* d (analysis/diagnosis)
   Rationale: There are many similarities between the demographics and clinical features of FMS and CFS; however, pain is primary in FMS, whereas fatigue predominates in CFS (Meredith & Horan, 2000).

6. *Answer:* b (assessment)
   Rationale: This is the only accurate statement about eliciting trigger and tender points; the others are false (Dunphy & Winland-Brown, 2001).

7. *Answer:* c (implementation/plan)
   Rationale: TCAs are used for promoting rest; narcotics and NSAIDs are avoided (Robinson, Kidd, & Rogers, 2000).

8. *Answer:* d (evaluation)
   Rationale: FMS is not a progressive or debilitating disease (Clark & Odell, 2000).

9. *Answer:* a (evaluation)
   Rationale: Pain control and maintenance of functional ability are primary goals of FMS management (Alarcon, 1999).

10. *Answer:* c (evaluation)
   Rationale: Follow-up after 1 month of management is appropriate (Clark & Odell, 2000).

FIFTH DISEASE *Denise Robinson*

OVERVIEW
Definition

Erythema infectiosum (Fifth disease) is a generally mild illness with few or no symptoms and a characteristic rash; however, pregnant women who contract fifth disease run a 1% to 3% risk of fetal hydrops and subsequent fetal loss. Fifth disease also can result in significant anemia in clients with chronic hemolytic anemia or clients who are immunocompromised.

Incidence

- Peak incidence is in the spring. The incubation period is 4 to 14 days. It is contagious before onset of illness but not after onset of rash.
- Approximately 60% of cases occur in children between the ages of 5 and 15.
- Approximately 40% of adults are seronegative.
- Approximately 1.5% of women are infected during pregnancy.

Pathophysiology

Humans are the only known host of human parvovirus (HPV-B19). Spread is by respiratory and blood routes. The characteristic "slapped cheeks" rash represents an immune response. The virus is a single-strand DNA that replicates in erythroid progenitor cells. The replication causes lysis of the cell with transient anemia.

ASSESSMENT: SUBJECTIVE/HISTORY
History of Present Illness

- Ask about symptoms and duration of symptoms.
- Ask about fever.
- Ask about the pattern of the rash.
- Ask about the following:
  - Immunization history

  - Environmental exposure (illness at home, work, school, day care)
  - Travel (to area with high incidence)
  - Communicable disease history

Symptoms

Approximately 50% of children have mild systemic symptoms, which include low-grade fever (100.4° F to 101.3° F [38° C to 38.5° C]), mild malaise, sore throat, cough, and conjunctivitis. A rash may be the first symptom or sign. Adolescents have similar presenting symptoms as those seen in children; they may also have symptoms of arthritis lasting for 2 to 3 weeks.

Past Medical History

- Determine whether there is any history of sickle cell or chronic hemolytic anemia.
- Is the client pregnant?
- Is there a history of immunocompromise?

Medications

Determine whether the client is taking any antibiotics or other medications at this time.

Family History

- Ask if any family members have a rash.
- Ask if anyone is the family is immunocompromised, has hemolytic anemia, or is pregnant.

ASSESSMENT: OBJECTIVE/PHYSICAL EXAMINATION
Physical Examination

In stage 1, erythematous cheeks have appearance of "slapped cheeks" because of redness. They may be warm and nontender, and they may itch. Rash may also be present on chin, forehead, and postauricular areas, but the area around the mouth is spared.

In stage 2 (1 to 2 days later), an erythematous, symmetric, maculopapular rash occurs on the trunk, neck, buttocks, or all three. Palms and soles are spared.

In stage 3, this rash fades with central clearing, leaving a distinctive lacy, reticulated rash that can last 2 to 40 days (average 2 weeks). Rash will recur with heat, exercise, bathing, or stress.

Diagnostic Procedures

No diagnostic tests are necessary. A CBC may reveal an initial leukopenia, followed by a leukocytosis and lymphocytosis.

DIAGNOSIS

This illness needs to be differentiated from the other childhood exanthems. The slapped cheeks rash and the mild course make it less like the other childhood illnesses. Scarlet fever produces more systemic signs and pharyngitis (Table 3-32).

THERAPEUTIC PLAN
Erythema Infectiosum

Nonpharmacologic treatment is supportive. Isolation is used for children with aplastic crisis.

Client Education

Symptomatic Treatment. Pregnant women should not be excluded from the workplace and children should not be excluded from school because once rash is present, children are not contagious.

Consultation

- Any client with sickle cell or hemolytic anemia
- Pregnant woman

Prevention

None available. Immunoglobulin M (IgM) is not effective, and quarantine is not helpful.

EVALUATION/FOLLOW-UP

Children (most likely adolescents) may have severe joint symptoms. Girls are more commonly affected than boys. It usually resolves without sequela.

Clients with chronic hemolytic anemia should be monitored closely. Fifth disease can cause a severe anemia in such clients. Those with immunosuppression illnesses such as acquired immune deficiency syndrome (AIDS) may develop anemia or pancytopenia. These clients should be isolated if in the hospital. Pregnant women should be monitored closely by ultrasound for evidence of hydrops and distress. Fetal death occurs in about 6% of cases, usually during the first 20 weeks (Levin, 1999).

TABLE **3-32**   Differential Diagnosis: Fifth Disease (Erythema Infectiosum)

DISEASE	RASH	LOCATION	SYMPTOMS	TIMING
Scarlet fever	Flushed face and pinpoint red papules, sandpaper-like rash	Initially on face and trunk then moves to extremities	Strawberry tongue, fever, sore throat, headache	Rash and symptoms occur simultaneously
Mononucleosis	Macular/papular red, morbilliform	Trunk and upper arms; may involve face	Headache, fatigue, sore throat	Rash occurs 4-6 days after symptoms occur
Rubella	Pinpoint to 1 cm oval or round pink macules and/or papules	Begins on face and neck; spreads rapidly to trunk and extremities; rash fades in 24-48 hr	Mild fever, headache, and malaise; Enlarged cervical lymph glands	Rash occurs at the height of enlarged lymph glands
Roseola	Pale pink oval macules	Begins on trunk and neck; becomes confluent	*High* fever, with few other symptoms	Rash occurs after fever resolves
Measles	Bright red to purple macules and papules; often becomes confluent	Begins behind the ears; spreads to trunk and extremities	Severe cough, fever, conjunctivitis, photophobia, and Koplik spots	Rash occurs 3-4 days after symptoms present
Fifth disease	Bright red confluent rash; pink to red confluent, lacy	Starts on face; open pattern on extremities	Mild fever, headache, sore throat, coryza	Rash occurs after systemic symptoms have resolved
Drug eruptions	Maculopapular red rash; may become confluent	Generalized; usually spares face	Possibly pruritic rash; symptoms of underlying illness	Rash begins 1-2 wk after starting medication

From Robinson, D., Kidd, P., & Rogers, K.M.: *Primary care across the lifespan*, St Louis, 2000, Mosby.

COMPLICATIONS

- Fetal death
- Severe anemia in immunocompromised clients

REFERENCES

Bartlett, J. G. (1996). *Pocket book of infectious disease therapy*. Baltimore: Williams & Wilkins.

Benenson, A. (1995). *Control of communicable diseases manual* (16th ed.). Washington, DC: American Public Health Association.

Committee on Infectious Diseases, American Academy of Pediatrics. (2000). In *1997 Red book: Report of the committee on infectious diseases* (25th ed.). Elk Grove Village, IL: AAP.

Cooper, L. (2000). Fifth's disease. In D. Robinson, P. Kidd, & K. Rogers (Eds.), *Primary care across the lifespan*. St. Louis: Mosby, 459-462.

Kirchner, J. (1994). Erythema infectiosum and other parovirus B19 infections. *American Family Physician, 54*, 335-340.

Levin, M. (1999). Infections: viral and rickettsial. In W. Hay, A. Hayward, M. Levin, & J. Sondheimer (Eds.), *Current pediatric diagnosis and treatment* (14th ed.). Norwalk, CT: Appleton & Lange, 984-987.

Merenstein, G. B., Kaplan, D. W., & Rosenberg, A. A. (1997). *Handbook of pediatrics* (18th ed.). Norwalk, CT: Appleton & Lange.

Review Questions

1. Which of the following descriptions is consistent with erythema infectiosum?
   a. Rash beginning on the body and going to the face
   b. Raised, red, maculopapular lesions on the cheeks
   c. Kopliks spots on the mucus membranes
   d. Maculopapular lesions on palms and soles

2. Who is most likely to be infected with erythema infectiosum?
   a. 2-year-old with fever
   b. 7-year-old with upper respiratory infection (URI) symptoms
   c. 25-year-old with sore throat
   d. 2-month-old with fever of 100.4° F

3. Mary calls because her son has just recovered from Fifth disease. She is concerned because his rash, which had been going away, is now prominent. Which of the following is the most likely scenario?
   a. He has become reinfected with the virus.
   b. He has developed aplastic anemia.
   c. He has likely been out in the sun.
   d. He now is likely to have scarlet fever.

4. Who is more at risk for developing complications from erythema infectiosum?
   a. 3-month-old baby
   b. 7-year-child with chronic hemolytic anemia
   c. 19-year-old with acne
   d. 10-year-old girl with stiff and painful joints

5. In the second stage of erythema infectiosum, the rash has central clearing of confluent lesions. This is most usually described as which of the following?
   a. A lace-like pattern
   b. Slapped cheeks appearance
   c. Annular lesion
   d. Flaky, irritated skin

6. When differentiating Fifth disease from the other childhood illnesses, which of the following best describes this illness when compared with measles?
   a. Fifth disease makes the child feel worse.
   b. In many cases, the slapped cheek appearance is the first clue it is present.
   c. Pharyngitis and systemic symptoms are more prominent.
   d. Lymphadenopathy is a common problem with Fifth disease.

7. If a woman is pregnant and contracts Fifth disease, routine follow-up is recommended. Which of the following is best for the client and baby?
   a. Monthly IgM levels
   b. Monthly CBC
   c. Routine ultrasound
   d. Isolation while hospitalized

8. Sally's mom has been called by the school for a suspected case of Fifth disease. Which of the following is correct advice pertinent to attendance at school?
   a. Sally should stay at home until the rash disappears.
   b. Sally is contagious once the rash appears.
   c. An increased temperature makes other children more susceptible to Fifth disease.
   d. Sally is not contagious once the rash appears.

Answers and Rationales

1. **Answer: b** (assessment)
   Rationale: The characteristic rash pattern of Fifth disease is the "slapped cheek" appearance (Levin, 1999).

2. **Answer: b** (analysis/diagnosis)
   Rationale: Children between 5 and 15 are more at risk for erythema infectiosum (Levin, 1999).

3. **Answer: c** (evaluation)
   Rationale: The rash of Fifth disease often reappears in response to local irritation, heat, sun, and stress (Levin, 1999).

4. **Answer: b** (evaluation)
   Rationale: Reticulocytopenia occurs in most clients, but in a person with chronic hemolytic anemia, it can result in severe anemia (Levin, 1999).

5. **Answer: a** (assessment)
   Rationale: As the rash fades and the center clears, a characteristic lacelike pattern appears (Levin, 1999).

6. **Answer: b** (analysis/diagnosis)
   Rationale: Because the illness is so mild, in many cases the first indication that the illness is present is the slapped cheek appearance (Cooper, 2000).

F

7. *Answer:* c (evaluation)

Rationale: The best way to monitor the status of the fetus for hydrops and distress is via routine ultrasound (Levin, 1999).

8. *Answer:* d (implementation/plan)

Rationale: Once the rash has appeared, the client is not contagious (Cooper, 2000).

FOLLICULITIS *Pamela Kidd*

OVERVIEW
Definition
Folliculitis is a minor inflammation of hair follicles with or without pustules.

Incidence
More common in men who shave.

Pathophysiology
Folliculitis has multiple causes, including the following:
- Gram-negative folliculitis may follow treatment of acne with antibiotics.
- Nonbacterial folliculitis may occur from use of oils.
- Folliculitis may be caused by occlusion.
- May occur as a response to the initiation of systemic steroids or in the tapering of a steroid dose.
- Pseudofolliculitis is caused by ingrown hairs.

Factors Increasing Susceptibility
- Shaving
- Use of hot tubs
- Public swimming pools
- Use of coconut butter or oils
- Tight clothing

Protective Factors
- Using depilatories
- Growing a beard

ASSESSMENT: SUBJECTIVE/HISTORY
Symptoms
- Itching
- Burning and slight tenderness of area
- Breakout of pimples

Past Medical History
- More common in diabetic clients
- Acne

Medication History
- Determine use of antibiotics. Gram-negative organisms may cause folliculitis during antibiotic treatment of acne.
- Determine use of corticosteroids. Topical or systemic use of corticosteroids can produce folliculitis.

Family History
Noncontributory.

Dietary History
Noncontributory.

ASSESSMENT: OBJECTIVE/PHYSICAL EXAMINATION
Physical Examination
Check the skin for pustules of hair follicles, usually in a hairy area, neck, head, face (male), thighs; inflammation may occur around the area, with the skin becoming red and crusting (sycosis).

Diagnostic Procedures
Gram stain and culture of a pustule is used to discriminate bacterial from nonbacterial forms.

DIAGNOSIS
Differential diagnoses include the following:
- Acne affects mainly adolescents. Includes comedones (black and white). Hair is usually oily.
- Miliaria (heat rash) is associated with heat and humidity. It is found in areas of sweat gland concentration (neck, axillae, shoulders, chest), and is more common in infants and children. There is a greater incidence in summer.

THERAPEUTIC PLAN
Nonpharmacologic Treatment
If caused by irritation, remove irritant (shaving is often the irritant).

Pharmacologic Treatment
Use antibiotics for bacterial form or if local treatment is not effective (Table 3-33): Clindamycin 150 to 300 mg qd PO.

Client Education
- Treatment may take weeks, so adherence to treatment plan is important.
- Cleanse areas twice daily with soap containing hexachlorophene.
- Avoid minor trauma and irritants to area (cosmetics, abrasive soaps).

TABLE **3-33**   Pharmacologic Treatment

DRUG	DOSE	COMMENT
Mupirocin (Bactroban) ointment	2%, apply bid × 10 days and cover with DSD	
Gentamicin Sulfate cream or ointment 0.1%	Apply to area bid-tid.	May be covered with gauze DSD if desired
Isoretinoin	0.5 to 1 mg/kg/day PO in divided doses	Used in gram-negative treatment of folliculitis
3% clioquinol and 0.5% hydrocortisone lotion or ointment	Apply to area bid-tid	Do not use in or around eyes
Anhydrous ethyl alcohol with 6.25% aluminum chloride	Apply tid before antibiotic ointment	

DSD, Dry sterile dressing.

- Be sure that hot tubs and swimming pools are adequately treated with chlorine.

Referral

Refer to a dermatologist recurrent cases that do not respond well to antibiotics.

Prevention

- Control blood glucose in diabetic client.
- Avoid hot tubs and public swimming pools.

EVALUATION/FOLLOW-UP

Follow-up is determined per flare-up. Most treatment requires at least 14 days.

COMPLICATIONS

Abscess formation from bacterial form.

REFERENCES

Berger, T. (2001). Skin, hair, and nails. In L. Tierney, S. McPhee, & M. Papadakis (Eds.), *Current medical diagnosis and treatment* (40th ed.). New York: McGraw-Hill.

Berger, T., Goldstein, S., & Odom, R. (1998). Skin and appendages. In L. Tierney, S. McPhee, & M. Papadakis (Eds.), *Current medical diagnosis and treatment* (36th ed.). Stamford, CT: Appleton & Lange.

Kidd, P. (2000). Folliculitis. In D. Robinson, P. Kidd, & K. Rogers (Eds.), *Primary care across the lifespan.* St. Louis: Mosby.

Review Questions

1. Which of the following factors increases the susceptibility for folliculitis?

- **a.** Growing a beard
- **b.** Using a depilatory
- **c.** Use of cologne
- **d.** Using a hot tub

2. In a client with coexisting illness, which of the following measures decreases the risk of folliculitis?

- **a.** Regulation of blood pressure
- **b.** Prescribing antibiotics
- **c.** Regulating blood sugar
- **d.** Prescribing NSAIDs

3. Which of the following statements indicates effective teaching of a client diagnosed with folliculitis?

- **a.** "I will add chlorine to my hot tub."
- **b.** "I will shave daily."
- **c.** "I will wash with an abrasive soap."
- **d.** "I will wash areas once daily."

4. Which of the following medications should the NP prescribe to treat folliculitis?

- **a.** Mupirocin (Bactroban) ointment
- **b.** Cephalexin (Keflex)
- **c.** Hydroxyzine (Atarax)
- **d.** Calamine lotion

Answers and Rationales

1. *Answer:* **d** (assessment)
Rationale: Shaving increases the likelihood of irritation. Coconut butter and oil have been associated with folliculitis, but cologne has not. Using a hot tub without adequate chlorination produces folliculitis.

2. *Answer:* **c** (implementation/plan)
Rationale: Uncontrolled blood sugar is associated with folliculitis. Depending on the type of antibiotics prescribed, antibiotics can even allow Gram-negative organisms to grow and cause folliculitis. NSAIDs and hypertension are not related to folliculitis.

3. *Answer:* **a** (evaluation)
Rationale: The client should wash twice, not once, a day with a nonabrasive soap. Shaving should be avoided. Chlorine kills organisms and prevents folliculitis.

F

4. *Answer:* **a** (plan)

Rationale: Oral antibiotics are not first-line agents in treating folliculitis and should only be used if local treatment is not effective. Itching may be present but is not severe enough to warrant systemic treatment and usually not even local treatment. The use of calamine lotion on the face (a frequent location for folliculitis) may decrease one's body image.

FOREIGN BODY/CORNEAL ABRASION   *Pamela Kidd*

OVERVIEW
Definition

Ocular foreign bodies (FBs) may be extraocular or intraocular. A corneal abrasion is a defect in the bulbar conjunctiva that extends through one or more layers of the conjunctiva.

Incidence

Corneal abrasion caused by an FB is the most common ocular emergency.

Pathophysiology

- Foreign bodies may be wood, metal, sand, or dust. May be imbedded in bulbar conjunctiva (white surface of eye), under lid (palpebral conjunctiva), intraocular, or removed with continued FB sensation.
- Possible sources of trauma include tree or bush limbs, mascara brush, paper, and infant fingernail.
- Contact lenses can cause trauma when worn improperly or are inadequately cleaned.

Factors Increasing Susceptibility
- Contact lens wearers
- High-risk occupations (welder, construction)

Protective Factors
- Eyeglasses
- Safety goggles

ASSESSMENT: SUBJECTIVE/HISTORY
Symptoms

Ask about time of onset, activity at time of injury, whether FB sensation persists, problems with visual acuity or photophobia, and drainage or bleeding from eye. Was FB from explosion, pounding metal, or other high-velocity projectile?

Past Medical History
- Diabetes
- Eye disease, including glaucoma
- Hypertension
- Last tetanus inoculation
- Contact lenses

Past Surgical History

Ask about corneal implants.

Medication History
- Inquire about drops for glaucoma.
- Determine allergies to the following:
  - Local anesthetics
  - Fluorescein stain
  - Antibiotics

Family History

Not relevant.

Dietary History

Not relevant.

ASSESSMENT: OBJECTIVE/PHYSICAL EXAMINATION
Physical Examination

A focused examination is indicated. Note the following:
- General: Look for signs of anxiety, fear, and pain.
- HEENT: Assess visual acuity. Inspect eye for globe penetration, corneal FB, hyphema, injected conjunctiva. Instill topical anesthetic and fluorescein stain. Examine eye with slit lamp, Wood's lamp, or other cobalt-blue light for abrasions. Abrasions show as pooling of stain under cobalt-blue light. Inspect the cornea, bulbar, and palpebral conjunctiva (underside of eyelids) for retained FB. Vertical linear abrasions are usually the sign of an FB under the upper lid.

Diagnostic Procedures

No diagnostic procedures are indicated.

DIAGNOSIS
- Intraocular FB
- Chemical injury (e.g., acid, alkali, solvents)
- Thermal burn
- Ultraviolet keratitis (welders, sunlamp, high-altitude snow)
- Extraocular FB
- Corneal abrasion (mechanical)

THERAPEUTIC PLAN
- Get baseline visual acuity before removal or treatment.
- Instill topical anesthetic (if client is not allergic).

Nonpharmacologic Treatment
- Perform fluorescein examination.

- Remove FB from cornea or bulbar conjunctiva with eye spud or 22- to 25-gauge needle used as spud.
- Remove FB from under eyelids with moist cotton swab.
- Instill broad-spectrum antibiotic ointment (erythromycin, gentamicin, or sulfacetamide) in eye.
- Do not patch affected eye unless abrasion is extensive. If patching is used, the affected eye should be double-patched, with possible referral to ophthalmologist. Patching is controversial. In some cases, such as with corneal abrasions from contact lens, there may be an increased risk of Pseudomonas infection post-patching (Parshall, 2000). An infected eye should *not* be patched.
- Recheck visual acuity.

Pharmacologic Treatment

- Prescribe pain medication. (Vicodin is not too strong.)

ᵠCAUTION: *Topical anesthetics should never be prescribed.*

Client Education

- Patch affects depth perception, so driving, operating machinery, and reading are not allowed.
- Client must wear patch for 24 hours.
- Teach about signs of early infection: white necrotic area around area with small amount of gray exudates (Riorda-Eva, 2001).

Referral

- If FB is metallic and rust ring has formed, refer to ophthalmologist for removal of ring with corneal bur.
- Ophthalmologic consult should be considered if there are multiple FBs, rust rings, if FB is in lens or iris (visual axis), or if mechanism is high velocity.
- Ophthalmologic follow-up if pain persists or if visual acuity is decreased after 24 hours with removal of patch.

Prevention

Use of eyeglasses or safety goggles.

EVALUATION/FOLLOW-UP

- Recheck client in office 24 hours later for corneal abrasion.
- Client should be pain free before being discharged.
- Visual acuity should be normal and client should be pain free 24 hours after treatment.

COMPLICATIONS

- Corneal erosion
- Intraocular infection
- Blindness

REFERNCES

Ghezi, K., & Renner, G. (1992). Ophthalmologic disorders. In P. Rosen (Ed.), *Emergency medicine concepts and clinical practice.* St. Louis: Mosby, 2434-2439.

Hancox, J. D. (2001). Corneal abrasion/foreign body. In D. Robinson, P. Kidd, & K. Rogers (Eds.), *Primary care across the lifespan.* St. Louis: Mosby.

Parshall, M. (2000). Eye conditions. In P. Kidd, P. Sturt, & J. Fultz (Eds.), *Emergency nursing reference* (2nd ed.). St. Louis: Mosby.

Riordan-Eva, P. (2001). Eye. In L. Tierney, S. McPhee, & M. Papadakis (Eds.), *Current medical diagnosis and treatment.* New York: McGraw-Hill.

Review Questions

1. When examining a client for a possible FB in the eye, the NP notices vertical linear abrasions under the cobalt-blue light after using fluorescein stain. This may indicate which of the following?
  a. Allergic reaction to the stain
  b. Removal of FB
  c. Overwearing of contact lens
  d. Retained FB under upper lid

2. When discharging a client treated for a corneal abrasion who had an eye patch applied, the NP should do which of the following?
  a. Refer the client to an ophthalmologist.
  b. Warn the client that pain may be present as long as 48 hours after treatment.
  c. Tell the client to wear an eye patch over the affected eye for 48 hours.
  d. Inform the client about impaired depth perception.

3. The NP should prescribe which of the following for the client with a corneal abrasion?
  a. Topical anesthetic agent
  b. Systemic antibiotic
  c. Saline eye drops
  d. Oral pain medication

4. Which of the following should be assessed in a client with a potential corneal abrasion?
  a. Visual acuity
  b. Extraocular movements
  c. Color acuity
  d. Amblyopia

5. Which eye patching technique should the NP use?
  a. Fold the eye patch in half and tape diagonally.
  b. Patch both eyes to prevent consensual movement.
  c. Double patch the affected eye.
  d. Patch the eye and the side of the face to minimize movement.

Answers and Rationales

1. *Answer:* d (assessment)
  Rationale: Vertical lines indicate a repeated rubbing of the conjunctiva by a foreign object.

2. *Answer:* d (implementation/plan)
  Rationale: Ophthalmologist referral is needed only if there are multiple FBs, a rust ring has formed, an FB is found in the

lens, or an abrasion from a high-velocity mechanism occurred. Both pain and the eye patch should disappear or be discontinued in 24 hours.

3. Answer: d (implementation/plan)

Rationale: Topical anesthetic and antibiotic ointment may be used during the client visit. Although topical antibiotics may be useful in some cases, systemic antibiotics are not normally used. Topical anesthetics may prevent the client from feeling and seeking treatment for an acute change in the eye. Oral pain medication is necessary.

4. Answer: a (assessment)

Rationale: Visual acuity should be checked and compared with acuity before injury. Extraocular movements are associated with a blow directly to the eye or with a neurologic condition. Color acuity and double vision are not associated with FBs.

5. Answer: c (implementation/plan)

Rationale: The eye should be double patched to prevent movement of the eyelid as well as movement of the pupil in relation to light.

FUNCTIONAL LIMITATIONS *Pamela Kidd*

OVERVIEW
Definition

Functional limitations include recent or progressive difficulties in performing or inability to perform various tasks that are necessary or highly desirable for independent living (Lachs, 1996). The impairments are relatively new, and the tasks were at one time within the capabilities of the older client.

Incidence

The incidence is unknown. The condition is often missed by clinicians and may be falsely attributed to normal aging.

Pathophysiology

The condition seldom occurs in isolation. Functional limitations may be signs and symptoms of a new underlying medical illness or of decompensating chronic disease. They may also suggest a change in environment. For example, incontinence may occur as a result of staying in a new home and having to go farther to reach the bathroom.

Factors Increasing Susceptibility
- New environment
- New drug
- Disruptions in usual routine
- Impaired mobility
- Sensory/cognitive deficit
- Incontinence
- Impaired nutritional status (Schuler, Huebscher, & Hallock, 2001)

Protective Factors
- General good health
- Consistent routine and environment

ASSESSMENT: SUBJECTIVE/HISTORY
Symptoms

The history is the most important tool in assessing functional limitations.

- Track limitations according to landmarks, such as holidays. This helps family assess when and for how long a functional limitation has been present, particularly in situations of gradual decline. Acute onset suggests an acute underlying medical condition. If the client and family cannot reach a consensus concerning onset, most likely the limitation is caused by the natural history of a chronic disease.
- When multiple limitations are present, assess the chronology of onset. These usually appear in the following order: (1) bathing, (2) dressing, (3) toileting, (4) transferring, and (5) feeding. Impairments in ADLs with normal instrumental ADLs (IADLs) suggest specific local problems (e.g., incontinence related to enlarged prostate).
- Distinguish capability from ability. Is the client unmotivated or depressed, rather than truly experiencing a functional limitation?
- Consider environmental factors as the basis for any limitations. Examples include obstacles in the home, a new dwelling, and change in caregiver or social services.

Past Medical History

Review all chronic diseases with the client. Functional limitations may appear in place of typical dyspnea or pain. Consider multiple coexisting conditions. The addition of a new condition to a chronic disorder may cause decompensation of the client.

Medication History

Medications, particularly drugs that produce vasodilation or anorexia, may cause functional decline. Diuretics increase the need to go to the bathroom, which may result in incontinence.

Family History

History of Alzheimer's disease if possibility of dementia as a chronic condition exists.

Dietary History

Not relevant.

ASSESSMENT: OBJECTIVE/PHYSICAL EXAMINATION
Physical Examination
Because clients tend to rate self-function higher than do family members, performance measures are more reliable.

The use of standardized tools allows measurement of changes from normal abilities and of treatment effectiveness. Examples include Katz ADLs, which assess toileting, bathing, dressing, and feeding abilities, and Lawton IADLs, which assess higher-order functions necessary for managing a home and household, such as shopping, balancing a checkbook, and telephone use.

- Personal performance tests allow the NP to assess psychomotor skills. For example, ask the client to put on a lab coat or to get up and go from a sitting position.
- Assess sources of pain that may be overlooked, such as mouth (dental problems), perineum (abscess), and feet (bunions).
- Assess general hygiene, dress, and nutritional status.
- Assess cognitive status with a formal tool (e.g., Mini-Mental State Exam) because functional limitations may represent disorientation or cognitive impairment.

Diagnostic Procedures
Electrolyte profiles, urinalysis, and CBC help rule out infection, anemia, and electrolyte shifts as a source of the decline. Radiographic films may help in assessing infection or abscesses as possible causes of decline.

DIAGNOSIS
Depression, infection, angina, diabetes, and arthritis are all common causes of functional decline and should be considered as precipitating factors. Drug side effects should also be considered in the differential diagnosis. Pain may also precipitate decline in function.

THERAPEUTIC PLAN
The NP focuses on preventing decline by anticipating and decreasing risk factors, promoting a rapid response to detected declines, and conducting periodic reassessment.

Nonpharmacologic Treatment
If no cause can be found and the client has decompensated to the state that assistance with caregiving is necessary, hospital admission may be necessary until social services can be obtained, particularly when family is not present.

Pharmacologic Treatment
Treat the precipitating cause of the decline (e.g., infection) as indicated.

Client Education
Caregiver may need information about the precipitating factors and immediate and long-term needs of the client.

Referral
A referral to and consultation with a physician or gerontologist and geriatric assessment team should always be made when no basis for the functional limitations can be identified. A consultation with a pharmacist can assist the provider in ascertaining the role medications may play in functional decline.

Prevention
Periodic assessment of medications by provider can prevent decline related to drug toxicity. Family and/or caregiver assessment of the elder residing in the home environment can prevent potential decline related to falls and improper diet.

EVALUATION/FOLLOW-UP
Follow-up phone calls should be made at 24 and 48 hours after the client visit to see whether improvements have occurred after treatment. If so, 2-week follow-up is indicated to prevent recurrence of the precipitating factor.

COMPLICATIONS
Impaired functional status and dependency in ADLs are better predictors of complications from hospital admissions, subsequent institutionalization, and services needed than are age or mental status (Gudmundsson & Carnes, 1996).

REFERENCES
Bernstein, E. (1996). Functional assessment, mental status, and case finding. In A. Sanders (Ed.), *Emergency care of the elder person*. St. Louis: Mosby.
Gudmundsson, A., & Carnes, M. (1996). Geriatric assessment: Making it work in primary care practice. *Geriatrics, 51,* 62.
Lachs, M. (1996). Functional decline. In A. Sanders (Ed.), *Emergency care of the elder person*. St. Louis: Mosby.
Shuler, P., Huebscher, R., & Hallock, J. (2001). Providing wholistic care for the elderly: Utilization of the Shuler Nurse Practitioner Practice Model. *Journal of the Academy of Nurse Practitioners, 13*(7), 297-303.

Review Questions

1. A daughter brings her mother to the NP because the mother is not able "to keep up anymore." To help assess the scope of this problem, the NP should do all the following, *except:*
   a. Try to determine whether one or multiple impairments are present.
   b. Have the client rate herself with respect to ADLs.

c. Determine the landmark time around when these changes began.

d. Make sure that the client has been able to perform the activities in the past.

2. When examining a client with functional limitations, the NP notes that IADLs are intact but toileting is impaired. Which of the following does this suggest?

a. More ADLs are disrupted.

b. The problem's cause is local, not systemic.

c. Cognitive impairments may exist.

d. Motivation is the problem.

3. In the differential diagnosis of functional limitations, which of the following should be considered?

a. Mental health problems

b. Sexually transmitted diseases

c. Occupational-related disorder

d. Biologic aging

4. When planning care for a client with functional limitations of unknown origin, the NP should do which of the following?

a. Consult with a physician.

b. Admit the client or arrange for hospital admission.

c. Refer the client to psychiatry.

d. Contact home health care.

5. When should initial evaluation of a client with functional limitations be done?

a. In the office within 24 hours

b. By phone within 1 week

c. By phone within 24 hours

d. Within 1 month

Answers and Rationales

1. **Answer: b** (assessment)
Rationale: Clients tend to overrate their abilities, and self-assessment is not reliable. Understanding the number of impairments and their onset, duration, and severity is important. If the client was never able to perform a task, the inability to perform it now may not be related to functional limitations.

2. **Answer: b** (assessment)
Rationale: If higher-order function is preserved, there is no cognitive impairment. This also suggests that a specific structural cause may be present. Motivation level should be assessed, but there is no reason yet to believe that it is the problem.

3. **Answer: a** (analysis/diagnosis)
Rationale: Depression may be a source of functional decline because of the lack of energy to perform ADLs. No specific occupational illnesses have been associated with functional limitations as initial presenting symptoms. Aging does not in itself produce functional limitations. Sexually transmitted diseases do not induce changes in ADLs. Only syphilis may produce neurologic symptoms and possible deterioration of IADLs.

4. **Answer: a** (implementation/plan)
Rationale: Functional limitations of unknown origin need further evaluation to ensure that an acute or chronic illness is not being missed. This evaluation may be done on an outpatient basis, depending on client status. Psychiatry is not needed initially unless a diagnosis of a mental health problem has been made. Home health care may not be necessary if adequate caregiving can be provided by the family or if functional changes are minor.

5. **Answer: c** (evaluation)
Rationale: Follow-up within 24 hours of the visit is necessary to assess whether severity has increased, perhaps as the result of an acute process. An office visit is not necessary, however, if the family's reports are reliable.

FURUNCLE AND CARBUNCLE *Pamela Kidd*

OVERVIEW
Definition

A furuncle is often called an *abscess* or *boil* and is a more extensive infection of the hair follicle. A carbuncle is an extensive infection of several adjacent hair follicles that form a mass with multiple drainage points.

Incidence

True incidence is not known.

Pathophysiology

- Most common pathogen is *Staphylococcus aureus.*
- May occasionally be caused by streptococcal organisms.

Factors Increasing Susceptibility

- Poor hygiene
- Use of body or hair oils
- Local skin trauma from friction of clothing
- Maceration from obesity

ASSESSMENT: SUBJECTIVE/HISTORY
Symptoms

- Inquire about onset, location, duration, appearance of lesions, and presence of pustules or drainage.
- Inquire about hygiene and shaving practices, past causes of skin irritation, recent change in soaps or skin products, and use of hair, bath, and suntan oils.
- Inquire about associated symptoms of pain, pruritus, fever, and chills.

- Inquire about past occurrence of similar lesions.
- Inquire about self-help measures and picking.

Past Medical History

- Inquire about general health and past dermatologic problems.
- Diabetes, HIV, and other immunosuppressive diseases may predispose a client to furuncle formation.

Medication History

Injection drug use.

Family History

Noncontributory.

Dietary History

A diet rich in sugars and fats.

ASSESSMENT: OBJECTIVE/PHYSICAL EXAMINATION
Physical Examination

- Inspect lesions. Determine location, distribution, erythema, pain, and the presence of pustules with central hair follicles or purulent drainage from more extensive lesions.
- Palpate for fluctuance, which indicates accumulation of purulent matter.
- Palpate for lymphadenopathy.
- Assess temperature to evaluate systemic involvement.
- A furuncle presents as walled-off mass that is filled with pus and is painful, firm, or fluctuant. Furuncles most often appear in sites of friction, such as the groin, waistline, axilla, and buttocks.
- A carbuncle occurs in areas of thick dermis, such as the back of the neck and lateral aspect of the thigh.

Diagnostic Procedures

- Take a culture of any drainage, especially in immunocompromised clients.
- Consider taking a culture of the nares to identify a chronic staphylococcal carrier.

DIAGNOSIS

Differential diagnoses include the following:
- Acne vulgaris is the most common form of acne in adolescents and young adults caused by androgenic hormones and *Propionibacterium acnes* in the hair follicle. Most commonly presents on the face, chest, and back.
- Hydradenitis is an inflammation and infection of the sweat glands. Old scars or sinus tracts and a negative culture are present.
- Epidermoid cyst is a common, benign, variable subcutaneous mass lined by keratinizing epithelium and filled with a cheesy material composed of sebum and epithelial debris.

THERAPEUTIC PLAN
Nonpharmacologic Treatment

- Warm, moist compresses promote spontaneous localization and drainage for furuncles and carbuncles.
- Incision and drainage is commonly required for furuncles and carbuncles.

Pharmacologic Treatment

- Systemic pharmacologic treatment for furuncles and carbuncles includes the following:
  - Keflex 250 mg PO q6h × 10 days; Children: 50 mg/kg/day in divided doses q6h, or
  - Biaxin 250 mg PO q12h × 7 to 14 days; Children: 15 mg/kg/day in divided doses q12h, or
  - Dicloxacillin 250 mg PO q6h × 10 days; Children: 25 mg/kg/day in divided doses q6h
- Staphylococcal carriers should be treated with 2% mupirocin to nares, axillae, and anogenital areas bid × 5 days.

Client Education

- Recurrent furuncles are common.
- Educate clients about the role of good hygiene.
- Recommend that antibacterial soap be used daily.

Referral

- Clients with cutaneous abscesses of the face, scalp, and neck should be referred to a dermatologist.
- Clients with recurrent abscesses should be cultured and referred to a physician for further evaluation for underlying conditions such as immunodeficiency, diabetes mellitus, alcoholism, malnutrition, and severe anemia.

Prevention

Family members and intimate contacts need evaluation of staphylococcal carrier state and treatment if appropriate.

EVALUATION/FOLLOW-UP

Follow-up depends on the client's general health, extensiveness of lesions, response to treatment, and recurrence.

COMPLICATIONS

A furuncle is a serious infection. Osteomyelitis and endocarditis can occur from manipulation of a furuncle. Fatal cavernous sinus thrombosis may occur following manipulation of a furuncle on the upper lip or near the nasolabial folds (Berger, 2001).

REFERENCES

Berger, T. (2001). Skin, hair, and nails. In L. Tierney, S. McPhee, & M. Papadakis (Eds.), *Current medical diagnosis and treatment* (40th ed.). New York: McGraw-Hill.

F

Hay, W. W., Groothuis, J. R., Hayward, A. R., & Levin, M. J. (1995). *Current pediatric diagnosis and treatment* (12th ed.). Norwalk, CT: Appleton & Lange, 404.

Kidd, P. (2000). Abcess, boil, furuncle. In D. Robinson, P. Kidd, & K. Rogers (Eds.), *Primary care across the lifespan*. St. Louis: Mosby.

Sauer, G. C., & Hall, J. C. (1996). *Manual of skin diseases*. Philadelphia: Lippincott-Raven, 158-159.

Review Questions

1. Which of the following diagnoses is consistent with the finding of a boil or abscess?

  a. Folliculitis
  b. Impetigo
  c. Carbuncle
  d. Furuncle

2. Which of the following factors increases susceptibility for furuncle and carbuncle formation?

  a. Poor hygiene
  b. Hypertension
  c. Diet rich in spicy foods
  d. African-American heritage

3. The NP suspects that the client with a furuncle is a chronic staphylococcal carrier. The NP should do which of the following?

  a. Perform a blood culture.
  b. Culture drainage from the lesion.
  c. Culture the nares.
  d. Obtain a CBC.

4. In treating a chronic staphylococcal carrier the NP should prescribe which of the following?

  a. Cephalexin (Keflex) 250 mg PO q6h
  b. Clarithromycin (Biaxin) 250 mg PO q12h
  c. 2% mupirocin ointment tid
  d. Dicloxacillin 250 mg PO q6h

Answers and Rationales

1. Answer: d (analysis/diagnosis)
  Rationale: A carbuncle is an extensive infection of several adjacent hair follicles that form a mass with multiple drainage points. A furuncle is an extensive infection of a hair follicle. Folliculitis is inflammation of multiple hair follicles that may be in multiple areas. Impetigo is an infection of the skin and does not affect hair follicles.

2. Answer: a (assessment)
  Rationale: No ethnicity is at higher risk for furuncle or carbuncle formation. A diet rich in sugar and fat increases risk. Immunosuppression also increases risk.

3. Answer: c (implementation/plan)
  Rationale: The lesion may contain staphylococcus without the client being a carrier. The presence of staphylococcus in the nares suggests an autoinoculation process. A CBC is nonspecific. A blood culture should only be used to help diagnosis moderate to severe systemic infection.

4. Answer: c (implementation/plan)
  Rationale: Antibiotics are used to treat furuncles and carbuncles when severe. Only local application of mupirocin to the nares, axillae, and anogenital areas is used to treat chronic staphylococcus states.

GALLBLADDER DISEASE *Cheryl Pope Kish*

OVERVIEW

Definition

Cholecystitis is an inflammation of the gallbladder caused by cystic duct irritation or obstruction. Such inflammation is caused by gallstones 90% of the time and may be either acute or chronic in nature. Acalculous cholecystitis, inflammation without gallstone formation, is associated with stressful situations or ischemia to the gallbladder.

Cholelithiasis refers to gallstone formation with or without obstruction. There are three types of gallstones: cholesterol, pigment, or mixed (most common).

Choledocholithiasis refers to the condition that occurs when a gallstone lodges in the common bile duct.

Gallbladder disease may be asymptomatic or may be accompanied by recurrent bouts of abdominal discomfort. With asymptomatic disease, there is a 20% or less probability that the pain of biliary colic will occur in a client who is 20 years old. When gallstones have formed, 18% to 33% of clients become symptomatic within 1 to 2 years of diagnosis.

Cholangitis is a bacterial infection and associated obstruction of the duct system.

Incidence

More than 25 million persons in the United States have gallbladder disease; this represents 10% of all adult men and 20% of women. More then 500,000 surgical procedures are performed for a diagnosis of gallbladder disease annually.

Gallbladder disease is more common in women than men, especially in overweight women older than 40 years of age; however, it can occur in young women of thin to normal weight. In those 65 years of age and older, men and women are affected equally.

Gallbladder disease is the most common cause of acute abdominal symptoms in older clients; acute cholecystitis is fatal in nearly 10% of elderly clients.

The incidence of gallbladder disease is highest in industrial countries and in certain native North American populations.

Pathophysiology

A change in bile composition and bile stasis related to irregular contractions of the gallbladder, spasms of the sphincter of Oddi, delayed emptying, and infections of the gallbladder predispose clients to gallstone formation. Subsequently, ischemia or obstruction of the cystic duct (by stones) causes symptoms. Cholesterol stones, common in the United States and Europe, are large, single, round or oval and pale yellow stones that form when cholesterol supersaturates bile in the gallbladder and crystals precipitate out. Pigment stones, multiple small dark brown or black stones with high bilirubin content, are more common in Asian countries in persons who have parasitic bile duct infections with medical conditions that increase breakdown of bilirubin (i.e., sickle cell anemia). Mixed gallstones consist of both cholesterol and bilirubin and tend to be multiple in number and dark brown.

Factors Increasing Susceptibility
- Obesity
- Rapid weight loss on a very low-calorie diet
- Exogenous estrogen (oral contraceptive pills [OCPs] and estrogen replacement therapy)
- Hyperlipidemia
- Diabetes mellitus
- Use of thiazide diuretics
- Cirrhosis
- Prolonged parental alimentation
- Pregnancy (transitory)

Other conditions that have also been considered to introduce some possible risk include spinal cord injury, pancreatic insufficiency, Crohn's disease, and ileal resection.

Protective Factors. A low-calorie, low-fat diet in an individual of normal weight who is not predisposed to gallbladder disease by genetics may offer some degree of protection. Being less than 40 years old also decreases the probability of gallbladder disease, although rare cases do occur.

ASSESSMENT: SUBJECTIVE/HISTORY
Symptoms

Acute cholecystitis causes abrupt severe abdominal pain of a colicky nature in the epigastrium or right upper quadrant (RUQ). The pain often radiates to the upper back or scapula on the right and often increases with movement and deep breathing and lasts 2 to 4 hours. Tenderness in the RUQ may last several days. Clients often notice the pain 1 to 6 hours after a large or fatty meal. Nausea and vomiting occur in 75% of clients. Anorexia, heartburn, bloating, belching, and, rarely, fever and jaundice may be clinical features.

Chronic cholecystitis is usually associated with less marked signs and symptoms including vague dyspepsia, intolerance to fried or fatty foods and dairy products, heartburn, bloating, and flatulence. Some clients report pale stools and dark urine. Clients may have gallbladder disease and be asymptomatic for long periods.

Cholangitis, bacterial infection of the gallbladder and biliary ductal system, may cause Charçot's triad of symptoms: fever/chills, jaundice, and RUQ pain.

Children rarely have gallbladder disease, but when they do the presentation is similar to that of an adult. Gallbladder disease is a common cause of abdominal pain in the elderly; in some, symptoms are typical, whereas for others symptoms are more vague and altered mental status may be part of the presentation.

A comprehensive description of the pain is essential. Determine location, radiation, duration, 0 to 10 pain scale quantification, relationship to eating particular foods, and alleviating and aggravating factors. Inquire about nocturnal awakening with pain and how position changes affect it.

Past Medical History

Inquire about a history of diabetes, recent rapid weight loss or total parenteral nutrition, or hyperlipidemia. Ask about previous symptoms. Determine if there is heart disease or risks for heart disease. Inquire about parity.

Medication History

Ask specifically about estrogen use in the form of hormone replacement or OCPs, and about thiazides. Ask about use of cholesterol-lowering drugs, which may increase risk.

Family History

Sometimes there is a positive family history.

Psychosocial History

Social intake of alcohol may decrease incidence of gallstones.

Dietary History

Ask about frequent dieting or starvation diets and/or high-caloric, high-fat intake.

ASSESSMENT: OBJECTIVE/PHYSICAL EXAMINATION

Objective findings depend on the degree of inflammation present. A thorough problem-based physical examination should be performed that focuses on the following:
- Assess general appearance and vital signs; determine height and weight.

- Assess the skin and mucous membranes for jaundice. Assess for icterus. In the present of vomiting, assess turgor and skin temperature.
- Assess the heart.
- Assess the lungs.
- Conduct a comprehensive abdominal assessment. Note contour, bulges, and pulsations. Auscultate bowel sounds. Percuss to determine organic structures and areas of tenderness, delaying to RUQ until last. Perform superficial and deep palpation, noting tenderness, guarding, rebounding, rigidity, organomegaly, and presence of Murphy's sign (respiratory pause with deep inspiration and palpation of gallbladder region). The gallbladder is palpable in less than 50% of clients.

Diagnostic Procedures

First-line diagnostic tests include the following:

- *Complete blood count (CBC) with differential:* Leukocytosis and left shift are commonly seen with cholecystitis.
- *Urinalysis:* Urine may be dark with urobilinogen.
- *Pregnancy test:* Provide if indicated, before treatment or invasive testing.
- *Blood chemistry panel such as SMA-7:* Assess liver function. Bilirubin levels may be elevated even if the common duct is not obstructed but is highly suggestive of cholangitis.
- *Transaminases (aspartate transaminase [AST] and alanine transaminase [ALT]):* Elevated levels indicate biliary obstruction.
- *Abdominal/gallbladder ultrasound:* Sensitive in confirming diagnosis of gallstones; stones in the common duct are not always visible. Dilated bile ducts suggest obstruction. Less sensitive test for diagnosing cholecystitis by showing edema.

Other tests are indicated by history and physical examination as follows:

- Alkaline phosphatase elevation indicates cholangitis.
- Obtain serum amylase and lipase levels to rule out pancreatitis.
- Perform electrocardiogram (ECG) in those older than 50 or at risk for heart disease.
- Obtain chest radiograph to rule out pneumonia.
- If ultrasonography indicates a normal gallbladder and signs and symptoms cannot be linked to other causes, a hepatobiliary (HIDA) scan, which is a radionuclide scan, is particularly helpful in diagnosing an obstructed cystic duct.
- Oral cholangiogram is not helpful in diagnosing acute gallbladder disease.
- Endoscopic retrograde cholangiopancreatography (ERCP) or percutaneous transhepatic cholangiography (PTC) may be necessary for definitive diagnosis.
- Radiographic examination of kidneys and upper bladder sometimes detects air in the wall of the gallbladder or emphysematous cholecystitis.

DIAGNOSIS

Differential diagnoses of RUQ pain include the following:

- Biliary disease, acute or chronic
- Pancreatitis
- Appendicitis
- Myocardial infarction (MI)
- Gastric or duodenal ulcer disease
- Gastritis
- Irritable bowel disease
- Gastric esophageal reflux disease (GERD) with or without hiatal hernia
- Hepatitis
- Pneumonia with pleurisy
- Radicular pain
- Nephrolithiasis

THERAPEUTIC PLAN
Pharmacologic Treatment

Nonsteroidal antiinflammatory drugs (NSAIDs) such as indomethacin have been shown to relieve pain and prevent stones and to prevent recurrence in some cases. For medical management of cholesterol stones with the use of ursodiol (Actigall), recurrence is a factor. Criteria for treatment of gallstones with ursodiol include clients with a functioning gallbladder, stones smaller than 15 mm in diameter, stones that float on oral cholecystogram or are lucent, who are poor candidates for surgery, with mild symptoms, a single stone, or multiple stones in a client receiving long-term NSAID therapy.

Antibiotics may be necessary; ampicillin and a third-generation cephalosporin are commonly used, with the addition of an aminoglycoside if sepsis is suspected. Analgesia is often needed; morphine sulfate is avoided because it contributes to spasm of the sphincter of Oddi and increases pain. Anticholinergics are not helpful.

Demonstrating the presence of gallstones is sufficient indication for surgical treatment. Refer client for definitive treatment. Treatment of choice is laparoscopic cholecystectomy. Use of medical therapies must be prescribed by a specialist; these are usually reserved for cases of high surgical risk or in which surgery is contraindicated.

Any suspicion that the source of pain is cardiac requires an immediate referral.

Client Education

- Advise that asymptomatic gallstones do not grow rapidly and rarely dissolve or pass spontaneously; surgery is not generally performed.
- Advise that one episode followed by a pain-free interval can be managed expectantly. Advise to report recur-

Straughn, A., & English, B. (1996). Oral rehydration therapy: A neglected treatment for pediatric diarrhea. *Maternal Child Nursing, 6*(5), 144-147.

Review Questions

1. Which of the following histories is most consistent with a diagnosis of traveler's diarrhea?

- **a.** Bloody diarrhea
- **b.** Travel to a third world country
- **c.** Large group picnic
- **d.** Family members with similar symptoms

2. Which of the following histories is consistent with a food-borne illness?

- **a.** Bloody diarrhea
- **b.** Travel to a third world country
- **c.** Large group picnic
- **d.** Family members with similar symptoms

3. Which of the following clients should have laboratory testing done for their AGE?

- **a.** A client with nausea, vomiting, and diarrhea for 18 hours
- **b.** A client with prolonged diarrhea for 5 days
- **c.** A client with mild abdominal cramping
- **d.** A client with a 2-ounce weight loss

4. It is important to differentiate viral diarrhea from bacterial diarrhea. In contrast to viral diarrhea, the characteristics of a diarrhea caused by a bacteria are which of the following?

- **a.** Diarrhea, mild fever, and vomiting
- **b.** Profuse watery diarrhea and vomiting
- **c.** Diarrhea accompanied by headache, malaise, chills, and myalgia
- **d.** Green, liquid stool and mild abdominal pain

5. Which of the following patient comments indicates a need for more teaching related to AGE?

- **a.** "I need to make sure all meat is well cooked."
- **b.** "I will go to a local farm and buy milk 'fresh' to avoid any organisms."
- **c.** "I should make sure all eggs are adequately cooked."
- **d.** "I will avoid eating unwashed produce."

6. What rationale do you give to a patient who wants to take medicine for her diarrhea?

- **a.** "The medicines may make you feel worse."
- **b.** "The medications are not effective if the diarrhea is caused by bacteria."
- **c.** "The medications are only appropriate for people 12 years of age and older."
- **d.** "The medications slow intestinal mobility and delay clearance of the organism."

7. Which of the following is the best way to rehydrate a child with AGE?

- **a.** Carbonated beverages
- **b.** Sport drinks
- **c.** Popsicles
- **d.** Rehydration solutions

8. Fecal impaction and AGE need to be differentiated. Compared with viral AGE, which of the following are characteristics of fecal impaction?

- **a.** Liquid diarrhea
- **b.** Family member with similar symptoms
- **c.** Abdominal discomfort
- **d.** Palpable stool in left lower quadrant (LLQ)

Answers and Rationales

1. *Answer:* **b** (assessment)

Rationale: Travel to a developing country is consistent with the development of traveler's diarrhea 3 to 5 days after entering the country (Robinson et al., 2000).

2. *Answer:* **d** (assessment)

Rationale: It is likely that food poisoning symptoms develop in family members (Robinson et al., 2000).

3. *Answer:* **b** (analysis/diagnosis)

Rationale: Prolonged diarrhea for 5 days indicates the need for testing for continuing diarrhea (Centers for Disease Center and Prevention [CDC], 2001b).

4. *Answer:* **c** (analysis/diagnosis)

Rationale: Diarrhea accompanied by headache, malaise, chills, and myalgia is characteristic of salmonella; the symptoms of viral AGE usually include nausea, vomiting, and, rarely, fever (CDC, 2001b).

5. *Answer:* **b** (evaluation)

Rationale: Going to a farm and buying fresh milk does not prevent food-borne illness if the milk is not pasteurized (CDC, 2001b).

6. *Answer:* **d** (implementation/plan)

Rationale: The antidiarrheal medications slow intestinal mobility and delay clearance of the organism and therefore are not recommended. In addition, these medications can increase the risk and severity of HUS (CDC, 2001b).

7. *Answer:* **d** (implementation/plan)

Rationale: Clear liquids do not contain the necessary electrolytes to correct dehydration (Robinson, 2000).

8. *Answer:* **b** (analysis/diagnosis)

Rationale: Symptoms of fecal impaction include abdominal discomfort and palpable stool in the LLQ. The fecal impaction may cause overflow fecal incontinence, which may be mistaken for AGE (Robinson, 2000).

G

GASTROESOPHAGEAL REFLUX DISEASE *Pamela Kidd*

OVERVIEW
Definition

Gastroesophageal reflux disease (GERD) is characterized by an abnormal reflux of gastroduodenal contents into the esophagus, which may result in esophageal inflammation. It is a chronic disease; without therapy, individuals are prone to have relapses.

Incidence

- Incidence is increasing in the United States, where more than 60% of the adult population have had "heartburn."
- From 70% to 80% of women who are pregnant report heartburn.
- More than 20% of affected adults have had symptoms for longer than 10 years.
- Approximately 10% of affected adults experience symptoms daily.
- Children may also be affected, usually in the first year of life.
- Males and females are affected equally.
- GERD causes complications in less than 2% of the general population.
- Without long-term therapy, 50% to 80% of persons with GERD have a relapse within 6 to 12 months of healing of the acute disease.
- An increasing number of individuals are observed to have GERD-induced asthma.

Pathophysiology

GERD is caused by a reflux of gastric contents into the esophagus, which may be caused by an abnormal antireflux barrier, defective esophageal clearance, increased gastric secretions, and delayed gastric emptying. The pathophysiology of the asthma–GERD connection is less clear. It is suggested that the esophageal bronchial reflux triggers bronchospasm, which promotes acid reflux, leading to further bronchospasms.

Factors Increasing Susceptibility
- Smoking
- Obesity
- Eating large meals
- Pregnancy: Progesterone lowers sphincter tone.

Protective Factors. Allow gravity to help by maintaining an upright posture after eating meals.

ASSESSMENT: SUBJECTIVE/HISTORY
Symptoms

- Burning substernal pain radiates upward, often called "heartburn," usually within 30 to 60 minutes of eating.
- Note frequency, onset, progression, and duration of pain.
- Pain is aggravated by large meals, lying down, or bending over.
- Pain is relieved by antacids or nonprescription doses of H_2-receptor antagonists.
- Dysphagia, cough, weight loss, or blood loss may suggest other problems.
- Regurgitation of fluid or food particles may occur.
- Reflux may trigger angina-like chest pain.
- Hoarseness, sore throat, and feeling of lump in throat may be symptoms of GERD.
- Wheezing, nocturnal coughing, and shortness of breath may suggest an asthmatic component.

Past Medical History

- Chronic diseases
- Similar episodes
- History of asthma

Medication History

Medications that reduce lower esophageal sphincter pressure are the following:
- Anticholinergics
- Progesterone
- Calcium channel blockers (nifedipine and verapamil)
- Calcium
- Theophylline
- Diazepam
- Meperidine
- Transdermal nicotine

Drugs that may injure the esophageal mucosa are the following:
- Doxycycline, quinidine, NSAIDs
- Bisphosphonate alendronate (Fosamax)

Note whether any prescribed, OTC, or herbal remedies are taken.

Family History

Noncontributory.

Dietary History

- Acidic foods: citrus fruit, spicy foods, tomato products, coffee
- Foods that delay gastric emptying or relax the gastric sphincter: alcohol, high-fat diets, chocolate, peppermint

ASSESSMENT: OBJECTIVE/PHYSICAL EXAMINATION
Physical Examination

A problem-oriented physical examination is necessary, with attention to vital signs, height and weight, and general appearance.

- Evaluate lungs for adventitious sounds.
- Check abdomen for bowel sounds, distention, obesity, masses, and pain.
- Perform rectal assessment for masses, tenderness, and occult blood.
- A comprehensive examination should be scheduled to evaluate other problems.

Diagnostic Procedures

- Usually no laboratory studies are required.
- Obtain a CBC with differential to rule out anemias and infections.
- Complete a chemistry profile to evaluate for other chronic problems, such as diabetes and liver problems.
- Procedures include endoscopy in the case of dysphagia, weight loss, blood loss, or treatment failure.
- Perform a guaiac evaluation of stool for occult blood.

DIAGNOSIS

Differential diagnoses include the following:
- Cardiac chest pain
- Peptic ulcer disease
- Esophageal infection (*Candida*, herpes, HIV, cytomegalovirus)
- Esophagitis from pill taking (e.g., doxycycline, ascorbic acid, quinidine)
- Esophageal carcinoma
- Asthma may coexist with GERD.

THERAPEUTIC PLAN

Management of GERD involves a stepped approach to care. Try nonpharmacologic strategies first.

Nonpharmacologic Treatment

Pediatric Clients. Gastroesophageal reflux is common in the first year of life. Symptoms include vomiting, weight loss, failure to thrive, and possibly apnea and bradycardia secondary to vagal response. The symptoms generally resolve by age 18 months. Placing the infant upright in a car seat 2 to 3 hours after feeding and thickening the feedings with rice cereal may help minimize symptoms. Surgical treatment may be indicated if there is apnea, persistent vomiting, or difficulty in breathing or swallowing.

Dietary Changes
- Possibly necessary lifestyle modifications include losing weight, stopping smoking, and reducing alcohol consumption; eat small, frequent meals and take no food 2 to 3 hours before bed.
- Raise head of bed 4 inches. (Do not use pillows because this may worsen problem.)

Pharmacologic Treatment

- In pediatric clients, Antacids and liquid H_2-receptor antagonists (Zantac syrup) are used to manage symptoms.

- Adult clients with erosive esophagitis and complications (see following discussion) should be treated initially with a proton-pump inhibitor (step 3).
- Step 1 pharmacologic treatment includes the following:
  - Take antacids (after meals and at bedtime).
  - Antacids can be used on an as-needed basis. Remember that magnesium-based antacids may cause diarrhea; aluminum-based antacids may cause constipation.
  - Take nonprescription (low-dose) H_2-receptor antagonist PO; H_2-receptor antagonist dosage may need to be lower if client has renal disease.

Cimetidine 200 mg bid
Ranitidine, nizatidine 75 mg bid
Famotidine 10 mg bid

- Step 2 pharmacologic treatment includes higher dose (prescribed) H_2-receptor antagonist PO as follows:
  - Take cimetidine (Tagamet), 400 mg bid (interacts with many drugs, such as theophylline, warfarin, and phenytoin).
  - Take ranitidine (Zantac), 150 mg bid
  - Take famotidine (Pepcid), 20 mg bid
  - Take nizatidine (Axid), 150 mg bid
- In step 3 pharmacologic treatment, proton-pump inhibitors (PPIs) may be used as follows:
  - Omeprazole (Prilosec), 20 mg/day
  - Lansoprazole (Prevacid), 30 mg/day
  - Esomeprazole (Nexium) 20 mg/day
  - Short-term therapy, 8 to 12 weeks
  - Long-term therapy, longer than 12 weeks to lifetime

Client Education

- Long-term maintenance therapy with an H_2-receptor antagonist and lifestyle modifications are essential to prevent exacerbation of GERD. Maintenance therapy is usually half the therapeutic dose taken at bedtime.
- Stop smoking.
- Elevate head of bed.
- Lose weight if more than 130% of ideal body weight.
- Avoid lying down immediately after meals.
- Eat smaller meals and a low-fat diet.
- Avoid foods that cause symptoms.
- Avoid alcohol and coffee.
- Avoid stooping, bending, and tight clothes.
- Avoid drugs that decrease lower esophageal sphincter pressure.
- Exercise daily.
- Refer client to local support groups if available.

Referral

Referral is usually to a gastroenterologist.

Adults
- Dysphagia, weight loss, blood loss, myocardial infarction

G

- Recurrence after full course of therapy with two different medications
- Clients receiving protein-pump inhibitors
- Pregnant women whose symptoms persist despite lifestyle modifications

Children
- Failure to thrive in children
- Persistent or worsening symptoms in children (apnea, vomiting, difficulty in swallowing or breathing)
- Weight loss and vomiting in children

Prevention

Pregnant Clients. Heartburn among pregnant women is worse in the first and second trimesters. Treatment is self-managed: frequent small meals, avoidance of meals 2 to 3 hours before lying down, and elevating the head of bed for sleeping.

EVALUATION/FOLLOW-UP
- Initial follow-up in 1 to 2 weeks to assess improvement; recheck in 4 weeks.
- At 8 weeks, adjust follow-up on the basis of recurring signs and symptoms.

COMPLICATIONS
- Reflux esophagitis results in inflammation in the esophageal wall, increasing capillary permeability, edema, tissue fragility, and erosion.
- Hiatal hernia is a possibility.
- Chronic GERD may be associated with strictures, hemorrhage, and increased risk of Barrett's esophagus (adenocarcinoma). Age increases the risk of malignancy.
- Asthma is a possible complication.

REFERENCES

Brady, W. M., & Ogorek, C. P. (1996). Gastroesophageal reflux disease. *Postgraduate Medicine, 100*(5), 76-89.

Clark, C. L., & Horwitz, B. (1996). Complications of gastroesophageal reflux disease. *Postgraduate Medicine, 100*(5), 95-113.

Dumont, J. A., & Richter, J. E. (1997). Gastroesophageal reflux masquerading as asthma. *Internal Medicine, February,* 19-37.

Larsen, R. (1997). Gastroesophageal reflux disease. *Postgraduate Medicine, 101*(2), 181-187.

Meierbachtol, D. (2000) GERD. In D. Robinson, P. Kidd, & K. Rogers (Eds.), *Primary care across the lifespan.* St. Louis: Mosby.

Review Questions

1. Which of the following is most indicative of GERD?
   a. Abdominal pain is relieved by bowel movement.
   b. Food intake makes the pain worse.
   c. Pain is relieved by food intake.
   d. Burning, substernal pain is noted 1 hour after eating.

2. Which of the following findings is common in a client with GERD?
   a. Abnormal liver function studies
   b. Normal physical findings
   c. Angina pectoris
   d. Occult blood

Situation: T.M., a 57-year-old man, seeks treatment for chest pain after eating. This symptom has been intermittent for 3 months. He uses antacids as needed, with relief. He smokes two packs of cigarettes per day, drinks two beers per night, and is 130% of his ideal body weight. He points to his chest and describes his chest pain as burning, substernal pain that moves upward. He takes no other medications and denies chronic diseases. He was last seen 1.5 years ago for a similar episode. He coughed frequently during the office visit. Results of his examination are normal. (Applies to questions 3 through 5.)

3. On the basis of this history, what is the most likely diagnosis for T.M.?
   a. GERD
   b. Inflammatory bowel disease
   c. Angina
   d. Peptic ulcer disease

4. What is the best treatment for this individual?
   a. H_2-receptor antagonist only
   b. Lifestyle changes and H_2-receptor antagonist
   c. Lifestyle modifications, dietary changes to lose weight, and antacids
   d. Beta-blocker only

5. When should T.M. return for follow-up?
   a. 8 weeks
   b. 1 to 2 weeks
   c. 3 months
   d. As needed

6. Which of the following percentages best describes the incidence of GERD?
   a. Eighty percent of pregnant women have symptoms.
   b. Eighty percent of adults have symptoms for more than 10 years.
   c. Seventy percent of those older than 70 years have GERD.
   d. GERD occurs in 20% of the adult population.

Situation: You are treating a 33-year-old client who is 4 months pregnant, a smoker, and reports heartburn. You suspect that she may have a weakened lower esophageal sphincter, which is a risk factor for GERD. (Applies to questions 7 and 8.)

7. You suspect lower esophageal sphincter relaxation is caused by which of the following?
   a. Pressure caused by increasing size of pregnancy
   b. Progestational hormones associated with pregnancy
   c. Not related to her pregnancy
   d. Foods she is eating

8. What would you recommend to alleviate symptoms?
   a. Omeprazole (Prilosec)
   b. H_2-receptor antagonist

c. Smoking cessation
d. Frequent, small meals

Answers and Rationales

1. *Answer:* d (assessment)
Rationale: Burning substernal pain 1 hour after eating is a classic definition of GERD. Pain relieved by bowel movements is associated with irritable bowel syndrome (IBS). Food often makes the pain worse for those with gastric ulcers, whereas pain may be relieved by food for those with duodenal ulcers.

2. *Answer:* b (assessment)
Rationale: Often, physical findings are normal and diagnostic tests are not required to make a diagnosis of GERD. If there is any question that the history is suggestive of angina, liver problems, or anemia, tests need to be done to rule out these conditions.

3. *Answer:* a (analysis/diagnosis)
Rationale: The condition is most likely GERD because of the nature and duration of the chest pain, especially when it is relieved by antacids. T.M.'s weight, alcohol intake, and smoking behavior increase his risk for symptoms of GERD; however, given his age and symptoms, heart disease, gastric ulcer disease, and malignancy also need to be ruled out.

4. *Answer:* c (implementation/plan)
Rationale: In a step approach, lifestyle modifications (e.g., stop smoking, eat small meals), dietary changes (to avoid selected foods and reduce types and amounts to lose weight), and antacids or nonprescription H_2-receptor antagonists are the appropriate first step. If this does not work, the second phase is to add H_2-receptor antagonists in conjunction with lifestyle and dietary modifications. Beta-blockers are commonly used to treat hypertension.

5. *Answer:* b (evaluation)
Rationale: This is a new client starting a new regimen of care. Follow-up in 1 to 2 weeks allows you to spot any changes in his heartburn and to provide support and reinforcement of the lifestyle changes and dietary modification. If symptoms are not better, you may want to add the H_2-receptor antagonist at this time. Follow-up intervals of 8 weeks and 3 months are both too long if the client is not getting better. As-needed follow-up may be interpreted by the client as a message not to come back. When implementing a plan involving lifestyle and dietary changes, "structured" or scheduled support visits may be reinforcing for the client.

6. *Answer:* a (assessment)
Rationale: Approximately 70% to 80% of women who are pregnant experience heartburn, one of the symptoms of GERD. Only 20% of adults have symptoms longer than 10 years. Of 70-year-old clients, 70% have diverticular disease. Both diverticular disease and IBS occur in 20% of the adult population.

7. *Answer:* b (analysis/diagnosis)
Rationale: There may be decreased pressure of the lower esophageal sphincter during pregnancy as a result of progestational hormones; pressure caused by increasing uterine size does not usually influence lower esophageal sphincter relaxation. You lack a dietary history to make any conclusions relating the cause to foods.

8. *Answer:* d (implementation/plan)
Rationale: Starting with frequent, small meals may reduce her symptoms. Omeprazole is a category C drug for pregnancy. H_2-receptor antagonists are category B drugs for pregnancy and could be prescribed; however, most providers encourage minimal or no prescription drug use during pregnancy.

GIANT CELL ARTERITIS/POLYMYALGIA RHEUMATICA *Pamela Kidd*

G

OVERVIEW
Definition

Giant cell (temporal) arteritis is a systemic panarteritis affecting medium- to large-size vessels. Polymyalgia rheumatica is an autoimmune condition of pain and stiffness of the joints (usually shoulder, hip, and pelvis).

Incidence

Not known.

Pathophysiology

Both conditions are considered as ramifications of one disease. They coexist in at least 50% of clients. The exact cause is not known, but they are considered autoimmune disorders. In giant cell arteritis, blindness is possible resulting from occlusion of the posterior branch of the ophthalmic artery.

Factors Increasing Susceptibility. Clients older than age 50.

Protective Factors. Intact immune system.

ASSESSMENT: SUBJECTIVE/HISTORY
Symptoms

Giant Cell Arteritis
- Dry cough
- Fever, with night sweats
- Painful paralysis of a shoulder
- Headache
- Scalp tenderness
- Visual changes
- Jaw claudication
- Throat pain
- Vague pain in tongue, head, neck, nose or ears

Polymyalgia Rheumatica

- Pain and stiffness of shoulder, hips, and pelvis
- Trouble combing hair
- Trouble dressing
- Joint swelling in some cases

Past Medical History

Autoimmune disorders.

Medication History

Corticosteroid use (helpful in planning treatment, does not predispose to condition).

Family History

Autoimmune disorders.

Dietary History

Noncontributory.

ASSESSMENT: OBJECTIVE/PHYSICAL EXAMINATION

Physical Examination

- Perform total body examination. Assess vital signs (high fever may be present).
- Assess head, eyes, ears, nose, and throat (HEENT). No funduscopic findings may be present in first 48 hours after blindness occurs.
- Assess cardiac functioning for asymmetry of radial and brachial pulses in the arms, aortic regurgitation murmur, and subclavian artery bruits (heard near clavicle).
- Assess the musculoskeletal system for knee and wrist sternoclavicular joint swelling; there will be *no* muscular weakness.

Diagnostic Procedures

- Erythrocyte sedimentation rate will be very elevated.
- Obtain CBC. Anemia may be present. White blood cell (WBC) count is frequently normal.
- In giant cell arteritis, temporal artery biopsy will show giant cells, lymphocytes, plasma cells (inflammation markers).

DIAGNOSIS

Differential diagnoses include chronic infection and malignancy.

THERAPEUTIC PLAN

Nonpharmacologic Treatment

Not helpful.

Pharmacologic Treatment

Both conditions respond to corticosteroids.

- Polymyalgia rheumatica: Prescribe low dose of corticosteroids (10 to 20 mg); if no improvement in 72 hours, doubt diagnosis.

- Giant cell arteritis: Prescribe high dose (40 to 60 mg); must be initiated immediately at 60 mg to prevent blindness.

Client Education

Stress that this is a chronic disease and emphasize the need for regular check-ups because of the severity of complications (see following).

Referral

Refer to rheumatologist promptly for confirmation of diagnosis, obtaining biopsy (if appropriate), and treatment.

Prevention

Adherence to treatment plan diminishes flare-ups. No prevention of initial disease is known.

EVALUATION/FOLLOW-UP

- Polymyalgia rheumatica requires 6 months to 2 years of steroid treatment. Slow tapering prevents relapse.
- Giant cell arteritis requires steroid treatment at 60 mg × 2 months before tapering; do not taper until erythrocyte sedimentation rate (ESR) is normal; frequently recurs.

COMPLICATIONS

- Blindness
- Higher incidence of thoracic aortic aneurysm even with treatment

REFERENCES

Hellmann, D. B., & Stone, J. H. (2001). Arthritis and musculoskeletal disorders. In L. Tierney, S. McPhee, & M. Papadakis (Eds.), *Current medical diagnosis and treatment* (40th ed.). New York: McGraw-Hill.

Review Questions

1. What differentiates the treatment of polymyalgia rheumatica from giant cell arteritis?
- **a.** Use of corticosteroids
- **b.** Dosage of corticosteroids
- **c.** Response to corticosteroids
- **d.** Slow tapering of corticosteroid dose

2. What clinical sign is used for tapering corticosteroids in giant cell arteritis?
- **a.** WBC count
- **b.** Peripheral blood smear results
- **c.** ESR
- **d.** Joint aspiration results

3. What major complication is associated with giant cell arteritis?
- **a.** Facial palsy
- **b.** Joint destruction

c. Blindness
d. Leukemia

4. Which of the following assessment data are common in the syndrome of polymyalgia rheumatica and giant cell arteritis?
a. Elevated heart rate
b. Asymmetry of radial pulses
c. Muscular weakness
d. Paresthesia

Answers and Rationales

1. **Answer: b** (analysis/diagnosis)
Rationale: Corticosteroids are used to treat both conditions. High dose corticosteroids are used in giant cell arteritis

and low dose corticosteroids are used in polymyalgia rheumatica. Corticosteroids are always tapered.

2. **Answer: c** (analysis/diagnosis)
Rationale: ESR should be normal before tapering corticosteroids. The other laboratory tests are not useful.

3. **Answer: c** (analysis/diagnosis)
Rationale: Blindness is caused by occlusion of the posterior branch of the ophthalmic artery resulting from inflammation.

4. **Answer: b** (assessment)
Rationale: Asymmetry of radial pulses as well as aortic regurgitation murmur and subclavian bruits may be present.

GLAUCOMA *Pamela Kidd*

OVERVIEW
Definition

Glaucoma is a condition in which the intraocular pressure (IOP) becomes increased and the optic nerve becomes cupped, leading to visual field loss. Elevated IOP is defined as a pressure greater than 21 mm Hg; however, higher pressures leave some clients unaffected, and some persons with normal pressures have optic nerve and visual field changes. Acute glaucoma is closed-angle glaucoma. Chronic glaucoma is open-angle glaucoma.

Incidence

● Glaucoma is the second most common cause of permanent blindness (after macular degeneration).
● An estimated 3 million persons in the United States have elevated IOP.
● Glaucoma occurs in as much as 15% of the older adult population.

Pathophysiology

Aqueous humor fills the posterior chamber of the eye, flows through the pupil and the anterior chamber, and leaves the eye through the trabecular meshwork, a connective tissue filter at the angle between the iris and the cornea. The aqueous humor passes out of the trabecular meshwork into Schlemm's canal. IOP is maintained by a balance between inflow and outflow of aqueous humor. Increased IOP is related to improper aqueous humor flow. Elevated IOP results in optic nerve damage. The exact mechanism of this damage is unknown but probably relates to ischemia.

Types of Glaucoma
● Primary open-angle glaucoma occurs from obstruction at the microscopic level in the trabecular meshwork or

from overproduction of aqueous humor in 90% of all cases.
● Acute closed-angle glaucoma results from obstruction of the trabecular network by the iris, by a narrow angle between the anterior iris and the posterior corneal surface, shallow anterior chambers, or a thickened or bulging iris. It is associated with pupillary dilation.
● Congenital glaucoma occurs rarely as a result of an autosomal-recessive gene.

Factors Increasing Susceptibility
● Eye inflammation or trauma
● Neoplasm
● Neovascularization
● Corticosteroid therapy
● Increasing age (prevalence 0.7% after age 40 years, 20% after age 60 years)
● Blacks older than 40 years (five times more likely than whites)
● Diabetes
● Hypertension
● Familial history of glaucoma
● Eye injury
● In closed-angle glaucoma:
  ● Pharmacologic mydriasis
  ● Anticholinergics
  ● Asian ancestry
  ● Hyperopic

ASSESSMENT: SUBJECTIVE/HISTORY
Open-Angle Glaucoma
● Bilateral symptoms
● No symptoms in early stages
● Slow loss of peripheral vision
● Tunnel vision
● Eventual loss of central vision

G

- Mild, dull ache in the eyes
- Halos around lights, blurred vision
- Headache

Closed-Angle Glaucoma

Closed-angle glaucoma may be precipitated by the following:

- Sitting in a darkened movie theater
- Stress leading to epinephrine excretion
- Unilateral symptoms
- Acute pain and pressure over one eye
- Decreased visual acuity
- Photophobia
- Halo around light
- Nausea and vomiting

Past Medical History

- Trauma to the eye
- Intraocular surgery
- Hypertension
- Diabetes
- Sarcoidosis
- Herpes zoster
- Myopia
- Migraine headache

Medication History

- Open-angle glaucoma: Steroid (topical, systemic, or inhaled) use may predispose the client to glaucoma.
- Closed-angle glaucoma: In certain cases glaucoma may be precipitated by the following:
  - Antihistamines
  - Stimulants
  - Vasodilators
  - Sympathomimetics
  - Cocaine
  - Clonidine

Family History

Persons with a first-degree relative with open-angle glaucoma are five times more likely to develop glaucoma than the general population.

ASSESSMENT: OBJECTIVE/ PHYSICAL EXAMINATION

Physical Examination

Both Types

- Diminished fields of vision
- Funduscopic examination may reveal the following:
  - Increased cup-to-disk ratio (greater than 1:3)
  - Large optic cup
- Tonometry reading
  - Higher than 24 mmHg (not always present)
  - Increasing tonometry readings

Open-Angle Glaucoma

- Bilateral symptoms
- Asymmetry of cup between eyes

Closed-Angle Glaucoma

- Unilateral symptoms
- Pupil dilated, nonreactive to light
- Cloudy cornea
- Decreased visual acuity
- Unilateral red eye

Diagnostic Procedures

- Tonometry (pressure measurement in anesthetized eyes)
  - Schiøtz sits on eye surface; often undermeasures pressures in early disease.
  - Applanation is more accurate but slightly difficult to use; done by ophthalmologist.
  - Air puff is done by ophthalmologist; no anesthesia is necessary.
  - Hand-held Tono-Pen is a new, easy to use diagnostic tool.
- Central visual field testing (difficult to perform accurately)

DIAGNOSIS

Differential diagnoses may include the following:

- Open-angle glaucoma (mostly symptom free): Presbyopia may be one of the few differential diagnoses. For diagnosis of open-angle, requires two of the following: abnormality in central visual field, optic nerve (cupping or cup-to-disk ratio), and IOP (normal IOP is 10 to 24 mm Hg).
- Closed-angle glaucoma
  - Conjunctivitis—usually bilateral, rare pain, no nausea, vomiting, A.M. matting
  - Uveitis
  - Corneal disorders

THERAPEUTIC PLAN

Nonpharmacologic Treatment

Not relevant.

Pharmacologic Treatment

Open-Angle Glaucoma. Medical management includes the following:

- Eyedrops
  - β-blocker eyedrops (timolol, betaxolol) given bid
  - Sympathomimetics (epinephrine)
  - Miotics (pilocarpine) given qid
  - Brimonidine (selective α_2 agonist) 0.2% solution bid can be used instead of β-blockers (presence of cardiopulmonary disease)

- Dorzolamide 2% (topical carbonic anhydrase inhibitor) can be used tid as a single agent or bid as adjunct therapy
- Systemic medications
  - Carbonic anhydrase inhibitors (acetazolamide), decrease aqueous humor production
  - β-blockers
- Surgery
  - Argon laser trabeculoplasty
  - Surgical trabeculectomy

Closed-Angle Glaucoma

✝**CAUTION:** *This is a medical emergency!*

- Immediate referral to an ophthalmologist is essential. Untreated acute glaucoma results in severe and permanent visual loss within 2 to 5 days after onset of symptoms.
- Surgery is almost always indicated.
- Medications may be instituted to reduce IOP while preparing for surgery.
- Prescribe miotic drugs: 4% pilocarpine solution, 1 drop every 20 minutes.
- Acetazolamide, a carbonic anhydrase inhibitor, is given 500 mg IV, followed by 250 mg qid.
- Osmotic diuretics, such as urea or mannitol, may be used.
- Iridectomy (laser or surgical) is often done prophylactically for the unaffected eye.

Client Education
Postoperative Care

- Give cycloplegic drops to relax ciliary muscle.
- Encourage early ambulation.
- Observe unaffected eye for symptoms.
- Avoid activities that increase IOP, such as straining, coughing, stooping, or lifting.

Referral

Closed-Angle Glaucoma. Immediate referral to an ophthalmologist is essential.

Open-Angle Glaucoma. Ophthalmologist referral is necessary for initial workup.

Prevention

Prevention is a better option than treatment. There is no cure for glaucoma. The primary care provider must be able to recognize early stages of optic nerve damage, symptoms of increased IOP, and especially acute, closed-angle glaucoma. Also, primary care providers need to be familiar with glaucoma medications and their possible impact on other chronic disease management.

EVALUATION/FOLLOW-UP

- Follow-up of IOP and visual field changes should be done weekly at first, then monthly.
- Compliance with the medical regimen is often difficult, requiring eyedrop use as often as qid.
- Monitor for side effects of drugs, especially with non-cardioselective β-blocker use. Even with topical use, bronchoconstriction may be a side effect of these drugs.

COMPLICATIONS

Blindness.

REFERENCES

Hahn, M. (1996). Common eye problems in primary care. *Advance for Nurse Practitioners, 4*, 3.

King, P. (2000). Glaucoma. In D. Robinson, P. Kidd, & K. Rogers (Eds.), *Primary care across the lifespan.* St. Louis: Mosby.

Riordan-Eva, P. (2001). Eye. In L. Tierney, S. McPhee, & M. Papadakis (Eds.), *Current medical diagnosis and treatment.* New York: McGraw-Hill.

Review Questions

1. Untreated or uncontrolled glaucoma damages the optic nerve. Which of the following symptoms is associated with optic nerve damage?
  - **a.** Loss of central vision
  - **b.** Dull ache behind the eyes
  - **c.** Decreased pigmentation of the iris
  - **d.** Floaters and flashing lights

2. Which of the following is a typical finding in closed-angle glaucoma?
  - **a.** Cloudy cornea
  - **b.** Pupillary constriction
  - **c.** Excessive tearing
  - **d.** Altered extraocular movements

3. Carbonic anhydrase inhibitors are sometimes used to treat glaucoma because they do which of the following?
  - **a.** Reduce aqueous humor production
  - **b.** Diminish pupillary dilation
  - **c.** Promote diuresis
  - **d.** Constrict the pupil

4. A 72-year-old man has a 1-day history of eye pain. He reports no visual disturbances. Eye examination reveals an injected conjunctiva, cup-to-disk ratio of 2:3, tonometry readings of 20 mm Hg, and visual acuity of 20/30. Which of the following should the NP do next?
  - **a.** Refer for ophthalmology evaluation.
  - **b.** Evert the eyelid to look for foreign bodies.
  - **c.** Instill anesthetic ophthalmic drops.
  - **d.** Correlate findings with vital signs.

G

5. When following up a client who has a family history of glaucoma, client education and evaluation should include which of the following?

    a. Yearly eye examination by primary care provider
    b. Review of symptoms of open-angle glaucoma
    c. Annual dilated pupil examination by an ophthalmologist
    d. Measurement of IOP of family members

6. An 88-year-old man with a history of hypertension and hyperlipidemia comes in for evaluation. You note that he seems to be in some respiratory distress, and he tells you that he has been having increasing problems with shortness of breath. A review of his medications reveals that he is using eyedrops prescribed by the ophthalmologist to treat glaucoma in addition to a variety of nonprescription drugs. Use of which of the following medications may be related to his symptoms?

    a. Pseudoephedrine (Sudafed)
    b. Timolol (Timoptic) eyedrops
    c. Acetazolamide (Diamox)
    d. Ibuprofen (Advil)

Answers and Rationales

1. *Answer:* **b** (assessment)
    Rationale: A dull ache in the eyes is not an uncommon finding in glaucoma, probably related to optic nerve ischemia.

Floaters and flashing lights are associated with retinal detachment. Loss of central vision is macular degeneration.

2. *Answer:* **a** (assessment)
    Rationale: A cloudy cornea is a classic finding in acute glaucoma. Pupillary dilation is common.

3. *Answer:* **a** (implementation/plan)
    Rationale: Acetazolamide results in decreased aqueous humor production.

4. *Answer:* **a** (implementation/plan)
    Rationale: The increased cup-to-disk ratio in the presence of a red eye and eye pain is a clear indicator of acute glaucoma, which is a medical emergency. The ophthalmologist will most likely recommend immediate surgery.

5. *Answer:* **a** (evaluation)
    Rationale: The primary care provider can be effective in detecting early glaucoma by a funduscopic examination. Dilating the pupils may precipitate acute glaucoma in selected individuals.

6. *Answer:* **b** (evaluation)
    Rationale: The most commonly prescribed eyedrops include noncardioselective β-blockers such as timolol. Systemic absorption of this drug could cause exacerbation of respiratory problems and other side effects common to beta-blockers.

GONORRHEA   *Cheryl Pope Kish*

OVERVIEW
Definition

Gonorrhea is a sexually transmitted disease (STD) caused by the organism *Neisseria gonorrhoeae*. It is acquired primarily by intimate sexual contact.

Incidence

There are approximately 600,000 new cases of gonorrhea each year in the United States. The highest incidence is among males 20 to 24 years old and females 18 to 24 years old. Most cases (85%) occur in black and Hispanic populations. At least 20% of newborns of infected women delivered vaginally acquire the disease. In some populations, there is a 40% coinfection with chlamydia trachomatis.

Pathophysiology

Gonorrhea is caused by a Gram-negative diplococcus with an incubation period of 2 to 7 days. It is transmitted through contact with secretions or exudates of infected mucous membranes.

Factors Increasing Susceptibility
- Sexual exposure to infected individuals
- Failure to use barrier protection during sexual contact
- Multiple sexual partners
- Infants born through infected birth canal
- Sexual abuse of child
- Presence of intrauterine device (IUD)

ASSESSMENT: SUBJECTIVE/HISTORY
Symptoms

Men are likely to seek treatment before serious sequelae occur because of symptoms; only 10% are asymptomatic, whereas as many as 80% of infected women are asymptomatic and at risk because they do not seek treatment.

The most common infection sites in men are the urethra, epididymis, prostate, rectum, and pharynx. Genitourinary symptoms include urethral burning and a milky discharge that may become mucopurulent over time. The most common infection sites in women are the urethra, endocervix, rectum, upper genital tract, and pharynx. Genitourinary symptoms include increased vaginal discharge, abnormal uterine bleeding, postcoital spotting, and dyspareunia.

Clinical findings of gonococcal pharyngitis include erythema and edema of tonsils and posterior pharynx. Disseminated gonococcal infection is associated with tenosynovitis, skin lesions, fever, and polyarthralgias.

History

History includes the following:
- Previous vaginal, urethral, and prostatic infections and treatments; those illnesses in sexual partner(s)

and whether a full course of treatment was completed before resumption of sexual relations

- Any chronic illnesses
- Sexual history (including specific practices)
- Type of contraceptive used
- Most recent sexual contact
- Any changes in menstrual flow or postcoital spotting
- HIV risk or exposure
- Current medications

Onset, duration, and characteristics of symptoms should be explored and considered in light of sexual practices and potential exposure.

ASSESSMENT: OBJECTIVE/PHYSICAL EXAMINATION
Physical Examination

- Female clients: Assess abdomen for guarding, tenderness, and rebound pain. On pelvic examination, inspect Skene's and Bartholin's glands and urethra. Evaluate cervix for friability and mucopurulent discharge from the endocervix. Attempt to demonstrate cervical motion tenderness and generalized pelvic tenderness on bimanual examination.
- Male clients: Assess for penile discharge and testicular tenderness or swelling. Perform rectal examination to evaluate the prostate.
- In both males and females, examine throat for tonsillar exudate, edema, and erythema.
- Check for fever; joint motion, effusion, and tenderness; and skin lesions (necrotic) if disseminated disease is suspected. (Two thirds of disseminated gonococcal cases are in women.)
- Pregnant woman: Consider gonococcal screening examination at first prenatal visit and reevaluate subsequently during pregnancy in those at risk.
- Newborns: Assess for ophthalmia neonatorum, conjunctivitis of the newborn, which can lead to blindness. Prophylactic eye treatment is required in all 50 states to prevent this disorder.

Diagnostic Procedures

- Perform saline wet prep to assess for increased WBC count and decreased normal vaginal flora.
- Culture sites of exposure using modified Thayer-Martin medium or DNA probe that would enable gonococcus and chlamydia concurrently.
- Nucleic acid amplification tests on first-voided urine samples are popular choices in men, who are uncomfortable with the thought of urethral cultures by swab.
- Cultures of the throat, urethra, and anus should also be considered, depending on sexual practices.
- With septic joint involvement, gonococci can be recovered from joint aspirate for culture.

DIAGNOSIS

Differential diagnoses include the following:

- Chlamydia
- Appendicitis
- Ectopic pregnancy
- Pelvic inflammatory disease (PID)

THERAPEUTIC PLAN
Pharmacologic Treatment

The Centers for Disease Control and Prevention (CDC) recommends the following drugs to treat gonorrhea; choice depends on compliance issues, allergy, contraindications, and cost. All of the following single-dose regimens are considered effective:

- Ceftriaxone (Rocephin) 125 mg IM (causes pain at injection site; side effects are diarrhea, rash) or
- Cefixime (Suprax) 400 mg PO as single dose (may cause GI upset, pruritus, rash, headache or dizziness) or
- Ciprofloxacin 500 mg PO as single dose (can cause dizziness, central nervous system stimulation, rash, eosinophilia, elevated liver enzymes, myalgia, photosensitivity, Stevens-Johnson syndrome) or
- Ofloxacin 400 mg PO as single dose (can cause rash, Stevens-Johnson syndrome, and local reactions)

An additional doxycycline or azithromycin regimen is effective against possible co-infection with chlamydia.

- Quinolones and tetracycline are contraindicated during pregnancy. Erythromycin and Ampicillin may be used in pregnant and lactating women, as can cefixime or spectinomycin 2 g IM as single dose.
- If pharyngeal infection is a concern, the client should be treated with either ceftriaxone or ciprofloxacin.

Newborns. For the prophylactic management of ophthalmia neonatorum, 1% silver nitrate, 0.5% erythromycin ophthalmic ointment, or 3.1% tetracycline ophthalmic ointment may be administered.

Client Education

- Advise that no test of cure is needed if treated with reliable regimens recommended by the CDC.
- Inform client of need for notification and treatment of all sexual partners with whom contact has been made within the previous 60 days.
- Advise sexual abstinence until both partners are fully treated. If a single-dose medication is used, abstinence for 7 days is warranted to ensure cure.

Prevention

- Responsible sexual practices that limit the number of exposures through abstinence, mutually monogamous relationships, and/or barrier protection aids in prevention.

- Prompt notification and treatment of all sexual contacts of infected persons helps control spread.
- Screening programs that include sexually active adolescents and 20- to 24-year-olds with new or multiple partners aids in prevention.
- An endocervical culture for gonococcus (and timely treatment) at the first prenatal visit in high-risk populations or high-prevalence areas helps prevent spread to the fetus.

Referral

- Clients who experience treatment failure despite compliance with recommended dosage regimens should be referred.
- Gonorrhea is a reportable disease; all positive results must be reported to Public Health Services.

EVALUATION/FOLLOW-UP

- Children diagnosed with gonorrhea should be evaluated for sexual abuse.
- Clients with disseminated gonococcal infections (bacteremia) may require hospitalization for parenteral antibiotics.
- Discuss the signs and symptoms of the complications, and encourage the client to seek care quickly if he or she exhibits any of the symptoms.
- Serologic testing for syphilis is recommended within 30 days.

COMPLICATIONS

- Women are at risk for PID, pelvic or Bartholin's gland abscess, infertility, and disseminated gonococcal infection.
- Pregnant women are at risk for spontaneous abortion, premature rupture of membranes, preterm delivery, and chorioamnionitis.
- Men are at risk for proctitis, infertility related to epididymitis, proctitis or seminal vesiculitis, ureteral stricture, and disseminated gonococcal infection.
- Neonates are at risk for ophthalmia neonatorum, sepsis, arthritis, meningitis, and scalp abscess.
- Men and women are at risk for meningitis, endocarditis, and gonococcal conjunctivitis and antibiotic-resistant strains.

REFERENCES

Cash, J. C., & Glass, C. A. (2000). *Family practice guidelines.* Philadelphia: Lippincott.
Gerrig, J. N. (1998). Preventing and recognizing STDs in the adolescent. *Lippincott Primary Care Practice, 2*(3), 312-314.
Hawkins, J. W., Roberto-Nichols, D. M., & Stanley-Haney, J. L. (1997). *Protocols for nurse practitioners in gynecologic settings.* New York: Tiresias Press.
Rawlins, S. (2001). Nonviral sexually transmitted infections. *Journal of Obstetric, Gynecologic, and Neonatal Nursing, 30*(3), 324-331.
Robinson, D., Kidd, P., & Rogers, K. M. (2000). *Primary care across the lifespan.* St. Louis: Mosby.
Shaffa, S. D. (1998). Vaginitis and sexually transmitted diseases. In E.Q. Youngkin & M.S. Davis (Eds.), *Women's health care: A primary care clinical guide* (2nd ed., pp. 265-300). Stamford, CT: Appleton & Lange.
Smith, M. A., & Shimp, L. A. (2000). *20 common problems in women's health care.* New York: McGraw-Hill.
Star, W. L., Lommel, L. L., & Shannon, M. T. (1995). *Women's primary health care: Protocols for practice.* Washington, DC: American Nurses Publishing.
Trotto, N. E. (1999). STDs: Are you up to date? *Patient Care, May 30,* 74-76, 81, 85-103.
Uphold, C. R., & Graham, M. V. (1998). *Clinical guidelines in family practice.* Gainesville, FL: Barmarrae Books.

Review Questions

1. Mike, a 9-year-old boy, is brought in from a foster home. He has a purulent urethral discharge. The foster parent present at the clinic denies sexual contact. A wet prep shows 15 WBC count/HPF. The next day the child's right knee is edematous, hot, and painful and he has chills and fever. What is the most likely cause?

- **a.** Gonorrhea
- **b.** Meningitis
- **c.** Chlamydia
- **d.** Mycoplasma hominis

2. Phyllis Snow is a 46-year-old who comes in for an employment physical. Which fact in her history justifies gonorrhea/chlamydia screening at this visit?

- **a.** She had an IUD in the past but has been on "the pill" for 8 years.
- **b.** She underwent an elective abortion at 17.
- **c.** She had a ruptured appendix at age 22.
- **d.** Two weeks ago, while drinking, she had intercourse with two men.

3. Which finding on physical examination is most consistent with a diagnosis of gonorrhea?

- **a.** "Fishmouth"-shaped cervical os
- **b.** Vulvar erythema and itching
- **c.** Mucopurulent discharge from cervical os
- **d.** Petechiae on vaginal mucosa and cervix

4. Which diagnostic test can be used to confirm gonorrhea?

- **a.** Saline wet prep
- **b.** Thayer-Martin culture
- **c.** Colposcopy
- **d.** Culdocentesis

5. Jill is a 14-year-old who was brought in by a social worker with Child Protective Services. She disclosed sexual abuse by her mother's live-in boyfriend over several months. A diagnosis of gonorrhea is suspected. Which medication regimen is most appropriate for Jill?

a. Erythromycin base 500 mg PO bid × 14 days and metronidazole 2 g PO
b. Doxycycline 100 mg bid × 7 days and Rocephin 125 mg IM stat
c. Azithromycin 1 g PO and Ampicillin 250 mg bid × 7 days
d. Procaine penicillin 2 million units and Flagyl 2 g PO

6. Jill asks why she needs two different medications for one infection. The NP gives which of the following explanations?

a. The two drugs treat gonorrhea and chlamydia, two infections that often co-exist.
b. Combination therapy is necessary because of the nature of the sexual abuse.
c. Two drugs are necessary because adolescents cannot tolerate adult-strength drugs.
d. The injectable drug protects against genital herpes.

7. Prophylactic management of ophthalmia neonatorum includes which of the following medications?

a. Bacitracin ophthalmic ointment
b. Silver nitrate aqueous solution
c. Sulfacetamide sodium (Sodium Sulamyd)
d. Prednisolone acetate and sulfacetamide sodium (Blephamide) ophthalmic solution

8. Which of the following symptoms is least indicative of gonorrhea?

a. Odorous, musty vaginal discharge
b. Dysuria
c. Abdominal pain
d. Asymptomatic presentation

9. Which of the following drugs for treating gonorrhea are contraindicated for pregnant women?

a. Cephalosporins
b. Quinolones
c. Spectinomycins
d. Antivirals

10. Which of the follow-up options is *not* necessary in the management plan of a client with gonorrhea?

a. Inform the client that reinfection may be prevented by ensuring that sexual contacts from the previous 60 days are treated.
b. Advise barrier contraception as a preventive measure.
c. Schedule test of cure 21 days after treatment.
d. Notify Public Health Services of positive results of gonorrhea testing.

Answers and Rationales

1. *Answer:* **a** (analysis/diagnosis)
Rationale: Child has symptoms suggestive of disseminated gonococcal infection. In a child this age, gonorrhea occurs as a result of sexual abuse (Robinson, Kidd, & Rogers, 2000).

2. *Answer:* **d** (assessment)
Rationale: Multiple partners without barrier protection increase the risk of gonorrhea and other STDs (Cash & Glass, 2000).

3. *Answer:* **c** (assessment)
Rationale: Mucopurulent discharge from the cervical os is a consistent finding in gonorrhea (Uphold & Graham, 1998).

4. *Answer:* **b** (assessment)
Rationale: Thayer-Martin culture or DNA probe is appropriate for diagnosing gonorrhea (Uphold & Graham, 1998).

5. *Answer:* **b** (analysis/diagnosis)
Rationale: Doxycycline offers protection against chlamydia; Rocephin as a single IM dose is effective for treating gonococcus (Uphold & Graham, 1998).

6. *Answer:* **a** (evaluation)
Rationale: In some populations, there is a 40% rate of coinfection with chlamydia and gonorrhea. This combination offers dual treatment (Robinson, Kidd, & Rogers, 2000).

7. *Answer:* **b** (implementation/plan)
Rationale: Silver nitrate drops or erythromycin ointment are commonly used as prophylactic medication to prevent ophthalmia neonatorum. The medication should be given within the first hour after delivery to offer optimum protection. The 1-hour delay allows the eye contact that is so important to maternal-infant bonding (Robinson, Kidd, & Rogers, 2000).

8. *Answer:* **a** (assessment)
Rationale: Dysuria, abdominal pain, and asymptomatic presentations are commonly associated with gonococcus. The odorous, musty discharge is associated with bacterial vaginosis (Uphold & Graham, 1998).

9. *Answer:* **b** (implementation/plan)
Rationale: Quinolones and tetracyclines are contraindicated in pregnancy (Robinson, Kidd, & Rogers, 2000).

10. *Answer:* **c** (implementation/plan)
Rationale: A test of cure is not required if the CDC-recommended drug regimens are used for treatment (Cash & Glass, 2000).

G

GOUT *Pamela Kidd*

OVERVIEW
Definition
Gout is an inflammatory arthritis, caused by deposition of monosodium urate (MSU) crystals in joints, because of an inborn error of purine metabolism and uric acid excretion.

Incidence
- Rare before puberty in males and before menopause in females. It is the most common cause of inflammatory arthritis in males older than 40.
- Incidence of gout is 3 times greater for hypertensive men taking diuretics (hyperuricemic effect) when compared with normotensive men. Increases as serum uric acid level rises as follows:
  - 0.1% with serum uric acid less than 7 mg/dL
  - 4.5% with levels at or higher than 9 mg/dL

Pathophysiology
Primary gout is caused by either decreased excretion or increased production of uric acid. Hereditary underexcretion is the most common cause of gout. After many asymptomatic years of chronic hyperuricemia (30 years mean), acute gout develops in 25% of these individuals.

Factors Increasing Susceptibility
- Obesity
- Alcohol intake
- Acute illness or surgery may alter uric acid levels and precipitate an attack.

Protective Factors.
Women are protected until menopause by estrogen because it promotes uric acid excretion.

ASSESSMENT: SUBJECTIVE/HISTORY
Symptoms
- Classic symptoms present with significant pain, erythema, usually of the great toe, followed by desquamation of the overlying skin. Onset of symptoms is rapid, increasing over a few hours and lasting a few days to weeks, with complete recovery.
- Ask about the onset, duration, and progression of symptoms. Note any history of previous attacks, including location, duration, type of treatment, and response to therapy.
- In adults, typical pain is severe and is generally confined to one joint of the foot or ankle in middle age or older males.
- In the elderly, women may have several joints affected, particularly in the hands. Males with gout have usually experienced at least one episode of acute arthritis, which may recur or progress to chronic joint changes over time.
- The metatarsophalangeal (MTP) joint, instep, or ankle is often the target of a first attack. MSU crystals are soluble at body temperature, and with the temperature of the great toe being lower, it predisposes the crystals to precipitate into the joint, thereby causing symptoms. Women often have more than one joint involved; 70% of women present with polyarticular, instead of monoarticular, symptoms of gout (hands most common). Low-grade fever is possible; no other systemic symptoms are usually present.

Past Medical History
- Secondary gout is caused by acquired conditions causing overproduction or underexcretion of uric acid.
  - Overproduction: polycythemia vera, leukemia, multiple myeloma, psoriasis, hemolytic anemias, disseminated carcinoma, hyperlipidemia and diabetes
  - Underexcretion: chronic renal insufficiency, lead poisoning, acidosis, drug ingestion (nicotinic acid, levodopa, pyrazinamide, ethambutol, cyclosporine, diuretics, low-dose salicylates)

Medication History
Any sudden change in uric acid levels can precipitate symptoms of gouty arthritis. Factors causing a rise in uric acid levels include diuretics, alcohol, and low-dose aspirin. Lowering of uric acid is attributed to sudden cessation of alcohol use, high-dose salicylates, or initiation of allopurinol or uricosuric drugs.

Family History
More common in Pacific Islanders. Twelve percent of gout sufferers have a positive family history of the condition.

Dietary History
Ask about ingestion of alcohol, especially beer, and intake of a diet high in purines such as meat, gravy, yeast products, and various vegetables such as peas, beans, spinach, and asparagus.

ASSESSMENT: OBJECTIVE/PHYSICAL EXAMINATION
Physical Examination
- Assess weight and vital signs with attention to temperature and blood pressure.
- Evaluate affected joints for redness, increased warmth, tenderness, effusion, and range of motion.
- Check for nonpainful tophi on achilles, extensor surfaces of the forearms, or less commonly on the helix

of the ear. In early stages, tophi may appear as small, superficial, yellow-white patches on the palmar and plantar surfaces of the hands and feet. Advanced tophi may ulcerate, leaving a white urate deposit on the skin surface.

- Look for joint deformity, particularly of the hands and feet, and check for joint stiffness.

Diagnostic Procedures

See Table 3-35.

DIAGNOSIS

Chronic gout or interval gout may affect multiple joints of the upper and lower extremities and can be confused with rheumatoid or osteoarthritis. The presence of Bouchard's and Heberden's nodes indicates osteoarthritis (McGovern, 2001). Primary differential diagnoses include pseudogout and septic joint infection (Table 3-36).

THERAPEUTIC PLAN

Nonpharmacologic Treatment

Asymptomatic Hyperuricemia. Treatment generally is not required for persons with uric acid levels lower than 9 to 10 mg/dL with normal renal function whose physical examinations are negative for tophi. Consider secondary causes of hyperuricemia in these individuals and follow up annually.

Pharmacologic Treatment

Treat the acute arthritis first, then the hyperuricemia. Sudden reduction of uric acid may produce another attack (Hellmann & Stone, 2001) (Table 3-37).

Client Education

- Avoid alcohol binges, fasting, or low-calorie diets because these can trigger an attack; gradual weight reduction is recommended.
- Generous fluid intake is important if at risk for kidney stones.
- Consider a low-purine diet. Authors differ in their opinions of the importance of a low-purine diet on reducing uric acid levels.

Referral

Consult with a physician when joint aspiration/injection is required and the NP is lacking technical expertise in these procedures.

Prevention

One attack of gout does not require continuous treatment with medication, but multiple attacks and/or development of tophi justify use of medication, which should be considered lifelong treatment (see Table 3-37).

TABLE **3-35**   Diagnostic Tests for Gout

DIAGNOSTIC TEST	DIAGNOSTIC VALUE	CONSIDERATIONS
Joint aspiration	Only confirmatory test for acute gout; find MSU crystals in phagocytes or free in tophi, seen under polarized microscope	Practitioner's technical experience with this procedure; consult or refer to physician. Use clinical judgment to omit test if symptoms classic.
Serum uric acid	Limited value: 20-30% of people with acute gout have normal values	Hyperuricemia common, but acute arthritis may not be due to gout in individual with elevated uric acid.
Creatinine, BUN	Will be elevated if renal insufficiency is an underlying problem	Order when uric acid elevated in young man or premenopausal woman to look for secondary cause.
24-hour urine for urate and creatinine	Order with serum uric acid and creatinine to look for secondary cause	These tests may help determine risk for kidney stones.
X-rays	Limited value in acute gout. Characteristic findings in advanced gout	Helps exclude other disorders.
CBC, ESR	+/- elevated with acute gout	Elevated with septic joint infection.
Gram stain and culture of synnovial fluid	WBC>50,000-100,000 cells/mm^3 increases likelihood of septic joint	Aspiration limited by practitioners experience with this procedure.

G

TABLE **3-36** Differential Diagnoses

GOUT	PSEUDOGOUT	SEPTIC JOINT INFECTION*
More common in men over 35-40	Only slightly more common in men, age over 60	Age not a factor, children affected
Acute and chronic arthritis	Acute and chronic arthritis	Acute arthritis
Affects MTP, ankle, instep	Generally affects the knee	Usually affects large joints, knee more common
Onset within hours	Onset occurs over days	Acute onset
Monosodium urate crystals in synnovial fluid	Calcium pyrophosphate dihydrate crystals present	Purulent joint aspirate, gram + (S. aureus common)
X-ray examination: acute normal; chronic asymmetric bony erosions	X-ray examination of knees, wrist, symphsis-chondrocalcinosis	X-ray examination may show joint destruction within 10 days

*Nongonococcal.

TABLE **3-37** Pharmacologic Treatment of Gout

DRUG	DOSE	COMMENTS
Colchicine	0.6 mg PO bid	Use qd in cases of coexisting renal and/or heart failure.
Probenecid (used for undersecretion of uric acid [24 hr uric acid <800 mg/dL])	0.5 PO qd; can increase to 2 g/day	Must maintain UO of 2000 mL/day to minimize precipitation of uric acid and stone formation.
Allopurinol (used for overproduction [>800 mg uric acid in 24 hr urine])	100 mg/dL for 1 week may require up to 300 mg PO qd to lower uric acid level	If on probenecid also, must lower dose of probenecid and raise dose of allopurinol to achieve desired effect.

EVALUATION/FOLLOW-UP

- Recheck within 48 hours if not responding to treatment for acute attack. Have client return in 4 to 8 weeks to discuss further treatment or evaluation.
- Refer to orthopedic surgeon or rheumatologist if concerned about septic joint, diagnosis is in question, or if unresponsive to therapy.

COMPLICATIONS

- Untreated chronic gout can lead to tophaceous destruction of bone and cartilage or gouty nephropathy.
- Increased risk of diabetes, hyperlipidemia, and renal disease

REFERENCES

American hospital formulary service drug information. (1997). Bethesda, MD: American Society of Health-Systems Pharmacists, Inc.

Bailey, E. (2000). Gout. In D. Robinson, P. Kidd, & K. Rogers (Eds.), *Primary care across the lifespan.* St. Louis: Mosby.

Emmerson, B. T. (1996). The management of gout. *New England Journal of Medicine, 334*(7), 445-452.

George, T. M., & Mandell, B. F. (1996). Individualizing the treatment of gout. *Cleveland Clinic Journal of Medicine, 63*(3), 150-155.

Hershfield, M. S. (1996). Gout and uric acid metabolism. In J. C. Bennett and F. Plum (Eds.), *Cecil textbook of medicine* (20th ed.). Philadelphia: W. B. Saunders.

Holland, N. W., & Agudelo, C. A. (1997). Hyperuricemia and gout. In R. Rakel (Ed.), *Conn's current therapy.* Philadelphia: W. B. Saunders.

McGovern, T. W. (2001). Digital distress. *Clinical Advisor,* June, 27-28.

Towheed, T. E., & Hochberg, M. C. (1996). Acute monoarthritis: A practical approach to assessment and treatment. *American Family Physician, 54*(7), 2239-2243.

Review Questions

1. Which of the following statements about gout is *true*?
   a. Gout is caused by joint deposition of pyrophosphate dihydrate crystals.
   b. Gout is more prevalent in men than in women.
   c. Gout is primarily a result of a poor diet high in purines.
   d. Most cases of gout are the result of secondary conditions.

2. Which of the following scenarios is most indicative of gout?
   a. 35-year-old woman with swollen, painful fingers
   b. 30-year-old man with MTP joint pain, iritis, and penile discharge

c. 55-year-old alcoholic man with recurrent instep pain and redness

d. 75-year-old hypertensive man with hip pain and limp

3. Which of the following statements best describes the pathophysiologic findings of gout?

   a. Gout is most commonly a result of increased uric acid production.

   b. The onset of gout is caused by a gradual change in uric acid levels.

   c. Secondary gout is a hereditary chronic disorder.

   d. The lower temperature of the toe causes precipitation of uric acid crystals.

4. Which one of the following statements is *not* true?

   a. Symptoms of gout evolve during a period of several days.

   b. Surgery may bring on an attack of acute gout.

   c. Gout can be confused with cellulitis.

   d. As gout resolves, skin over the joint desquamates.

5. Which statement is *not* correct regarding the treatment of gout?

   a. Any NSAID can be given to relieve symptoms.

   b. With renal insufficiency, corticosteroids are an alternative treatment.

   c. Colchicine provides good relief and is well tolerated.

   d. Intraarticular injections should be preceded by joint aspiration.

6. Which statement about the long-term treatment of recurrent gout is *not* true?

   a. Serum uric acid–lowering agents should be started immediately after an attack.

   b. Allopurinol can cause a sensitivity reaction with rash and fever.

   c. Uricosuric drugs require intake of large quantities of fluid.

   d. Colchicine can be given to reduce recurrence of gout symptoms.

7. Which of the following client education teaching points about gout is *incorrect*?

   a. Binge drinking of alcohol can bring on an attack.

   b. Only high doses of aspirin can bring on symptoms of gout.

   c. Medication for acute gout should reduce pain within 48 hours.

   d. A low-purine diet has limited impact on uric acid levels.

Answers and Rationales

1. Answer: b (assessment)

   Rationale: Gout is primarily a disease of adult men. MSU crystals are found in gout; pyrophosphate dihydrate crystals are found in pseudogout. Dietary sources are responsible for only 10% of blood purines, which has limited impact on gout. Gout is primarily caused by an inborn error of metabolism and less often by secondary diseases.

2. Answer: c (assessment)

   Rationale: Gout is more common after the fifth decade of life and is associated with alcohol use. The instep is a common site of inflammation. The hip is a rare location for gout. Symptoms in women are rare before menopause; findings described suggest rheumatoid arthritis. The 30-year-old man's triad points to Reiter's syndrome.

3. Answer: d (analysis/diagnosis)

   Rationale: Uric acid is soluble in serum at body temperature, but at lower temperatures uric acid precipitates into a joint. Only 10% of gout is caused by overproduction of uric acid. Onset of gout symptoms is caused by a rapid change in uric acid levels. Secondary gout is caused by an acquired disease and is not hereditary.

4. Answer: a (assessment)

   Rationale: Gout evolves rapidly, usually during a period of hours or a day.

5. Answer: c (implementation/plan)

   Rationale: Colchicine does provide good relief for gout symptoms but often must be discontinued because of GI tract side effects.

6. Answer: a (implementation/plan)

   Rationale: Serum uric acid–lowering agents should be delayed until at least 1 month after an acute attack for gout. Sudden reduction can precipitate another attack of gout. During this time, antiinflammatory medication is started to prevent recurrence when the serum uric acid–lowering agents are initiated.

7. Answer: b (implementation/plan)

   Rationale: Both high and low doses of aspirin can trigger symptoms of acute gout.

G

GYNECOLOGIC CANCERS   *Cheryl Pope Kish*

OVERVIEW
Definition

Gynecologic (GYN) cancer refers to malignancies affecting the reproductive organs. The most common GYN malignancies are endometrial, cervical, ovarian, and vulvovaginal cancers, in order of incidence.

Incidence

- Cancers of the genital tract account for approximately 20% of cancer in women and 10% of cancer deaths.
- Endometrial cancer represents 50% of all GYN cancers. There are approximately 36,000 cases and 6000 deaths annually in the United States attributable to endometrial cancer. Although 25% of cases occur in premenopausal women, the mean age at diagnosis is 60 years.
- Cervical cancer has an annual incidence in the United States of 13,550 cases, with 6000 deaths annually. The death rate has decreased significantly with Pap smear screening for cervical cancer. Cervical cancer peaks at 25 to 45 years of age for carcinoma in situ and again after age 60. It is often considered preventable because annual Pap screening identifies cancer precursors, which often can be successfully treated. Details about Pap screening and follow-up are provided later. Because of early detection, most women with cervical cancer present in their twenties and thirties.
- Ovarian cancer is the fourth most common cause of cancer death in women, with a lifetime risk of 1:70. This type of cancer increases after the age of 45 and peaks in the sixth decade of life. The prognosis in ovarian cancer is poor; 49% of all GYN cancer deaths occur from ovarian cancer because in 75% of cases the cancer has spread significantly before the woman becomes symptomatic.
- Vaginal cancer is extremely rare; its peak incidence is 50 to 70 years of age. Vaginal cancer is more common in whites, extremely rare in blacks, and almost nonexistent in Jewish women. Vulvar cancer represents 5% of all GYN cancer.

Pathophysiology

Endometrial Cancer. Columnar cells in the uterine endometrium become malignant. The precursor lesion is endometrial hyperplasia that progresses to invasive disease. Estrogen exposure without progesterone to counterbalance its effects is often a causative factor in endometrial hyperplasia.

Factors Increasing Susceptibility. Any factor that increases estrogen exposure increases the risk of endometrial cancer. These factors include the following:

- Hormone replacement therapy (HRT) that includes unopposed estrogen in a woman with an intact uterus
- Early menarche
- Late menopause (after 52 years of age)
- Nulliparity
- Infertility
- Polycystic ovary disease (chronic anovulation)
- Obesity
- Tamoxifen therapy for breast cancer

Endometrial cancer has a strong association with diabetes mellitus, hypertension, and gallbladder disease.

Protective Factors
- Multiparity
- OCP use
- Smoking

Cervical Cancer. Cervical cancer arises from single cell precursors found in the transformation zone of the endocervix. Virtually all cases of cervical cancer are now considered to be caused by human papillomavirus (HPV); the strongest link is with subtypes 16 and 18, but other subtypes of HPV are also considered to cause some cervical cancers.

Factors Increasing Susceptibility
- Failure to undergo routine Pap testing increases risk. Half of all cervical cancers in the United States are in women who were never screened; a person who has never been screened is 50 to 60 times more likely to have cervical cancer than someone who has been screened in the past 3 years.
- Multiple sex partners increases risk. Risk is greater if the client's partners also have multiple partners.
- Early first coitus (younger than 18 years old) increases risk.
- STD history, especially HPV and herpes simplex virus (HSV), increases risk.
- Smoking increases risk threefold.

Protective Factors
- Barrier contraception with spermicide
- Avoidance of high-risk sexual behaviors
- Not smoking
- Good general health for positive immune system
- Annual Pap test in high-risk populations

Ovarian Cancer. The origin of ovarian cancer is unknown. Because early symptoms are nonexistent or vague, in 75% of women the disease has spread significantly at the time of diagnosis. Hence, it has a high mortality rate. Most cases of ovarian cancer are considered sporadic; however, 5% to 10% of cases are associated with an inherited trait for the disease. Ovarian cancer tends to occur earlier in this group of women; the trait may be transmitted in both maternal and paternal lineage.

Factors Increasing Susceptibility
- Low parity
- Delayed childbearing
- Multiple ovulation/infertility treatment
- Menarche later than 14 years old
- Menopause before 45 years old
- High-fat diet (possible relationship)
- Talc on perineum (possible relationship)

Protective Factors
- OCP use
- Multiparity
- Prolonged lactation

Vaginal and Vulvar Cancer. The cause commonly cited for vaginal cancer is intrauterine diethylstilbestrol (DES) exposure; women were given DES during pregnancy between the years of 1938 and 1971, so DES-daughters are at risk for vaginal cancer. Other risk factors for vaginal cancer include multiple pregnancies, syphilis, uterine prolapse, and pessary use. Vaginal cancers have often spread from cervix or uterus. Vulvar cancer appears to be associated with HPV. Risk factors for vulvar cancer include HPV, smoking, and an immunocompromised state.

ASSESSMENT: SUBJECTIVE/HISTORY

The predominant role for the NP in assessing women for GYN cancers is in general screening. Effective cancer screening requires a knowledge base about risk factors for the various types of GYN cancer and an ability to sensitively ask questions about these risks. An effective screening history for GYN cancer includes the following components:
- Review of systems
- History of present illness
- Past medical history, including evidence of appropriate screening tests and results
- Family history, including questions about first-degree male and female relatives with breast, ovarian, or colon cancer
- Obstetrical history
- Sexual history that includes behaviors associated with risk and treatment of STDs
- Medication history, including birth control measures, HRT, and ovulation induction
- Psychosocial history with questions about drug use and cigarette smoking

Common Symptoms

Endometrial Cancer. Abnormal uterine bleeding, especially postmenopausal bleeding, is the primary presenting sign of endometrial cancer. Pain is a late sign.

Cervical Cancer. Often asymptomatic, cervical cancer occasionally presents with abnormal uterine bleeding (menometrorrhagia) and vaginal discharge. Pain is a late symptom. Postcoital bleeding should raise the index of suspicion.

Ovarian Cancer. Symptoms of ovarian cancer are vague with an indefinite onset. There is rarely pain until late in the disease; the pain is not related to the menstrual cycle or defecation. There may be dyspareunia. Early symptoms include increasing abdominal girth, vague GI complaints such as heartburn, bloating, early satiety, constipation, postprandial fullness, and excess gas. As the tumor grows, symptoms may relate to pressure on adjacent structures, for example shortness of breath and urinary symptoms.

Vaginal and Vulvar Cancer. Vaginal cancer is generally asymptomatic. Women with vulvar cancer may complain of prolonged irritation, pruritus, local discomfort, and a slightly bloody vaginal discharge.

ASSESSMENT: OBJECTIVE/PHYSICAL EXAMINATION
Physical Examination

Women may present with symptoms of or concerns about GYN cancer that direct a focused physical examination, or evidence of GYN cancer may be found on routine examination in asymptomatic women. A complete physical examination is important to diagnosing GYN cancer that is still localized to the reproductive tract or late signs such as pain, weight loss, and anemia. The focal examination also includes a comprehensive GYN examination that includes inspection and palpation of external structures, including inguinal nodes, a speculum examination, and a bimanual examination.

Endometrial Cancer. There are no definitive objective findings of endometrial cancer evident on pelvic examination. Endometrial biopsy is diagnostic.

Cervical Cancer. A cervical lesion may be visible as a tumor or ulceration, but there may not be visible cervical changes. Pap smear is diagnostic.

Ovarian Cancer. Pelvic examination is not specific for ovarian cancer. There is no guarding, cervical motion tenderness (CMT), or focal signs. Sometimes a mass can be palpated; some women have firm nodules notable along the uterosacral ligaments or cul de sac. There may be

G

adnexal fullness and decreased mobility of the uterine structures. Rectovaginal examination may be necessary to palpate an ovarian mass. A palpable ovary in a postmenopausal woman is suspicious.

Vaginal and Vulvar Cancer. Annual examinations are needed on DES-daughters, with Pap separately for the cervix and the surface of the upper vagina. Inspection and palpation of the vaginal walls may reveal lesions, masses, or tenderness.

Changes in pigmentation (including leukoplakia), skin thickness, and symmetry are often associated with vulvar cancer. Early disease may appear to be a dermatologic disorder; later findings may include a mass, exophytic growth, or a firm ulcerated area. Area may be painful to palpation. Any localized atypical vulvar lesion, including white patches, need to be biopsied. The NP can "Pap" the lesion and send the specimen for cytologic evaluation, carefully noting location and characteristics of the lesion for the referral.

Diagnostic Procedures

Endometrial Cancer. Although occasional cancerous endometrial cells are noted on Pap smear, the Pap test is not reliable for identifying endometrial cancer. Endometrial sampling through suction aspiration endometrial biopsy is diagnostic. The American Cancer Society recommends endometrial biopsy for all high-risk women at menopause. Transvaginal ultrasound to assess the size of the endometrial stripe (thickness) helps confirm endometrial hyperplasia and the need for biopsy.

Cervical Cancer. The definitive diagnosis of cervical cancer is through a Pap smear. Details about Pap testing for diagnosis of precancerous lesions and cervical cancer are provided later in this chapter.

Ovarian Cancer. There are no specific diagnostic tests for ovarian cancer. The CA-125 is a nonspecific test that increases (more than 35 units) in most women with late ovarian cancer and many in early disease. It also increases in pregnancy, infection, and endometriosis and cannot be used as a reliable screening test for ovarian cancer. Transvaginal ultrasound, especially when augmented by color Doppler imaging, can help in confirming an ovarian mass. A magnetic resonance imaging (MRI) scan or laparoscopy may be necessary for confirmation.

Vaginal and Vulvar Cancers. Diagnosis of vaginal cancer is made on the basis of biopsy findings performed during a culdoscopic evaluation. Vulvar cancer is also diagnosed by biopsy of suspicious lesions.

DIAGNOSIS
Differential Diagnosis

Endometrial Cancer. The differential diagnoses include benign tumors such as leiomyoma and adenomyosis, preg-

nancy, endometriosis, and adhesions.

Cervical Cancer. Differential diagnoses for cervical cancer include cervicitis, abnormal uterine bleeding, and cervical polyps.

Ovarian Cancer. When ruling out ovarian cancer, the NP must consider other differential diagnoses, including ovarian cysts, chronic pelvic pain, endometriosis, and bowel disease.

Vaginal and Vulvar Cancers. When considering vaginal cancer, differential diagnosis includes STDs. Differentiation in cases of vulvar cancer include differential diagnoses of lymphogranuloma venereum, condyloma, and neurofibromatosis.

THERAPEUTIC PLAN

All cases of suspected GYN cancer should be immediately referred for substantiation of the diagnosis and treatment. Treatment generally depends on staging of the cancer and is the province of a gynecologist or oncologist. Inclusion of the age- and population-appropriate screening tests into daily practice is an important measure for preventing GYN cancer in many cases or of finding it early enough to allow for optimal treatment.

Prevention

Endometrial cancer might be preventable with prompt endometrial biopsy in women with anovulatory uterine bleeding and in women with postmenopausal bleeding. In addition, progesterone to counterbalance unopposed estrogen when hormone replacement is ordered for a woman with an intact uterus may prevent some cases of endometrial cancer by avoiding the precursor endometrial hyperplasia.

Cervical cancer might be prevented by sexual behavior that avoids risks of HPV and by timely screening by Pap testing beginning at the age of first coitus or 18 years, whichever occurs first.

There are no known preventive approaches to ovarian cancer. Women with the genetic trait may minimize their risk by careful follow-up. Women at particularly high risk are often encouraged to have bilateral oophorectomy at age 35 or when childbearing ends as a preventive approach.

The probability of vaginal cancer may be decreased by timely follow-up when there has been intrauterine DES exposure. Preventing HPV exposure decreases the risk of vulvar cancer.

Client Education

One of the NP's important roles is in educating women about the risk factors and protective strategies for GYN cancer and about the screening tests that allow early diagnosis. Early diagnosis and treatment is consistently strongly correlated with increasing life expectancy in cases of GYN cancer.

HEADACHE   *Pamela Kidd*

OVERVIEW
Definition

Headache is an acute or chronic diffuse pain in different portions of the head, not confined to any nerve distribution area. It is usually a benign symptom and only occasionally is a manifestation of a serious illness. A migraine headache interferes with daily functioning (Primary Care Network, 2000).

Incidence

- Headache is the most common complaint experienced by humans.
- Disabling headaches are experienced annually by at least 40% of the world population, accounting for a significant proportion of visits to health care providers and approximately 2.5% of visits to emergency departments.
- Headache affects 30% of children and teens (ages 5 to 17) and 34% of adults (ages 25 to 44).

Migraine Headache
- Higher incidence in children and younger adults
- Greater occurrence in women than in men
- Equal occurrence in boys and girls
- Typical onset in the second and third decades, between ages 10 and 25
- Peak prevalence around age 40 in women and age 35 in men

Tension-Type Headache
- Tension-type headache accounts for 20% to 30% of headaches that occur more than once a month.
- There is female-to-male ratio of 1:1 until puberty, and after puberty there is a ratio of 5:4.

Cluster Headache
- Cluster headaches account for less than 1% of headaches.
- Cluster headaches can begin at any age and are more prevalent in men with a male to female ratio of 6:1 to 8:1.

Pathophysiology

A headache can be a symptom indicating another disease, rather than representing a disease in itself. Headache can originate from activation of peripheral nociceptors in the presence of a normally functioning nervous system or as a result of injury or activation of the CNS or peripheral nervous system.

Headaches may arise from dysfunction, displacement, or encroachment on pain-sensitive cranial structures. Headaches can occur as the result of (1) distention, traction, or dilation of intracranial or extracranial arteries; (2) traction or displacement of large intracranial veins or their dural envelope; (3) compression, traction, or inflammation of cranial and spinal nerves; (4) spasm, inflammation, and trauma to cranial and cervical muscles; (5) meningeal irritation and raised intracranial pressure; and (6) disturbance of intracerebral serotonergic projections.

Headaches are broadly classified into the categories of primary (benign or idiopathic) headache disorders and secondary (organic or malignant) headache disorders.

Primary headaches include common tension-type (muscle-contraction) headaches, migraine headaches, and cluster headaches. These types of headaches constitute 99% of headache complaints. Current thoughts indicate that tension-type headaches and migraine headaches occur together along a continuum with tension-type headache at one end and migraine at the other end.

Secondary headaches are due to some underlying pathophysiologic condition, are responsible for less than 1% of headache complaints, and include such precipitants as cerebrovascular lesions, meningeal irritation, intracranial pressure changes, arteritis, infections, and facial (trigeminal neuralgia), cervical (osteoarthritis), systemic, or traumatic causes.

Factors Increasing Susceptibility. Factors that trigger migraine headaches include the following:
- Stress and mental tension
- Excessive sleep and lack of sleep
- Irregular eating habits
- Alcohol
- Hormonal changes
- Hypoglycemia
- Bright lights
- Exercise
- Orgasm
- Weather changes

Factors that trigger tension-type headaches include the following:
- Stressful events
- Emotional upset
- Depression

Factors that trigger cluster headaches include the following:
- Changes in length of daylight can trigger cluster headaches.
- Alcohol and nitroglycerin may trigger an attack once the cluster has started.

In general, the following applies:
- Women have headaches more often than men.
- Headache is a frequent complaint of older adults.

H

Protective Factors
- Male gender

ASSESSMENT: SUBJECTIVE/HISTORY
Symptoms

Gather the following information about the characteristics of the client's headache:

- Age at onset
- Duration (range)
  - Without treatment
  - With treatment
- Frequency
- Location (unilateral, bilateral)
  - If unilateral, does it alternate sides?
  - Quality of pain (pulsating or constant steady ache)
- Prohibit usual daily activities
- Aggravated by mild physical activity (e.g., walking around, climbing stairs)
- Presence of associated features such as nausea, vomiting, photophobia, or phonophobia
- Presence of an aura
  - If yes, describe the aura
  - Duration of the aura
  - Relation to onset of pain
- Potential Precipitating Factors
  - Relationship to menses
  - Frequent strenuous activity (e.g., jogging, aerobics)
- Nonpharmacologic therapies tried (e.g., biofeedback, hot or cold compresses, sleep); note effectiveness

The following is a description of the symptoms of the most common types of primary headaches:

Primary Headaches
Migraine Headache

Migraine without Aura (Common Migraine). Usually a moderate to severe, throbbing, unilateral headache in the temple region or around the eye in persons with a family history of migraine

Migraine with Aura (Classic Migraine). In addition to the symptoms associated with migraine without aura, migraine with aura is characterized by typical neurologic symptoms preceding the headache: visual scotomata (flashing lights), visual field defects (hemianopsia: blindness in one half of the visual field; quadrantanopsia: diminished visual acuity in one fourth of the visual field), fortification scintillations (zig-zag lines or waves), vertigo, and, rarely, aural or olfactory hallucinations.

Usually the symptoms of an aura cease soon after the headache starts and have no lasting impairment.

Tension-Type Headache
- A tension-type headache can be episodic or chronic.
- Usually is a bilateral, steady aching pain of mild to moderate intensity that lasts from minutes to days.
- The pain gradually builds with time.

Cluster Headache (Migrainous Neuralgia)
- Pain begins unilaterally, usually in or around the eye or anywhere on one side of the head.
- The pain quickly progresses to involve the whole side of the head and is described as a severe and boring mixture of jabs and pressure.
- Radiation of the pain to the teeth on one side may occur.
- The eye on the side of the pain tears and turns red, and sometimes the lid droops.
- Attacks of pain are associated with extracranial vasodilation, increased cerebral blood flow, and internal carotid artery changes.
- Each attack lasts anywhere from 10 minutes to 3 hours.
- Individuals may experience one to three attacks per day with many of the attacks occurring at night, especially approximately 90 minutes after onset of sleep.
- The cluster period lasts an average of 2 months and appears to be related to seasonal photoperiod changes (length of daylight), which often occur in the spring or fall with remission periods between clusters.

Past Medical History
- Asthma
- Peptic ulcer
- Anxiety
- Raynaud's disease
- Depression
- Insomnia

Medication History
- Oral contraceptive pills (OCPs)
- Anticoagulants
- Drugs tried for symptomatic relief of headache (both over-the-counter [OTC] and prescription medications; include highest dose reached and reason for discontinuation)
- Current medications used for the treatment of headache (include dose, length of time the drug has been taken, and effectiveness)
  - Symptomatic
  - Prophylactic
- Medications used for reasons other than headache

Family History
- Headaches
- Polycystic kidney disease
- Coarctation of the aorta

Dietary History
- Determine history of tyramine and nitrite sensitivity.
- Food triggers usually include aged cheese, red wine, monosodium glutamate (MSG), chocolate, caffeine (DeRaps, 1999).

ASSESSMENT: OBJECTIVE/PHYSICAL EXAMINATION

Physical Examination

Perform a problem-oriented physical examination that includes all body systems, with emphasis on the vital signs, head, neck, ear, eyes, and neurologic aspects of the examination. The physical examination results are usually normal. Components of the physical examination to be performed are the following:

- Height, weight
- *Vital signs:* temperature, blood pressure, pulse, respirations
- Skin
- Head
- Ears
- Eyes
- Face
- Nose
- Mouth
- Neck, including lymph nodes
- Thorax and lungs
- Cardiovascular systems
- Peripheral vascular systems
- Abdomen
- Musculoskeletal
- Neurologic
  - Cranial nerves I through XII
  - Eyegrounds (fundus of the eye)
  - Reflexes
  - Muscle strengths
  - Breast, genitalia, and rectal examinations can be deferred.

Diagnostic Procedures

Most individuals with headache have normal or unrelated diagnostic findings.

Laboratory Studies

- CBC to rule out inflammatory and infectious conditions
  - White blood cell (WBC) count and differential high in meningitis; WBC left shift if bacterial meningitis
  - Viral syndrome: moderately elevated WBC count and lymphocytosis
- When human immunodeficiency virus (HIV) is suspected: WBC and CD_4 count
- Thyroid function test to rule out hyperthyroidism
- Lumbar puncture if meningitis or subarachnoid hemorrhage is suspected
- Erythrocyte sedimentation rate (ESR) if suspected temporal arteritis (levels higher than 80% usually supports the diagnosis)
- Glucose tolerance test to detect significant metabolic abnormalities causing headaches

- Arterial blood gas (ABG) level to rule out hypoxia and hypercapnia

Radiologic Studies

- Radiologic tests are indicated only if an individual describes an atypical headache pattern, changes in headache pattern, or recent onset of persistent headaches.
- Computed tomography (CT) scan of head is preferred when intracranial lesions are suspected or sinusitis is not responsive to antibiotics.
- Magnetic resonance imaging (MRI) is preferred when suspected posterior fossa lesions or craniospinal lesions are suspected.

Other Studies

- Temporal artery biopsy is indicated in older adults with a tender temporal artery and an elevated ESR.
- EEG is indicated for headaches with seizures.

DIAGNOSIS

Diagnostic Criteria for Migraine without Aura

The International Headache Society (IHS) (1988) diagnostic criteria are as follows:

1. Headache attack lasts 4 to 72 hours
2. At least five attacks fulfilling two to four of the following:
   a. Unilateral location
   b. Pulsating quality
   c. Moderate or severe intensity (inhibits or prohibits activities of daily living [ADLs])
   d. Aggravated by walking stairs or similar routine physical activity
3. During headache, at least one of the following occurs:
   a. Nausea or vomiting
   b. Photophobia or phonophobia
   c. No evidence of organic disease or, if organic disorder present, migraine attack not temporally related.

Diagnostic Criteria for Migraine with Aura

The IHS (1988) diagnostic criteria for migraine with aura are in addition to the criteria for migraine without aura:

1. At least two attacks fulfilling criterion 2.
2. At least three of the following characteristics:
   a. One or more fully reversible aura symptoms indicating focal cerebral, cortical, or brain stem dysfunction:
      (1) Homonymous visual disturbance
      (2) Unilateral paresthesias and/or numbness
      (3) Unilateral weakness
      (4) Aphasia or unclassified speech difficulty
   b. At least one aura symptom that develops gradually during a period of more than 4 minutes or two or more symptoms that occur in succession

H

c. No aura symptoms that last more than 60 minutes; if more than one aura symptom present, accepted duration proportionally increased

d. Headache before, concurrent with, or following aura in less than 60 minutes

3. No evidence of organic disease, or if organic disorder present, migraine attack not temporally related

Diagnostic Criteria for Episodic Tension-Type Headache

The IHS (1988) diagnostic criteria for episodic tension-type headache are as follows:

1. At least 10 previous headache episodes fulfilling criteria 2 through 4; number of days with headache more than 180 per year or more than 15 per month

2. Headache lasting from 30 minutes to 7 days

3. At least two of the following pain characteristics:
   a. Pressing/tightening (nonpulsating) quality
   b. Mild or moderate intensity (may inhibit but does not prohibit activities)
   c. Bilateral location
   d. No aggravation by walking stairs or similar routine physical activity

4. Both of the following:
   a. No nausea or vomiting (anorexia may occur)
   b. Photophobia and phonophobia absent, or one but not the other present

5. May include one of the following:
   a. Increased tenderness of pericranial muscles demonstrated by manual palpation of pressure algometer
   b. Increased EMG level of pericranial muscles at rest during physiologic tests

6. No evidence of organic disease or organic condition present, tension-type headache, not temporally related

Diagnostic Criteria for Chronic Tension-Type Headache

1. Average headache frequency 15 days per month (180 days per year) for 6 months fulfilling criteria 2 through 4

2. At least two of the following pain characteristics:
   a. Pressing/tightening quality
   b. Mild or moderate severity (may inhibit but does not prohibit activities)
   c. Bilateral location
   d. No aggravation by walking stairs or similar physical activity

3. Both of the following:
   a. No vomiting
   b. No more than one of the following: nausea, photophobia, or phonophobia

4. No evidence of organic disease or, if comorbid, no temporal relation

Diagnostic Criteria for Cluster Headache

The IHS (1988) diagnostic criteria for cluster headache are as follows:

1. At least five attacks fulfilling criteria 2 through 4

2. Severe unilateral orbital, supraorbital, and/or temporal pain lasting 15 to 180 minutes untreated

3. Headache associated with at least one of the following signs, which must be present on the side of the pain
   a. Conjunctival injection
   b. Lacrimation
   c. Nasal congestion
   d. Rhinorrhea
   e. Forehead and facial sweating
   f. Miosis
   g. Ptosis
   h. Eyelid edema

4. Frequency of attacks from one every other day to eight per day
   a. Episodic cluster headache: At least two periods of headache (cluster periods) lasting (untreated) from 7 days to 1 year, separated by remissions of at least 14 days
   b. Chronic cluster headaches: Attacks occurring for more than 1 year without remission or with remission lasting less than 14 days

5. No evidence of organic disease or if organic disease present, cluster headache not temporally related

Secondary Headaches

Many organic causes can produce secondary headaches of varying types, characteristics, and location. (The most common and potentially lethal causes are discussed here.)

- Cerebrovascular Lesion: Headache depends on location, type, and extent of vascular lesion.
- Subarachnoid Hemorrhage
  - Approximately 98% to 100% associated with headache
  - Can occur at any age; average age about 51
  - Sudden onset; described as the worst headache of life; referred to as the thunderclap headache
  - May have a sentinel headache (the sudden, unusual headache)
  - Occasional family history of polycystic kidney disease or coarctation of the aorta
  - Nuchal rigidity in approximately 75% of cases
  - Neurologic abnormalities common, but may be absent
  - CT scan can be falsely negative (15%)
  - Cerebrospinal fluid (CSF) bloody; electrocardiogram (ECG) results abnormal; may have leukocytosis, albuminuria/glycosuria
- Intraparenchymal Hemorrhage
  - More than 50% of cases associated with headache

- Occurs in 3% to 10% of all strokes
- Hypertension in more than 50%
- Sudden onset of profound ataxia in cerebellar hemorrhage
- Ischemia Cerebrovascular Disease
  - Headache frequency of 17% to 54%
  - Headache generally mild to moderate in intensity
- Carotid Artery Dissection
  - Rare, usually occurs in young adult
  - Headache present in more than 80% of cases
  - Ipsilateral Horner's syndrome (ptosis, myosis, anhydrosis) a diagnostic clue
  - Infarcts in approximately one third of individuals
- Hypertension
  - Hypertension usually does not cause pain unless diastolic pressure is greater than 120 mm Hg.
  - When headache is present, it is generally mild and occurs on waking but improves on rising.
- Cervical Disease
  - Most common cause of headache that begins to occur in middle to late life; wide variety of cervical (neck) disease processes involved
  - Pain usually occipital, frequently asymmetric, nonthrobbing aching quality and associated with shoulder and lower back pain
  - Course chronic and relapsing
- Drug Overuse or Withdrawal
  - Drug overuse or withdrawal may contribute to as many as 20% of chronic headache syndromes.
  - Medications that may cause withdrawal and rebound headaches include barbiturates, opioids, ergotamine tartrate compounds, benzodiazepines, and caffeine-containing analgesic preparations.
- Infectious Diseases
  - Headache is common and predominant in bacterial meningitis.
  - Severe headache is the most frequent symptom in viral meningitis.
  - Headache is common and prominent with fever.
  - Severe headache is common with acute sinusitis (a dull, nonpulsating aching headache); the location depends on the sinus involved.
- Inflammatory Disease
- Temporal Arteritis
  - Usually seen in women (four times more than in men) older than 50
  - Typically a new kind of headache for the individual
  - Focal pain unvarying in location, at the temporal artery (tenderness in this area) and behind the eye
  - Possible sudden blindness without warning; visual impairment in one third to one half of individuals

- ESR elevated with a mean of 100 mm/hr
- Malaise, fever, weight loss, and jaw claudication early symptoms; symptoms associated with polymyalgia rheumatica
- Neoplastic Disease
  - Headache associated with a brain tumor is usually deep, aching, nonthrobbing, often generalized, and intermittent.
  - Headache is occasionally associated with vomiting and may be worse with exertion (e.g., coughing or straining) by increasing intracranial pressure.
- Trigeminal Neuralgia (Tic Douloureux)
  - This severe, disabling, lancinating pain in distribution of cranial nerve V (trigeminal) division 1 or 2 lasts a few seconds to minutes interspersed with a minute or so of relief.
  - Pain may recur several times per day and become more frequent.
  - Exposure to environmental irritants such as wind and cold may precipitate pain.
- Ophthalmologic Disorders
  - Eyestrain (refractory errors): When pain is present, it is increased with use of the eyes.
  - Narrow-angle glaucoma
  - Episodic pain in and around the eye
  - A severe, boring ache centered in the eye (though may be diffused on that side of the head)
  - Possible nausea and vomiting
  - Can cause blindness if not treated
  - Optic Neuritis: The pain is in or behind the eye and may be exacerbated by pressure over the eye or by ocular movement.
  - Tolosa-Hunt Syndrome: Single or recurrent attacks of unilateral retroorbital continuous boring pain are followed by ophthalmoplegia.
  - Otalgic Pain: Headache from ear pain may originate from external canal foreign bodies, external otitis, external or middle ear neoplasia, otitis media, acoustic neuroma, and external/middle ear trauma.
- Spinal Puncture
  - Headache occurs in 10% to 30% of individuals who receive a spinal puncture. It usually begins 15 minutes to 4 days after the procedure and lasts 4 to 8 days. The female-to-male ratio is 2:1.
  - The pain is described as either frontal, occipital, or diffuse, which is a pounding or a dull ache. The pain is present when the individual is in the upright position, and the pain is relieved when the individual is lying flat.
- Temporomandibular Joint Dysfunction
  - Localized facial pain, limitation of jaw motion, muscle tenderness, and temporomandibular joint crepitus

H

- Pain in front of and behind ear of affected side; may radiate over cheek and face; "full" feeling in ear possible
- Toxic and Metabolic Causes
  - Toxic causes (carbon monoxide, hypercapnia, and acute mountain sickness): A gradual intensification of headache is followed by impaired consciousness.
  - Chinese Restaurant Syndrome: Caused by the ingestion of MSG by individuals who are sensitive to it. Symptoms include headache, nausea, lightheadedness, and numbness and burning of head, chest, and arms.
  - Chronic Hemodialysis: Individuals receiving long-term dialysis therapy frequently have headaches.
  - Endocrine Disorders: Headache occasionally occurs in individuals with endocrine disorders such as hormonal disorders associated with the menstrual cycle and use of birth control pills, diabetes, hyperthyroidism, and adrenal and pituitary abnormalities.
- Trauma
  - Hematomas: Conscious individuals with epidural or acute hematomas without exception complain of headache. In subacute or chronic subdural hematoma, headache occurs in up to 60% of individuals. The headache is more severe than that associated with brain tumor. Suspect a hematoma in individuals with headache who are alcoholic, uncontrolled epileptics, older than 60, or receiving dialysis or anticoagulant therapy or in those who have a history of a fall or blow to the head.
  - Head Injury: An immediate transient headache follows almost all head injuries. Prevalence of chronic posttraumatic headache varies from 33% to 83%.

THERAPEUTIC PLAN

When a secondary headache is diagnosed, the goal is treatment of the organic cause of the headache or cure of the illness associated with the headache, with referral for medical or surgical interventions. The goal of treatment of primary headaches is pain alleviation, prevention, and the limitation of dysfunction.

Nonpharmacologic Treatment

- Adequate nutrition with regular meals and adequate fluid intake
- Avoidance of trigger foods and situations
- Adequate rest
- Regular exercise
- Proper posture
- Topical heat or cold applications
- Stress-reduction techniques: Work and home stresses discussed and reduced if possible

- Individual and family counseling
- Lifestyle: Lifestyle modifications implemented before considering medications

Pharmacologic Treatment

- Pharmacologic treatment consists of abortive (symptomatic) therapy and prophylactic (preventive) therapy as follows:
  - Abortive therapy is used to treat symptoms once they occur or to prevent headaches after warning signs (such as an aura) have appeared.
  - Prophylactic therapy should be considered for the individual who has at least one headache per week that interferes with ADLs.
- The choice of therapy is guided by the type of headache, previous and concurrent use of typical medication, the client's preference and needs as to route of delivery, concurrent symptoms or problems, cost, and length of treatment.
- Prescribe the least potent and least addictive analgesic medication that relieves most of the pain. Opioids and barbiturates have a tendency for addiction.
- Caffeine or ergotamine contribute to rebound headaches. Rebound headaches result from too frequent dosing with analgesics, particularly those that contain caffeine and ergotamine. The client must be weaned from these medications before proper management can be initiated. Refer to a neurologist for evaluation.
- Older adults are more susceptible to the cardiovascular effects of the prophylaxis headache medications. Older adults are also more likely to be receiving other medications; therefore drug interactions must be anticipated. Thus medication therapy should be initiated at low dosages and titrate increases slowly.

Abortive Therapy
Migraine Headache

- Analgesics/NSAIDs
  - Aspirin or acetaminophen 325 mg (2 tablets q4 to 6h)
  - Naproxen 250 to 750 qd or 250 mg bid
  - Ibuprofen 300 to 600 mg tid
- Analgesic combinations
  - Aspirin/butalbital/caffeine (Fiorinal) 1 to 2 tablets/caplets q4h (maximum 6/24 hours)
  - Acetaminophen/isometheptene/dichloralphenazone (Midrin) 2 caplets, then 1 caplet qh (maximum 5 in 12 hours)
- Narcotics/opioids
  - Acetaminophen/codeine (various fixed dosages) 1 to 2 tablets q4h
  - Butorphanol nasal spray (very addictive) 1 spray unilateral to headache, can repeat once in 3 to 5 hours
- Ergot alkaloids

- Ergotamine/caffeine (Cafergot, Wigraine) tablets: 2 tablets, then 1 q30 min up to a maximum of 6 tablets per attack
- Ergotamine/caffeine rectal suppositories: one at onset, then may repeat once in 1 hour
- Dihydroergotamine mesylate (DHE, 45) for severe pain 1 ml IV/IM at onset, then every hour (maximum 2 ml IV or 3 ml IM per attack)
- Serotonin receptor agonist
  - Sumatriptan (Imitrex) 6 mg/0.5 ml SC, may repeat once (maximum 2 injections/24 hours)
  - Sumatriptan (Imitrex) tablets: 25 to 100 mg (maximum 300 mg/24 hours, 200 mg if SC injection used initially)
- Antiemetics
  - Prochlorperazine (Compazine) 5 to 25 mg
  - Metoclopramide (Reglan) 5 to10 mg

Tension-Type Headache
- Analgesics/NSAIDs
  - Same as for migraine headache
- Analgesic combinations
  - Aspirin/butalbital/caffeine (Fiorinal): Same as for migraine headache
  - Acetaminophen/isometheptene/dichloralphenazone (Midrin) 1 to 2 tablets q4h (maximum 6/24 hours)
- Antidepressants
  - Amitriptyline (Elavil) 50 to 100 mg hs
  - Buspirone (Buspar) 15 to 80 mg qd
  - Sertraline (Zoloft) 50 to 200 mg qd
- Muscle relaxant
  - Cyclobenzaprine (Flexeril) 10 to 40 mg qd

Cluster Headache
- Oxygen therapy
  - 100% oxygen at 7 L/min via face mask (first line of treatment)
- Ergot alkaloids
  - Ergotamine sublingual or medihaler: Inhaled at the onset of attack, then may be repeated 3 times at 5 minutes apart if needed
  - Ergotamine/caffeine (Cafergot, Wigraine) 2 tablets, then every 30 minutes (maximum 6 tablets per attack)
  - Dihydroergotamine mesylate 1 ml IV/IM at onset, then every hour (should be reserved for emergency department use; maximum 2 ml IV or 3 ml IM per attack)
- Serotonin receptor agonist
  - Sumatriptan: Same as for migraine headache
- Lidocaine
  - Viscous lidocaine 4% intranasally on side of headache, 1 inhalation qh

Prophylactic Therapy
Migraine Headache
- Beta-adrenergic blockers
  - Propranolol (Inderal) 40 to 100 mg qd

- Timolol (Blocadren) 10 to 30 mg bid
- Nadolol (Corgard) 20 to 40 mg qd
- Atenolol (Tenormin) 50 mg qd
- Calcium channel blockers
  - Verapamil (Calan) 40 to 120 mg tid
  - Nifedipine (Procardia) 10 to 30 mg tid
- Antidepressants
  - Amitriptyline (Elavil) 50 to 200 mg qd
  - Sertraline (Zoloft) 50 to 200 mg qd
  - Buspirone (Buspar) 15 to 80 mg qd
  - Imipramine (Tofranil) 75-200 mg qd
- Serotonin inhibitors
  - Methysergide (Sansert) 2 to 4 mg bid (maximum 8 mg/day)
  - Cyproheptadine (Periactin) 4 to 20 mg qd

Tension-Type Headache
- Antidepressants
  - Amitriptyline (Elavil) 25 to 200 mg qd
  - Nortriptyline (Aventyl, Pamelor) 75 to 150 mg qd
- Muscle relaxant
  - Cyclobenzaprine (Flexeril) 10 to 40 mg qd
- NSAIDs
  - Naproxen (Naprosyn) 250 mg bid
  - Ibuprofen (e.g., Advil, Motrin) 200 mg bid

Cluster Headache
- Calcium channel blocker
  - Verapamil (Calan, Isoptin) 120 mg tid
- Antidepressant
  - Lithium carbonate (Lithium) 300 mg tid
- Ergot alkaloid
  - Methysergide (Sansert) 4 to 8 mg qd
- Corticosteroid
  - Prednisone 40 mg qd in divided doses

Client Education
Instruct older adults that frequency and severity of migraine diminishes as one ages.
- Instruct the client to recognize triggers and early warning signs of headaches.
- Instruct the client to use protective or preventive factors against headache.
- Migraine headaches are made more severe by lying down and are relieved by standing or sitting.

Referral
Any of the following presentations should be referred to a neurologist or a physician:
- "First or worst" headache, particularly with acute onset or abnormal neurologic findings
- Headache (particularly in those older than age 50) with subacute onset that progressively worsens over days or weeks
- Headache related with fever, nausea, and vomiting that cannot be explained by a systemic disorder
- Headache associated with focal neurologic findings
- No obvious identifiable headache etiologic factor

H

- Clients requiring "rescue" medication to treat pain (and therefore not responding to initial treatment) more than once a month (Primary Care Network, 2000)

Prevention

- No preventive measures have been clearly indicated for individuals at risk for migraine and tension-type headaches.
- The use of the following can reduce the incidence of tension-type headache:
  - Use of glare screen on computer terminals
  - Use of proper ergonomics at work stations to reduce neck strain
  - Use of good ventilation systems at work sites with exposure to chemical fumes
  - Use of stress-reducing behaviors
- No protective factors for cluster headaches have been identified.
- Discuss with the client protective factors for secondary types of headaches as appropriate to the individual case (e.g., wearing of seat belts and safety helmets to prevent head injury).
- Client needs to seek clinician input early when therapies do not work.
- Advise the client to keep a headache diary.
- Inform the client of available resources for managing treatment of headaches.
- Ensure the client understands the benefits, proper use, and side effects of medications and other treatments.
- Provide the client with information on headaches, need for stress reduction, and dangers of drug overuse.

EVALUATION/FOLLOW-UP

Clients with chronic headaches should be monitored regularly (monthly) to evaluate the headache diary, effectiveness of medications, and client's compliance in taking medication and for counseling, education, and support in maintaining the treatment plan.

COMPLICATIONS

Complications arise from failure to treat the underlying disorder that is producing secondary headaches. These include but are not limited to stroke, death, blindness, and disability.

REFERENCES

Coutin, I. B., & Glass, S. F. (1996). Recognizing uncommon headache syndromes. *American Family Physician, 54*(7), 2247-2252.

DeRaps, P. K. (1999). Migraine management. *ADVANCE for Nurse Practitioners. 7*(5), 51, 53-55.

Dodick, D. (1997). Headache as a symptom of ominous disease. *Postgraduate Medicine, 101*(5), 46-64.

Headache Classification Committee of the International Headache Society (1988). Classification and diagnostic criteria for headache disorders, cranial neuralgia and facial pain. *Cephalagia 8*(Suppl 7), 1-96.

Porter, B. (2000). Headaches. In D. Robinson, P. Kidd, & K. Rogers (Eds.). *Primary care across the lifespan*. St. Louis: Mosby.

Primary Care Network. (2000). Patient-centered strategies for effective management of migraine. Retrieved Fall 2001, from www.headachecare.com.

Review Questions

1. Which of the following symptoms are suggestive of a secondary type of headache?
   a. Moderate pulsating pain on the right side of the head for more than 24 hours, nausea, and phonophobia
   b. Approximately four episodes per day of 30 minutes of severe pain on the left side of the head in and around the eye, nasal congestion, and conjunctival infection
   c. Pain in the right temporal area and behind the right eye, fever, and jaw claudication
   d. Bilateral, nonpulsating, moderate, steady aching pain for more than 48 hours; no aggravation by performance of routine physical activities

2. Mrs. Smith, a 30-year-old housewife has a severe pulsating pain on the left side of the head, which has been present more than 48 hours with nausea and phonophobia; she has some numbness on the left side of the face. Mrs. Smith reports "having this type of headache since she was 18 years old and usually has one headache per month." Mrs. Smith's physical examination results are normal. Which of the following types of primary headache is Mrs. Smith most likely experiencing?
   a. Cluster headache
   b. Episodic tension-type headache
   c. Chronic tension-type headache
   d. Migraine headache

3. Which of the following statements regarding the use of pharmaceuticals for alleviating pain in migraine headaches is *not* correct?
   a. "NSAIDs have been found to be as effective as the ergotamine-caffeine preparations in relieving migraine headaches."
   b. "The use of metoclopramide (Reglan) and phenothiazines enhances the effectiveness of analgesics in the treatment of migraine headache."
   c. "Narcotic analgesics should be used with caution in the treatment of migraine headache."
   d. "Administration of 7 L of oxygen by face mask should be given as early as possible after the onset of a migraine headache."

4. Mrs. Webb, a 40-year-old woman, is being treated for chronic tension-type headaches. She should receive follow-up on a regular basis for all the following *except:*
   a. Continuity of care
   b. Instructions on various triggers of headaches and how to avoid them

   c. Instructions on relaxation and stress-reduction techniques
   d. Routine CBC and urinalysis

5. Mr. Douglas, a 32-year-old white man, is being treated for headaches. He has been asked to keep a diary of his headaches, sleep patterns, diet, anger, and other possible contributing factors for 1 month and bring the diary with him on his follow-up visit. The purpose of a diary is which of the following?
   a. Provide information for establishing the specific type of headache.
   b. Assist the health care provider to get to know the client personally.
   c. Provide a form of therapy for the client.
   d. The diary is not necessary.

6. Which of the following triggers differentiates migraine from tension headaches?
   a. Stress
   b. Lighting
   c. Excessive sleep or lack of sleep
   d. Alcohol

7. What statement indicates adequate client education about prevention of rebound headaches?
   a. "I will wait until the pain increases to start treatment."
   b. "I will use Cafergot prophylactically."
   c. "I will use up to 6 Cafergot tablets per attack."
   d. "I will wait at least 30 minutes before using another Cafergot tablet during an attack."

Answers and Rationales

1. Answer: c (assessment)
Rationale: Moderate pulsating pain on right side of the head for more than 24 hours, nausea, and phonophobia are more indicative of a moderate migraine headache without an aura, whereas approximately four episodes per day of 30 minutes of severe pain on the left side of the head in and around the eye, nasal congestion, and conjunctival injection are more likely to occur with a cluster headache. Bilateral, nonpulsating, moderate, steady pain not aggravated by performance of routine physical activities is identified as a tension-type headache.

2. Answer: d (analysis/diagnosis)
Rationale: Cluster, episodic tension-type, and chronic tension-type headaches should be considered as the differential diagnosis for the symptoms presented. Typically with migraine headache, the individual has a unilateral moderate to severe pulsating pain that may last from 4 to 72 hours and may be accompanied by nausea, vomiting, phonophobia, or photophobia.

3. Answer: d (implementation/plan)
Rationale: NSAIDs have been found to be as effective as the ergotamine-caffeine preparations in relieving migraine headaches; the use of metoclopramide (Reglan) and phenothiazines enhances the effects of analgesics; and narcotic analgesics should be used with caution in treatment of migraine headaches because of possible addiction. Administration of oxygen is the first line of treatment for cluster headaches.

4. Answer: d (evaluation)
Rationale: Clients with headaches should be followed regularly to ensure continuity of care; provide instructions on participator factors, relaxation and stress reduction techniques, and effects and side effects of medications; counseling; and support.

5. Answer: a (evaluation)
Rationale: A diary of when the headache starts, duration, events occurring before headache, sleep patterns, stress, anger, environmental irritants exposure, diet, and other factors, assist in the establishment of the specific type of headache an individual is experiencing.

6. Answer: c (analysis/diagnosis)
Rationale: Excessive sleep or lack of sleep may trigger migraine headaches but is not associated with tension headaches. Lighting changes may affect both migraine and tension headaches. Bright lights may trigger a migraine, whereas change in length of daylight may trigger tension-type headaches. Alcohol and stress may trigger both.

7. Answer: d (evaluation)
Rationale: Ergot alkaloids and caffeine (such as Cafergot) are abortive agents used during an attack or impending attack (warning signs are present). It is not a prophylactic agent because of its vasoconstrictive properties. Rebound headaches are produced by too frequent dosing of analgesics, particularly those containing caffeine (e.g. Fioricet) and ergotamine, and drugs containing caffeine and ergotamine.

H

HEARING LOSS *Pamela Kidd*

OVERVIEW
Definition

Hearing loss is the decreased ability to hear sounds. Presbycusis is the slowly progressive symmetrical loss of predominantly high-frequency hearing associated with aging.

Incidence

Hearing loss occurs in 25% to 30% of persons aged 65 and older, and in nearly 50% of those older than 75. Approximately 28 million Americans are affected by hearing loss. Only approximately 20% of people wear hearing aids.

Pathophysiology

Conductive hearing loss results from dysfunction of the middle ear, with a resulting impairment of the passage of sound vibrations to the middle ear. These are caused by obstruction (cerumen impaction), middle ear effusion, otosclerosis, and ossicular disruption. Conductive hearing loss is generally correctable.

Sensory Hearing Loss results from deterioration of the cochlea, usually because of the loss of hair cells from the organ of Corti. Examples of causes include noise trauma, aging, and ototoxicity. Sensory hearing loss is not correctable but may be prevented or stabilized.

Neural Hearing Loss results from lesions of the eighth cranial nerve, auditory nuclei, or auditory cortex. It is the least common cause of hearing loss. Disorders that may cause neural hearing loss include neuroma, multiple sclerosis, and cerebrovascular disease.

Factors Increasing Susceptibility. Occupational and recreational noise.

Protective Factors. Use of hearing protection.

ASSESSMENT: SUBJECTIVE/HISTORY
Symptoms

Clients may present with complaints of difficulty hearing or family members may identify an inability of the client to hear. May exhibit the following symptoms:
- Complains of feeling stressed or tired during conversations.
- Frequently asks people to repeat themselves.
- Avoids social situations.
- Frequently denies hearing problems.
- Turns up television so loudly that others complain.
- Complains of nausea/vomiting, tinnitus.
- Loses ability to "pop" ears.
- Has a sense of fullness in ears.
- Pulls at ears.
- Loses equilibrium.
- May complain of foreign body in the ear.
- Ask about involvement of one ear or both.

- Determine whether the onset was gradual or sudden.
- Determine whether hearing has fluctuated since the hearing loss began.
- Determine whether there are associated symptoms of tinnitus, vertigo, otalgia, otorrhea, or facial weakness.

Children
- Makes few attempts to communicate by 12 months.
- Unable to use more than 8 to 10 words at 18 months.
- Uses two-word combinations for most of talking at age 2½.
- Difficult to understand at age 3½.

Past Medical History

Ask about the following:
- Hypertension
- Mumps
- Neurologic problems
- Head trauma
- Diabetes
- Hypothyroidism
- Syphilis
- Frequent colds, congestion, allergies or ear infections as child

Medication History

Ask about use of the following:
- ASA (high dose)
- Antibiotics: aminoglycosides (gentamicin, streptomycin)
- Diuretics (Loop: furosemide)
- Quinine

Family History

Ask about a family history of hearing loss.

Dietary History

Noncontributory.

ASSESSMENT: OBJECTIVE/PHYSICAL EXAMINATION
Physical Examination

The examination should concentrate on the head and neck.
- *HEENT:* Evaluate for an upper respiratory infection (URI).
- *Ear:* Evaluate tympanic membrane (TM), external canal.
  - Complete pneumatic otoscopy: check for TM movement
  - Tympanogram

- *Neurologic examination:* Check sensation of face, note if facial movement is symmetrical, note presence of any rapid alternating movements (RAMs).
- *Hearing examination:* Have client repeat aloud words presented in a soft whisper, normal speaking voice or a shout. Have the opposite ear occluded, then repeat on other side.
  - Children: 0 to 3 months: responds to noise
    - 3 to 5 months: child turns to sound
    - 6 to 10 months: child responds to name
    - 10 to 15 months: child imitates simple words

- *Weber:* Place the tuning fork on the forehead or front teeth. Have the client indicate where it is heard the best.
- *Rinne:* The tuning fork is placed alternately on the mastoid bone and in front of the ear canal.

Diagnostic Procedures

See Table 3-38.

DIAGNOSIS

Differential diagnosis includes the information presented in Table 3-39 and hearing tests and hearing loss are discussed in Tables 3-40 and 3-41.

TABLE **3-38**   Diagnostic Tests for Hearing Loss

DIAGNOSTIC TEST	FINDING/RATIONALE
Audiometric studies	Hearing test is conducted in sound proof room. Pure-tone thresholds in dB are obtained over the ranges of 250-8000 Hz for both air and bone conduction. All clients with hearing loss should be referred for audiometric testing unless the cause is easily remediable (e.g., impacted cerumen). Clients can be referred directly to an audiologist.
Speech discrimination testing	Evaluates the clarity of hearing. Results are reported as percentage correct.
Tympanogram	Used to detect fluid in the middle ear and to determine the mobility of the TM. An electroacoustic device is used to measure the compliance of the TM. Results are displayed in a graphic form. It is most reliable in children younger than 6 months.
Audiogram	Small, hand held audioscopes can provide a rough indication of hearing impairment. Usually 4 pure tones are emitted in sequence. This test can be affected by background noise, so the examination room must be quiet.

dB, Decibel; *Hz,* hertz; *TM,* tympanic membrane.

TABLE **3-39**   Differential Diagnosis of Hearing Loss

DIAGNOSIS	DATA SUPPORT
Conductive loss	Rinne test shows AC less than BC; Weber test lateralizes to the involved ear. The whisper is abnormal if more than 40 dB loss is present.
Cerumen impaction	Occlusion of the external ear canal by cerumen. Usually self-induced via attempts at cleaning.
Serous otitis media	Dull TM, hypomobile TM, air bubbles may be seen in the middle ear, with a conductive hearing loss present.
Otosclerosis	Progressive disease with a familial tendency that affects bone surrounding the inner ear.
TM perforation	Perforation of the TM may result in decreased hearing abilities. The perforation may occur from trauma or as the result of increased pressure with otitis media. Spontaneous healing occurs in the majority of cases.
Sensorineural loss	In Rinne, both AC and BC are decreased; Weber localizes to the uninvolved ear; the whisper test is abnormal if more than 40 dB loss is present.
Presbycusis	Progressive, mainly high frequency hearing loss of aging. Frequently with genetic predisposition. Clients complain of an inability to hear well (speech discrimination) in a noisy environment.
Noise trauma	Second most common cause of hearing loss. Sounds louder than 85 dB are potentially damaging to the cochlea, especially with prolonged exposure. The loss typically occurs in the high frequencies (4000 Hz) and progresses to involve sounds in the normal speech frequencies. Sounds that have the potential to cause damage include industrial machinery, loud music, and weapons.
Ototoxicity	Hearing loss can be caused by substances that affect both the auditory and vestibular systems. Common causes include salicylates, aminoglycosides, loop diuretics and antineoplastic agents, and especially cisplatin.

AC, Air conduction; *BC,* bone conduction; *dB,* decibel; *Hz,* hertz; *TM,* tympanic membrane.

H

TABLE **3-40**   Classification of Hearing Test and Type of Hearing Loss

CLASSIFICATION	RINNE	WEBER
Normal: Both ears	AC louder than BC	Midline
Conductive loss		
Right ear	Right ear: BC louder than AC	Lateralized to right ear
	Left ear: AC louder than BC	
Left ear	Right ear: AC louder than BC	Lateralized to left ear
	Left ear: BC louder than AC	
Both ears	Right ear: BC louder than AC	Lateralized to poorer ear of the two
	Left ear: BC louder than AC	
Sensorineural loss		
Right ear	AC louder than BC in both ears	Lateralized to left ear
Left ear	AC louder than BC in both ears	Lateralized to right ear
Both ears	AC louder than BC in both ears	Lateralized to better ear

AC, Air conduction; *BC,* bone conduction.

TABLE **3-41**   Hearing Loss

CATEGORY OF HEARING LOSS	DB LEVEL
Mild hearing loss	26-40 dB
Moderate hearing loss	41-55 dB
Moderately severe hearing loss	56-70 dB
Severe hearing loss	71-90 dB
Profound hearing loss	More than 91 dB

dB, Decibel.

THERAPEUTIC PLAN

Nonpharmacologic Treatment

- Depends on cause of hearing loss
- Hearing aids:
  - Can assist those people with sensorineural and conductive hearing loss.
  - Can increase the intensity of sounds up to about 70 dB.
  - Can be obtained only after an evaluation by a health care provider. Medicare and most insurance companies do not pay for hearing aids.
  - Three types of hearing aids are available (Table 3-42).
  - Four basic models of hearing aids are available:
  - Behind-the-ear hearing aids fit in ear and behind the ear, connected by a loop that wraps around the top of the ear.
  - In-the-ear hearing aids are slightly smaller, fit just inside the ear and sit flush with the outer ear.
  - In-the-canal hearing aids fit into the ear canal and show only slightly on the outside of the ear.
  - Completely-in-the-canal hearing aids fit deep in the ear canal with a tiny sensor wire that protrudes from the ear.

Pharmacologic Treatment

None.

Client Education

Use the following to assist with speech:
- Face people while talking.
- Obtain their attention before speaking.
- Use gestures.
- Speak at a moderate pace.
- Use adequate lighting.
- Minimize background noise if possible.
- Ask what can be done to facilitate hearing.
- Use telecommunications device for the deaf (TDD) phone.
- Use television with a closed captioning feature.

Referral

- Ear, nose, and throat (ENT) specialist for conductive hearing loss
- Audiologist

Prevention

- Wear ear plugs or ear muffs (cotton balls won't do the job).
- Keep volume low when wearing headphones.
- See noise levels listed in Table 3-43.

EVALUATION/FOLLOW-UP

- If hearing loss is caused by acute disease, check for resolution in 1 to 2 weeks.
- Recheck hearing abilities to determine improvement.

COMPLICATIONS

- Deafness

TABLE **3-42** Types of Hearing Aids

TYPE OF HEARING AID	HOW THEY WORK	COST
Conventional/traditional	Amplify sound using preprogrammed circuits	$600 and up
Programmable (analog sound processing)	Use tiny computer chips that can be programmed to different settings, environments, background noise, types of noise; these can be reprogrammed as hearing loss changes	$850-$2000
Digital sound processing	Use the latest technology with clear sound, sophisticated circuits, front and rear microphones, voice versus nonvoice sensors to make sound audible without discomfort	$2000-$3200

TABLE **3-43** Examples of Noise Levels

NOISE LEVEL IN DECIBELS	EXAMPLES
SAFE HEARING LEVELS	
20 dB	Whispered voice
40 dB	Refrigerator humming
60 dB	Normal conversation
LEVELS AT WHICH HEARING LOSS CAN OCCUR:	Prolonged exposure to noise louder than 90 dB can cause gradual hearing loss.
90 dB	Lawn mower
100 dB	Wood shop—**no more than 15 minutes of unprotected exposure is recommended**
110 dB	Chain saw, some video arcades, head phones, stereos—**regular unprotected exposure longer than 1 minute at this decibel level or higher risks permanent hearing loss**
120 dB	Loud cars, snowmobiles, rock concerts
130 dB	Some lawn mowers, leaf blowers, power tools
140 dB	Firecrackers
150 dB	Gunshot or some toy guns shot from 1 foot away

Source: National Institute on Deafness and Communication Disorders.

REFERENCES

Jackler, R., & Kaplan, M. (2001). Ear, nose, throat. In L. Tierney, S. McPhee, M. Papadakis.(Eds.), *Current medical diagnosis and treatment* (40th ed.). New York: McGraw Hill.

Robinson, D. (2000). Hearing loss. In D. Robinson, P. Kidd, & K. Rogers (Eds.), *Primary care across the lifespan*. St. Louis: Mosby.

Review Questions

1. Which of the following best describes conductive hearing loss?

   a. Conductive hearing loss is irreversible.
   b. Results from damage or injury to eight cranial nerve.
   c. Results from deterioration of the cochlea.
   d. Results from dysfunction of the middle ear.

2. Which of the following assessment data would help discriminate hearing loss from other differential diagnoses?

   a. Pulling at the ears
   b. Tinnitus
   c. Avoidance of social situations
   d. Client turns up the television volume

3. All of the following drugs may produce hearing loss *except:*

   a. Aspirin
   b. NSAIDs
   c. Loop diuretics
   d. Streptomycin

4. When assessing a 15-month-old child for the complaint of hearing loss, the nurse practitioner (NP) notes that the child turns to sound but does not imitate words. Which of the following statements applies to this finding?

H

  a. This finding is normal.
  b. This finding represents sensory hearing loss.
  c. This finding indicates the need for further evaluation.
  d. This finding indicates cerumen impaction.

5. When performing the Rinne and Weber test in a client with suspected conductive hearing loss in the right ear, the NP expects which of the following findings?

  a. Bone conduction greater than air conduction in the right ear, lateralization to the left ear
  b. Air conduction greater than bone conduction in the right ear, lateralization to the right ear
  c. Bone conduction greater than air conduction in the right ear, lateralization to the right ear
  d. Air conduction greater than bone conduction in the right ear, lateralization to the left ear

Answers and Rationales

1. **Answer: d** (analysis/diagnosis)
  Rationale: Sensory hearing loss is not reversible and is produced by deterioration of the cochlea. Neural hearing loss results from lesions of the eight cranial nerve.

2. **Answer: d** (assessment)
  Rationale: Pulling at the ears may be present with otitis media. Tinnitus may be a temporary side effect of medications. Avoidance of social situations may be symptomatic of depression.

3. **Answer: b** (analysis/diagnosis)
  Rationale: Furosemide and aspirin are commonly associated with hearing loss. Aminoglycosides (gentamycin, streptomycin) are also associated with hearing loss.

4. **Answer: c** (analysis/diagnosis)
  Rationale: A diagnosis of the type of hearing loss or cause of hearing loss cannot be determined by this symptom alone. It must be confirmed by physical examination or diagnostic testing. At 15 months, the child should be imitating simple words if the child's hearing is normal.

5. **Answer: c** (evaluation)
  Rationale: In conductive hearing loss, bone conduction is better than air conduction of sound. Lateralization occurs to the affected ear.

HEART SOUNDS *Pamela Kidd*

GENERAL RULES FOR HEART MURMURS

- For murmurs originating in the left side of the heart (e.g., mitral), roll the client onto left side.
- Lean client forward for aortic murmurs.
- Midsystolic murmurs usually originate in semilunar valves (tricuspid and mitral).

- Pansystolic murmurs are usually associated with regurgitation.
- Middiastolic/presystolic murmurs are associated with atrioventricular valves (pulmonic, aortic).
- Murmurs originating in the right side of the heart (e.g., pulmonic, tricuspid) change more with respiration.

Abnormal Heart Sounds

SOUND	LOCATION	SIGNIFICANCE
Split S_1	LLSB	Heard elsewhere or with split S_2 split may indicate right bundle-branch block and premature ventricular contractions
Split S_2	Second, third left ICS	Normal if accentuated by inspiration, absent with expiration or sitting up. Widens with pulmonic valve closure delays. Fixed with atrial septal defect and right ventricular failure. Paradoxical with left bundle-branch block.
Systolic click	LLSB, medial to apex Diaphragm, midsystole	Mitral valve prolapse.
Opening snap	LLSB, medial to apex Diaphragm, early diastole	Mitral valve stenosis.
S_3	Apex, left lateral position. Louder on inspiration.	Rapid ventricular filling, healthy children. Ventricular gallop: overloaded left ventricle as in mitral or tricuspid regurgitation.
S_4	Apex, left lateral position.	Normal athletes and aged. Atrial gallop: represents increased resistance to ventricular filling as in hyperparathyroidsm, coronary artery disease, aortic stenosis.

ICS, Intercostal space; *LLSB*, left lateral sternal border.

Systolic Heart Sounds

CONDITION	SYMPTOMS, IF PRESENT	MOST SUSCEPTIBLE	PATHOLOGIC CONDITION	EXAMINATION	CLUES IN HISTORY	DIAGNOSIS	TYPE OF MURMUR
Mitral regurgitation Malfunction of papillary muscles or wall of ventricle or calcification of mitral valve. Keeps it from closing during systole.	Depends on severity; as worsens, symptoms of CHF occur	Occurs most frequently in 60-70 year range. Rare in children.	Causes regurgitation of blood flow backward from left ventricle to left atrium.	Best position for auscultation is the client rolling partly on the left side. Also may have a S_3.	Chronic CHF	Echo	Plateau murmur, pansystolic in nature. No gap between murmur and heart sounds.
Tricuspid regurgitation		Rare following rheumatic heart disease.	Allows blood flow backward into right ventricle from right atrium.	Jugular venous distention may be present. May be associated with S_3 systolic pulsation of the liver.	Right ventricular failure (cor pulmonale) COPD	Echo	Blowing holosystolic murmur in fourth and fifth parasternal spaces.
Mitral valve prolapse	Most asymptomatic Some may c/o c/p, palpitations or dizziness	Five percent of young adults. More common in women	Abnormal ballooning of part of mitral valve into the left atrium.	May include S_3. Best heard in standing or squatting position, systolic click	Familial tendencies	Echo	Loudest at apex. May be transmitted to axillae, high pitched blowing quality.
Innocent systolic ejection murmur Also known as Still's murmur		Children and adolescents; heard from age 2 to adolescence.	Contractile force of the heart results in greater blood flow velocity.	Auscultate second and third ICSs while client breathes quietly and then deeply.		Chest radiograph, ECG to rule out pathologic condition.	Left lower sternal border. Musical or vibratory, short high-pitched grade I-III early SEM. Loudest when the client is in the supine position; it diminishes when the client sits or during Valsalva. It may be louder in clients with fever or tachycardia.

Continued

Systolic Heart Sounds—cont'd

CONDITION	SYMPTOMS, IF PRESENT	MOST SUSCEPTIBLE	PATHOLOGIC CONDITION	EXAMINATION	CLUES IN HISTORY	DIAGNOSIS	TYPE OF MURMUR
Ventricle septal defect	Acyanosis, dyspnea, exercise intolerance	Most common form of congenital heart disease 20-25% overall.	Smaller defect may create greater resistance to pressure and louder murmur. Congenital hole between left and right ventricle.	Best heard at fourth, fifth, and sixth intercostal spaces at left sternal border.	Frequent respiratory infections	Echo	Short in duration, softer than other systolic murmurs. High pitched hard, may be accompanied by a thrill.

CHF, Congestive heart failure; *c/o,* complain of; *COPD,* chronic obstructive pulmonary disease; *c/p,* chest pain; *ECG,* electrocardiogram; *ICS,* intercostal space; *SEM,* systolic ejection murmur.

Diastolic Heart Sounds

CONDITION	SYMPTOMS IF PRESENT	MOST SUSCEPTIBLE	PATHOLOGIC CONDITION	EXAMINATION	CLUES IN HISTORY	DIAGNOSIS	TYPE OF MURMUR
Aortic insufficiency	Unusual to have symptoms, except in severe disease. Increased sweating, heat intolerance, dyspnea.	More severe in men and blacks.	Abnormal backflow of blood from aorta or volume overload.	Have client lean forward in deep expiration, listen at second through fourth intercostal space. Use diaphragm of stethoscope, wide pulse pressure, bounding peripheral pulses.	Rheumatic heart disease Congenital valve disease	Echo	Diastolic murmur that begins loud in early diastole and then fades (decrescendo) high pitched and blowing.
Mitral stenosis	Exercise increases fatigue and the murmur intensity, as the stenosis worsens, orthopnea, PND.	Usually found in adults.	Produced by blood flow from left atrium to left ventricle.	Best heard when client turns onto left side at point of maximal impulse. With exhalation use bell of stethoscope. Loud first heart sound.	Rheumatic heart disease Congenital valve disease	Echo, a cardiac catheterization can quantify the degree of obstruction. Considered mitral stenosis if 25% of orifice is available.	Middiastolic murmur. Low pitched and rumbling may have increased, first heart sound "opening click."

PND, Paroxysmal nocturnal dyspnea.

Heart Sounds that are Diastolic and Systolic in Nature

CONDITION	SYMPTOMS IF PRESENT	MOST SUSCEPTIBLE	PATHOLOGIC CONDITION	EXAMINATION	CLUES IN HISTORY	DIAGNOSIS	TYPE OF MURMUR
Venous hum		Children. Usually heard after age of 3.	Produced by turbulent blood flow in internal jugular veins.	Heard best over supra-clavicular spaces, particularly right side with client sitting up and turning head to left and slightly upward. Heard best with bell of stethoscope.		Can be stopped by applying gentle pressure over internal juggler vein between trachea and sternocleidal mastoid muscle at level of thyroid cartilage, also disappears when the client is placed in supine position.	Continuous low pitched hum, described as musical quality.
Patent ductus arteriosus	Failure to thrive, fatigue. Severity of symptoms depends on severity of defect.	Infants and children, account for 2%-5% of symptomatic cardiac disease seen in first 28 days after birth.	Open channel between aorta and pulmonary artery.	Listen at second intercostal space, bounding pulses, wide pulse pressure, hyperactive precordium		Echo	Continuous murmur, loudest in late systole, may radiate to left clavicle.
Pericardial friction rub			Inflammation of pleural sac makes sound with respiration.	Best heard with diaphragm of stethoscope. Have client lean forward, may increase with exhalation.	Lower respiratory infection, fever, cough	Chest radiograph may demonstrate pulmonary problem.	Scratchy, scraping sound best heard in third intercostal space left of sternum.

Review Questions

1. When assessing an infant who is not gaining weight as expected, the NP auscultates a continuous murmur, loudest in late systole, that radiates to the left clavicle. The NP charts this as which of the following?

  a. Venous hum
  b. Pericardial friction rub
  c. Suspicious of patent ductus arteriosus
  d. Systolic ejection murmur

2. A pericardial friction rub can be differentiated from other heart sounds by which of the following?

  a. Change in intensity throughout the heart cycle
  b. Radiation to the neck
  c. Scratchy, scraping sound
  d. Blowing, whistling quality

3. A client with exercise fatigue and a history of rheumatic heart disease presents for an examination. Based on the history, the NP should use which of the following auscultation techniques?

  a. Lean forward.
  b. Listen at the second through fourth intercostal space.
  c. Have client hold breath.
  d. Have client turn onto left side and listen at point of maximal impulse (PMI).

4. A client diagnosed with angina has a pansystolic, loud, decrescendo–crescendo murmur. The NP anticipates the need for an echocardiogram to assess for the presence of which of the following?

  a. Aortic stenosis
  b. Pulmonic stenosis
  c. Mitral regurgitation
  d. Tricuspid regurgitation

5. An adolescent presents for a sports physical examination. He has a family history of premature cardiac death. He is non-symptomatic and appears in good health. The NP should use which technique during the examination to help determine the presence of abnormal heart sounds?

  a. Have client perform Valsalva's maneuver.
  b. Have client lean forward.
  c. Have client lay on his left side.
  d. Have client hold his breath.

Answers and Rationales

1. *Answer:* **c** (analysis/diagnosis)
  Rationale: Failure to thrive is a classic indicator of patent ductus arteriosus (PDA). The murmur does go throughout both diastole and systole. A venous hum is low pitched and does not change in character. A pericardial friction rub is associated with a lower respiratory infection. A systolic ejection murmur is not usually detected until age 2.

2. *Answer:* **c** (assessment)
  Rationale: A pericardial friction rub does not change throughout systole and diastole. It is a scratchy, scraping sound, heard best in the third intercostal space and it does not radiate.

3. *Answer:* **d** (assessment)
  Rationale: This history suggests mitral stenosis, a murmur produced as a result of blood flow from the left atrium to the left ventricle. Leaning the client forward helps to hear aortic murmurs.

4. *Answer:* **a** (analysis/diagnosis)
  Rationale: Pulmonic stenosis is associated with a softer murmur that radiates to the shoulder and neck. Mitral regurgitation produces a plateau murmur (no change in intensity). Tricuspid regurgitation produces a blowing holosystolic murmur.

5. *Answer:* **a** (assessment)
  Rationale: In hypertrophic cardiomyopathy, a murmur may not be present but performing Valsalva's maneuver will accentuate the murmur if present.

HEMORRHOIDS *Cheryl Pope Kish*

OVERVIEW
Definition

Hemorrhoids are distended venous varicosities and stretched mucosal and submucosal tissue that may prolapse through the anal canal, causing swelling and pain or becoming thrombosed.

Internal hemorrhoids are dilations of veins within the superior hemorrhoidal plexus occurring above the anal sphincter that are lined with nonsensitive rectal mucosa. External hemorrhoids occur below the anal sphincter and are covered by well-innervated anal mucosa. They originate from the inferior hemorrhoidal plexus. Hemorrhoids are only clinically significant when they cause symptoms.

Incidence

Hemorrhoids are the most common anorectal problem seen in primary care practice, occurring in both men and women and increasing in prevalence in the population older than age 50. As many as 50% to 80% of the adult population has problems but may not seek care because of anxiety about the examination or the findings. Up to one third of women experience hemorrhoids during the second and third trimesters of pregnancy.

Pathophysiology

Venous cushions are part of normal anatomy and physiology of the anal canal that serve to guide stool out of the rectum during defecation. Constipation and frequent straining during defecation contributes to these thin-wall venous cushions becoming permanently dilated and inflamed and sometimes prolapsed or thrombotic.

Increased intraabdominal pressure, engorgement, stretching of supportive connective tissue, including age-associated decreased muscle tone, predisposes to prolapse and entrapment of hemorrhoids by the internal anal sphincter. Prolapse occurs secondary to the shearing force associated with the passage of a large, firm stool; increased venous pressure from pregnancy, congestive heart failure, or portal hypertension in cirrhosis; straining that occurs with heavy lifting or Valsalva's maneuver in defecation.

Pregnancy predisposes to hemorrhoids because of increased pelvic congestion, vascular engorgement, pressure from the gravid uterus, laxity of connective tissue, and constipation secondary to decreased intestinal motility and exogenous iron intake.

Hemorrhoids become clinically significant when the vascular submucosa protrudes through the congested anal canal or an external hemorrhoid becomes thrombosed.

Protective Factors. Hemorrhoids rarely occur in those less than 20 years old except during pregnancy. Regular bowel habits may also provide protection.

Factors Increasing Susceptibility

- Chronic constipation or diarrhea associated with straining during defecation
- Current pregnancy
- Obesity
- Multiparity
- Sedentary lifestyle and occupations requiring prolonged sitting (e.g., truckers)
- Diets deficient in fiber
- Anal sex
- Previous episiotomy, third or fourth degree perineal laceration during childbirth
- Portal hypertension
- Heavy lifting with poor body mechanics
- Hereditary propensity
- Age older than 50 years

ASSESSMENT: SUBJECTIVE/HISTORY
Symptoms

Hemorrhoids may be asymptomatic. Internal hemorrhoids may cause painless, bright red bleeding with defecation that streaks the toilet tissue or stains toilet water. Signs and symptoms of external hemorrhoids include the following:

- Perianal itching from mucus discharge
- History of rectal soiling
- Bleeding
- Rectal burning or pain with defecation
- Sensation of a perianal lump or visible mass

Hemorrhoids can prolapse during straining, becoming trapped and compressed by the anal sphincter. This causes sudden extreme pain.

Traumatic passage of stool can contribute to a thrombosis. A thrombosed hemorrhoid presents as an acutely painful, extremely tender, shiny bluish subcutaneous nodule at the anus.

Past Medical History

Ask about previous symptoms of hemorrhoids, recent pregnancy, childbirth that included third or fourth degree perineal laceration, cirrhosis, anorectal surgery, and bowel disease associated with chronic diarrhea or constipation.

Medication History

Inquire about medication that predisposes to constipation (e.g., oral iron, codeine). Ask about use of enemas, laxatives, stool softeners, or bulk forming agents.

Family History

There may be a familial predisposition to hemorrhoids.

Psychosocial History

Inquire about career or leisure activities associated with prolonged sitting, inability for timely response to the urge to defecate, and heavy lifting or straining. Note sexual practice that includes anal intercourse or sex toys.

Dietary History

Inquire about the amount of fiber and fluid in the diet. Question alcohol use.

ASSESSMENT: OBJECTIVE/PHYSICAL EXAMINATION
Physical Examination

- Visual inspection of the perianal region is best accomplished with the client in the left lateral position, standing and leaning forward onto the examination table, or, for women, in lithotomy position; anoscopy may be required for ideal visualization.
- Perform a lubricated digital examination.

Diagnostic Procedures

No diagnostic procedures are routinely indicated. A hematocrit may be ordered in cases of excessive bleeding. In clients at risk, to rule out colon cancer, despite obvious hemorrhoids, a sigmoidoscopy, colonoscopy, or barium enema may be appropriate.

DIAGNOSIS

Hemorrhoids generally are diagnosed through history and clinical examination. The following differential diagnoses must be considered:

- Anal skin tags
- Condyloma acuminata

- Pruritus ani
- Rectal bleeding related to the following:
  Cancer
  Anorectal fistula
  Rectal polyps
  Anal fissures
  Irritable bowel syndrome
  Diverticulitis

THERAPEUTIC PLAN
Pharmacologic Treatment

- Advise OTC bulk forming agents such as psyllium (Metamucil), methylcellulose (Citrucel), or calcium polycarbophil (FiberCon) to prevent constipation.
- Recommend one of the following to control discomfort. Suggest use of a finger cot or latex or plastic glove for application inside the anus.
  - Anusol HC-1 ointment (OTC) applied 3 to 4 times daily for 7 days
  - Preparation H ointment (OTC) applied 4 times daily.

(Suppositories may be used instead of ointment but are less effective.)

Client Education

- Prevent constipation with increased fluid, fiber, and exercise.
- Sitz baths for 15 to 20 minutes 1 to 2 times daily (not when bleeding excessively).

NOTE: *Cold compresses are more comforting for some than heat.*

- Use witch hazel compresses (client can make own compresses or purchase Tucks or Tucks gel OTC) applied to painful area up to 6 times daily.
- Clean perianal region gently with soap and water daily and after bowel movement (BM); pat dry, do not rub.
- Use lubricated, gloved finger or finger cot to gently reduce hemorrhoid with digital pressure held in place for 60 seconds.
- Use good body mechanics when lifting heavy objects.
- Decrease weight if obese.
- Avoid prolonged sitting when possible. Avoid prolonged sitting on toilet as well.
- Avoid "doughnut" pads for sitting because these cause congestion in area.
- Notify provider if pain is extreme or continuous bleeding occurs.
- Prop feet on footstool during defecation to minimize strain on the perineal/perianal area.

Hemorrhoids often can be prevented by avoiding constipation or responding to diarrhea quickly. Suggest the following to prevent constipation:

- Drink 8 to 10 glasses of water daily
- Increase fiber in diet (whole grain breads and cereals; brown rice and oats; baked potato with skin; five fruits and vegetables daily, especially carrots, beans, peas, apples, strawberries, and citrus fruits).
- Regular exercise

Referral

Refer clients with thrombosed hemorrhoids for excision and evacuation of clot within 48 hours. For severe symptoms or those nonresponsive to treatment, refer client to a surgeon for treatment (rubber band ligation, infrared coagulation, sclerotherapy, or hemorrhoidectomy).

EVALUATION/FOLLOW-UP

- Follow-up is needed only if symptoms persist or recur.
- Without treatment, hemorrhoids may cause additional pain or itching and may be associated with blood loss. A thrombosed hemorrhoid should be excised within 48 hours; after 48 hours, the thrombus begins to organize and evacuation is generally unsuccessful.

REFERENCES

Cash, J. C., & Glass, C. A. (2000). *Primary care guidelines.* Philadelphia: Lippincott.

Dunphy, L. M., & Winland-Brown, J. E. (2001). *Primary care: The art and science of advanced practice nursing.* Philadelphia: F.A. Davis.

Haussain, J. N. (1999). Hemorrhoids. *Primary Care: Clinics in Office Practice, 26*(1), 35-51.

Hicks, T. C., & Stamos, M. J. (1998). Practical approaches to common anorectal problems. *Patient Care, 32*(14), 24-26, 35, 38.

Meredith, P. V., & Horan, N. M. (2000). *Adult primary care.* Philadelphia: W.B. Saunders.

Robinson, D., Kidd, P., & Rogers, K. M. (2000). *Primary care across the lifespan.* St. Louis: Mosby.

Schaeffer, D. C. (1998). Constipation in the elderly. *American Family Physician, 58*(4), 907-914.

Star, W. L., Shannon, M. T., Lommel, L. L, & Gutirrez, Y. M. (1999). *Ambulatory obstetrics.* San Francisco: University of California San Francisco Nursing Press.

Uphold, C. R., & Graham, M. V. (1998). *Clinical guidelines in family practice.* Gainesville, FL: Barmarrae.

Review Questions

1. Mr. Dent, age 35, presents with rectal pain and bleeding. Which subjective finding is consistent with a diagnosis of internal hemorrhoids?

  a. Occupation as an international pilot for a parcel delivery service
  b. Raising vegetables as a hobby
  c. History of military duty
  d. History of thrombophlebitis

H

2. Which of the following symptoms supports a diagnosis of internal hemorrhoids in Mr. Dent?

    a. An anal skin tag found during a shower

    b. Rectal burning after defecation

    c. Bright blood noted in the toilet bowl with defecation

    d. Mucus drainage from the rectum that causes itching

3. Which of the following medical conditions is *not* a common comorbidity with hemorrhoids?

    a. Peripheral neuropathy

    b. Cirrhosis of the liver

    c. Crohn's disease

    d. Congestive heart failure

4. Which test is most appropriate for confirming a diagnosis of hemorrhoids?

    a. Sigmoidoscopy

    b. Colonoscopy

    c. Barium enema

    d. Physical visualization with anoscopy

5. In which of the following situations is a hematocrit appropriately ordered for a diagnosis of hemorrhoids?

    a. The client notices more perianal itching than in the past.

    b. The client reports rectal bleeding as continuous.

    c. An external hemorrhoid becomes thrombosed.

    d. The client is 27 weeks pregnant.

6. The NP lists differential diagnoses for Mr. Dent. Which of the following does not belong on that list?

    a. Prostatitis

    b. Irritable bowel syndrome

    c. Rectal polyps

    d. Colon cancer

7. The NP teaches Mr. Dent about the relationship between constipation and hemorrhoids and how to prevent future constipation. Which comment by Mr. Dent indicates that further instruction is needed?

    a. "I will eat a raw apple instead of applesauce."

    b. "I should drink at least eight glasses of fluid daily."

    c. "I need to eat bran cereal or wheat bread daily."

    d. "I will ask my wife to prepare more mashed potatoes and noodles for me."

8. Grace is in the 27th week of her first pregnancy and has hemorrhoids. Which comment she makes about treatment possibilities should definitely be corrected by the NP?

    a. "Sitz baths at least twice daily may help my rectal discomfort."

    b. "I have read that Tucks used on my rectal area several times daily will likely be soothing."

    c. "One of my neighbors suggested I take milk of magnesia every day or two to prevent constipation."

    d. "Propping my feet on a low stool while using the toilet may minimize the straining during a BM."

9. Which of the following clients with hemorrhoids should be referred to a physician?

    a. Mrs. Hampton, an 80-year-old with painful hemorrhoids

    b. Mrs. Lashley, who notices occasional "brief spotting" after anal intercourse

    c. Mr. Todd, whose hemorrhoids are worse despite treatment

    d. Mrs. Johnson, who delivered her first child 4 weeks ago

10. Which of these objective findings in a client with hemorrhoids justifies referral to a physician?

    a. A prolapsed hemorrhoid that cannot be reduced easily in a pregnant 22-year-old

    b. A shiny, blue protrusion from the anus that is exquisitely tender in a woman in extreme pain

    c. A skin tag at the external anal sphincter of a elderly male

    d. Some bright blood when the anoscope is removed from the anus after an examination

---

Answers and Rationales

1. *Answer:* **a** (analysis/diagnosis)

    Rationale: Occupations or leisure activities that involve prolonged sitting and inability to respond to urges to defecate exacerbate hemorrhoids (Meredith & Horan, 2000).

2. *Answer:* **c** (analysis/diagnosis)

    Rationale: Internal hemorrhoids are associated with painless blood loss; external hemorrhoids cause pain (Hicks & Stamos, 1998).

3. *Answer:* **a** (analysis/diagnosis)

    Rationale: Cirrhosis and congestive heart failure increase venous pressure whereas Crohn's disease is associated with diarrhea; all of these are associated with hemorrhoid formation. Peripheral neuropathy is not associated with hemorrhoid formation (Hicks & Stamos, 1998).

4. *Answer:* **d** (analysis/diagnosis)

    Rationale: Hemorrhoids are diagnosed on the basis of the clinical examination. No diagnostic tests are necessary for diagnosis (Uphold & Graham, 1998).

5. *Answer:* **b** (implementation/plan)

    Rationale: In cases of continual hemorrhoidal bleeding, a hematocrit should be ordered to assess for anemia (Uphold & Graham, 1998).

6. *Answer:* **a** (analysis/diagnosis)

    Rationale: The client is experiencing rectal bleeding. Choices b, c, and d are all associated with rectal bleeding. Choice a, prostatitis, is not (Robinson, Kidd, & Rogers, 2000).

7. *Answer:* **d** (evaluation)

    Rationale: Mashed potatoes and noodles are not foods with increased fiber. Dietary mentioned in options a, b, and c all increase fiber (Robinson, Kidd, & Rogers, 2000).

8. Answer: c (evaluation)

Rationale: Laxatives may actually exacerbate the problem because they cause straining. Moreover, laxatives can stimulate uterine contractions in pregnancy; this client is not at or near term and labor stimulation is contraindicated (Starr, Shannon, Lommel, & Gutierriz, 1999).

9. Answer: c (evaluation)

Rationale: A client whose symptoms become worse despite treatment should be referred to a physician for evaluation and treatment (Hicks & Stamos, 1998).

10. Answer: b (evaluation)

Rationale: A client with a thrombosed hemorrhoid should be referred for excision (Hicks & Stamos, 1998).

HEPATITIS *Pamela Kidd*

OVERVIEW

Definition

Hepatitis is a general term denoting inflammation of the liver. It can be caused by viral or bacterial sources or by chemical damage.

Hepatitis A virus (HAV) is found in infected water and food and is common in crowded situations, such as low-income housing, schools, and dormitories.

Hepatitis B virus (HBV) is common among individuals exposed to needle punctures or blood products and those who engage in unprotected sexual intercourse.

Hepatitis C virus (HCV) is an RNA virus that mutates frequently preventing recognition by the immune system and contributing to the inability to develop antibodies or effective vaccine.

Incidence

- HAV is always limited to an acute infection. Ranks sixth among the top 10 causes of foodborne illness in the United States (Shovein, Damazo, & Hyams, 2000).
- HBV has the highest incidence among users of intravenous drugs and men who are homosexual. Health care workers who are not vaccinated for HBV have an incidence of 15% to 30%. When a pregnant woman has HBV, a cesarean section is performed to protect the infant. Chronic HBV occurs in more than 90% of neonates infected with HBV at birth.
- HBV is responsible for almost 80% of the primary cases of hepatoma worldwide.
- HCV is the leading cause of posttransfusion hepatitis, and individuals receiving repeated blood transfusions therefore have a higher incidence. There are 30,000 new cases reported annually.
- Hepatitis D occurs only in conjunction with HBV, with the same routes of transmission.
- Hepatitis E viral infection is rare in the United States; it is usually a mild disease in clients older than 15 years. Hepatitis E carries a considerable (10% to 20%) mortality rate in pregnant women and does not progress to chronic liver disease.

Pathophysiology

The liver performs numerous metabolic and regulatory functions. It is the largest gland in the body and normally weighs approximately 1.4 kg (3 pounds). The liver processes nearly every nutrient class absorbed from the GI tract. It is able to withstand and repair damage remarkably. Complete regeneration can take place even when 70% of the liver is destroyed. Cirrhosis is due to necrosis of the hepatic cells, leading to fibrosis of hepatic tissue, loss of hepatic architecture, and eventual loss of hepatic function.

The physiologic function of the liver can be divided into the following six categories:

1. Metabolism of carbohydrates, proteins and lipids, some hormones, and vitamins A, D, and K; conservation of iron salvaged from destruction of red blood cells (RBCs); regulation of temperature; major role in regulating plasma cholesterol
2. Excretion of bile salts and bile pigment, heavy metals, and dyes; conversion of ammonia into urea to be excreted
3. Phagocytic abilities of the Kupffer cells in removing specific pathogens; prevention of intravascular coagulation
4. Detoxification of drugs, endotoxins, alkaloids, steroids, alcohol, among others
5. Storage of glycogen, vitamins, and iron; packaging fatty acids into forms for storage or transportation
6. Circulatory functions are systemic and portal transfer of blood, regulation of blood volume, and production of lymphatic fluid

Transmission

- HAV infection is transmitted through the fecal–oral route and person-to-person contact (lower possibility). Incubation period is 2 to 6 weeks.
- HBV infection is transmitted through blood and body fluids. Incubation period is 6 weeks to 6 months. Detectable in blood, breast milk, saliva, tears, nasal secretions, menstrual fluid, urine, semen, and blood-sucking insects that have bitten infected individuals.

H

HBV may occasionally exist in a quiescent nonhepatotoxic state (chronic carrier state).
- HCV infection is transmitted through blood and body fluids, organ transplantation, IV drug use, perinatally, occupational exposure (sharps), and body piercing and tattooing. Incubation period is 5 to 10 weeks.
- Hepatitis D viral infection is present as a coinfection with HBV only. Concurrent infection results in a more virulent manifestation than if the individual had HBV alone.
- Hepatitis E viral infection is transmitted through the fecal–oral route. Incubation period is 2 to 9 weeks.

Factors Increasing Susceptibility
- HAV. Persons who work at day care centers and institutions (such as those caring for mentally challenged individuals), individuals engaging in foreign travel
- HBV. Users of intravenous drugs who share needles, homosexual men, individuals on hemodialysis, persons with hemophilia, health care personnel (such as nurses, laboratory personnel, surgeons, and personnel performing hemodialysis), sexually promiscuous persons (the same high-risk groups for hepatitis D), those with tattoos and body piercing
- HCV. Individuals receiving frequent blood transfusions, men who are homosexuals, health care workers, and those with tattoos and body piercing

Protective Factors. Because hepatitis can become a chronic disease with severe complications, the best protective factor is prevention. See prevention strategies following.

ASSESSMENT: SUBJECTIVE/HISTORY
Symptoms
- Ask about sexual practices, recreational use of drugs, or other habits or occupations that place the individual at risk for viral hepatitis infection.
- For HAV it is important to determine whether other contacts have demonstrated the same illness. With food contamination, events (such as weddings or other gatherings), school cafeterias, or any other common source should be identified.
- Signs and symptoms of HAV appear at the end of prodromal period and include fatigue, weakness, and mild GI disturbances. A striking aversion to cigarettes may occur. Some may have joint pain, fever, hepatomegaly, lymphadenopathy, and jaundice.
- Symptoms of HBV are general malaise, joint swelling, rash pruritus, hepatomegaly, and GI symptoms. Jaundice is seen with more nausea and vomiting.
- HCV involves acute illness with fever, chills, malaise, nausea, abdominal pain, anorexia, and vomiting. Eighty-five percent of cases become chronic.

The following applies to all hepatitis viruses:

- Assess for presence of weight loss, cough, dyspnea, and history of yeast infections, which is significant to help rule out HIV.
- Assess for history of menorrhagia in females or constipation in both genders; may help rule out hypothyroidism.

Past Medical History
The individual may remember the exposure to the viral agent.

Medication History
Noncontributory.

Family History
Family member with history of hepatitis.

Dietary History
May be useful in determining source of HAV exposure.

ASSESSMENT: OBJECTIVE/PHYSICAL EXAMINATION
Physical Examination
- A general skin examination should note jaundice, rashes (mononucleosis), dryness (hypothyroidism), and spider angiomas.
- Conduct a HEENT examination to rule out mononucleosis. Oral lesions or lymphadenopathy may indicate HIV infection.
- Abdominal examination is imperative to assess liver size and tenderness, splenomegaly, and presence of ascites.
- A neurologic examination helps rule out thyroid dysfunction.
- Presence of occult blood loss should be evaluated with a stool specimen, optimally obtained by voluntary evacuation because there is a percentage of false-positive results with a digital rectal examination specimen.

Diagnostic Procedures
- Do Monospot test to rule out mononucleosis.
- Perform thyroid screen (thyroid-stimulating hormone, triiodothyronine, thyroxine) to rule out hypothyroidism. Thyroid-stimulating hormone will be elevated and free thyroxine will be low in hypothyroidism.
- Electrolytes, renal panel, and liver function tests are important because of the hepatic involvement. Aspartate aminotransferase (AST) is maximally elevated in the acute phase of hepatitis (greater than 1000 IU/L) then tapers off. Remember that AST and alanine transaminase (ALT) levels do not always correlate with the degree of liver damage. Total and direct bilirubin is elevated with hepatitis. Jaundice is usually detectable, with a total bilirubin level higher than 2 mg/dL. Jaundice does not reflect the severity of the illness.
- Do HIV screen to rule out HIV infection.

- Liver biopsy determines the extent of the disease but is not usually performed until the disease is believed to be chronic, as defined by clinical history of unresolved symptoms with AST and ALT elevations for 6 months or longer. This test does not provide useful prognostic value in the acute phase of hepatitis.
- CBC with differential provides information regarding anemia and possible infection. Lymphocytosis with more than 10% atypical cells is characteristic for Epstein-Barr, and leukopenia is common with HAV.
- Chest radiograph examination can be delayed until the serologic test results are known; however, if the history and physical examination strongly indicate a cytomegaloviral infection, a chest radiograph is useful. If cytomegaloviral infection is present, the radiograph may demonstrate bilateral, diffuse white infiltrates.
- Hepatitis screening determines which viral infection is responsible for the illness and the stage of the infection (Table 3-44).

Hepatitis A

- Immunoglobulin (Ig)M–anti-HAV assay is diagnostic for HAV infection. It is usually detectable at the time of clinical presentation and persists for several months.
- Detectable serum IgG–anti-HAV confirms HAV immunity (think G for gone).
- Detectable IgM-anti HAV means acute case is confirmed (think M for miserable).

Hepatitis B

- HBV e antigen (HBeAg) is present when the liver is making large quantities of HBV core antigen (HBcAg) during viral replication. When HBeAg is present for longer than 6 months, a chronic HBV state is likely (Fu, 2001). HBeAg is used to manage the client in the chronic state and signifies ongoing viral replication and liver damage. Antibody to HBeAg is associated with resolution of the infection.

Hepatitis C

- Enzyme immunoassay, recombinant immunoblot assay, and polymerase chain reaction assay (most sensitive) are used to detect the presence of the virus. HCV antibodies indicate resolved or current infection.

Hepatitis D (Delta)

- Hepatitis D virus causes infection only in coinfection with HBV.
- Hepatitis D viral superinfection usually correlates to a more severe and rapid progression of HBV infection.
- Serum anti–hepatitis D virus proteins are diagnostic for hepatitis D virus infection.

DIAGNOSIS

Differential diagnoses include the following:
- Anemia
- Cytomegaloviral infection
- Epstein-Barr virus
- Viral infection
- Hepatitis
- Chronic fatigue syndrome
- Acquired hypothyroidism
- Depression

THERAPEUTIC PLAN

The main therapeutic plan is to track the liver enzyme levels and closely observe symptoms.

Nonpharmacologic Treatment

The following applies to all hepatitis viruses:
- Rest
- Avoid alcohol

Hepatitis A
- Eat frequent small, low-fat meals.

Pharmacologic Treatment

Hepatitis A. HAV infection commonly requires no treatment. If an epidemic of HAV is noted in the community from a common source of food or water contamination, close contacts should be offered passive immunity with serum Ig (Gamastan, Gammar), 0.02 ml/kg IM. This vaccine is safe and inexpensive. Usually, casual contacts such as coworkers do not need to be vaccinated. Individuals expecting to be exposed to HAV (e.g., travelers, institutional workers, day care employees, military personnel) should receive an inactivated HAV vaccine (Havrix). Clients ages 2 to 18 years receive two IM injections of 360 enzyme-linked immunosorbent assay (ELISA) units (0.5 mL) given 1 month apart. Adults receive one dose of 1440 ELISA units. Both populations should receive a booster injection at 6 months.

TABLE **3-44** Laboratory Interpretation of Hepatitis Tests

HBSAG	ANTI-HBS	ANTI-HBC	IGM	INTERPRETATION
+	–	–	–	Early acute HBV infection
+	–	+	+	Acute HBV infection
+	–	+	–	Chronic HBc carrier
–	–	+	+/–	Early convalescence, HBV
–	+	+	–	Recover/immunity to HBV
–	+	–	–	Immunity to HBV infection

HBsAg, Hepatitis B surface antigen; *Anti-HBs,* antibody to HBsAg; *Anti-HBc,* antibody to hepatitis B core antigen; *HBV,* hepatitis B; *IgM,* immunoglobulin M.

H

Hepatitis B. HBV treatment consists of observation of liver enzymes and hepatitis markers to identify individuals who may benefit from interferon therapy. The icteric phase lasts 2 to 6 weeks; it peaks in 14 days with a variable period of disappearance. Interferon is used to eradicate viral replication and end chronic hepatitis infection. Common side effects of interferon are flulike symptoms, especially at initiation of treatment, which tend to decrease with continued therapy. The flulike symptoms can be minimized by keeping the client well hydrated and administering the dose at bedtime. Acetaminophen 30 minutes before the interferon dose may also help. Interferon alpha 5 million IU daily, or 10 million IU 3 times a week IM or Sub-c for 16 weeks are possible pharmaceutical therapies. The side effects of interferon therapy are numerous and uncomfortable. They include flulike symptoms, headache, mental disturbances. Leukopenia may develop (Fu, 2001).

Hepatitis C. For clients age 18 and older with no symptoms of active liver disease, prescribe the following:

- Ribavirin 1000 to 1200 mg/dL PO plus subcutaneous interferon alfa 2b (3 million units 3 times a week) for 12 months.

Client Education
Hepatitis A
- Transmitted through fecal–oral route.
- Do not cook for others or share finger foods for at least 7 days after the onset of jaundice.
- Usually has a 6-week course of illness with a high recovery rate.
- HAV has no carrier state and no chronic state.

Hepatitis C
- Seroconversion may not occur for as long as 6 months.

In general, fatigue is a common symptom of hepatitis, and the client should be educated about appropriate behavioral management. Assist the client in assessing the home and work situations to identify where energy can be conserved. Give permission to ask for assistance and to take the needed rest breaks.

Referral

If the liver function test results remain elevated or progressively elevate, the client should be referred to a gastroenterologist for a possible liver biopsy to assess the extent of hepatic damage.

Prevention

Safe sexual practices should be reviewed because HBV, HCV, and hepatitis D are sexually transmitted. Condom use should be encouraged.

Hepatitis A
- Preventive measures include handwashing. Pooled human immune serum globulin (0.02 mg/kg IM) is effective only when administered within 2 weeks of the exposure.
- Vaccination especially for children who frequently transmit the disease because of poor hygiene, for those living in countries, states, and communities with high rates (usually Western states) and before international traveling (Shovein, Damazo, & Hyams, 2000).

Hepatitis B. Immunoprophylaxis for HBV can be achieved by both passive (high-titered antibody to hepatitis B surface antigen [anti-HBs] Ig [HBIG]) and active immunization (Hep B/HBV vaccine; Recombivax HB, Engerix-B). Prophylaxis before exposure consists of three deltoid IM injections of HBV vaccine at 0, 1, and 6 months. Dosage depends on the formulation of the vaccine. Immunocompromised individuals should receive a higher dose.

Active immunization (Hep B) vaccine should be administered to household members and sex partners of HBsAg positive persons, persons with recently diagnosed sexually transmitted diseases (STDs), health care workers, hemodialysis clients, and to all anti-HCV positive persons.

Prophylaxis for unvaccinated individuals exposed to HBV should be with both HBIG and HBV vaccine. Adult dosage of HBIG is 0.06 ml/kg IM, followed by a complete course of HBV vaccine. Another dose of HBIG can be repeated 1 month later. This is the same protocol used for infants born to hepatitis B surface antigen (HBsAg)–seropositive mothers or for sexual contacts of persons seropositive for HBsAg.

When the previously vaccinated individual is exposed to HBsAg-positive blood or body fluids, serum anti-HBs titers should be obtained. If the antibody level is less than 10 mIU/ml, the individual should be treated the same as an unvaccinated person.

Prompt administration of HBIG and HBV vaccine to neonates is highly effective in prevention of vertical transmission of HBV. This protocol is also recommended for accidental needle sticks or splashes.

Hepatitis C
- Cannot be prevented by vaccination (Buckhold, 2000).
- Handle contaminated needles carefully, immediately discard in disposal container and do not recap needle.
- Wash hands after removing gloves.
- Wear personal protective equipment (e.g., goggles, gloves, gowns)

EVALUATION/FOLLOW-UP

Follow-up should be on a monthly basis to assess disease progression. If the client has an increase in severity of symptoms, the follow-up will be more frequent. Blood work should be done every 2 months, more frequently if the symptoms worsen.

COMPLICATIONS

- Death: For example, Fulminant HAV is infrequent; however, when it does occur, it has a 50% mortality rate.
- Occasionally it progresses to an active ongoing hepatocellular necrosis (chronic active hepatitis) and eventually cirrhosis, with a dramatically increased risk for hepatocellular carcinoma (hepatoma).
- Chronic liver disease is seen in approximately 10% to 40% of individuals with HCV infection.
- Half of the individuals who acquire posttransfusion HCV develop chronic hepatitis, with potential for cirrhosis.
- Hepatitis D: Associated with a higher rate of fulminant hepatitis and a high fatality rate. There is also a substantially higher risk for development of chronic HBV liver disease.

REFERENCES

Buckhold, K. (2000). Who's afraid of hepatitis C? *American Journal of Nursing 100*(5), 26-31.

Fu, H. C. (2001). Individualizing care of hepatitis B in older adults and Asians. *Journal of the American Academy of Nurse Practitioners 13*(5), 215-222.

Rushman, K. (2000). Hepatitis. In D. Robinson, P. Kidd, & K. Rogers (Eds.), *Primary care across the lifespan.* St. Louis: Mosby.

Shovein, J., Damazo, R., & Hyams, I. (2000). Hepatitis A: How benign is it? *American Journal of Nursing 100*(3), 43-47

Zeldis, J. B., & Friedman, L. S. (1997). Acute and chronic viral hepatitis. In R. E. Rakel (Ed.), *Conn's current therapy* (pp. 488-495). Philadelphia: W. B. Saunders.

Review Questions

Situation: Rose is a 36-year-old female who has had a history of tiring easily for 2 months. She is able to work all day as a secretary but needs to rest as soon as she gets home. She has no energy left for family activities and her libido is low. (Questions 1 through 4 relate to this situation.)

1. Which of the following findings rules out chronic fatigue syndrome?

    a. The fact that Rose is female
    b. Her age
    c. Unknown cause with 2-month duration
    d. Fatigue resolution with bed rest

2. Which of the following diagnostic tests will best assist you in narrowing your diagnosis for Rose?

    a. Liver enzymes, liver biopsy, HIV
    b. HIV, liver enzymes, chest radiograph
    c. CBC, chest radiograph, liver enzymes
    d. Liver enzymes, HIV, Monospot

3. With the history, you have narrowed the diagnosis down to one of the hepatitis infections. Rose's laboratory results are as follows: hemoglobin 15.6, hematocrit 43.1, WBC count 7.4 cells/mm³, AST 60 IU/L, ALT 121 IU/L, alkaline phosphatase within normal limits, total bilirubin 2 mg/dL, anti-HBs negative, HBsAg positive, and HBcAg positive. Your diagnosis is which of the following?

    a. Acute HBV infection, resolving
    b. Acute HCV infection
    c. Chronic HBV infection
    d. Acute HAV infection

4. As a NP, your role in caring for Rose, a 36-year-old woman, would include all the following *except:*

    a. Referral to a gastroenterologist as soon as possible for a liver biopsy
    b. Education related to the disease process and possible treatment options
    c. Following Rose's progress on a periodic basis to determine disease progression
    d. Assistance in identifying resources and offering support in notifying spouse

5. Elmer has a diagnosis of HCV. His level of function has not changed in the past 6 months. Although he has been able to carry out ADLs, his AST and ALT levels have remained elevated. Your next best interaction would be which of the following?

    a. Monitor Elmer for 6 more months; monitor his disease progress for 2 more months.
    b. Initiate interferon therapy and prophylactically medicate him before therapy.
    c. Refer Elmer to a gastroenterologist for a liver biopsy.
    d. Advise Elmer that the disease continues to destroy hepatic cells and that there is nothing else to be done.

6. Mary is a nurse who just stuck herself with an HBV-contaminated needle. She has received her full course of HBV vaccine but does not know her titers. Mary washes the puncture with copious amounts of soap and water. She asks you what else needs to be done. What is your response?

    a. Mary needs to have a booster of HBV vaccine.
    b. Mary needs to have a titer level drawn, and if it is 10 mIU/mL, she should receive a regimen of HBIG and HBV vaccine.
    c. Mary should receive a dose of HBIG.
    d. Mary should receive no further treatment because she received the full course of HBV vaccine.

7. All the following are true about HAV viral infection *except:*

    a. Found in infected food, it often runs its course without diagnosis.
    b. It has a chronic carrier state.
    c. It is common in crowded situations.
    d. IgM antibody (anti-HAV) denotes active infection.

8. A client diagnosed with HBV has elevated transaminases for 7 months since diagnosis. The NP interprets this finding as which of the following?

    a. Indicative of acute infection.
    b. Denotes chronic carrier state.
    c. Indicates chronic infection.
    d. Suggests need for liver biopsy.

H

Answers and Rationales

1. *Answer:* d (assessment)
Rationale: One of the defining characteristics of chronic fatigue syndrome is fatigue unresolved with rest.

2. *Answer:* d (analysis/diagnosis)
Rationale: Liver biopsy is inappropriate as a work-up test. A chest radiograph is not useful in narrowing down a diagnosis, and the only answer that has useful tests is d.

3. *Answer:* a (analysis/diagnosis)
Rationale: On the basis of HBsAg and HBcAg, the diagnosis has to be narrowed to HBV infection. Anti-HBs would have to be present for it to be a chronic infection, so this is therefore an acute HBV infection.

4. *Answer:* a (implementation/plan)
Rationale: Liver biopsy is not appropriate in the acute stage. Education and assistance in identifying resources and offering support is always a correct approach, as is periodic assessment to determine progression.

5. *Answer:* c (evaluation)
Rationale: Six-month duration is the definition of chronic hepatitis infection. Rose should be evaluated by a gastroenterologist who can conduct a liver biopsy. Initiating interferon therapy is premature, and there is no foundation to tell her that the disease is continuing to destroy liver cells.

6. *Answer:* b (implementation/plan)
Rationale: If titer is low, the person is treated as though he or she has not received vaccine.

7. *Answer:* b (analysis/diagnosis)
Rationale: HAV is never a chronic infection. IgM denotes active whereas IgG denotes recovery and immunity stages. The mnemonics "it has me" (IgM) for active and "it's gone" (IgG) for recovery may help the provider remember the correct interpretation of lab tests.

8. *Answer:* d (analysis/diagnosis)
Rationale: Acute infection is denoted by large quantities of HBcAg. HBeAG indicates chronic infection. Liver biopsy is indicated when enzymes have been elevated for 6 months.

HERNIA, ABDOMINAL (INGUINAL, UMBILICAL, FEMORAL) *Pamela Kidd*

OVERVIEW
Definition
A hernia is the result of an abnormal opening or weakness of the abdominal musculature allowing protrusion of the abdominal viscera.

Types
- Inguinal
- Femoral
- Umbilical
- Incisional
- Epigastric

Classification
- Reducible
- Nonreducible or incarcerated
- Strangulated

Incidence
- Inguinal hernias are responsible for 99% of all groin hernias in children younger than 3 years of age.
- Inguinal hernias are more common in boys.
- There is a 1% prevalence rate among term infants.
- Between 13% and 30% prevalence rate among premature infants.
- One third of inguinal hernias are diagnosed before 6 months of age.
- A unilateral inguinal hernia is more likely to develop on the right.

- Between 10% and 15% of infants and children will have bilateral hernias.
- Umbilical hernias are very common and are considered a normal variant of development.
- Umbilical hernias are more common in black children, with a prevalence of between 40% and 60%; white children have a prevalence rate of 4%.
- Most umbilical hernias close spontaneously and by 1 year of age the prevalence rate drops to 12% for black children and 2% for white children.
- Umbilical hernias are present in boys and girls equally.
- Femoral hernias are more common in women and very rare in children.

Pathophysiology
- Congenital defect may cause a hernia.
- Secondary to conditions that cause increased intraabdominal pressure such as chronic coughing, obesity, pregnancy, chronic constipation with straining, and jobs or hobbies that require heavy lifting.

Factors Increasing Susceptibility
- Prematurity
- Pregnancy
- Obesity

Protective Factors
- Gender (female)
- Ethnicity (Caucasian)

ASSESSMENT: SUBJECTIVE/HISTORY
Symptoms
- Inquire about onset and duration of symptoms.
- Inquire specifically about the presence of a bulge, swelling, or lump in the abdomen, umbilicus, groin, or scrotum if applicable.
- Inquire about softness and reducibility.
- Inquire about pain, nausea, vomiting, and abdominal cramping.
- Inquire as to whether the swelling is constant or intermittent.
- Inquire about work conditions (requiring heavy lifting or straining).

Past Medical History
- Inquire about past surgery in the area and the presence of a scar.
- Inquire about underlying medical conditions.
- Determine presence of chronic constipation.

Medication History
Laxative use may suggest chronic constipation as cause.

Family History
Noncontributory.

Dietary History
Low fiber diet and inadequate fluid intake may contribute to constipation and straining.

ASSESSMENT: OBJECTIVE/PHYSICAL EXAMINATION
Physical Examination
- Assess abdomen for bowel sounds and lymphadenopathy.
  - Inspect for protruding subcutaneous mass. Ask client to lift head.
  - Assess for tenderness and reducibility. Assess for scars.
  - Palpate femoral pulses. Assess for tenderness and mass.
  - *A strangulated hernia will present as discolored and painful. Do not reduce.*
- In men, examine the genitourinary system, assessing the scrotum and testes for size and consistency.
  - Transilluminate the scrotum if mass present.
- Assess for inguinal hernia by invaginating the scrotum and advancing the finger into the inguinal canal. Ask the client to cough or bear down. Assess for bulge on the tip or side of finger.
- In women, attempt to locate the inguinal ring between the inguinal ligament and os pubis. Place hand over inguinal ring and ask the client to bear down.

Diagnostic Procedures
- Abdominal ultrasound may be indicated if uncertain about abdominal mass.
- Inguinal hernias may or may not be visible. When visible, may present as a soft swelling in the groin or scrotum. Inguinal hernias are difficult to identify in females. An inguinal mass and a hydrocele in an infant is most likely an inguinal hernia.
- Femoral hernias present with pain and swelling over femoral canal. The swelling or mass is more medial and higher in the proximal thigh. Pulse can be palpated.
- Umbilical and incisional hernias are diagnosed by the location of the bulge or mass.

DIAGNOSIS
Differential diagnoses are located in Table 3-45.

THERAPEUTIC PLAN
Nonpharmacologic Treatment
- Inguinal hernias, including femoral hernias in clients of all ages, should be surgically repaired. The timing depends on the presence of complications.
- Umbilical hernias often resolve spontaneously and do not pose a significant risk of incarceration or strangulation. Surgical repair is often cosmetic.

Pharmacologic Treatment
Usually not helpful.

Client Education
- Educate client about aggravating and alleviating factors.
- Educate client about signs and symptoms of incarceration/strangulation.
- Client may need pre- and postoperative instructions.

TABLE **3-45**   Differential Diagnoses

DIAGNOSIS	SYMPTOM
Hydrocele	A hydrocele is a collection of fluid between the two layers of the tunica vaginalis in the scrotum. Swelling progresses throughout the day and resolves at night. Hydroceles usually resolve spontaneously.
Varicocele	Varicocele is the result of the dilation of veins in the spermatic cord in the scrotum. Rare before puberty.
Testicular tumor	May present as a slow growing, painless mass that is firm and free of fixation. The tumor usually replaces the testicle.
Lymph node	Enlarged and sometimes painful lymph nodes can easily be palpated in the inguinal area of children and in adults. May be indicative of an infection.

H

- Lifestyle modifications may include no heavy lifting.
- Educate parents about umbilical hernias as a normal variant.

Referral

Refer to surgeon.

Prevention

- Avoid heavy lifting and straining.
- Avoid constipation.

EVALUATION/FOLLOW-UP

- Inguinal hernias require postoperative follow up.
- Umbilical hernias can be monitored at well-child examinations.

COMPLICATIONS

- Incarceration: The risk of incarceration of an inguinal hernia is greatest in children younger than 1 year of age. Incarcerated hernias may cause pain, nausea, and vomiting. Most incarcerated hernias (95%) can be reduced.
- Strangulated hernias are a surgical emergency because of the risk of vascular compromise. Pain and discoloration may be present.

REFERENCES

Dershewitz, R. A. (1998). *Ambulatory pediatric care* (pp. 500-503). Philadelphia: J. B. Lippincott.

Dunn, S. A. (1998). Hernia, abdominal. In S. A. Dunn (Ed.), *Mosby's primary care consultant* (pp. 276-277). St. Louis: Mosby.

Hoekelman, R.A. (1997). *Primary pediatric care* (3rd ed., pp. 1638-1639, 1102-1104). St. Louis: Mosby.

Rogers, K. (2000). Hernia. In D. Robinson, P. Kidd, & K. Rogers (Eds.), *Primary care across the lifespan*. St. Louis: Mosby.

Review Questions

1. Which of the following assessment data are associated with inguinal hernias in children?

- **a.** Inguinal hernias in children usually occur on the left side.
- **b.** Bilateral hernias are more frequent than unilateral.
- **c.** They are more common in girls.
- **d.** They are associated with prematurity.

2. Which of the following statements indicates a parent understands the teaching received about her child's umbilical hernia?

- **a.** "My child will most likely need surgery to repair the hernia."
- **b.** "It is considered a normal variant."
- **c.** "My child has a hernia because he is a boy."
- **d.** "It should close spontaneously by his fifth birthday."

3. Which of the following actions decreases the likelihood of hernia formation in an adult?

- **a.** Lift heavy objects slowly.
- **b.** Eat a low fiber diet.
- **c.** Increase fluid intake to 2 to 3 L/dL.
- **d.** Strain gently.

4. A NP is caring for a client with a strangulated inguinal hernia. The NP should do which of the following?

- **a.** Attempt to reduce the hernia.
- **b.** Transilluminate the area.
- **c.** Apply pressure.
- **d.** Refer to a surgeon immediately.

Answers and Rationales

1. *Answer:* **d** (assessment)
Rationale: They are more common in boys, and tend to occur on the right side. Only 15% of children have bilateral inguinal hernias. There is a 30% prevalence rate among premature infants compared with a 1% prevalence rate in term infants.

2. *Answer:* **b** (evaluation)
Rationale: Umbilical hernias occur equally in girls and boys. They tend to close by the first year of life and rarely need surgery. It is considered a normal finding.

3. *Answer:* **c** (implementation/plan)
Rationale: Constipation contributes to hernia formation in adults. Increased fluid intake helps prevent constipation. A high-fiber, not a low-fiber, diet is beneficial. Straining and heavy lifting, whether done slowly or gently, still predisposes to hernia formation.

4. *Answer:* **d** (implementation/plan)
Rationale: A strangulated hernia is a surgical emergency because of lack of blood supply. No attempt to reduce it or apply pressure should be made because perforation is possible. Transillumination is useful in assessing an unknown mass only.

HERPES SIMPLEX VIRUS TYPE 1: NONGENITAL HERPES *Denise Robinson*

OVERVIEW
Definition

Herpes simplex refers to cutaneous infections with the herpes simplex virus (HSV); HSV-1 is usually associated with oral infections and HSV-2 with genital infections. Nongenital HSV infection, whether primary or recurrent, is characterized by grouped vesicles arising on an erythematous base on keratinized skin or mucous membrane.

Incidence

Herpes simplex occurs most commonly in young adults but affects all ages. Incubation period is 2 to 20 days.

Pathophysiology

- Transmission is usually skin-to-skin, skin-to-mucosa, or mucosa-to-skin contact.
- Increased HSV-1 transmission is associated with crowded living conditions. After exposure, the virus replicates in epithelial cells, causing lysis of infected cells. After inoculation, herpes ascends peripheral sensory nerves and enters sensory nerve root where latency is established (Fitzpatrick, Johnson, Wolff, Suurmond, 2001).
- Incubation is 2 to 20 days (average 6).
- Risk factors for herpes include the following:
  - Skin or mucosal irritation (ultraviolet radiation)
  - Altered hormonal milieu (menstruation)
  - Fever
  - The common cold
  - Altered immune states
  - Site of infection
  - Neonates
  - Occupational exposure
  - Previous HSV
  - Immunocompromising factors: HIV infection, malignancy, transplantation, chemotherapy, systemic corticosteroids, irradiation, immunosuppressive drugs

ASSESSMENT: SUBJECTIVE/HISTORY
History of Present Illness

- Ask about location, onset, duration, and appearance of lesions.
- Ask whether pain, burning, or paraesthesia was present before eruption.
- Ask about associated symptoms of fever, myalgia, or malaise.
- Ask about previous occurrence.
- Ask about exposure to infected persons.

Past Medical History

Ask about immunocompromised state.

Symptoms
Primary Episode

- Many persons have no symptoms or have only minor symptoms with primary herpes.
- If present, symptoms may include regional lymphadenopathy, intense itching, pain, fever, headache, malaise, and myalgia peaking within 3 to 4 days of onset.
- Gingivostomatitis (sore throat, fever, and vesicles on pharynx and oral mucosa) is the most common symptom in children.

Recurrent Episode. Recurrent herpes may have prodrome of tingling, itching, or burning often 1 to 2 days before outbreak.

ASSESSMENT: OBJECTIVE/PHYSICAL EXAMINATION
Physical Examination

- Examine lesions for characteristic location, distribution, and appearance.
- Check for cervical lymphadenopathy.

Skin Findings. Erythema is often noted initially, followed by grouped, often umbilicated vesicles, which may evolve into pustules. These may become eroded and may enlarge into ulcers. They may heal in 2 to 4 weeks. Vesicles on the end of fingers are characteristic of herpetic whitlow. The defects will heal in 2 to 4 weeks (Fitzpatrick et al. 2001).

General Findings
- Fever is often present
- Gingivostomatitis
- Regional lymphadenopathy

Diagnostic Procedures
- Tzanck smear
- Viral culture

DIAGNOSIS

Differential diagnoses include the following:
- Erythema multiforme
- Pemphigus
- Aphthous ulcers
- Herpangina
- HFM disease

THERAPEUTIC PLAN
- Treatment is primarily supportive.
- Administer lidocaine 2% for lesions of the mouth and lip directly to lesion or as a rinse.

- For oral lesions, apply hydrocortisone acetate (Orabase Hca).
- Diphenhydramine (Benadryl) may also be used as a rinse.
- For lip lesion, apply ice, Blistex, and sunscreen.
- Administer acetaminophen (Tylenol) for pain.
- Acyclovir ointment (Zovirax) can be applied using finger cot or glove q3h for 7 days (by prescription).
- Docosanol (Abreva) is a new product available OTC for oral facial herpes simplex. It should be applied 5 times daily until lesion is healed. It should be applied at earliest symptom.
- Acyclovir (Zovirax) and famciclovir (Famvir) are antivirals approved to treat herpes in immunosuppressed persons.

Client Education

- Warn client about the transmittability of lesions by direct contact (e.g., kissing). This includes oral sex.
- Make sure client knows the natural history of the disease, with emphasis on potential for recurrent episodes, and asymptomatic viral shedding.
- Encourage good hand washing.
- Health care providers should use gloves to care for clients with lesions.

Referral/Consultation

Consult with infectious disease or HIV specialist for the client who is immunocompromised with herpes.

Prevention

- Good handwashing is preventative.
- Avoid contact with those who have active lesions.

COMPLICATIONS

- Systemic dissemination can occur in immunocompromised clients; mortality can range from 10 to 50% (Fitzpatrick et al, 2001).

EVALUATION/FOLLOW-UP

No follow-up is indicated for herpes simplex infection unless secondary infection occurs.

REFERENCES

Barker, L. R., Burton, J. R., & Zieve, P. D. (1999). *Principles of ambulatory medicine* (5th ed.). Baltimore: Williams & Wilkins.

Fitzpatrick, T. B., Johnson, R. A., Wolff, K., & Suurmond, D. (2001). Color atlas and synopsis of clinical dermatology (4th ed.). New York: McGraw-Hill.

Robinson, D., Kidd, P., Rogers, K. (2000). *Primary care across the lifespan,* St. Louis: Mosby.

Solomon, A., Smith, S. (1997). Understanding herpes simplex virus: diagnosis, treatment, transmission and management. *Female Patient 22,* 37-43.

Review Questions

1. The skin lesions most suggestive of herpes are which of the following?
   - a. Thick, crusted plaques, varying in size
   - b. Erythematous papular rash
   - c. Topical, grayish white burrows of varying lengths
   - d. Erythematous, vesicular rash

2. A cardinal symptom of herpes simplex and zoster is which of the following?
   - a. Burning sensation on trunk
   - b. Nocturnal itching
   - c. Generalized itching
   - d. Painful vesicles

3. Which of the following is not included in a list of differential diagnoses when herpes is suspected?
   - a. Drug eruption
   - b. HFM disease
   - c. Pediculosis
   - d. Erythema multiforme

4. Which of the following is not a product that can be used for herpes lesions on the lips (cold sore)?
   - a. Amantadine (Symmetrel)
   - b. Abreva
   - c. Acyclovir
   - d. Famciclovir

5. Bill has cancer of the lung. He has vesicular lesions scattered all over his body. Which of the following actions is appropriate for the NP to do at this time?
   - a. Begin Acyclovir 800 mg 5 times a day.
   - b. Consult with Bill's oncologist.
   - c. Begin treatment with Burow's solution.
   - d. Provide supportive treatment only.

6. Transmission of herpes simplex occurs through which of the following?
   - a. Droplet
   - b. Skin-to-skin contact
   - c. Bloodborne contact
   - d. Fomites

7. Which of the following comments by a client with herpes simplex indicates a need for further teaching?
   - a. "I need to let my partner know I have herpes."
   - b. "Acyclovir will cure my herpes."
   - c. "I should use Zovirax when I have tingling around my mouth."
   - d. "Sun makes my cold sores worse."

8. Which of the following is *not* appropriate to be discussed with a client who has oral herpes?
   - a. Do not have oral sex because the virus can be transmitted.
   - b. Avoid the sun because it may make it worse.

c. A soft diet will be more comfortable while the lesion is present.

d. Kissing does not transmit the herpes virus.

Answers and Rationales

1. *Answer:* d (assessment)

Rationale: The diagnosis of herpes is suggested by finding an erythematous, vesicular rash (Fitzpatrick et al. 2001).

2. *Answer:* d (assessment)

Rationale: A cardinal symptom of herpes infections is painful lesions (Fitzpatrick et al. 2001).

3. *Answer:* c (analysis/diagnosis)

Rationale: Pediculosis does not have erythematous, vesicular lesions (Fitzpatrick et al. 2001).

4. *Answer:* a (implementation/plan)

Rationale: Amantadine is an antiviral, but it is used for influenza and for Parkinson's disease. All the other products are appropriate for herpes simplex (Fitzpatrick et al. 2001).

5. *Answer:* b (implementation/plan)

Rationale: Consultation with the oncologist is the appropriate action. Because Bill is immunosuppressed, he may need higher doses of medication (Robinson, Kidd, & Rogers, 2000).

6. *Answer:* b (analysis/diagnosis)

Rationale: Herpes is spread by skin-to-skin contact (Fitzpatrick et al. 2001).

7. *Answer:* b (evaluation)

Rationale: Herpes is never cured. The virus always remains in the nerve ganglion, even after treatment (Robinson et al. 2000).

8. *Answer:* d (implementation/plan)

Rationale: Kissing is skin-to-skin contact and does spread the herpes virus (Fitzpatrick, et al. 2001).

HERPES SIMPLEX VIRUS TYPE 2: GENITAL HERPES *Cheryl Pope Kish*

OVERVIEW
Definition

Herpes simplex is a recurring viral disease transmitted through direct contact with infected secretions or mucous membranes of an infected individual who is shedding the virus. HSV-1 is usually associated with lesions above the waist, including those on the mouth, and HSV-2 with genital infections, but the reverse may also be true.

Incidence

Although bacterial STDs are declining in the United States, genital herpes is increasing in incidence; 1 of 5 individuals and 1 of 20 women of childbearing age are infected in the United States. In the United States, there are 600,000 new cases annually. Nearly 2000 newborns are affected each year.

Pathophysiology

Transmission of HSV-2 generally occurs from oral–genital or genital–genital contact with a double-stranded DNA virus. Viral particles enter skin or mucus membranes through traumatic microscopic fissures incurred during intercourse. The virus attacks the neural ganglia, causing an acute infection followed by remission. Reactivation occurs at unpredictable intervals. The incubation period for HSV-2 is 3 to 7 days; lesions generally heal within 5 to 10 days without scarring. There is no cure.

Factors Increasing Susceptibility
- Late adolescent and young adult age groups
- Previous or concurrent STDs
- Multiple sexual partners
- Early age at first coitus

Trigger Factors for Recurrence or Reactivation
- Menstruation
- Emotional stress
- Physical trauma
- Pregnancy
- Vigorous sexual activity
- Exposure to ultraviolet light
- Fever

ASSESSMENT: SUBJECTIVE/HISTORY
History of Present Illness
- Ask about location, onset, duration, and appearance of lesions, and aggravating and relieving factors. Determine if this is the primary case or a recurrence.
- Ask whether pain, burning, itching or paraesthesia was present before eruption as a prodrome.
- Ask about associated symptoms of fever, myalgia, or malaise.
- Ask about exposure to infected persons.

Symptoms

Many persons have no symptoms or have only minor symptoms with primary herpes. In many cases, the initial episode includes a flulike syndrome occurring several days after exposure: fatigue, malaise, fever, headache, and myalgia. Classically, there are painful genital vesicles that coalesce and break down to form ulcerated areas. Often symptoms include regional lymphadenopathy, intense

H

itching, pain, fever, headache, malaise, and myalgia peaking within 3 to 4 days of onset. Gingivostomatitis (sore throat, fever, and vesicles on pharynx and oral mucosa) is the most common symptom in children. Recurrent herpes may have prodrome of tingling, itching, or burning. Sometimes 1 or 2 vesicles occur and ulcerate within 12 hours. These lesions tend to be less painful than the primary case.

ASSESSMENT: OBJECTIVE/PHYSICAL EXAMINATION

Physical Examination

A problem-oriented physical assessment focuses on the site of the lesion.

- Examine lesions for characteristic location, distribution, and appearance. The physical examination can be extremely uncomfortable for women. In men, lesions are commonly seen on the penis, buttocks, and thighs; in women they may appear on the labia, buttocks, vagina, cervix, and nipples, depending on the sexual contact of exposure. Erythema is often noted initially, followed by grouped, often umbilicated vesicles, which may evolve into pustules. These may become eroded and may enlarge into ulcers. They may heal in 2 to 4 weeks. Vesicles on the end of fingers are characteristic of herpetic whitlow.
- Check for regional lymphadenopathy.
- Assess for fever.
- Inspect the mouth for gingivostomatitis.

Diagnostic Procedures

- Viral culture is standard for diagnosis. Vesicular fluid is obtained by unroofing the ulcer and swabbing with a cotton-tipped or Dacron applicator within days of appearance of lesions. Place in appropriate transport medium. Refrigerate until transport. Results take 5 days.
- Tzanck smear is less expensive. Scrape base of ulcer with number 15 blade, affix cells to glass slide, and stain with Wright's or Giemsa stain. Multinucleated giant cells support diagnosis of HSV.

DIAGNOSIS

The most common differential diagnoses include the following:

- Primary syphilis
- Chancroid (painful ulcer and tender inguinal adenopathy)
- Lymphogranuloma venereum (initial ulcer or vesicle, often unnoticed; enlarged lymph nodes; secondary invasion: draining abscesses [buboes] and lymphedema)
- Folliculitis
- Granuloma inguinale (large, unsightly ulcers of genitalia, anus, and inguinal area)

THERAPEUTIC PLAN

Pharmacologic Treatment

The Centers for Disease Control and Prevention (CDC) recommends the following treatment regimens:

Primary Episodes

- Acyclovir (Zovirax) 200 mg PO 5 times/day for 7 to 10 days or 400 mg PO tid for 7 to 10 days (pregnancy category C: register pregnant clients; side effects: nausea, vomiting, headache, vertigo, rash, malaise, and fatigue)
- Famciclovir (Famvir) 125 mg PO tid for 7 to 10 days; some sources recommend 500 mg tid for 7 days with dosing dependent on creatinine clearance (side effects: headache, fatigue, GI upset; pregnancy category B: register pregnant clients; not recommended for children)
- Valacyclovir (Valtrex) 1 g PO bid/tid for 7 days with dosing schedule dependent on creatine clearance (side effects: headache, GI upset, dizziness, abdominal pain; pregnancy category B: register pregnant clients; not recommended for children).

Recurrent Episodes. Begin with prodromal symptoms.

- Acyclovir 400 mg PO tid for 5 days or 200 mg PO 5 times/day for 5 days or 800 mg PO bid for 5 days
- Famciclovir 125 mg PO bid for 5 days
- Valacyclovir 500 mg PO bid for 5 days

Suppressive Therapy (If More Than 6 to 8 Episodes/Year)

- Acyclovir 400 mg PO bid
- Famciclovir 250 mg PO bid
- Valacyclovir 250 mg PO bid or 500 mg PO qd or 1 g PO qd

Nonpharmacologic Treatment

This avenue of treatment focuses on comfort measures, minimization of recurrences, and education to prevent spread of infection to sexual partners or the fetus of an infected mother.

Client Education

- Advise notification of sexual partners to enable maximal protection against transmission.
- Recommend condom use with new or uninfected partners and abstinence when lesions or prodromal symptoms are present. Because transmission is associated with direct contact with lesion, not body fluids, condoms are not 100% effective; lesions may occur on areas of the genitals not covered by a condom during intercourse.
- Inform to avoid oral–genital sex with a partner with cold sores.

- Suggest tepid Sitz baths with plain water or Betadine for comfort. If voiding is painful, suggest voiding directly into water.
- Recommend avoiding tight clothing and allowing air to circulate onto vulva as often as possible.
- Suggest drying perineal area with hair dryer set on cold setting.
- Suggest wearing cotton-lined panties and pantyhose.
- Suggest use of topical lidocaine (Xylocaine) on lesions for comfort several times daily. Caution about use near urethra. Cool wet tea bags applied to lesions may also promote comfort.
- Advise of need to wash hands after toileting.
- Advise yearly Pap smear.
- Recommend avoiding factors that trigger recurrences if possible.

Pregnant Clients
- Infection in first trimester contributes to spontaneous abortion, intrauterine growth retardation, and preterm delivery. Schedule ultrasonography at 18 weeks and in 3rd trimester to assess fetal size.
- Instruct client to report outbreaks during pregnancy. Avoid sexual intercourse during the last weeks in pregnancy because sex can trigger recurrence; active lesions necessitate Cesarean childbirth. Notify provider immediately of rupture of membranes; with active lesions, Cesarean is scheduled within 6 hours to minimize likelihood of transmission to fetus.
- Infants born to infected mothers may have mild illness, but are at risk for CNS involvement and disseminated disease with 80% mortality; survivors can have long-term neurologic damage. Antiviral acyclovir can decrease risk.
- Risk of intrapartum problems increases with active herpetic lesions, premature rupture of membranes (PROM), and application of a fetal scalp electrode.
- Breastfeeding is contraindicated in presence of herpetic lesions on the breasts only.

Prevention
The risk of infection can be minimized by responsible sexual behavior and consistent use of condoms. Antivirals reduce the duration of symptoms and of viral shedding.

Referral
- Children with herpes should be evaluated for sexual abuse.
- Those nonresponsive to therapy should be referred, as well as those with secondary infection complicating lesions.
- Refer clients with bladder distention related to dysuria.

EVALUATION/FOLLOW-UP
Follow up on a weekly basis until primary lesions are healed. Schedule annual physical examinations and for women Pap smears because of the association of cervical herpes and cervical dysplasia.

The emotional response to genital herpes and fear related to transmission requires provider support and comprehensive client education.

COMPLICATIONS
- Secondary infection of lesions
- Keratitis (may be preventable by keeping hands away from eyes when active lesions are present)
- Meningitis
- Encephalitis
- Pneumonia
- Rare sensory neurogenic bladder that requires parenteral antivirals and suprapubic catheter.

REFERENCES
Cash, J. C., & Glass, C.A. (2000). *Family practice guidelines.* Philadelphia: Lippincott.

Diagnosing and managing genital ulcers. (1999). *Women's Health in Primary Care 2*(2), 121-125.

Emmert, D. H. (2000). Treatment of common cutaneous herpes simplex virus infections. *American Family Physician 61*(6), 1697-1704.

Hawkins, J. W., Robert-Nichols, D. M., & Stanley-Haney, J. L. (1997). *Protocols for nurse practitioners in gynecologic settings.* New York: Tiresias.

Miller, K. E., & Graves, J. C. (2000). Update on the prevention and treatment of sexually transmitted diseases. *American Family Physician 61*(2), 379-386.

Nettina, S. M. (1998). Herpes genitalis. *Lippincott Primary Care Practice, 2*(3), 303-306.

Robinson, D., Kidd, P., & Rogers, K. M.(2000). *Primary care across the lifespan.* St. Louis: Mosby.

Sandhaus, S. (2001). Genital herpes in pregnant and nonpregnant women. *The Nurse Practitioner 26*(4), 15-33.

Uphold, C. R., & Graham, M. V. (1997). *Clinical guidelines in family practice* (3rd ed.). Gainesville, FL: Barmarrae Books.

Youngkin, E., Davis, M. (1998). *Women's health: A primary care clinical guide.* Stamford, CT: Appleton & Lange.

Review Questions

1. Heather, a 23-year-old secretary, presents with " a sore on my bottom." Which of the following lesions is consistent with genital herpes?
   a. Thick, crusted plaques, varying in size
   b. Umbilicated erythematous papules
   c. Topical, grayish white burrows of varying lengths
   d. Vesicles on an erythematous base

2. Which of the following clinical findings is common in the prodromal phase of recurrent genital herpes?

    a. Increased cheesy vaginal discharge
    b. Itching, tingling, or burning of the perineum
    c. Tender, enlarged inguinal nodes
    d. Chills and fever

3. Richard, a 26-year-old, reports that during recent intercourse with a woman known to have genital herpes, the condom broke. A week later, he had painful blisters on his penis that lasted 8 days. There are currently no lesions. He asks to be tested for genital herpes. Which action by the NP is most appropriate?

    a. Perform a Tzanck smear.
    b. Swab the urethral meatus for cells for viral culture.
    c. Draw blood for a rapid plasma reagin (RPR).
    d. Explain that lesions must be present for the test.

4. Which finding on a Tzanck smear confirms genital herpes?

    a. Multinucleated giant cells
    b. Intracellular nonmotile parasites
    c. Coated epithelial cells
    d. Presence of WBCs

5. The NP wishes to differentiate between the lesion of genital herpes and the chancre of primary syphilis. Which of the following is the major difference?

    a. Herpetic lesions are pustules and chancres are umbilicated papules.
    b. Herpetic lesions are vesicular, whereas chancres are necrotic.
    c. Chancres are painless and herpetic lesions are painful.
    d. Chancres heal without scarring and herpetic lesions produce a large scar.

6. Joe, a client with genital herpes, makes all of the following statements. Which is incorrect and deserves clarification by the NP?

    a. "My doctor has prescribed acyclovir to cure my herpes."
    b. "I need to use condoms consistently during sex because shedding of the virus is unpredictable."
    c. "Reducing stress in my job may help prevent recurrence."
    d. "Symptoms of recurring outbreaks are usually less severe than the first outbreak."

7. For which of the following clients is daily suppressive therapy for genital herpes recommended?

    a. A 15-year-old who was recently diagnosed.
    b. A 30-year-old whose primary outbreak was 4 years ago.
    c. A 25-year-old who has outbreaks after every menstrual period.
    d. A 40-year-old whose primary outbreak included both oral and genital lesions.

8. The NP has provided Gail with education about living with genital herpes. Which of the following comments made by Gail indicates a need for further teaching?

    a. "Since I can't sunbathe I am going to join a spa with a tanning bed."
    b. "Warm sitz baths may make me more comfortable during outbreaks."

    c. "I'll need yearly Pap smears to check for cervical problems."
    d. "I should advise any new sexual partners about my condition."

9. Which of the following drugs is appropriate for treatment of genital herpes?

    a. Metronidazole
    b. Nizoral
    c. Acyclovir
    d. Zostrix.

10. Vickie is a pregnant woman with a history of genital herpes. How will her management during pregnancy be different because of this history?

    a. Weekly viral titers are required.
    b. Monthly ultrasonography is necessary to assess fetal growth.
    c. Cesarean delivery will be scheduled if she has active genital lesions.
    d. Antiviral drugs will be administered parentally during labor.

Answers and Rationales

1. *Answer:* **d** (analysis/diagnosis)
    Rationale: Genital herpes causes vesicles, which coalesce into groups and ulcerate, then heal without scarring (Robinson, Kidd, & Rogers, 2000).

2. *Answer:* **b** (assessment)
    Rationale: Itching, burning, and tingling are common prodromal symptoms for recurrent outbreaks of HSV-2 (Robinson, Kidd, & Rogers, 2000).

3. *Answer:* **d** (implementation/plan)
    Rationale: A lesion must be present which can be unroofed to obtain vesicular fluid for viral culture. Tzanck smear requires scraping cells from the base of the legion (Cash & Glass, 2000).

4. *Answer:* **a** (analysis/diagnosis)
    Rationale: The Tzanck smear shows multinucleated giant cells of herpes (Robinson, Kidd, & Rogers, 2000).

5. *Answer:* **c** (analysis/diagnosis)
    Rationale: Chancres are generally painless ulcers whereas herpetic lesions are tender and painful (Robinson, Kidd, & Rogers, 2000).

6. *Answer:* **a** (evaluation)
    Rationale: Herpes is not a curable disease; it is a disease of remissions and exacerbations (Cash & Glass, 2000).

7. *Answer:* **c** (implementation/plan)
    Rationale: Suppression therapy is appropriate for clients who experience more than 6 outbreaks annually (Robinson, Kidd, & Rogers, 2000).

8. *Answer:* **a** (evaluation)
    Rationale: Ultraviolet light can be a precipitating factor in recurrences of genital herpes (Cash & Glass, 2000).

9. Answer: c (implementation/plan)

  Rationale: Acyclovir, famciclovir, and valacyclovir are drugs of choice in treating HSV-2 (Sandhaus, 2001).

10. Answer: c (implementation/plan)

  Rationale: Because of the risk of vertical transmission, a Cesarean delivery is performed for women with active lesions or prodromal symptoms at delivery (Sandhaus, 2001).

HERPES ZOSTER *Denise Robinson*

OVERVIEW
Definition

Herpes zoster, or shingles, is an acute dermatomal infection. It is characterized by unilateral pain and a vesicular or bullous eruption limited to dermatomes innervated by a corresponding sensory ganglion.

Incidence

More than 66% of those affected are older than 50 years; only 5% of cases occur in children younger than 15 years of age. Herpes zoster occurs in 10% to 20% of the population at some time, equally in males and females.

Pathophysiology

Herpes zoster is associated with reactivation of varicella-zoster virus (VZV) that has been dormant in a dorsal root ganglion.

  Factors Increasing Susceptibility. The most common risk factor is diminishing immunity with advancing age, with most cases occurring in those older than 55.
- Malignancy
- Immunosuppression
- Radiotherapy
- HIV-infected individuals have a 20 times increased incidence of zoster.

  Protective Factors
- Youth
- Immunocompetence

ASSESSMENT: SUBJECTIVE/HISTORY
Symptoms
- Ask about when and how the eruption began and about appearance and distribution of the lesions.
- Ask whether there was preeruption pain, itching, or burning in the affected dermatome several days before the eruption.
- Ask about immunosuppressed status.

  Prodromal Stage
- Headache, malaise, and fever occur in 5% of affected persons.
- Tenderness, neuritic pain, or paresthesia (itching, tingling, or burning) in the involved dermatome precedes cutaneous eruption by 3 to 5 days, but can have a range of 1 to 14 days.

- Pain is described as stabbing, pricking, boring, penetrating, or shooting.
- Allodynia, which is a heightened sensitivity to mild stimuli, may also be reported.

  Active Vesiculation
- Headache, malaise, and fever
- Lasts 3 to 5 days
- Neuritic pain
- Pain in the involved skin
- Crust formation occurs from days to 2 to 3 weeks.

  Chronic Postherpetic Neuralgia
- Depression is common.
- Burning pain can persist for weeks, months, or even years after the cutaneous involvement has resolved.

Past Medical History
- Diabetes
- HIV
- Cancer and its treatment (chemotherapy, radiation therapy)
- Transplant recipient

Medication History
- Immunosuppressive drugs (transplant recipients)
- Corticosteroids

Family History

Determine whether family members have had varicella (chicken pox).

Dietary History

Chronic alcohol use.

ASSESSMENT: OBJECTIVE/PHYSICAL EXAMINATION
Physical Examination
- Examine skin for characteristic lesions and distribution.
- Determine whether there is ophthalmic involvement.

  Skin Lesions
- Assess type. Lesions progress from papules (24 hours) to vesicles and bullae (48 hours) to pustules (96 hours) to crusts (7 to 10 days). New lesions continue to appear for as long as 1 week. Necrotic and gangrenous lesions may also occur.

H

- Assess color. Lesions have erythematous, edematous base, with superimposed clear or hemorrhagic vesicles.
- Assess shape. The vesicle or bulla is oval or round, and may be umbilicated.
- Assess arrangement. Herpetiform clusters of lesions are characteristic.
- Assess distribution. Distribution is unilateral and dermatomal. Two or more contiguous dermatomes may be involved. Noncontiguous dermatomal zoster is rare. Hematogenous dissemination to other skin sites occurs in 10% of healthy individuals.
- Assess sites of predilection. Site is thoracic in 50%, trigeminal in 10% to 20%, and lumbosacral and cervical in 10% to 20%. In HIV-infected persons, lesions may be multidermatomal or recurrent.
- Assess mucous membranes. Vesicles and erosions occur in mouth, vagina, and bladder, depending on dermatome involved.
- Assess lymphadenopathy.
- Regional nodes draining the area are often enlarged and tender.
- Assess for sensory or motor nerve changes.
- Changes are detectable by neurologic examination. Sensory defects and motor paralysis may occur.
- Assess eyes. In ophthalmic zoster, nasociliary branch involvement of the trigeminal nerve occurs in about one third of cases and is heralded by vesicles on the side and tip of the nose.

Diagnostic Procedures

- In addition to tests specific for herpes zoster and to rule out other conditions, consider HIV testing.
- Obtain Tzanck smear. Smear of vesicle base or fluid shows giant or multinucleated epidermal cells.
- Perform VZV antigen detection. Direct fluorescent antibody detects VZV antigen in smear of vesicle base or fluid. The test is specific and very sensitive.
- Obtain viral culture for isolation of VZV.

DIAGNOSIS

Differential diagnosis is different for the prodromal and the dermatomal eruption phases.

Prodromal Phase

- Migraine
- Cardiac or pleural disease
- Acute abdomen
- Vertebral disease

Dermatomal Eruption

- Varicella
- HSV
- Cellulitis
- Poison oak or poison ivy
- Contact dermatitis
- Erysipelas

- Bullous impetigo
- Necrotizing fasciitis

NOTE: *Herpes zoster is not pruritic and does not present with systemic signs (e.g. fever, infection). These two factors can help rule out the above diagnoses.*

THERAPEUTIC PLAN

Suppression of pain, inflammation, and infection is goal of therapy.

Nonpharmacologic Treatment

- Use NSAIDs for pain and fever.
- Wet compresses with Burrow's solution or cool tap water can be applied for as long as 30 minutes several times a day.
- Calamine or starch shake lotions may be applied.
- Isolate client from neonates, pregnant women, people who have not had chickenpox, and immunosuppressed persons because the active lesions are potentially infectious, although such infection is rare.

Pharmacologic Treatment

- Antiviral therapy is indicated for herpes zoster in any immunosuppressed person, adults at greatest risk for postherpetic neuralgia (older than age 55), and younger clients with acute pain.
  - Acyclovir, 800 mg 5 times per day for 5 to 7 days if client seeks treatment within first 72 hours of neuralgic symptoms OR
  - Valacyclovir 1 g tid for 7 days
  - Famvir 500 mg tid for 7 days if client seeks treatment within 72 hours of symptom onset
- Corticosteroids reduces acute pain and can be used for immunocompetent client. A 60 mg/dL initial dose tapered over 3 weeks should be used (Berger, 2001).

Postherpetic Neuralgia

- After all vesicles have resolved, topical capsaicin cream may be used qid for 21 days for postherpetic neuralgia.
- Regional nerve blocks can be used as appropriate for the location of pain. Corticosteroids may be added to the injection.
- Amitriptyline (25 to 75 mg) qhs may also be used.

Client Education

Instruct that if a flare-up occurs, early treatment (within 72 hours) is best to avoid postherpetic neuralgia.

Referral

Refer all clients with eye or facial involvement or dissemination beyond two dermatomes to an ophthalmologist or an infectious disease specialist.

Prevention

For family member and contacts who have not had chicken pox, varicella vaccine should be administered.

EVALUATION/FOLLOW-UP

- Follow up in 7 days, or in 2 to 3 days for clients who are immunosuppressed, elderly, or debilitated.
- Monitor renal function in people taking acyclovir.

Complications

- In ophthalmic zoster (trigeminal nerve involvement), complications include uveitis, keratitis, conjunctivitis, retinitis, optic neuritis, glaucoma, proptosis, cicatricial lid retraction, and extraocular muscle palsies.
- Postherpetic neuralgia is possible.
- Scarring is possible.

REFERENCES

Bechtle, M. (1999). Herpes zoster. In D. Robinson, P. Kidd, & K. Rogers (Eds.), *Primary care across the lifespan.* St. Louis: Mosby.

Berger, T. (2001). Skin, hair, and nails. In L. Tierney, S. McPhee, & M. Papadakis (Eds.), *Current medical diagnosis and treatment* (40th ed.). New York: McGraw-Hill.

Fitzpatrick, T. B., Johnson, R. A., Wolff, K., Polano, M. K., & Suurmond, D. (1997). *Color atlas and synopsis of clinical dermatology* (3rd ed.). New York: McGraw-Hill.

Review Questions

1. The skin lesions most suggestive of herpes zoster are which of the following?

   a. Thick, crusted plaques, varying in size

   b. Erythematous papular rash

   c. Topical, grayish white burrows of varying lengths

   d. Erythematous, vesicular rash

2. Which of the following is a cardinal symptom of herpes zoster?

   a. Burning sensation on trunk

   b. Nocturnal itching

   c. Generalized itching

   d. Painful vesicles

3. Which of the following is the treatment of choice for herpes zoster?

   a. Acyclovir 800 mg 5 times a day

   b. Prednisone 40 mg/day

   c. Burow's solution q4h

   d. Hydrocodone (Vicodin) 1 tablet q4h for pain

4. Mr. Smith, a 66-year-old man with lung cancer, reports persistent pain on the face where he had herpes zoster 4 weeks ago. These symptoms sound like which complication of herpes zoster?

   a. Chronic pain syndrome

   b. Postherpetic neuralgia

   c. Chronic cutaneous herpes

   d. Drug-seeking behavior

Answers and Rationales

1. *Answer:* d (assessment)

   Rationale: The diagnosis of herpes is suggested by finding an erythematous, vesicular rash. Impetigo has crusted plaques. Contact dermatitis would have erythematous papules. Burrows are associated with scabies.

2. *Answer:* d (assessment)

   Rationale: A cardinal symptom of herpes infections is painful lesions. Itching is more frequently associated with contact dermatitis and varicella.

3. *Answer:* a (implementation/plan)

   Rationale: Although the other medications help with symptoms of herpes zoster, acyclovir is a viral inhibitory agent that hastens healing and decreases viral shedding.

4. *Answer:* b (evaluation)

   Rationale: Postherpetic neuralgia occurs in approximately 40% of clients older than 60 years. The incidence is even higher when the zoster is ophthalmic.

HIRSCHSPRUNG'S DISEASE   *Denise Robinson*

H

OVERVIEW

Definition

Hirschsprung's disease is also known as megacolon or congenital aganglionic megacolon. Hirschsprung's disease results from an absence of ganglion cells in the colon causing abnormal innervation of the bowel.

Incidence

- Accounts for 15% to 20% of neonatal intestinal obstruction; 1 of 5000 live births.
- More common in boys by 4 to 1.
- Unlikely in preterm infants.
- Ten percent to fifteen percent of clients also have Down syndrome.

- Also associated with other congenital defects, including Laurence-Moon-Bardet-Biedl and cardiovascular abnormalities.

Pathophysiology

This is a congenital condition in which there is failure of the nerve cells to migrate to the mesodermal layers. This process most often affects the rectum (30%) or the rectosigmoid (44%). Involvement of the entire colon occurs in 8% of cases. The section of the colon affected is narrowed, with dilation of the segment of normal colon, which is proximal. The mucosa of the dilated segment becomes thin and inflamed resulting in diarrhea, bleeding and protein loss. Enterocolitis is a common result of the stasis, which allows proliferation of bacteria.

ASSESSMENT: SUBJECTIVE/HISTORY

- Earliest sign is lack or delayed meconium stool passage (99% of all newborns pass meconium within 48 hours of birth).
- Ask about problems with constipation, distention, and vomiting (newborn) in the first weeks of life.
- In later infancy, alternating constipation and diarrhea is a warning sign.
- In older children, look for constipation, with offensive, ribbonlike stool.
- Ask about fever; approximately 50% of newborns with this disease have fever, explosive diarrhea, and prostration. These episodes may lead to perforation and sepsis.
- Ask about weight gain.
- Ask about feeding patterns (breastfed babies do not present with as severe disease as formula fed infants).
- Ask about bowel patterns; may have ribbonlike stools.
- Ask about prenatal course, any genetic testing.

Past Medical History

- Failure to thrive
- Hypochromic anemia
- Hypoproteinemia
- Fecal impaction/intestinal obstruction

Family History

There is a familial pattern for Hirschsprung's disease, particularly total colonic aganglionosis.

ASSESSMENT: OBJECTIVE/PHYSICAL EXAMINATION

Physical Examination

- Perform a thorough physical examination, with particular attention to the GI tract.
- Obtain vital signs, weight, head circumference, length (may see fever).
- In a newborn, assess abdominal distention, vomiting.
- In an older child, assess for enlarged abdomen, prominent veins, more visible peristaltic waves, and palpable fecal masses.
- Perform a rectal examination. No stool may be present even though fecal impaction is seen on radiograph and normal rectal tone is present.

Diagnostic Procedures

- Rectal manometry and rectal suction biopsy are the easiest and most reliable indicator of Hirschsprung's disease (Wyllie, 1996).
- Test for aganglionic cells in the submucosal and muscular layers of the involved bowel.
- Abdominal radiograph shows dilated proximal colon and absence of gas in the pelvic colon.
- Barium enema demonstrates the narrowed segment.

DIAGNOSIS

Differential diagnoses (Table 3-46):

- Retentive constipation
- Functional constipation
- Celiac disease

TABLE **3-46** Distinguishing Features of Hirschsprung's Disease and Functional Constipation

Variable	Functional	Hirschsprung's disease
History		
Onset	After 2 years of age	Birth
Encopresis	Common	Uncommon
FTT	Uncommon	Common
Enterocolitis	None	Possible
Abdominal pain	Common	Common
Examination		
Abdominal distention	Rare	Common
Poor weight gain	Rare	Common
Anal tone	Normal	Normal
Rectal examination	Stool in ampulla	Ampulla empty
Lab		
Anorectal manometry	Distention of the rectum causes relaxation of the internal sphincter	No sphincter or paradoxical relaxation or increase in pressure
Rectal biopsy	Normal	No ganglion cells, increased ACTH staining
Barium enema	Massive amounts of stool, no transition zone	Transition zone, delayed evacuation (longer than 24 hr)

From Wyllie, R. (1996). Motility disorders and Hirschsprung disease. In R. Behrman, R. Kliegman, & W. Arvin (Eds.), *Nelson textbook of pediatrics* (15th ed., p. 1071). Philadelphia: W. B. Saunders.
ACTH, Adrenocorticotropic hormone.

THERAPEUTIC PLAN
Nonpharmacologic Treatment

Treatment is surgical. Initially, a colostomy or ileostomy is performed proximal to the aganglionic segment. The resection is completed when the child is 6 months or older. The aganglionic section is resected.

Pharmacologic Treatment

Not applicable.

Prevention

None.

EVALUATION/FOLLOW-UP

- Immediate follow-up is done by surgeon.
- The NP should be aware of the surgery and follow up on the child's bowel patterns.

COMPLICATIONS

- Chronic constipation
- Fecal incontinence
- Anastomotic breakdown or stricture
- Enterocolitis in approximately 15% of cases

REFERENCES

Harjai, M. M, (2000). Hirschsprung's disease: revisited. *Journal of Postgraduate Medicine 46*(1), pp. 52-54.

Sondheimer, J. (1999). Gastrointestinal tract. In W. Hay, A. Hayward, M. Levin, &. J., Sondheimer, (Eds.), *Current pediatric diagnosis and treatment* (14th ed., pp. 535-536). Norwalk, CT: Appleton & Lange.

Wyllie, R. (1996). Motility disorders and Hirschsprung disease. In R. Behrman, R. Kliegman, & W. Arvin. (Eds.), *Nelson textbook of pediatrics* (15th ed., pp. 1070-1072). Philadelphia: W. B. Saunders.

Review Questions

1. The triad of constipation, abdominal distention, and vomiting are characteristic of what disease in children?
   a. Functional constipation
   b. Irritable bowel disease
   c. Hirschsprung's disease
   d. Irritable bowel syndrome

2. Which of the following historical data are *not* consistent with a diagnosis of Hirschsprung's disease?
   a. Little interest in feeding
   b. Alternating constipation and diarrhea
   c. Refusal to toilet train
   d. Hypochromic anemia

3. Which of the following is the appropriate treatment for Hirschsprung's disease?
   a. Surgical resection of the bowel
   b. Bowel retraining program
   c. Daily enemas
   d. Daily stool softener

4. Which of the following examination findings are consistent with the diagnosis of Hirschsprung's disease?
   a. Large fecal mass palpable in abdomen but no stool in rectal vault
   b. Large amount of stool in rectal vault
   c. Fluid wave of abdomen
   d. Hepatosplenomegaly

5. When Hirschsprung's disease is suspected, it needs to be differentiated from functional constipation. Unlike Hirschsprung's disease, characteristics of functional constipation include which of the following?
   a. Onset after 2 years of age
   b. Abdominal pain
   c. Normal rectal tone
   d. Failure to thrive

Answers and Rationales

1. **Answer: c** (analysis/diagnosis)
   Rationale: The newborn typically presents with abdominal distention, nausea, and vomiting. Delayed passage of meconium is also a sign of Hirschsprung (Wyllie, 1996).

2. **Answer: c** (assessment)
   Rationale: The lack of refusal to toilet train is not a common symptom seen in Hirschsprung (Wyllie, 1996).

3. **Answer: a** (implementation/plan)
   Rationale: Surgical resection of the bowel is the treatment for Hirschsprung's disease (Sondheimer, 1999).

4. **Answer: a** (assessment)
   Rationale: A large mass of feces may be palpated through the abdomen, but no stool is found in the rectal vault. This is different from functional constipation in that in functional constipation a large amount of stool is found in the rectum (Wyllie, 1996).

5. **Answer: a** (analysis/diagnosis)
   Rationale: The onset of functional constipation is later than Hirschsprung's disease. The onset of Hirschsprung's disease is typically found at birth when the child does not pass meconium (Wyllie, 1996).

H

HUMAN IMMUNODEFICIENCY VIRUS/ACQUIRED IMMUNE DEFICIENCY SYNDROME *Denise Robinson*

OVERVIEW

Definition

Human Immunodeficiency Virus Type 1. Human immunodeficiency virus type 1 (HIV-1) is the virus that is recognized as the agent that induces acquired immune deficiency syndrome (AIDS). This illness consists (usually) of a number of years of asymptomatic infection, followed by repeated episodes of illness of varying and increasing severity as immune function deteriorates.

Human Immunodeficiency Virus Type 2. HIV type 2 (HIV-2) is closely related to but less virulent than HIV-1, and is epidemic only in West Africa.

AIDS is a transmissible retroviral disease caused by infection with HIV and is manifested by depression of cell-mediated immunity, with a CD_4 count lower than 200 cells/mm³. The outcome of this process is an increase in opportunistic infections with bacterial, fungal, protozoan, or viral pathogens.

Incidence

- About 1 in 250 persons in the United States is infected with HIV.
- Worldwide, as of December 2001, approximately 40 million people have been infected with HIV. Three million people with AIDS died in 2001 (CDC, 2002).
- Approximately 90% of cases occur in the developing world.
- AIDS onset is most common in the age range of 20 to 50, with the peak incidence between 30 and 39 years.
- Occupationally transmitted HIV has been documented in 95 definite and 191 possible cases (probably under-reported).
- The overall seroprevalence estimate for childbearing women in the United States is 0.15%, which reflects approximately 6000 births per year to infected women. The efficiency of vertical transmission of HIV transmission from mother to infant is approximately 12% to 39%.

AIDS Indicator Conditions

- HIV-seropositivity with CD_4 cell count lower than 200 cells/mm³ or a percentage of CD_4 cells lower than 14%
- Candidiasis of bronchi, trachea, or lungs
- Candidiasis of esophagus
- Cervical cancer, invasive
- Coccidioidomycosis, disseminated or extrapulmonary
- Cryptococcosis, extrapulmonary
- Cryptosporidiosis, chronic intestinal (longer than 1 month in duration)
- CMV disease (other than liver, spleen, or nodes)
- CMV retinitis (with loss of vision)
- Encephalopathy, HIV-related
- Herpes simplex: Chronic ulcers (1 month duration), bronchitis, pneumonitis, or esophagitis
- Histoplasmosis, disseminated or extrapulmonary
- Isosporiasis, chronic intestinal (longer than 1 month duration)
- Kaposi's sarcoma
- Lymphoma, Burkitt's (or equivalent term)
- Lymphoma, immunoblastic (or equivalent term)
- Lymphoma, primary, of brain
- Mycobacterium avium complex or Mycobacterium kansasii, disseminated or extrapulmonary
- Mycobacterium tuberculosis (TB), any site (pulmonary or extrapulmonary)
- Mycobacterium, other species or unidentified species, disseminated or extrapulmonary
- Pneumocystis carinii pneumonia (PCP)
- Pneumonia, recurrent
- Progressive multifocal leukoencephalopathy
- Salmonella septicemia, recurrent
- Toxoplasmosis of brain
- Wasting syndrome from HIV

Table 3-47 presents the revised classification system used by the CDC for individuals with HIV infection and AIDS.

Pathophysiology

The major target for HIV is the CD_4 T lymphocyte; macrophages and monocytes may also be infected. The virus attaches to the CD_4 cell, enters the cytoplasm, and uncoats. By means of the viral enzyme reverse transcriptase, a DNA copy of the viral RNA genome is transcribed and duplicated. This new DNA integrates into the DNA of the host cell. This process generates viral buds that separate from the host cell, thereby initiating viral replication. HIV is transmitted by sexual exposure, by contamination in intravenous drug use (IDU), through contaminated blood and blood products, and from mother to fetus. Within 2 to 6 weeks after exposure and lasting approximately 1 to 2 weeks, there are symptoms indicative of acute retroviral conversion in approximately 50% to 70% of those exposed. These symptoms, characteristic of infectious mononucleosis or flulike in character, include fever, arthralgias, myalgias, and fatigue. Physical examination may reveal a diffuse, erythematous rash and generalized adenopathy. This clinical presentation coincides with high levels of viral replication, which are measured by HIV RNA and the presence of p24 antigen. CD_4 cell counts drop dramatically and CD_8 cell counts generally rise in response to the virus. Seroconversion generally takes 6 to 12 weeks after transmission. The levels of HIV RNA are sharply reduced and CD_4 counts return to higher

TABLE **3-47**   CDC 1993 Revised Classification System for HIV Infection and Expanded AIDS Surveillance Case Definition for Adolescents and Adults

CD4 + T-CELLS CATEGORIES (CELLS/MM3)	Clinical Categories		
	(A), ASYMPTOMATIC, ACUTE (PRIMARY)HIV, OR PGL	(B), SYMPTOMATIC, NOT (A) OR (C) CONDITIONS	(C), AIDS INDICATOR CONDITIONS
(1) >500	A1	B1	C1
(2) 200-499	A2	B2	C2
(3) <200 AIDS-indicator T cell count	A3	B3	C3

From Centers for Disease Control and Prevention. (1992). 1993 Revised classification system for HIV infection and expanded surveillance case definition for AIDS among adolescents and adults. *MMWR: Morbidity and Mortality Weekly Report 44*(RR-17), 1-19.
Shaded areas indicate AIDS.
PGL, Persistent generalized lymphadenopathy.

levels, but generally not to preinfection levels. This stage is followed by a prolonged stage of asymptomatic clinical latency. During this stage, there is a large viral reservoir actively replicating in the lymphoid tissues. As this clinical latency continues and disease progresses, the framework of the lymph tissue disintegrates, accounting for the rise of viral burden detectable in the plasma. Immunologic damage increases, and opportunistic infections develop unabated. The rate of disease progression is outlined in Figure 3-7.

Clients for Whom HIV Testing Is Recommended

- Persons who have STDs should be tested for HIV.
- Persons in high-risk categories should be tested. The major risk factor for HIV is unprotected heterosexual or homosexual intercourse. Persons with history of IDU, persons with hemophilia, and regular sexual

partners of persons in these categories are considered high-risk. People with STDs are high-risk (there is a two to five times greater risk of HIV infection among people with STDS). Lower risk categories include prostitutes and persons who received blood or artificial insemination during the years 1978 through 1985.
- Persons who consider themselves at risk or request testing should be tested.
- Women at risk who are of childbearing age should be tested; risk factors include IDU; prostitution; living in a high-prevalence community; birth in a high-prevalence country; blood transfusion between 1978 and 1985; and male sexual partner with history of IDU, bisexual relationships, or HIV infection.
- All pregnant women should be tested.
- Clients with clinical or laboratory findings suggestive of HIV infection should be tested.

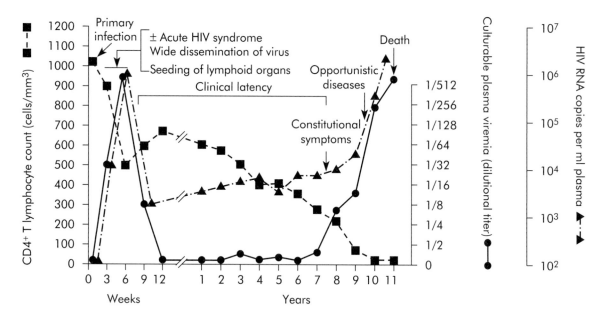

FIGURE **3-7**   Typical course of HIV infection without therapy. (From Bartlett, J.G., & Finkbeiner, A. [1996]. The Johns Hopkins Hospital guide to medical care of patients with HIV infection. Baltimore: Williams & Wilkins.)

- Clients with active TB should be tested.
- Recipients who receive blood or body fluid exposures should be tested.
- Health care workers who perform exposure-prone invasive procedures should be tested.
- Clients between 15 and 45 years old who have been admitted to the hospital in facilities where seroprevalence is 1% or the AIDS case rate is 1 case per 1000 discharges should be tested.
- Donors of blood, semen, and organs should be tested. (This is the only category in which testing is mandatory in all states.)

ASSESSMENT: SUBJECTIVE/HISTORY
History of Present Illness

Ask specifically about the following symptoms:
- Fatigue
- Malaise
- Fevers without cause with oral temperatures of 100° F
- Night sweats
- Swollen or painful lymph nodes
- Unexplained loss of 10% of body weight
- Loss of appetite, painful or difficult swallowing, nausea, vomiting, or diarrhea
- Cough, shortness of breath (SOB), chest tightness, orthopnea, tachypnea, or history of TB or positive purified protein derivative (PPD) of tuberculin testing, change in exercise tolerance
- Oral candidiasis (thrush)
- Changes in CNS function, including headaches, changes in mental status, stiff neck, seizures, and cognitive, motor, change in vision, and behavioral changes, difficulty thinking, depression, muscle weakness, loss of sensation
- Skin rashes: new or pigmented lesions, bruises, itching
- Herpes zoster (shingles)
- Allergies to foods, pets, or environment
- STDs, including gonorrhea, chlamydia, syphilis, condylomata, hepatitis, herpes simplex
- Sexual preference and safe sex practices
- In women, pregnancy history, Pap smear history, vaginal infections, contraceptive use
- In children, gestational history, including drug exposure, labor and delivery history, gestational age at birth, and weight at birth; growth patterns, feeding patterns, developmental milestones, history of illnesses
- Substance abuse
- Smoking
- Ongoing high-risk behavioral exposures that may place the client at risk for opportunistic infections or risk of HIV transmission to others
- Client's perception and knowledge about HIV infection—has the client ever known anyone infected with HIV; ever taken care of anyone with HIV infection or AIDS?

Medication History

Medication history should include prescribed and OTC drugs and herbs, vitamins, and other nontraditional therapies.

Family History

- Cardiopulmonary disease
- Diabetes
- GI disease
- Cancer
- Depression
- Suicide
- Substance abuse
- Whether the client's family is aware of the diagnosis, and, if not, whether they will be informed
- Previous family experiences with HIV infection

Psychosocial History

- Signs and symptoms of depression
- Suicidal ideation
- Previous psychologic or psychiatric care
- Support network of family and friends
- Current employment status and medical and dental benefits

ASSESSMENT: OBJECTIVE/PHYSICAL EXAMINATION
Physical Examination

A summary of physical examination findings and considerations for clients with AIDS is presented in Table 3-48.

Diagnostic Procedures

- Obtain HIV serology. Test results are reported as negative, positive, or indeterminate. A positive HIV serologic result requires both a positive ELISA and the confirmatory positive Western blot. If the test result is questionable because of the client's history, repeated testing is warranted. Pre- and posttest counseling is required in most states. If clients want true anonymity for the test, they should go to an anonymous test site.
- Obtain CD_4 count. Results of the CD_4 count direct initiation and use of prophylactic antiretrovirals, treatment for opportunistic infections, and diagnostic tests. The test is done initially and repeated every 6 months.
- CBC is done initially then every 3 to 6 months.
- The HIV RNA test is used primarily for disease staging and monitoring of the response to antiretroviral therapies. Frequency of testing should coincide with CD_4 screening.
- Venereal disease research laboratory test (VDRL) or RPR test should be done initially and yearly if client is sexually active.
- Obtain chemistry panel initially and when warranted by disease status or adverse drug reaction.

TABLE **3-48** Physical Examination of Clients with HIV/AIDS

AREAS	SYMPTOMS/FINDINGS	DIFFERENTIAL DIAGNOSES
Mouth	Whitish coating on tongue, gums, roof of mouth	Oral candidiasis
	Fine lines or ridges on sides of tongue	Hairy leukoplakia
	Purple spots or lesions	Kaposi's sarcoma
	Bleeding gums	ITP
	Lesions	Herpes simples, aphthous ulcers
Eyes	Cotton-wool spots, exudate plus hemorrhage	Cytomegalovirus retinitis
Neck	Swollen, painful lymph nodes	Lymphadenopathy
	Nuchal rigidity	Cryptococcosis
Lungs	Auscultation for extraneous sounds (rales, wheezes, rhonchi)	PCP
	Cough	*Pneumococcus Mycobacterium tuberculosis* Bacterial pneumonia
Abdomen	Abnormal tenderness	ITP
	Enlarged liver/spleen	Hepatitis
		Cirrhosis
		Cancers
Genitourinary/rectal	Warts	Venereal warts
	Whitish coating of membranes	Candidal infection
	Ulcers/lesions	Herpes simplex
		Syphilis
Skin (entire body examination)	Purple lesions	Kaposi's sarcoma
	Vesicular lesions	Herpes simplex or zoster
	Bruising	ITP
	Dry, flaking skin	Seborrheic dermatitis
	Rashes	Drug reactions
	Warts/papules	Syphilis
		Disseminated disease
		Molluscum/HPV
Neurologic	Memory loss	Cryptococcosis
	Personality changes	Toxoplasmosis
	Decreased cognitive function	Central nervous system lesions
	Decreased or increased reflexes	HIV dementia
	Neuropathies	Progressive multifocal leukoencephalopathy
Gynecologic	Yeast/white discharge	Vaginal candidiasis
	Papular lesions	STD
	Vesicles	Condylomata acuminatum
		Herpes
		Syphilis

From Robinson, D., Kidd, P., & Rogers, K. M. (2000). *Primary care across the lifespan.* St. Louis: Mosby.
HPV, Human papillomavirus; *ITP,* idiopathic thrombocytopenic purpura; *PCP, Pneumocystis carinii* pneumonia; *STD,* sexually transmitted disease.

- Test for hepatitis. The choice of diagnostic test is determined by client history. HBV immunization status can be determined.
- The PPD test, done initially and yearly, should be repeated in nonreactors with suspected TB or exposure to TB. Induration of 5 mm is considered a positive result.
- Chest radiograph should be done when clinically warranted.
- Pap smear should be done initially and repeated every 6 to 12 months according to client's immune status.

- Toxoplasmosis serology should be done initially and when client is severely immunocompromised (CD$_4$ of 100 cells/mm^3).

DIAGNOSIS

- Differential diagnoses include numerous and varied possibilities, depending on client history and physical examination. Most common are the following:
  - Persistent generalized lymphadenopathy
  - Cytopenias: anemia, leukopenia, thrombocytopenia

H

- Pulmonary symptoms suggesting PCP
- Kaposi's sarcoma
- Candidiasis: vaginal, esophageal, oral
- Constitutional symptoms: weight loss, night sweats, fatigue, chronic fever or chronic diarrhea for 30 days
- Bacterial infections, primarily pulmonary
- TB
- STDs
- Neurologic syndromes
- HIV-associated dementia: difficulty concentrating, memory loss, mental slowing
- Peripheral syndrome: Pain and paresthesia of the feet

THERAPEUTIC PLAN

Physician Consult Preferably in AIDS Treatment Center

Client returns in 2 weeks to discuss laboratory results. The plan of care is reviewed with the client at that time, allowing client involvement and questions.

Pharmacologic Treatment

- Medication selection according to clinical and laboratory profile of the client is at present highly controversial and subjective, and is constantly changing with new developments. Therefore all recommendations must be periodically reviewed and modified.
- Indications to treat include a CD_4 count less than 500 cells/mm^3 (Bartlett, 1996); it is likely that future strategies will consider initiation of treatment with higher CD_4 counts and viral burden of 20,000 to 75,000 copies/dL as a possible independent indicator of treatment.
- Monotherapy is generally not advocated, although some considerations may justify exceptions. Drug regimens of zidovudine and another nucleoside analogue reduce the risk of new AIDS defining illnesses compared against zidovudine alone, although adverse effects were more common with two drug regimens (Wilkinson, Phillips, & Johnson, 2001). In addition, taking a protease inhibitor and two nucleoside analogue drugs cuts the risk of new AIDS disease and death in half over 1 year compared with two nucleoside analogue drugs alone.
- Discussion of early versus deferred antiretroviral therapy has not been answered. All clinical trials were done when zidovudine was the only drug available. No trials have compared the efficacy of two- or three-drug regimens (Table 3-49).

TABLE **3-49**   Combination Drug Therapy: Select a Protease Inhibitor to Be Administered with One of the Nucleoside Analogs

DRUG	DOSE	COMMENTS	COST
PROTEASE INHIBITOR			
Saquinavir (Invirase; new formulation: Fortovase)	600 mg tid with meals	Pregnancy: B Indinavir (C) GI intolerance	$573/200 mg (270)
Indinavir (Crixivan)	800 mg tid between meals	Nephrolithiasis ↑ Indirect bilirubin	$336/200 mg (270)
Ritonavir (Norvir)	600 mg bid with meals	GI intolerance Peripheral paraesthesia → Transaminase levels	$146/100 mg (100)
NUCLEOSIDE ANALOG:			
Zidovudine (Retrovir, AZT)	100 mg 3-5 × daily	Pregnancy: C GI intolerance/headache/malaise	$155/100 mg (100)
Didanosine (Videx, ddI)	≤ 60 kg 200 mg bid ≥ 60 kg 125 mg bid	Peripheral neuropathy/pancreatitis	$89/100 mg (60)
Zalcitabine (Hivid, ddC)	0.75 mg tid	Peripheral neuropathy	$230/0.750 mg (100)
Stavudine (Zerit, d4T)	40 mg bid	Peripheral neuropathy	$233/40 mg (60)
Lamivudine (Epivir, 3TC)	150 mg bid	GI intolerance/headache	$230/150 mg (60)
SELECT A PROTEASE INHIBITOR FROM ABOVE LIST TO GIVE WITH 3TC AND AZT:			
3TC AZT	See above	Side effects of combined drug therapy are additive; see above	See costs above

From Bartlett, J. G. (1996). *The Johns Hopkins Hospital guide to medical care of patients with HIV infection.* Baltimore: Williams & Wilkins.
GI, Gastrointestinal.

Pregnant Women

- 3'-Azido-3'-Deoxythymidine (AZT) is initiated at 14 to 34 weeks' gestation and carried through to delivery.
  - Labor: AZT IV infusion
  - Neonate: AZT beginning 8 to 12 hours after birth
- HIV transmission occurs in utero, at delivery, and with breastfeeding. AZT reduces the rate of transmission from 25% in those untreated to 9% in those receiving AZT.
- Postexposure prophylaxis in health care workers includes the following:
  - Treatment with several antiretroviral drugs is more likely to be effective than treatment with zidovudine alone (Wilkinson, Phillips and Johnson, 2001). HIV infection is less likely in people who received postexposure prophylaxis than those who did not. The risk of seroconversion increased with severity of exposure; for example, a penetrating injury with a hollow needle carried the greatest risk.

Prevention of Opportunistic Disease

Tuberculosis. HIV and AIDS have substantially increased the prevalence of TB in the United States, as well as of isoniazid (INH)- and rifampin-resistant strains. This represents a significant health threat to those who live and work in crowded facilities and communities. Indications for therapy are as follows:

- PPD of 5 mm
- Previous positive PPD result without INH prophylaxis
- High-risk exposure

Treatment is as follows:

- INH and pyridoxine (vitamin B_6) for 12 months
- Liver function tests at 1 and 3 months after initiating INH to screen for hepatitis, a risk of INH

***Pneumocystis Carinii* Pneumonia.** PCP is the major AIDS-defining diagnosis and the major identifiable cause of death in persons with AIDS. Indications for therapy are as follows:

- Previous PCP
- CD_4 of 200 cells/mm^3
- Thrush

Treatment is as follows:

- Trimethoprim-sulfamethoxazole (Bactrim DS)
- Adverse reactions: rash, fever, nausea and vomiting, neutropenia, and hepatitis

Toxoplasmosis. Toxoplasma gondii is a protozoan organism that is ubiquitous in nature. Cats are the primary host and reservoir. Symptoms for clients with immunocompromise include headache, confusion, fever, lethargy, and seizures. Indications are CD_4 count less than 100 cells/mm^3 and positive T gondii serologic result. Treatment is Bactrim DS.

***Mycobacterium Avium* Complex.** *Mycobacterium avium* complex refers to a group of atypical mycobacteria, of which *M. avium* and *Mycobacterium intracellulare* are the most important. They are widely isolated from the soil and water and are a threat to those who are immunocompromised. The indication is a CD_4 count of 75 cells/mm^3. Treatment is clarithromycin, azithromycin, or rifabutin.

Psychosocial Considerations

- Determine the interest and need for psychologic counseling for the client and those close to him or her. Depression and suicide risk must be assessed by qualified staff.
- Review the natural history of HIV infection and course of disease.
- Assess client's involvement and desired level of participation in health care decisions.
- Notify sexual partners and needle-sharing partners of risk status. Physicians and dentists involved in care should be informed.

Client Education

- Provide resources for education, client services, National Institutes of Health clinical trials, financial aid services, community support groups, and national organizations.
- Review lifestyle behaviors associated with disease prevention, including stopping smoking, reducing alcohol intake and stopping other substance abuse, increasing exercise, and using safe sex practices (e.g., using condoms even if both partners are positive because this exposes both partners to the other's opportunistic organisms).
- Household pets are a concern because they may carry microbes that cause diarrhea. If a pet has diarrhea, veterinary care should be sought for the pet. Litter boxes should be cleaned daily and pets should be kept indoors and should not be fed raw meat. Wash hands frequently and thoroughly; preferably pet care is done by someone other than HIV-positive client.
- Discuss food preparation. Avoid raw eggs and undercooked poultry, seafood, and meat. Wash produce. Keep utensils used with raw meat washed and keep countertops and cutting boards washed and clean.
- During travel, avoid contaminated food and water. Review immunization needs for travel.
- Provide immunizations. Pneumococcal vaccine should be given early in the disease. HBV vaccine should be given; live attenuated vaccines such as oral polio, typhoid, yellow fever and varicella should not be given. The measles vaccine has been shown to be safe in children and can be given following the normal immunization schedule.

H

- Discuss occupational risks. Major occupational settings that pose risks for HIV-infected individuals are health care settings, day care settings, and animal shelters.

EVALUATION/FOLLOW-UP

- Repeat CBC and HIV RNA testing every 6 months when CD$_4$ count is 500 cells/mm^3.
- Provide the following immunizations.
  - Pneumovax vaccine initially and consider boosters every 5 to 7 years
  - Influenza vaccine yearly
  - Tetanus-diphtheria toxoid vaccine every 10 years
  - Canine herpesvirus in a series of three
- Frequency of subsequent visits is determined by laboratory data, clinical response, and emotional well-being of the client.

REFERENCES

Bartlett, J. A. (1996). *Care and management of patients with HIV infection.* Durham, NC: Glaxo Wellcome.

Bartlett, J. G., & Finkbeiner, A. (1996). *The Johns Hopkins Hospital guide to medical care of patients with HIV infection.* Baltimore: Williams & Wilkins.

Carpenter, C. C. J., Fischl, M. A., Hammer, S. M., Hirsch, M. S., Jacobsen, D. M., Katzenstein, D. A., Montaner, J. S. G., Richmond, D. D., Saag, M. S., Schooley, R. T., Thompson, M. A., Vella, S., Yeni, P. G., & Volberding, P. A. (1996). Antiretroviral therapy for HIV infection. *Journal of the American Medical Association 276*(2), 146-154.

Centers for Disease Control and Prevention (1992). 1993 Revised classification system for HIV infection and expanded surveillance case definition for AIDS among adolescents and adults. *MMWR: Morbidity and Mortality Weekly Report 44* (RR-17), 1-19.

Centers for Disease Control and Prevention (1995). USPHS/IDSA guidelines for the prevention of opportunistic infections in persons infected with human immunodeficiency virus: A summary. *MMWR: Morbidity and Mortality Weekly Report 44*(RR-8), 1-34.

Centers for Disease Control and Prevention (2002). *International Statistics.* Retrieved July 31, 2002, from www.cdc.gov.

Kesner, S. (2000). HIV. In D. Robinson, P. Kidd, & K. Rogers (Eds.) *Primary care across the lifespan* (pp.582–591). St. Louis Mosby.

Minkoff, H., DeHovitz, J. A., & Duerr, A. (1995). *HIV infection in women.* New York: Raven Press.

Saag, M. S., Holodniy, M., Kuritzkes, D. R., O'Brien, W. A., Coombs, R., Poscher, M. E., Jacobsen, D. M., Shaw, G. M., Richman, D. D., Volberding, P. A. (1996). HIV viral load markers in clinical practice. *Nature Medicine 2*(6), 625-629.

Wilkinson, D., Phillips, A., & Johnson, M. (2001). HIV infection. In S. Barton (Ed). *Clinical Evidence 5,* 481-489.

Review Questions

1. All the following clients should be advised to seek HIV testing except:
   a. Persons who have any STD
   b. Recipients of blood transfusion since 1990
   c. All pregnant women
   d. Clients with active TB

2. When auscultating the lungs of a client with HIV and suspected PCP, which of the following is consistent with a diagnosis of HIV?
   a. Crackles and dry rales
   b. Wheezing
   c. Pleural rub
   d. Stridor

3. HIV-infected pregnant women should be counseled for all the following except:
   a. HIV transmission occurs in utero, at delivery, and during breast-feeding
   b. All HIV-infected women must bottle-feed their infants
   c. AZT significantly reduces HIV transmission
   d. AZT therapy for the neonate continues for the first year of life

4. The workplace can harbor communicable disease exposure. All the following should be of concern for the HIV-infected individual except:
   a. Chickenpox and individuals recently vaccinated
   b. TB
   c. Salmonella
   d. Esophageal candidiasis

5. If two partners have HIV, what recommendation would you give regarding condom/protection for sexual intercourse?
   a. No condoms are needed.
   b. Condoms should be worn.
   c. Abstinence is the best policy.
   d. Withdrawal on ejaculation.

6. Which of the following illnesses are possible for those HIV clients who have cats?
   a. Toxoplasmosis
   b. *M. avium*
   c. PCP
   d. Salmonella

7. June is getting a 4-year well child check. Which of the following immunizations is contraindicated when you find out her mother is HIV-positive
   a. Diphtheria and tetanus toxoids and acellular pertussis (DtaP) vaccine
   b. Influenza vaccine
   c. Varicella vaccine
   d. Inactivated polio vaccine (IPV)

8. Which of the following descriptions is consistent with Kaposi's sarcoma?
   a. Ecchymoticlike macule that evolves into papules
   b. Frecklelike macules

TABLE **3-50** Topical Treatments for Genital Warts

DRUG AND DOSAGE	INSTRUCTIONS FOR ADMINISTRATION	IMPLICATIONS FOR CLIENT EDUCATION
Podofilox (Condylox) 0.5%: Client-administered; available as solution or gel. Total treatable area should be no greater than 10 cm² and total volume of drug used should not exceed 0.5 mL/day	Gel is easier to apply to confined space on skin than solution. **Do not apply to mucous membranes—for use on external warts only.** Apply bid, once in A.M. and once in P.M., for 3 consecutive days/week, followed by 4 consecutive days of no treatment. Discontinue if no visible wart tissue remains. Continue cycle up to 4 weeks if lesion remains. Use cotton-tip applicator packaged with drug to apply solution or use finger	Pregnancy Category: C **Contraindicated during pregnancy and lactation.** Local erythema is common. Local reactions may include erosion of mucosal surfaces especially in uncircumcised men. Allow treated area to dry before allowing it to touch other skin areas. Do not treat more often than 3 days/week. If treatment for 4 weeks does not remove warts, follow-up is needed.
Imiquimod cream 5% (Aldara): Client-administered. Available as single-use 250 mg sachets, which is enough to cover an area of 20cm². Should not be used for larger area.	Apply thin layer of cream and rub in thoroughly until no visible cream remains. (Usually 1/3 of packet is enough for one treatment.) Use hs 3 times/week and leave on for 6 to 10 hours. Wash off in morning with mild soap and lukewarm water. Use maximum of 16 weeks Wash hands thoroughly after application.	Do not cover treated area with occlusive bandage. Do not engage in sexual contact while cream remains on skin. Follow-up every 4 weeks; client should see results in 8 to 10 weeks. Local skin reactions usually mild: erythema, erosion, itching, and rarely pain. Inflammatory reaction in 1 week to 1 month expected sign that drug is working. Client should report significant skin reactions.
Podophyllin resin 10% to 25% solution in tincture of benzoin (Podocon-25 is 25% solution): Provider-administered	Petroleum jelly may be used to protect area of skin around wart from medication. Apply small amount to wart and allow to air dry. Have client wash off in 1 to 4 hours. Repeat once per week. Limit application to no more than 0.5 mL of agent and no more than 10 cm² of warts per treatment session.	Some experts advise against use of this agent because of its carcinogenic potential. Still listed in 1998 CDC treatment guidelines but discontinued in many settings. Cannot be used on mucosa because of systemic absorption and toxicity. Caustic substance produces intense, painful local reaction that may last 1 week or longer. Takes 1 to 4 applications to see evidence of response. **Contraindicated in those with diabetes, poor circulation, or taking steroids, with inflamed or irritated wart surrounding skin. Contraindicated in pregnancy and lactation.**
Trichloroacetic acid 50%: provider-administered	Cover entire wart completely but sparingly with agent once each week using cotton-tipped applicator. Do not apply to areas that are not healed. Do not allow excess medication to run onto unprotected skin. A white coating appears on treated warts. Can be used for both internal and external warts. Causes significant burning on external warts. Local anesthetic such as lidocaine/prilocaine cream or 20% benzocaine may help.	Fair skinned clients are often extremely sensitive to this agent. **May be used in pregnancy.**
Bichloracetic acid	Apply as noted previously.	No data available on effectiveness.

- Reassure the client that although the virus is extremely common, the risk for cervical cancer is low, especially with conscientious Pap smears annually and early treatment of precancerous lesions if they occur.
- Advise clients to improve their immune status by eating a healthy diet, limiting alcohol, getting adequate rest, exercising regularly, and not smoking.
- Explain that HPV is a sexually transmitted infection that may persist even when visible lesions no longer exist. Inform clients that exposure to HPV may have occurred in relationships in their past and not in the current relationship. Recommend screening for other STDs.
- Recommend abstinence or condom use until lesions have disappeared or treatment has ended. Make sure that clients know that condoms do not totally prevent infection; lesions may occur on areas not covered by a condom. Explain that warts may resolve spontaneously or recur unpredictably.
- Reinforce need for follow-up to assess progress of treatment and check for side effects of medications.
- Explain that partners might benefit from being examined and counseled about their risks of infection.
- Pregnancy may cause genital warts to proliferate or become friable. Even without treatment, they may resolve spontaneously by the time of the postpartum visit at 4 to 6 weeks. During pregnancy, warts may be treated by TCA or BCA. Cautious cryotherapy (by a physician) may also be used. Client-administered agents are contraindicated during pregnancy. Genital warts during pregnancy are rarely associated with laryngeal papillomas in the newborn. Cesarean delivery is required only if the vaginal area is totally obscured by warts.

Referral

The following situations warrant referral by the NP:
- Need for vulvar biopsy to confirm diagnosis in situations of uncertainty.
- No response to standard treatment in 3 months.
- In children, the presence of genital warts indicates sexual abuse.
- Immunocompromised clients should be referred.
- Treatment required or preferred by client is beyond the scope of the NPs training or scope of legal practice.
- Treatment of warts on cervix, urethra, anus.

Prevention

The only known methods for preventing acquisition of HPV is sexual abstinence or avoidance of intimate contact with an individual known to be infected. Condoms offer limited protection because lesions may occur on areas not covered by a condom during sexual intimacy.

EVALUATION/FOLLOW-UP

One of every five clients with genital warts has recalcitrant lesions or lesions that recur promptly. They need to be followed carefully. Women need annual Pap smears; more frequent examinations or colposcopy is not indicated for genital lesions. A follow-up visit after warts have disappeared is not mandatory but does allow documentation that warts have cleared. Recurrences are most likely within 3 months.

COMPLICATIONS

Unlike bacterial STDs, which are widely preventable with consistent condom use, individuals harbor the HPV virus, often without knowing it, and experience periodic recurrences. Because warts may occur on body surfaces not covered by a condom, that barrier protection minimizes but does not guarantee 100% safety. Clients must appreciate that they can remain infectious even after visible warts have resolved.

Women exposed to the oncogenic forms of HPV are at risk for cervical cancer (see Cervical Cancer for further examination of this topic).

REFERENCES

Association of Reproductive Health Professionals (ARHP) Clinical Proceedings. (2001). *Human papillomavirus and cervical cancer.* Washington, DC: Author.

ARHP Clinical Proceedings. (2001). *Human papillomavirus and cervical cancer: Quick reference guide to patient questions about HPV.* Washington, DC: Author.

Carter, J. F., & Soper, D. E. (1998). Strategies for managing external genital warts. *Women's Health in Primary Care 1*(4), Reprint.

Cash, J. C., & Glass, C. A. (2000). *Family practice guidelines.* Philadelphia: Lippincott.

Chopra, K., & Tyring, S. (1999). Human papillomavirus: A growing epidemic. *The Clinical Advisor* June, 62-67.

Hawkins, J. W., Roberto-Nichols, D. M., & Stanley-Haney, J. L. (1997). *Protocols for nurse practitioners in gynecologic settings* (6th ed.). New York: Tiresias.

McFadden, S. E., & Schumann, L. (2001). The role of human papillomavirus in screening for cervical cancer. *Journal of the American Academy of Nurse Practitioners, 13*(3), 116-125.

New approaches to management of external genital warts: A supplement to patient care for the nurse practitioner. (1999). Montvale, NJ: Medical Economics Company.

Richart, R. M. (2000). Genital warts: A clinical and management challenge. Supplement to Medical Economics, Fall.

Thomas, D. J. (2001). Sexually transmitted viral infections: Epidemiology and treatment. *Journal of Obstetric, Gynecologic, and Neonatal Nursing, 30*(3), 316-323.

Review Questions

1. Grace, a 26-year-old factory worker, presents with complaints of "a bump down there" as she points toward her pubic area. She has been married for 1 year. Which information from Grace's history indicates a risk of HPV infection?

  a. Use of birth control pills since age 18 for cycle control
  b. History of oral sex with her current partner
  c. Allergy to spermicide nonoxynol 9
  d. Occasional oral ulcers when she is unduly stressed

2. Which of the following descriptions of the visible lesions is most consistent with genital warts?

  a. Three small, fluid-filled extremely tender vesicles grouped on the left labia
  b. Papular skin-colored lesion with indentation at the center that contains curdy white material
  c. Raised beefy red nodule with sharply defined borders on the vaginal wall
  d. Flesh-colored cauliflowerlike lesion on the moist surface at the right vaginal introitus

3. Which diagnostic test is appropriate at this visit, assuming that none has been done in the preceding 12 months?

  a. Darkfield examination of fluid from lesion
  b. Tzanck smear
  c. Pap smear
  d. Microhemagglutination assay (MHA-TP)

4. When the NP informs Grace of a suspected diagnosis of genital warts, a sexually transmitted infection, she begins to cry. She says her husband has already accused her of "playing around." She says she has been faithful throughout her marriage and had only one previous sexual partner. Which understanding should the NP have about this scenario?

  a. Grace is obviously not being completely truthful about her sexual history.
  b. Grace's husband undoubtedly has genital warts that she has not noticed.
  c. Either Grace or her husband might have become infected in a previous relationship without their knowledge.
  d. Grace must have acquired the virus from a nonsexual source.

5. After careful consideration, the decision is made to treat Grace's genital warts with TCA. Which of the following statements about this topical agent is *true*?

  a. TCA will be liberally applied to the lesion in gel form and washed off 4 hours later.
  b. TCA is effective for external warts but not those on the vaginal mucosa.
  c. TCA is contraindicated in pregnancy.
  d. TCA is applied once per week during an office visit.

6. Brad has been diagnosed with HPV. He has several small lesions on his penile shaft and the decision is made to treat them with podofilox 0.5%. The NP provides instructions and demonstrates the first application during Brad's clinic visit. Which comment made by Brad after the instruction demonstrates a need for *further* instruction?

  a. "I will apply the solution morning and night for 3 days, then use none for the next 4 days."
  b. "I will wash the medication off my penis 6 to 10 hours after it is applied."
  c. "I should not have intercourse during this treatment."
  d. "A local irritation is common with this medication."

7. Donna, a pregnant client with a genital wart, is provided with extensive information about the infection and treatment by her NP. Which information indicates that Donna has understood the instructions provided?

  a. She asks for a prescription for imiquimod cream 5%, which she plans to apply herself.
  b. She tells her parents that the infection means she must have a Cesarean delivery.
  c. She informs her husband that their baby is very likely to have respiratory problems because of her infection.
  d. She tells her husband that the wart may resolve spontaneously after delivery.

8. Jim is an NP who works in a free clinic where podophyllin continues to be used to treat genital HPV. For which client is podophyllin contraindicated?

  a. An uncircumcised man
  b. A man with a history of seizures
  c. A lactating woman
  d. A woman allergic to nickel

9. Which follow-up is appropriate for a woman whose genital warts have resolved?

  a. Pap smears every 6 months for 1 year
  b. Colposcopic examination within the next 3 months
  c. Reevaluation in 3 months
  d. Weekly visits for 4 weeks

10. Which statement about transmission of genital warts is accurate?

  a. Consistent use of condoms with spermicide prevents transmission.
  b. Once lesions have been surgically excised, there is no possibility of transmission.
  c. Sexual partners of infected women should be presumptively treated.
  d. Abstinence is the only certain way of preventing transmission.

H

Answers and Rationales

1. *Answer:* **a** (assessment)
  Rationale: OCPs increase susceptibility to HPV (Richart, 2000).

2. *Answer:* **d** (analysis/diagnosis)
  Rationale: Condyloma acuminata, a cauliflower-type lesion, is a classic type of HPV genital wart.

3. *Answer:* **c** (analysis/diagnosis)
  Rationale: If the client has not had a Pap smear within the preceding year, one should be performed at this visit. There are types of HPV virus that cause cervical dysplasia, noted by Pap smear (Chopra & Tyring, 1999).

4. *Answer:* c (analysis/diagnosis)

Rationale: HPV is a virus that has a long incubation, an asymptomatic course in many clients, and the potential for reactivation (ARHP, 2000).

5. *Answer:* d (implementation/plan)

Rationale: TCA is a provider-administered treatment that is applied once per week.

6. *Answer:* b (evaluation)

Rationale: Podofilox is not washed off; imiquimod is applied at bedtime and washed off the next morning 6 to 10 hours after application (Richart, 2000).

7. *Answer:* d (evaluation)

Rationale: Although genital warts may become larger and more friable during pregnancy, they generally resolve before the postpartum checkup at 4 to 6 weeks (Richart, 2000).

8. *Answer:* c (implementation/plan)

Rationale: Podophyllin resin continues to be used in some clinics because it remains on the CDC list of treatments; however, it is contraindicated in pregnancy, lactation, immunocompromised clients, and those with poor circulation (Richart, 2000).

9. *Answer:* c (implementation/plan)

Rationale: Women with genital warts do not need more frequent Pap smears or colposcopy as a result of their genital lesions. They should be followed at 3 months because recurrence of warts is most common in the first 3 months (Richart, 2000).

10. *Answer:* d (evaluation)

Rationale: The only certain preventive strategy is abstinence (Richart, 2000).

HYPERLIPIDEMIA *Pamela Kidd*

OVERVIEW
Definition

Hyperlipidemia is excessive accumulation of one or more of the lipoproteins in the blood. Primary hyperlipidemia is hereditary or spontaneous genetic disorder of metabolism. Secondary hyperlipidemia is caused by disease (e.g., diabetes mellitus, renal disease, hypothyroid). Clinical trials have clearly demonstrated a relationship between high cholesterol levels and coronary artery disease (CAD). Reduction of cholesterol levels reduces the incidence of cardiac events.

Incidence

- In the United States, approximately 120 million people have cholesterol at 200 mg/dL or higher.
- Hypercholesterolemia incidence is 1 in 500.
- Prevalence increases with age.
- The condition is more common in men than in women.

Pathophysiology

Hyperlipidemia results from excessive production of lipids, defective removal of lipids, or both excessive production and defective removal.

Factors Increasing Susceptibility

- History of coronary heart disease (CHD), such as myocardial infarction (MI) or angina
- At least two of following:
  - Male gender
  - Family history of CAD (e.g., MI, sudden death of parent or sibling younger than 55 years)
  - Cigarette smoking

- Hypertension
- Low high-density lipoprotein (HDL) cholesterol levels (lower than 35 mg/dL in men, lower than 45 mg/dL in women)
- Diabetes mellitus
- History of cerebrovascular accident (CVA) or peripheral vascular disease
- Obesity (more than 30% above desirable weight)
- Sedentary lifestyle
- Stress
- Heredity

Emerging Risk Factors

NOTE: *At time of publication, homocysteine level higher than 15 mmol/L and lipoprotein (a) levels higher than 30 mg/dL for whites and Asians (McCormick & Deeg, 2000) are additional risk factors, although not commonly measured.*

- Impaired fasting glucose (National Cholesterol Education Program [NCEP], 2001)

Protective Factors
- Exercise
- Estrogen
- HDL higher than 40 mg/dL

ASSESSMENT: SUBJECTIVE/HISTORY
Symptoms

No symptoms are pathognomic for hypercholesterolemia; however, 35% to 55% of affected persons may report abdominal pain. These episodes are related to marked elevations of triglyceride levels (higher than 1000 mg/dL). Client may also have nausea, vomiting, borborygmi, and diarrhea.

Past Medical History

- Ask about past history of elevated cholesterol, exercise, smoking, and stress.
- Determine CHD or CHD risk equivalents: Diabetes, peripheral artery disease, abdominal aortic aneurysm, carotid artery disease, hypertension blood pressure higher than 140/90 or taking antihypertensive agent, low HDL (lower than 40 mg/dL), family history of premature CHD (in men, first degree relative younger than 55 years; in female, first degree relative younger than 65 years), age of client (men 45 or older, women 55 or older) (NCEP, 2001).

Medication History

OCPs, anabolic steroids, and corticosteroids can decrease HDL and increase low-density lipoproteins (LDLs).

Family History

Ask about family history of elevated cholesterol and CHD. Age at occurrence in first-degree relative (see previously noted CHD risk equivalent).

Dietary History

- High intake of saturated fatty acids increases risk.
- High intake of dietary cholesterol increases risk.
- High intake of total calories resulting in obesity increases risk.
- Inquire about diet. Consider 24-hour diet recall or diet diary. Caffeine may increase cholesterol.

ASSESSMENT: OBJECTIVE/PHYSICAL EXAMINATION

Physical Examination

A problem-oriented physical examination should be conducted, with particular attention to vital signs, weight (obesity), and general appearance. Note the following:

- Skin: xanthomas
- Eyes: arcus senilis in clients younger than 50 years (congested fundi)
- Cardiovascular: carotid bruits, peripheral vascular insufficiency

Diagnostic Procedures

Initial evaluation should include the following:

- Fasting lipid profile (total cholesterol, triglyceride, LDL, and HDL)
- To rule out underlying disease that may have elevated lipid levels, obtain the following:
  - Fasting blood glucose level
  - Glycosylated hemoglobin (HbA1c) level
- Thyroid-stimulating hormone level (hyperthyroidism can increase cholesterol level)

- Creatinine kinase level
- Liver function tests

Results. Cholesterol level lower than 200 mg/dL is desirable, 201 to 239 mg/dL is borderline, and higher than 240 mg/dL is high.

- HDL: higher than 40 mg/dL is desirable
- LDL:
  - Very high is 190 mg/dL or higher
  - High LDL 160 mg/dL to 189 mg/dl
  - Borderline: 130 to 159 mg/dL
  - Optimal: below 100 mg/dL

Triglycerides levels lower than 200 mg/dL is desirable, 200 to 400 mg/dL is borderline high, 400 to 1000 mg/dL is high, and higher than 1000 mg/dL is very high. Needs to be fasting specimen.

Children

Screening should be done for children who have a family history of premature CAD (younger than 55 years) or parental hypercholesterolemia (levels higher than 240 mg/dL).

DIAGNOSIS

- Accurate diagnosis is important. Consider secondary lipoprotein disorders.
- LDL level higher than 190 mg/dL indicates genetic form of hypercholesterolemia. Refer to specialist.
- For elevated triglycerides (higher than 200 mg/dL), treat as if LDL were high.
- In the case of low HDL (less than 40 mg/dL), strive for reaching target goal of LDL, focus on weight reduction and increase exercise.

THERAPEUTIC PLAN
Nonpharmacologic Treatment

A therapeutic plan for treatment of hyperlipidemia is shown in Table 3-51.

Cholesterol Reduction in Older Adults

The benefit of lowering cholesterol in older adults has not been clearly defined. Research shows a decreased mortality among persons (up to age 75) with CAD who follow a low-cholesterol diet and take medications.

Cholesterol Reduction in Children

- Dietary changes appear to reduce LDL levels in children with familial elevated cholesterol levels. However, long-term benefits of cholesterol reduction in children are unclear. Studies are ongoing to determine long-term benefits and medication safety and efficacy.
- Dietary management is first line of defense.
- Step One diet is recommended by the American Heart Association as "prudent" for the U.S. population.
- Step Two diet decreases cholesterol and fat intake further (Table 3-52).

H

TABLE **3-51**   Therapeutic Plan for Treatment of Hyperlipidemia

TREATMENT	INITIATION LDL LEVEL	GOAL LDL LEVEL
DIETARY TREATMENT		
Without CHD with no or one risk factor*	160 mg/dL or higher	160 mg/dL or lower
Without CHD but more than two risk factors and 10-year risk of 20% or less	130 mg/dL or higher	160 mg/dL or lower
If 3 month of diet changes alone is ineffective, drug therapy may be initiated to achieve goal with CHD or CHD risk equivalents	100 mg/dL or higher	100 mg/dL or lower
DRUG TREATMENT PLUS DIET		
Without CHD with no or one risk factor†	190 mg/dL or higher	160 mg/dL or lower
Without CHD but more than two risk factors and 10-year risk between 10% and 20%	130 mg/dL or higher	130 mg/dL or lower
and 10-year risk less than 10%	160 mg/dL or higher	130 mg/dL or lower
With CHD or CHD risk equivalents	130 mg/dL or higher	100 mg/dL or lower

*To calculate percent of risk of development of CHD over time, risk factors are assessed using the Framingham risk scoring method, which includes age, total cholesterol, HDL level, systolic blood pressure, cigarette smoking adjusted for gender.
†Severe risk factor (smoking, poorly controlled hypertension, very low HDL, strong family history of premature CHD), or 10 year risk approaching 10%.
From Expert Panel on Detection, Evaluation, and Treatment of High Blood Cholesterol in Adults. (2001, May). *Third report of the National Cholesterol Education Program.* National Institutes of Health Publication No 01-3670.
CHD, Coronary heart disease; *LDL,* low-density lipoprotein.

TABLE **3-52**   Dietary Management of Hyperlipidemia

RECOMMENDED GUIDELINES	STEP ONE	STEP TWO
Total fat	Less than 30% of total calories	Less than 30% of total calories
Saturated fatty acids	Less than 10% of total calories	Less than 7% of total calories
Polyunsaturated fatty acids	10% or less of total calories	10% or less of total calories
Monounsaturated fatty acids	10% to 15% of total calories	10% to 15% of total calories
Carbohydrates	55% or more of total calories	55% or more of total calories
Protein	15% of total calories	15% of total calories
Cholesterol	Less than 300 mg/dL/day	Less than 200 mg/dL/day

Modified from U.S. Preventive Services Task Force (1996). *Guide to clinical preventive services* (2nd ed.). Baltimore: Williams & Wilkins.

- Saturated fats should be less than 7% of total calories consumed, and cholesterol level should be lower than 200 mg/dL. Reduce consumption of trans-fatty acids.
- Use plant stanols/sterols (2 g/dL) (Benecol, Take Charge). These agents impede absorption of cholesterol.
- Consume 10 to 25 g/day of fiber.
- Regular exercise enhances fatty acid oxidation and glycogen storage, increasing HDL formation, triglyceride clearance, and insulin sensitivity. These changes cause reductions in serum lipid levels. HDL levels rise approximately 20% and LDL levels may decrease as much as 10%.
- Smoking cessation is important. Individuals who smoke tend to have lower HDL and higher very-low-density lipoproteins (VLDLs) levels. All clients with hyperlipidemias should be counseled to stop smoking.

Pharmacologic Treatment

Pharmaceutical agents should be tried if client does not respond to 3 months of intensive dietary therapy. Dietary therapy should continue during drug therapy. For those older than age 75 with CAD, consider pharmacologic therapy if necessary to achieve targets if client is physically and socially active with few or no comorbidities.

Statins inhibit cholesterol synthesis in the liver. They may increase liver enzymes. Baseline liver enzyme levels are obtained and again after starting or increasing the dose. If they elevate (defined as three times the upper limit of normal on two separate occasions with at least 1 week between measurements) with statin use, discontinue the drug to avoid the increased risk of liver cancer.

Four categories of medication are available for reduction of cholesterol levels (Table 3-53).

Combination Drug Therapy. If response with one drug and diet is inadequate, consider adding a second drug. Statins are first line drug; if, after 6 weeks, goal has not been reached, increase dose or add bile acid sequestrant or nicotinic acid. If, after 12 weeks, goal has not been reached, refer to lipid specialist.

TABLE **3-53**   Comparison of Pharmacologic Agents in Treating Hyperlipidemia

CLASS	LDL LEVEL EFFECT	HDL LEVEL EFFECT	TRIGLYCERIDE LEVEL EFFECT	CONSIDERATIONS
Fibric acids (gemfibrozil)	5% to 15% decrease	14% to 20% increase	20% to 50% decrease	Perform baseline liver function tests. Take 30 minutes before meals. Warfarin (Coumadin) levels may increase, monitor closely.
Niacin (nicotinic acid)	10% to 25% decrease	15% to 35% increase	20% to 50% decrease	Perform baseline liver function tests. May take with aspirin 30 minutes before to decrease flushing. Use cautiously with insulin resistance and type 2 DM because may increase insulin resistance. May worsen gout.
Bile acid sequestrants (colestipol)	10% to 20% decrease	3% to 5% decrease	May increase	Perform baseline liver function tests. Take other medications 1 hour before or 4 hours after using this drug. Use cautiously in type 2 DM because of effect on triglycerides. Increase fiber in diet when using to avoid constipation.
Statins (Lipitor)	20% to 60% decrease	5% to 15% increase	10% to 40% decrease	Perform baseline liver function tests. Drugs that inhibit Cytochrome P-450 (calcium channel blockers, azole antifungals) increase serum stain concentration and can produce rhabdomyolysis.

DM, Diabetes mellitus; *HDL*, high-density lipoproteins; *LDL*, low-density lipoprotein.

H

Other Drug Therapy. Estrogen may increase HDL levels and lower LDL levels. Estrogens have been shown to be beneficial to postmenopausal women with preexistent CHD. They may increase triglyceride levels and predispose to breast cancer. The increase of triglycerides is less with the transdermal form.

Client Education

- For clients 20 to 70 years old, measure cholesterol level every 5 years.
- Discuss healthy diet; encourage use of diet diary, exercise, smoking cessation.
- Statins should be taken in the evening when cholesterol synthesis is at its highest.
- Fasting lipoprotein profile should be obtained every 5 years in adults age 20 and older.
- Alcohol intake for men should be limited to two beers or two glasses of wine or two shots of spirits/d; intake for women should be limited to one beer or one glass of wine or one shot of spirit/d.

NOTE: *Total calories must be adjusted to reflect this intake to prevent weight gain (Lichenstein, Ornish, Rippe, & Willett, 1999).*

- Teach portion size.

Referral

- Referral may be made to lipid specialists if target goal has not been reached within 12 weeks. Those with genetic hyperlipidemias should be followed up by specialists. Refer to dietitian.

Prevention

Hyperlipidemia can be prevented by lowering lipid levels. If lipid levels are lower, CAD is reduced by 37% and coronary death is reduced by 42% (McCormick & Deeg, 2000).

EVALUATION/FOLLOW-UP

- After drug therapy is started, lipids should be checked in 4 weeks and at 3 months.
- Once target goals of LDL and cholesterol have been achieved, total cholesterol should be measured every 4 months, with a full lipid analysis every year.

Complications

- CHD
- Coronary death

REFERENCES

American Heart Association. Dietary guidelines. Dallas, TX: Author.

Lichenstein, A., Ornish, D., Rippe, J., & Willett, W. (1999). The best diet for healthy adults. *Patient Care for the Nurse Practitioner* 2(11), 30-31, 34, 37-40, 43-44, 47-48, 51-52.

McCormick, J., & Deeg, M. (2000). Pharmacologic treatment of dyslipidemia. *American Journal of Nursing. 100*(2), 55-60.

National Cholesterol Education Program (NCEP). (2001). *Expert panel on detection, evaluation, and treatment of high blood cholesterol in adults. Third report of the National Cholesterol Education Program (NCEP)*. National Heart, Lung, and Blood Institute: May 2001. National Institutes of Health Publication No. 01-3670.

United States Preventive Services Task Force (1996). *Guide to clinical preventive services* (2nd ed.). Baltimore: Williams & Wilkins.

Review Questions

1. Calvin Smith (47 years old) had an MI 2 years ago. His cholesterol level is 245 mg/dL, with LDL of 159 mg/dL and HDL of 45 mg/dL. The treatment goal for his LDL cholesterol level should be which of the following?:

  a. 190 mg/dL
  b. 160 mg/dL
  c. 130 mg/dL
  d. 100 mg/dL

2. Which of the following subjective factors should most influence your choice for treatment for hyperlipidemia?

  a. Obesity
  b. Sedentary lifestyle
  c. Family history of elevated cholesterol
  d. High intake of dietary cholesterol

3. Cardiovascular risk and treatment goals related to hyperlipidemia are determined by which factor?

  a. Total cholesterol
  b. LDL
  c. HDL
  d. VLDL

4. Which of the following physical examination findings would lead you to suspect hyperlipidemia?

  a. Increased liver size
  b. Xanthoma of inner canthus of both eyes
  c. Obesity
  d. Decreased peripheral vision

5. All of the following would be the initial treatment prescribed for a 40-year-old woman, cholesterol 297 mg/dL, LDL 189 mg/dL, triglycerides 400mg/dL, and who is in general good health without preexisting conditions *except:*

  a. Lifestyle changes
  b. Step Two dietary plan of the American Heart Association
  c. Estrogen therapy
  d. Use of pharmaceutical agents

6. What is the most appropriate recommendation for screening of cholesterol in children?

  a. Screen all children.
  b. Screen children who have family members with elevated cholesterol levels.
  c. Only obese children should be screened.
  d. Because treatment for elevated cholesterol in children is controversial, no children should be screened.

7. Bev, a 50-year-old woman with a history of elevated cholesterol (340 mg/dL), LDL of 220 mg/dL, and a history of recent angioplasty, has been started on a 3-hydroxy-3-methylglutaryl coenzyme A (statin) drug. What information is crucial to obtain before beginning this drug?

- **a.** CBC
- **b.** Renal panel
- **c.** Liver panel
- **d.** Thyroid-stimulating hormone

8. Bev has been taking the statin drug for 1 month. She reports muscle weakness and has noticed brown discoloration of her urine. What is the appropriate action for the NP to take at this time?

- **a.** Continue her antilipemic, but check her laboratory values.
- **b.** Stop her antilipemic and encourage increased hydration.
- **c.** Increase her antilipemic dosage.
- **d.** Send her to the emergency department.

Answers and Rationales

1. *Answer:* **d** (analysis/diagnosis)
Rationale: Any client with known CAD should have as a treatment goal reduction of LDL levels to lower than 100 mg/dL (NCEP, 2001).

2. *Answer:* **c** (assessment)
Rationale: Clients who have a family history are more likely to require pharmacologic treatment to reduce their hyperlipidemia (NCEP, 2001).

3. *Answer:* **b** (implementation/plan)
Rationale: Treatment for and risk of CAD are determined by the client's LDL level.

4. *Answer:* **b** (assessment)
Rationale: Xanthomas are dermatologic indications of elevated cholesterol. They are commonly seen in the inner canthus of the eyelids, as well as behind the knees, skin folds, and scars. Enlarged liver can be secondary to liver disease. Obesity predisposes one to hyperlipidemia but it does not indicate high cholesterol.

5. *Answer:* **c** (implementation/plan)
Rationale: Initial treatment for most clients consists of dietary changes and exercise. Clients with no or one risk factor and LDL higher than 160mg/dL should be started on pharmacologic therapy in conjunction with diet (NCEP, 2001). Estrogen increases HDLs but may also increase triglycerides (this client's triglycerides are already elevated). Estrogen has been shown to be beneficial in postmenopausal women with CHD only. This woman is most likely premenopausal.

6. *Answer:* **b** (analysis/diagnosis)
Rationale: Only children who have family members with elevated cholesterol levels or family member with premature CAD (younger than 55 years at time of diagnosis) should be screened. The long-term benefit of cholesterol reduction in children is unclear; however, for those who have known elevated cholesterol levels, dietary changes can be initiated.

7. *Answer:* **c** (implementation/plan)
Rationale: Statins may cause elevated hepatic function tests (in approximately 1% of clients.) A baseline liver function test is essential before starting therapy.

8. *Answer:* **b** (evaluation)
Rationale: Statins can cause myopathy in approximately 0.1% of clients. The myopathy is reversible if the drug is discontinued and hydration is encouraged. If the drug is not stopped, severe myopathy (rhabdomyolysis) can occur.

HYPERTENSION *Pamela Kidd*

OVERVIEW
Definition

Primary (Essential) Hypertension. Primary hypertension is an elevation of blood pressure of higher than 140 mm Hg systolic and higher than 89 mm Hg diastolic on the average of two or more readings taken at each of two or more visits.

Urgent Hypertension. Urgent hypertension is an elevated diastolic blood pressure (DBP) between 120 and 160 mm Hg without symptoms or acute retinopathy.

Severe, Accelerated, or Malignant Hypertension. Severe, accelerated, or malignant hypertension is an elevation of DBP to higher than 120 mm Hg with evidence of target-organ damage such as retinal hemorrhages, exudates, or papilledema, left ventricular hypertrophy or dysfunction, and renal or cerebrovascular injury.

Isolated Systolic Hypertension. Isolated systolic hypertension (ISH) is persistently elevated systolic blood pres-

sure (SBP) higher than 160 mm Hg, with DBP less than 90 mm Hg.

Hypertensive Crisis. A hypertensive crisis is severe elevation of DBP higher than 120 to 130 mm Hg; this is considered an emergency in the presence of acute or ongoing target-organ damage (rapid or progressive deterioration of the CNS, myocardial, hematologic, or renal function).

Incidence

Approximately 50 million Americans have elevated blood pressure that requires monitoring or drug therapy. The prevalence increases with age and is greater for blacks than for whites.

Pathophysiology

Hypertension results from an increase in the total peripheral resistance caused by arteriolar constriction. This may be due to a primary problem with blood pressure regulation in which there is no identifiable cause. In some cases,

H

the arteriolar constriction may be due to some secondary underlying disorder.

The central and autonomic nervous systems regulate blood pressure through the stimulation of alpha and beta receptors on the arterioles and venules. The kidneys also provide a humoral response to maintain blood pressure in the presence of decreased blood flow to the kidneys, which results in the release of renin and its subsequent vasoconstrictors, angiotensin and aldosterone. Pathologic disruption in any of these systems can lead to hypertension.

Factors Increasing Susceptibility

- Age
- Ethnicity
- Less educated
- Lower socioeconomic status
- Cigarette smoking
- Sedentary lifestyle
- Obesity

Protective Factors

- Not smoking
- Low-fat, low sodium diet
- Genetics

ASSESSMENT: SUBJECTIVE/HISTORY
Symptoms

- Ask about smoking, employment and family status, educational level, leisure and exercise activities, and stress management.
- Symptoms may include the following:
  - Blurred vision
  - Chest pain
  - Claudication
  - Dizziness
  - Dyspnea
  - Fatigue
  - Flushing
  - Headaches
  - Hematuria
  - Muscle cramps
  - Palpitations
  - Tingling or cold extremities
  - Weakness, usually as a result of end-organ damage or the underlying primary disorder
- Clients with early primary hypertension are usually free of symptoms.

Past Medical History

- Hyperlipidemia
- Diabetes mellitus
- Cardiovascular disease (angina, MI, heart failure)
- Cerebrovascular disease (transient ischemic attack [TIA], CVA, or seizures)

- Secondary causes for hypertension include the following:
  - Polycystic kidneys
  - Renovascular disease
  - Aortic coarctation
  - Cushing's disease
  - Pheochromocytoma
  - OCPs
  - Chronic alcohol abuse
  - Gout
  - Toxemia of pregnancy

Medication History

OCPs, steroids, NSAIDs, nasal decongestants, cold remedies, appetite suppressants, sodium bicarbonate products (antacids), licorice, tricyclic antidepressants, monoamine oxidase inhibitors, cyclosporine, and erythropoietin can increase blood pressure or interfere with blood pressure therapy.

Family History

- There is a higher incidence in children who exhibit other risk factors for cardiovascular disease or have hypertensive parents.
- Ask about anyone in the family with a history of the following:
  - Premature CAD
  - Peripheral vascular disease
  - Diabetes mellitus
  - Hypertension
  - Stroke, TIA, or seizures
  - Renal disease
  - Dyslipidemia

Dietary History

- Diet (especially sodium, cholesterol, and fat intake)
- Alcohol use

ASSESSMENT: OBJECTIVE/PHYSICAL EXAMINATION
Physical Examination

- Evaluate blood pressure per the following:
  - Obtain two or more blood pressure readings at least 2 minutes apart in supine or seated positions and after standing for 2 minutes.
  - The client should not drink coffee or smoke cigarettes within the 30 minutes preceding the evaluation.
  - Check blood pressure in both arms on at least one occasion to verify that results are equivalent.
  - The appropriate cuff size should have the bladder encircle at least 80% of the arm above the antecubital space.
  - Record pulse pressure, particularly in older clients. This is the difference between SBP and DBP (denotes arterial stiffness).

- Record height and weight measurements.
- Perform funduscopic examination of the eyes for arteriolar narrowing, nicking, hemorrhages, exudates, and papilledema.
- Examine the neck for carotid bruits, distended veins, or thyromegaly.
- Examine the heart for increased rate, size, precordial heave, clicks, murmurs, arrhythmias, and S_3 or S_4.
- Examine the abdomen for bruits, enlarged kidneys, masses, or abnormal aortic pulsations.
- Examine the extremities for decreased or absent peripheral arterial pulsations, bruits, or edema.
- Perform a neurologic assessment.

Diagnostic Procedures

Laboratory testing may be used to assess cardiovascular risk factors as well as evaluate end organ function or secondary cause of hypertension. Tests may include the following:

- Urinalysis
- Lipid profile
- Comprehensive metabolic panel (potassium, calcium, creatinine, uric acid, magnesium)
- ECG
- Fasting blood glucose
- Thyroid-stimulating hormone
- CBC

DIAGNOSIS

- Differential diagnosis should focus on distinguishing true primary hypertension from pseudohypertension caused by faulty blood pressure reading and from secondary hypertension.
- Suspect underlying pathologic condition for secondary hypertension in the following cases:
  - Drug therapy is ineffective in the compliant client.
  - Elevated blood pressure occurs in individuals younger than 25 or older than 60 years in the absence of family history.
  - Associated symptoms occur (edema, abnormal pulses or heart sounds, hirsutism, stria, palpitations, perspiration, and dizziness).
- Classification of hypertension: The various levels of blood pressure for adults, including four stages of hypertension, are discussed below.

Hypertension in Children and Adolescents

Children and adolescents with a persistently elevated blood pressure (higher than 95th percentile for children of the same age and sex) are at risk for development of the same complications as in adults. Secondary hypertension is more common in children than in adults. Secondary hypertension is seen most often in infancy and late childhood.

THERAPEUTIC PLAN
Overall Plan

Normal
- SBP less than 130 mm Hg, DBP less than 85 mm Hg
- Recheck in 2 years (Grimm, 2001)

High Normal
- SBP 130 to 139 mm Hg, DBP 85 to 89 mm Hg
- Lifestyle modification
- Recheck in 1 year

Stage 1
- SBP 140 to 159 mm Hg, DBP 90 to 99 mm Hg
- One or more risk factors (not including diabetes)
- No target organ damage

NOTE: *Target organ damage is left ventricle hypertrophy, angina, previous MI, coronary revascularization, heart failure, stroke, TIA, neuropathy, peripheral artery disease, and retinopathy.*

- No cardiovascular disease
- Drug therapy initiated if lifestyle modifications not effective within 6 months; recheck/confirm in 2 months (Grimm, 2001)

Stage 1 with Diabetes, Target Organ Damage, Cardiovascular Disease
- Start drug therapy in conjunction with lifestyle modification immediately.

Stage 2
- SBP 160 to 179 mm Hg, DBP 100 to 109 mm Hg
- Lifestyle modification
- Initiate drug therapy
- Follow-up within 1 month

Stage 3
- Severe
- SBP 180 to 209 mm Hg, DBP 110 to 119 mm Hg
- Lifestyle modification
- Drug therapy initiated
- Two or three agents if necessary
- Follow-up within 1 week

Stage 4
- Very severe
- SBP higher than 210 mm Hg, DBP higher than 120 mm Hg
- Lifestyle modification
- Initiate drug therapy
- Often necessary to start with two or three agents
- Follow-up in 1 week

If target-organ disease is present, consider hospitalization with immediate drug therapy. Hospitalization is

H

almost always required for DBP higher than 130 mm Hg. Therapeutic goals are 125/75 mm Hg in clients with proteinuria (usually diabetic); 130/85 mm Hg in clients who are diabetic or have renal disease.

Nonpharmacologic Treatment

Treatment in Adults
- Lose weight if overweight.
- Limit alcohol intake to less than 1 ounce ethanol/day (24 ounces beer, 8 ounces wine, or 2 ounces 100-proof whiskey) for men or 0.5 ounces for women.
- Perform daily aerobic exercise for 30 to 45 minutes.
- Reduce sodium intake to less than 2.4 g sodium.
- Maintain adequate dietary intake of potassium, calcium, and magnesium.
- Stop smoking and decrease dietary saturated fat and cholesterol.
- Reducing fat intake decreases caloric intake for weight control.

Treatment in Children
- The underlying cause, severity, and potential complications should determine intensity and type of therapy required.
- Lifestyle modifications can be used as initial therapy.

Pharmacologic Treatment

Adult Treatment
- Diuretics and beta-blockers are preferred because they have shown a reduction in cardiovascular morbidity and mortality in controlled clinical trials.
- Calcium-channel antagonists, angiotensin-converting enzyme (ACE) inhibitors, alpha^1-receptor blockers and alpha-beta blockers are also effective in reducing blood pressure, although no long-term studies have been done on mortality and morbidity.
- Monotherapy is used for 4 months; if goal has not been reached, add another drug in a different class. If client needs a larger reduction than 14/10 mm Hg to reach goal, start with combination therapy (Arnow, Bakris, & Weart, 2000).

Special Considerations (Table 3-54)
- For hypertension and heart failure or nephropathy, use diuretic and ACE inhibitor or angiotensin receptor blocker (ARB).
- For hypertension and previous MI, use diuretic and beta-blocker.
- For hypertension and hyperlipidemia, use ACE inhibitor and statin.
- For hypertension and diabetes (no proteinuria), use ACE inhibitor and low dose diuretic.
- For hypertension and diabetes (with proteinuria) and hypertension (with or without proteinuria in blacks), use ACE inhibitor and calcium channel blocker.
- Blacks respond better to diuretics and calcium channel antagonists than to beta-blockers or ACE inhibitors. Older adults respond to all classes. No differences in treatment response have been found between genders.
- Undesirable side effects of drug therapy may worsen quality of life and play a role in noncompliance.
- Costs of drug therapy, routine laboratory tests, follow-up office visits, and time off from work should be considered in selecting therapy.
- Choose medications that may help treat coexisting disease.
- For the pregnant client, use aldomet.

Treatment in Children
- Drug therapy should be reserved for clients with blood pressure higher than the 99th percentile or those who do not respond to lifestyle modifications.
- Children with insulin-dependent diabetes mellitus and primary renal disease should be treated with drug therapy to slow disease progression.
- Agents used in adults are also effective in young persons.

TABLE **3-54** Special Considerations in Antihypertensive Therapy

COMORBID CONDITIONS	DRUG TO USE	DRUG TO AVOID
Heart failure	ACE inhibitor, ARB, diuretic	Beta-blocker, calcium antagonist (non-DHP)
Diabetes	ACE inhibitor, calcium antagonist, low dose diuretic	Beta-blocker
Dyslipidemia	Alpha-blocker	Beta-blocker (non-ISA), high-dose diuretic
Prostatism	Alpha-blocker	None
Gout	None more favorable	Thiazide diuretic
Osteoporosis	Thiazide diuretic	None
Migraine	Beta-blocker (non-ISA) calcium antagonist (non-DHP)	None

Non-ISA atenolol, metoprolol may have greater effect on heart rate and peripheral vasoconstriction,
Non-DHP verapamil, diltiazem inhibits sinus and atrioventricular node automaticity and conductivity.
Modified from Ross, B., & Fischer, R. (1998). Pharmacologic management of hypertension. *ADVANCE for Nurse Practitioners* 6(4), 27-28, 31-35.
ACE, Angiotensin-converting enzyme; *ARB,* angiotensin receptor blocker; *DHP,* dihydropyridine; *ISA,* intrinsic sympathomimetic activity.

Client Education

- Educate on side effects of drugs (e.g. erectile dysfunction).
- Instruct to make postural changes slowly.

Referral

Refer to hypertension specialist in the following cases:
- Refractory hypertension
- When secondary hypertension is suspected (DBP rises to 100 mm Hg after age 60, resistance develops in a previously effective regimen, renal dysfunction increases, spontaneous hypokalemia occurs [Aronow, Bakris, & Weart, 2000])

Prevention

- Attain ideal weight.
- Do not abuse tobacco.
- Drink alcohol moderately (as defined previously).
- Engage in regular aerobic exercise (as defined previously).
- Eat low fat, low sodium diet (as defined previously) (Ross & Fischer, 1998).

EVALUATION/FOLLOW-UP

The scheduling of follow-up should be modified by reliable information about past blood pressure measurements, other cardiovascular risk factors, or target-organ damage.

Once the client's blood pressure has stabilized, follow-up should be at 3- to 6-month intervals. Normotensive clients should be evaluated every 1 to 2 years. Annual evaluations should be performed for those clients with hereditary or medical risks.

COMPLICATIONS

Clients with hypertension are at risk for development of CHD, peripheral vascular disease, stroke, renal disease, and retinopathy.

REFERENCES

Aronow, W., Bakris, G., & Weart, C. (2000). Aiming for lower than 140/90 mm Hg. *Patient Care for the Nurse Practitioner 3*(4), 60-62, 65-66, 69-70, 74-76, 79-80.

Grimm, R. (2001). Cardiovascular risk factor management. A self-study supplement. *Clinician Reviews 11*(9), 4-9.

Joint National Committee on Detection, Evaluation and Treatment of High Blood Pressure (1997). *The sixth report of the Joint National Committee on detection, evaluation and treatment of high blood pressure.* Bethesda, MD: National Institutes of Health, U. S. Department of Health and Human Services. National Institutes of Health Publication No 98-4080.

Noyes, K. (2000). Hypertension. In D. Robinson, P. Kidd, & K. Rogers (Eds.), *Primary care across the lifespan.* St. Louis: Mosby.

Ross, B., & Fischer, R. (1998). Pharmacologic management of hypertension. *ADVANCE for Nurse Practitioners 6*(4), 27-28, 31-35.

Schumann, L., & Emerson, B. (1998). Diagnostic evaluation for hypertension. *Journal of the American Academy of Nurse Practitioners 10*(6), 269-280

United States Public Health Service, United States Department of Health and Human Services. (1997). Put prevention into practice. *Nurse Practitioner 9*(1), 27-31.

Review Questions

1. Which of the following diagnostic tests is *not* appropriate for a hypertension work-up?
   a. ECG
   b. CBC
   c. Sedimentation rate
   d. Urinalysis

2. The differential diagnosis for true primary hypertension includes which of the following?
   a. Pseudohypertension
   b. Polycystic kidneys
   c. Cushing's disease
   d. Pheochromocytoma

3. Which of the following *does not* suggest a secondary cause for hypertension?
   a. Drug therapy is ineffective in the compliant client.
   b. No associated symptoms are found.
   c. Elevated blood pressure occurs in client younger than 25 or older than 60 years.
   d. Family history is positive for stroke and hypertension.

4. Which of the following medications should not interfere with blood pressure therapy?
   a. OCPs
   b. Antibiotics
   c. Nasal decongestants
   d. NSAIDs

5. Once their blood pressure has stabilized, how often should hypertensive clients should be evaluated?
   a. Every 1 to 2 weeks
   b. Every 2 to 3 weeks
   c. Every 2 to 3 months
   d. Every 3 to 6 months

6. Which physical finding is *not* characteristic of hypertensive end-organ disease?
   a. Funduscopically visible hemorrhages
   b. Carotid bruits
   c. Cardiac hypertrophy Cushing's disease
   d. Pulmonary rhonchi

7. Which of the following statements is true?
   a. Drug therapy should be used as initial therapy for all children with diagnoses of hypertension.
   b. Concomitant disease should have no impact on the drug therapy selected.
   c. Blacks respond better to beta-blockers and ACE inhibitors.
   d. If a therapeutic response is inadequate, you may increase the dose or change to another agent.

H

8. A client in stage 2 hypertension should have which therapeutic plan?

    a. Lifestyle changes plus one drug class
    b. Lifestyle changes plus two or three drug classes
    c. Hospitalization
    d. Lifestyle changes, with drug therapy in 6 months if not effective

Answers and Rationales

1. *Answer:* **c** (assessment)
    Rationale: ECG, CBC, and urinalysis are appropriate diagnostic tests to assess for cardiovascular and renal function; they may exhibit end-organ damage as a result of hypertension.

2. *Answer:* **a** (evaluation)
    Rationale: Hypertension may be caused by faulty blood pressure readings as seen in pseudohypertension or because of secondary underlying pathologic conditions. The remaining options are secondary causes of HPT.

3. *Answer:* **b** (analysis/diagnosis)
    Rationale: Secondary hypertension usually is seen with other associated symptoms.

4. *Answer:* **b** (assessment)
    Rationale: Antibiotics do not have any vasoconstrictive properties with respect to the neural and humoral mechanisms that control blood pressure. OCPs, decongestants, and NSAIDs have been documented to interfere with these mechanisms.

5. *Answer:* **d** (evaluation)
    Rationale: Once their condition has been stabilized, hypertensive clients should be evaluated at 3- to 6-month intervals.

6. *Answer:* **d** (assessment)
    Rationale: Funduscopically visible hemorrhages, carotid bruits, and cardiac hypertrophy are indications of end-organ damage. Pulmonary rhonchi are not associated with hypertension.

7. *Answer:* **d** (implementation/plan)
    Rationale: Lifestyle modifications should be initial therapy for all children. Only children with blood pressures higher than the 99th percentile or who do not respond to lifestyle modifications should be considered for drug therapy. Concomitant disease, quality of life, and economic constraints should be considered in selecting drug therapy. Blacks respond better to diuretics and calcium channel antagonists.

8. *Answer:* **a** (implementation/plan)
    Rationale: Stage 1 can be managed with lifestyle modifications for 6 months. Stage 2 is managed with lifestyle and drug therapy (one agent). Stage three is managed with lifestyle, and may progress to 2 or 3 drug classes. Stage 4 is managed with lifestyle, and starts with 2 or 3 drug classes; hospitalization is a consideration if target-organ disease is present.

IMPETIGO   *Denise Robinson*

OVERVIEW
Definition

Impetigo is a contagious superficial infection of the epidermis caused by *Staphylococcus aureus* and *streptococcus pyogenes*. It also can extend into the dermis (ecthyma).

Incidence

- Impetigo is the most common skin infection in children.
- *S. aureus* is the most common cause of impetigo.

Pathophysiology

The infection begins as a primary infection in minor superficial breaks in the skin or as a secondary infection of preexisting conditions. Streptococcal disease typically produces crusted lesions and staphylococcal disease produces bullae. The incubation period is up to 3 days. Impetigo is communicable up to 48 hours after treatment is begun.

    Factors Increasing Susceptibility
- Warm temperature
- High humidity
- Presence of skin disease (especially atopic dermatitis)
- Age of client
- Crowded living conditions
- Poor hygiene
- Neglected minor trauma
- Previous antibiotic therapy
- Ecthyma (lesion of neglect that develops in areas of excoriations, insect bites, or minor trauma in people with diabetes, elderly clients, soldiers, and alcoholics)

ASSESSMENT: SUBJECTIVE/HISTORY
History of Present Illness

- Ask about the duration of the lesions (impetigo—days to weeks and ecthyma—weeks to months).
- Ask about itching, pain, and tenderness.
- Ask about recent minor trauma.
- Ask about exposure to others with skin rashes.

Past Medical History

Ask about recent chickenpox, scabies, insect bites, or atopic dermatitis.

Medications

Ask about recent antibiotic use.

Family History

Determine whether another member in the home recently has had impetigo.

Psychosocial History

Ask about living conditions.

Associated Symptoms

Fever may accompany impetigo.

ASSESSMENT: OBJECTIVE/PHYSICAL EXAMINATION

Physical Examination

- *Skin:* Superficial small vesicles or pustules that rupture, resulting in erosions (Fitzpatrick, 2001). A crust develops. Honey-yellow crusts often are seen but are not pathognomic. They are 1 to 3 cm in size. The lesions most often involve the face, nose and perioral and exposed areas. The lesions are scattered and discrete.
- Bullous impetigo consists of vesicles and bullae containing clear yellow fluid. With rupture the bullous lesions compress. This is most common in intertriginous sites.
- Ecthyma is ulceration with thick adherent crust, usually on distal extremities.
- Check the entire body for lesions.
- Check the lymph for regional lymphadenopathy.

Diagnostic Procedures

- Laboratory tests are not usually necessary.
- Culture reveals a gram-positive *cocci*, usually *s. aureus*.

DIAGNOSIS

- Impetigo: herpes simplex, scabies, contact dermatitis, chickenpox
- Bullous: contact dermatitis, herpes simplex, herpes zoster, thermal burns, bullous pemphigus, folliculitis
- Ecthyma: chronic ulcers, excoriated insect bites, venous stasis, atherosclerotic lesions

THERAPEUTIC PLAN

Pharmacologic Treatment

- Topical treatment: mupirocin ointment (Bactroban), use tid for 10 days on involved skin and to the nares for 10 to 14 days (works for 90% of cases)
- Systemic treatment for *S. aureus*:
  - Dicloxacillin 250 to 500 qid for 10 days
  - Cephalexin (Keflex) 250 to 500 qid for 10 days (in children, 40 to 50mg/kg/day for 10 days)
  - Amoxicillin with clavulanic acid (Augmentin) 20mg/kg tid for 10 days

- Systemic treatment for group A streptococcus:
  - Penicillin VK: 250mg qid for 10 days
  - Benzathine pcn 600,000 units IM in children younger than 6 and 1.2 million units in children older than 7.
- Systemic treatment for a client who is sensitive to penicillin:
  - Erythromycin 1 to 2 g/day qid for 10 days (in children, 40 mg/kg/day qid for 10 days)

Client Education

- Remove crusts by gentle washing with warm water and antibacterial soap.
- Wash linen and towels separately.
- Trim fingernails to minimize scratching.
- If left untreated, impetigo can lead to systemic infection (scarlet fever, glomerulonephritis) with serious complications.
- Children should not return to school until the lesions are clear or the client has been receiving antibiotics for 48 hours.
- Check all family member for lesions.
- Recurrent *s. aureus* can occur by recolonization from a family member or dog.

Referral/Consultation

- If the lesions appear in a newborn or infant, refer the client to a physician if there are symptoms of acute glomerulonephritis.
- Refer if there is no improvement in 4 days.

Prevention

Washing with benzoyl peroxide may help prevent impetigo.

EVALUATION/FOLLOW-UP

Client should follow-up by phone in 24 hours.

COMPLICATIONS

- Untreated impetigo can progress to ecthyma.
- Lesions can progress to invasive infection such as cellulitis or septicemia.
- Group A streptococcus can lead to guttate psoriasis, scarlet fever, and glomerulonephritis.
- Recurrence may result from failure to eradicate the disease from a family member.

REFERENCES

Fitzpatrick, T., Johnsen, R., Wolff, K., & Suurmond, D. (2001). *Color atlas & synopsis of clinical dermatology* (4th ed.). New York: McGraw Hill.

O'Dell, M. (1998). Skin and wound infections: an overview. *American Family Physician, 59.* Retrieved May 22, 2002, from http://www.aafp.org/afp/980515ap/odell.html.

Review Questions

1. Adam is a 7-year-old boy with a complaint of a skin lesion. It is a honey-crusted lesion located near his right nares. Which of the following historical data is consistent with a diagnosis of impetigo?

   a. He has many allergies.
   b. He scratched himself in the same area several days ago.
   c. His family has a history of early acne.
   d. Poor hygiene is a contributing factor.

2. Which of the following objective findings, in addition to a honey-colored crust, is typical of impetigo?

   a. Transient small vesicles that rupture, resulting in erosions
   b. Well-demarcated plaques of erythema and edema on which are imposed nonumbilicated vesicles
   c. Papules, flat topped, 1 to 10 mm, sharply defined, with white lines
   d. Scaling, sharply marginated plaques with or without pustules, usually at margins

3. Which of the following clients is most likely to contract impetigo?

   a. Steve, 47-year-old banker
   b. Gloria, a 22-year-old swimmer
   c. Ethan, a 7-year-old 2nd grader
   d. George, a 66-year-old farmer

4. Which of the following terms describes a superficial infection of the skin extending into the epidermis?

   a. Impetigo
   b. Ecthyma
   c. Pyoderma
   d. Tinea corporis

5. Which of the following organisms is most likely to cause impetigo?

   a. *Staphylococcus aureus*
   b. *Pseudomonas*
   c. *Streptococcus pneumoniae*
   d. *Escherichia coli*

6. Which of the following diagnostic tests are first line in cases of impetigo?

   a. Skin biopsy
   b. Gram stain or culture
   c. Cell pathology
   d. Wood's lamp illumination

7. Which of the following drug choices is the most appropriate for impetigo?

   a. Mupirocin (Bactroban)
   b. Erythromycin
   c. Macrolide antibiotic
   d. Hydrogen peroxide cleansing tid

8. The nurse practitioner (NP) discusses the need for prevention related to impetigo. Which of the following is an appropriate way to prevent impetigo?

   a. Good handwashing
   b. Avoiding small cuts
   c. Washing with benzoyl peroxide
   d. Applying antibiotic ointment prophylactically

Answers and Rationales

1. *Answer:* **b** (assessment)
   Rationale: Impetigo frequently arises as a primary infection in minor superficial breaks in the skin (Fitzpatrick, Johnsen, Wolff, & Suurmond, 2001).

2. *Answer:* **a** (assessment)
   Rationale: Impetigo starts as small vesicles that rupture, and then erosions develop. Honey-colored crusts are pathognomic of impetigo, but they are not always present. B describes contact dermatitis; c describes lichen planus, and d describes tinea corporis (Fitzpatrick, Johnsen, Wolff, & Suurmond, 2001).

3. *Answer:* **c** (assessment)
   Rationale: Children are most likely to contract impetigo (Fitzpatrick, Johnsen, Wolff, & Suurmond, 2001).

4. *Answer:* **a** (analysis/diagnosis)
   Rationale: Impetigo is a superficial infection of the epidermis. Ecthyma is an infection that extends into the dermis. Pyoderma is a general term addressing infections of the skin. Tinea is a dermatophyte infection of the skin (Fitzpatrick, Johnsen, Wolff, & Suurmond, 2001).

5. *Answer:* **a** (analysis/diagnosis)
   Rationale: *Staphylococcus aureus* is the most common organism to cause impetigo. It also can be caused by *streptococcus pyogenes* (Fitzpatrick, Johnsen, Wolff, & Suurmond, 2001).

6. *Answer:* **b** (analysis/diagnosis)
   Rationale: A Gram stain identifies whether the bacteria is gram positive or negative. The culture identifies the organism, and it usually includes a sensitivity to antibiotics. A cell biopsy is not needed for this diagnosis, nor is the Wood's lamp, which is useful in dermatophyte infestations. (Fitzpatrick, Johnsen, Wolff, & Suurmond, 2001).

7. *Answer:* **a** (implementation/plan)
   Rationale: Bactroban is an effective treatment for impetigo in 90% of cases (O'Dell, 1998).

8. *Answer:* **c** (implementation/plan)
   Rationale: Benzoyl peroxide wash is an effective way to prevent impetigo. Family members should be checked for signs of impetigo as well (Fitzpatrick, Johnsen, Wolff, & Suurmond, 2001).

INFERTILITY *Cheryl Pope Kish*

OVERVIEW
Definition

Infertility is the inability to achieve fertilization and pregnancy after 1 year of unprotected sexual intercourse. Primary infertility is used to describe couples who have never been able to conceive; secondary infertility describes those who have conceived at least once but are now experiencing difficulty achieving a pregnancy. Sterility is the inability to reproduce.

Incidence

- Infertility affects as many as 1 in 6 couples.
- From 1% to 2% of couples are involuntarily sterile.

Pathophysiology

To be fertile the following conditions must be present:

- Males must be able to produce normal quantity and quality of sperm that are transported through a nonobstructed genital tract to be deposited in the ejaculate at the woman's cervix during intercourse.
- Females must ovulate and have the ovum transported through a patent fallopian tube, where fertilization occurs, to a uterine cavity, where the endometrium is sufficiently developed to allow for implantation. Cervical mucus must be favorable for sperm to enter the reproductive tract.

Factors Affecting Fertility

- As a woman ages, her fertility decreases. The tendency to delay pregnancy until a woman is in her 30s and 40s means that fertility is naturally declining when pregnancy is first attempted. Endometriosis, which increases with age, also can affect fertility. As people age, they also are more likely to have chronic illness that may negatively affect fertility (e.g., diabetes, conditions requiring antihypertensive medication).
- Increasing rates of sexually transmitted diseases (STDs) that contribute to pelvic inflammatory disease (PID) and its sequelae also may affect a woman's ability to become pregnant.
- Increasing environmental exposure to toxins such as lead and pesticides and lifestyle exposure to drugs, tobacco, and alcohol affect fertility also.

Etiology. Female-related factors account for 40% of infertility cases; the most common female-related causes are ovulation disorders, problems related to tubal patency, and endometriosis. Male-related factors account for another 40% of infertility cases. Disordered sperm production, reproductive tract abnormalities, and endocrine disorders are common causes of male infertility. Couple factor infertility, such as coital frequency and timing,

sperm–cervical mucus interaction, and antisperm antibodies, accounts for 20% of infertility. In 5% to 10% of cases, the cause of infertility never is determined.

Overview of the Evaluation of Infertility

- The evaluation of infertility proceeds systematically from least invasive to more invasive diagnostic testing.
- Testing is time intensive (3-month minimum) and expensive (rarely covered by insurance).
- Evaluation involves candid discussion of private lives and aspects of sexual intimacy not always easily shared with strangers.
- Timing of testing is sometimes inconvenient and uncomfortable.
- Investigation of infertility involves answering five basic questions—the answers to which diagnose 90% of cases:
  - Does the woman ovulate? (This question is answered by evaluation of basal body temperature [BBT] measurement, cervical mucus changes, progesterone assays, endometrial biopsy, and laparoscopy to view the corpus luteum.)
  - Does the man produce normal sperm? (This question is answered by evaluation of a semen analysis. If the answer is "no," the male is referred to a urologist for further workup.)
  - Is the woman's cervical mucus conducive to sperm survival and motility in the reproductive tract? (This question is answered by evaluation of postcoital cervical mucus with the Sims-Huhner test.)
  - Is the woman's reproductive tract patent? (This is evaluated with a hysterosalpingogram.)
  - Is the uterine endometrium hormonally prepared to support an implantation? (This is evaluated by endometrial biopsy.)

ASSESSMENT: SUBJECTIVE/HISTORY
Female Partner

- Last menstrual period and menstrual history (age at menarche, interval, duration, quality, dysmenorrhea, intermenstrual or premenstrual spotting, and molimina)
- Previous contraceptive and obstetric history (full review of previous pregnancies and outcomes)
- History of abdominal or pelvic pain, endometriosis, or dyspareunia
- Intrauterine exposure to diethylstilbestrol (DES)
- History of pubertal and sexual development
- Previous surgeries, especially pelvic surgery (including for ruptured appendix and adnexal or ovarian mass or cyst) and voluntary abortion
- Previous infection, including STDs, PID, and cervicitis
- Sexual history as it relates to risk behavior

- Endometriosis
- Eating disorders
- Abnormal Pap smear, abnormal cone biopsy sample, cryosurgery, or loop electrosurgical excision procedure
- Leiomyomas
- Thyroid disease
- Hirsutism, galactorrhea, hot flushes, or severe psychologic stress
- General health (diet, weight stability, medications, exercise, and alcohol consumption)
- Use of nicotine, alcohol, and illegal substances, such as marijuana and other street drugs
- Excessive exercise now or in the past
- Current medications—prescription, herbal/supplements, and over-the-counter (OTC)
- Environmental exposure (chemical or radiation in work or leisure)

Male Partner

- Intrauterine DES exposure
- Congenital abnormalities, including hypospadias
- Previous paternity
- Sexual history as it relates to risk behavior
- Exposure to environmental toxins, drugs, alcohol, or tobacco
- Previous surgery on reproductive tract, including testicular, prostate, or hernia repair surgery
- Urologic history
- Erectile or ejaculatory dysfunction
- Previous infections and treatments, including STDs and postpubertal mumps
- Drugs and medications, including genital radiation, chemotherapy, and anabolic steroids
- Excessive exposure to heat (e.g., hot tubs, saunas), toxic chemicals, and pesticides
- General health (diet, medications, exercise, review of systems)
- Details of pubertal development
- Current medications: prescription, herbal/supplements, and OTC

Both Partners

- Determine length of time conception has been attempted.
- Determine frequency of intercourse and timing in cycle.
- Determine use of lubricants or douches (can be spermicidal).
- Determine whether dyspareunia or ejaculatory dysfunction exist.
- Determine how the lack of conception is affecting the couple's relationship. Infertility is considered a crisis by many couples whose coping skills are sorely tested by the involuntary childlessness, the diagnostic requirements, expense, inconvenience, and inherent strain on their relationship. Infertility is fraught with decreased self-esteem, blame (both self and partner),

guilt, and a sense of loss and grief. At times, the sex act becomes mechanical in search of pregnancy. Mutual respect and open communication between the two is essential or the relationship may be compromised permanently.

ASSESSMENT: OBJECTIVE/PHYSICAL EXAMINATION
Physical Examination

- Note age, height, weight, and vital signs.
- Perform complete physical examination, including notation of the overall body habitus and hair distribution in the appropriate pattern for the gender plus evidence of secondary sexual characteristics.
- Palpate thyroid gland for evidence of enlargement or nodules.
- Note breast development in women and the presence of gynecomastia in men.
- Inspect abdomen and genitals for scars from previous reproductive surgery.
- In men, note Tanner staging, testicular descent, size, consistency; examine the epididymis and vas deferens; check for penile lesions.
- In women, examine external genitalia for signs of infection, lesions, or anomalies; perform pelvic examination and bimanual examination for masses, tenderness, and anomalies.

Diagnostic Procedures

The most common causative factors in infertility can be evaluated by semen analysis, documentation that ovulation occurs, a postcoital test, and evaluation of tubal patency. A semen analysis can be done at any time; however, other testing is coordinated around the woman's menstrual cycle. If she has regular menses and molimina, ovulation is presumed. If not, BBT assessment continues throughout the cycle to document ovulation. Postovulation temperatures are increased by 0.4x F to 0.8x F under the influence of progesterone. Temperatures typically remain elevated until menstruation. The postcoital examination is performed at midcycle around the anticipated time of ovulation. An endometrial biopsy is scheduled 1 to 2 days before the expected menses, whereas a hysterosalpingogram is performed after menstruation but before the next ovulation. Ovulation induction in an anovulatory woman must precede the postcoital test or endometrial biopsy but follow semen analysis and the hysterosalpingogram.

In addition to the physical examination, both men and women should have testing for gonorrhea and chlamydia. Women should also undergo a Pap smear to rule out cervical dysplasia and a wet prep for evidence of trichomoniasis, candidal infection, and bacterial vaginosis. Additional testing for male and female factors when seeking a cause of infertility are shown in Tables 3-55 and 3-56.

TABLE **3-55**   Diagnostic Testing: Seeking Cause for Female Factor Infertility

DIAGNOSTIC TEST	SUMMARY INFORMATION
Serum progesterone	Evaluated 7 days after presumed ovulation Values >15 ng/mL: consistent with ovulation Values <5 ng/mL: consistent with anovulation
Serum FSH, LH	Evaluate hypothalamic–pituitary–ovarian axis dysfunction Elevated LH to FSH ratio—especially with symptoms of hirsutism, obesity, and amenorrhea—consistent with PCOS Elevated FSH: consistent with ovarian failure Decreased FSH and LH: consistent with anovulation
Serum prolactin	Elevated levels: consistent with pituitary adenoma
Serum TSH	Elevated levels: consistent with hypothyroidism
Urinary LH ovulation predictor test	Based on LH surge, precedes ovulation by 20-48 hours. Evaluated midcycle. False-positive result associated with PCOS, menopause, and pregnancy
Antisperm antibody test	Evaluated with serum or cervical mucus analysis Presence: consistent with potential impairment of sperm/cervical mucus interaction
Cervical mucus test	Evaluated for ferning pattern noted microscopically: consistent with ovulation
BBT	Evaluated for signs of ovulation: decrease of 0.4 degrees followed by sustained increase of 0.4 degrees remainder of cycle using BBT thermometer on arising and before any activity Biphasic temperature record: consistent with thermogenic effects of progesterone at ovulation. If increased temperature occurs <10 days, then suspect luteal phase deficiency (inadequate secretion of progesterone)
Pelvic ultrasonography	Allows definition of pelvic contents and documents cystic pathologic conditions Can be performed using abdominal or vaginal transducer
Postcoital (Sims-Huhner) test	Evaluates for sperm/cervical mucus interaction Requires 48 hours of ejaculatory abstinence before test Timed to coincide with 48-72 hours of cervical mucus receptivity to sperm at ovulation 2-8 hours after coitus, endocervical mucus is aspirated and examined to identify quality or ability to sustain sperm survival and numbers of viable, motile sperm Normal: Abundant, thin, clear mucus Spinnbarkeit >8 cm 5-10 progressively motile sperm/hpf noted on microscopic examination

Continued

TABLE **3-55** Diagnostic Testing: Seeking Cause for Female Factor Infertility—cont'd

DIAGNOSTIC TEST	SUMMARY INFORMATION
Endometrial biopsy	Allows histologic determination of ovulation by evaluation of uterine lining under influence of progesterone Timing: 1-2 days before expected menses Procedure: cervix stabilized with tenaculum. Uterus sounded to determine size. Sample aspirated by suction curette May cause uterine cramping and spotting Risk: uterine perforation Secretory endometrium: consistent with ovulation
Hysterosalpingogram	Evaluates patency of uterine cavity and fallopian tubes by fluoroscopic visualization as contrast medium is instilled transcervically and outlines uterus and tubes Normal: medium flows without obstruction through uterus, into fallopian tubes and out the fimbriated ends Timing: performed after menstruation but before next ovulation Risks: uterine perforation and allergy to contrast May cause uterine cramping, bleeding, dizziness, and nausea
Hysteroscopy	Evaluates uterine cavity by direct visualization May cause moderate discomfort. With vagal response as the cervix is manipulated, may cause mild bradycardia, diaphoresis, and hypertension May enable lysis of intrauterine adhesions secondary to Asherman's syndrome
Diagnostic laparoscopy	Defines characteristics of internal reproductive organs Surgical procedure associated with anesthesia risk and discomforts such as sore throat from placement of an endotracheal tube and abdominal pain, nausea and vomiting, and shoulder discomfort (secondary to insufflation of the abdomen with carbon dioxide) In addition to a diagnostic function, this test may enable lysis of adhesions, vaporization of endometrial implants, correction of certain anatomic defects, and removal of damaged fallopian tube

BBT, Basal body temperature; *FSH*, follicle-stimulating hormone; *hpf*, high-powered field; *LH*, luteinizing hormone; *PCOS*, polycystic ovary syndrome; *TSH*, thyroid-stimulating hormone.

TABLE **3-56**   Diagnostic Testing: Seeking Cause for Male Factor Infertility

DIAGNOSTIC TEST	SUMMARY INFORMATION
Serum FSH and LH	Low levels may indicate hypothalamic or pituitary dysfunction
	Elevated levels may indicate testicular failure
Serum testosterone levels	Indicates level of hormone production
Serum prolactin	Increased level associated with pituitary adenoma
Sperm antibodies	Presence may occur secondary to vasectomy or STD
Semen analysis	Requires 48 hours of ejaculation abstinence before test
	Fresh ejaculate examined within 2 hours of collection; abnormal initial test followed by two additional tests 2 weeks apart before diagnosis
	Normal:
	Volume: 2-5 mL
	Liquefication: 30-60 minutes
	pH: 7.2-7.8
	Sperm count: >20million/mL
	Motility: >50%
	Morphology: >50%
Sperm penetration assay	Indicates functional ability of sperm to penetrate hamster eggs
Testicular biopsy	Evaluation of testicular failure versus obstruction
	Requires referral to surgeon
	Discomfort from local anesthetic and biopsy

STD, Sexually transmitted disease.

DIAGNOSIS

Refer to Table 3-57 for possible causes of infertility in men and women. These will guide the differential diagnosis.

THERAPEUTIC PLAN

The major role for the NP in primary care includes the following priorities:

- Help in identifying the cause of infertility
- Client education and anticipatory guidance throughout evaluation
- Correction of disease states, where possible
- Treatment of infection
- Referral to qualified specialists
- Ongoing emotional support

Depending on qualifications, those in family practice settings may participate in treatment with ovulation induction with clomiphene (Clomid, Serophene) and treatment of endometriosis with gonadotropin releasing hormone agonists (Synarel, Lupron) or danazol (Danocrine), but most infertility treatment requires referral to specialists. The family NP may have a role in the following:

- Coordinating infertility testing. This may entail collaboration between NPs in primary care and those in specialty practice, physicians, and other providers. The couple's choices about infertility testing (and ultimate treatment) depend on the intensity of their feelings about childlessness, perception of benefits/risks, and their financial situation. For those advancing in reproductive age, time limits are also a factor.
- Referring clients to RESOLVE, the national support group for infertile couples.
- Providing basic education on reproductive physiology, including appropriate frequency and timing of sexual intercourse and sexual practices to enhance fertility. In their desperation to achieve pregnancy, many couples engage in coitus too frequently; the best sperm counts and sperm motility occur with coital intervals of 36 hours. Encourage a healthy lifestyle: nutritious diet, regular exercise, stress reduction, smoking cessation, alcohol moderation, and elimination of any environmental toxins and drugs.
- Discussing with clients the following factors known to influence the probability of conception:
  - Frequent ejaculations from coitus or masturbation dilute sperm.
  - Alcohol, tobacco, and drugs decrease sperm count.
  - Douching and lubricants have antisperm properties and change the cervical mucus.
  - Ideal testicular temperatures favorable to conception can be achieved by wearing loose clothing, including boxer-type underwear; minimizing use of saunas and hot tubs; and not engaging in strenuous exercise.

TABLE **3-57** Causes of Infertility

MALE FACTOR INFERTILITY (40%)	FEMALE FACTOR INFERTILITY (40%)
DISORDERS OF SPERMATOGENESIS Mumps orchitis Chromosomal abnormalities Cryptorchidism Varicocele Environmental exposure (chemical agents, radiation, alcohol, sulfa drugs, nitrofurantoin) **DISORDERS OF SPERM MOTILITY** Varicocele Antibody formation **ANATOMICAL ABNORMALITIES** Obstruction of vas deferens Congenital anomalies of reproductive organs **SEXUAL DYSFUNCTION** Retrograde ejaculation Decreased libido/impotence **ENDOCRINE DISEASE** Pituitary failure (tumor, surgery, radiation) Hyperprolactinemia (tumor or drug) Thyroid disease Adrenal disease Endogenous androgens	**DISORDERS OF OVULATION** Anovulation Excessive exercise, eating disorders Drug induced (hormonal contraception, marijuana, tranquilizers) Pituitary adenoma (prolactin secreting) Small cell cancer of lung **ANXIETY, STRESS** PCOS Chronic disease (e.g., tuberculosis, uremia, type 1 diabetes, hemochromatosis, thyroid disease, liver disease, androgen excess) Premature ovarian failure **ANATOMIC ABNORMALITIES** Intrauterine DES exposure Müllerian duct abnormality Hypoplastic uterine cavity Infection PID (tubal obstruction) Endometriosis **UTERINE DISORDERS** Asherman's syndrome Leiomyoma Surgical adhesions

DES, Diethylstilbestrol; *PID,* pelvic inflammatory disease; *PCOS,* polycystic ovary syndrome.

- Depositing the semen pool nearer the cervical os is facilitated when the woman elevates her hips on a pillow during and after coitus and maintains her position for a full 20 minutes afterward. Male-superior position accomplishes the same goal. This is important because most sperm are in the first drops of ejaculate.
- Providing information on artificial insemination, if appropriate
- Referring clients to a reproductive endocrinologist for assisted reproductive technology. The following are the current options, which require complex stimulation protocols. They are appropriate in cases of advancing reproductive age, tubal factors, male factors, and lack of success with more conventional treatments:
  - Artificial insemination with donor sperm (AID)
  - Artificial insemination with homologous (partner's) sperm (AIH)
  - Intracytoplasmic sperm injection (ICSI)–single sperm directly injected into cytoplasm of selected oocyte
  - Gamete intra-fallopian transfer (GIFT)
  - Intrauterine insemination (IUI)
  - In-vitro fertilization with embryo transfer (IVF/ET)
  - Zygote intra-fallopian transfer (ZIFT)

- Assisted hatching (manual or chemical treatment of zona pellucida to create opening for dividing embryo to hatch and implant)
- Providing information about adoption

Referral

Depending on the expertise of the NP in primary care, referral to various specialists likely will be appropriate. Knowing the qualifications of various specialists (endocrinologist, urologist, infertility specialist) is a valuable resource. The NP might be the constant in the coordination of infertility evaluation and care.

Prevention

Some infertility is preventable by safe sexual practices to preclude exposure to STDs or by protection against exposure to environmental toxins and unhealthy lifestyles. Timely, appropriate treatment of factors contributing to infertility, such as chronic disease, may prevent some causes. Most cases of infertility, however, are not preventable; a cause is never found for up to 10% of infertility cases.

EVALUATION/FOLLOW-UP

Most infertility evaluations occur during the course of 12 to 18 months. Follow-up visits during that time are based on the menstrual cycle.

COMPLICATIONS

Infertility itself is not associated with complications; however, many causes of infertility can have complicated courses. Failure to treat infertility appropriately has the potential to waste the couple's time, money, and efforts and to intensify the emotional crisis they experience. Some relationships do not survive infertility.

REFERENCES

Cash, J., & Glass, C. (2000). *Family practice guidelines.* Philadelphia: Lippincott.

Guzick, D. S. (2000). When infertility can't be explained. *Contemporary OB/GYN, 45*(9), 102-108.

Hawkins, J. W., Roberto-Nichols, D. M., & Stanley-Haney, J. L. (1997). *Protocols for nurse practitioners in gynecologic settings* (6th ed.). New York: Tiresias.

Johnson, C. L. (1996). Regaining self-esteem: Strategies and interventions for the infertile woman. *Journal of Obstetric, Gynecologic, and Neonatal Nursing, 25*(4), 291-295.

Keltz, M. D., Tekin, B., & Arici, A. (1997). Clomiphene citrate: Review and management update. *The Female Patient, 22,* 49-55.

Kennedy, H. P., Griffin, M., & Frishman, G. (1998). Enabling conception and pregnancy. Midwifery care of women experiencing infertility. *Journal of Nurse Midwifery, 43*(3), 190-207.

Martin, M. C. (1994). Infertility. In A. H. De Cherney & M. L. Pernoll, *Current obstetric and gynecologic diagnosis and treatment* (pp. 996-1006). Norwalk, CT: Appleton & Lange.

Mastroianni, L., Morrell, K., & Sokol, R. (1997). Helping infertile patients. *Patient Care, October 15,* 103-121.

Matteson, P. S. (2001). *Women's health during the childbearing years: A community based approach.* St. Louis: Mosby.

Morell, V. (1997). Basic infertility assessment. *Primary Care, 24*(1), 195-205.

Robinson, D., Kidd, P., & Rogers, K. M. (2000). *Primary care across the lifespan.* St. Louis: Mosby.

Smith, R. P. (1997). *Gynecology in primary care.* Baltimore: Williams & Wilkins.

Stansberry, J. (1996). The infertile couple: An overview of pathophysiology and diagnostic evaluation for the primary care clinician. *Nurse Practitioner Forum, 7*(2), 76-86.

Schoener, C. J. (1996). The comfort and discomfort of infertility. *Journal of Obstetric, Gynecologic, and Neonatal Nursing, 25*(2), 167-172.

Trantham, P. (1996). The infertile couple. *American Family Physician, 54*(3), 1001-1110.

Youngkin, E. Q., & Davis, M. S. (1998). *Women's health—a primary care clinical guide* (2nd ed). Stamford, CT: Appleton & Lange.

Review Questions

1. Which of the following symptoms is more indicative of a male infertility factor?

- **a.** DES exposure
- **b.** Pituitary insufficiency
- **c.** Thyroid disease
- **d.** Mumps orchitis

2. Which of the following physical findings on a pelvic examination might be significant in terms of an infertility evaluation?

- **a.** A retroflexed uterus
- **b.** An enlarged, irregular uterine contour
- **c.** A mobile uterus
- **d.** Bacterial vaginosis

3. Infertility is defined as which of the following?

- **a.** The inability to conceive with multiple sexual partners
- **b.** The inability to conceive for 9 months of unprotected intercourse when both partners are younger than 30 years
- **c.** The inability to conceive after 1 full year of unprotected intercourse
- **d.** The state of voluntary childlessness

4. The definition of sterility is which of the following?

- **a.** Unexplained infertility
- **b.** The inability to reproduce
- **c.** A decrease in the ability to conceive
- **d.** Infertility greater than 1 year

5. A referral to a reproductive endocrinologist for infertility is appropriate for which of the following?

- **a.** To advise on assisted reproductive technologies
- **b.** To advise on basic infertility workup
- **c.** To advise on an adoption plan
- **d.** To advise on the treatment of PID

6. Sperm antibodies can be found in all the following except:

- **a.** Serum
- **b.** Semen
- **c.** Tissue
- **d.** Cervical mucus

Answers and Rationales

1. *Answer:* **d** (assessment)
Rationale: DES exposure, pituitary insufficiency, and thyroid disease are both male and female factors. Mumps orchitis, however, is specific to male infertility (Martin, 1994).

2. *Answer:* **b** (assessment)
Rationale: A retroflexed uterus or mobile uterus are both normal findings. Bacterial vaginosis is a common, easily treated infection that is not typically significant in terms of an infertility evaluation. An enlarged, irregular uterine contour may be indicative of uterine fibroids and warrants further evaluation (Trantham, 1996).

3. *Answer:* **c** (analysis/diagnosis)
Rationale: Infertility is defined as the inability to conceive after 1 full year of unprotected intercourse.

4. *Answer:* **b** (analysis/diagnosis)
Rationale: Sterility is the inability to reproduce, whereas infertility implies a decrease in the ability to conceive in a certain time frame, with the potential for conception remaining a possibility (Smith, 1997).

5. *Answer:* a (implementation/plan)

Rationale: The primary care provider is responsible for the basic workup, treatment of infections (including PID), and advising the couple on options such as adoption. A reproductive endocrinologist is an appropriate referral if a couple's infertility is unexplained or if the couple could benefit from advanced assisted reproductive technologies.

6. *Answer:* c (implementation/plan)

Rationale: Sperm antibodies can be found in serum, semen, and cervical mucus and may impair the sperm's ability to penetrate an egg. Tissue is not identified as a location of sperm antibodies.

INFLAMMATORY BOWEL DISEASE *Denise Robinson*

OVERVIEW
Definition

Inflammatory bowel disease (IBD) in general refers to any chronic, inflammatory condition of the small or large bowel. Specifically, the two most common types of IBD are ulcerative colitis and Crohn's disease. These two entities share many features secondary to bowel inflammation such as diarrhea, pain, fever, and blood loss, but they differ in terms of distribution of disease, histologic findings, incidence and type of extraintestinal symptoms, response to medications and surgery, and prognosis.

Incidence
Ulcerative Colitis
- Occurs at a rate of 4 to 15 per 100,000 in the general population
- Familial tendency
- More common in young adulthood; peak age 20 to 40 years
- Almost equal between the sexes
- More prevalent among people of Jewish descent
- Less likely to develop in cigarette smokers

Crohn's Disease
- Occurs at a rate of 1 to 8 per 100,000 in the general population
- Common age of onset is 15 to 40 years of age
- Three to five times more common among European or North American Jews
- Equal to slightly higher rate among females compared with males
- Smokers are more likely affected and are more likely to have recurrences
- Familial tendency

Pathophysiology

The cause of IBD is unknown. Research has focused on many variables, immune factors, genetic factors, infectious agents, food allergies, collagen disorders, and psychosocial factors.

Ulcerative colitis affects only the colon. It usually extends upward from the rectum. It generally affects the mucosa and submucosa of the colon and rectum. Initially the colon is friable, with a tendency of the mucosa to bleed when touched. As the lesions progress, frank ulceration and exudation occur uniformly over the involved areas. Fissures and fistula rarely are seen.

Crohn's disease can occur anywhere in the gastrointestinal (GI) tract, from the anus to the mouth. It may involve all layers of the bowel wall, the mesenteries, and associated lymph nodes. It is characterized by "skip" lesions in which normal mucosa is interspersed with areas of inflammation. Areas of aphthous ulcers and ulcerations are adjacent to normal tissue. Fissures and fistulas are common.

ASSESSMENT: SUBJECTIVE/HISTORY
History of Present Illness

- The most prominent features of ulcerative colitis are rectal bleeding and diarrhea.
- Severity ranges from intermittent bleeding, mild diarrhea with no systemic involvement to marked diarrhea, bleeding severe enough to cause anemia, abdominal cramping, tenderness, anorexia, and weight loss.
- Associated systemic manifestations of ulcerative colitis include skin lesions, eye lesions, arthritis, and liver disease.
- Early Crohn's disease presents with vague and episodic symptoms. These initial manifestations include general malaise, anorexia, fever, mild abdominal discomfort, and diarrhea. As the disease progresses, so do the most consistent symptoms: abdominal pain and diarrhea.
- Rectal bleeding is not as common with Crohn's disease as with ulcerative colitis.
- Perianal disease is common with Crohn's disease and may present as an edematous skin tag; a wide, painless fissure; an abscess; an anal ulcer; or anal stenosis.
- Nutritional deficiencies are common in Crohn's disease, secondary to malabsorption and stricture formation.
- Associated systemic manifestations of Crohn's disease include joint problems, skin lesions, ocular disorders, and aphthous ulcers of the mouth. Other systemic disorders associated with Crohn's disease include kidney stones, gallstones, osteoporosis, liver disorders, vascular problems, and psychiatric disorders.
- Children and adolescents may experience growth retardation and/or delayed sexual development.

Past Medical History
- Ask about past episodes of diarrhea and abdominal pain.

- Ask about autoimmune disorders, food allergies or intolerances, and GI disorders.

Medication History

- Ask about all prescription drugs and OTC medications.
- Ask about herbal remedies.
- Ask about antidiarrheal medications.

Psychosocial History

- Determine the client's ethnic origin.
- Ask about psychosocial stressors and methods of coping.
- Ask about past psychiatric disorders and treatment.

Family History

Ask about family history of IBD and GI disorders.

ASSESSMENT: OBJECTIVE/PHYSICAL EXAMINATION

Physical Examination

A complete physical examination often is indicated to rule out extraintestinal involvement. The examination should pay attention to the following:

- Assess vital signs, height, and weight.
- Assess abdomen for bowel sounds, pain, guarding, rebound, masses, and distention.
- Assess rectum for tone, integrity, abscess, mass, and guaiac for occult blood.

Diagnostic Procedures

- Evaluate complete blood count (CBC) for anemia, infection.
- Evaluate guaiac stool for occult blood.
- Perform culture and sensitivity testing on stool to evaluate for bacterial infection.
- Evaluate serum albumin and total protein levels; decreased with advanced disease and malnutrition.
- Evaluate vitamin B_{12} levels; decreased with distal ileitis.
- Evaluate liver function studies for liver disease.
- Evaluate folic acid levels; may be reduced.
- Perform x-ray examination of the abdomen to rule out dilation or obstruction.
- Perform barium studies and upper GI testing to evaluate for mucosal irregularities, ulcers, fissures, cobblestoning, skip lesions, stenosis, stricture (barium enema is contraindicated in acute ulcerative colitis).
- Perform endoscopy to evaluate mucosal irregularities, ulcers, fissures, biopsy (colonoscopy is contraindicated during acute ulcerative colitis because of the risk of perforation; sigmoidoscopy can be performed).
- Perform biopsy for diagnosis and to rule out malignancy.
- Perform computerized tomography of the abdomen to evaluate mesenteric abnormalities, thickening of the bowel wall, and abscess and fistula formation.

DIAGNOSIS

Differential diagnoses include the following:

- Ulcerative colitis versus Crohn's disease (Table 3-58)
- Irritable bowel syndrome (IBS)
- Peptic ulcer disease
- Gastroenteritis
- Pseudomembranous enterocolitis
- Diverticulitis
- Cholecystitis
- Pancreatitis

THERAPEUTIC PLAN
Pharmacologic Treatment

- The goal of treatment is to decrease inflammation and suppress the immune system's response.
- Loperamide (Imodium) increases colonic water absorption. Cholestyramine (Questran) is helpful for clients who develop bile salt-induced diarrhea after ileal resection.
- Sulfasalazine (Azulfidine) is a combination salicylate/sulfonamide and is most commonly prescribed for maintenance for both ulcerative colitis and Crohn's disease. Common side effects include nausea and headache, which can be avoided if titration is done slowly.
- If the client is allergic to sulfa compounds, a topical antiinflammatory agent such as mesalamine or 5-aminosalicylic acid (5-ASA; Asacol, Pentasa, Rowasa) can be given.
- Initiate sulfasalazine therapy with corticosteroids because it may take 2 weeks to achieve therapeutic results. The corticosteroids are used during acute exacerbations to suppress inflammation.
- Hydrocortisone enemas (Cortenema) and rectal foam (Cortifoam) are used to alleviate symptoms of the lower colon and anogenital area.
- Regarding antibiotics, bacterial flora play a role in the pathogenesis of IBD. Most studies have been done in clients with Crohn's disease.
- Metronidazole (Flagyl) is an anaerobic antiinfective agent used for fistulas or perianal involvement in Crohn's disease. Ciprofloxacin (Cipro) is also effective in clients with Crohn's disease and can be combined with Flagyl.
- Immunosuppressant agents are for clients with intractable IBD. They have fewer side effects and are better tolerated than long-term corticosteroid therapy.
- Azathioprine (Imuran) and mercaptopurine (Purinethol) are helpful for IBD clients. Their effects may not be seen for as long as 3 months.
- Methotrexate (Rheumatrex) also has been used for severe IBD, as has cyclosporine (Sandimmune).
- Leukotriene synthetase inhibitors, currently in Phase III drug trials, act on an important intestinal inflammatory pathway. Zileuton (Zyflo) has been shown to be effective in IBD.

TABLE **3-58**   Distinguishing Ulcerative Colitis from Crohn's Disease

MEANS OF ASSESSMENT	ULCERATIVE COLITIS	CROHN'S DISEASE
SYMPTOMS		
Abdominal pain	Unusual	Usual
Hemorrhage	Usual	Unusual
Fistula formation	Very unusual	Not rare
Anal changes	Unusual	Usual
Palpable intestinal mass	Never	Often
Involvement of rectum	Almost always	Not so often
SCOPE		
Rectoscopy	No normal mucous membrane	Quite normal, or islands of normal mucous membrane
X-RAY EVALUATION		
Spreading	Continuous	Discontinuous
Strictures	No	Often
Mucosal appearance	Granulomatous, superficial ulcerations	Deep, undetermined ulcerated fissures
Shortened, arched colon	Often	No
EVALUATION BY PATHOLOGY		
Mucosa	Largely lacking, superficial ulcerations	Discrete ulcerations, fissures, cobblestone appearance
Connective tissue	Increased, the intestine generally somewhat constricted, no strictures, less length	Normal amount of connective tissue, normal or dilated intestine between stricturing parts
Fistula	None	Often
Involved terminal ileum	Never	Often
Inflammation	Mucosa and submucosa	All layers
Lymph nodes	Reactive, hyperplasia	Sarcoid, conglomerate

Adapted from Cooke, D.M. (1991). Inflammatory bowel disease: primary health care management of ulcerative colitis and Crohn's disease. *The Nurse Practitioner, 16*: 27–39.

- Monoclonal antibodies to tumor necrosis factor and other inflammatory cytokines are future treatments for IBD.
- Antidiarrheal agents include the following:
  - Psyllium products for bulking effect on watery diarrhea
  - Diphenoxylate (Lomotil) and iopromide (Imodium)

Nonpharmacologic Treatment

Surgery frequently is indicated for clients with ulcerative colitis to relieve strictures, but surgery also is indicated in emergency situations in which the disease is unresponsive to medical measures, the client has intractable bleeding, or an unresponsive megacolon has developed. The surgery generally done for ulcerative colitis is proctocolectomy with ileostomy. This procedure is considered curative for ulcerative colitis.

Surgical intervention in Crohn's disease can be therapeutic, but there is a significant recurrence rate. Indications for surgery include intestinal obstruction, abscess formation, fistula of the bladder or vagina, or colon failure with intractable bleeding. Typically the procedure used is resection of the diseased bowel, with reanastomosis.

Diet

- No single diet causes or corrects IBD; however, a special diet may be helpful in clients with active symptoms.
- IBD frequently is accompanied by lactose deficiency.
- A low-fiber, low-residue diet is recommended.
- Bolus obstructions can result from nuts, popcorn, tough meat, raw fruit, corn, coleslaw, and uncooked vegetables.
- IBD clients are at risk for protein deficiencies, and a diet high in calories and protein is advisable.
- A deficiency of fat-soluble vitamins (A, D, E, and K) can occur.
- Vitamin B_{12} deficiencies can occur, and vitamin B_{12} injections should be considered.

Referral/Consultation

- Refer the following clients to an internist or gastroenterologist:
  - Newly diagnosed clients
  - Clients with uncontrollable symptoms
  - Clients with acute exacerbation of symptoms
  - Clients needing screening for colorectal cancer
- Refer clients for psychosocial evaluation and counseling as indicated.

- Refer clients for support and self-help groups as indicated.

EVALUATION/FOLLOW-UP

- Most clients follow a cyclic course of remission and flare-up.
- Overall mortality for ulcerative colitis is between 12% and 15% because of the risk for serious complications such as hemorrhage, perforation, and toxic megacolon.
- An estimated 50% to 65% of clients with Crohn's disease undergo surgery at some point in their lives for intestinal resection or colectomy.
- The overall prognosis remains modest with Crohn's disease, unlike ulcerative colitis, which can be cured by a colectomy.

REFERENCES

Botoman, V., Bonner, G., & Botoman, D. (1998). Management of inflammatory bowel disease. *American Family Physician, 57*(1), 57-68.

Chutkin, R. K. (2001). Inflammatory bowel disease. *Primary Care, 28*(3), 539-556.

Fishman, M. (2001). Diagnosis and classification of inflammatory bowel disease. *Canadian Journal of Gastroenterology, 15*(9), 627-628.

Hastings, G. & Weber, R. (1993a). Inflammatory bowel disease: Part 1. Clinical features and diagnosis. *American Family Physician, 47*(3), 598-608.

Hastings, G. & Weber, R. (1993b). Inflammatory bowel disease: Part 2. Medical and surgical management. *American Family Physician, 47*(4), 811-818.

Kurina, L. M., Goldacre, M. J., Yeates, D., & Gill, L. E. (2001). Depression and anxiety in people with inflammatory bowel disease. *Journal of Epidemiology and Community Health, 55*(10), 716-720.

Rogers, K. (2000). Inflammatory bowel disease. In D. Robinson, P. Kidd, & K. Rogers (Eds.). *Primary care across the lifespan* (pp. 635-640). St. Louis: Mosby.

Tremaine, W. J., Sandborn, W. J., Loftus, E. V., Kenan, M. L., Petterson, T. M., Zinsmeister, A. R., & Silverstien, M. D. (2001). A prospective cohort study of practice guidelines in inflammatory bowel disease. *American Journal of Gastroenterology, 96*(8), 2401-2406.

Review Questions

1. Close follow-up is important for IBD. Ulcerative colitis needs close follow-up for which specific problem?
- **a.** Weight loss
- **b.** Colorectal cancer
- **c.** Breast cancer
- **d.** Pancreatitis

2. Which of the following findings is most consistent with IBD?
- **a.** Frequent abdominal pain and constipation
- **b.** Weight gain, bloating
- **c.** Diarrhea and weight loss
- **d.** Lactose intolerance

3. IBS needs to be differentiated from IBD. In contrast to IBS, IBD is characterized by which of the following?
- **a.** Left lower quadrant pain after meals
- **b.** Left lower quadrant pain with bloody diarrheal stools
- **c.** No detectable pathologic cause, generalized abdominal pain
- **d.** Intermittent abdominal pain with diarrhea for 3 months

4. Gary has Crohn's disease. Which of the following historical data is consistent with Crohn's disease?
- **a.** Constipation
- **b.** Excessive alcohol consumption
- **c.** Eastern European Jewish descent
- **d.** Nonsmoker

5. Which of the following comments by the client regarding IBD education indicates a need for further teaching?
- **a.** Lactose intolerance causes my symptoms.
- **b.** Smoking may help decrease recurrences of Crohn's disease.
- **c.** A low-fiber diet may help improve my symptoms.
- **d.** Taking vitamins may help prevent deficiencies.

6. Allen has a complaint of abdominal pain for the last 3 months. He has had diarrhea, anorexia, and weight loss. He has a painful area around the anus. On examination, he has diffuse abdominal tenderness and a erythematous area in the right perirectal area. Which of the following is the most likely diagnosis?
- **a.** IBS
- **b.** Crohn's disease
- **c.** Ulcerative colitis
- **d.** Lactose intolerance

7. Which of the following comments by the client indicates attainment of a realistic goal for IBD?
- **a.** "I am taking 1 g of sulfasalazine twice daily."
- **b.** "I need to continue the corticosteroid medications now."
- **c.** "I am taking azathioprine (Imuran) for my symptoms."
- **d.** "Cyclosporine is the drug that works for me."

8. A client presents with a 6-month history of diarrhea, blood in stool, and weight loss of 30 lb. She has had an intermittent fever. On examination, she looks ill; there is generalized abdominal tenderness with no rebound. A sigmoidoscopy reveals a friable rectal mucosa with multiple bleeding points. The most likely diagnosis in this client is which of the following?
- **a.** Ulcerative colitis
- **b.** Crohn's disease
- **c.** Irritable bowel syndrome
- **d.** Diverticulitis

Answers and Rationales

1. *Answer:* **b** (evaluation)

Rationale: Ulcerative colitis is associated with increased risk of colon cancer. The risk of malignancy is related to the extent and duration of the disease (Botoman, Bonner, & Botoman, 1998).

2. *Answer:* **c** (analysis/diagnosis)
Rationale: Weight loss and diarrhea are the hallmark symptoms of IBD (Rogers, 2000).

3. *Answer:* **b** (analysis/diagnosis)
Rationale: Bloody diarrhea is a hallmark of IBD. IBS has no pathologic or organic cause (Rogers, 2000).

4. *Answer:* **c** (assessment)
Rationale: Eastern European Jews are more at risk to develop Crohn's disease (Botoman, Bonner, & Botoman, 1998).

5. *Answer:* **a** (evaluation)
Rationale: Lactose has no effect on the activity of IBD. Lactose consumption does not need to be limited. The symptoms of IBD and lactose malabsorption can be confused (Botoman, Bonner, & Botoman, 1998).

6. *Answer:* **b** (analysis/diagnosis)
Rationale: Rectal fistulas, perianal abscesses, and rectal fissures are common in Crohn's disease (Rogers, 2000).

7. *Answer:* **a** (evaluation)
Rationale: Cyclosporine, azathioprine (Imuran), and corticosteroids are used only for intractable disease. Sulfasalazine is the drug of choice for maintenance of IBD (Botoman, Bonner, & Botoman, 1998).

8. *Answer:* **a** (analysis/diagnosis)
Rationale: This client most likely has ulcerative colitis. This disease usually reveals friability with easy bleeding and granularity on sigmoidoscopy (Rogers, 2000).

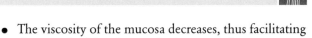

INFLUENZA *Pamela Kidd*

OVERVIEW
Definition

Influenza is an acute, febrile, viral illness associated with upper and lower respiratory involvement.

Incidence

- Influenza occurs worldwide in pandemics, and epidemics occur every 2 to 3 years.
- Approximately 20,000 to 40,000 people die each year of influenza and associated complications (Kennedy, 1998).
- Influenza peaks in winter months in temperate climates.
- Influenza affects healthy children at a rate of 10% to 40%, with a hospitalization rate of 1%.
- The risk of complications from lower respiratory tract infection ranges from 0.2% to 25%.
- Neonates with influenza have a higher morbidity rate secondary to sepsis, apnea, and lower tract disease.
- Children who have sickle cell disease, bronchopulmonary dysplasia, asthma, cystic fibrosis, malignancies, diabetes, or chronic renal failure have a higher rate of complications from influenza secondary to bronchitis and pneumonia.

Pathophysiology

- Influenza viruses are orthomyxoviruses.
- There are three types of viruses: Type A, B, and C, each with many strains.
- Types A and B produce clinically indistinguishable infections, whereas type C is usually a minor illness.
- The virus is transmitted by direct contact person to person, by large droplet infection, or by articles contaminated by nasopharyngeal secretions.
- The virus penetrates the surface of upper respiratory tract mucosal cells, producing lysis and destruction of the ciliated epithelium.

- The viscosity of the mucosa decreases, thus facilitating the spread of the virus to the lower respiratory tract.
- Inflammation and necrosis of the bronchiolar and alveolar epithelium result, filling the alveoli with an exudate containing leukocytes, erythrocytes, and hyaline membrane.
- Influenza resembles many other febrile illnesses, but it always is accompanied by a cough.
- It is most infectious in the 24 hours before the onset of symptoms and during the period of peak symptoms.
- Viral shedding in the nasal secretions usually ceases within 7 days of the onset of illness.
- The incubation period is 1 to 3 days.

Factors Increasing Susceptibility. Influenza is highly contagious and can spread rapidly, especially in the following situations:

- Persons of age or with a diminished immune system
- Persons working in health care agency
- Persons living in a nursing home
- Children and adolescents in schools and colleges, especially among those living in dormitories or residential facilities or members of athletic teams

Protective Factors
- Adequate rest
- Regular exercise
- Well-balanced diet
- Vitamin C (debatable effect)

ASSESSMENT: SUBJECTIVE/HISTORY
History of Present Illness

- Inquire about sudden onset of fever, chills, rigor, headache, malaise, diffuse myalgia, and a dry cough.
- Inquire about progression of respiratory symptoms, which may include sore throat, rhinitis, nasal conges-

tion, a prominent cough, and substernal soreness. Malaise may progress to prostration.

- Inquire about associated symptoms of conjunctivitis, abdominal pain, nausea, and vomiting.
- Influenza is usually self-limiting with acute symptoms lasting 2 to 7 days followed by a convalescent period of about a week.
- Confirm the age of the client. Infants, young children, and the elderly are at greatest risk for complications. Pregnant women are also at risk for complications. Complications are pneumonia, bronchitis, exacerbation of asthma, pericarditis, Reye's syndrome, and Guillain-Barré–type peripheral neuropathy.

Past Medical History

- Inquire about general health and any underlying medical problems–specifically ask about a history of cardiac disease including rheumatic heart disease, pulmonary disease including asthma, diabetes, renal disease, malignancies, and HIV/AIDS.
- Influenza can alter the metabolism of certain medications, such as theophylline, which can result in toxicity from elevated serum concentrations.
- Ask about immunosuppression.
- Ask about a history of chronic cardiopulmonary disease.
- Determine if child has asthma.
- Adults or children who have metabolic conditions (e.g., diabetes, renal dysfunction, blood dyscrasias) are all considered high risk.

Medication History

Determine if client has used OTC medications for symptom relief.

Family History

Not relevant.

Dietary History

Not relevant.

ASSESSMENT: OBJECTIVE/PHYSICAL EXAMINATION
Physical Examination

- Perform general observation.
- Obtain vital signs, especially temperature and respiration.
- Upper and lower respiratory assessment: pharyngeal injection, flushed face, anterior cervical adenopathy, and conjunctival redness are common signs of influenza. Assess for lower respiratory involvement, including crackles and rhonchi.

Diagnostic Procedures

- For viral culture, if used, nasopharyngeal swabs should be obtained within the first 72 hours of illness because the quantity of virus shed decreases rapidly.

- Leukopenia is common. Conversely, an elevated white blood count may indicate a secondary bacterial infection. Hemoglobin and hematocrit may be elevated.

DIAGNOSIS

- Influenza resembles many other mild febrile illnesses and can be difficult to diagnosis in the absence of an epidemic.
- Rhinosinusitis or the common cold may be incorrectly diagnosed. Differentiating data include pressure on bending over or on palpation of face in rhinosinusitis and insidious onset of symptoms in cold.

THERAPEUTIC PLAN
Pharmacologic Treatment

- Amantadine and rimantadine (Table 3-59) are Food and Drug Administration-approved for prophylaxis against influenza A infections in adults. Only amantadine is approved for treatment in children.
- Antiviral prophylactic therapy, if indicated, should be initiated within 48 hours of onset of symptoms and continued for 2 to 5 days or for 24 to 48 hours after the client becomes asymptomatic.
- Amantadine and rimantadine are not effective against influenza B and are not approved for infants less than 1 year of age. Dosage should be reduced in the elderly and in clients with significant renal insufficiency. Elderly clients are more likely to have central nervous system and GI side effects. Amantadine is classified as pregnancy category C. Rimantadine is recommended in clients with renal failure. Rimantadine is also available as a syrup (50 mg/mL). Dosage adjustments are based on creatinine clearance.
- Zanamivir (Relenza) should be used within 48 hours of symptom onset. Take two doses separated by at least 2 hours on the first day of use. Use 10 mg (2 inhalations) q12h for 5 days. Zanamivir is dispensed as a disk inhale.
- Antipyretics such as acetaminophen are recommended. Children and adolescents should not receive salicylates secondary to the risk of Reye's syndrome.
- Antitussives may help reduce cough.
- Antibiotics may be indicated for secondary bacterial infections.
- Aerosolized ribavirin with oxygen for 12 to 18 hours a day for 3 to 7 days has been associated with a modest shortening of clinical symptoms.

Client Education

- Encourage fluids and rest.
- Educate client about medications and course of illness.
- Instruct client to return to the clinic if fever persists for more than 4 days or if cough becomes productive. (Along with an elevated white blood cell count, this may indicate a bacterial infection).

TABLE **3-59** Recommended Doses for Amantadine* and Rimantadine

	AGES 1-9	AGES 10-65	AGE 65 AND OLDER
Treatment	5 mg/kg/day, maximum dose 150 mg/day, in one or two divided doses	Weight <40 kg: 5 mg/kg/day in one or two divided doses Weight >40 kg: 200 mg/day in one or two divided doses	100 mg/day Dosage reduced in clients with impaired renal function.
Prophylaxis	100 mg/day for children weighing >20 kg and adults	100 mg bid	100 mg qd

*Only amantadine is recommended for treatment in children (>1 year of age); rimantadine is used for prophylaxis and not treatment in children.

Referral

Referral may be necessary for high-risk clients or those with complications. Consider a cardiologist, pulmonologist, or neurologist, based on the situation.

Prevention

See Table 3-60 for an influenza vaccination schedule.

- The influenza vaccine provides partial immunity (approximately 85% efficacy) for a few months to 1 year. The composition is changed periodically and is based on prevalent strains of the preceding year.
- Annual vaccination with the trivalent influenza virus vaccine 0.5 mL intramuscularly is recommended each October or November for persons 65 years of age and older; children and adolescents receiving aspirin therapy; nursing home residents; and those with chronic lung or heart disease or other debilitating illnesses including immunosuppressive disorders, diabetes, renal disease, and sickle cell anemia.
- Immunization of adults in contact with children at high risk may be an important means of protection for these children. This includes health care workers and family members. Conversely, children who are members of households with high-risk adults should be vaccinated for the same reasons.
- Split-virus vaccines are recommended for children younger than 13 years of age.
- The influenza vaccine is strongly recommended for all women who are pregnant in their second and third trimester during the influenza season. Immunization is considered safe at any stage of pregnancy.
- The vaccine is contraindicated in clients with hypersensitivity to chicken or egg protein.
- Side effects include local redness, induration, and tenderness. Myalgias and fever are rare but possible.
- Consider amantadine or rimantadine prophylaxis (2-week course of therapy with daily medication) during peak period of influenza activity in the community for high-risk people who cannot receive the influenza vaccine.

EVALUATION/FOLLOW-UP

- Monitor closely infants, children, the elderly, and the chronically diseased client (24-hour call-back).

TABLE **3-60** Influenza Vaccination Schedule

AGE	VACCINE	DOSE	NUMBER OF DOSES
6-35 mo	Split virus	0.25 mL IM	1-2*
3-8 yr	Split virus	0.5 mL IM	1-2*
9-12 yr	Split virus	0.5 mL IM	1
>12 yr	Whole virus	0.5 mL IM	1

*Infants and children receiving the influenza vaccine for the first time should receive two doses administered 1 month apart.

- Report to local health department.

COMPLICATIONS

- Sinusitis
- Otitis media
- Bronchitis
- Pneumonia (especially influenza Type A)
- Reye's syndrome (especially influenza Type B)
- Pericarditis
- Guillain-Barré–type peripheral neuropathy

REFERENCES

American Academy of Pediatrics. (1997). Influenza. In: G. Peter. (Ed.). *1997 Red Book: Report of the Committee on Infectious Diseases* (24th ed., pp. 307-315). Elk Grove Village, IL: American Academy of Pediatrics.

Kennedy, M. (1998). Influenza viral infections: presentation, prevention and treatment. *The Nurse Practitioner, 23*(9), 17, 21-22, 25-26, 28, 35-37.

Rogers, K. M. (2001). Influenza. Chapter 101. In D. Robinson, P. Kidd, & K. Rogers. (Eds.). *Primary care across the lifespan.* St. Louis: Mosby.

Review Questions

1. Which of the following statements explains the complication of pneumonia postinfluenza?

    a. It is transmitted through nasopharyngeal secretions.

    b. The viscosity of the mucus increases.

    c. The virus penetrates mucosal cells producing lysis.

    d. Viral shedding occurs.

2. Which of the following findings helps the NP diagnose influenza?

   a. Nonproductive cough
   b. Fever
   c. Pain on palpation of face
   d. Insidious onset of symptoms

3. What is an appropriate treatment to prevent influenza in an exposed, high-risk child?

   a. Administer flu vaccine.
   b. Prescribe antibiotics.
   c. Administer pneumovax vaccine.
   d. Prescribe amantadine.

4. Which of the following remarks indicates a need for further client teaching?

   a. "I should return if I my fever lasts more than 4 days."
   b. "I should get the flu shot next year."
   c. "I should call the clinic if my cough remains dry."
   d. "I should avoid people for the next week."

5. Who should receive the influenza vaccine?

   a. A person hypersensitive to egg protein
   b. A child receiving aspirin therapy
   c. A 45-year-old adult with osteoarthritis
   d. A woman in the first trimester of pregnancy

Answers and Rationales

1. ***Answer:*** **b** (analysis/diagnosis)
   Rationale: Increased viscosity means less expectoration and greater opportunity for bacterial growth in the mucus. All of the other factors are true but would not increase the incidence of pneumonia directly.

2. ***Answer:*** **a** (analysis/diagnosis)
   Rationale: Influenza always is accompanied by a dry cough. Fever may be present with any upper respiratory infection. Pain on palpation is associated more frequently with rhinosinusitis. A cold has an insidious onset of symptoms; influenza has a sudden onset of symptoms.

3. ***Answer:*** **d** (implementation/plan)
   Rationale: The child has been exposed, so the flu and pneumovax vaccine will not help. Antibiotics should be reserved for secondary infection.

4. ***Answer:*** **c** (evaluation)
   Rationale: One should return for care if the fever lasts more than 4 days or the cough turns productive in nature. For a 67-year-old client (or any client older than age 65 years), it would be wise to get the flu vaccine in the future. Depending on when the client sought care, viral shedding lasts 1 week.

5. ***Answer:*** **b** (analysis/diagnosis)
   Rationale: A child receiving aspirin therapy is at high risk for consequences from influenza (such as Reye's syndrome). Clients with immunosuppressive diseases and chronic heart or lung disease should receive the flu vaccine, but clients with osteoarthritis should not receive the vaccine. Pregnant women who are in their second or third trimester during the flu season should receive the vaccine. It is contraindicated in clients with an allergy to chicken or egg protein.

IRRITABLE BOWEL SYNDROME *Denise Robinson*

OVERVIEW
Definition

Irritable bowel syndrome (IBS) is a functional disturbance of intestinal mobility characterized by both diarrhea and constipation (constipation is predominant), bloating, and abdominal and rectal pain. There is a high correlation between emotional factors and signs and symptoms. IBS sometimes is referred to as mucous colitis, spastic bowel, or spastic colitis. IBS often becomes chronic, with varying symptoms.

Incidence

- There is an estimated incidence of 7% to 20% of the adult population.
- Of middle-school and high-school students, 6% to 14% have symptoms of IBS.
- The incidence is unknown in children and adolescents; it is thought to be relatively uncommon or possibly underdiagnosed.
- The syndrome is predominant in ages 20 to 35 years; it rarely is seen after age 50.

- In the United States, women are twice as likely as men to have IBS, whereas men are more frequently afflicted in other parts of the world.
- Because of the concern for organic disease, IBS accounts for 50% of the referrals to gastroenterologists.
- There is a familial pattern.

Pathophysiology

It is believed that IBS is a functional disturbance in motor activity and visceral perception of the bowel. It is not explained by organic causes. Triggers include psychologic factors and luminal irritants. Motor-activity abnormalities (decreased or excessive contractility) account for the diarrhea and constipation. Excessive sensitivity of the viscera may explain the abdominal and rectal pain caused by pressure of stool or bloating.

Factors Increasing Susceptibility

- Individuals with persistent symptoms have been found to have a greater prevalence of situational stress, which is thought to modify the underlying pathophysiology and influence the severity of symptoms.

- Intraluminal factors that cause bloating and diarrhea include lactose (in dairy products), fructose (in citrus fruits), and sorbitol (often found in "sugar-free" candies and gum).

ASSESSMENT: SUBJECTIVE/HISTORY
History of Present Illness

- Continuous or recurrent symptoms for at least 3 months
- Abdominal pain and cramps, often relieved by bowel movement
- Diarrhea or constipation, or alternating between both (note frequency and consistency of stool)
- Abdominal pain, possibly in left lower quadrant
- Diet (note whether milk products, citrus fruit, and sugar-free products with sorbitol make symptoms worse)
- No change in appetite
- Mucus in stool; no blood in stool
- Bloating and distention; often flatulence, especially after meals
- Stressful life events exacerbate symptoms
- Possible depression (e.g., loss of appetite, lack of energy, poor concentration, insomnia)
- No weight loss with IBS
- No temperature elevations
- Urinary frequency
- Travel, camping history (or any possibility of drinking contaminated water)
- Usually does not wake client at night with abdominal pain; organic causes are more likely if wakes at night

Past Medical History

- Client may "physician hop" because of unrelieved symptoms or lack of "cure."
- Note any previous episodes with similar clinical course.
- Note any chronic disease or food or drug allergies.
- Clients often have other somatic complaints, such as tension headaches, fibromyalgia, noncardiac chest pain, chronic fatigue, and chronic pelvic pain.
- Ask about sexual or domestic abuse (past or current). Sensitive information may not be revealed until the client feels trust for the provider. Determine if there has been a history of sexual abuse in child.
- Ask about previous abdominal surgeries, such as cholecystectomy or other abdominal surgery. Find out the indications and the response to surgery. The persistence of presurgical symptoms suggests the possibility of functional symptoms.

Psychosocial History

- Determine stress level and how it is managed.
- Ask about past or current counseling.

Medication History

Note all medications currently being taken (prescription, OTC, vitamins, or herbal therapies), including use of laxatives or enemas.

Family History

Determine if there is a family history of IBS or other GI problems. In children:

- Assess growth parameters. Any child who does not follow his or her weight and height curves may be experiencing malabsorption.
- School-age children may present and describe abdominal pain but may be less likely to describe change in bowel habits.
- Assess a school-age child for whether he or she will use the bathroom at school. Many children will hold stool and urine at school because of lack of privacy and time constraints.

ASSESSMENT: OBJECTIVE/PHYSICAL EXAMINATION
Physical Examination

- A problem-oriented physical examination should include vital signs, height, and weight.
- Assess abdomen for bowel sounds, distention, pain, and organomegaly; note any surgical scars.
- Perform rectal examination; assess for tenderness and masses, and assess stool for occult blood.
- Schedule a comprehensive examination to rule out other pathologic causes.

Diagnostic Procedures

- The history is the cornerstone of the diagnosis of IBS. The NP should consider the possibility of organic causes while balancing the risk and expense of testing.
- Obtain CBC with differential and sedimentation rate (to rule out anemia, infection, and inflammatory causes).
- Obtain chemistry panel (to identify any other pathologic causes, such as diabetes or abnormal liver function). Elevated magnesium may indicate diuretic or laxative abuse.
- Test stool (guaiac, usually six times), maybe ova and parasites (usually three times), or culture (to rule out bowel symptoms caused by other pathologic conditions, malignancy, bacterial infections, or parasites).
- If indicated, obtain abdominal x-ray examination (flatplate and upright). If symptoms are severe (excessive bloating pain, rule out obstruction), procedures include barium enema, abdominal ultrasonography or flexible sigmoidoscopy, and possible colonoscopy (to rule out diverticular disease, inflammatory bowel disease, or malignancy). These may be indicated for clients older than age 50 years.

- For those with diarrhea-predominant IBS, a breath hydrogen test to detect evidence of lactose malabsorption should be performed.

DIAGNOSIS

Consider IBS if the following are present:
- Abdominal pain is recurrent or continuous for 2 to 3 months.
- Pain is relieved with defecation.
- Bowel changes such as diarrhea or constipation are seen. The diagnosis is made by careful history and the absence of clinical findings. Use caution so as not to overuse medical services (see previous diagnostic procedures).

Diagnostic criteria have been developed for IBS. These are the Rome II Diagnostic criteria. At least 12 weeks to 12 months of abdominal discomfort or pain that has at least two of the following features must be present:
- Relief with defecation
- Onset associated with a change in frequency of stool
- Onset associated with a change in form (appearance) (Hyams, 2001)

Differential diagnoses includes the following:

- Inflammatory bowel disease (ulcerative colitis, Crohn's disease)
- Carbohydrate intolerance: lactose, fructose, sorbitol
- Diverticulosis
- Chronic appendicitis
- Malignancy
- Diabetes (may be seen as diarrhea)
- Obstruction
- Celiac disease
- Medication side effects
- Parasites (giardiasis)
- Psychologic pathologic condition
- Further evaluation in the presence of warning signs such as blood in the stool, weight loss, vomiting, extraintestinal symptoms, travel to areas noted for enteric pathogens, recent antibiotic therapy, or family history of IBD

THERAPEUTIC PLAN

Comprehensive care emphasizing client–provider relationships is critical to the management of this syndrome.

Pharmacologic Treatment

- No single agent has proved effective.
- Take bulk-producing agents such as psyllium (Metamucil) bid or tid, 1 tablespoon (helps with constipation and diarrhea).
- Take loperamide (Imodium) 2 mg PO or diphenoxylate (Lomotil) 2.5 to 5.0 mg after each unformed stool.
- Take antispasmodics and anticholinergics such as dicyclomine (Bentyl, Levsin), 10 to 20 mg bid to qid with meals, for postprandial cramping. Warn the client of

possible side effects: dry mouth, blurred vision, and urinary retention.
- Take LactAid, 1 to 3 caplets with meals, for lactose intolerance.
- Relieve bloating and flatulence with simethicone (Mylicon), 80 mg, with meals and at bedtime.
- Consider anticholinergic agent amitriptyline (Elavil) 50 to 100 mg at bedtime for depressed clients with diarrhea. Anticholinergic agents also are significantly better than placebo to help reduce abdominal pain (small doses such as 10 to 20 mg/d are helpful).
- Use fluoxetine (Prozac) 20 mg/day, for depressed clients with constipation.

Nonpharmacologic Treatment

- Tell client that there is not a cure, but relief can be obtained through a long-term process.
- Heat to abdomen may help (contraindicated if inflammation such as appendicitis or diverticulitis is suspected).
- Biofeedback may help.
- Stress reduction may help.
- Avoid straining with bowel movements, and respond promptly to urges to defecate.
- Teach the need for patience and tolerance to find out what will work best for the client.
- Validate client's symptoms.

Diet

- Increase fiber intake up to 25 g/day. To avoid bloating and flatus, increase the fiber gradually. Warn the client of potential side effects.
- Avoid intraluminal factors (lactose, fructose, and sorbitol) in foods (milk products, citrus fruits and juices, and sugar-free candies and gums) if they increase symptoms.
- Products that contain caffeine or alcohol can increase the diarrheal symptoms for some clients.
- Avoid large meals and spicy and fatty foods.
- Increase fluid intake (water) to 2000 mL/day.
- A food diary may be needed.

Exercise

Encourage 20 to 45 minutes of walking at least four or five times a week.

Client Education

- Find out if the client has sought help because of fear of cancer.
- Determine what the client's goals are for treatment.

Referral

- For uncontrolled IBS, refer to primary care physician or gastroenterologist.
- For psychopathologic conditions (anxiety, depression, posttraumatic stress disorder) refer for counseling and stress relief.

- If the symptoms interfere with the client's quality of life, consider mental health services.
- Consider referral for nutrition counseling.
- Consider referring to self-help and support groups.

Consultation

- Newly diagnosed
- Worsening IBS

Prevention

A high-fiber diet may help prevent IBS.

EVALUATION/FOLLOW-UP

- Initial follow-up is done in 1 to 2 weeks to assess improvement.
- Every 1 to 3 months, adjust follow-up on the basis of recurring signs and symptoms.
- Consider more frequent visits or develop a support group to establish client–provider relationship.

COMPLICATIONS

- Continued diarrhea/constipation
- Frequent medical visits/hopping
- Decreased quality of life

REFERENCES

Bonis, P. & Norton, R. (1996). The challenge of irritable bowel syndrome. *American Family Physician, 53*(3), 1229-1239.

Carlson, E. (1998). Irritable bowel syndrome. *Nurse Practitioner, 23* 82-93.

Cerda, J., Drossman, D., & Scherl, E. (1996). Effective, compassionate management of IBS. *Patient Care, 30*(1), 131-142.

Dalton, C. B. & Drossman, D. A. (1997). Diagnosis and treatment of irritable bowel syndrome. *American Family Physician, 55*(3), 875-880.

Hancock, L. & Selig, P. (1994). Irritable bowel disease. In E. Youngkin & M. Davis (Eds.). *Women's health—a primary care clinical guide* (pp. 609-611). Norwalk, CT: Appleton & Lange.

Hurst, J. W. (1996). *Medicine for the practicing physician.* Norwalk, CT: Appleton & Lange.

Hyams, J. (2001). Diarrhea/constipation: when it is irritable bowel syndrome. *Consultant, 41*(8): 1089-1096.

Johnson, T. R. & Apgar, B. (1995). Irritable bowel syndrome. *The Female Patient, 20,* 48-58.

Lonergan, E. (Ed.). (1996). *Geriatrics: A clinical manual.* Norwalk, CT: Appleton & Lange.

Lynch, J. & Wright, R. (1999).*Update on the management of IBS.* AANP symposium highlights, AANP.

Verne, G. & Cerda, J. (1997). Irritable bowel syndrome: streamlining the diagnosis. *Postgraduate Medicine, 102,* 197-208.

Review Questions

1. Which of the following symptoms are most indicative of IBS?
   a. Fever, nausea, and diarrhea for 10 days
   b. Right lower quadrant abdominal pain with fever
   c. Left lower quadrant abdominal pain with bloody diarrheal stools
   d. Intermittent abdominal pain with diarrhea for 3 months

2. Which of the following findings are most likely to be observed in a client with IBS?
   a. No detectable pathologic condition, generalized abdominal pain
   b. Elevated sedimentation rate
   c. Splenomegaly
   d. Positive guaiac test result

Situation: M.J. is a 28-year-old woman with a history of rape 6 months ago. She seeks treatment with vague symptoms of abdominal pain and bloating after meals for the past 3 months. Her abdominal pain is relieved by a bowel movement. She denies diarrhea or constipation. (Refers to questions 3 and 4.)

3. Which of the following diagnoses is most appropriate for this woman?
   a. Posttraumatic stress disorder
   b. Probable IBS
   c. Probable peptic ulcer
   d. Early stages of ulcerative colitis

4. The client states that the symptom that is causing the most problem is bloating. Which of the following pharmaceutical agents is likely to be most therapeutic?
   a. Dicyclomine (Bentyl)
   b. Loperamide (Imodium)
   c. Simethicone (Mylicon)
   d. Fluoxetine (Prozac)

5. It is important to differentiate between IBS and organic abdominal pain. Which of the following is characteristic of organic abdominal pain?
   a. Pain accompanied by bloating
   b. Pain that radiates to the back
   c. Pain accompanied by diarrhea
   d. Pain that wakes a person from sleep

6. What would you do for an individual with "cramping" after meals associated with IBS?
   a. Amitriptyline (Elavil), 50 mg at bedtime
   b. Dicyclomine (Bentyl), 10 mg qid with meals
   c. Simethicone (Mylicon), 80 mg with meals and at bedtime
   d. Psyllium (Metamucil), bid

7. For clients with IBS, it is important to teach which of the following?
   a. Respond to urges to defecate immediately.
   b. Avoid exercises such as walking.
   c. Eat large meals to create bulk.
   d. Avoid alcohol.

8. Which of the following tests used during a workup for IBS is most expensive?
   a. Stool hematocrit
   b. Echocardiogram
   c. Colonoscopy
   d. Flat-plate and upright abdominal x-ray examination

Answers and Rationales

1. Answer: d (assessment)
Rationale: Fever, bloody stools, nausea, right lower quadrant pain, and diarrhea for short durations are more like an inflammatory or infectious condition, such as appendicitis. Criteria for diagnosis of IBS include continuous or recurrent abdominal pain and a change in bowel habits (diarrhea, constipation, or both) for a 2- to 3-month period (Dalton & Drossman, 1997).

2. Answer: a (assessment)
Rationale: IBS features symptoms of abdominal pain and altered bowel habits with no detectable pathologic condition. Elevated sedimentation rates, splenomegaly, and a positive guaiac result are indicative of infection, of inflammatory disorders, or of a malignancy, all of which/which require further follow-up (Cerda, Drossman, & Scherl, 1996; Dalton & Drossman, 1997).

3. Answer: b (analysis/diagnosis)
Rationale: This individual fits the profile of a person vulnerable to IBS: female, age 28, with previous experience with sexual violence. Her symptoms are typical of IBS, more so than of any other listed diagnoses. Additional information is required to rule out the other diagnoses listed (Dalton & Drossman, 1997).

4. Answer: c (implementation/plan)
Rationale: Simethicone is an antiflatulent, which will help with symptoms of bloating. Dicyclomine is an antispasmodic; loperamide is a constipating agent; and fluoxetine is given for

individuals with depression who have constipation (Rogers, 2000).

5. Answer: d (analysis/diagnosis)
Rationale: Pain that awakens the client from sleep is more likely organic in nature. IBS abdominal pain does not wake the client from sleep. All the other descriptions are characteristic of IBS (Rogers, 2000).

6. Answer: b (implementation/plan)
Rationale: Dicyclomine is an antispasmodic and anticholinergic agent suitable for relief of postprandial cramping. Amitriptyline is an anticholinergic agent used at night for clients with depression and diarrhea. Simethicone is an antiflatulent agent, and psyllium is a bulk-producing agent (Lynch and Wright, 1999).

7. Answer: a (implementation/plan)
Rationale: It is important to promote bowel habits that minimize problems associated with constipation and promote normal bowel function, so responding promptly to urges to defecate is important. Exercise (such as walking) should be encouraged for general health, and it is not contraindicated. Alcohol in moderation (if tolerated) is not contraindicated. Small meals rather than large meals are encouraged (Rogers, 2000).

8. Answer: c (implementation/plan)
Rationale: Colonoscopy is the most expensive procedure. It may be used to rule out diverticular disease, inflammatory bowel disease, or malignancy. Stool hematocrit is the least expensive. An x-ray examination is moderately expensive. Echocardiograms are expensive and are not part of an IBS workup (Hyams, 2001).

JUVENILE RHEUMATOID ARTHRITIS *Denise Robinson*

OVERVIEW
Definition

Juvenile rheumatoid arthritis (JRA) is a disease or group of diseases characterized by chronic synovitis and associated with a number of extraarticular symptoms (Schaller, 1996). Persistent arthritis must be present at least 6 consecutive weeks for the diagnosis of JRA. The outcome is unpredictable: some children may have mild arthritis causing little disability, whereas others may have severe arthritis that progresses to joint destruction and permanent deformity. Patients with rheumatoid factor positive polyarthritis have the worst prognosis for joint function.

JRA has three major presentations, following:
1. *Acute febrile form* with salmon macular rash, arthritis, splenomegaly, leukocytosis, and polyserositis
2. A *polyarticular pattern* (five or more joints involved) that resembles adult disease, with chronic pain and swelling of many joints. Two subgroups include rheumatoid factor positive group and rheumatoid factor negative group. The positive group is characterized by onset in late childhood, more severe arthritis, rheumatoid nodules, and occasional rheumatoid vasculitis. The negative group has symptoms that occur at any time, gen-

erally with milder course. More girls than boys are affected in both groups.
3. *Pauciarticular disease* (less than five joints) characterized by chronic arthritis of a few joints, often the large weight-bearing joints, in asymmetric distribution. There are two types: type I is the most common form of JRA. The disease usually occurs in girls before the fourth birthday. Up to 30% of children 1 to 16 years old with this form of disease develop iridocyclitis, which can cause blindness if untreated. Type II mainly affects boys who are usually older than 8 years at onset. Large joints are affected, especially those of the lower extremities. Hip girdle involvement is common.

Incidence

- Approximately 250,000 children are affected in the United States.
- Five percent of all cases of arthritis begin in childhood.
- The onset of JRA occurs between 2 and 4 years of age.
- The rate of JRA in girls is almost twice that of boys.
- Polyarticular onset occurs in 35% of children with JRA.
- Pauciarticular onset is the most common, occurring in 30% to 40% of children.

J

- Acute febrile onset occurs in 10% of children, boys equal to girls.

Pathophysiology

- The cause of JRA is unknown.
- Hypothesis of cause is that the disease results from an infection with an unidentified microorganism that results in hypersensitivity or an autoimmune reaction.
- Immunodeficiency may predispose the child to JRA; the onset may follow an acute systemic illness or physical trauma to a joint.
- Rheumatoid arthritis is characterized by the following:
  - Chronic nonsuppurative inflammation of synovium is present.
  - The affected tissues are infiltrated with lymphocytic and plasma cells, causing swelling. The thickened synovial tissue protrudes into joint spaces, becoming adherent to cartilage.
  - With chronic synovitis, the joint structures can become eroded and progressively destroyed.
- Damage with JRA occurs later than with adult-onset RA.
- Rheumatoid nodules occur less commonly in children than adults.
- Children exhibit different immunogenic traits compared with adult RA patients.
- In JRA, human leukocyte antigen (HLA)-DR5 is associated with iritis and the production of antinuclear antibody (ANA), whereas HLA-DR4 is found in seropositive, polyarticular disease. Tumor necrosing factor (TNF) may be the cytokine that promotes continuation of the inflammation.

ASSESSMENT: SUBJECTIVE/HISTORY
History of Present Illness

There are three patterns of presentation in JRA.

Acute Febrile Form

- Fever, high and intermittent, usually occurs in the morning and evening, sometimes with shaking chills.
- Salmon pink macular rash occurs on the trunk and proximal extremities but can occur anywhere on the body; it usually occurs during febrile periods.
- One third of children have pleuritis or pericarditis, often subclinical.
- Joint symptoms include swelling in the midcarpal and midtarsus bones.

Polyarticular Pattern. The polyarticular pattern resembles adult RA, as follows:

- Gradual, insidious onset of joint stiffness, swelling, and loss of motion occurs. Affected joints are swollen and warm, but rarely red. Joints first involved are the knees, ankles, wrists, and elbows. Arthritis of the neck occurs in approximately 50% of patients, as does hip involvement.
- Chronic pain and swelling of many joints in symmetric fashion, including small joints of the hand may be present.
- Fatigue may be present.
- Low-grade fever may be present.
- Rheumatoid nodules may be present.

Pauciarticular Disease

- Four or fewer joints are involved in the first 6 months.
- Chronic arthritis of a few joints may occur, including in the weight-bearing joints, asymmetric distribution; knees, ankles, elbows.
- Inflammation of the eye may occur; symptoms include redness, pain, photophobia, decreased visual acuity.
- Mild systemic signs are fever, malaise, lymphadenopathy.

Past Medical History

Ask about joint swelling, intermittent fevers, and eye problems such as pain, redness, and decreased acuity.

Family History

Ask about a family history of arthritis, ankylosing spondylitis, Reiter's syndrome, or acute iridocyclitis.

ASSESSMENT: OBJECTIVE/PHYSICAL EXAMINATION
Physical Examination

Conduct a problem-oriented physical examination, keeping in mind potential systemic manifestations of RA (e.g., dermatologic, pleurisy, splenomegaly, ocular manifestations) that might necessitate a complete physical examination.

- Pay attention to vital signs, weight, blood pressure, and pulse.
- Note general appearance, gait, and activity level.
- Pay particular attention to eye, looking for redness, inflammation, and photophobia. A slit lamp examination is recommended for those patients in whom iridocyclitis is suspected.
- Perform abdominal examination; check for hepatomegaly and splenomegaly.
- Perform musculoskeletal examination, doing the following:
  - Inspect affected joints for deformities, nodes, numbers of affected joints, symmetry of affected joints, and erythema.
  - Observe affected joints in active/passive range of motion (ROM).
  - Palpate affected joints for warmth, tenderness, crepitus, and edema.
  - Assess muscle strength.
  - Assess joint stability.

Diagnostic Tests

- Hemoglobin to check for anemia of chronic disease
- Complete blood count (CBC) to check for leukocytosis
- Rheumatoid factor
- ANA
- Erythrocyte sedimentation rate (ESR) may be normal
- Culture of joint fluid
- Magnetic resonance imaging (MRI) to possibly show joint damage earlier in the course of disease than other methods

DIAGNOSIS

- Monoarticular arthritis (pain in the hip is often seen in childhood cancers such as leukemia)
- Bacterial arthritis
- Rheumatic fever
- Orthopedic causes resulting from increased physical activity

THERAPEUTIC PLAN

Objectives are to restore function, relieve pain, and maintain joint motion.

Pharmacologic Treatment

- Nonsteroidal antiinflammatory drugs (NSAIDs), such as naproxen and ibuprofen, are approved for use with children.
- Drug-modifying agents include the following:
  - Methotrexate can be used if NSAIDs fail.
  - Sulfasalazine is showing promise with some patients with JRA.
  - Etanercept (Enbrel) is a tumor necrosis factor (TNF) receptor blocker that is showing promise in patients with rheumatoid arthritis.

Nonpharmacologic Treatment

- Range-of-motion exercises
- Muscle-strengthening exercises
- Night splints may be helpful in preventing and correcting deformities.

Education

- Bed rest is avoided unless in the most acute stages.
- Children should lead as normal a life as possible.
- Parents and children need to know realistically what to expect and to be treated optimistically.
- Children should be able to lead active lives, attend school, and participate in usual activities.

Referral/Consultation

Iridocyclitis should be followed by an ophthalmologist. Screening should be done every 3 months for the first 4 years.

EVALUATION/FOLLOW-UP

- In the primarily articular forms of JRA, the disease activity diminishes with age and stops in about 95% of cases by teen years.
- Cases presenting in the teen years are more likely to be similar to adult RA.
- Functional classifications:
  - I: Performs all activities
  - II: Performs adequately with some limitations
  - III: Limited activity, self-care only
  - IV: Wheelchair-bound or bedridden
- Children should report any visual changes or problems.
- Eye examinations should occur at every visit; children with pauciarticular disease should have examinations four times a year.

COMPLICATIONS

- Blindness
- Deformities, activity-limiting disease

REFERENCES

Hollister, J. (1999). Rheumatic disease. In W. Hay, A. Hayward, M. Levin, & J. Sondheimer (Eds.), *Current pediatric diagnosis and treatment*. Stamford, CT: Appleton Lange, 715-717.

Lovell, D. J., Giannini, E. H., Reiff, A., Cawkwell, G. D., Silverman, E. D., Nocton, J. J., Stein, L. D., Gedalia, A., Dowite, N. T., Wallace, C. A., Whitmore, J., & Finck, B. K. (2000). Etanercept in children with polyarticular juvenile rheumatoid arthritis. *New England Journal of Medicine, 342*, 763-769.

Rosenberg, A. (1996). Treatment of juvenile rheumatoid arthritis: Approach to patients who fail standard therapy. *Journal of Rheumatology, 23*, 9-13.

Schaller, J. (1996) Juvenile rheumatoid arthritis. In W. Nelson, R. Behrman, R. Kliegman, & A. Arvin (Eds.), *Nelson textbook of pediatrics*. Philadelphia: W. B. Saunders, 661-670.

Tibbits, G. (1994). Juvenile rheumatoid arthritis: Old challenges, new insights. *Postgraduate Medicine, 96*, 75-80.

Review Questions

1. Carly is a 9-year-old girl who has been diagnosed with juvenile rheumatoid arthritis. Which of the following historical data is consistent with a diagnosis of JRA?
- **a.** Carly plays tackle football.
- **b.** Carly is wheelchair bound.
- **c.** Carly complains of joint stiffness in the morning when she wakes up.
- **d.** Carly reports that her knee pain started after she played soccer.

2. Which of the following symptom descriptions provided by Sara, in addition to joint pain and stiffness, is typical of JRA?
- **a.** "My hands and feet are swollen."
- **b.** "I can't get up the steps."

J

c. "I have noticed that my urine has a stronger odor and is darker in color."
d. "I am unable to tell red from green when I look at things."

3. During the physical assessment, which of the following findings are consistent with JRA?

a. Eczema
b. Erythema migrans
c. Monoarticular joint involvement
d. Hepatosplenomegaly

4. What are the first-line tests in cases of JRA?

a. Rheumatoid factor, ANA, MRI
b. Bone scan, blood culture
c. Viral culture, CBC
d. Tissue biopsy, genital culture

5. JRA must be differentiated from Lyme disease. Compared with JRA, Lyme disease is associated with which of the following?

a. Fewer than four joints involved, flulike illness, episodic recurrent symptoms
b. Monoarticular, joint hot, swollen, painful, red
c. Severe bone and joint pain, night pain
d. Transient arthritis, often polyarticular

6. Which of the following drug choices is the best choice for JRA?

a. NSAID
b. ASA
c. Gold therapy
d. Chronic corticosteroids

7. Gina is a 6-year-old girl with pauciarticular onset disease JRA. Which of the following is critical for the nurse practitioner to screen for regularly?

a. Urine culture every 6 months
b. MRI every month to check for bone destruction
c. Slit lamp examination every 3 months
d. CBC every 6 months

8. What comment by the parents of a child with JRA indicates the need for more teaching?

a. "Karen should see her eye doctor every 3 months."
b. "Steve cannot participate on the debate team because of his JRA."
c. "JRA waxes and wanes during childhood."
d. "Marvion should take his Ibuprofen every day."

Answers and Rationales

1. *Answer:* **c** (assessment)
Rationale: Joint stiffness in the morning is a frequent complaint of kids with JRA (Schaller, 1996).

2. *Answer:* **a** (assessment)
Rationale: The underlying pathophysiologic process of JRA includes swelling of the synovial tissue, leading to swelling (Schaller, 1996).

3. *Answer:* **d** (assessment)
Rationale: Hepatosplenomegaly is common in all forms of JRA. Erythema migrans is the lesions characteristic of Lyme disease; monoarticular joint involvement is more characteristic of septic arthritis or trauma. Eczema is not associated with JRA (Schaller, 1996).

4. *Answer:* **a** (implementation/plan)
Rationale: ANA, rheumatoid factor, and MRI are all important in the diagnosis of JRA. They help determine what the course of the illness will be. Viral culture is important for Lyme disease; bone scan and blood culture are usual tests for osteomyelitis. Tissue biopsy would be important if malignancy were a differential. Genital culture would be needed if septic arthritis were a consideration (Schaller, 1996).

5. *Answer:* **a** (analysis/diagnosis)
Rationale: Lyme disease usually involves fewer than four joints, with episodic and recurrent symptoms. Erythema migrans is a characteristic skin lesion seen in Lyme disease. Severe bone and joint pain is associated with childhood malignancy. A monoarticular joint that is hot, swollen, and painful is symptomatic of septic arthritis. A transient arthritis involving more than five joints is characteristic of viral arthritis (Schaller, 1996).

6. *Answer:* **a** (implementation/plan)
Rationale: NSAIDs are the drugs of choice for JRA. ASA use is not recommended because of the possibility of Reye syndrome. Gold therapy is also not used as frequently for JRA patients. Corticosteroids should only be used during acute episodes of inflammation and should be immediately tapered and discontinued (Schaller, 1996).

7. *Answer:* **c** (evaluation)
Rationale: Children with pauciarticular onset JRA are at risk of developing iridocyclitis. They should be screened every 3 months for the first 5 years of the disease regardless of the activity of joint disease (Schaller, 1996).

8. *Answer:* **b** (evaluation)
Rationale: Children with JRA can lead active lives; activities can include sports, just not strenuous activities. Bed rest and long inactive periods are not recommended (Schaller, 1996).

KAWASAKI DISEASE   *Denise Robinson*

OVERVIEW
Definition

Kawasaki disease is a febrile illness with an acute onset from inflammation of the arteries, particularly the coronary arteries. Also known as mucocutaneous lymph node syndrome and infantile polyarteritis.

Incidence

- Boys are affected more than girls (1.5:1).
- The greatest incidence is between age 18 and 24 months.
- Approximately 80% of affected children are younger than 5.
- The highest risk is among Asian children, especially those of Japanese or Korean ethnicity.
- It is the leading cause of acquired heart disease in the United States.
- From 20% to 25% of untreated children develop coronary artery abnormalities, which may resolve or persist.
- It occurs more often in winter and spring.
- Incidence rates in the United States and Canada are 6 to 11 cases per 100,000 children younger than 5 (Taubert & Shulman, 1999).
- Incidence in Japan is 90 cases per 100,000 children younger than 5 years old. More than 1% of affected children had a family history of sibling Kawasaki disease.

Pathophysiology

The cause is unknown, but it is believed to be associated with the dust mite. It is a type III hypersensitivity reaction with depositing of immune complexes. These complexes increase blood viscosity and produce aneurysm formation. It may also be caused by a superantigen secreted by *Staphylococus aureus.*

The disease has four stages:
- Stage 1 (11 days): signs and symptoms of fever (fever persisting at least 5 days), conjunctivitis, irritability, rash, cervical lymph node enlargement, elevated erythrocyte sedimentation rate (ESR)
- Stage 2 (10 to 14 days): cardiac complications, fever irritability, desquamation of fingers and toes
- Stage 3 (6 to 10 weeks): conjunctivitis and aneurysms of peripheral vessels
- Stage 4 (duration unknown): coronary complications in adulthood, thrombosis, myocardial infarction, dysrhythmias, congestive heart failure

Factors Increasing Susceptibility
- Living by bodies of water
- Recently shampooed rugs

ASSESSMENT: SUBJECTIVE/HISTORY
History of Present Illness

- Rash
- Fever greater than 5 days' duration unresponsive to antibiotics
- Diarrhea in infants
- Irritability
- Cough
- Joint pain
- Conjunctivitis

Past Medical History
- Recent respiratory illness
- Recent streptococcal infection

Medication History
Antibiotics.

Family History
Not usually significant in the United States, but in Japan frequently a sibling also has Kawasaki disease.

Psychosocial History
Recent exposure to dust and dust mites.

Associated Symptoms
- Arthralgia
- Erythema and induration at recent BCG inoculation site

ASSESSMENT: OBJECTIVE/PHYSICAL EXAMINATION
Physical Examination

A physical examination should be performed with attention to the following:
- *General appearance:* Note irritability in infants; assess vital signs to rule out fever.
- *Head, eyes, and ears:* In the ears, the tympanic membrane (TM) may be pink. The eyes may have poor light reflex, concomitant otitis media, bilateral tearing without exudate, and injection of conjunctiva, which is usually painless.
- *Lymph:* Usually the anterior cervical chain is enlarged, with at least one lymph node of 1.5 cm or greater, usually unilateral enlargement, nodes firm and slightly tender.
- *Throat:* Enlarged, erythematous tonsils without exudate may be present.
- *Mouth:* Strawberry tongue and dry, erythematous, cracked lips may be present; ulcers are not seen.
- *Skin:* Indurative edema or erythema of the soles and palms, desquamation of hands and feet beginning in

the fingertips, nonvesicular diffuse, polymorphous rash mostly on the trunk within 5 days of onset of fever (no bullae or vesicles are seen); Beau's lines (white lines across the fingernails) appear 1 to 2 months after the onset of fever.
- Cardiac: May hear murmur of mitral valve regurgitation or friction rub.

Diagnostic Procedures

- Complete blood count (CBC): leukocytosis with shift to the left (neutrophils in immature format); thrombocytosis, anemia
- Urinalysis: proteinuria
- Erythrocyte sedimentation rate (ESR): elevated
- C reactive protein: positive
- Liver enzymes: elevated
- Chest radiograph: pulmonary infiltrates and cardiomegaly possible
- Electrocardiogram (ECG): dysrhythmia
- Echocardiogram: mitral insufficiency, aneurysms; pericardial effusion

DIAGNOSIS

- Scarlet fever
- Measles
- Toxic shock syndrome
- Stevens-Johnson syndrome
- Classic diagnostic criteria more often lacking in infants younger than 6 months old

THERAPEUTIC PLAN
Pharmacologic Treatment

- For best effect, treatment needs to take place within the first 10 days of illness, especially in children younger than 1 year.
- Hospitalization is required for administration of intravenous (IV) gamma globulin and monitoring of cardiac status.
- Dipyridamole and warfarin therapy may be started if the child develops coronary artery aneurysm.
- Corticosteroids are contraindicated and have been associated with aneurysm formation.
- In addition, acetylsalicylic acid (ASA) is given 80 to 100 mg/kg/day in four divided doses (stopped if varicella or flu is present to prevent Reye syndrome); it is continued into the convalescent phase at 3 to 5 mg/kg/day in a single dose.

Nonpharmacologic Treatment

Depending on the degree of cardiac involvement, activity may be limited.

Client Education

- Parents should be taught that administration of live virus (e.g., varicella, typhoid, yellow fever, and measles) should be delayed after administration of IV gamma globulin.
- Parents should be taught that coronary artery damage may not manifest itself until adulthood; therefore echocardiograms should be repeated throughout adolescence.

Consultation/Referral

Children suspected of having Kawasaki disease should be evaluated by a pediatric cardiologist and followed by the cardiologist if complications are present.

Prevention

- Avoid newly shampooed rugs.
- Limit exposure to dusty environments.

EVALUATION/FOLLOW-UP

- Beware of the development of aneurysms in unusual places, such as the hepatic, axillary, and brachial arteries.
- Clients should be followed throughout all stages: initially in 1 week, then in 1 month, then in 6 months, and annually.

COMPLICATIONS

- Coronary artery aneurysms are possible.
- Myocardial infarction is the principal cause of death, usually 1 year or later after the illness.
- Congestive heart failure is possible.

REFERENCES

Fredriksen, M. (1998). An infant with persistent fever. *Clinical Review, 8*, 129-136.

McKenzie, C. (1998). A 3-year-old girl with a rash. In D. Robinson (Ed.). *Clinical decision making for nurse practitioners: A case study approach*. Philadelphia: Lippincott, 291-298.

Rubin, B., & Cotton, D. (1998). Kawasaki disease: A dangerous acute childhood illness. *Nurse Practitioner, 23*, 34-48.

Taubert, K., & Shulman, S. (1999). Kawasaki disease. *American Family Physician*, June. Retrieved July 31, 2002, from www.aafp.org/990600ap/3093.html

Review Questions

1. Which of the following is consistent with historical data for Kawasaki disease?
- **a.** Bilateral conjunctivitis
- **b.** Pharyngitis
- **c.** Diarrhea
- **d.** Syncope

2. Which of the following symptoms should make the nurse practitioner suspicious of Kawasaki disease in a child?
- **a.** Nausea and vomiting
- **b.** Prolonged fever for 5 or more days

c. Syncope
d. Anemia

3. Which of the following tests is crucial to the child with Kawasaki disease?

a. CBC
b. ESR
c. Chest radiograph
d. Echocardiogram

4. When is the development of coronary artery aneurysms likely to develop in Kawasaki disease?

a. At onset
b. In the first week
c. Within the first 2 to 3 weeks
d. After 2 months

5. The treatment of choice for a child with Kawasaki disease is which of the following?

a. Penicillin
b. IV gamma globulin
c. Azathioprine (Imuran)
d. Corticosteroids

6. After hospitalization for Kawasaki disease, which of the following therapy treatments should be started?

a. Oral gamma globulin
b. Acetaminophen
c. Aspirin
d. Nitroglycerine

7. Which of the following children is more at risk for development of coronary artery disease?

a. Girls less than 1 year of age
b. Children with a fever lasting longer than 4 weeks
c. Children who have a low-grade fever
d. Children with a normal ESR

8. Which of the following historical data is consistent with the diagnosis of Kawasaki disease?

a. 10-year-old African-American boy
b. 3-year-old Asian boy
c. 5-year-old Russian girl
d. 14-year-old American girl

Answers and Rationales

1. *Answer:* **a** (assessment)
Rationale: Bilateral conjunctivitis occurs in 90% of children who have Kawasaki disease, along with a fever, rash, and lym-phadenopathy, which occurs in 50% of children (Rubin & Cotton, 1998).

2. *Answer:* **b** (analysis/diagnosis)
Rationale: Clients with Kawasaki disease have a prolonged spiking fever, which lasts longer than 5 days. It is unresponsive to antibiotics and is unexplained by any symptoms (Rubin & Cotton, 1998).

3. *Answer:* **d** (implementation/plan)
Rationale: The echocardiogram is crucial to the evaluation of the child with Kawasaki disease. It is important to obtain a baseline echo at the onset of the disease (Rubin & Cotton, 1998).

4. *Answer:* **c** (evaluation)
Rationale: Coronary artery aneurysms usually develop during stage II of the illness, during the second to third weeks after onset. The echocardiogram should be repeated during the second to third week of the illness and 1 month later (Rubin & Cotton, 1998).

5. *Answer:* **b** (implementation/plan)
Rationale: The treatment of choice for Kawasaki disease is IV gamma globulin. The goal of treatment is to prevent the development of coronary artery aneurysm and thrombosis by reduction of inflammation. This treatment is given while the child is hospitalized (Rubin & Cotton, 1998).

6. *Answer:* **c** (implementation/plan)
Rationale: ASA is started after hospitalization to help decrease coronary artery inflammation and prevent thrombosis (Rubin & Cotton, 1998).

7. *Answer:* **b** (evaluation)
Rationale: Those children who have had a fever lasting longer than 4 weeks are more at risk for development of coronary artery disease (CAD). Boys less than 1 year of age and children with a high ESR are also more at risk for development of CAD (Rubin & Cotton, 1998).

8. *Answer:* **b** (assessment)
Rationale: Kawasaki disease is more prevalent in young children under the age of 5. It is more common in children of Asian descent (Rubin & Cotton, 1998).

KNEE INJURIES   *Denise Robinson*

OVERVIEW
Definition

An injury to one of the ligamentous structures of the body is called a *sprain*. A *strain* is trauma to a muscle or musculoskeletal unit of the body from an excessive forcible stretch. Loss in continuity in the substance of the bone is called a *fracture*.

Anatomy. The knee joint includes four bones: the distal femur, the patella, the proximal fibula, and the proximal tibia. Soft, pliable cartilage, the medial and lateral menisci, lie within the tibiofemoral joint and function to reduce stress and act as a cushion between the femur and tibia.

Intraarticular ligaments called the anterior cruciate ligament (ACL) and the posterior cruciate ligament (PCL) stabilize the knee in an anterior and posterior fashion. The extraarticular ligaments, the medial collateral ligament (MCL) and the lateral collateral ligament (LCL), maintain varus and valgus stability of the knee. The extensor mechanism of the knee is maintained by the quadriceps ligament, the patella, and the patellar tendon (Figure 3-8).

Incidence

- Knee trauma is responsible for an estimated 1.3 million visits to emergency departments in the United States.

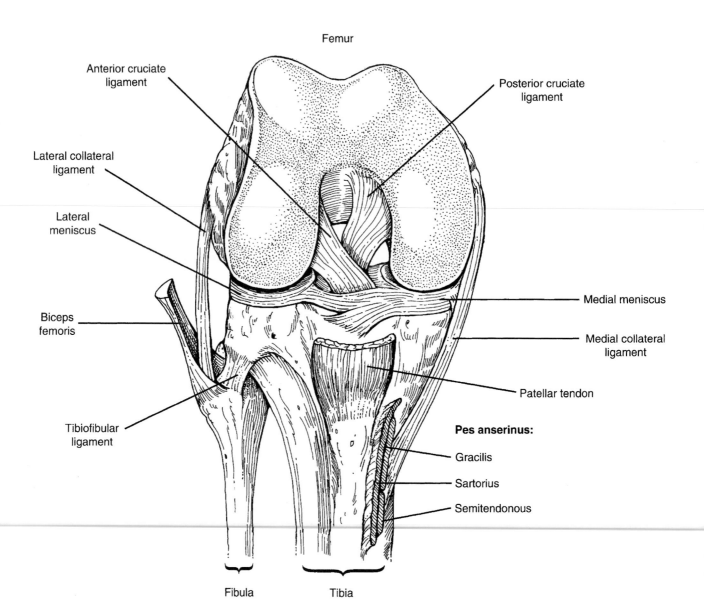

FIGURE **3-8**   Anterior view of the knee. (From Scuderi, G. R., McCann, P. D., & Bruno, P. J. (1997). *Sports medicine: Principles of primary care*. St. Louis, Mosby.)

- Women appear to be more susceptible to ACL injuries than men, they are injured 2 to 8 times more frequently.
- ACL, PCL, MCL, and LCL injuries are uncommon in children.
- Growth plate fractures are more common in children.

Pathophysiology

Sprain. Ligaments, which connect bones together, can sustain injuries. Ligamentous injuries are classified as first degree, second degree, or third degree, depending on the extent of injury. A completely torn ligament is classified as a third-degree sprain, whereas a mildly stretched ligament is classified as a first-degree sprain.

Fractures. Fractures are classified as either open or closed. Open fractures are exposed to the environment and are highly prone to serious infection. Description of a fracture includes anatomic location as well as degree of displacement, translation, or shortening. Fractures into the joint are called *intraarticular fractures*. Fracture patterns are described as transverse, oblique, spiral, comminuted, or greenstick. Salter-Harris classification is commonly used to describe growth plate fractures in children.

Common Injuries/Fractures. *Meniscus* injuries usually result from a tear in either the lateral or medial meniscus secondary to some type of sport involvement. They are unusual in children younger than 12 years of age.

Ligament injuries involving the ACL, PCL, MCL, and LCL commonly occur during high-impact injuries to the knees.

ASSESSMENT: SUBJECTIVE/HISTORY
History of Present Illness

- Exact mechanism of injury
- Timing of injury
- Description/location of pain
- Radiation
- Quality
- Timing
- Severity
- Aggravation/relief
- Previous treatment

Symptoms

- Swelling: If swelling occurs quickly after an injury (within 4 hours), there is a high likelihood of a major osseous, ligamentous, or meniscal injury (Johnson, 2000).
- Deformity may be present.
- Masses may be present.
- Paralysis may occur.
- Gait changes may be present.

Past Medical History
- Previous injuries
- Surgery
- Exercise history
- Allergies

Medication History
Ask about recent or present use of pain medications, non-steroidal antiinflammatory drugs (NSAIDs), and other medications.

Family History
Inquire about orthopedic problems.

Psychosocial History
- Occupational job description
- Smoking
- Alcohol intake
- Conditioning history

History of Common Injuries/Fractures
- Meniscus injuries occur in all age groups and often are associated with athletic activity in which a hyperextension, hyperflexion, or rotational injury occurs. A twisting of the knee is a common complaint with meniscal injuries. The client may describe swelling, clicking, locking, and pain with rotational movements.
- Collateral ligament injuries occur as a result of varus or valgus stress to the knee. ACL injuries occur with twisting motion, a quick stop, or a hyperextension.
- ACL injuries are also associated with an audible pop. Eighty-five percent of clients who have an ACL tear are immediately disabled and are not able to continue their activity. Clients often describe a feeling of "giving way" and report hearing or feeling a "pop" at the time of injury (Ballas, Tytko, & Mannarino, 1998).
- PCL injuries are associated with a direct blow to the anterior portion of the tibia. They occur less commonly than ACL injuries. The typical mechanism of injury is a blow to the anterior proximal tibia with the knee flexed, such as striking the dashboard in an automobile accident. Less instability and less swelling is seen with PCL than with ACL injuries.
- Knee fractures are more likely in clients who were involved in a high-velocity collision, reported occurrence of a "pop" at time of injury, are older than 55, and have an inability to bear weight after the injury.

ASSESSMENT: OBJECTIVE/PHYSICAL EXAMINATION
Physical Examination

A problem-oriented physical examination should be conducted, with particular attention to vital signs, general assessment, musculoskeletal area of complaint, adjacent musculoskeletal areas, and neurovascular status distal to the injury.

- Vital signs should be relatively normal with common, non-life-threatening injuries.
- General assessment should note the client's response to pain, gait, and how the client holds the injured extremity.
- Musculoskeletal assessment should observe for swelling and effusion, palpation of adjacent and actual areas of injury, evaluation of range of motion (ROM), and special physical testing to diagnose specific conditions.
- Inspect the knee in both flexed and extended positions, noting the major landmarks. Palpate the popliteal space, noting any swelling or tenderness. The joint should feel firm and smooth, without tenderness, bogginess, or crepitus.
- Neurovascular assessment should be performed distal to the injury. Check pulses, sensation, and capillary refill.

Specific Physical Findings of Common Injuries/ Fractures

- Meniscus injuries are characterized by mild swelling, joint line tenderness, and positive results from a McMurray test (Figure 3-9). The client is unable to hop or squat because of pain.

- MCL injuries are associated with joint line pain, mild swelling, +/1 joint effusion, pain, and/or laxity with valgus stress (Figure 3-10).
- LCL injuries include joint line pain, +/1 swelling or effusion, and pain and/or laxity with varus stress (Figure 3-11).
- ACL injuries often include a joint effusion with a positive anterior drawer sign or positive Lachman's test (Figures 3-12 and 3-13).
- PCL injuries are associated with minimal swelling but a positive posterior drawer sign or a positive sag sign of Godfrey (Figure 3-14).
- Physical examination findings suggestive of fracture include a tense effusion, deformity, crepitation, and ecchymosis.

Diagnostic Procedures

Consider x-ray examinations with significant pain, swelling, effusion, or contusion. Obtain radiographs when there is significant swelling, pain, or high-impact injury. Always obtain multiple views, including anteroposterior and lateral. Oblique views may be necessary for tibial plateau fractures. Obtain a sunrise view of the patella if trauma occurred directly to the patella.

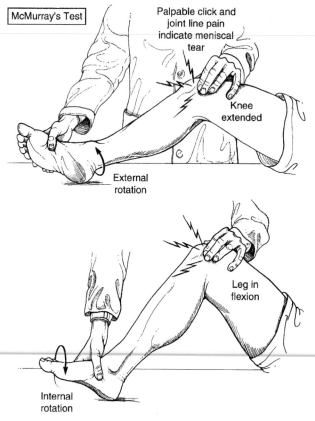

FIGURE **3-9** McMurray's test. The leg in flexion is moved from valgus, external rotation, to varus, internal rotation. Alternatively, the knee can be extended during the maneuver. A meniscal tear is suspected with a palpable click or joint line pain. (From Scuderi, G. R., McCann, P. D., & Bruno, P. J. (1997). *Sports medicine: Principles of primary care*. St. Louis, Mosby.)

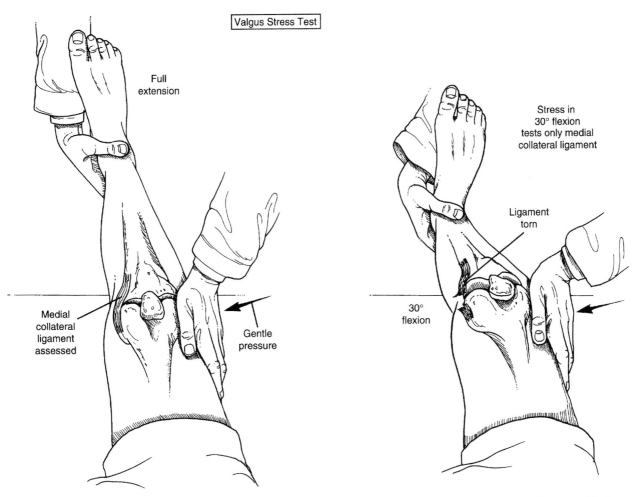

FIGURE **3-10** The valgus stress test is performed *A*, at full extension to assess secondary restraints and *B*, at 30 degrees of flexion to assess medial collateral ligament. (From Scuderi, G. R., McCann, P. D., & Bruno, P. J. (1997). *Sports medicine: Principles of primary care.* St. Louis, Mosby.)

Radiographic Findings of Common Injuries/Fractures.
Soft tissue injuries (ACL, MCL, PCL, LCL, and meniscus injuries) usually reveal normal findings on radiograph films, with the exception of a visible joint effusion or soft tissue swelling. Occasionally, a ligament rupture reveals a small avulsion fracture.

DIAGNOSIS

The differential diagnoses include the following:
- Sprain
- Strain
- Fracture
- Tendinitis: microscopic tears of the involved muscles with inflammation; no swelling, normal ROM
- Osteoarthritis (OA): articular deterioration and bony overgrowth of the joint surface
- Rheumatoid arthritis (RA): multiple joints, morning stiffness, swelling, heat, and stiffness
- Gout
- Gonococcal arthritis
- Overuse syndromes
- Infections
- Bursitis: limitation of movement caused by swelling, point tenderness; most common site prepatellar bursae in the knee

THERAPEUTIC PLAN
Nonpharmacologic Treatment

- Follow RICE procedure: rest, ice, compression, and elevation.
- Rest any injured part of the musculoskeletal system. Rest time varies according to the seriousness of the injury.
- Ice all musculoskeletal injuries in an attempt to control swelling. Continue ice application as long as swelling exists. Ice can be applied for 15 minutes at a time.
- Compression controls edema and provides comfort and support. Compression can be accomplished with elastic bandages, neoprene braces, custom-made splints, and commercially made splints.
- Elevate all injured extremities.

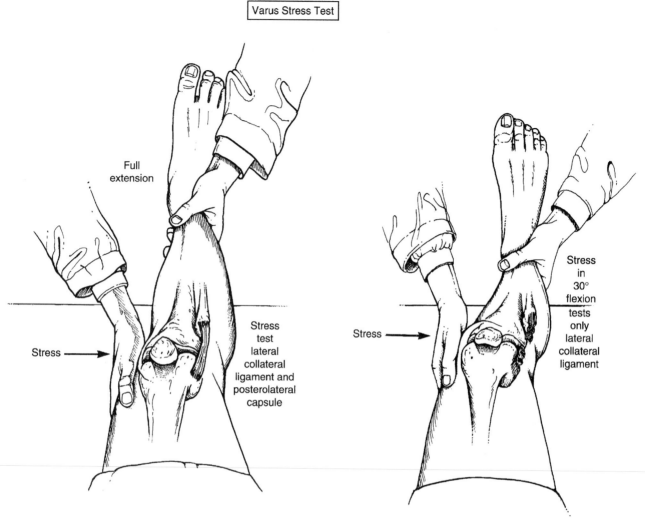

FIGURE **3-11**   The varus stress test is performed *A*, at full extension to assess secondary restraints and *B*, at 30 degrees of flexion to assess the lateral collateral ligament. (From Scuderi, G. R., McCann, P. D., & Bruno, P. J. (1997). *Sports medicine: Principles of primary care*. St. Louis, Mosby.)

- Surgery is the best option for athletes with an ACL tear who want to continue activities requiring twisting or rapid changes in direction. In nonathletes or older clients, the decision should be based on the client's activity level and expectations regarding activities. In these clients, alteration of lifestyle and use of a support or brace may represent a preferred alternative (Ballas, Tytko, & Mannarino, 1998).

Joint Protection/Immobilization

- The injured joint should be protected with application of a splint.
- Splinting allows for postinjury swelling.
- Never apply a circumferential cast to an acutely injured extremity.
- Use crutches for lower extremity injuries.

- Many splints are commercially made, and easy-to-apply custom-made splinting material includes plaster and fiberglass.
- Immobilization assists in pain control.

Splints for Knee Injuries. Commercially available knee immobilizers apply compression and immobilize the knee in full extension. If a commercial knee brace is not available, the knee can be adequately immobilized in full extension with a bulky wrap or Kerlex rolls and elastic bandages. Crutches should be used for knee injuries.

Pharmacologic Treatment

- Antiinflammatory drugs and muscle relaxants are the drugs of choice for musculoskeletal injury.
- NSAIDs are indicated for musculoskeletal injury. NSAIDs inhibit prostaglandin synthesis, which

Anterior Drawer Test

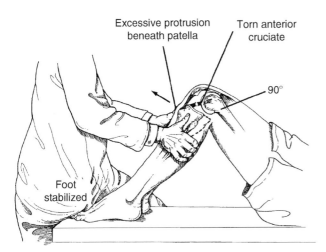

FIGURE **3-12**   The anterior drawer test is performed at 90 degrees of flexion with anteriorly directed force applied to the proximal tibia. (From Scuderi, G. R., McCann, P. D., & Bruno, P. J. (1997). *Sports medicine: Principles of primary care.* St. Louis, Mosby.)

Lachman's Test

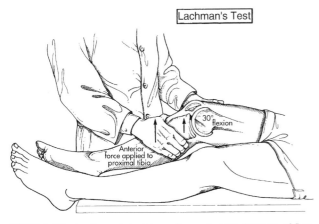

FIGURE **3-13**   Lachman's test is performed at 30 degrees of flexion with an anteriorly directed force applied to the proximal tibia while the opposite hand stabilizes the thigh. (From Scuderi, G. R., McCann, P. D., & Bruno, P. J. (1997). *Sports medicine: Principles of primary care.* St. Louis, Mosby.)

decreases pain. Common NSAIDs include ibuprofen (Motrin), naproxen (Naprosyn), etodolac (Lodine), and diclofenac (Voltaren). Do not prescribe NSAIDs to clients with peptic ulcer disease, allergy to NSAIDs/aspirin, renal dysfunction, or pregnancy. NSAIDs should be used with caution in congestive heart failure (CHF).

- Myorelaxants are indicated for pain related to muscle spasm. Common muscle relaxants include cyclobenzaprine (Flexeril) and chlorzoxazone (Parafon Forte). Muscle relaxants should be prescribed for short periods (3 to 5 days).
- Over-the-counter (OTC) analgesics such as acetaminophen are used for less severe pain and for clients who are unable to take NSAIDs.

Posterior Drawer Test

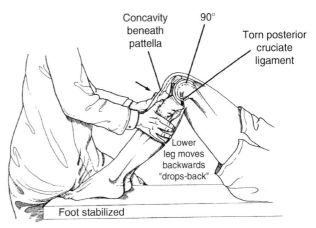

FIGURE **3-14**   Posterior cruciate ligament deficiency results in a posterior sag (sign of Godfrey) in the resting position, which can be appreciated at 90 degrees of flexion by comparing the contour of the anterior knee with that of the opposite side. Further posteriorly directed force produces the posterior drawer test to assess the extent of laxity. (From Scuderi, G. R., McCann, P. D., & Bruno, P. J. (1997). *Sports medicine: Principles of primary care.* St. Louis, Mosby.)

- Narcotic analgesics are indicated only for severe pain and should be given for several days only.

Client Education

- RICE: Emphasize the importance of rest, ice application, use of splints or elastic bandages, and elevation. These measures tend to decrease swelling and help control pain.
- Pathophysiology: Explain injury pathophysiology with expected outcomes.
- Cast/splint care: Give detailed information concerning splint care, including bathing instructions, removal and application procedure if indicated, and observation for signs of neurovascular compromise.
- Medications: Include potential medication side effects and instructions for administration. Advise the client to take NSAIDs with food to avoid abdominal discomfort. Muscle relaxants/narcotic analgesics may cause drowsiness; advise the client not to operate machinery or work above ground level.

Prevention

- Strength training of muscles around the knee can help decrease the likelihood of injury by keeping the knee more stable. Strength in the hamstrings has been shown to protect the ACL from excessive strain; women tend to be stronger in the quadriceps muscle, creating an injury-prone imbalance.
- Jump training strengthens leg muscles and can help avoid knee injury.
- Balancing training by building up the muscles around the knee can help. These muscles serve as shock

absorbers, reducing the force that gets transferred from the ACL and protecting against excessive rotation of the knee joint. Working on a balance board for 20 minutes a day over 6 weeks can help improve coordination of the hamstrings and the calf muscles (Smith, 2000).

- Physical conditioning through warm-up and cooldown also promotes knee stability.

Referral

- Immediate referral to an orthopedic surgeon is necessary for long-bone fractures, displaced fractures, intraarticular fractures, all fractures with neurovascular compromise, and knee injuries with significant effusion and/or instability.
- Three- to five-day referral to an orthopedic surgeon is recommended for simple, nondisplaced fractures and grade II to III ankle sprains of the ankle and knee after appropriate splinting and client education.
- Referral to an orthopedic surgeon should be made for all minor injuries that do not respond to conservative management.

EVALUATION/FOLLOW-UP

- Recheck all minor injuries and sprains in 1 week. For those that do not show improvement, consider a referral to an orthopedic surgeon.
- Begin rehabilitation for minor injuries and sprains as soon as possible to prevent contractures and loss of conditioning.
- Continue prescribing NSAIDs with food.

COMPLICATIONS

- Laxity of knee joint
- Inability to walk or run based on extent of knee problems
- ACL injury: early degenerative joint disease, as well as subsequent damage to other structures of the knee

REFERENCES

Alonso, J. (1996). Ankle fractures. In V. Masear (Ed.), *Primary care orthopedics*. Philadelphia: W. B. Saunders, 122-127.

Anderson, B. (1995). *Office orthopedics for primary care*. Philadelphia: W. B. Saunders.

Andrish, J. (2001). Anterior cruciate ligament injuries in the skeletally immature patient. *American Journal of Orthopedics, 30*(2), 103-110.

Balano, K. (1996). Anti-inflammatory drugs and myorelaxants. Pharmacology and clinical use in musculoskeletal disease. *Primary Care, 23*(2), 329-334.

Ballas, M., Tytko, J., & Mannarino, F. (1998). Commonly missed orthopedic injuries. *American Family Physician*. Retrieved July 31, 2002, from

Dvorkin, M. (1993). *Office orthopedics*. Norwalk, CT: Appleton & Lange.

Garth, W. (1996). Knee injuries in sports. In V. Masear (Ed.), *Primary care orthopedics*. Philadelphia: W. B. Saunders, 88-101.

Jacoby, D. (2000). Musculoskeletal injuries: Knee. In D. Robinson, P. Kidd, & K. Rogers (Eds.), *Primary care across the lifespan*. St. Louis: Mosby.

Johnson, M. (2000). Acute knee effusions: A systematic approach to diagnosis. *American Family Physician, 61*, 2391-2400.

Martin, J. (1996). Initial assessment and management of common fractures. *Primary Care, 23*(2), 405-409.

Meislin, R. (1996). Managing collateral ligament tears of the knee. *The Physician and Sports Medicine, 24*(3), 67-80.

Paluska, S., & McKeag, D. (2000). Knee braces: Current evidence and clinical recommendations for their use. *American Family Physician, 61*, 411-418, 423-424.

Savage, P. L. (1996). Casting and splinting techniques. In V. Maeser (Ed.), *Primary care orthopedics*. Philadelphia: W. B. Saunders, 337-346.

Smith, I. (2000). On bended knee. *Time, 156*(20), 120.

Swenson, E. J. (1995, June). Diagnosing and managing meniscal injuries in athletes. *The Journal of Musculoskeletal Medicine*, 35-45.

Tandeter, H., Shvartzman, P., & Stevens, M. (1999). Acute knee injuries: Use of decision rules for selective radiograph ordering. *American Family Physician, 60*, 2599-2608.

Torburn, L. (1996). Principles of rehabilitation. *Primary Care, 23*(2), 335-343.

Review Questions

1. ACL knee injuries usually show which one of the following radiograph findings?

- **a.** No radiographic findings
- **b.** Soft tissue swelling or effusion
- **c.** Tibial plateau fractures
- **d.** Distal fibula avulsion fractures

2. Which of the following knee injuries is associated with a "pop" that is either felt or heard?

- **a.** PCL injuries
- **b.** ACL injuries
- **c.** MCL injuries
- **d.** LCL injuries

3. Which finding seen during the physical examination is consistent with an ACL injury?

- **a.** Effusion
- **b.** Joint line tenderness
- **c.** Crepitus on movement
- **d.** Varus/valgus pain

4. Which of the following tests is expected to be abnormal with a meniscal injury?

- **a.** McMurray test
- **b.** Drawer test
- **c.** Varus/valgus stress
- **d.** Lachman's

5. Steve fell on his knee yesterday while running across a parking lot. Which radiograph is appropriate in this case?

- **a.** Anteroposterior view
- **b.** Anteroposterior and lateral view

c. Anteroposterior and lateral view with sunrise of knee
d. Anteroposterior and oblique views

6. Which of the following is *not* considered standard of care treatment for knee injuries?
   a. Arthrocentesis
   b. Knee immobilizer
   c. RICE
   d. Non–weight-bearing with crutches

7. Which of the following best describes the mechanism of action for NSAIDs?
   a. NSAIDs inhibit H_2 receptors in the gastric mucosa.
   b. NSAIDs alter pain receptors in the brain by altering serotonin release.
   c. NSAIDs inhibit prostaglandin synthesis, thereby decreasing pain.
   d. NSAIDs relax skeletal muscle by decreasing stimulation along the axons.

8. Which of the following historical data is suggestive of a knee fracture?
   a. Falling down the steps
   b. 10-year-old boy
   c. Auto accident
   d. Able to walk on leg after injury

Answers and Rationales

1. ***Answer:* b** (analysis/diagnosis)
   Rationale: Radiographs are routinely obtained with suspected ACL tears. Routine findings usually include only soft tissue swelling or effusion. Occasionally an avulsion fracture is visible (Garth, 1996).

2. ***Answer:* b** (analysis/diagnosis)
   Rationale: The client with an ACL injury may give a history of a shifting sensation of the knee with a pop being felt or heard (Garth, 1996).

3. ***Answer:* a** (assessment)
   Rationale: ACL injuries often exhibit effusion of the involved knee. Joint line pain is more indicative of meniscal injuries. Varus/valgus pain is more indicative of collateral ligament injury (Johnson, 2000).

4. ***Answer:* a** (analysis/diagnosis)
   Rationale: McMurray test indicates meniscal injury. Drawer and Lachman's tests determine the integrity of the ACL, and varus/valgus stress tests the collateral ligaments (Jacoby, 2000).

5. ***Answer:* c** (analysis/diagnosis)
   Rationale: Anteroposterior and lateral views are always done for knee injuries. If there is direct trauma to the patella, a sunrise view is appropriate.

6. ***Answer:* a** (implementation/plan)
   Rationale: Treatment for knee injuries includes RICE, crutches, and a knee immobilizer. Arthrocentesis is not a routine part of care for all knee injuries (Johnson, 2000).

7. ***Answer:* c** (implementation/plan)
   Rationale: NSAIDs decrease prostaglandin synthesis via inhibition of cyclooxygenase. Prostaglandins are associated with the development of pain after trauma (Balano, 1996).

8. ***Answer:* c** (assessment)
   Rationale: Fractures of the knee are more likely to occur in those who are older than 55 years of age, with a "pop" heard at the time of injury, an inability to bear weight after the injury, and a high-velocity accident (Johnson, 2000).

LEAD POISONING   *Denise Robinson*

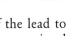

OVERVIEW
Definition
Lead poisoning is defined as a blood lead level of 10 mg/dL.

Incidence
Children
- Lead poisoning is primarily a problem for children younger than age 6 years because of the increased absorption (approximately 50%) of lead to which they are exposed.
- Children ages 6 to 36 months are at greatest risk.
- More than 4% of children in the United States have lead levels higher than 10 mg/dL.

Adults. Adults generally absorb 10% of the lead to which they are exposed, usually as a result of occupational exposure.

Pathophysiology
Lead is absorbed primarily through the respiratory and gastrointestinal (GI) tracts. After lead is absorbed into the bloodstream most of it is bound to red blood cells (RBCs). The highest concentrations are found in the liver, bone, teeth, lungs, brain, kidneys, and spleen. Lead in blood has a half-life of 35 days, in soft tissue of 40 days, and in bone of 20 to 30 years. Lead is substituted for calcium in the bone matrix; this lead is a source for remobilization and continued toxicity. Lead is excreted very slowly from the body (biological half-life of 10 years).

Lead is a protean poison; it causes cellular disturbances in most body tissues and organs. It interferes with hemesynthesis, causing an anemia that mimics iron-deficiency anemia. The major effect in young children is on the developing nervous system by interference with nerve pathways.

Children absorb approximately 50% of the lead they ingest. Adults absorb only 10% of the lead they ingest.

Primary Sources of Lead Exposure. Sources and pathways of lead exposure include the following:

- *Lead-Based Paint.* Lead-based paint remains the most common high-dose source of lead exposure for children 6 years old and younger. Many homes built before 1950 were painted with paint containing 50% or more lead. It is ingested in the form of paint chips or, more frequently, lead dust. Lead was not banned from paint until 1978. Lead-painted surfaces in poor repair offer the greatest risk.
- *Pica.* The repeated ingestion of nonfood substances has been implicated in cases of lead poisoning. This includes paint chips, dust, and soil contaminated with lead from paint that flaked or chalked as it aged or was disturbed during home maintenance or renovation. These substances usually are ingested during normal, repetitive, hand-to-mouth activity.
- *Soil and Dust.* Lead is deposited from paint, gasoline, and industrial sources in soil and dust, where it can serve as a significant source of lead exposure for children.
- *Drinking Water.* The 1986 Safe Drinking Water Act amendments banned the use of lead in public drinking water distribution systems and limited the lead content of brass used for plumbing to 8%. Lead pipes still are found in residences built before the 1920s. Pipes made of copper and soldered with lead came into general use in the 1950s. In general, lead in drinking water is not the predominant source for lead poisoning in children. Some water coolers and fountains have been found to have lead-soldered or lead-lined tanks. Patterns of intermittent water use from these fountains result in the water standing in the tanks longer than in typical residential situations, which can increase the amount of lead leached from the tanks. Several babies have been poisoned when hot tap water, which then was boiled (resulting in concentration of the lead), was used to make baby formula.
- *Parental Occupations and Hobbies.* "Take-home" exposures may result when workers wear their work clothes home or wash them with the family laundry or when they bring scrap or waste material home from work. Some industries in which workers commonly are exposed to lead are as follows:
  - Secondary smelting and refining of nonferrous metals

- Plumbing fixture fittings and trim
- Vehicle parts and accessories (tire weights for balancing)
- Pottery
- Automotive repair
- Industrial machinery and equipment
- Batteries
- Glass products
- *Airborne Lead.* Although lead use in gasoline has been reduced markedly, previous use has resulted in widespread contamination of soil and dust. However, airborne lead exposure is still minimal.
- *Food.* The quantity of lead in the U.S. diet has decreased markedly in recent years. Improperly fired ceramic ware, leaded crystal, pewter ware, and lead-soldered cans result in lead leaching into foods. Some food-handling practices can increase the lead content of foods.
- *Other Sources.* Lead exposure also may come from "traditional" or folk medicines, cosmetics, casting ammunition, fishing weights, toy soldiers, making stained glass, making pottery, refinishing furniture, burning lead-painted wood, and some plastic household blinds.

Factors Increasing Susceptibility
- Age younger than 6
- Exposure to lead hazard
- Low blood hemoglobin, hematocrit, and iron
- Pica behaviors
- Poor diet
- Poor handwashing
- Children of black race
- Children from low-income family
- Children in urban area

ASSESSMENT: SUBJECTIVE/HISTORY
History of Present Illness

Ask the client (or parents) about the following:
- Presence or absence of clinical symptoms, including fatigue, irritability, distractibility, inability to concentrate, unusual sleep patterns, poor appetite, nausea, vomiting, coordination problems (however, most children with lead poisoning will be asymptomatic)
- Child's ability to concentrate and developmental history with attention to language development
- Mouthing activities, including pica behaviors, use of a pacifier, bottle drinking, or thumb sucking
- Nutritional status
- Use of folk remedies
- Use of pottery

Past Medical History

Ask the client (or parents) about the following:
- Past blood lead levels

- History of anemia
- History of developmental delay
- History of GI, hematologic, renal, reproductive, and neurologic problems
- Medication use
- Vitamins or any prescription or nonprescription drugs taken

Family History

Ask about any family history of lead poisoning.

Environmental History

- Characteristics of home: age, location, condition of paint, recent remodeling or restoration, pipes
- Parents' occupation
- Others in the home with lead poisoning

Diet History

- Iron and calcium intake
- Infant formula: type and amount
- Meal frequency
- Amount of fat in diet (a high-fat diet is associated with increased lead absorption)

ASSESSMENT: OBJECTIVE/PHYSICAL EXAMINATION

Physical Examination

Signs and symptoms as stated earlier may be noted during examination. Because symptoms usually do not occur until the child has had significant lead exposure, the presence of any symptoms should be treated as a medical emergency.

- Determine vital signs. Determine growth parameters including height, weight, head circumference, as plotted on growth charts.
- Assess general appearance, paying particular attention to the neurologic examination; psychosocial skills, cognition, language, and behavior should be observed.

Diagnostic Procedures

- Determine blood lead level.
- Screen high-risk children by 6 months of age. The Centers for Disease Control and Prevention (CDC) recommends that all children have lead screening done by 12 months of age.
- Perform x-ray examination of kidneys and upper bladder (KUB) (positive if presence of paint chips in abdomen).
- Check hemoglobin level.

DIAGNOSIS

Differential diagnoses include the following:

- Attention deficit disorder
- Learning disabilities
- Central nervous system (CNS) tumor
- Anemia
- Developmental delay
- Colic
- Metabolic disorders

THERAPEUTIC PLAN

The following guidelines are adopted from the 1991 CDC risk classification for children without symptoms:

Class I

- This class has a blood lead level higher than 9 mg/dL.
- Assess risk factors at every well-child visit (at least yearly) until the child is 3 years old. A child who is at high risk because of housing or family history of lead poisoning should have a lead level checked every 6 months until 3 years of age.

Class IIa

- This class has a blood lead level of 10 to 14 mg/dL.
- Rescreen clients in this class every 6 months.
- Assess risk factors for sources of lead exposure.
- Provide education about diet as follows:
  - Increase high-calcium foods. (Lead is absorbed more efficiently in the presence of low calcium.)
  - Increase iron-containing foods (e.g., organ meats, red meat, green leafy vegetables, dried fruit).
  - Eat a low-fat diet to reduce absorption and retention of lead.
  - Provide education about cleaning (recommend wet-mopping with trisodium phosphate solution found in many dishwashing detergents).
  - Discuss ways to protect child from lead hazards, such as decreasing hand-to-mouth behaviors.

Class IIb

- This class has a blood lead level of 15 to 19 mg/dL.
- Rescreen every 3 months.
- Assess risk factors for sources of lead.
- Provide education about diet, cleaning, and the like.
- Consider environmental investigation with a paint and water lead testing kit, found in most hardware stores, or call the health department for professional testing.
- Some states require home evaluation by the health department at this level.

Class IIIa

- This class has a blood lead level of 20 to 24 mg/dL.
- Perform complete medical assessment with KUB and long bone x-ray examination.
- Identify and eliminate environmental lead.
- Provide education about diet, cleaning, and the like.
- Refer to the local health department for environmental investigation.
- Rescreen after 1 month.
- Refer to lead poisoning program, if available.

Class IIIb

- This class has a blood lead level of 25 to 44 mg/dL.
- Treat as in IIIA, plus start oral chelating treatment. Give succimer, 10 mg/kg or 350 mg/m² PO q8h for 5 days. Reduce to 10 mg/kg or 350 mg/m² q12h for 2 weeks.
- A child receiving succimer should have blood lead level, complete blood count (CBC), ferritin level, total iron-binding capacity, calcium level, liver enzymes, aspartate transaminase (AST), blood urea nitrogen, creatinine, and medical evaluation done initially, 1 week after starting the medication, and on completion of the course of treatment (total 19-day treatment).
- The course can be repeated after a 3-week interval if lead level has not dropped significantly.
- In young children who cannot swallow capsules, succimer can be administered by separating the capsule and sprinkling the medicated beads on a small amount of soft food or putting them in a spoon and following with fruit drink.
- Identification of the source of lead in the child's environment and abatement of this source are critical to a successful therapy outcome. Chelation therapy is not a substitute for preventing further exposure to lead and should not be used to permit continued exposure to lead.

Class IV

- This class has a blood lead level of 45 to 69 mg/dL.
- Treat as in classes IIIa and IIIb; however, admit child to the hospital for treatment with ethylenediaminetetraacetic acid (EDTA) in the following cases:
  - Client has symptoms.
  - Client is younger than 3 years old and lead level is higher than 60 mg/dL.
  - KUB is positive.

Class V

- This class has a blood lead level of 70 mg/dL.
- It is a medical emergency.
- Treatment options include chelation therapy with the following:
  - EDTA
  - Dimercaprol (BAL) and EDTA
  - Dimercaptosuccinic acid (DMSA)

Client Education

Provide detailed education for parents, including the following key points:

- Most homes built before 1950 contain lead paint, and many homes built between 1950 and 1978 contain lead paint.
- Check home for peeling paint, especially around door and window frames.
- Wet-mop floors with trisodium phosphate solutions, contained in most dishwashing detergents.

- Consider buying a simple lead testing kit for paint and water (available from most hardware stores).
- Never attempt to remove lead paint yourself. Regular vacuuming, sanding, and scraping tend to stir up more lead into the air. Lead must be removed by a professional.
- Wash hands frequently (extremely important).
- Increase calcium and iron in the child's diet. Deficiencies increase absorption of lead.

Referral

- Refer all clients with blood lead levels higher than 44 mg/dL by venous sample confirmation.
- Refer any child with an elevated lead level that is symptomatic.

Consultation

- Consult with an appropriate health professional for treatment of language, behavior, developmental delay, or attention disorders.
- Report cases of occupational lead poisoning to the health department.

Prevention

- Lead poisoning may be prevented by inspection of homes built before 1978 for lead paint.
- High suspicion of potential for lead poisoning also may help prevent it.
- The condition also may be prevented by screening on a regular basis for lead poisoning.

EVALUATION/FOLLOW-UP

Lead levels may drop to less than 20 mg/dL within a few months of chelating treatment. Some children with higher levels of lead may take much longer and need to undergo chelation several times. Lead moves from storage in the bones back into the circulating blood, creating a "rebound" phenomenon. It is important to inform parents of this phenomenon so that they do not become discouraged when lead levels rebound. Follow-up is determined by lead levels.

COMPLICATIONS

Complications associated with lead poisoning include the following:

- Complications associated with treatment failure
- Chronic anemia, mild to severe
- Mental retardation or seizures
- Learning disabilities, behavior disorders, sleep disorders, or developmental delay

REFERENCES

American Academy of Pediatrics Committee on Environmental Health. (1998). Screening for elevated blood lead levels. *Pediatrics 101*, 1072-1078.

Centers for Disease Control and Prevention. (1991). *Preventing lead poisoning in young children: A statement by the Centers for Disease Control.* Atlanta: CDC.

Centers for Disease Control and Prevention. (1997). *Screening young children for lead poisoning: Guidance for state and local public health officials.* Atlanta: CDC, National Center for Environmental Health, U.S. Department of Health and Human Services, Public Health Service.

Ellis, M., & Kane, K. (2000). Lightening the lead load in children. *American Family Physician 62*, 545-554, 559-560.

Glotzer, D. E., Weitzman, M., Aschengrau, A., & Freedberg, K. A. (1997). Economic evaluation of environmental interventions for low-level childhood lead poisoning. *Ambulatory Child Health Journal 3*, 255-267.

Illinois Department of Public Health. (1996). *Guidelines for the detection and management of lead poisoning for physicians and health care providers.* Springfield, IL: Illinois Department of Public Health.

Mendelsohn, A. L., Dreyer, B. P., Fierman, A. H., Rosen, C. M., Legano, L. A., Kruger, H. A., Lim, S. W., Barasch, S., Au, L., Courtlandt, C. D. (1998). Low-level lead exposure and behavior in early childhood. *Pediatrics, 101*:E10.

Needham, D. D. (1994). Diagnosis and management of lead poisoned children: The pediatric nurse practitioner in a specialty program. *Journal of Pediatric Health Care 8*(6), 268-273.

Rooney, B. L., Hayes, E. B., Allen, B. K., & Strutt, P. J. (1994). Development of a screening tool for prediction of children at risk for lead exposure in a midwestern clinical setting. *Pediatrics 93*, 183-187.

Schaffer, S. J., Szilagyi, P. G., & Weitzman, M. (1994). Lead poisoning risk determination in an urban population through the use of a standardized questionnaire. *Pediatrics 93*, 159-163.

Wright, R. O., Shannon, M. W., Wright, R. J., & Hu, H. (1999). Association between iron deficiency and low-level lead poisoning in an urban primary care clinic. *American Journal of Public Health 89*, 1049-1053.

Review Questions

1. Lead poisoning is primarily a problem for children younger than age 6 years for which of the following reasons?

   a. Adults absorb less lead into their systems than do children.
   b. Adults are better handwashers.
   c. Children are more prone to pica.
   d. Children do more hand-to-mouth activity.

2. The most common high-dose source of lead exposure for children is which of the following?

   a. Drinking water
   b. Pica
   c. Paint
   d. Soil

3. Lead poisoning is diagnosed when the blood lead is at what level?

   a. 10 mg/dL
   b. 15 mg/dL

   c. 20 mg/dL
   d. 25 mg/dL

4. If a child with lead poisoning has symptoms, the treatment should be which of the following?

   a. Treat as a medical emergency.
   b. Assess risk factors and recheck in 1 month.
   c. Educate parents on how to check home for lead.
   d. Encourage calcium- and iron-rich foods.

5. Homes built before which of the following years should be assessed for lead paint?

   a. 1978
   b. 1980
   c. 1983
   d. 1984

6. If a parent suspects that the home's water distribution system contains lead, it is recommended that the parent do which of the following?

   a. Use hot water from the faucet to make formula.
   b. Use cold water to make formula.
   c. Boil hot water form the faucet for 5 minutes to make formula.
   d. Boil hot water from the faucet for 10 minutes to make formula.

7. Lead pipes still can be found in homes built before which date?

   a. 1920
   b. 1930
   c. 1940
   d. 1950

8. A parental occupation that may cause "take-home" lead exposure is which of the following?

   a. Pencil manufacturing company
   b. Cigarette manufacturing company
   c. Automotive repair shop
   d. Print shop

Answers and Rationales

1. *Answer:* **a** (assessment)
   Rationale: Adults only absorb approximately 10% of the lead to which they are exposed, whereas children absorb as much as 50% of the lead to which they are exposed (CDC, 1991).

2. *Answer:* **c** (assessment)
   Rationale: The most common source of lead for children is lead in paint (Illinois Department of Public Health, 1996).

3. *Answer:* **a** (assessment)
   Rationale: Blood lead level of 10 mg/dL is considered lead poisoning (Needham, 1994).

4. *Answer:* **a** (implementation/plan)
   Rationale: The presence of any symptoms of lead poisoning should be treated as a medical emergency (CDC, 1991).

5. *Answer:* **a** (assessment)

   Rationale: Lead-based paint still was used in homes built before 1978. In 1978 a ban was placed on this type of paint (CDC, 1991).

6. *Answer:* **b** (implementation/plan)

   Rationale: Water sitting in an old water tank can absorb lead from the tank or other parts of the distribution system. Heating or boiling water concentrates the lead. Using cold water from the faucet to make formula is the safest course (CDC, 1991).

7. *Answer:* **a** (assessment)

   Rationale: Lead pipes still can be found in homes built before the 1920s (CDC, 1991).

8. *Answer:* **c** (assessment)

   Rationale: Parents who work in automotive repair shops can bring home lead on their clothes (Illinois Department of Public Health, 1996).

LEIOMYOMAS *Cheryl Pope Kish*

OVERVIEW
Definition

Leiomyomas, also referred to as fibroids and uterine myomas, are benign tumors of the female reproductive tract that arise from the uterine musculature and grow under the influence of estrogen.

Incidence

Leiomyomas, because they are responsive to estrogen, are least common at the extremes of reproductive life: among adolescents and menopausal women. They occur in 30% of women of reproductive age with a 3 to 9 times greater occurrence in black women. The average age of occurrence for black women is 37.5 years, whereas the average age is 41.6 years for white women. Leiomyomas regress at menopause.

Pathophysiology

The leiomyoma is a discrete firm tumor, often occurring in multiples, composed of smooth muscle and connective tissue. They most often grow in the uterine fundus but may be found elsewhere. Uterine myomas are classified by their anatomic location within the uterus: (1) subserous—under the outside lining of the uterus, growing outward; (2) intramural—within the uterine or myometrial wall; (3) submucous—beneath the endometrial lining; and (4) intraligamentous—beneath the folds of the round ligaments. A submucous myoma may become pedunculated and descend through the cervix into the vagina; it also may undergo torsion, causing acute pain.

Factors Increasing Susceptibility
- Black ethnicity
- Sedentary lifestyle
- Obesity
- Nulliparity
- Age older than 35 years
- Nonsmoker
- Family history
- History of infertility
- Oral contraceptive use
- Intrauterine device use

Protective Factors. Adolescent and menopausal women have the least risk of leiomyoma.

ASSESSMENT: SUBJECTIVE/HISTORY
History of Present Illness

- Leiomyomas are asymptomatic in 50% of women; in these women, the fibroids are identified on incidental routine gynecologic examination. The most common presenting complaint is heavy, prolonged menses (10% to 40%).
- Obtain description of onset, progression, and duration of symptoms; associated complaints; and factors that make symptoms better and worse.
- Obtain a careful description of all symptoms and their effect on lifestyle.
- Attempt to quantify amount of bleeding with pad count and degree of saturation. Have client compare current menstrual pattern with usual pattern since menarche.

Symptoms
- Excessive, prolonged uterine bleeding (menorrhagia)
- Irregular periods
- Lower abdominal pain (pain is an infrequent symptom, often associated with menorrhagia; also can occur when a fibroid outgrows its blood supply and undergoes acute degeneration)
- Dysmenorrhea
- Constipation, bloating, and GI discomfort
- Urinary frequency and nocturia
- Backache
- Pelvic pressure
- Flank pain
- Dyspareunia
- Increasing abdominal girth
- Recurring spontaneous abortion
- Infertility

Past Medical History

- Inquire about a family history of fibroids.
- Inquire about previous pregnancy.

Medication History

- Identify current medications.
- Ask about birth control method.

Dietary History

In cases of heavy bleeding and anemia, ask about sources of iron in diet.

ASSESSMENT: OBJECTIVE/PHYSICAL EXAMINATION
Physical Examination

- The physical examination focuses on the abdominal and pelvic bimanual examination. To avoid confusing the uterine mass with a full bladder, have the woman void before the examination.
- Note abdominal girth.
- Auscultate bowel sounds.
- Palpate abdomen for ascites, tenderness, and evidence of mass.
- During the pelvic examination, when using the speculum, note cervical lesions, polyps, and discharge.
- On bimanual examination, estimate the uterine size compared with gestational size. Note presence of discrete mass and its characteristics. Determine shape and contour of uterus (fibroids generally cause an irregular contour). Determine if the mass moves with cervical motion to differentiate from the adnexal mass, which does not move with cervical motion. Note tenderness of uterus and cervical motion tenderness (leiomyomas do not generally cause uterine tenderness).
- Assess adnexa. If fibroid precludes assessment of adnexa, transvaginal ultrasonography can be done to rule out ovarian neoplasm.

Diagnostic Procedures

- Obtain a urine pregnancy test if period has been missed. If the woman has missed a period, cannot date her last menstrual period, or describes her last menses as different than usual, perform qualitative beta human chorionic gonadotropin.
- Perform a Pap smear.
- Obtain cervical cultures if indicated by history and physical.
- Obtain CBC or hemoglobin and hematocrit when client has a history of menorrhagia.
- Perform pelvic ultrasonography to confirm presence of leiomyoma, location, number, and size. Definitive diagnosis usually is made on the basis of ultrasound findings. Diagnosis also can be confirmed by dilation and curettage (D&C), hysteroscopy, or laparoscopy.

DIAGNOSIS

Differential diagnoses include the following:
- Intrauterine pregnancy
- Abdominal mass
- Ovarian cyst
- Adnexal mass
- Uterine or cervical polyps
- Adenomyosis
- Irritable bowel syndrome or diverticular mass
- Interstitial cystitis
- Cancer
- Tuboovarian inflammatory mass
- Ectopic pregnancy
- Constipation

THERAPEUTIC PLAN

- The treatment approach depends on the woman's age, her desires for fertility, the size and rate of growth of the fibroid, and the severity of symptoms. Only 10% to 20% of clients require treatment. If the woman is pregnant, fibroids may increase in size because of the increased estrogen, primarily in the first trimester. Careful follow-up is necessary. There is a minimal risk of spontaneous abortion or premature labor. Analgesics may be required. During pregnancy, analgesics and rest are appropriate if pain occurs.
- In the nonpregnant client, a leiomyoma that causes uterus smaller than 12-week gestational size may be observed for 3 to 6 months to determine if it is growing or creating troublesome symptoms. This is an expectant management approach, and the woman undergoing this management approach should know to report increasing symptoms in advance of the next scheduled follow-up appointment.
- Those clients with a uterus larger than 12-week size and who have discomforting pressure or excessive bleeding necessitate treatment and possibly referral. Surgical treatment includes myomectomy performed with open laparotomy or with laparoscopy or hysteroscopy; hysterectomy; endometrial ablation; and uterine artery embolization by an intervention radiologist. Myomectomy is the procedure of choice for those who wish to maintain fertility.

Pharmacologic Treatment

- Nonsteroidal antiinflammatory drugs (NSAIDs) are appropriate for pain control (ibuprofen 600 mg PO q6h or naproxen sodium as Aleve, Anaprox, or Naprosyn 500 mg PO bid); they have the additional benefit of decreasing blood loss by 30% to 50%. Iron therapy is commonly necessary to treat anemia. Ferrous sulfate 325 mg PO once to tid commonly is prescribed for that purpose.
- Medical management usually involves the gonadotropin-releasing hormone (GnRH) analogues for short-term use (8 to 12 weeks). These drugs function by

decreasing follicle-stimulating hormone and luteinizing hormone to produce a hypoestrogenic or menopauselike effect. Sometimes these drugs are used preoperatively to shrink the fibroids enough to enable vaginal hysterectomy; they may shrink the tumor enough (60%) to eliminate the need for surgery. They have the additional preoperative benefit of reducing anemia, possibly decreasing the need for blood transfusions during surgery. In women who do not have surgery, when the drug is discontinued, the fibroid will return to its original size within 3 to 6 months. Treatment with GnRH agonists can be administered as follows:

- Leuprolide (Lupron) 0.5 mg SC daily for 8 to 12 weeks or depot leuprolide (Lupron) 3.75 mg IM every 28 days. If the subcutaneous option is preferred, the woman must be taught to self-administer the injection or a willing friend or family member may be taught this skill.
- Nafarelin (Synarel) 200mg/spray intranasally into one nostril in the morning and the other nostril in the evening.
- Goserelin (Zoladex) is a small biodegradable cylinder inserted SC each month.
- The GnRH agonists are expensive and have adverse effects: hot flashes, vaginal dryness, mood swings, depression, weight gain, insomnia, diminished libido, reduction in bone density, and elevated cholesterol levels. Because the adverse effects are poorly tolerated and osteoporosis is a concern, add-back therapy with estrogen/progesterone may be used. Women need to understand that although they may experience amenorrhea as a result of these drugs, pregnancy may be possible and barrier contraception is necessary.
- Danazol (Danocrine) used for 6 months is an option selected by many physicians for decreasing myoma size. This drug also produces hypoestrogenic effects and has androgenic properties as well. Common side effects include weight gain, fluid retention, decreased breast size, acne, oily skin, facial hair growth, atrophic vaginitis, hot flashes, muscle cramps, and emotional lability.

Client Education

- Educate client about the nature of leiomyoma, treatment of symptomatic leiomyomas only, possible therapy options, and the low risk of malignancy (less than 0.5%). Inform client of signs and symptoms, and advise when to report changes to provider. Reinforce importance of adhering to scheduled follow-up.
- Recommend NSAIDs as needed for comfort, advising clients about taking with food to minimize risk. Advise that NSAIDs are contraindicated for those with allergy to the agents or a history of peptic ulcer disease.

- Encourage women who are experiencing excess menses related to fibroids to decrease activity during days of heavy flow.
- Educate women taking iron therapy about changes in stool color and possible GI side effects (constipation, diarrhea, bloating). Teach to optimize bioavailability of iron by taking it on an empty stomach (unless it causes nausea) with orange juice or other form of ascorbic acid and avoiding milk, tea, or antacid for at least 60 minutes before and after dose.
- Educate all women with excess menses about ways to increase iron in their daily diet.
- Advocate for clients in fully appreciating the treatment options available and their rights to participate actively in decisionmaking about medical and surgical treatment.

Referral

Women who experience symptomatic or rapidly growing fibroids should be referred for evaluation and possibly medical management with GnRH analogues or surgery. Elective myomectomy can be scheduled if needed to preserve the uterus for future childbearing. Urgent surgery is needed only when significant pressure is exerted on uterus, bladder, or bowel, or hemorrhage occurs. Large cervical or pedunculated fibroids are generally surgically removed. Surgical therapy is curative. Hysteroscopic or laparoscopically assisted surgery is often possible, minimizing the risks associated with open surgical procedures. Uterine artery embolization as a treatment measure is being used in some centers.

Prevention

No preventive measures have been identified.

EVALUATION/FOLLOW-UP

Women with small and asymptomatic fibroids are scheduled for follow-up every 3 months for two visits, then every 6 months to determine increase in fibroid size with pelvic examination and possibly ultrasonography. When fibroids are larger than 12-week gestational size or growing more than 1 to 2 cm/year, women should be referred. Women experiencing menorrhagia should be monitored for anemia; treatment is warranted if the hemoglobin level is lower than 10 gm/dL or the hematocrit is lower than 30%. Fibroids may regress after pregnancy or menopause.

COMPLICATIONS

Quality of life can be affected negatively for women who experience symptomatic fibroids. Hemorrhage and its sequelae represent a complication for many. An acute pain episode is possible with torsion of a pedunculated fibroid. The risk of malignancy (sarcoma) from fibroids is low—less than 0.5%. Unusual uterine bleeding or rapid uterine growth may signal malignancy. Pregnancy loss, although rarely caused by fibroids, is a concern because growing tumors crowd the intrauterine space.

REFERENCES

Brown, K. (2000). *Management guidelines for women's health nurse practitioners.* Philadelphia: F. A. Davis.

Davidson M. (2001). Managing uterine fibroids: new approaches to treatment. *Clinical Review 11*(6), 78-85.

Grabo, T. N., Fahs, P. S., Nataupsky, L. G., & Reich, H. (1999). Uterine myomas: Treatment options. *Journal of Obstetric Gynecologic and Neonatal Nursing 28*(1), 23-31.

Hutchins, F. L. (1998). Fibroids in primary care. *Clin Advisor* Sept, 26-29.

Lucas, B. D. (1999). Five reasons to consider a hysterectomy. *Patient Care Sept,* 15, 34-36, 41-44, 47, 50.

Meredith, P. V., & Horan, N. M. (2000). *Adult primary care.* Philadelphia: W. B. Saunders.

Stewart, E. A., & Faur, A. (2000). The future of fibroid therapy. *Contemporary OB/Gyn, July*:28-38.

Tierney, L. M., McPhee, S. J., & Papadakis, M. A. (2001). *Current medical diagnosis and treatment.* New York: Lange Medical Books/McGraw-Hill.

Youngkin, E. Q., & Davis, M. S. (1998). *Women's health: A primary care clinical guide.* Stamford, CT: Appleton & Lange.

Review Questions

1. Patricia Coleman is a 38-year-old who presents with clinical findings of leiomyoma. Which factor related to Mrs. Coleman is not associated with increased risk of leiomyoma?

  a. Black heritage
  b. History of nulliparity
  c. Heavy cigarette smoking
  d. Family history

2. Which finding is most consistent with a diagnosis of leiomyoma?

  a. Dyspareunia
  b. Constant pelvic pain
  c. Diarrhea
  d. Heavy, prolonged menses

3. Which objective finding is most consistent with a diagnosis of leiomyoma?

  a. Irregular contour of uterus
  b. Cervical polyps
  c. Increased leukorrhea
  d. Extreme uterine tenderness

4. A fibroid may be differentiated from an adnexal mass by which of the following?

  a. Abdominal ultrasonography only
  b. Magnetic resonance imaging (MRI) only
  c. Movement of the mass noted with movement of cervix
  d. Immobility of mass

5. Which diagnostic test offers an appropriate first-line confirmation of leiomyoma?

  a. Computed tomography (CT) scan
  b. Hysteroscopy
  c. Ultrasound
  d. MRI

6. Which of the following responses is not an expected effect of Lupron, a GnRH analogue used for leiomyoma treatment?

  a. Vaginal dryness
  b. Hot flashes
  c. Decreased bone density
  d. Breast tenderness

7. Gwen has a fibroid less than 2 cm in size. She complains of new-onset pelvic pressure and reports that her menses was heavier and longer last month. Which intervention is most appropriate?

  a. Immediate referral to a gynecologist
  b. Ibuprofen 600 mg PO q6h during menses
  c. Advice about the likelihood of impending surgery
  d. Danazol 200 mg PO bid

8. Donna, who has a small fibroid, has become anemic. The nurse practitioner (NP) orders ferrous sulfate 325 mg PO tid and provides detailed instructions about this medication's expected and untoward effects and how to administer it for optimal effect. Which comment, if made by Donna, indicates that the teaching has been effective?

  a. "This medicine will cause my urine to turn dark amber and I will need to drink more water."
  b. "Taking this medicine with milk or yogurt will prevent it from burning my stomach."
  c. "Drinking tea within 1 hour before or after this drug causes it not to work as effectively."
  d. "To tell if this drug is working as it should, I should have follow-up blood tests every 2 weeks."

9. Donna is educated about ways to increase her dietary intake of iron. Which menu choice has the most iron?

  a. Roast beef, mashed potatoes, broccoli, dried apricots, and lemonade
  b. Cream cheese and pineapple wedges on bagel, tossed salad, apple, and milk
  c. Bacon, lettuce, and tomato sandwich on white toast; carrot and celery sticks; and grape drink
  d. Green salad with tomato, lettuce, cucumber, and peppers; crackers; cantaloupe; and coffee

10. Connie has a small, asymptomatic fibroid first noted on routine gynecologic examination. How often should she be scheduled for follow-up by the NP?

  a. Every 2 to 3 weeks
  b. Monthly
  c. Every 3 to 6 months
  d. Annually

Answers and Rationales

1. *Answer:* c (assessment)
Rationale: Nonsmokers are more likely to have leiomyoma than heavy smokers. This finding is likely related to smoking's association with decreased circulating estrogen (Youngkin & Davis, 1998).

2. *Answer:* d (assessment)
Rationale: Heavy prolonged menses (menorrhagia/hypermenorrhea) is a classic symptom of leiomyoma (Davidson, 2001).

3. *Answer:* a (assessment)
Rationale: Examination of a woman with a leiomyoma generally reveals a uterus with a firm irregularity in its contour; the uterus often is enlarged and is usually nontender (Youngkin & Davis, 1998).

4. *Answer:* c (assessment)
Rationale: During examination, movement of the cervix generally causes movement of the fibroid, whereas an adnexal mass would remain immobile with motion exerted to the cervix (Youngkin & Davis, 1998). If confirmation of an adnexal mass cannot be done on bimanual examination, a transvaginal ultrasound is an appropriate test (Grabo, Fahs, Nataupsky, & Reich, 1999). Leiomyoma can be confirmed by hysteroscopy, D&C, laparoscopy, MRI, and ultrasonography. Because ultrasonography is the least expensive and least invasive, it is an appropriate first-line measure (Davidson, 2001).

5. *Answer:* c (assessesment)
Rationale: Ultrasonography confirms the presence of a fibroid (Youngkin & Davis, 1998)

6. *Answer:* d (implementation/plan)
Rationale: GnRH analogues are antiestrogen drugs and consequently cause menopauselike symptoms, such as vaginal dryness, declining bone density, hot flashes, mood changes, and decreased libido. Breast tenderness, often associated with estrogen excess, is not an expected finding (Youngkin & Davis, 1998).

7. *Answer:* b (implementation/plan)
Rationale: NSAIDs are generally effective for pelvic pressure and mild to moderate pain and may decrease menstrual flow (Youngkin & Davis, 1998; Davidson, 2001).

8. *Answer:* c (evaluation)
Rationale: The tannic acid in tea binds with iron and causes it to be less effective. Consequently, drinking tea and taking oral iron preparations should be separated by at least 1 hour to promote maximum effect of the drug (Youngkin & Davis, 1998).

9. *Answer:* a (implementation/plan)
Rationale: Roast beef, broccoli, and dried apricots are all sources of iron (Youngkin & Davis, 1998).

10. *Answer:* c (evaluation)
Rationale: Follow-up at 3 months for two visits then every 6 months is appropriate for a women with small asymptomatic fibroids (Grabo, et al., 1999).

LEUKEMIA *Denise Robinson*

OVERVIEW
Definition

Leukemia is a proliferation of immature white blood cells (WBCs) originating in the bone marrow.

Incidence

Incidence of all types of leukemia is approximately 13 cases in 100,000 population per year. In general, males are affected more than females and whites more than blacks.

Acute Lymphocytic Leukemia
- Abnormal proliferation of immature lymphocytes in the bone marrow
- Approximately 4 cases per 100,000 children every year
- Approximately 3500 new cases each year in the United States
- Peak incidence is at 3 to 5 years old
- Males outnumber females (1.3:1)
- Acute lymphocytic leukemia (ALL) accounts for 75% to 80% of all childhood leukemias

Acute Myelogenous Leukemia
- Abnormal proliferation of immature myeloid stem cells in the bone marrow

- Ratio of acute myelogenous leukemia (AML) to ALL is 1:4
- Accounts for 15% to 25% of childhood leukemia
- Approximately 10% of childhood AML in infants younger than 2 years
- Relatively constant incidence from birth through adolescence

Chronic Lymphocytic Leukemia
- A persistent absolute lymphocytosis for at least 3 months
- The most common type of leukemia in the United States
- Males outnumber females (2:1 to 3:1)
- Approximately 75% of chronic lymphocytic leukemia (CLL) cases occur in persons 60 years old or older

Chronic Myelogenous Leukemia
- Abnormal proliferation of differentiating myeloid cells in blood and bone marrow
- Juvenile chronic myelogenous leukemia (CML)
    - Rare in children.
    - CML accounts for 1% to 5% of all childhood leukemias.

- If seen in children, almost always seen in infants younger than 2 years.
- Has a relatively rapid course.
- Cytogenetic marker is the Philadelphia chromosome.
- Adult CML
  - Median age of onset is 45 years.
  - Natural course of disease: progresses from chronic, to accelerated, and then to the blast phase.

Leukemia in Pregnancy
- Fewer than 1 case in 100,000 pregnancies annually
- Limited studies done
- Two large studies (Antonelli et al, 1996) of 72 cases of leukemia from 1975 to 1988 found types and incidences:
  - AML, 61%
  - ALL, 28%
  - CML, 7%

Pathophysiology
- The overproliferation of immature WBCs in the bone marrow can replace completely the normal bone marrow precursors, leading to a decrease in RBCs, platelets, and granulocytes. Leukemic cells also may proliferate in other reticuloendothelial tissues and in other extramedullary sites, such as the central nervous system, testes, bones, or skin (Lampkin, 1997).
- The cause is theorized to be ecogenetic. A genetic transformation of the progenitor (stem) cell occurs in response to environmental agents.

Factors Increasing Susceptibility
- Genetic predisposition
  - Diamond Blackfan anemia: increased risk of AML
  - Down syndrome (trisomy 21): from 10 to 20 times increased incidence
  - Bloom syndrome and Fanconi's anemia: increased risk of AML
- AML
  - Ataxia-telangiectasia
  - Identical twins: a 25% increased risk of ALL
  - Nontwin siblings: increased risk of ALL
  - History of fetal loss
  - Advanced maternal age
- Possible environmental factors
  - Ionizing radiation
  - Chronic chemical exposure: benzene
  - Previous malignancy treated with alkylating agents
  - Exposure to electromagnetic fields
  - Herbicides and pesticides
  - Maternal use of alcohol, contraceptives, diethylstilbestrol, or cigarettes

- Viral infections
  - Human T-cell leukemia/lymphoma virus (HTLV)-I: linked to adult T-cell leukemia lymphoma
  - HTLV-II: linked to hairy cell leukemia
  - HTLV-III: linked to Kaposi's sarcoma
  - Epstein-Barr virus: associated with L3 subtype of ALL
- Immunodeficiency
  - Chronic use of immunosuppressive drugs
  - Wiskott-Aldrich syndrome
  - Congenital hypogammaglobulinemia
  - Ataxia-telangiectasia

ASSESSMENT: SUBJECTIVE/HISTORY
Symptoms
- In acute leukemias, symptoms are present 1 to 2 weeks before diagnosis.
- In chronic leukemias, symptoms are chronic and less obvious.

Anemia. Anemia is present at diagnosis in most cases. Symptoms include malaise, weakness, dyspnea, irritability, fatigue, anorexia, pallor, and heart murmur.

Thrombocytopenia. Thrombocytopenia is present in 75% of cases of childhood leukemia. Symptoms include petechiae, easy bruising, epistaxis, menorrhagia, GI and intracranial hemorrhage, and hematuria.

Neutropenia. Fever at diagnosis is present in 60% of cases of childhood leukemia. Other symptoms include persistent infections and abscesses.

Central Nervous System Involvement. CNS involvement is present in less than 10% of cases. Symptoms include headache, vomiting, and visual disturbances.

Bone Pain. Bone pain is present at diagnosis in approximately 23% of cases. Pain is from the overproliferation of leukemia cells within the bone marrow space and possibly from bony destruction by leukemic infiltration.

Gastrointestinal Symptoms. GI symptoms result from proliferation of leukemic cells in the abdominal viscera, liver, and spleen. Symptoms include anorexia, weight loss, abdominal pain, and hepatosplenomegaly.

Generalized Lymphadenopathy. Generalized lymphadenopathy is common at diagnosis as a result of infiltration by leukemic cells.

Genitourinary Symptoms. In males, testicular ALL can be seen with a painless, firm, unilateral, or bilateral enlargement, with or without discoloration.

Acute Lymphocytic Leukemia and Acute Myelocytic Leukemia. Most common presenting symptoms include pallor, bleeding, fever, and pain. These signs and symptoms are due to bone marrow infiltration and failure.

Chronic Myelocytic Leukemia. Most cases of CML are diagnosed during the chronic phase. Symptoms at diagnosis may include splenomegaly, hepatomegaly, fever, night sweats, pallor, weight loss, bone pain, and lymphadenopathy. If hyperleukocytosis is present, complications include focal or diffuse neurologic findings, respiratory distress, metabolic disturbances, and priapism.

Juvenile Chronic Myelocytic Leukemia. This condition usually affects children younger than age 2 years. Symptoms include cutaneous lesions (eczema, xanthomata, and café au lait spots), generalized lymphadenopathy, marked splenomegaly, hepatomegaly, and hemorrhagic problems. A facial rash (erythematous, maculopapules, or desquamative) is common and may have been present for months before diagnosis. Respiratory symptoms, including cough, expiratory wheezing, and tachypnea, also may be present.

Chronic Lymphocytic Leukemia. Most cases are diagnosed during the chronic phase. Symptoms at diagnosis include malaise, increased fatigability, generalized lymphadenopathy, and splenomegaly. As the disease progresses, hypogammaglobulinemia may develop.

Past Medical History

- Exposure to HTLV-I virus
- Family history of cancer
- Recent history of viral illness
- History of previous illnesses or surgery
- Allergies
- Immunizations and screening tests

Medication History

- Exposure to cytotoxic drugs, benzene, chloramphenicol
- Medications, including home remedies, over-the-counter (OTC) drugs, vitamin and mineral supplements, and borrowed medicines
- Tobacco, alcohol, or drug use

Family History

- Genetic abnormalities
- Family history of cancer

Psychosocial History

Ask about home situation and significant others, including family and friends.

ASSESSMENT: OBJECTIVE/PHYSICAL EXAMINATION

Physical Examination

Perform a complete physical examination, with increased attention to the following:

- Vital signs
- Weight
- Signs and symptoms of infection
- General appearance
- Skin: excessive bruising, petechiae, pallor, rashes, infections, leukemia cutis (leukemic skin infiltration associated mostly with AML)
- Lymphatic system: neck, axilla, supraclavicular, infraclavicular, epitrochlear, and inguinal nodal enlargement
- Head, eyes, ears, nose, and throat: fundi, papilledema
- Chest: murmurs from anemia, wheezing and decreased breath sounds from a possible mediastinal mass
- Abdomen: hepatosplenomegaly
- Male genitourinary (GU): Check testes for unilateral or bilateral firm, painless enlargement, with or without scrotal discoloration

Diagnostic Procedures

- Perform CBC with differential.
  - WBCs are higher than 50,000 cells/mm^3 in 20% of clients with ALL.
  - Initial WBC is single most important predictor of prognosis.
  - Low absolute neutrophil count is present.
  - Hgb is less than 10 g/dL.
  - Thrombocytopenia (platelets less than 100,000 cells/mm^3) is present at diagnosis in 75%.
  - Blast cells may or may not be seen on differential. Bone marrow may be "packed" before blasts are seen on peripheral smear.
- Bone marrow aspiration shows 25% blasts; cytogenetics, immunophenotyping, and special stains are done to differentiate type of leukemia.
- Bone marrow biopsy is done.
- Lumbar puncture should be done to rule out CNS involvement.
- Obtain chest x-ray film to check for mediastinal mass.
- Serum immunoglobulin levels are low at diagnosis in 30% of clients with ALL.
- Increased serum uric acid levels can lead to uric acid nephrology and renal failure.
- Liver function test results are elevated.
- Evaluate calcium phosphate.
- Take blood cultures if client is febrile.

Prognostic Factors

- Initial WBC count: high risk if WBC count is higher than 50,000 cells/mm^3.
- Age at diagnosis: poor prognosis for children younger than 2 or older than 10 years.
- Hgb level: poorer prognosis if low.
- Platelet count: poorer prognosis if low.
- Ethnicity: Blacks have poorer prognosis.
- Presence of mediastinal mass, organomegaly, or lymphadenopathy: More tumor burden requires more intense chemotherapy.

DIAGNOSIS

- Differential diagnoses include the following:
  - Aplastic anemia
  - Marrow infiltration with a solid tumor
  - Autoimmune pancytopenia
  - Immune thrombocytopenia
  - Severe megaloblastic anemia
  - Overwhelming infection
  - Rheumatoid arthritis
  - Marrow suppression related to drugs, toxins, or infections
- Children: Most likely diagnosis is ALL, then AML.
- Adults: Most likely diagnosis is CML or CLL.
- Pregnant client: Most likely diagnosis is AML, then ALL; least likely is CML.

THERAPEUTIC PLAN

Refer client if CBC, differential, history, and physical examination lead to suspicions of leukemia. The goal of treatment is to eradicate leukemic blast cells so that normal cells can regrow.

Acute Lymphocytic Leukemia

Treatment consists of combination chemotherapy, often according to specific multicenter protocols. Cranial-spinal radiation is used if there is CNS involvement. Length of the treatment is 2 years plus a few months for girls and 3 years plus a few months for boys.

Acute Myelocytic Leukemia

Treatment consists of extremely intense combination chemotherapy. Duration of treatment is shorter than for ALL. Cranial-spinal radiation is used if there is CNS involvement. Bone marrow transplantation (BMT) is performed if a complete match is found. Most treatment is done in the hospital.

Chronic Myelocytic Leukemia

- *Juvenile Type.* Generally this disease is resistant to therapy. Median survival is less than 9 months from diagnosis. BMT is the only possible curative treatment.
- *Adult Type.* Goal of treatment is to provide symptomatic relief by lowering the WBC count and reducing liver and spleen size. Hydroxyurea or busulfan, given as single agents, can be used to regulate leukocytosis. BMT is the only possible curative treatment.

Chronic Lymphocytic Leukemia

Stable, symptom-free clients, with or without lymphadenopathy or splenomegaly, do not require treatment. Symptoms (weight loss, malaise, anemia, thrombocytopenia) are treated with alkylating agents (chlorambucil) and prednisone.

Leukemia in Pregnancy

- AML or ALL requires immediate and aggressive treatment with combination chemotherapy.
- If AML or ALL is diagnosed in the first trimester, prognoses for both mother and child are extremely poor.
- If AML or ALL is diagnosed and treated in the second or third trimester, there is a 75% chance of remission and only a 1.5% incidence of congenital anomalies.
- CML has a slow, indolent course.

Client Education

- Client and family should be knowledgeable about diagnosis and treatment plan.
- Client and family should be knowledgeable about expected and toxic side effects of chemotherapy.
- Supportive care guidelines should be clear for family and primary care provider.
- Both the provider and family should know the following:
  - Hold all immunizations during treatment. Immunizations may be resumed 6 months to 1 year after treatment.
  - Avoid live virus vaccines (e.g., measles-mumpsrubella, oral polio).
  - Siblings of clients also need to avoid live virus vaccines.
  - Varicella-zoster immunoglobulin can be given within 72 to 96 hours of varicella exposure in non-immune children.
  - Prophylactic trimethoprim-sulfamethoxazole (Bactrim) can be given to prevent *Pneumocystis carinii*, 5 mg/kg/day 3 days/week.
  - Monthly use of intravenous (IV) or aerosolized pentamidine is suggested if client is allergic to Bactrim.
  - Use broad-spectrum antibiotics empirically for fever and neutropenia.
  - There should be no IM injections.
  - There should be no rectal temperatures or suppositories.
  - Do not use tampons.
  - Use soft toothbrush or toothettes for oral care.
  - If central line access is in place, administer antibiotic prophylaxis before dental work.

- If client is febrile, always check a CBC with differential as soon as possible to rule out fever from neutropenia.

Prevention

Avoidance of risk factors may help prevent leukemia, although there is no guarantee of avoiding the development of leukemia.

EVALUATION/FOLLOW-UP

- Client should be referred to a hematology/oncology specialist in a timely manner.
- Complications related to delays in referral are to be avoided.
- Communication between hematology/oncology specialist and primary care provider should be clear, concise, and current.
- Follow-up by specialists on a regular basis should be ensured, especially for children who are cancer survivors.

COMPLICATIONS

- Death
- Development of other cancers

REFERENCES

Abramson, N., & Melton, B. (2000). Leukocytosis: basics of clinical assessment. *American Family Physician 62*, 2053-2060.

Altman, A. J., & Wolff, L. (1997). The prevention of infection. In A. R. Abline (Ed.) *Supportive care of children with cancer* (2nd ed.). Baltimore: Johns Hopkins University Press.

Antonelli, N. M., Dotters, D. J., Katz, V. L., & Kuller, J. A. (1996). Cancer in pregnancy: a review of the literature. Part II. *Obstetrical and Gynecological Survey 51*(2), 135-142.

Baer, M. R. (1993). Management of unusual presentations of acute leukemia. In C. D. Bloomfield, G. P., Herzig (Eds.). *Hematology/oncology clinic of North America: management of acute leukemia*. Philadelphia: W. B. Saunders.

Bates, B. (1995). *Physical exam and history taking* (2nd ed.). Philadelphia: Lippincott.

Bennetts, G. A. (1993). Immunization of patients with malignant disease. In A. R. Abline (Ed.), *Supportive care of children with cancer*. Baltimore: Johns Hopkins University Press.

Black, S. (2000). Leukemia. In D. Robinson, P. Kidd, & K. Rogers (Eds.), *Primary care across the lifespan* (pp. 658-664). St. Louis: Mosby.

Cohen, D. G. (1993). Leukemia in children and adolescents—acute lymphocytic leukemia. In G. V. Foley, D. Fochtman, & K. H. Mooney (Eds.), *Nursing care of the child with cancer,* 2nd ed. Philadelphia: W. B. Saunders.

Lampkin, B. (1997). Acute lymphoblastic leukemia. In R. J. Arceci (Ed.), *Hematology/oncology/stem cell transplant handbook* (2nd ed.). Cincinnati: Hematology/Oncology Division, Children's Hospital Medical Center.

Panzarella, C., Aitken, T., Patterson, K. et al (1993). *Pediatric oncology nursing study guide*. Skokie, IL: Association of Pediatric Oncology Nurses.

Reynoso, E. E., Shepherd, F. A., Messner, H. A., Farquharson, H. A., Garvey, M. B., & Baker, M. A. (1987). Acute leukemia during pregnancy: The Toronto leukemia study group experience with long-term follow-up of children exposed in utero to chemotherapeutic agents. *Journal of Clinical Oncology 5*, 1098-1106.

Sambrano, J. (1997). Chronic myelogenous leukemia. In Arceci, R.J. (Ed.), *Hematology/oncology/stem cell transplant handbook* (2nd ed.). Cincinnati: Hematology/Oncology Division, Children's Hospital Medical Center.

Skidmore-Roth, L. (1995). *Mosby's nursing drug reference*. St. Louis: Mosby.

Waterburg, L., & Zieve, P. D. (1999). Selected illnesses affecting lymphocytes: Mononucleosis, chronic lymphocytic leukemia, and the undiagnosed patient with lymphadenopathy. In L. R. Barker, J. R. Burton, & P. D. Zieve (Eds.), *Principles of ambulatory medicine* (5th ed.). Baltimore: Williams & Wilkins.

Wiley, F. M. (1993). Leukemia in children and adolescents: acute myelogenous leukemia. In G. V. Foley, D. Foctman, & K. H. Mooney (Eds.), *Nursing care of the child with cancer* (2nd ed.). Philadelphia: W. B. Saunders.

Young, G., Toretsky, J., Campbell, A., & Eskenazi, A. E. (2000). Recognition of common childhood malignancies. *American Family Physician, 61*, 2144-2154.

Review Questions

1. The most common presenting symptoms in childhood ALL are which of the following?
- **a.** Lymphadenopathy, fever, and night sweats
- **b.** Pallor, bleeding, fever, and pain
- **c.** Headache, vomiting, and visual disturbances
- **d.** Anorexia, abdominal pain, and weight loss

2. Jenny, a 6-year-old with ALL diagnosed 1 year ago, is away from home visiting her aunt. She had a temperature of 102° F last night. Her aunt knows that Jenny is on a "maintenance" chemotherapy regimen consisting of prednisone, 5 day pulses/month, 6 mercaptopurine pills/day, and methotrexate pills once per week. Jenny also takes trimethoprim-sulfamethoxazole (Bactrim) for *P. carinii* prophylaxis. On physical examination, Jenny has no obvious site of infection and is now afebrile and playing. What should you do for Jenny?
- **a.** Send her home with instructions to take acetaminophen (Tylenol) q4h as needed.
- **b.** Give her amoxicillin, 250 mg PO tid for 10 days.
- **c.** Obtain a CBC with differential to rule out neutropenia.
- **d.** Tell her to hold chemotherapy until she sees her oncologist.

3. Onute is diagnosed with acute myelocytic anemia. Which of the following historical data is consistent with the diagnosis?
- **a.** Pallor
- **b.** Increased moles
- **c.** Nausea/vomiting
- **d.** Weight loss

4. John, a 70-year-old male whose CLL was diagnosed 3 years ago, has been symptom free until recently. He now has weight loss, malaise, anemia, and thrombocytopenia. His oncologist begins treating John with chlorambucil and prednisone. Parameters for evaluating the efficacy of this treatment include all the following except:

   a. John and family are able to state possible side effects of medications.
   b. John's weight stabilizes or increases, and symptoms improve.
   c. John keeps his follow-up appointments with his oncologist.
   d. John seeks information about his disease.

5. Which of the following statements is true?

   a. CML is the most common type of leukemia in the United States.
   b. CLL usually affects males older than 60 years.
   c. The median age of onset for adult CML is younger than 30 years.
   d. The ratio of AML to ALL is 4:1.

6. Risk factors in development of leukemia include all the following except:

   a. Chronic use of immunosuppressive drugs
   b. Twin with leukemia
   c. Chronic chemical exposure, especially benzene
   d. Chronic aspirin use

7. Which of the following physical signs is *not* consistent with a diagnosis of leukemia?

   a. Petechiae
   b. Murmur
   c. Alopecia
   d. Lymphadenopathy

8. June is getting a 4-year well-child check. Which of the following immunizations is contraindicated when you find out her sister is undergoing treatment for leukemia?

   a. DtaP
   b. Influenza vaccine
   c. Mumps, measles, rubella (MMR)
   d. Inactivated polio vaccine (IPV)

Answers and Rationales

1. **Answer: b** (assessment)
   Rationale: Pallor, bleeding, fever, and pain are early symptoms in the course of the disease and may be present 1 to 2 weeks before the actual diagnosis. These symptoms reflect bone marrow replacement with leukemic cells, resulting in anemia, thrombocytopenia, neutropenia, and pain from bone marrow "packing" with leukemic replacement (Cohen, 1993).

2. **Answer: c** (evaluation)
   Rationale: It is critical to obtain a CBC with differential to determine Jenny's ability to fight infection. An absolute neutrophil count higher than 500 cells/mm^3 plus a temperature of 100.5° F could necessitate a hospital admission, complete with blood cultures and IV antibiotics.

3. **Answer: a** (assessment)
   Rationale: Pallor is one of the most common symptoms of acute leukemia (Black, 2000).

4. **Answer: d** (evaluation)
   Rationale: Although seeking information about the disease is important, it does not indicate the efficacy of the treatment. Knowing the side effects of the medications, increasing weight, and keeping follow-up appointments all help in evaluating the effectiveness of treatment (Black, 2000).

5. **Answer: b** (diagnosis/analysis)
   Rationale: CLL usually affects men older than age 60. It is the most common type of leukemia. The median onset for adult CML is 45. The ratio of AML to ALL is 1:4 (Lampkin, 1997).

6. **Answer: d** (diagnosis/analysis)
   Rationale: Aspirin may cause adverse hematologic reactions, such as increased prothrombin time, partial thromboplastin time, and bleeding time. It also can cause thrombocytopenia, agranulocytosis, leukopenia, neutropenia, and hemolytic anemia (Black, 2000).

7. **Answer: c** (assessment)
   Rationale: Alopecia is not a symptom seen in leukemia. Petechiae, murmur, and lymphadenopathy are all symptoms seen with leukemia (Black, 2000).

8. **Answer: c** (plan/intervention)
   Rationale: Live virus immunizations are contraindicated for children with leukemia during treatment. They are also contraindicated for the siblings of children being treated for leukemia. Live virus immunizations include oral polio and MMR (Black, 2000).

LICE   *Denise Robinson*

OVERVIEW
Definition

Pedicular infestation of the skin or hair is caused by a species of blood-sucking lice capable of living as external parasites on the human host. There are three types of lice that inhabit the human host:

- *Pediculus humanis corporis:* The body louse infests the body but actually emerges from the lining or seams of infested clothing, upholstery, or bedding to bite the human host.
- *Pediculus humanis capitis:* The head louse infests the scalp and head hair.
- *Phthirus pubis:* The crab louse infests the genital region. Referred to as pediculosis pubis, *P. pubis* infestation also may affect the hair of the axilla, chest, abdomen, thighs, and eyelashes.

Incidence

- From 6 to 12 million cases occur annually in the United States.
- Of all cases of lice infestation, 50% to 75% occur in children younger than 12 years old.
- Lice can be epidemic in day care, kindergartens, and schools.
- Lice occurs in all ages, races, and socioeconomic groups and in all geographic regions.
- It can occur in any season but is most common August through November.

Pediculosis Capitis. Infestation occurs most commonly in 5- to 12-year-olds, more often in girls. It may spread to family members. It occurs in less than 1% of blacks because the structure of their hair shaft is less conducive. Head lice are acquired through personal contact.

Pediculosis Corporis. Infestation occurs most commonly in crowded living conditions, situations of poverty, and where laundering is limited, such as in the homeless population. It is rare in children, except in colder climates when changing clothes is infrequent.

Pediculosis Pubis. Infestation is highly contagious (90% acquisition rate per contact). Transmission occurs during intimate personal or sexual contact. Infestation can occur in children who have been sexually abused.

Pathophysiology

Lice are ectoparasites that, when spread by direct or fomite contact, pierce the skin to feed. When they bite, they infuse saliva to prevent clotting and probe for a vessel. The louse lays 100 to 300 eggs (nits) during a lifetime. Nits are attached to the hair shaft by a cementlike structure, which makes them difficult to remove. They can remain viable on clothes for up to 1 month. Lice cannot live away from a human host for more than 48 hours. It is the saliva of the louse that creates symptoms through a histamine response.

Protective Factors

- Clean hair and good hygiene do not prevent infestation with lice.
- A lifestyle that does not include behaviors and situations that provide exposure will help prevent lice infestation.
- Black race reduces the likelihood of lice infestation.

Factors Increasing Susceptibility
Pediculosis Capitis

- Childhood, especially with enrollment in day care, school, or camp
- Family member with infestation
- Sharing of combs, brushes, hair decorations, and other objects that touch the head where lice are present

Pediculosis Corporis

- Homelessness
- Poor hygiene
- Infrequent laundering
- Close contact in crowded situations with individuals who are infested with lice
- Sharing of clothing or bedding that is contaminated

Pediculosis Pubis. Sexual contact with individual infected with pubic lice increases transmission risk.

ASSESSMENT: SUBJECTIVE/HISTORY
History of Present Illness

- Intense itching (the hallmark of lice), often worse at night
- With *P. capitis,* itching at the occipital hairline and the postauricular area
- Known exposure

Symptoms

- Sleeplessness
- Irritability
- Difficulty concentrating in school because of itching

Family History

Inquire about infestation in any family member.

Psychosocial History
Pediculosis Capitis

- Child enrolled in day care, kindergarten, school, or camp
- Sharing of clothing or hairbrushes, combs, barrettes, and other hair care items

- Participation in sports in which equipment is shared
- Participation in activities in which wigs and borrowed clothes are shared

Pediculosis Corporis
- Living in crowded environment, being homeless, or otherwise being unable to bathe, shampoo, and launder clothing as needed
- Sharing clothing, pillows, and bedding
- Purchasing clothing (and not laundering it before use) from yard sales or thrift shops
- Wearing clothing found or from lost-and-found sites

Pediculosis Pubis
- Multiple sexual partners
- Child: sexual abuse by an adult or older child with lice infestation

It is important to assess client, parent, and family perceptions of the problem of lice because there are many misconceptions about infestation. A stigma exists concerning lice infestations.

ASSESSMENT: OBJECTIVE/PHYSICAL EXAMINATION
Physical Examination
Strong lighting and a magnifying lens facilitate identification of lice and nits. The examiner always should wear gloves when examining for lice.

Skin and Hair
- Visualize lice on hair shaft. Lice are smaller than a sesame seed, 3 to 4 mm, and gray-brown; they quickly move away from light and hide.
- Identify nits. Nits are teardrop shaped, 0.8 mm, and cream colored; empty ova shells are white. They are attached near the base of hair shafts at the scalp or pubic area. Dandruff and hair product artifacts usually blow or fall away, whereas a nit must be pulled along the hair shaft.
- Note pinpoint red bites or black specks (lice feces).
- Look for erythema at the nape of the neck and postauricular areas.

Lymph and Femoral Lymphadenopathy
- Lesions of secondary infection from scratching may be present.
- Cervical lymphadenopathy may occur with secondary infections associated with head lice.
- Symptoms of other sexually transmitted diseases (STDs) may coexist with *pediculosis pubis.*

Diagnostic Procedures
- A louse may be removed for examination under a microscope for confirmation if desired.

- A Wood's lamp may be used because lice fluoresce. This is normally not necessary for diagnosis.

DIAGNOSIS
Confirm the type of lice infestation. Rule out hair artifacts (e.g., spray, gel), dandruff, seborrhea, psoriasis, and tinea capitis.

THERAPEUTIC PLAN
Nonpharmacologic Treatment

NOTE: *No pediculicide is 100% ovicidal. Nit removal is essential.*

- There are commercial preparations, such as Step 2, that assist in nit removal. A 50/50 white vinegar and water solution also may be used to loosen nits. A nit comb (metal combs work best) is used to remove all nits from the hair shafts. This can be a time-consuming process.
- To treat lice-infested eyelashes, apply petrolatum 2 times a day for 10 days.

Pharmacologic Treatment
Pediculicides are required to kill lice and nits. Most are contraindicated in children younger than 2 years and in pregnant and lactating women. During use the client's eyes should be covered and shut.

Types of Pediculicides
- Pyrethrins (with piperonyl butoxide) 0.3% (A200, RID, Triple X): Leave shampoo on for 10 minutes, then rinse thoroughly. Reapplication may be needed in 7 to 10 days. Products are available OTC.
- Permethrin 1% cream rinse (Nix, Elimite): This is the drug of choice because it has a 97% to 99% cure rate and minimal side effects. Apply after shampooing hair, leave on for 10 minutes, and rinse thoroughly. Do not shampoo for 24 hours after use. Reapplication is not usually necessary. These products are available OTC.
- Lindane (Kwell): Prescription is required. Product comes as 1% lotion, 1% cream, and 1% shampoo. Shampoo, leave on for 4 minutes, then rinse. Repeat in 1 week. Product must be used with caution because it may cause neurotoxicity. Lindane should not be used on acutely inflamed skin or scalp.

Client Education
- Reassure the client and family that pediculosis is curable, does not cause long-term effects, and is a common problem in all socioeconomic groups.
- Because person-to-person transmission occurs, educate children and parents about mode of transmission and preventive measures, such as not sharing combs, brushes, hair decorations, hats, scarves, helmets, headphones, bedding, and sleeping bags. Coats

and hats should be hung separately, not touching those of others. Sleeping mats should be individually labeled and kept separately in plastic bags, not stacked.

- Teach how to disinfect the personal articles of the infested individual and how to clean the environment, reinforcing that lice do not jump or fly but spread through crawling.
  - Machine wash all washable clothing and bedding used within the last 48 hours with hot water and detergent (water should be hotter than 125° F).
  - Dry clothing and bedding on as high heat as possible in a clothes dryer for at least 20 minutes.
  - Dry clean clothing and personal items that cannot be washed. Upholstered furniture, pillows, and stuffed animals may be ironed with a hot iron.
  - Soak brushes, combs, barrettes, and similar hair items in 2% disinfectant or pediculicide for 1 hour (items can be boiled on stove for 10 minutes if they are not plastic).
  - Clean other objects that have been in contact with infested hair within the last 48 hours, such as curlers, headphones, earpieces or glasses, helmets, and car seats.
  - Place other items that have been exposed to infestation in a plastic bag and keep it closed for 2 weeks; lice will die of starvation.
- Recommend that all family members and close contacts be examined for presence of infestation and treated at the same time as the identified client.
- Advise parents to inform school authorities about infested children.
- Reinforce the importance of exposing all lice and nits to pediculicide and destroying or removing all nits from infested hair. Hair should be separated into multiple sections, with each part of the scalp exposed, examined, and methodically treated. Nits are removed with a nit comb. A different comb should be used for each infested person, and combs should be cleaned frequently during the removal process. Vinegar or a nit removal product may be used to loosen nits from the hair shaft for easier removal.

Referral

Referral to a physician is necessary for the following:
- Children younger than 2 years of age
- Pregnant and lactating women
- Treatment failures
- Lice in eyelashes that persist despite treatment
- Coexisting dermatologic conditions

If *pediculosis pubis* is seen in a child, appropriate authorities should be notified regarding the potential for child sexual abuse.

Prevention

Lice can be prevented by avoiding head-to-head contact and changing and cleaning clothes on a regular basis.

EVALUATION/FOLLOW-UP

During lice season, the parent should check the child's hair every 3 days. Once treated for lice, the individual should be reexamined at least by a family member several days after treatment. Reapplication of pediculicide 7 to 10 days after the initial treatment is often necessary. In the case of *pediculosis pubis*, all sexual contacts for the past month should receive treatment.

COMPLICATIONS

- Chronic infestation of the body with lice results in "vagabonds" skin, which are lichenified, scaling, hyperpigmented papules, most commonly on the trunk.
- Chronic infestation of the hair can lead to multiple pyodermas of the scalp, particularly in tropical areas.

REFERENCES

Copeland, L. (1995). *The lice-buster book.* New York: Warner Books.

Crain, E. F., & Gershel, J. C. (1997). *Clinical manual of emergency pediatrics.* New York: McGraw-Hill.

Fenstermacher, K., & Hudson, B. T. (1997). *Practice guidelines for family nurse practitioners.* Philadelphia: W. B. Saunders.

Fitzpatrick, T. B., Johnson, R. A., Wolff, K., & Suurmond, D. (2001). *Color atlas and synopsis of clinical dermatology* (4th ed.). New York: McGraw-Hill.

Forsman, K. E. (1995). Pediculosis and scabies: What to look for in patients who are crawling with clues. *Postgraduate Medicine 98*(6), 89-100.

Hawkins, J. W., Roberto-Nichols, D. M., & Stanley-Haney, J. L. (1995). *Protocols for nurse practitioners.* New York: Tiresias Press.

Kish, C. (2000). Lice. In D. Robinson, P. Kidd, & K. Rogers (Eds.), *Primary care across the lifespan* (pp. 665-670). St. Louis: Mosby.

Lichtman, R., & Papera, S. (1990). *Gynecology—Well woman care.* Norwalk, CT: Appleton & Lange.

Millonig, V. L. (1991). Back to school signals—head lice season. *Journal of the American Academy of Nurse Practitioners 3*(3), 136-137.

Sokoloff, F. (1994). Identification and management of pediculosis. *Nurse Practitioner, 19*(8), 62-64.

Star, W. L., Lommel, L. L., & Shannon, M. T. (1995). *Women's primary health care: Protocols for practice.* Washington, DC: American Nurses Publishing.

Uphold, C. R., & Graham, M. V. (1994). *Clinical guidelines in family practice.* Gainesville, FL: Barmarrae Books.

Wong, D. (1995). *Nursing care of infants and children* (5th ed.). St. Louis: Mosby.

Youngkin, E. O., & Davis, M. S. (1994). *Women's health: A primary care clinical guide.* Norwalk, CT: Appleton & Lange.

Review Questions

1. Which symptom associated with *pediculosis capitis* is least likely to be reported by Megan, a 7-year-old female, or her mother?

  a. Difficulty sleeping
  b. Problems concentrating on school work
  c. Headache
  d. Irritability

2. The NP suspects that Megan has *pediculosis capitis.* What diagnostic measure can provide additional supportive evidence?

  a. Use of Wood's lamp
  b. Eosinophil count
  c. Sedimentation rate
  d. WBC count

3. Which of the following individuals is most likely to have *pediculosis corporis*?

  a. Older, homeless woman
  b. Black transportation executive
  c. Middle-aged wheat farmer
  d. Hispanic high-school librarian

4. In cases of *pediculosis capitis,* in what area of the head are findings most evident?

  a. Frontal hair, such as bangs
  b. Crown of head
  c. Occipital hairline
  d. Preauricular region

5. How can lice and nits in the eyelashes be treated?

  a. Soak lashes bid in permethrin for 3 days.
  b. Coat lashes with petrolatum bid for 1 week.
  c. Apply hot, moist cloths tid for 7 days.
  d. Brush lashes with a gauze dipped in disinfectant.

6. What is the appropriate approach in the event of initial treatment failure for *pediculosis capitis*?

  a. Reapply pediculicide daily for 1 week.
  b. Shave the hair.
  c. Initiate oral pediculicide.
  d. Reapply pediculicide 7 to 10 days after initial treatment.

7. Mr. Ludlum is a 33-year-old male with *pediculosis pubis.* Which additional associated diagnosis does not need to be considered?

  a. Gonorrhea
  b. Human immunodeficiency virus (HIV) infection
  c. Chlamydial infection
  d. Orchitis

8. *Pediculosis capitis* needs to be differentiated from dandruff. Which of the following characteristics makes lice distinguishable from dandruff?

  a. Lice is a different color than dandruff.
  b. Dandruff blows or falls away from the hair shaft.
  c. Dandruff causes itching.
  d. Dandruff is white and attached to the hair shaft.

Answers and Rationales

1. *Answer:* **c** (assessment)
Rationale: Sleeplessness, difficulty concentrating, and irritability commonly are associated with lice infestation (Sokoloff, 1994).

2. *Answer:* **a** (assessment)
Rationale: Lice fluoresce under the Wood's lamp (Fitzpatrick, Johnson, Wolff, & Suurmond, 2001).

3. *Answer:* **a** (analysis/diagnosis)
Rationale: Homeless populations are at particular risk for body lice infestations because of compromised hygiene and laundering (Forsman, 1995).

4. *Answer:* **c** (assessment)
Rationale: Although any part of the head may itch and have lice present, the occipital hairline and postauricular area generally are most affected (Millonig, 1991).

5. *Answer:* **b** (implementation/plan)
Rationale: Petrolatum applied to lashes bid for 7 to 10 days effectively removes lice and nits (Uphold & Graham, 1994).

6. *Answer:* **d** (implementation/plan)
Rationale: Ovicides may need to be reapplied in 7 to 10 days to kill nits (Forsman, 1995).

7. *Answer:* **d** (analysis/diagnosis)
Rationale: In the presence of *pediculosis pubis,* other STDs must be considered as possible coexisting diagnoses (Fitzpatrick, et al 2001).

8. *Answer:* **b** (assessment)
Rationale: Dandruff falls or blows away from the hair shaft. Nits are attached firmly to the hair shaft and cannot blow away. They need to be removed from the hair shaft (Kish, 2000).

LOWER BACK PAIN   *Pamela Kidd*

OVERVIEW
Definitions

Lumbosacral Strain. Lumbosacral strain (LBS) is defined as stretching or tearing of muscles, tendons, ligaments, or fascia of the lumbosacral area secondary to trauma or mechanical injury. Acute lower back pain is defined as symptoms of less than 3 months duration.

Herniated Nucleus Pulposa. Herniated nucleus pulposa (HNP) is rupture of an intervertebral disc with herniation of nucleus pulposa into the spinal canal. Sciatica refers to pain and paresthesias extending down the leg in a dermatomal pattern; the most common cause is HNP at L_{4-5} and L_5S_1.

Incidence

- Of working adults, 50% are affected every year and 15% to 20% seek health care. For people older than age 45 years, low back problems are the most common cause of disability. Only approximately 10% of clients with low back pain experience herniated nucleus pulposa.
- Children: Strains of the ligaments/muscles of the back are unusual in children unless they occur as a result of trauma, infection, inflammation, or malignancies.

Pathophysiology

The cause of LBS is unclear; herniation occurs with tears in annulus fibroses, which allows contents of pulposa to protrude.

Factors Increasing Susceptibility
- Overweight
- Mechanical disorders (e.g., scoliosis, kyphosis)
- Nonmechanical disorders (e.g., ankylosing spondylitis, prostate cancer, pelvic and renal disease)
- Occupational strain
- Leg-length differences
- Poor posture
- Poor body mechanics with lifting

Protective Factors
- Proper body mechanics
- Appropriate weight maintenance
- Conditioned state

ASSESSMENT: SUBJECTIVE/HISTORY
Symptoms

- Inquire regarding duration of symptoms and any known trauma.

- In children, inquire regarding trauma, infection, inflammation, and malignancy.
- In adults and the elderly, ask about occupation, leisure/hobby activities, and underlying physical conditions.

Common Symptoms

Lumbosacral Strain. For LBS, determine mechanism of injury, if known. Symptoms include the following:

- Pain that has increased over time and accompanied by stiffness and soft-tissue swelling
- Pain located primarily in back, but may radiate to buttocks or thighs
- Pain increased with movement and relieved with rest
- Muscle spasms in lower back

In elderly people, symptoms are less severe. Elderly women may confuse low back pain with vertebral fractures; assess for presence of severe pain and limited activity.

Herniated Nucleus Pulposa
- Radicular pain (shooting, electrical) below the knee
- Paresthesia or numbness along sensory distribution of nerve root

In the elderly, the nucleus pulposa is more fibrotic, making the incidence and/or symptoms much less common.

Past Medical History

- Inquire about previous history of back pain or other painful conditions, treatment measures, compliance, and outcome.
- Ask about use of alcohol and tobacco products.
- Before any radiologic tests, ask about last menstrual period, in consideration of pelvic inflammatory disease and ectopic pregnancy.
- Inquire about history of weight loss, systemic disease, or malignancy.
- Ask about previous history of affective disorders.

Medication History

- Recent use of acetaminophen, NSAIDs or other OTC preparations with responses
- Other current medications

Family History

Inquire about family history of back problems, treatment, outcome, and malignancies.

Dietary History

Inquire as to overall nutrition pattern, and emphasize weight reduction, if needed, and a balanced diet.

ASSESSMENT: OBJECTIVE/PHYSICAL EXAMINATION

Physical Examination

The physical examination should be conducted with attention to vital signs, weight, general appearance, and systems other than musculoskeletal to rule out mechanical, systemic, or psychosocial causes for back pain. The examination should be conducted in a systematic head-to-toe fashion incorporating standing, sitting, and lying positions of the client.

Gait

- Assess client's gait walking to examination room, removing shoes, and getting on the examination table, noting flexion or other difficulties performing these functions.
- Note activity level in affected children.

Standing

- Client should be undressed with back exposed.
- Note posture in bare feet.
- Walk on heels (L_{4-5}) and toes (S_{1-2}); if there is nerve root irritation, the client will be unable to perform this.

Back

- Examine spinal column from front, back, and side. Note any scoliosis and abnormalities of expected S curvature. Lumbar lordosis may be seen in acute LBS.
- Note that level of shoulder tips, scapular ranges, iliac crests, gluteal folds, and popliteal creases should be equal. In LBS, unequal levels may be present.
- Perform spinal range of motion (ROM), including flexion, extension, lateral bending, and rotation. Severe guarding may support a diagnosis of fracture, spinal infection, or tumor.
- Palpate paravertebral muscles for spasm and/or tenderness; this may be seen in acute LBS.

Sitting

- Check lung sounds for signs of pleural effusion or consolidation.
- Note heart rate, rhythm, and any signs of recent cardiac event (rub, effusion).
- Check deep tendon reflexes of knees (L_4) and Achilles (S_1), Babinski. Observe for bilaterally equal responses. If unequal responses, consider nerve root irritation. Test strength, vibratory, and proprioceptive sensation bilaterally (should be equal). Weakness in dorsiflexion of ankle or great toe (L_{4-5}) suggests nerve root dysfunction.
- Check light touch sensation of medial (L_4), dorsal (L_5), and lateral (S_1) aspects of foot.
- Perform sitting straight-leg raise (SLR). Knee should extend without radiation of pain below knee; this is also one way to check for malingering behavior because results should equal those of SLR performed in lying position.

- Check for ankle and toe (L_5) dorsiflexion strength bilaterally; they should be equal.

Supine

- Check abdomen for tenderness of peptic ulcer disease, bruits, and enlargement of dissecting aortic aneurysm.
- Check extremities for flexion, abduction, external rotation (FABER or Patrick test) of hips: decreased ROM may indicate hip or sacroiliac joint problem.
- With standard SLR, normally the hip can be flexed to 80 degrees without pain, except in thigh. A positive test is one that elicits shooting, sharp, or electrical pain that radiates below the knee on the affected side at 30 degrees flexion or less.
- Crossed SLR is SLR of the unaffected leg; a positive test is when the SLR of the unaffected leg causes radicular pain in the affected leg to be reproduced.
- Perform sensory assessment of buttocks and perineum to rule out saddle anesthesia of cauda equina syndrome (compression of nerves at L_{4-5} level, which needs emergency surgical decompression).

Indicators for Pelvic Examination

- Reports of abdominal pain, dyspareunia, vaginal discharge
- Rest of examination equivocal

Indicators for Rectal Examination

- Men older than age 50
- Rest of examination equivocal

Specialized Examination Techniques for Malingering Behavior. "Pain behaviors" of distress such as amplified grimacing, distorted gait or posture, or rubbing of painful body parts may cloud the picture. Interpreting inconsistencies or pain behaviors as malingering may not be useful because they could be viewed as a plea for help. The goal is to facilitate recovery and avoid the development of chronic low back disability. However, there may be times when malingering behavior must be ruled out. The following tests may be used in these cases:

- Waddell's signs: a standardized group of nonorganic physical signs
  - Tenderness: nonanatomic or superficial
  - Simulation: simulate movement without actually performing it
  - Axial loading: pressure to top of head should not produce pain
  - Distraction: examine SLR in sitting and supine position and compare results
  - Regionalization: inappropriate location of pain from normal neuroanatomy

- Overreaction: disproportionate verbalization, facial expression, or tremor
- Magnuson's test: Mark areas that were tender when palpated; return to the marked areas later in the examination to see if pain can be reproduced. With malingering behavior, those marked areas are not likely to reproduce pain.
- Hoover's test: Put examiner's hands under both heels. (Client can be standing, sitting, or lying.) Ask client to raise affected leg. If the pain is real, the heel on the other leg will push into the examiner's hands.

Diagnostic Procedures

Radiographs and laboratory testing are generally *not* necessary at the initial visit unless there is a history of trauma or suspicion of systemic or structural changes.

DIAGNOSIS

- See Table 3-61.
- The NP should consider discogenic causes, malignancies, vascular lesions, infections, intraabdominal or pelvic causes, neurologic complications, congenital causes, trauma, and metabolic bone diseases as possible causes of lower back pain.
- Children: Because pain caused by sprains of ligaments and muscles is unusual in children, inflammation, infections, tremors, and trauma must be considered.
- See Table 3-62.

THERAPEUTIC PLAN

Nonpharmacologic Treatment

- Adjunct therapies, such as ultrasound and massage, have no effect on outcome but provide symptomatic relief and may be used for 3 weeks or less.
- Chiropractic manipulation, if used in the first month, has been found to be safe and effective.

- Bed rest is reserved for those clients with rare severe leg pain and should not exceed 2 to 4 days. The emphasis for other clients is on maintaining physical activity.
- Local application of ice may help initially in decreasing edema and/or pain; after 2 to 3 days either ice or heat may be applied.
- Explore community resources available (e.g., exercise programs, swimming pools, physical therapists, walking trails).

Pharmacologic Treatment

- Nonprescription drugs such as acetaminophen, aspirin, or NSAIDs (ibuprofen, naproxen, ketoprofen) provide relief for most people. If a NSAID from one class is not tolerated or does not provide relief, another NSAID within the same or different class may be prescribed.
- Muscle relaxants do not appear to be more effective than NSAIDs and should be reserved for those in whom NSAIDs do not help or those in whom NSAIDs are contraindicated. If muscle relaxants are used, they should be limited to a course of 1 to 2 weeks; they should be avoided, or used in reduced dosages, in older clients who are at risk of falling.
- Opiates are *not* necessary in the management of acute LBS; if they are used for more severe pain, they should be taken for a short time only. Poor client tolerance, drowsiness, clouded judgment, decreased reaction time, and the potential for misuse (dependence) may occur.

Client Education

- Aerobic conditioning exercises (e.g., walking, swimming, stationary biking, light jogging) may be recommended to avoid debilitation. If a person was sedentary before this event, walking is preferred; if they were more active, light jogging is permitted.

TABLE **3-61**   Primary Differential Diagnoses of Low Back Pain

TYPE	SYMPTOMS	FINDINGS
Acute LBS	Pain with movement and relieved with rest	Painful gait
	Minimal pain initially and increasing over time	Lumbar lordosis
	Stiffness	Asymmetry
	Radiation to buttocks/thigh	Muscle spasm or tenderness
	Negative genitourinary symptoms	Normoreactive DTR
		Negative SLR and crossed SLR
HNP	Radicular pain below knee	Unable to walk on heels or toes
	Numbness or paresthesia	Unequal DTR
	Sleep disturbance	Decreased unilateral strength, vibratory
	Difficulty getting comfortable	sensation, proprioception
	Pain with defecation	Positive SLR and crossed SLR
	Negative genitourinary symptoms	

DTR, Deep tendon reflexes; *HNP,* herniated nucleus pulposa; *LBS,* lumbosacral strain; *SLR,* straight-leg raise.

TABLE **3-62** Secondary Differential Diagnoses

DIAGNOSIS	DATA SUPPORT
PID	Cervical/vaginal discharge Lower abdominal pain Cervical motion tenderness Laboratory evidence with *Neisseria gonorrhea* or *Chlamydia trachomatis*
Prostate tumor	Prostatic induration on prostate examination Elevation of PSA Asymptomatic
Prostate infection	If acute: fever, irritative voiding symptoms, perineal or suprapubic pain, exquisite tenderness on examination, positive urine culture If chronic: irritative voiding symptoms, perineal or suprapubic discomfort (may be dull and poorly localized), positive EPS/culture
Malingering behavior	Inconsistencies with history and examination, overexaggeration of symptoms, conflicting examination results, positive Waddell sign
Spinal cord disease	Back pain (may precede neurologic signs) Back pain aggravated by lying down, bearing weight, sneezing/coughing Progressive weakness, recent weight change Sensory loss, usually in lower extremities Late findings include bowel/bladder dysfunction Back pain may be local, root, or both
Osteoporosis	Back pain may be asymptomatic or severe Spontaneous fractures Demineralization, especially of spine, hip, pelvis
Vertebral body metastasis	Smoker, older than age 50, weight loss, positive cancer history, back pain unrelieved by supine position
Osteoarthritis	Morning stiffness longer than 30 minutes Pain relieved by rest Minimal articular inflammation Radiographic findings (narrowed joint space, osteophytes, bony cysts, lipping of marginal bone)

EPS, Expressed prostatic secretions; *PID,* pelvic inflammatory disease; *PSA,* prostate specific antigen.

- Exercises may increase the pain, but clients must work through the pain unless it is intolerable.
- Back braces and belts, transcutaneous electrical nerve stimulation units, shoe lifts (unless leg-length discrepancy), biofeedback, and traction have not been shown to be beneficial.
- If client must stand, they should rest one foot on low stool to relieve pressure on back. Every 5 to 15 minutes, they should switch the foot they are resting on the stool.
- Continuation of daily activities is preferred.
- A goal is to return to light work in 4 to 7 days and to normal duty within 1 to 2 weeks.
- Sleeping is facilitated by lying on either side with knees flexed; if client sleeps on his or her back, pillows under the knees and a small pillow under the lower back may increase comfort.
- Men should lift no more than 20 pounds if pain is severe and 60 pounds if mild; women should lift no more than 20 pounds if pain is severe and no more than 35 pounds if pain is mild.
- Client should sit no longer than 20 minutes if back pain is severe and up to no longer than 50 minutes if no back pain without getting up and walking around for 5 to 10 minutes.

Referral

Children
Because strains of the back are uncommon in children and may be related to trauma, malignancies, infections, or inflammation, many children require referral.

Adults
- Refer those in whom herniated nucleus pulposa, fractures, malignancies, aortic aneurysms, cauda equina syndrome, spinal cord disease, or renal colic are suspected. Consider consulting with the physician about any client in whom you suspect infection,

malingering, previous treatment failures, or current treatment failure.

- Chiropractor referral may be appropriate.
- Physical therapist referral may be appropriate.

Prevention

- Discuss ergonomic issues involved in work, home, or leisure activities and ways to remedy any problems identified.
- Teach proper body mechanics.
- Promote overall muscular conditioning.
- Encourage weight loss, if appropriate.

EVALUATION/FOLLOW-UP

- Most episodes of acute lumbosacral strain resolve spontaneously within 4 weeks.
- Consider scheduling a return visit in 2 weeks with instructions to call or return if questions or no improvement.

COMPLICATIONS

A herniated disk may occur.

REFERENCES

Birchfield, P. (2000). Low back pain. In D. Robinson, P. S. Kidd, & K. Rogers (Eds.), *Primary care across the lifespan.* St. Louis: Mosby.

Cherkin, D., Deyo, R., Battie, M., Street, J., & Barlow, W. (1998). A comparison of physical therapy, chiropractor manipulation, and provision of an educational booklet for the treatment of patients with low back pain. *New England Journal of Medicine 339,* 1021-1029.

Deen, H. G. (1996). Concise review for primary care physicians. *Mayo Clinic Proceedings 71,* 283-287.

Gillette, R. D. (1996). Behavioral factors in the management of back pain. *American Family Physician 53,* 1313-1318.

Gillette, R. D. (1996). A practical approach to the patient with back pain. *American Family Physician 53,* 670-676.

Hellmann, D., & Stone, J. (2001). Arthritis and musculoskeletal disorders. In L. M. Tierney, S. J. McPhee, & M. A. Papadakis (Eds.), *Current medical diagnosis and treatment* (40th ed.). New York: McGraw Hill.

McIntosh, E. (1997). Low back pain in adults. Guidelines for the history and physical exam. *ADVANCE for Nurse Practitioners 5*(8), 16-8, 23-5.

Review Questions

1. Which of the following symptoms are more indicative of acute LBS?
   a. Paresthesia, numbness
   b. Pain that increases over time as soft-tissue swelling occurs
   c. Radicular pain
   d. Severe pain at onset

2. A client with a chief complaint of lower back pain who was unable to walk on heels or toes would be suspected of having which of the following?
   a. Nerve root irritation
   b. Acute LBS
   c. Spinal column stenosis
   d. Structural abnormality

3. The SLR and crossed SLR tests are used to help diagnose:
   a. Acute LBS
   b. Soft-tissue injury to the leg
   c. HNP
   d. Prostate infection

4. In which of the following conditions, in a client with a herniated lumbar disk, is emergency surgical treatment required?
   a. Cauda equina syndrome
   b. Sciatica
   c. Diabetic peripheral neuropathy
   d. L_5 radiculopathy

5. Which of the following statements about the use of medications in the treatment of acute LBS is *false?*
   a. Muscle relaxant use should be limited to 2 weeks.
   b. Opiates generally are not indicated.
   c. Muscle relaxants are as effective as NSAIDs.
   d. NSAIDs, with rapid onset of action, are preferred.

6. A complaint of lower back pain often interferes with sleep. The client may experience pain when sleeping on the back. The NP should suggest which of the following?
   a. The client could switch to sleeping on the side that is most comfortable.
   b. The client could sleep propped up with two to three pillows.
   c. Pillows under the head make pain increase.
   d. Pillows under the knees and lower back may help.

7. Most episodes of acute LBS resolve spontaneously in:
   a. 6-8 weeks
   b. 2 weeks
   c. 4 weeks
   d. More than 8 weeks

8. In assessing a client for low back pain, which of the following tests, if positive, indicates legitimate low back pain?
   a. Waddell's signs
   b. Magnuson's test
   c. Patrick's test
   d. Hoover's test

Answers and Rationales

1. Answer: b (assessment)
Rationale: Pain that increases with movement, is relieved with rest, and increases over time as soft-tissue swelling occurs is more indicative of LBS.

2. Answer: a (assessment)
Rationale: Heel walking (L_5) and toe walking (S_1) cannot be accomplished if there is nerve root irritation.

3. Answer: c (analysis/diagnosis)
Rationale: The SLR is considered sensitive for HNP, and the crossed SLR is more specific for HNP. Normally the hip can be flexed to 80 degrees without pain, except in the thigh. A positive test is one that elicits shooting, sharp, or electrical pain that radiates below the knee on the affected side at 30 degrees flexion or less. Crossed SLR involves SLR of the *un*affected leg; a positive test is when the SLR of the unaffected leg causes radicular pain in the affected leg to be reproduced.

4. Answer: a (implementation/plan)
Rationale: Sensory assessment of buttocks and perineum is performed to rule out saddle anesthesia. Cauda equina syndrome is compression of nerves at L_{4-5} level, which needs emergency surgical decompression.

5. Answer: c (implementation/plan)
Rationale: NSAIDs appear to be more effective than muscle relaxants.

6. Answer: d (implementation/plan)
Rationale: Pillows under the knees and lower back reduce the strain of muscles and consequently reduce pain, making sleeping on the back better tolerated.

7. Answer: c (evaluation)
Rationale: With a diagnosis of acute LBS, recovery should occur within 4 weeks; if recovery does not occur, additional assessment, examination, and diagnostic testing should be performed.

8. Answer: d (assessment)
Rationale: Patrick's test involves flexion, abduction, and external rotation of the hip. A positive test indicated by decreased ROM denotes a hip or sacroiliac joint problem. Waddell's signs are a standardized grouping of nonorganic physical signs:
- Tenderness: nonanatomic or superficial pain is present.
- Simulation: simulate movement without actually performing it.
- Axial loading: pressure to top of head should not produce pain.
- Distraction: examine SLR in sitting and supine position and compare results.
- Regionalization: inappropriate location of pain from normal neuroanatomy is present.
- Overreaction: disproportionate verbalization, facial expression, or tremor is present.

Magnuson's test involves marking areas that were tender when palpated; return to the marked areas later in the examination to see if pain can be reproduced. With malingering behavior, those marked areas are not likely to reproduce pain. Hoover's test is conducted by putting the examiner's hands under both heels. (Client can be standing, sitting, or lying.) Ask client to raise affected leg. If the pain is real, the heel on the other leg will push into the examiner's hands.

LYME DISEASE   *Pamela Kidd*

OVERVIEW
Definition

Lyme disease is an infection caused by *Borrelia burgdorferi,* a spirochete; it is the most common arthropod-borne disease in the United States. It is transmitted by prolonged attachment of 2 days or more by an infected tick.

Incidence

- Highest incidence in the northeast, upper midwest, and northern California; however, cases have been reported in all 50 states.
- Prevalence is associated with increased deer population in endemic areas. Most infections occur between the months of May to August in most of the United States, and in January through May in the Pacific Northwest.

Pathophysiology

Lyme disease is a multisystem disorder involving passage of spirochetes from tick into human host.

Protective Factors
- Weed control
- Proper clothing when in high-risk areas
- Insect repellent

Factors Increasing Susceptibility. Exposure to tick-infested areas, particularly during May through August.

ASSESSMENT: SUBJECTIVE/HISTORY
Symptoms

- Symptoms include malaise, fatigue, headache, fever, chills, stiff neck, muscle and joint pain, lymphadenopathy, backache, anorexia, nausea and vomiting, abdominal pain, and rash. Ask about duration of symptoms.
- Ask about possible exposure to tick bites, such as recent camping trips, hiking, or working in yard.
- Ask about occupation, such as farming, logging, or landscaping.

- Ask client to describe duration and characteristics of any skin lesions.
- Ask about recent occurrence of headache, fatigue, fever, or myalgias.
- Less than 50% of clients with Lyme disease recall a preceding tick bite.

Past Medical History

- Any history of arthritis, systemic lupus erythematosus (SLE), recent viral syndrome
- History of Lyme disease and any treatment

Medication History

Inquire about current and recent medication therapy to rule out any recent infections, such as syphilis, or the existence of any chronic problem, such as arthritis or SLE, that the client may not have included in past medical history.

Family History

- Ask if there are any family members with similar symptoms.
- Ask about family history of rheumatoid arthritis.

Diet History

Ask about recent ingestion of inadequately cooked meat or possibly contaminated water to rule out *Tularemia*.

ASSESSMENT: OBJECTIVE/PHYSICAL EXAMINATION

Physical Examination

- Carefully inspect skin for lesions, such as *erythema migrans*, a skin lesion at the sight of tick bite that begins as a red bull's eye with central clearing that enlarges over days to weeks. Lesions more than 5 cm in diameter are most specific for diagnosis of Lyme disease. *Erythema migrans* does not occur in all cases; in some clients, arthritis is the first and only sign.

- Palpate for lymphadenopathy.
- Perform a thorough cardiac examination for secondary carditis, which occurs in 6% to 10% of untreated cases, manifested by atrioventricular conduction abnormalities and left ventricular dysfunction (shifted point of maximal impulse [PMI], presence of S_3 or S_4).
- Inspect joints, particularly knee, shoulder, hip, elbow, and ankle, for swelling, tenderness, or erythema.
- Perform neurologic examination; 10% to 20% of untreated cases result in neurologic complications including meningitis (headache and neck pain), encephalitis (sleep disturbances, poor memory, irritability, dementia), and cranial neuropathies (Bell's palsy, decreased sensation, weakness, loss of reflexes).

Diagnostic Procedures

Diagnostic procedures include detection of IgM and IgG antibodies to *B. Burgdorferi* with an enzyme-linked immunosorbent assay (ELISA) followed by Western blot assay for confirmation.

DIAGNOSIS

For diagnosis of Lyme disease the following must be present (CDC, 2000):
- Endemic area: *erythema migrans* larger than 5 cm in diameter with at least one late manifestation and laboratory confirmation of infection
- Nonendemic area: *erythema migrans* larger than 5 cm in diameter with involvement of two or more organs and laboratory confirmation of infection

Differential Diagnosis

See Table 3-63.

Stages of Lyme Disease

See Table 3-64.

TABLE **3-63** Differential Diagnoses

Syphilis	Chancre
	Nonpruritic rash (maculopapular) to trunk, palms, and soles
	Increased mononuclear cells and protein and decreased glucose in cerebrospinal fluid
	Diagnostic tests: VDRL, RPR, more sensitive, or FTA-ABS test
Rheumatoid arthritis	Joint swelling, particularly PIP and MCP joints, wrists
	Synovial cysts
	Diagnostic tests: CMC, HCT 30% to 34%, HgB may be decreased, normocytic-normochromic, WBC count normal, ESR elevated
Viral syndrome	Abrupt onset, fever (as high as 106° F)
	Malaise, headache, clear nasal discharge, cough
SLE	Photosensitivity, oral ulcers, persistent proteinuria, seizures

CBC, Complete blood count; *ESR,* erythrocyte sedimentation rate; *FTA-ABS,* fluorescent treponemal antibody absorption; *HCT,* hematocrit; *HgB,* hemoglobin; *MCP,* metacarpophalangeal; *PIP,* proximal interphalangeal; *RPR,* rapid plasma reagin; *SLE,* systemic lupus erythematous; *VDRL,* venereal disease research laboratory; *WBC,* white blood cell.

TABLE **3-64** Stages of Lyme Disease

	STAGE 1	STAGE 2	STAGE 3
Skin	Rash (*erythema migrans*)	Cutaneous patches in axillae, groin, trunk	Sclerodermalike lesions
Cardiac	None	AV blocks, left ventricular dysfunction	None
Systemic	Malaise, low-grade fever	High fever, malaise, fatigue	None
Musculoskeletal	Myalgia	Pain in joints, muscles, tendons	Arthritis of knees
Neurologic	Headache, stiff neck	Bell's palsy, aseptic meningitis, encephalitis	Memory loss, difficulty concentrating, sleep disturbance, distal paresthesia
Timing	Days to weeks after bite	Weeks to month after bite	Weeks to months after bite

AV, Atrioventricular.

THERAPEUTIC PLAN
Pharmacologic Treatment

Adults (Including Nonpregnant, Nonlactating Females, and Children Older than 8 Years)
- Doxycycline 100 mg bid × 10 to 21 days OR
- Tetracycline 250 to 500 mg qid × 10 to 21 days OR
- Erythromycin 250 mg qid × 10 to 21 days for clients allergic to penicillin or tetracycline
- For pregnant or lactating women and for children younger than age 8 years, amoxicillin 250-500 mg tid × 10-21 days is the preferred treatment.

Children
- Amoxicillin 25 to 50 mg/kg/day in divided doses, maximum dose 1 to 2 g/day
- Erythromycin 30 mg/kg/day divided into q6h dosing for children younger than age 8 who are allergic to penicillin

NOTE: *Consult physician about treatment of clients with cardiac or neurologic manifestations.*

- Intravenous therapy of penicillin 20 million IU/day OR ceftriaxone 2 g/day for 14 days is recommended. Doxycycline bid or amoxicillin tid for 30 days is effective for clients with arthritis.
- NSAIDS may be used as an analgesic in arthritis.

Client Education
- Inspect entire body following potential exposure.
- Use tweezers to remove attached tick, and place the tick in a jar with a small amount of alcohol. Label jar with date, location on body where removed, and geographic area where tick was acquired.
- Watch for rash and other symptoms for 8 weeks.

- Most ticks removed are not infected with *B burgdorferi;* therefore prophylactic antimicrobial therapy is not recommended.
- No data exist to document resistance to reinfection following treatment.

Referral
- Any clients with cardiac or neurologic manifestations should be referred to physician.
- Follow-up by cardiologist or neurologist may be indicated.

Prevention
- Avoid exposure to ticks by wearing light-colored clothes so ticks are easily detected.
- Wear long pants tucked into socks and a long-sleeved shirt tucked at waist.
- Use insect repellent (e.g., DEET) that is safe for all ages; read precautions on container.
- Avoid tick-infested areas during May through August.
- Keep the area around the house and yard free of brush and tall grass.
- Suggest Lymerix vaccine for use in people 15 to 70 years old who live in high-risk geographic areas and perform high-risk activities (e.g., hunting, logging).

EVALUATION/FOLLOW-UP
Follow-up evaluation at end of treatment (2 to 3 weeks) is adequate for uncomplicated cases. Clients with more severe symptoms, such as cardiac or neurologic manifestations, should be seen more frequently.

COMPLICATIONS
See Table 3-65.

TABLE **3-65**   Complications of Lyme Disease

COMPLICATIONS	FINDINGS
Palpitations with AV conduction Abnormalities Presence of S_3, S_4	Lyme carditis
Headache, nausea, vomiting, fatigue, depressed consciousness, impaired concentration, neck pain	Lyme meningitis (present in 80% of those with neurologic problems associated with Lyme disease) Diagnostic test: cerebrospinal fluid may have mild to moderate mononuclear pleocytosis (<500) with elevated protein and normal glucose concentrations
Sixth nerve palsy, facial (Bell's) palsy	Facial nerve paralysis
Sleep disturbances, poor memory, irritability, dementia	Lyme encephalitis
Diffuse arthralgia; synovial fluid with WBC counts >25,000 cells/mm³; arthritis manifested in knees, shoulder, hip, ankle, and elbow	Lyme arthritis

AV, Atrioventricular; *WBC,* white blood cell.

REFERENCES

Angelov, L. (1996). Unusual features in the epidemiology of Lyme borreliosis. *European Journal of Epidemiology 12*(l), 9-11.

Bartlett, C. R., & Brown, J. W. (1996). New and emerging pathogens, part 2: Tick, tick, tick, tick. . . boom! The explosion of tick-borne diseases. *MLO: Medical Laboratory Observer 28*(3), 44-52.

Centers for Disease Control and Prevention. (2000). Surveillance for Lyme Disease. United States, 1992-1998. *MMWR: Morbidity and Mortality Weekly Report* (Publication No. 49 SS03, pp 1-11). Atlanta: CDC.

Deltombe, T., Hanson, P., Boutsen, Y., Laloux, P., & Clerin, M. (1996). Lyme borreliosis neuropathy: A case report, *American Journal of Physical Medicine and Rehabilitation 75*(4), 314-316.

Dennis, D., Fikrig, E., & Schaffner, W. (1998). Now you can prevent Lyme disease. *Patient Care for the Nurse Practitioner 2*(6), 20-26, 29-32, 35-36.

Sornson, B. (2000). Lyme disease. In D. Robinson, P. Kidd, & K. Rogers (Eds.). *Primary care across the lifespan.* St. Louis: Mosby.

Herman, L., Robinson, T. T., & Birrer, R. B. (1996). Lyme disease: Ready cure, but a challenging diagnosis. *Journal of the American Academy of Physician Assistants 9*(10), 39-40, 43-44, 47-48.

Meyers, J. (1998). Lyme disease: A challenge and an opportunity for nurse practitioners. *Journal of the American Academy of Nurse Practitioners 10,* 315-319.

Verdon, M. E., & Sigal, L. H. (1997). Recognition and management of Lyme disease. *American Family Physician 56*(2), 427-436, 439-440.

Wright, D. (2001). Lyme disease. *Journal of the American Academy of Nurse Practitioners 13,* 223-226.

Ziska, M. H., Donta, S. T., & Demarest, F. C. (1996). Physician preferences in the diagnosis and treatment of Lyme disease in the United States. *Infection 24*(2), 182-186.

Review Questions

1. Which of the following sets of symptoms is most indicative of Lyme disease?
   a. Fatigue and headache
   b. Fever and stiff neck
   c. Joint stiffness and erythematous skin lesions
   d. Lymphadenopathy and malaise

2. Which of the following diseases results in false-positive results of the ELISA test for Lyme disease?
   a. Meningitis
   b. Tularemia
   c. SLE
   d. Rocky Mountain spotted fever

3. Which sign or symptom is most specific for the diagnosis of Lyme disease?
   a. Erythematous macular lesion with central clearing
   b. Positive indirect fluorescent antibody test result
   c. Persistent fatigue
   d. Adenopathy and pharyngitis

4. The treatment of choice for an 11-year-old boy with a presenting symptom of a 5-cm *erythema migrans* lesion and a positive ELISA test result is which of the following?
   a. Doxycycline, 100 mg bid for 14 days
   b. Erythromycin, 250 mg qid for 14 days
   c. Amoxicillin, 500 mg tid for 14 days
   d. Trimethoprim-sulfamethoxazole (Bactrim), 1 tablet bid for 14 days

5. A client with Lyme disease has been prescribed doxycycline, 100 mg bid for 10 days. The client should be instructed to return for follow-up:
   a. After 3 days of antibiotic therapy
   b. At the end of treatment

c. 1 month after completion to ensure that symptoms have resolved
d. Follow-up is not necessary.

6. Which of the following clients should receive Lymerix vaccine?
   a. Pregnant woman in her third trimester
   b. A renal transplant recipient
   c. A logger in Oregon
   d. A 65-year-old client with chronic obstructive pulmonary disease

Answers and Rationales

1. Answer: c (assessment)
   Rationale: Erythema migrans is the most specific symptom for Lyme disease; however, it does not occur in all cases. Many clients have arthritic symptoms as the first and only sign.

2. Answer: c (assessment)
   Rationale: SLE, viral infections, and rheumatoid arthritis also may result in a positive ELISA result.

3. Answer: a (assessment)
   Rationale: Fatigue, adenopathy, and pharyngitis are nonspecific symptoms of numerous disease processes; *erythema migrans* is most specific for Lyme disease.

4. Answer: a (implementation/plan)
   Rationale: Doxycycline is the drug of choice for all adults who are not pregnant or lactating and for children older than age 8 years.

5. Answer: b (evaluation)
   Rationale: For first-time cases or those without severe secondary symptoms, follow-up is recommended at the end of treatment.

6. Answer: c (implementation/plan)
   Rationale: Lymerix vaccine should be used in people 15 to 70 years old who live in high-risk geographic areas and engage in high-risk activities. Immunosuppression and pregnancy does not increase susceptibility. There are no pulmonary complications from Lyme disease.

LYMPHOMA *Denise Robinson*

OVERVIEW
Definition

Lymphoma is a malignant disease of the lymphoid tissue, considered to be either Hodgkin's or non-Hodgkin's lymphoma. Usually it is a painless, unilateral, enlarging, firm, neck mass (70% of cases are located in the neck), often in the upper third of the neck. Non-Hodgkin's lymphoma is a malignant disease of the lymphoid tissue with no Reed-Sternberg cells present.

Incidence

- Hodgkin's lymphoma incidence is 3.5 cases per 100,000 population.
- Approximately 7500 cases a year occur in the United States; it occurs more often in males than in females.
- Non-Hodgkin's lymphoma has an incidence of 9 cases per 100,000 population, with peak incidence at 7 to 11 years of age.

Children
- Birth to 6 years: Lymphoma is one of the top four malignancies.
- Younger than 12 years: Hodgkin's lymphoma is one of the top two malignancies.
- Older than 12 years: Hodgkin's lymphoma is the most frequent malignancy of the head and neck.

Pathophysiology

Malignant transformation of an uncertain progenitor cell leads to the Reed-Sternberg cell or other malignant cell. Disease spreads to lymphoid tissue and eventually to non-lymphoid tissue (Table 3-66).

Factors Increasing Susceptibility
- Autoimmune disease
- Immunodeficiency
- Onset before 1 month of age

TABLE **3-66** Staging of Hodgkin's Disease

STAGE	CHARACTERISTICS	SURVIVAL
Stage I	Single node group	90% at 5 years
Stage II	Two or more groups on same side of diaphragm	90% at 5 years
Stage III	Node groups on both sides of diaphragm	75% at 10 years
Stage IV	Dissemination involving nonlymphatic organs	66% at 10 years
Subclassification	A, Asymptomatic	Better prognosis
	B, Symptomatic	

ASSESSMENT: SUBJECTIVE/HISTORY
Symptoms

- Painless, enlarged lymph nodes
- Fever
- Night sweats
- Weight loss
- Fatigue
- Anorexia

Past Medical History

- Ask about recent infections that may have caused enlarged lymph nodes and about exposure to someone who is ill.
- Ask about exposure to unusual or uncommon animals, ingestion of unpasteurized milk, or travel to exotic lands.
- Ask about congenital/acquired dysfunction of the immune system.
- Ask about history of blood product use.
- Determine if the client has risk factors for HIV.

Medication History

Ask about chronic treatment with phenytoin (increased risk of lymphoma).

Family History

Ask about family history of lymphoma or other malignancies.

ASSESSMENT: OBJECTIVE/PHYSICAL EXAMINATION
Physical Examination

- A problem-oriented physical examination should be conducted with particular attention to vital signs, weight, general appearance, and growth parameters in children.
- Lymph: check neck, axilla, and groin for enlarged nodes. Evaluate for size, shape, consistency, location, fixation, and duration and rate of change.
- Abdomen: check for liver and spleen enlargement.

Diagnostic Procedures
Laboratory Tests
- CBC with differential
- Chemistry
- Sedimentation rate

Special Tests
- Liver and renal function tests
- Chest x-ray film
- CT or MRI scan
- Lymph node biopsy: excisional; Reed-Sternberg cell is diagnostic for Hodgkin's lymphoma.
- Lymphangiogram
- Exploratory laparotomy, with splenectomy in some clients
- Bone marrow biopsy

DIAGNOSIS

- Differential diagnosis includes the following:
  - Other lymphomas
  - Mononucleosis
  - Sarcoidosis
  - Acquired immunodeficiency syndrome (AIDS)
  - Autoimmune disease
- Lymphadenopathy is a condition involving a painless lymph node that is larger than 10 mm in size (except epitrochlear [larger than 5 mm] and inguinal [larger than 15 mm]).
- Adenitis is inflammation of a lymph node, usually caused by staphylococci or streptococci.
- Cat-scratch fever also causes enlarged lymph nodes.
- Enlarged lymph nodes are common with viral infections in children. Some systemic illnesses, such as mononucleosis, AIDS, and Kawasaki syndrome, can cause generalized lymphadenopathy.

THERAPEUTIC PLAN
Nonpharmacologic Treatment

Subtotal or total nodal irradiation may be used.

Pharmacologic Treatment

The chemotherapeutic regimen is called MOPP (**m**echlorethamine [nitrogen mustard], vincristine [**On**covin], **P**rocarbazine, **p**rednisone).

Client Education

- Discuss the effect of therapy on gonads and consideration of sperm banking.
- Inform clients of the risk of secondary malignancies.

Referral

All clients should be referred to a surgeon for excisional biopsy and then to an oncologist if the disease is malignant.

REFERENCES

Barker, L., Burton, J., & Zieve, P. (1999). *Principles of ambulatory medicine* (5th ed.). Baltimore: Williams & Wilkins.

Ferrer, R. (1998). Lymphadenopathy. *American Family Physician 59,* 1313-1320.

Hardell, L., & Eriksson, M. (1999). A case-control study of non-Hodgkin lymphoma and exposure to pesticides. *Cancer 85,* 1353-1360.

Robinson, D., Kidd, P., & Rogers, K. (2000). *Primary care cross the lifespan.* St. Louis: Mosby.

Young, G., Toretsky, J., & Campbell, A. (2000). Common childhood malignancies. *American Family Physician 61,* 2144-2154.

Review Questions

1. All the following may cause generalized lymphadenopathy except:

a. AIDS
b. Mononucleosis
c. Cat-scratch fever
d. Streptococcal infection

2. The most frequent site of a palpable lesion in lymphoma is which of the following?

a. Neck
b. Groin
c. Extremity
d. Abdomen

3. A client comes in with fever, weight loss, and fatigue. Differential diagnosis would include all except which of the following?

a. Chronic fatigue syndrome
b. Lymphoma
c. AIDS
d. Tuberculosis

4. A risk factor for lymphoma elicited in the past medical history is which of the following?

a. Lupus
b. Mononucleosis
c. Splenectomy
d. Lyme disease

5. When an enlarged, painless, firm node is discovered in the client's neck, the NP should do which of the following?

a. Order a soft-tissue film of the neck.
b. Perform an incision and drainage of the lesion, and culture the drainage.
c. Refer the client to a surgeon for biopsy.
d. Order a chest x-ray examination.

6. Which of the following characteristics should make the NP suspicious of malignancies in an enlarged lymph node?

a. Painless enlarged node of neck larger than 12mm
b. Painful node larger than 10 mm
c. Enlarged groin node 10 mm in size
d. Painful occipital node

7. A lymph node excision has been sent for biopsy. Which of the following is associated with Reed-Sternberg cells?

a. Non-Hodgkin's lymphoma
b. Hodgkin's lymphoma
c. Cat-scratch fever
d. Lymphadenopathy

Answers and Rationales

1. *Answer:* d (analysis/diagnosis)
Rationale: Streptococcal infection usually causes inflammation of a particular lymph node or nodes in a specific area related to a local infection. The other diagnoses are associated with generalized lymphadenopathy (Barker, Burton, & Zieve, 1999).

2. *Answer:* a (assessment)
Rationale: Approximately 70% of lymphomas are first seen as a painless, unilateral, enlarging, firm neck mass (Barker, Burton, & Zieve, 1999).

3. *Answer:* a (analysis/diagnosis)
Rationale: Chronic fatigue syndrome does not have fever or weight loss associated with it. The other choices have all three symptoms (Barker, Burton, & Zieve, 1999).

4. *Answer:* a (assessment)
Rationale: Autoimmune diseases increase the risk of lymphoma. Lupus is the only autoimmune disease listed (Robinson, Kidd, & Rogers, 2000).

5. *Answer:* c (implementation/plan)
Rationale: A soft-tissue film of the neck might give better parameters for the size of the lesion, but it will not help diagnose the source of the lesion. A firm lesion does not have drainage and should not be excised until it has been sampled for biopsy. Neither biopsy nor excision is within the normal NP scope of practice. A chest radiograph is helpful in staging the disease or before surgery (Barker, Burton, & Zieve, 1999).

6. *Answer:* a (assessment)
Rationale: Lymphoma is a painless enlargement of a lymph node, usually in the neck (Robinson, Kidd, & Rogers, 2000).

7. *Answer:* b (analysis/diagnosis)
Rationale: Reed-Sternberg cells are associated with Hodgkin's lymphoma (Robinson, Kidd, & Rogers, 2000).

MENIERE'S DISEASE   *Pamela Kidd*

OVERVIEW
Definition

Meniere's disease (MD) is an idiopathic disease characterized by hearing loss, tinnitus, and episodic vertigo. The hearing loss is fluctuating, usually low frequency, sensorineural, and associated with tinnitus. The vertigo is a spontaneously occurring sensation of movement that is accompanied by unsteadiness, lasts from minutes to hours, and is frequently accompanied by nausea and vomiting (Slattery & Fayad, 1997).

Incidence

MD primarily affects whites, with a prevalence of approximately 1 per 1000 of population. The disease occurs in children, but the peak onset is between 20 and 50 years of age. Approximately 85% of people have only one ear affected.

Pathophysiology

The principal underlying pathology is endolymphatic hydrops. There are several theories regarding the development of MD; it is probably a multifactorial process. Several of the factors are listed as follows:

- Structural abnormalities of the temporal bone exist.
- Immunologic: Immune complex deposition has been found in the endolymphatic sac.
- Viral: There is a possible role of neurotropic viruses.
- Vascular: Association between migraines and MD suggests a vascular pathogenesis.
- Metabolic: Exposure of the hair cells with chronic loss of hair cell motility is present.

Factors Increasing Susceptibility
- Upper respiratory infection (URI)

Protective Factors. None.

ASSESSMENT: SUBJECTIVE/HISTORY
Symptoms

- The early symptom is vertigo. This is usually described as a sensation of motion when there is no motion, or an exaggerated sense of motion in response to a bodily movement associated with nausea and vomiting. The episode is often preceded by an aura of fullness or pressure in the ear lasting from 20 minutes to several hours. Between attacks, the hearing is normal.
- Hearing loss fluctuates and is finally lost, affecting lower pitches first.
- Patients may present with complaints of difficulty hearing, or family members may identify an inability of the patient to hear.
- Patient may present with the following complaints:
  - Nausea or vomiting
  - Tinnitus
  - Loss of ability to "pop" ears
  - Sense of fullness in ears
  - Pulling at ears
  - Loss of equilibrium
  - Foreign body in the ear
- Ask about involvement of one ear or both.
- Determine whether the onset was gradual or sudden.
- Determine whether the hearing has fluctuated since the hearing loss began.
- Determine whether there are associated symptoms of tinnitus, vertigo, otalgia, otorrhea, or facial weakness.

Past Medical History

Ask about the following:
- Hypertension (HTN)
- Mumps
- Neurologic problems
- Head trauma
- Diabetes
- Hypothyroidism
- Syphilis
- Migraine

Medication History

Ask about use of the following:
- Acetylsalicylic acid (ASA, high-dose aspirin)
- Antibiotics: aminoglycosides (gentamicin, streptomycin)
- Diuretics (loop-furosemide)
- Quinine

Family History

- Ask about a family history of hearing loss.
- Ask about a familial disposition to Meniere's disease.

Dietary History

Noncontributory.

ASSESSMENT: OBJECTIVE/PHYSICAL EXAMINATION
Physical Examination

- The examination should concentrate on the head and neck.
- Evaluate head, eyes, ears, nose, and throat (HEENT) for an URI.
- Evaluate ears–tympanic membrane (TM), external canal.
- Complete pneumatic otoscopy: Check for TM movement.
- Perform a tympanogram.
- Perform neurologic examination, checking for sensation of face; note if facial movement is symmetrical, rapid alternating movements
- Do a Romberg test.
- Evaluate gait.
- Check for nystagmus. Perform Nylen-Barany maneuver (limited use when the patient is able to visually fixate).
- A Fukuda test (patient walks in place with eyes closed) can detect subtle defects. A positive response is when the patient rotates toward the diseased labyrinth.
- Assess hearing. Have patient repeat aloud words presented in a soft whisper, normal speaking voice, or a shout. Occlude one ear, then repeat on the other side.

Children
- Child 0 to 3 months responds to noise.
- Child 3 to 5 months turns to sound.
- Child 6 to 10 months responds to name.
- Child 10 to 15 months imitates simple words.
- Perform a Weber test. Place the tuning fork on the forehead or front teeth. Have the patient indicate where it is heard the best.
- Perform a Rinne test. The tuning fork is placed alternately on the mastoid bone and in front of the ear canal.

Diagnostic Procedures

See Table 3-67 for diagnostic procedures.

DIAGNOSIS

See Table 3-68 for differential diagnoses.

TABLE **3-67** Diagnostic Tests

DIAGNOSTIC TEST	FINDINGS/RATIONALE
RPR	Should be done to rule out syphilis, a known cause of MD.
Audiometric studies	Hearing test conducted in soundproof room. Pure-tone thresholds in dB are obtained over the ranges of 250 to 8000 Hz for both air and bone conduction. All patients with hearing loss should be referred for audiometric testing unless the cause is easily remediable (impacted cerumen). Patients can be referred directly to an audiologist. The location of an accredited audiologist can be obtained by calling the American Speech-Language Association at 1-800-638-8255.
Speech discrimination testing	Evaluates the clarity of hearing. Results are reported as percentage correct.
Tympanogram	Used to detect fluid in the middle ear and to determine the mobility of the TM. An electroacoustic device is used to measure the compliance of the TM. Results are displayed in a graphic form. It is most reliable in children older than 6 months.
Audiogram	Small handheld audioscopes can provide a rough indication of hearing impairment. Usually four pure tones are emitted in sequence. This test can be affected by background noise, so the examination room must be quiet.
Glycerol dehydration test	Measures the audiometric response to an oral dose of glycerol. Improvement in scores for hearing low frequency and discriminating speech is diagnostic because there is no other condition in which this change is observed.
Caloric testing	Reveals loss or impairment of nystagmus induced with cold substance in involved ear.
Electrocochleography	Presents with a highly characteristic waveform of MD, although the results may give negative results in the early and late stages of the disease.
Electronystagmography	Objective recording of the nystagmus induced by head and body movements. It helps to quantify the degree of vestibular dysfunction.

dB, Decibels; *Hz,* hertz; *MD,* Meniere's disease; *RPR,* rapid plasma reagin; *TM,* tympanic membrane.

M

TABLE **3-68** Differential Diagnosis of Meniere's Disease

DIAGNOSIS	DATA SUPPORT
Conductive loss	Rinne shows air conduction worse than bone conduction, Weber test lateralizes to the involved ear. The whisper is abnormal if more than 40 dB loss is present.
Cerumen impaction	An occlusion of the external ear canal by cerumen; usually self-induced via attempts at cleaning.
Serous otitis media	Dull TM, hypomobile TM; air bubbles may be seen in the middle ear, with a conductive hearing loss present.
Acoustic neuroma	Hearing loss, vertigo, nausea and vomiting, and deterioration of speech discrimination may be present.
Otosclerosis	Progressive disease with a familial tendency that affects bone surrounding the inner ear.
TM perforation	Perforation of the TM may result in decreased hearing abilities. The perforation may occur from trauma or as the result of increased pressure with otitis media. Spontaneous healing occurs in most cases.
Sensori-neural loss	Rinne test: both AC and BC are decreased; Weber localizes to the uninvolved ear; the whisper test will be abnormal if more than 40 dB loss is present.
Presbycusis	Progressive, mainly high-frequency hearing loss of aging. Frequently with genetic predisposition. Patients complain of an inability to hear well (speech discrimination) in a noisy environment.
Noise trauma	Second most common cause of hearing loss. Sounds louder than 85 dB are potentially damaging to the cochlea, especially with prolonged exposure. The loss typically occurs in the high frequencies (4000 Hz) and progresses to involve sounds in the normal speech frequencies. Sounds that have the potential for damage include industrial machinery, loud music, and weapons.
Ototoxicity	Hearing loss can be caused by substances that affect both the auditory and vestibular systems. Common causes are salicylates, aminoglycosides, loop diuretics, and antineoplastic agents, especially cisplatin.

AC, Air conduction; *BC,* bone conduction; *dB,* decibel; *TM,* tympanic membrane.

THERAPEUTIC PLAN

- Treatment is currently empirical. No treatment has modified the clinical course and prevented the progressive hearing loss.
- The vertigo eventually disappears in approximately 70% of patients. Nonsurgical treatment is considered effective in approximately 80% of patients.

Nonpharmacologic Treatment

- Eat low-salt diet (less than 2 g per day) to lower endolymphatic pressure.
- Restriction of caffeine, nicotine, and alcohol is suggested.
- Bedrest may reduce the severity of vertigo in an acute attack.
- In chronic vertigo, exercise is one of the most important therapies. It enhances the ability of the central nervous system (CNS) to compensate for labyrinth dysfunction. The patient should begin body conditioning exercises after the nausea and vomiting has resolved. Exercise should be performed until vertigo occurs.

- Specific exercises to promote adaptation of the vestibular system may be prescribed by the otolaryngologist.
- Surgical options include procedures that are not destructive to hearing: endolymphatic sac surgery (effective in approximately 80% to control vertigo), vestibular nerve section (effective in 90% to 95% to control vertigo; however, the surgery is major in that the posterior cranial fossa is opened), sacculotomy, cryosurgical treatment, and insertion of tympanostomy tubes. Other surgeries destroy any remaining hearing: labyrinthectomy, cochleosacculotomy, and vestibulocochlear neurectomy. Cochlear implantation is an option; end-stage Meniere's disease is a recognized indication for implantation.

Pharmacologic Treatment

Acute Attack. The aim is to sedate the vestibulobrain stem, use for 2 weeks only, and gradually wean. See Table 3-69 for pharmacologic treatment information.

TABLE **3-69** Pharmacologic Treatment of Meniere's Disease

DRUG	DOSE	COMMENTS
Prochlorperazine (Compazine)	5 to 10 mg 3 to 4 times per day or 15 to 30 mg spansule qam or 10 mg spansule q12h (sustained release)	Considered antidopaminergic agent Side effects: drowsiness, lowered seizure threshold, amenorrhea, photosensitivity, extrapyramidal reactions
Promethazine (Phenergan)	25 mg PO q6h Children: 12.5 to 25 mg Supp: 12.5, 25, 50 mg	Antihistamine, anticholinergic Side effects: sedation, sleepiness, dry mouth, lowered seizure threshold

Diazepam (Valium)	2 to 5 mg PO tid/qid	Vestibular suppressant
		  Drug of choice for acute vertigo
		  Many people with vertigo, particularly elderly, respond well to decreased dose and frequency
		Side effects: dizziness, drowsiness, dry mouth, orthostatic hypotension

Glycopyrrolate (Robinul)	1 to 2 mg PO qd/bid	Anticholinergic when combined with diazepam is very helpful in controlling inner ear symptoms of nausea and vomiting Side effects: dry mouth, distorted visual acuity, or increase symptoms of BPH. Contraindications: glaucoma, symptomatic BPH
Dimenhydrinate (Dramamine)	50 to 100 mg tid/qid	Recommended for refractory cases Side effects: drowsiness, blurring of vision, dry mouth, constipation
Meclizine (Antivert)	25 mg PO tid/qid	Used for vertigo; slower onset and longer duration of action than most other antihistamines Recommended for refractory cases Side effects: drowsiness, fatigue, dry mouth, blurred vision
Hydrochlorothiazide (HCTZ)	50 to 100 mg daily	To reduce endolymphatic pressure

BPH, Benign prostatic hypertrophy; *Supp,* suppository.

Maintenance. The aim is to attempt to modify the endolymphatic hydrops itself by lowering endolymphatic pressure. Long-term maintenance therapy is usually not recommended because of the fluctuant nature of the disease. Maintenance therapy usually includes diet modifications combined with pharmacologic interventions. See Table 3-70 for pharmacologic maintenance information. Medical options include intratympanic aminoglycosides to control vertigo.

Ablative Therapy. Use of aminoglycosides to control vertigo via vestibulotoxic effects. Partial ablation of the labyrinth is recommended to control the severity of ataxia and perhaps stabilize hearing. Administration of low doses of intramuscular streptomycin is the treatment of choice (1 g 5 days/week until ablation occurs). Ablation is demonstrated via absence of ice water caloric test. Ablation should be done by an ear, nose, and throat (ENT) specialist.

Client Education

- Completely explain the disorder, indicating the expected course of the disease and medications.
- Discuss the need to live with unpredictable illness.

Referral

A variety of options for medical and surgical treatment are available if the patient is referred to an otolaryngologist.

Prevention

Exercise (see Nonpharmacologic Treatment section).

EVALUATION/FOLLOW-UP

- Usually done by otolaryngologist.
- Improvement in vertigo with preserved hearing ability is the goal.

COMPLICATIONS

- Falls
- Dehydration from vomiting
- Hearing loss

REFERENCES

Arts, H., Kileny, P., & Telian, S. (1997). Diagnostic testing for endolymphatic hydrops. *Otolaryngology Clinics of North America 30*(6), 987-1005.

Clendaniel, R., & Tucci, D. (1997). Vestibular rehabilitation strategies in Meniere's disease. *Otolaryngology Clinics of North America 30*(6), 1145-1158.

Derebery, M. (1997). The role of allergy in Meniere's disease. *Otolaryngology Clinics of North America 30*(6), 1007-1016.

Gibson, W., & Arenberg, I. (1997). Pathophysiologic theories in the etiology of Meniere's disease. *Otolaryngology Clinics of North America, 30*(6), 961-967.

Grant, I., & Welling, D. The treatment of hearing loss in Meniere's disease. *Otolaryngology Clinics of North America 30*(6), 1123-1144.

Jackler, R., & Kaplan, M. (2001). Ear, nose, and throat. In L. Tierney, S. McPhee, & M. Papadakis (Eds.), *Current medical diagnosis and treatment* (40th ed.). New York: McGraw-Hill.

Quaranta, A., Marini, F., & Sallustio, V. (1998). Long-term outcome of Meniere's disease: Endolymphatic mastoid shunt versus natural history. *Audiology and Neurootolaryngology 3*(1), 54-60.

TABLE **3-70** Pharmacologic Maintenance of Meniere's Disease

DRUG	DOSE	COMMENTS
Furosemide (Lasix)	20 to 80 mg qd	K supplementation needed Side effects: GI upset, electrolyte imbalance, rash, photosensitivity
Amiloride (Midamor)	5 mg qd	K sparing diuretic Side effects: H/A, GI upset, hyperkalemia, muscle cramps, dizziness, impotence
HCTZ*	12.5 to 50 mg qd	K supplementation usually needed Side effects: electrolyte disorders, orthostatic hypotension, GI disturbances
HCTZ and triamterene (Dyazide)*	One tablet qd	Provides diuretic action with need for K supplementation
Betahistine (Serc)	8 mg tid	Clinical studies have revealed this histamine analogue helpful in improving hearing loss, vertigo, and tinnitus in the short term (not available in United States) Betahistine with or without diuretic is the recommended maintenance; be aware of future developments regarding this drug
Nimodipine (Nimotop)	30 mg bid	Used for patients who have failed diuretic therapy (use in refractory cases) Side effects: GI upset
Eriodictyol glycoside (lemon bioflavonoid extract)	2 mg capsule tid for a trial period of 6 months	May act as a blocking agent for histidine decarboxylase

*Preferred initial maintenance therapy.
K, Potassium, *GI,* gastrointestinal; *H/A,* headache, *HCTZ,* hydrochlorothiazide.

Rodgers, G., & Telischi, F. (1997). Meniere's disease in children. *Otolaryngology Clinics of North America 30*(6), 1101-1104.

Saeed, S. (1998). Fortnightly review: Diagnosis and treatment of Meniere's disease. *British Medical Journal 316*(7128), 368-372.

Silverstein, H., Isaacson, J. E., Olds, M. J., Rowan, P. T., Rosenberg, S. (1998). Dexamethasone inner ear perfusion for the treatment of Meniere's disease: A prospective, randomized, double-blind, crossover trial. *American Journal of Otolaryngology, 19*(2), 196-201.

Slattery, W., & Fayad, J. (1997). Medical treatment of Meniere's disease. *Otolaryngology Clinics of North America 30*(6), 1027-1037.

Review Questions

1. When assessing a client with vertigo, the nurse practitioner (NP) should perform which test?

  a. Romberg
  b. Brudzinski
  c. Phalen's
  d. Patrick's

2. Which diet should a client with Meniere's disease follow?

  a. Low fat
  b. Low salt
  c. Low carbohydrate
  d. Low protein

3. The goal of acute therapy in Meniere's disease is which of the following?

  a. Sedating the vestibulobrain stem
  b. Lowering endolymphatic pressure
  c. Restoring hearing
  d. Relieving pain

4. Untreated Meniere's disease may result in which of the following?

  a. Hearing loss
  b. Tinnitus
  c. Inability to hear high pitches
  d. Roaring in the ears

5. What is the best way to describe vertigo?

  a. Sensation of motion when there is no motion
  b. Unsteadiness
  c. Spontaneous movement
  d. Dizziness

Answers and Rationales

1. *Answer:* a (assessment)
  Rationale: Romberg test assesses cerebellar functioning by maintaining balance with the eyes closed. Patrick's test is used to diagnose degenerative hip joint disease. Phalen's maneuver is used to diagnose carpal tunnel syndrome. Brudzinski's sign is used to assess meningeal irritation. Refer to Chapter 2 for more information.

2. *Answer:* b (implementation/plan)
  Rationale: A low-salt diet is used to reduce endolymphatic pressure.

3. *Answer:* a (implementation/plan)
  Rationale: Lowering endolymphatic pressure is the goal of maintenance therapy. Pain is not a symptom in Meniere's disease. Hearing restoration occurs as vertigo subsides and the vestibulobrain stem is sedated.

4. *Answer:* a (analysis/diagnosis)
  Rationale: Tinnitus is an early symptom of Meniere's. Low-pitched sounds are not heard, but eventually complete hearing loss occurs if left untreated.

5. *Answer:* a (analysis/diagnosis)
  Rationale: Vertigo may be associated with unsteadiness and may produce dizziness. It is not actual movement, but rather a sensation of movement.

MENINGITIS *Denise Robinson*

OVERVIEW
Definition

Meningitis is an inflammation of the meninges of the brain caused by an infectious agent, either viral or bacterial. *Neisseria meningitidis* remains a major health problem in much of the developing world.

Incidence

- In infants, 20 to 100 per 100,000 live births contract bacterial meningitis during the newborn period.
- Meningitis occurs most often in the very young or elderly and debilitated patients.
- Men account for 55% of cases.
- Twenty-nine percent of cases occur in children younger than 1 year of age.
- Forty-six percent of cases occur in children younger than 2 years of age.
- Twenty-five percent of cases occur in people older than 30 years of age.
- Highest attack rates are during the winter and early spring.

Pathophysiology

Organisms that have entered the meningeal space multiply and spread throughout the cerebrospinal fluid (CSF). Infection may also affect nearby cranial nerves or contribute to parenchyma abscesses. A fibrous exudate, which may accompany the inflammatory response, may impede cerebrospinal fluid flow; accumulation can block the narrow Sylvian duct, leading to hydrocephalus. Inflammatory swelling may exert pressure on the hypopituitary gland, stimulating excess secretion of antidiuretic hormone and secondary cerebral edema.

The most common organism causing meningitis before the 1990s was *Haemophilus influenza*. Now *Streptococcus pneumoniae* and *Neisseria meningitidis* are the leading causes of bacterial meningitis (see Table 3-71).

Factors Increasing Susceptibility
- Sickle cell anemia, diabetes, alcoholism
- basilar skull fracture
- Indwelling CSF shunting device
- Debilitated or institutionalized
- Contact with others who have had meningitis

ASSESSMENT: SUBJECTIVE/HISTORY
History of Present Illness

Bacterial and aseptic meningitis present similarly: there is no reliable symptom that readily distinguishes one from the other.

Neonates. Onset is usually acute: hypothermia, hypotonia, weak or absent cry, fretfulness, weak sucking response, vomiting, diarrhea, respiratory distress, and seizures.

Young Infants. Onset is generally acute with nonspecific symptoms of temperature instability or hypothermia, irritability, lethargy, poor feeding, unusual cry, jitters, or hypotonia. Because neonates usually do not have meningismus, a change in affect or state of alertness is one of the most important signs (Tunkel & Scheld, 1997).

Older Infants, Children, Adults. Onset is usually acute, although sometimes it is subacute. A prodromal febrile illness rapidly progresses to vague complaints of irritability, listlessness, or general malaise; older children and adults may complain of photophobia, myalgia, headaches, and stiff neck and vomiting. Seizures may also occur.

Elderly. The presentation may be insidious, with lethargy or obtundation, no fever, and variable signs of meningeal irritation.

Associated Symptoms

A diffuse macular, maculopapular, or purpuric rash may occur, depending on the type of infection. Abdominal pain and diarrhea may also be present if the offending agent is enterovirus.

Past Medical History

Inquire about the following:
- Recent infections (especially ear and respiratory or partially treated meningitis)
- Facial or cranial injuries or surgery
- Immunization status

ASSESSMENT: OBJECTIVE/PHYSICAL EXAMINATION
Physical Examination

Physical examination should focus on the following:
- *Vital signs:* Temperature, heart rate, blood pressure may help to identify septicemic shock.
- *General appearance:* Pay particular attention to mental status.
- *Skin:* Inspect/palpate for presence of rash, petechiae, purpura (fever with purpura is associated with meningococcal infections, even though the patient may not appear acutely ill at the time).
- *Head:* Inspect/palpate for bulging or enlarged fontanels in infants; a marked increase in head circumference may also be present.
- *Eyes:* Inspect for papilledema (this is a late sign).
- *ENT:* Inspect for sources of inflammation/infection; palpate for lymphadenopathy (oropharyngeal vesicles suggest enterovirus).
- *Cardiovascular system:* Assess capillary refill and peripheral pulses and turgor.
- *Neurologic:* Assess cranial nerves, muscle strength/tone, motor coordination and sensory status,

TABLE **3-71**   Bacterial Meningitis Incidence and Pathogens

	NEONATES	OLDER INFANTS/CHILDREN	ADULTS	POSTSURGICAL/POSTTRAUMATIC
Incidence	100 per 100,000 live births	90% before age 6 After 1 mo, 50 per 100,000 6 to 8 mo, 80 per 100,000	Extremely rare	
Pathogen	Group B *Streptococcus, S. pneumoniae,* gram-negative enteric	*Haemophilus influenzae B,* Neisseria meningitidis, S. pneumoniae*	*Listeria monocytogenes S. pneumoniae N. meningitidis*	*S. aureus,* Gram-negative bacilli

*The introduction of the *H. influenzae B* vaccine has dramatically reduced the influence of *H. influenzae* meningitis.

reflexes, and meningeal irritation (Kernig and Brudzinski's signs).

- Kernig: When the patient is supine with hip and knee flexed toward abdomen, extension of knee elicits pain.
- Brudzinski's sign: When the patient is supine, passive flexion of the neck elicits flexion of the knees and hip.
- Other: Symptoms of tachycardia, delayed capillary refill, hypotension, and oliguria may accompany septicemia.

Diagnostic Procedures

- Complete blood count (CBC) with differential
- Lumbar puncture with CSF analysis (see Table 3-72)
- Latex agglutination to detect the antigens of the common meningeal pathogens
- Chest X-ray examination
- Blood cultures
- CSF cultures

DIAGNOSIS
Differential Diagnosis

- Bacterial meningitis
- Aseptic (viral meningitis)
- Reye syndrome
- CNS occupying lesion: mass/infection

THERAPEUTIC PLAN

- Immediate medical consultation/referral, hospitalization, and prompt initiation of a broad-spectrum antibiotic are warranted if meningitis is suspected (within 30 to 60 minutes is optimal).
- CSF analysis is preferred before the initiation of antibiotics; however, there is a direct relationship between early treatment and positive outcomes in bacterial meningitis, so therapy should *not* be postponed for analysis if the patient appears ill or is deteriorating rapidly.

Pharmacologic Treatment

Antibiotic treatment is empiric based on the age of the patient, history, and the likely causative agent (see Table 3-73).

Client Education

- Discuss the seriousness of the illness and the need for aggressive supportive care.
- Discuss the availability of the meningococcal polysaccharide vaccine (Menomune), which is effective for most strains of meningococcus. The vaccine is helpful in adults and children older than 2 years old.
- Prophylactic antibiotics should be prescribed for those residing with the patient or spending 4 or more hours with the patient 5 to 7 days before the onset of the illness. This includes household members, classmates, and day care or preschool workers. The treatment should be administered as soon as possible, preferably within 24 hours. Drugs used for preventive treatment include rifampin (Rifadin), ciprofloxacin (Cipro), and ceftriaxone (Rocephin).

Referral/Consultation

Meningococcal disease is a medical emergency because of its rapid progression and poor outcomes. It is imperative to consult with a physician if you are suspicious of this disease. The goal of emergency departments is to have the first dose of the antibiotic given within 1 hour of arrival because of the seriousness of this illness. Do not postpone the patient's transfer to a tertiary setting to administer the medication.

Prevention

- Immunization against *H. influenza* has decreased the incidence of meningitis.
- Immunization of college students with protection against *N. meningitidis* is recommended for college freshman who are living on campus (Centers for Disease Control and Prevention [CDC], 1999).

EVALUATION/FOLLOW-UP

Observe for neurologic and developmental sequelae. Refer for multidisciplinary evaluation and treatment if necessary.

COMPLICATIONS

Approximately 3000 cases of meningococcal disease occur each year in the United States, and 10% to 13% of patients die despite receiving antibiotics early in the ill-

TABLE **3-72** Cerebrospinal Fluid Analysis

	NEONATE NORMAL	OLDER THAN 1 MO NORMAL	BACTERIAL	ASEPTIC
Appearance	Clear	Clear	Turbid	Clear
White blood cells	Less than 30	Less than 10	Higher than 500	Higher than 500
Organisms	Absent	Absent	Positive Gram stain	Negative Gram stain
Protein	Less than 90 mg/dL	Less than 40 mg/dL	Higher than 100 mg/dL	Less than 100 mg/dL
Glucose	70 to 80 mg/dL	50 to 60 mg/dL	Elevated	Decreased

TABLE **3-73** Bacterial Pathogens in Meningitis and Empiric Therapy by Age Group*

AGE GROUP	LIKELY ORGANISMS	EMPIRIC THERAPY (DRUG OF CHOICE IN BOLD)
Neonate	Group B and D *Streptococcus, Escherichia coli,* and other gram organisms, *Listeria monocytogenes*	Ampicillin plus gentamicin *or* ampicillin (50 mg/kg IV q8h) plus cefotaxime (100 mg/kg q12h IV)
1 to 3 mo	Group B *Streptococcus* (late onset), *Streptococcus pneumoniae,* and rarely, *L. monocytogenes*	Vancomycin with either ampicillin plus gentamicin *or* ampicillin (50-100 mg/kg IV q8h) plus cefotaxime (150 mg/kg IV q12h) or ceftriaxone plus dexamethasone 0.4 mg/kg q12h for 2 days or 0.15 mg/kg q6h; first dose 15 to 20 min before first dose of antibiotic; chloramphenicol, vancomycin, plus dexamethasone is alternate therapy.
3 mo to 7 yr	*S. pneumoniae, H. influenza,* and *Neisseria meningitidis*	Cefotaxime (150 mg/kg IV q 12h) or ceftriaxone (75 mg/kg initial dose, then 100 mg/kg/day q12h) (vancomycin is used for ceftriaxone-resistant *S. pneumoniae*) plus dexamethasone first dose 15 to 20 min before first dose of antibiotic. 0.4 mg/kg q12h for 2 days or 0.15 mg/kg q6h for 4 days
7 to 50 years	*S. pneumoniae, N. meningitidis, Listeria,* and occasionally, *Haemophilus influenzae*	Cefotaxime (2 g q4h IV) or ceftriaxone (2 g q12h IV) plus dexamethasone before first dose of antibiotic 0.4 mg/kg q12h for 2 days plus ampicillin 50 mg/kg q6h IV
Older than 50	*S. pneumoniae* most common; rare *H. influenzae, Listeria, Pseudomonas aeruginosa, N. meningitidis*	Ampicillin 50 mg/kg IV plus cefotaxime or ceftriaxone plus dexamethasone (doses as above)

*Empiric use of vancomycin must be customized, depending on the incidence of *S. pneumoniae* resistance to penicillin and cephalosporins in the community.

ness. Of those who survive, an additional 10% have severe aftereffects of the disease, including mental retardation, hearing loss, and loss of limbs.

REFERENCES

American Academy of Pediatrics (AAP), Committee on Infectious Diseases. (2000). *The red book report of the Committee on Infectious Diseases* (24th ed.). New York: AAP.

Booy, R., & Kroll, J. (1998). Bacterial meningitis and meningococcal infection. *Current Opinions in Pediatrics 10*(1), 13-18.

Centers for Disease Control and Prevention (CDC). (1997). Control and prevention of meningococcal disease and control and prevention of serogroup C meningococcal disease: Evaluation and management. *MMWR: Morbidity and Mortality Weekly Report 46*(RR-5), 1-21.

Herf, C., Nichols, J., Fruh, S., Holloway, B., Andersen, C. U. (1998). Meningococcal disease: Recognition, treatment and prevention. *Nurse Practitioner 23*(8), 30-46.

Luszcak, M. (2001). Evaluation and management of infants and young children with fever, *American Family Physician 64,* 1219-1226.

Michelow, I. C., Nicol, M., Tiemessen, C., Chezzi, C., Pettifor, J. M. (2000). Value of cerebrospinal fluid leukocyte aggrega-

tion in distinguishing the causes of meningitis in children. *Pediatric Infectious Disease Journal 19,* 66-72.

Niemer, L. (2000). Meningitis. In D. Robinson, P. Kidd, & K. Rogers (Eds.), *Primary care across the lifespan.* St. Louis: Mosby, 725-729.

Norris, C., Danis, P., & Gardner, T. (1999). Aseptic meningitis in the newborn and young infant. *American Family Physician 58,* 245-250.

Phillips, C., & Simor, A. (1998). Bacterial meningitis in children and adults: Changes in community-acquired disease may affect patient care. *Postgraduate Medicine 103*(3), 102-104.

Tunkel, A., & Scheld, W. (1997). Issues in the management of bacterial meningitis, *American Family Physician 56*(5), 423-434.

Review Questions

1. The NP suspects meningococcemia in a child. The treatment plan should include which of the following?

a. Erythromycin

b. Acyclovir

c. Immediate consultation

d. Beginning intravenous (IV) access and administering a corticosteroid and antibiotic

2. Which of the following historical data is most consistent with a diagnosis of meningitis in a child?

  a. Change in level of consciousness
  b. Vomiting and diarrhea
  c. Headache
  d. Fever

3. During the physical assessment of an adult with meningitis, which of the following is consistent with meningeal irritation?

  a. Patrick's sign
  b. Kernig's sign
  c. Positive straight leg raise
  d. Tinnell's sign

4. Which of the following constellation of symptoms is classic for meningitis?

  a. Fever and cough
  b. Decreased appetite, nausea, and fever
  c. Fever, headache, and stiff neck
  d. Visual changes, headache, and fever

5. A 2-year-old child is admitted to the hospital for bacterial meningitis. Her parents call you regarding the concern that they also may be at risk for meningitis. What is your reply?

  a. "Meningitis is not contagious; let me know if you have any symptoms similar to your daughter's."
  b. "A vaccine for meningitis is appropriate at this time."
  c. "If you have been immunized as a child, this protects you from meningitis."
  d. "Close contacts of a patient with meningitis should be treated prophylactically."

6. Josie is an 18-year-old who is going to college next month and will live on campus. Her parents are worried about meningitis because a student died of the disease at this college last year. What recommendation do you give to Josie's parents?

  a. "The chance of getting meningitis at college is very small and nothing to worry about."
  b. "Childhood immunizations protect most people unless she is immunocompromised."
  c. "A vaccine for meningitis is available and is recommended for students going to college who stay in the dorms."
  d. "Immunoglobulin is helpful in case of an outbreak."

7. Marisa was admitted to the hospital for fever and headache. A lumbar puncture revealed the following results: clear fluid, negative Gram stain, low protein, and low glucose. These results are consistent with what diagnosis?

  a. Bacterial meningitis
  b. Viral meningitis
  c. Encephalitis
  d. Space-occupying lesion

8. Steve is a 6-month-old child. He has had a fever and is not eating well. His parents became concerned when they noticed purplish spots on his body. What type of spot is consistent with the diagnosis of meningitis?

  a. Contact dermatitis
  b. Herpes simplex
  c. Purpura
  d. Petechiae

Answers and Rationales

1. **Answer: c** (implementation/plan)
  Rationale: Meningococcemia is a medical emergency and requires IV antibiotics with hospital admission, so immediate consultation is needed. (Niemer, 2000).

2. **Answer: a** (assessment)
  Rationale: A change in consciousness or affect is the best predictor for a child with meningitis. Vomiting and diarrhea may be present, as is fever, but these are very nonspecific signs (Tunkel & Scheld, 1997).

3. **Answer: b** (assessment)
  Rationale: Kernig's sign is present in approximately 50% of people with meningitis. Patrick's sign is a test for hip function, Tinnell's sign is a test for carpal tunnel, and straight leg raise is used to test for low back pain and nerve involvement (Tunkel & Scheld, 1997).

4. **Answer: c** (analysis/diagnosis)
  Rationale: The classic triad of symptoms for meningitis is fever, headache, and stiff neck (Tunkel & Scheld, 1997).

5. **Answer: d** (evaluation)
  Rationale: Close contacts (e.g., household members, school contacts, day care workers) should all be treated prophylactically with an antibiotic, preferably within 24 hours (Niemer, 2000).

6. **Answer: c** (evaluation)
  Rationale: A vaccination is available and recommended for college students who will live on campus (Niemer, 2000).

7. **Answer: b** (analysis/diagnosis)
  Rationale: CSF analysis with low protein and low glucose is consistent with viral or aseptic meningitis. Bacterial CSF would be turbid, high white blood cell (WBC) count, positive Gram stain, elevated protein, and glucose (Niemer, 2000).

8. **Answer: c** (assessment)
  Rationale: Purpura has a high association with meningitis, even though the patient may not exhibit classic symptoms of the illness (Niemer, 2000).

MOLLUSCUM CONTAGIOSUM *Pamela Kidd*

OVERVIEW
Definition
Molluscum contagiosum is a benign epidermal neoplasm.

Incidence
Common in infants, young children, immunocompromised persons, and sexually active adolescents.

Pathophysiology
Caused by pox virus. Pox virus causes the epidermis to proliferate and form papules.

Protective Factors
- Intact immune system
- Condoms

Factors Increasing Susceptibility
- Immunosuppression, chronic illness
- Unprotected sex

ASSESSMENT: SUBJECTIVE/HISTORY
Symptoms
- Onset usually insidious.
- Single skin-colored lesion noticed.

Past Medical History
- Previous sexually transmitted diseases
- HIV infection
- Substance abuse

Medication History
Noncontributory

Family History
Noncontributory.

Dietary History
Noncontributory.

ASSESSMENT: OBJECTIVE/PHYSICAL EXAMINATION
Physical Examination
- Skin: Begins as skin-colored lesions, progressing to discrete pearly white or yellowish lesion that is umbilicated, dome-shaped papule (white curdlike core).
- Size is 2 to 5 mm in diameter.
- May have multiple papules.
- Center is filled with a cheesy substance.
- Common locations are trunk, face, arms, and genitalia.
- If on genitalia in child, consider sexual abuse.

Diagnostic Procedures
- Not necessary.
- Microscopic examination of scraping shows basophilic epidermal cells.

DIAGNOSIS
See Table 3-74.

THERAPEUTIC PLAN
Nonpharmacologic Treatment
Remove each lesion with a sharp curette, electrosurgery, or cryotherapy (apply liquid nitrogen to lesion).

Pharmacologic Treatment
See Table 3-75.

Client Education
- Teach that lesions usually subside without treatment in 6 to 9 months (but may last for years).

TABLE **3-74** Differential Diagnoses of Molluscum Contagiosum

DIAGNOSIS	DATA SUPPORT
Acne	More common in adolescents. Hair may be oily. Includes comedones both black and white.
Wart	Flat lesion with pinpoint depression. More common in females ages 12 to 16.

TABLE **3-75** Pharmaceutical Treatment of Molluscum Contagiosum

DRUG	DOSE	COMMENT
Trichloroacetic acid	30%; apply to base of each lesion.	Avoid surrounding skin.
Salicylic Acid	Apply thin layer to lesion qd; cover with tape.	Remove tape in 12 hours.
Tretinoin gel (Retin A)	0.01%; apply to lesions qd.	Keep away from eye, nares, mouth; avoid exposure to ultraviolet light; may worsen acne; ***do not use in children younger than age 12.***

- Removal may produce scarring.
- Teach the signs and symptoms of secondary infection from touching lesions.
- Teach that contact with a lesion can spread to another person.

Referral

Refer to a dermatologist if multiple lesions are unresponsive to treatment.

Prevention

Condom use.

EVALUATION/FOLLOW-UP

- Recheck in 1 week.
- Decrease number of lesions.
- No secondary infection should be present.

COMPLICATIONS

Scarring may occur.

REFERENCES

Berger, T. (2001). Skin, hair, and nails. In L. Tierney, S. McPhee, & M. Papadakis (Eds.), *Current medical diagnosis and treatment* (40th ed.). New York: McGraw-Hill.

Boynton, R., Dunn, E., & Stephens, G. (1998). *Manual of ambulatory pediatrics* (4th ed.). Philadelphia: Lippincott.

Burkhart, C. (2001). Dermatology clinic. *Clinical Advisor 4*(6), 33-34.

Review Questions

1. Which agent produces molluscum contagiosum?
   a. Yeast
   b. Fungus
   c. Pox virus
   d. Herpes virus

2. Which of the following indicates adequate client education regarding molluscum contagiosum?
   a. "I will wear condoms to prevent reoccurrence."
   b. "I will not let my child go to school until lesions leave."
   c. "Removal of the lesions will prevent scarring."
   d. "The lesions will be gone in about 1 month if I leave them alone."

3. A child presents with molluscum in the genitalia area. The NP should do which of the following?
   a. Suspect child abuse.
   b. Anticipate poor hygiene.
   c. Assume that the child is not continent.
   d. Anticipate that it has been spread by scratching.

Answers and Rationales

1. **Answer: c** (analysis/diagnosis)
   Rationale: Yeast produces seborrhea. Fungus causes tinea. Herpes produces varicella. Pox virus produces molluscum contagiosum.

2. **Answer: a** (evaluation)
   Rationale: Molluscum can be transmitted sexually. The lesions will subside without treatment, usually within 9 months, but it may take years. A child does not need to be isolated with molluscum. Removal of the lesions may produce scarring.

3. **Answer: a** (analysis/diagnosis)
   Rationale: Sexual abuse should be considered because molluscum is transmitted sexually. Scratching may produce a secondary infection but will not spread the lesions. Hygiene is not a factor in molluscum transmission.

MONONUCLEOSIS   *Denise Robinson*

OVERVIEW
Definition

Infectious mononucleosis refers to the presence of an abnormally high number of mononuclear leukocytes in the body.

Incidence

- Approximately 12% to 30% of the total cases of infectious mononucleosis occur among university students and military cadets.
- By adulthood, most individuals have had at least one infection with Epstein-Barr virus (EBV).
- Infectious mononucleosis occurs most often in adolescents from higher socioeconomic groups and college students.

- The peak incidence in boys is ages 16 to 18 years old and in girls is 14 to 16 years old.
- Infectious mononucleosis is rare in children younger than 5 years, but infection occurs early in life among lower socioeconomic groups and in developing countries.

Pathophysiology

Infectious mononucleosis results from a viral syndrome caused by EBV. The virus is introduced when the prospective host comes into close contact with an individual who is shedding EBV in the oropharynx. Infectious mononucleosis is frequently called the "kissing disease" because of the close contact needed for transmission. The virus replicates in epithelial cells of the pharynx and salivary glands.

A localized inflammatory response produces the pharyngeal exudate. The virus is then carried through the lymphatics to the lymph nodes. Local and generalized lymphadenopathy develop. The incubation period is 30 to 50 days.

ASSESSMENT: SUBJECTIVE/HISTORY
Common Symptoms
- Fever and fatigue for 1 week
- Sore throat (may be described as the worst the client has ever had)
- Dysphagia
- Swelling of lymph nodes, especially posterior cervical lymph nodes
- In clients younger than 10 years and older than 50 years, atypical presenting symptoms of rash and nonspecific gastrointestinal complaints

Associated Symptoms
- Anorexia
- Headache
- Abdominal pain
- Jaundice (rare)

Past Medical History
- Exposure to person with infectious mononucleosis, history of URI in past
- History of recent streptococcal sore throat (coexists in approximately 26%)
- Last menstrual period for females
- Allergies

Medication History
Inquire about recent use of antibiotics and any other medications.

Family History
Ask about other family members who may be sick.

Psychosocial History
- Smoking history
- Ability to perform normal activities; extent to which fatigue has interfered with work or school expectations
- Ability to cope with interference with activities of daily living

Dietary History
Ask about the type of diet the client usually eats.

ASSESSMENT: OBJECTIVE/PHYSICAL EXAMINATION
Physical Examination
A problem-oriented physical examination should be conducted, with particular attention to the following:

- Check vital signs, weight, and general appearance
- Check skin for maculopapular rash.
- Assess HEENT for erythema of pharynx and exudate.
  - Petechiae at the junction of hard and soft palate occurs in 25% of cases.
  - Facial edema, especially eyelid edema, is rarely encountered in young adults and is suggestive of infectious mononucleosis.
- Assess lymph nodes. Significant lymphadenopathy is almost always present in the cervical and epitrochlear nodes; if not, question diagnosis.
- Assess abdomen for hepatomegaly (50%) and splenomegaly (75%).
- In children, assess for dehydration and activity level.

Diagnostic Procedures
- CBC with differential (more than 10,000 to 20,000); lymphocytes more than 50% with numerous atypical lymphocytes and monocytes
- Immunoglobulin M antibodies
- Monospot result positive after 7 to 10 days of illness
- Streptococcal screen
- Liver function tests: mild elevation

DIAGNOSIS
Differential diagnoses include the following:
- Streptococcal pharyngitis
- Measles
- Viral exanthems
- Viral hepatitis
- Cytomegalovirus (CMV)

THERAPEUTIC PLAN
Nonpharmacologic Treatment
- Bed rest for fatigue
- Maintenance of adequate fluid intake
- Anesthetic lozenges for pain relief
- Salt water gargles
- Soft diet

Pharmacologic Treatment
- Symptomatic treatment includes only acetaminophen for fever and pain relief. Approximately 20% of clients may also need antibiotics for concomitant streptococcal pharyngitis. Avoid ampicillin because it causes a rash in 80% of clients treated.
- Prednisone may be appropriate if the tonsils and lymphoid tissue are very enlarged and the potential for airway compromise exists.

Client Education
- Teach the client to prevent splenic rupture by avoidance of minor trauma, heavy lifting, overexertion, and contact sports for 1 to 2 months.

- Teach the client strategies to avoid constipation because this causes increased pressure on the spleen.
- Illness is self-limiting, and isolation is unnecessary.

Referral

- Marked splenomegaly
- Respiratory compromise
- Excessively enlarged tonsils and difficulty swallowing
- Jaundice
- Hyperbilirubinemia

Prevention

Good handwashing.

EVALUATION/FOLLOW-UP

- Promptly report abdominal pain and upper quadrant pain radiating to the shoulder.
- If the client experiences shortness of breath or inability to swallow, emergency services should be accessed immediately.
- Assess splenomegaly weekly until it no longer persists.

COMPLICATIONS

Splenic rupture.

REFERENCES

Gwaltney, J., & Segriti, J. (1996). Rationale management of sore throat. *Patient Care 30*(15), 76-80, 82, 88-89.

Hickey, S., & Strasburger, V. (1997). What every pediatrician should know about infectious mononucleosis in adolescents. *Pediatric Clinics of North America 11*(6), 1540-1556.

Perkins, A. (1997). An approach to diagnosing acute sore throat. *American Family Physician 55*(1), 131-138.

Robinson, D. (1996). Mononucleosis. In M. Sommers & S. Johnson (Eds.), *Davis's manual of nursing therapeutics for diseases and disorders.* Philadelphia: F. A. Davis, 696-699.

Robinson, D. (2000). Mononucleosis. In D. Robinson, P. Kidd, & K. Rogers (Eds.), *Primary care across the lifespan.* St. Louis: Mosby, 749-751.

Review Questions

1. What symptoms would make you most suspicious of infectious mononucleosis in a 21-year-old college student?

- **a.** Sore throat, fatigue, and cough
- **b.** Abdominal pain and sore throat
- **c.** Rash, sore throat, and fever
- **d.** Headache, jaundice, and sore throat

2. Which of the following objective findings, if not present, would make you reconsider the diagnosis of infectious mononucleosis?

- **a.** Throat erythematous, no exudate
- **b.** Maculopapular rash
- **c.** Facial edema
- **d.** Lymphadenopathy

3. Sarah is a 20-year-old college student. She reports a sore throat for 2 weeks, enlarged glands in her neck, and a fever. In addition to infectious mononucleosis, what diagnosis needs to be considered?

- **a.** Rubella
- **b.** Streptococcal pharyngitis
- **c.** Viral hepatitis
- **d.** CMV

4. Treatment for mononucleosis should include which of the following?

- **a.** Ampicillin, 250 mg bid for 10 days
- **b.** Symptomatic treatment
- **c.** Interferon
- **d.** Acyclovir

5. Sarah, a 20-year-old college student, had infectious mononucleosis diagnosed 2 weeks ago. She is now reporting abdominal pain. When should she be seen for follow-up?

- **a.** Sarah should be seen as soon as possible.
- **b.** Sarah should be followed up in 1 week.
- **c.** She should return for follow-up in 1 month.
- **d.** Follow-up is not needed because she has been feeling better.

6. In addition to the HEENT examination, what other system is crucial to examine in a patient with suspected mononucleosis?

- **a.** Respiratory
- **b.** Cardiovascular
- **c.** Abdomen
- **d.** Neurologic

7. Which of the following comments by the patient with infectious mononucleosis indicates a need for further teaching?

- **a.** "I should take it easy based on how I feel."
- **b.** "I will feel tired for a few weeks."
- **c.** "Infectious mononucleosis is cured by antibiotics."
- **d.** "I should report any abdominal pain."

8. A CBC was run on a patient complaining of severe sore throat. Which of the following findings is consistent with a diagnosis of mononucleosis?

- **a.** Positive rapid strep test
- **b.** Positive blood culture
- **c.** Decreased hemoglobin
- **d.** Lymphocytosis

Answers and Rationales

1. *Answer:* **c** (assessment)

Rationale: Jaundice and cough are not usual in infectious mononucleosis. Abdominal pain may occur; however, it would not lead you to suspect infectious mononucleosis. A rash occurs in 25% of clients (Robinson, 2000).

2. *Answer:* **d** (assessment)

Rationale: The localized inflammatory response produces the lymphadenopathy that is almost always present in infectious mononucleosis. Although usually present in infectious mononucleosis, the rash, facial edema, and sore throat could also occur with other illnesses. Their absence does not make one question the diagnosis (Robinson, 2000).

3. ***Answer:*** **b** (analysis/diagnosis)

Rationale: Sarah's symptoms are those commonly encountered with streptococcal pharyngitis. This occurs in approximately 20% of clients with infectious mononucleosis (Robinson, 2000).

4. ***Answer:*** **b** (implementation/plan)

Rationale: The treatment for infectious mononucleosis is rest and fluids, along with symptomatic care, such as antipyretics for fever or pain. Ampicillin commonly causes a rash when given to clients with infectious mononucleosis. Interferon and acyclovir have no place in the treatment of infectious mononucleosis (Robinson, 2000).

5. ***Answer:*** **a** (evaluation)

Rationale: Because splenic rupture is a possibility, as a result of splenomegaly during IM, Sarah should be seen as soon as possible to rule it out (Robinson, 2000).

6. ***Answer:*** **c** (assessment)

Rationale: Approximately 50% to 75% of patients with infectious mononucleosis have hepatosplenomegaly. It is important to determine if the patient has enlarged organs during the physical examination (Hickey & Strasburger, 1997).

7. ***Answer:*** **c** (evaluation)

Rationale: Antibiotics do not help in infectious mononucleosis unless the patient also has strep throat. Otherwise, treatment is symptomatic: rest, antipyretics for fever, and reporting any onset of abdominal pain (Robinson, 2000).

8. ***Answer:*** **d** (analysis/diagnosis)

Rationale: In mononucleosis, the WBC count is increased, with lymphocytes higher than 50% with numerous atypical lymphocytes (Robinson, 2000).

M

MULTIPLE SCLEROSIS *Denise Robinson*

OVERVIEW
Definition

Multiple sclerosis (MS) is a chronic inflammatory demyelinating disease of the CNS associated with periods of disability (relapsing/flares) alternating with periods of recovery (remission), which often results in progressive neurologic disability. MS may affect all parts of the CNS and produces a multiplicity of symptoms.

There are two phases of disease:
1. In the exacerbating-remitting phase, the client averages one attack per year.
2. After several years, most individuals enter the chronic-progressive phase (50% within 10 years; 60% within 15 years).

Incidence

- Approximately 250,000 to 350,000 Americans, with increasing incidence both nationally and worldwide
- Thirty per 100,000 prevalence in high-risk areas: northern Europe, United States, Canada, southern Australia, New Zealand
- Low prevalence around equator
- Most common neurologic disease in individuals younger than 40; average age 30; diagnosed as young as 10 years of age; can occur as late as 60 to 70
- Women: two to three times the rate of men
- Factors associated with adverse outcome are the following:
  - Older age at onset
  - Male
  - Cerebellar involvement
  - Persisting deficits in brain stem
  - Higher frequency of attacks in first 2 years after onset
  - High levels of disability

- Short first interattack interval (accelerated deterioration)

Pathophysiology

- Cause unknown; autoimmune disease
- Theories of four possible causes:
  1. Genetics: presence of genes that code for certain histocompatibility leukocyte antigen genes
  2. Environmental factors: documented occurrences of clusters and epidemics required to reinforce this hypothesis; however, no identified environmental factor
  3. Immunologic factors: decreased suppressor T lymphocytes; excess immunoglobulin; high levels of IgG secreted; loss of suppressor cell inducers
  4. Viruses: most widely accepted causal agent; exposure in adolescence that triggers autoimmune response penetrating blood–brain barrier and causing structural lesions in the CNS
- Hormonal factors possibly implicated in the disease; cyclic increase in symptoms associated with menstrual periods, during climacteric, and/or pregnancy, suggesting that hormones may be involved.

ASSESSMENT: SUBJECTIVE/HISTORY

- No characteristic clinical pattern; symptoms are extremely variable.
- Requires careful history with focus on the *temporal profile* of the neurologic deficit, which usually starts unilaterally or focally and eventually becomes bilateral and progressive.

Family History

Ask about family history of multiple sclerosis or other autoimmune diseases.

Symptoms

Most common symptoms are the following:

- Fatigue
- Limb weakness
- Paresthesia
- Aching pain
- Double vision
- Monocular impairment of vision
- Slurred speech
- Urgency
- Constipation
- Imbalance
- Impotence
- Depression
- Temperature lability

Less common symptoms are the following:

- Facial weakness
- Hearing loss
- Trigeminal neuralgia
- Euphoria
- Confusion
- Nystagmus

Uncommon symptoms are the following:

- Severe apraxia or aphasia
- Extrapyramidal movement disorders
- Seizures
- Perineal pains
- Hypersomnolence

ASSESSMENT: OBJECTIVE/PHYSICAL EXAMINATION

Physical Examination

Most common signs are the following:

- Asymmetric weakness
- Sensory loss
- Pale optic discs
- Nystagmus
- Positive Babinski sign
- Spastic gait
- Ataxia
- Diminished visual acuity

Less common signs are the following:

- Hyporeflexia
- Writhing facial muscles
- Afferent pupillary defect
- Deafness
- Muscle atrophy
- Significant dementia

Uncommon signs are the following:

- Aphasia
- Apraxia

Diagnostic Procedures

- The diagnosis of MS is primarily clinical because confirmatory tests are nonspecific; however, the following

tests may increase diagnostic sensitivity and should be evaluated in the clinical context:

- Magnetic resonance imaging (MRI) is gold standard; multiple (two to three) white matter lesions are clinically definitive.
- CSF: Cell count less than 40 WBCs; protein lower than 100 mg/dL; oligoclonal immunoglobulin (Ig) bands (+); IgG index higher than 0.70 (not specific for MS).
- Evoked potential (visual, auditory, somatosensory, motor) studies: Identifies subclinical areas of disease.

DIAGNOSIS

MS is difficult to diagnose because many symptoms mimic those of other diseases. Diagnosis is generally made by observation of the temporal clinical course in conjunction with a neurologic examination and laboratory tests.

The differential diagnoses include the following:

- Systemic lupus erythematosus
- Benign myalgic encephalomyelitis/chronic fatigue syndrome
- Lyme disease
- CNS lesions/tumors
- Acquired immune deficiency syndrome (AIDS)
- Seizure disorder
- Peripheral neuropathy

THERAPEUTIC PLAN

The goal is to (1) treat acute exacerbations, (2) manage chronic symptoms, and (3) delay progression of disease.

Pharmacologic Treatment

- For acute exacerbations prescribe adrenocorticotropic hormone and methylprednisolone.
- Chronic symptoms use the following:
  - Spasticity: baclofen (Lioresal) drug of choice; diazepam (Valium); dantrolene (Dantrium)
  - Fatigue: amantadine (Symmetrel); tricyclic antidepressants; selective serotonin reuptake inhibitors
  - Bladder dysfunction: urgency, frequency–oxybutynin (Ditropan); urinary retention–prazosin (Minipress); nocturia–desmopressin (DDAVP)
  - Ataxia: carbamazepine (Tegretol); isoniazid; less effective–Clonazepam (Klonopin), valproic acid (Depakene), beta-blockers
  - Pain: nonsteroidal antiinflammatory drugs; amitriptyline
  - Reduce rate of relapse, slow progression: azathioprine, cyclophosphamide (Cytoxan), cyclosporine, methotrexate, interferon beta-1b (Betaseron), Interferon beta-1a (Avonex)–fewer exacerbations
- Treatment currently under study includes the following:

- Copolymer 1 to desensitize myelin sheath
- Plasma exchange: mixed results

Treatment Recommendations

- Mild relapse of remitting: none
- Moderate-severe relapse of remitting: IV high-dose methylprednisolone infusion (500 mg qd for 5 days)
- Recent accelerated deterioration in chronic progressive disease: same as previous
- Sustained deterioration in severe chronic progressive disease refractory to IV methylprednisolone: oral low-dose methotrexate

Client Education

- Neurologic: Promote health/maintenance: physical therapy, exercise, group therapy, individual counseling.
- Inform about safety issues in the home related to leg spasticity, decreased visual acuity, and changes in balance.
- Provide information about illness; treatment is palliative and course is unpredictable.
- Provide current research on multiple sclerosis, medications, and side effects.
- Provide family planning services; pregnancy is not contraindicated; exacerbations are found in postpartum period.
- Encourage to avoid excessive fatigue; maintain well-balanced diet.

Referral

- Multifaceted disease often requires care from neurologists, urologists, physical therapists, home health nurses, and psychologists. Management of acute exacerbations, hospitalizations, and chronic symptoms should be coordinated by a neurologist.
- A positive finding on the neurologic examination requires referral to a neurologist.
- Pregnancy requires referral to an obstetrician.
- Bladder dysfunction requires referral to a urologist.
- Spasticity requires referral to a physical therapist.
- The primary care provider is in an ideal position to care for the client by coordinating services, offering emotional support, and managing episodic illness.
- Additional support can be obtained from the Multiple Sclerosis Society.

Prevention

Because the cause is unclear, no prevention is available.

EVALUATION/FOLLOW-UP

- Annual laboratory tests: CBC, chemistry profile, urinalysis, screening tests, influenza vaccinations, along with thorough examination to assess the client's condition

- Episodic illness: Increased risk of sinusitis; pseudoexacerbations resulting from fever and infection. Interferon beta-1b may cause depression of WBCs and elevation of liver function tests. Follow monthly for 3 months, then every 3 months.

COMPLICATIONS

Continued progression of disease.

REFERENCES

Brod, S. A., Lindsey, J. W., & Wolinsky, J. S. (1996). Multiple sclerosis: Clinical presentation, diagnosis and treatment. *American Family Physician 54*(4), 1309-1311.

Ford, H. L., & Johnson, M. H. (1995). Telling your patient he/she has multiple sclerosis. *Postgraduate Medical Journal 71*(838), 449-452.

Kaufman, M. D. (1996). Multiple sclerosis. In R. T. Rakel (Ed.), *Saunders manual of medical practice*. Philadelphia: W. B. Saunders, 1058-1060.

Pender, M. P. (1996). Recent advances in the understanding, diagnosis and management of multiple sclerosis. *Australia and New Zealand Journal of Medicine 26*, 157-161.

Poser, C. M. (1994). The epidemiology of multiple sclerosis: A general overview. *Annals of Neurology 36*(S2), S180-S193.

Reeve, K. (2000). Multiple sclerosis. In D. Robinson, P. Kidd, & K. Rogers (Eds.), *Primary care across the lifespan* (pp. 752-758). St. Louis: Mosby, 752-758.

Swain, S. E. (1996). Multiple sclerosis: Primary health care implications. *Nurse Practitioner 21*(7), 40, 43, 47-50.

Thompson, A. J. (1995). Multiple sclerosis: Symptomatic treatment. *Journal of Neurology 243*, 559-565.

van Oosten, B. W., Truyen, L., Barkhof, F., Polman, C. H. (1995). Multiple sclerosis therapy. A practical guide. *Drugs 49*(2), 200-212.

Review Questions

1. A poorer prognosis is associated with the development of MS in which of the following ages?

    a. 10 years old
    b. 30 years old
    c. 40 years old
    d. 60 years old

2. Major presenting symptoms occurring in MS include all *except* which of the following?

    a. Bladder and bowel dysfunction
    b. Visual dysfunction
    c. Dizziness
    d. Fatigue

3. Which of the following symptoms is relatively uncommon but highly indicative of multiple sclerosis?

    a. Paresthesia
    b. Seizures
    c. Constipation
    d. Slurred speech

4. All *except* which of the following signs are associated with MS?

   a. Ataxia
   b. Decreased visual acuity
   c. Increased motor strength
   d. Spastic gait

5. Which of the following tests is considered the gold standard in the diagnosis of MS?

   a. MRI
   b. CSF cell count
   c. Evoked potential
   d. Urine assay

6. One of the most common clinical findings in an individual with MS is which of the following?

   a. Aphasia
   b. Asymmetric weakness of the legs
   c. Apraxia
   d. Deafness

7. The single most important feature in diagnosing MS is which of the following?

   a. IgG bands in CSF
   b. Temporal profile of neurologic deficit
   c. Presence of single lesion on MRI
   d. Evoked potential abnormalities

8. In making the diagnosis of MS, which of the following conditions is *not* a differential diagnosis to consider?

   a. Systemic lupus erythematosus
   b. AIDS
   c. Peripheral neuropathy
   d. Diabetes

Answers and Rationales

1. *Answer:* **d** (evaluation)
   Rationale: Late-onset disease is usually more severe and progresses more quickly (Swain, 1996).

2. *Answer:* **c** (assessment)
   Rationale: Dizziness is a symptom of benign myalgic encephalomyelitis/chronic fatigue syndrome, which is often erroneously called MS on the basis of a single lesion visualized on MRI (Poser, 1994).

3. *Answer:* **b** (assessment)
   Rationale: Seizures are uncommon and highly indicative of MS, whereas the other choices are all common symptoms of numerous abnormalities (Thompson, 1996).

4. *Answer:* **c** (assessment)
   Rationale: Decreased motor strength is associated with MS (Swain, 1996).

5. *Answer:* **a** (analysis/diagnosis)
   Rationale: MRI scan shows areas of white matter demyelination within the CNS in 95% of clients with clinically definite MS (van Oosten, Truyen, Barkhoff, & Polman, 1995).

6. *Answer:* **b** (assessment)
   Rationale: Common findings on examination include decreased motor strength in the legs (Swain, 1996).

7. *Answer:* **b** (analysis/diagnosis)
   Rationale: The single most important feature in diagnosing inflammatory demyelination of the CNS is the temporal profile of the neurologic deficit (Pender, 1996; Brod, Lindsey, & Wolinsky, 1996).

8. *Answer:* **d** (analysis/diagnosis)
   Rationale: Because of the variability of MS symptoms, recognizing clinical symptoms is challenging. Important illnesses to include in the differential diagnosis include systemic lupus erythematosus, AIDS, and peripheral neuropathy (Swain, 1996).

MUMPS *Denise Robinson*

OVERVIEW
Definition

Mumps is a systemic viral disease characterized by swelling of the salivary glands, but it can involve multiple organs and be moderately debilitating.

Incidence

Peak incidence is in the late winter and spring. Incubation period is 16 to 18 days. Mumps is contagious 1 to 2 days before and 3 to 7 days after the development of swelling. Complications are worse in adults (50% of all deaths occur in this group). Vaccine and illness confer lifelong immunity. Serologic studies show that more than 85% of unimmunized adults have had a mumps infection.

Pathophysiology

Spread is by direct contact and the respiratory route. Aseptic meningitis occurs in 50% of cases. Orchitis and epididymitis occur in 15% to 35% of adults. Infertility is rare. Pancreatitis may occur because salivary gland secretion elevates serum amylase level.

ASSESSMENT: SUBJECTIVE/HISTORY
History of Present Illness

- History is usually 1 to 2 days of fever, headache, malaise, and swelling of the "jaw area."
- Sour foods cause pain as a result of stimulation of salivary flow.

- Some patients present with symptoms of aseptic meningitis: headache, fever, and stiff neck.
- Orchitis (usually unilateral) occurs in 20% to 30% of postpubertal males.

Past Medical History

Ask about the following:
- Immunization history
- Environmental exposure (illness at home, work, school, day care)
- Travel (to area with high incidence)
- Communicable disease history

Family History

Ask about any recent illness of household members and the immunization status of family members.

ASSESSMENT: OBJECTIVE/PHYSICAL EXAMINATION

Physical Examination

- Examine HEENT. Observe the parotid gland. Swelling occurs in the parotid gland, which obscures the angle of mandible, pushes the earlobe upward and outward, and causes pain with pressure on the gland.
- There is swelling and redness of Stensen's duct (yellow drainage with no pus).
- The submandibular or sublingual gland may be involved. Rarely, one of these glands is swollen and not the parotid.
- Observe genitals for orchitis, epididymitis, or oophoritis. Local tenderness and swelling may occur.

Diagnostic Procedures

- Diagnosis is made on clinical grounds.
- Serologic tests can confirm the diagnosis because mumps is now a rare infection.
- The virus can be isolated from saliva, blood, urine, and CSF during the acute phase of the disease. Skin tests are unreliable.

DIAGNOSIS

- Cervical adenitis: The angle of the jaw may be obscured, but the earlobe is not displaced and Stensen's duct is normal.
- Bacterial parotitis: Pus is present in Stensen's duct; systemic toxicity is seen.

THERAPEUTIC PLAN

Nonpharmacologic Treatment

Nonpharmacologic treatment is supportive, with fluids, analgesics, and scrotal support for orchitis.

Diet

- Determine diet as tolerated.
- Encourage fluids.
- Sour foods increase the pain in the gland, so they should be avoided.

Client Education

- Exclude an affected child from school for 9 days after onset of swelling.
- Immunization should be given routinely as a part of the MMR (measles, mumps, rubella) vaccine at 12 to 15 months of age, and again at 4 to 6 years. Mild fever without upper respiratory symptoms is not a contraindication to vaccination.
- Vaccine given after exposure will not prevent illness.

Referral/Consultation

- Women who become pregnant within 3 months after receiving mumps vaccine or who are infected during pregnancy should be referred to an obstetrician.
- Unimmunized children with severe egg allergies should be referred to an allergist for immunization.

Prevention

Immunization with MMR per schedule.

EVALUATION/FOLLOW-UP

Male adult clients with mumps should be seen in 1 to 2 weeks for genital examination.

COMPLICATIONS

- Arthritis, renal involvement, thyroiditis, mastitis, pancreatitis, and hearing impairment are all possible.
- Aseptic meningitis occurs in 50% of cases.

REFERENCES

Bartlett, J. G. (1996). *Pocket book of infectious disease therapy.* Baltimore: Williams & Wilkins.

Chin, J. (2000). *Control of communicable diseases manual* (17th ed.). Washington, DC: American Public Health Association.

Committee on Infectious Diseases, American Academy of Pediatrics. (2000). *2000 red book: report of the Committee on Infectious Diseases* (25th ed.). Elk Grove Village, IL: CID/AAP.

Cooper, L. (2000). Mumps. In D. Robinson, P. Kidd, & K. Rogers (Eds.), *Primary care across the lifespan* (pp. 759-760). St. Louis: Mosby.

Hay, W. W., Hayward, A. R., Levin, M. J., & Sondheimer, J. (1999). *Current pediatric diagnosis and treatment* (14th ed.). Norwalk, CT: Appleton & Lange.

Merenstein, G. B., Kaplan, D. W., & Rosenberg, A. A. (1997). *Handbook of pediatrics* (18th ed.). Norwalk, CT: Appleton & Lange.

Review Questions

1. A patient has been diagnosed as having mumps. Which of the following historical data is most consistent with a diagnosis of mumps?

   a. Severe sore throat
   b. Swelling of jaw area
   c. URI symptoms
   d. Cough lasting more than 7 days

2. Which of the following symptom descriptions provided by Steve, in addition to pain in the jaw, is typical of mumps?

   a. Pain when sour foods are eaten
   b. Fever
   c. Rash
   d. Sore throat

3. Which of the following is affected when the patient has mumps?

   a. Parotid gland
   b. Bartholin's duct
   c. Mastoid
   d. Lymph node

4. Appropriate treatment for mumps includes all *except* which of the following?

   a. Fluids
   b. Analgesics
   c. Avoidance of sour foods
   d. Antibiotics such as amoxicillin

5. Males who contract mumps after puberty are at high risk for involvement of which body system?

   a. Meninges
   b. Gonads
   c. Hearing
   d. Cardiovascular

Answers and Rationales

1. *Answer:* **b** (assessment)
   Rationale: Patients with mumps complain of a swelling in the jaw area, along with fever, headache, and malaise (Cooper, 2000).

2. *Answer:* **a** (assessment)
   Rationale: Patients with mumps complain of pain when sour food is eaten; the food causes stimulation of salivary flow from the parotid gland (Cooper, 2000).

3. *Answer:* **a** (analysis/diagnosis)
   Rationale: Mumps affects the salivary glands, including the parotid gland, which is most commonly involved. Stensen's duct is also affected. Bartholin's duct is in the perineal area of women. Lymph nodes are involved because of the illness, but not directly affected by the virus. The mastoid process is not involved in mumps (Chin, 2000).

4. *Answer:* **d** (implementation/plan)
   Rationale: Treatment for mumps is supportive, including fluids, rest, analgesics, and avoidance of sour foods. Antibiotics are not effective in mumps (Chin, 2000).

5. *Answer:* **b** (evaluation)
   Rationale: Males who contract mumps after puberty are likely to have involvement of the gonads. Approximately one third of postpubertal males have epididymitis and orchitis (Chin, 2000).

NEURAL TUBE DEFECTS   *Denise Robinson*

OVERVIEW

Definition

Neural tube defects include a variety of malformations, including anencephaly, spina bifida, myelomeningocele, sacral agenesis (also called caudal regression syndrome), sacral lipomas, and other spinal dysraphisms.

Spina Bifida Occulta. Spina bifida occulta consists of a midline defect of the vertebral bodies without protrusion of the spinal cord or meninges. Most are asymptomatic and lack neurologic signs.

Meningocele. A meningocele is formed when the meninges herniate through a defect in the posterior vertebral arches. The spinal cord is usually normal.

Myelomeningocele. A myelomeningocele represents the most severe form of dysraphism involving the vertebral column. Problems include paralysis of the lower extremities, hydrocephalus, and postural abnormalities including clubfeet and subluxation of the hips. Gastrointestinal and genitourinary problems also may be present.

Incidence

- Myelomeningocele accounts for most congenital abnormalities of the central nervous system; spina bifida and anencephaly are the most common of the neural tube defects.
  - Myelomeningocele incidence is 1: in 1000 live births; the mortality rate is 10% to 15%, with most deaths occurring before 4 years of age.
  - At least 70% of people with a myelomeningocele have normal intelligence, but learning problems and seizures are more common than in the general population.

- The incidence of neural tube defects has decreased by 20% since the mandatory addition of folic acid to bread in 1998.

Pathophysiology

- Myelomeningocele results from failure of the neural tube to close spontaneously between the third and fourth week of fetal development.
- Factors that may influence normal prenatal development include:
  - Radiation exposure
  - Drug use during pregnancy (valproic acid causes neural tube defects in 1% to 2% of pregnancies if taken during pregnancy)
  - Malnutrition
  - Chemical exposure
  - Genetic determinants

ASSESSMENT: SUBJECTIVE/HISTORY
Symptoms

The symptoms of neural tube defects range from no observable signs to multiple neurologic defects depending on the location of the myelomeningocele. Some symptoms include the following:

- Fluid-filled sac
- Hemangioma
- Asymmetric buttock creases
- Flaccid paralysis of the lower extremities
- Lack of response to touch and pain
- Absence of deep tendon reflexes (DTRs)
- Postural abnormalities: clubfeet, subluxation of the hips
- Urinary dribbling
- Relaxed anal sphincter
- Increasing neurologic deficits if the myelomeningocele goes higher into the thoracic region

Infants with the myelomeningocele in the upper thoracic or cervical region have minimal neurologic deficit and do not usually have hydrocephalus.

Past Medical History

If a child has had a neural tube defect, inquire as to past testing and treatment.

Family History

- Ask about folic acid supplementation before and during pregnancy.
- Ask about valproic acid ingestion during pregnancy.
- Ask about other siblings with similar problems.

Psychosocial History

The birth of a child with neural tube defects is devastating.

ASSESSMENT: OBJECTIVE/EXAMINATION
Physical Examination

- A thorough physical examination should take place with emphasis on the neurologic system.
- Skin: Look for patches of hair, a lipoma, or discoloration of the skin in the midline of the low back.
- Cardiovascular: Assess for murmurs.
- Lungs: Assess for pulmonary function.
- Neurologic: Assess DTRs, sensation, muscle strength, and response to pain and touch; evaluate for hydrocephalus (dilated scalp veins, bulging anterior fontanel, setting sun appearance of the eyes, irritability, and vomiting) and increased head circumference (more often occurs after closure of the back).
- Abdomen: Assess for neurogenic bowel and bladder.

Diagnostic Procedures

Perform x-ray examination, ultrasound, computed tomography scanning, or magnetic resonance imaging to determine the extent of neural tube involvement and associated anomalies.

DIAGNOSIS

Assess for abnormalities such as clubfoot or subluxation of the hip.

THERAPEUTIC PLAN
Nonpharmacologic Treatment

Those children with meningocele with leaking cerebrospinal fluid (CSF) or a thin skin covering should undergo immediate surgical treatment to prevent meningitis. Those children with myelomeningocele may have surgery within the first several days (unless there is a CSF leak). This gives the parents time to adjust to the shock of having a child with this devastating condition.

Pharmacologic Treatment

Pharmacologic treatment depends on the conditions that exist.

Client Education

- Provide information pertaining to myelomeningocele and what to expect.
- Inform the parents that once the back is closed, a hydrocephalus may develop; parents need to know the signs and symptoms of increased intercranial pressure.
- The parents need to know how to catheterize the child, and eventually the child will need to catheterize himself or herself.
- Bowel-training programs are completed to help with stool continence.

- The child's ability to walk depends on the level of the lesion.
- Children with spina bifida and urinary tract anomalies have a significant risk for type I allergic reactions to latex. The symptoms may range from urticaria to anaphylaxis. Avoidance of latex products is essential. The incidence of this condition frequently increases with age.
- Periodic multidisciplinary follow-up is required for life.
- Parents and patient should know that genetic counseling is recommended because there is a recurrence rate of 2% to 3%.
- Screening of future pregnancies is recommended.
- Folic acid and multivitamin supplementation is recommended before becoming pregnant. A mother who has had a child with a neural tube defect should take 4.0 mg of folic acid per day when pregnancy is planned.

Referral

Referral to a spina bifida or neural tube multispecialty clinic is recommended.

Prevention

- Intake of folic acid before pregnancy has reduced the number of neural tube defects.
- Identification of neural tube defects through prenatal testing is available.

EVALUATION/FOLLOW-UP

Close follow-up is recommended for all neural tube defects. Even those children with no appreciable deficits may have, for example, tethered spinal cords that require frequent monitoring.

COMPLICATIONS

Some complications of neural tube defects include the following:

- Complications associated with treatment failure
- Paralysis of lower extremities
- Hydrocephalus
- Diminished intellectual capacity
- Death caused by renal problems

REFERENCES

Haslam, R. (1996). The nervous system. In Behrman, R., Kliegman, R., & Jenson, H. (Eds.), *Nelson textbook of pediatrics* (16th ed., pp. 1667-1680). Philadelphia: W. B. Saunders.

Hernandez-Diaz, S., Werler, M. M., Walker, A. M., & Mitchell, A. A. (2000). Folic acid antagonists during pregnancy and the risk of birth defects. *New England Journal of Medicine 343*, 1608-1614.

Honein, M. A., Paulozzi, L. J., Mathews, T. J., Erickson, J. D., Wong, L. Y. (2001). Impact of folic acid fortification of the US food supply on the occurrence of neural tube defects, *Journal of the American Medical Association 285*(23), 2981-2986.

Knowledge and use of folic acid among women of reproductive age–Michigan 1998. (2001). *MMWR: Morbidity and Mortality Weekly Report 50*(10), 185-189.

Pace, B., Glass, R. (2001). Spina bifida. *Journal of the American Medical Association 285*(23), 3050.

Sujansky, E., Stewart, J., Manchester, D. (1999). Genetics and dysmorphology. In W. Hay, A. Hayward, M. Levin, J. M., Sondheimer (Eds.), *Current pediatric diagnosis and treatment* (14th ed., pp. 881-916). Stamford, CT: Appleton & Lange.

Review Questions

1. What is the most important thing a woman can do to prevent the development of neural tube defects?
- **a.** Eat a healthy diet.
- **b.** Exercise moderately.
- **c.** Take a multivitamin.
- **d.** Take a folic acid supplement before and during pregnancy.

2. Testing to determine the presence of neural tube defects during pregnancy includes all but which of the following?
- **a.** Serum alpha-fetoprotein level
- **b.** Rh factor
- **c.** Ultrasound
- **d.** Amniocentesis

3. Children who have spina bifida or other neural tube defects are at risk for which of the following?
- **a.** Frequent otitis media
- **b.** Speech delay
- **c.** Latex allergy
- **d.** Hymenoptera allergies

4. If the patient has a diagnosis of myelomeningocele, what clinical findings is the NP likely to find in the assessment?
- **a.** Flaccid lower extremities
- **b.** Myopia
- **c.** Otitis media
- **d.** Cataracts

Answers and Rationales

1. *Answer:* **d** (implementation/plan)
   Rationale: Taking folic acid before a planned pregnancy reduces the incidence of neural tube defects (Hernandez-Diaz, Werler, Walker, et al. 2000).

2. *Answer:* **b** (analysis/diagnosis)
   Rationale: All the tests except Rh factor can identify neural tube defects in utero.

3. *Answer:* **c** (evaluation)
   Rationale: Latex allergy is present in up to 40% of children with spina bifida (Sujansky, Stewart, & Manchester, 1999).

4. *Answer:* **a** (assessment)
   Rationale: The defects present with myelomeningocele vary, but in most cases there is paralysis of the lower extremity with absent DTRs and lack of response to touch and pain (Haslam, 1996).

OBESITY AND OVERWEIGHT *Denise Robinson*

OVERVIEW
Definition

- Being overweight is defined as having a body mass index (BMI) of 25 to 29.9 kg/m.
- Obesity is identified when BMI is greater than 30 kg/m². A BMI of 30 is approximately 30 pounds overweight.
- Overweight and obesity are not mutually exclusive because obese persons are also overweight.

Incidence

- Of U.S. adults older than 20, 54.9% are overweight.
- Obesity is higher in certain ethnic populations, particularly in women.
- Of black women older than 20, 44% are overweight.
- Of Hispanic women older than 20, 39% are overweight.
- Of prepubertal children, 25% to 30% are obese, and 18% to 25% of adolescents are obese.
- Of Hispanic children, 56% are overweight, and 41% of black children are overweight compared with 28% of white children (Hellmich, 1992). Obesity (BMI greater than 85th percentile) is 29% among Navajo children and 40% among Pueblo Indians (Davis et al., 1993).

Pathophysiology

- Obesity is a significant and independent predictor of coronary heart disease (CHD) morbidity and mortality; even mild to moderate weight gain has a significant influence in the morbidity and mortality because of associated chronic illness (Willett et al., 1995).
- Obesity is negatively related to high-density lipoprotein (HDL)2 and HDL3 cholesterol, and positively correlated with plasma total cholesterol, low-density lipoprotein (LDL) cholesterol, and triglyceride levels. The prevalence of diabetes, hypertension, and hyperlipidemia is three times higher in overweight adults. Obesity also increases the risk of certain types of cancer, including colon, rectal, prostate, gallbladder, breast, cervix, endometrium, ovary, and biliary tract cancers.
- The location of body fat depots, rather than body weight, is associated with type 2 diabetes mellitus and CHD, elevated concentrations of very-low-density lipoproteins (VLDLs), LDLs, apoprotein (APO) B-100, insulin resistance, and hypertension (Bjorntorp, 1990, 1992).
- Central (abdominal) fat distribution ("apple" shape) has been shown to be related to elevated blood glucose, plasma insulin, VLDL cholesterol and triglycerides, and low concentrations of HDL cholesterol (Kaplan, 1989).

Protective Factors. Prevention of overweight and obesity is the most successful method of achieving long-term health.

Factors Increasing Susceptibility

- Binge dieting increases susceptibility.
- Weight loss efforts are not without risk. The weight loss produced by dietary restriction is a result of the loss of both fat and lean body tissue (fat-free mass [FFM]). This contributes to the dilemma of weight cycling when the individual gains weight while eating less.
- Binge eaters account for 40% of obese participants in weight control programs (Delvin, Walsh, & Spitzer 1992; Hakala, 1994). Approximately half of obese individuals in treatment have nonpurging bulimia: they binge eat two to three times a week, have feelings of lack of control over eating behavior, and have significant concern with body weight and shape (Foryet & Goodrick, 1991).
- Some obese individuals have food dependence, similar to substance dependence.

Risk of Obesity in Children

- Parental obesity: Overweight parents increase the risk of an overweight child.
- Excessive weight of siblings: Assess sibling weight.
- Mother's preference for a chubby baby: Assess cultural values regarding weight gain for infant, appearance of a "chubby" baby.
- BMI greater than 95th percentile identifies child in need of treatment.
- BMI greater than 85th percentile with psychosocial problems identifies child in need of treatment.
- High infant birthweight: Assess infant's birthweight and mother's weight gain during pregnancy.

ASSESSMENT: SUBJECTIVE/HISTORY
History of Present Illness

Adults/Elderly. Determine the length of overweight and obesity; for example, has the client been overweight since childhood? Was the weight gain related to pregnancy? Menopause? Retirement? Stressful life change event such as a move or job change?

Children

- Determine the emotional impact of overweight and obesity on the child. Children often engage in inappropriate weight loss efforts in secret.
- Determine their perceptions of themselves, whether they consider themselves to be fat, slim, or just right.

Common Symptoms

- Determine the body image and self-esteem of the obese client.
- Some women from certain ethnic groups do not necessarily equate overweight and obesity with being unattractive.

Associated Symptoms

Determine associated symptoms the client may be experiencing, such as hyperglycemia, gastrointestinal (GI) disturbances, musculoskeletal disorders, and activity intolerance.

Past Medical History

Heart disease, diabetes, angina, hypertension, hyperlipidemia, pancreatic disorders, and musculoskeletal disorders may be reported. Determine if the obesity has caused limited mobility and physical endurance.

Medication History

Determine use of over-the-counter (OTC) medications, medications used for weight loss, sleep assistance, prescription medications.

Family History

Diabetes, congenital heart disease, hypertension, angina, hyperlipidemia., overweight/obesity.

Psychosocial History

Determine addictive behaviors, substance abuse, emotional disorders, psychiatric treatment. Determine if the client has experienced economic, social, or job discrimination related to obesity.

Lifestyle Assessment

Adults. Obtain dietary recall, pattern of weight loss/gain, bingeing, purging, amount and frequency of physical activity, length of time engaging in physical activity, both chronology and duration.

Children

- Obtain dietary recall, pattern of weight loss/gain, bingeing, purging, amount and frequency of physical activity, length of time engaging in physical activity, both chronology and duration.
- Parental/child knowledge and values: Assess the child/family for the following:
  - Assess parental knowledge of nutrition, including balance of fat, protein, and carbohydrates.
  - Assess duration of breastfeeding and introduction of solid foods.
  - Determine whether parents use food as reward or a comfort measure. Assess parental interpretation of infant cues.
- Family lifestyle: Assess the family situation for the following:

- Lower socioeconomic status: Assess food choices and resources for shopping and nutritional choices.
- Mother's marital status (single parent): Assess mother's social support resources.
- Several caretakers in childbearing: Assess feeding choices for caregivers.
- Assess snack food choices and foods available for nutrition in the home.
- Physical inactivity: Assess number of hours of TV and videos watched; amount, frequency, and duration of child's physical activity.

ASSESSMENT: OBJECTIVE/PHYSICAL EXAMINATION

Physical Examination

A thorough examination, including vital signs, should be conducted to determine the extent of overweight/obesity and the concurrent conditions that occur. See Tables 3-76 and 3-77 for physical examination components for adults and children.

- Adult/elderly: A BMI equal to or greater than 27.8 and 27.3 (kg/m²), for males and females, respectively, has been equated with obesity (The National Institutes of Health [NIH] Consensus Development Conference Statement, 1993).
- A weight-to-height ratio greater than 1.0 in men and 0.9 in women is associated with substantial increase in risk for hypertension, stroke, and diabetes.
- Child: Using the BMI, the child is classified as overweight when the index is equal to or exceeds the 85th percentile. The definition of obesity in children, using a triceps skinfold measurement, is thickness greater than or equal to 85th percentile and weight for height, age, and sex greater than or equal to the 85th percentile (Harsha, 1978). The 85th percentile corresponds roughly to 120 percent of ideal body weight and is the accepted definition of obesity in children (The NIH Consensus Development Conference Statement, 1993).

Diagnostic Procedures

- Total cholesterol, including HDL, LDL, VLDL
- Thyroid-stimulating hormone (TSH)
- Fasting plasma glucose

DIAGNOSIS

Differential diagnoses to consider include the following:

- Hypothyroidism
- Diabetes mellitus, type 2

THERAPEUTIC PLAN

Pharmacologic Treatment

Drugs may be used as part of a comprehensive weight loss program, including dietary and physical activity for clients with BMI greater than 30 with no concomitant obesity-related risk factors or diseases, and for clients with BMI

TABLE **3-76** Physical Examination: Adults

TEST	FINDINGS/RATIONALE
BMI	The BMI is an expression of body weight relative to height. BMI is calculated as weight (in Kg) divided by the square of height m^2. Use of BMI is limited for reflecting body fat because it does not distinguish fat weight from nonfat weight.
	A BMI equal to or greater than 27.8 and 27.3 (kg/m^2), for males and females, respectively, has been equated with obesity.
	Individuals with high BMI should be further examined for fat distribution and health risks associated with overweight and obesity, such as blood lipids.
Weight-to-height ratio	Determines an individual's relative weight to height.
Fat distribution	Measuring where fat is deposited on the body is an important dimension of the assessment of body fat because of its relationship to morbidity and mortality outcomes.
	WHR is the simplest method for determining regional fat and describes the anatomic distribution of fat tissue on the waist and hips.
	The waist circumference is measured at the narrowest spot between the ribs and hips, or when a narrow point is not evident, the midpoint between the lowest rib and the iliac crest.
	The hip circumference is measured at the widest circumference over the great trochanters. The WHR is calculated by dividing the waist measurement by the hip measurement. A WHR greater than 1.0 in men and 0.9 in women is associated with substantial increase in risk for hypertension, stroke, and diabetes.

BMI, Body mass index; *WHR,* waist-to-hip ratio.

TABLE **3-77** Physical Examination: Children

TEST	FINDINGS/RATIONALE
Weight-for-age methods	Although widely used, weight-for-age percentiles are inadequate to assess overweight because the contributions of stature and lean tissue are not taken into account (Himes & Dietz, 1994).
	Another method considers weight relative to the weight-for-age percentile that corresponds to the stature-for-age percentile; however, the percentiles of weight for stature are more narrow than weight for age, resulting in overestimation of the target weight (Himes & Dietz, 1994).
BMI	Using the BMI, the child is classified as overweight when the index is equal to or exceeds the 85th percentile. The percentiles are age and gender specific: for example, in children ages 12-14, the 85th percentile for boys is >23, for girls >23.4; for 15-17 year old males >24.3, for girls >24.8 (Harlan, 1993). In adolescents, the BMI is significantly associated with subcutaneous and total body fatness and is highly specific for those individuals with the greatest amount of body fat, making it a useful approach for measurement of fatness in this age group (Himes & Dietz, 1994).
	It is important to note that specific cutoff points of the BMI, which are associated with morbidity and mortality in children and adolescents, have not been adequately established.
Skinfold Measurements	Some investigators advocate the use of anthropometric (skinfold) measurements as a particularly practical approach for field measurement in children and adolescents (Lohman, 1992). Using this technique, special calipers grasp a skinfold, which is held between the tester's thumb and fingers to provide a measurement in millimeters for a double fold of skin and subcutaneous fat (Lohman, 1984).

BMI, Body mass index.

greater than 27 with concomitant obesity-related risk factors (e.g., hypertension [HTN], dyslipidemia, CHD, type 2 diabetes, and sleep apnea). Weight-loss drugs should never be used without lifestyle modifications. Continual assessment of drug therapy for efficacy and safety is necessary.

Drugs prescribed for weight loss for those people who are at a BMI of 30 or higher or a BMI of 27 or more with obesity-related risk factors include the following:

- To reduce energy intake: Benzphetamine (Didrex), Diethylpropion (Tenuate), Phendimetrazine (Bontril); side effects include high potential for abuse, central nervous system (CNS) overstimulation, and dry mouth.

- To affect the serotonin system: Sibutramine (Meridia), Phentermine (Ionamin); side effects include dry mouth, anorexia, insomnia, constipation, and HTN.
- Lipase inhibitor: Orlistat (Xenical) acts in the GI tract to decrease fat absorption. Side effects include steatorrhea, flatus, fecal incontinence, abdominal bloating, and oily spotting. These side effects are increased with the consumption of fatty foods, and they cause many clients to stop taking the drug.

Nonpharmacologic Treatment

Exercise

Adults

- Physical activity is particularly important in aiding and sustaining weight loss through increased total energy expenditure, preservation of lean body mass, and changes in metabolism (King & Tribble, 1991).
- The energy equation of energy intake and expenditure needs to be a major consideration in weight-loss efforts. It is the combination of exercise and caloric restriction that contributes to success of weight loss and maintenance (Avila & Hovell, 1994; Blair, 1993; Foryet & Goodrick, 1991; Ballor & Poehlman, 1994).
- Exercise is most advantageous in weight loss because it maintains the resting metabolic rate (RMR) and the TEF; in addition, exercise produces a favorable effect on plasma lipids and carbohydrate metabolism (Calles-Escandon & Horton, 1992). It is not only the amount of exercise, but also the intensity of the exercise that may be important in weight loss.

Children

- The goal of weight reduction in children is to achieve sustained weight loss of fat tissue without affecting BMI or linear growth. There is no generally accepted standard for the effective treatment of obesity in children. Interventions may address either prevention of overweight or treatment of the problem.
- The focus of most weight reduction interventions and research has been on coupling physical activity and moderate caloric restriction during the growth period.
- The main methods of treatment of childhood obesity are modification of diet, exercise, diet and exercise together, and child-oriented or family-based behavior modification programs.
- The interventions include parent education in behavioral techniques and problem-solving techniques and mothers' attendance at weight-loss classes.
- Exercise is an important adjunct to weight loss and subsequent reduction of unfavorable lipoproteins in children.
- Behavioral modification such as recognition of stimuli related to eating, behavioral substitution, goal setting, and self-monitoring with contracts are techniques that have been successful. Program interventions such as

"Shapedown" focuses on the child's cognitive behavioral and affective elements of weight management.

- Rather than using restrictive diets, emphasize healthy eating habits, exercise behavior, and communication skills in both prevention and reduction efforts.
- Efforts should be made to assist the child to normalize, not restrict food, increase physical activity, and gain a feeling of empowerment.

Diet

Adults

- Dietary restriction is the most commonly used strategy for weight loss and maintenance, and includes primarily two levels of calorie restriction.
  - The low-calorie diet (LCD) is 1000 to 1500 calories (12 to 15 Kcal/kg body weight). The very-low-calorie diet (VLCD) is approximately 800 calories (6 to 19 Kcal/kg body weight). Weight loss using the VLCD averages 1.5 to 2.5 kg/week; after 12 to 16 weeks, the average loss is 20 kg. The use of the VLCD has been associated with adverse complications such as ventricular arrhythmias or dysrhythmias, but it is generally safe when used under proper supervision in moderate and severely obese clients.
- The VLCD produces rapid short-term weight loss, with approximately one half of clients regaining more than one half of their lost weight after 1 year (Holden, Darga, Olson, Stettner, Ardito & Lucas, 1992; Kern, Trozzolino, Wolfe & Purdy, 1994).
- Other strategies of dietary restriction include changes in dietary proportions of fat, protein, and carbohydrates, for example, 30% of total caloric intake as fats.
- An initial goal of diet and exercise is for the client to lose 10% from initial body weight. Ongoing treatment then focuses on sustaining lifestyle changes to produce further weight loss, maintaining the desired weight, and ultimately avoiding future weight gain (Lyznicki, Young, Riggs, & Davis, 2001).

Children

- Dietary restrictions in infants, young children, and even adolescents are unsafe and may retard both physical and mental growth and development. Moderate dietary nutrition coupled with exercise does not contribute to a decrease in linear growth.
- Weight-reduction therapy should be focused primarily on those children and adolescents who have obesity-related morbidity. These include those with a BMI greater than the 95th percentile or those with a BMI greater than the 85th percentile who perceive their adiposity to be a significant psychosocial problem.
- Finally, identify "problem" foods such as cookies and chips, which are habitual. Encourage the reduced consumption of "problem" foods, rather than worry about the occasional pizza or ice cream treat.
- Enlist parental assistance to plan and structure healthy meals and snacks.

Client Education

- Behavior modification is the most widely recognized and studied approach to weight loss; management includes behavior modification elements.
- Programs using behavior approaches involve the systematic examination of factors preceding and following the target behavior (eating). The core of behavioral approaches is self-monitoring (Foryet & Goodrick, 1993a).
- Stimulus control is based on the concept of controlling the environment and modifying cues that lead to inappropriate eating or exercise (Foryet & Goodrick, 1993a). For example, altering behavior topology, such as the speed at which one eats, has been successful (Foryet & Goodrick, 1993a).
- Contracts, which focus on increasing healthy behaviors associated with weight loss, are used with contingency management in which the individual receives a reward for appropriate behavior (Foryet & Goodrick, 1993a). These weight-loss methods include alterations in cognitive-behavioral patterns. Thinking patterns that are reframed away from self-rejection and toward self-acceptance have been effective in therapy for binge eating (Foryet, 1993).

Family Impact

- The family role in weight loss efforts cannot be overemphasized. Esteem support is demonstrated by such things as verbal reinforcement, using behavioral techniques along with the participant, and attendance at meetings with the participant.
- Informational support includes assistance with monitoring the participant's weight-loss activities and prompting appropriate eating behavior. Instrumental support includes refraining from criticism of the participant's progress (Black, Gleser, & Kooyers, 1990).
- Family involvement in childhood weight management is important. In long-term management of obesity in children, successful programs include those with parents as active participants, family support to encourage behavior changes, and family motivational structures.

Referral/Consultation

Morbidly obese individuals, particularly those with accompanying risks, such as hypertension, and co-morbid chronicity, such as DM, should be referred to specialists.

EVALUATION/FOLLOW-UP

- It is necessary to encourage the weight-loss efforts beyond 20 weeks and provide frequent support to the client in his or her weight management attempts (Perri, Nezu, Patti, & McCann, 1989).
- Recognize that treatment for obesity is generally unsuccessful. Most weight loss attempts are self-directed and are usually the most successful at long-term success: 72% of people who maintained a significant weight loss did so on their own, whereas 20% enrolled in commercial programs, 3% used diet pills, and 5% enrolled in a medical-based program.
- Identify your own personal experiences and beliefs about body image, attractiveness, and the benefits of weight loss.
- The goal of weight loss should be to prevent the associated risks factors related to end-stage organ damage.

REFERENCES

Avila, P., & Hovell, M. F. (1994). Physical activity training for weight loss in Latinas: A controlled study. *International Journal of Obesity Related Metabolic Disorders, 18*(7), 476-482.

Ballor, D. L., & Poehlman, E. T. (1994). Exercise-training enhances fat-free mass preservation during diet-induced weight loss: A meta-analytical finding. *International Journal of Obesity Related Metabolic Disorders, 18,* 35-40.

Berke, E., & Morden, N. (2000). Medical management of obesity. *American Family Physician, 62,* 419-426.

Bjorntorp, P. (1990). "Portal" adipose tissue as a generator of risk factors for cardiovascular disease and diabetes. *Arteriosclerosis, 10,* 493-496.

Bjorntorp, P. (1992). Regional obesity. In P. Bjorntorp & B. N. Brodoff (Eds.), *Obesity.* Philadelphia: Lippincott.

Black, D. R., Gleser, L. J., & Kooyers, K. J. (1990). A meta-analytic evaluation of couples weight-loss programs. *Health Psychology, 9*(3), 330-347.

Blair, S. N. (1993). Evidence for success of exercise in weight loss and control. *Annals of Internal Medicine, 119*(7, pt. 2), 702-706.

Calles-Escadon, J., & Horton, E. S. (1992). The thermogenic role of exercise in the treatment of morbid obesity: A critical evaluation. *American Journal of Clinical Nutrition, 55,* 533s-537s.

Davis, S., Gomez, Y., & Lambert, L. (1993). Primary prevention of obesity in American Indians. *Annals of the New York Academy of Sciences, 699,* 167-180.

Delvin, M. J., Walsh, B. T., & Spitzer, R. L. (1992). Is there another binge eating disorder? A review of the literature on overeating in the absence of bulimia nervosa. *International Journal of Eating Disorders, 11,* 333-337.

Foreyt, J. P., & Goodrick, G. K. (1993a). Evidence for success of behavior modification in weight loss and control. *Annals of Internal Medicine, 119*(7, pt. 2), 698-701.

Foreyt, J. P., & Goodrick, G. K. (1993b). Weight management without dieting. *Nutrition Today 28*(2), 4-9.

Foreyt, J. P., & Goodrick, G. K. (1991). Factors common to successful therapy for the obese patient. *Medical Science and Sports Exercise, 23*(3), 292-297.

Hakala, P. (1994). Weight reduction programs at a rehabilitation center and a health center based on group counseling and individual support: Short- and long-term follow-up study. *International Journal of Obesity Related Metabolic Disorders, 18*(7), 483-489.

Harlan, W. R. (1993). Epidemiology of childhood obesity. *Annals of the New York Academy of Sciences, 699,* 1-5.

Hellmich, N. (1992). Today's kids weigh in heavier. *USA Today,* Sept. 25, 1D.

Himes, J. H., & Dietz, W. H. (1994). Guidelines for overweight in adolescent preventive services: Recommendations from an expert committee. *American Journal of Clinical Nutrition, 9,* 307-316.

Holden, J. H., Darga, L. L., & Olson, S. M. Stettner, D. C., Ardito, E. A., Lucas, C. P. (1992). Long-term follow-up of clients attending a combination very low calorie diet and behaviour therapy weight loss programme. *International Journal of Obesity, 16,* 605-613.

House, T. (1997). Obesity in women: Examining today's issues. *Advanced Nurse Practitioners, 5*(11), 55-59.

Kaplan, N. M. (1989). The deadly quartet: Upper body obesity, glucose intolerance, hypertriglyceridemia, and hypertension. *Archives of Internal Medicine, 149,* 1514-1520.

Kern, P. A., Trozzolino, L., & Wolfe, G. (1994). Combined use of behavioral models and very low calorie diets in weight loss and maintenance. *American Journal of Medicine and Science, 307,* 325-328.

King, A. C., & Tribble, D. L. (1991). The role of exercise in weight reduction in nonathletes. *Sports Medicine, 11*(5), 331-349.

Lohman, T. G. (1992). Advances in body composition assessment. In *Current Issue of Exercise, Science Service* (monograph #3). Champaign, IL: Human Kenetics.

Lyznicki, J., Young, D., Riggs, J., Davis, R. M. (2001). Obesity: Assessment and management in primary care. *American Family Physician, 63,* 2185-2196.

National Institutes of Health and National Heart, Lung, and Blood Institute. (1998). *Clinical guidelines on the identification, evaluation, and treatment of overweight and obesity in adults.* Washington, DC: NIH.

National Institutes of Health Consensus Development Conference Statement. (1983). Health implications of obesity. *Annals of Internal Medicine, 103*(6), 1073-1077.

Perri, M. G., Nezu, A. M., & Patti, E. T., & McCann, K. L. (1989). Effect of length of treatment on weight loss. *Journal of Consulting Clinical Psychology, 57*(3), 450-452.

White, J. H. (1984). The process of embarking on a weight control program. *Health Care for Women International, 5,* 77-91.

Willett, W. C., Manson, J. E., & Stampfer, M. J. (1995). Weight, weight change, and coronary heart disease in women. *Journal of the American Medical Association, 273,* 461-465.

Review Questions

1. Which of the following is the definition for obesity in adults?

   a. Being 20 pounds over optimal weight
   b. Staying within 10% of weight at 18 years of age
   c. BMI greater than 27 kg/m²
   d. BMI greater than 25 kg/m²

2. Obese adults have an increased incidence of which of the following?

   a. Diabetes mellitus, type 2
   b. Depression
   c. Arthritis
   d. Headaches

3. Which of the following is *not* recommended as part of a weight-loss program?

   a. Nutritionally balanced diet
   b. Exercise program
   c. Restricting calories to approximately 500 calories/day less than maintenance
   d. Following a very low calorie diet (i.e., approximately 1,000 calories/day less than maintenance)

4. Which of the following is a serious complication of very low calorie diets?

   a. Ventricular arrhythmias
   b. Gallstones
   c. Decreased metabolism
   d. Urinary tract infections

5. Susan is a client who has been following a low calorie and exercise program. She has lost 10 pounds so far (BMI 27, weight 140). Has she reached the initial goal in weight loss suggested by Lyznicki?

   a. Yes, she should reevaluate how much weight she needs to lose.
   b. It depends on whether her BMI has decreased.
   c. No, she needs to lose 4 more pounds to reach a 10% loss from initial weight.
   d. No, she needs to lose 10 more pounds to reach the 10% loss from initial weight.

6. For which of the following clients is it appropriate to use weight-loss drugs?

   a. Sue, a 45-year-old whose BMI is 27
   b. Steve, a 30-year-old whose BMI is 30
   c. Rhonda, age 20, whose BMI is 22
   d. George, age 38, whose BMI is 24

7. You have prescribed sibutramine (Meridia) for a client. When she returns for follow-up, you observe one of the big side effects of this drug. Which of the following is a reason to discontinue the drug?

   a. Dry mouth
   b. Constipation
   c. Blood pressure (B/P) increase to 148/100
   d. Insomnia

8. A client has been prescribed orlistat (Xenical). Which of the following side effects may cause clients to stop taking the drug?

   a. Oily spotting and steatorrhea
   b. Headache
   c. Interaction with warfarin (Coumadin)
   d. Dry mouth

Answers and Rationales

1. *Answer:* c (analysis/diagnosis)
   Rationale: The National Institutes of Health has identified a BMI greater than 30 kg/m² as being obese (NIH and National Heart, Lung, and Blood Institute, 1998).

2. *Answer:* a (evaluation)
   Rationale: Obesity is associated with an increased incidence of diabetes mellitus, type 2. Obesity is also a risk factor for coronary artery disease, HTN, congestive heart failure, and angina.

3. *Answer:* **d** (implementation/plan)

Rationale: Weight-loss programs recommend a nutritional diet, with approximately 500 kcal/ day less than maintenance. Also, decreasing the amount of fat in the diet is helpful. Very low calorie programs help people lose weight in the short term, but most clients gain the weight back within a year.

4. *Answer:* **a** (evaluation)

Rationale: Most clients who die while following a severe calorie-restricted diet do so because of ventricular arrhythmias or dysrhythmias.

5. *Answer:* **c** (evaluation)

Rationale: The initial goal recommended for weight loss is 10% of initial body weight. Once this goal is achieved, then other goals can be identified.

6. *Answer:* **b** (implementation/plan)

Rationale: Weight-loss drugs should only be used as part of an overall treatment plan, including diet, exercise, and behavior therapy. Current recommendations limit the use of these drugs to people with BMI greater than 30 or BMI greater than 27 with obesity-related risk factors (Lyznicki et al., 2001).

7. *Answer:* **c** (evaluation)

Rationale: All answers are considered side effects of the drug Meridia. Hypertension is a concern, and the drug should be stopped if it raises B/P above a normal level (Berke & Morden, 2001).

8. *Answer:* **a** (evaluation)

Rationale: Orlistat's side effects includes steatorrhea, flatus, fecal incontinence, abdominal bloating, and oily spotting. Clients have more difficulty with symptoms when they consume fatty foods. These side effects cause many clients to stop the medication (Berke & Morden, 2001).

OSGOOD-SCHLATTER DISEASE   *Denise Robinson*

OVERVIEW
Definition

- Osgood-Schlatter (OS) disease is a condition that involves inflammation and pain over the tibial tuberosity.
- Also referred to as epiphysitis or apophysitis of the knee.

Incidence

- OS disease is most common in athletic adolescents or preadolescents and accounts for approximately 28% of musculoskeletal conditions seen in a primary care office.
- It is very common is children ages 10 to 14 who are participating in sports on a regular basis.
- It is more common in males than females.

Pathophysiology

The condition results when tendinitis of the anterior patellar tendon occurs. The patella is embedded in this tendon, and recurrent strain of this tendon results in associated osteochondrosis of the tibial tubercle. In its mildest state, there is avascular necrosis in the region of the tibial tubercle, and hypertrophic cartilage forms in the distal tendon itself in an attempt to repair the injury. Ossicles that are separate from the tubercle have occasionally been found. Severe cases of OS disease may result in an epiphyseal separation of the tibial tubercle.

Protective Factors. Stretching before exercise may be beneficial in that it may limit excessive strain of a tight tendon. Delayed or limited athletic participation until later in adolescence may allow for a longer period of growth and development of tendons, ligaments, and the quadriceps muscles and may help reduce stress of the patellar tendon.

Factors Increasing Susceptibility

- Excessive athletic endeavors, particularly at a young age, increase susceptibility.
- Activities requiring excessive running, jumping, lateral movement of the knees, and contraction of the quadriceps often contribute to the development of OS disease.

ASSESSMENT: SUBJECTIVE/HISTORY
History of Present Illness

- Presents as gradually increasing pain and swelling over the tibial tubercle.
- Pain occurs during or immediately after activity or after direct trauma to the area.
- Pain decreases with cessation of the activity.
- Sudden pain may indicate that there is a pathologic fracture through an area of ischemic necrosis.

Common Symptoms

Pain and swelling over the tibial tuberosity are the cardinal symptoms.

Associated Symptoms

Nighttime leg cramps may occur.

Past Medical History

Noncontributary.

Medication History

Ask what medications, if any, have been taken to decrease the pain.

Family History

No specific correlation between family members has been shown.

Psychosocial History

The client may give a history of increasing athletic participation, trying out for a team, or increasing mileage in runners.

ASSESSMENT: OBJECTIVE/PHYSICAL EXAMINATION

Physical Examination

Tenderness of the tibial tuberosity is present. Mild inflammation may be visible. After long-standing disease, the tibial tuberosity becomes prominent.

Diagnostic Procedures

X-ray examination of the tibia and fibula confirms the enlargement of the tibial tubercle.

DIAGNOSIS

Differential diagnoses include the following:
- Avascular necrosis of the tibial tubercle
- Growing pains
- Hip abnormalities

THERAPEUTIC PLAN

Pharmacologic Treatment

- Nonsteroidal antiinflammatory drugs (NSAIDs) are not usually beneficial, but they may help by providing an analgesic effect.
- Corticosteroids are not recommended because they may weaken the quadriceps tendon and produce local cutaneous thinning and depigmentation.

Nonpharmacologic Treatment

- Rest and avoiding activity that causes repetitive contraction of the quadriceps, or deep-knee bending, may be helpful. In rare cases, a knee immobilizer splint may be helpful.
- Strengthening surrounding muscles, particularly the quadriceps, has been found to be beneficial in some cases. (This can be done with simple lifting exercises that involve placing 1-pound objects such as canned vegetables or dried beans in each of two tube socks tied together and draped across the ankle. The athlete gradually increases repetitions of extension of the lower legs.)
- Recurrent conditions, or those resulting in severe pain, may require a rest period of 6 to 8 weeks.

- Surgery may be required in rare cases for removal of the ossicle.

Client Education

- Rest
- Ice after sports
- Compression with a knee immobilizer (in severe cases)
- Stretching before exercise

Referral/Consultation

- Casting per an orthopedist may be indicated only in very severe cases to allow for full rest. Surgery has been shown to provide relief for clients with ossicle development, but this step is rarely indicated unless long-term conservative therapy is not successful.
- The clinician will want to consult if there is a fracture or the probability of occult fracture (sudden onset of acute pain).
- Also consult for conditions that are unresponsive to standard therapy.

EVALUATION/FOLLOW-UP

- The nurse practitioner (NP) should work with the client to help determine the degree of stress or athletic participation that may be undertaken without significant pain. Clients need to understand how to minimize stress (stretching, supporting muscle strengthening exercises), how to prevent pain (post-participation icing of the tubercle), and how to treat pain (usually NSAIDs).
- Complete resolution of symptoms through physiologic healing (physeal closure) of the tibial tubercle usually takes 12 to 24 months.
- See the client in the office in 1 to 2 weeks after the initial presentation to monitor symptoms and effectiveness of therapy.
- Further follow-up is indicated for acute exacerbation of symptoms or significant changes in symptoms.

REFERENCES

de Inocencio, J. (1998). Musculoskeletal pain in primary pediatric care: Analysis of 1000 consecutive general pediatric visits. *Pediatrics, 102*(6), E63.

Osgood-Schlatter disease: A cause of knee pain in children. (1995). *American Family Physician, 51*(8), 1897-1899.

Kaeding, C. C., & Whitehead, R. (1998). Musculoskeletal injuries in adolescents. *Primary Care, 25*(1), 211-223.

King, P. (2000). Osgood Schlatter. In D. Robinson, P. Kidd, & K. Rogers (Eds.), *Primary care across the lifespan.* St. Louis: Mosby, 817-819.

Szer, I. S. (2000). Musculoskeletal pain in adolescents: "Growing pains" or something else? Part 2. *Consultant, 40*(6), 1061-1065.

Wall, E. J. (1998). Osgood-Schlatter disease: Practical treatment for a self-limiting condition. *Physical Sports Medicine, 26*(3), 29-30, 32-34, 85-86.

Review Questions

1. Dean has been diagnosed with OS disease. Which of the following historical data statements is consistent with this disease?

    a. "I play on a select soccer team."
    b. "I hit my knee while playing softball."
    c. "My left knee has always hurt when I am active."
    d. "I twisted my knee while playing basketball."

2. Which of the following comments by a client with OS disease is consistent with the diagnosis?

    a. "My knee hurts when I run or jump."
    b. "My knee hurts all the time, even when I am not moving."
    c. "My knee only hurts when I twist it."
    d. "My knee only hurts when I try to straighten it."

3. Which of the following physical findings is consistent with OS disease?

    a. Positive varus/valgus test
    b. Positive McMurray test
    c. Localized tenderness and swelling over tibial tubercle
    d. Effusion of the involved knee

4. OS disease must be differentiated from osteochondritis. In comparison with OS disease, osteochondritis is associated with which of the following?

    a. Localized tenderness and swelling over tibial tubercle
    b. Pain at the medial femoral condyle
    c. Positive McMurray's test
    d. Decreased ability to flex knee

5. Of the following people, who is most at risk to develop OS disease?

    a. Teenage girl
    b. Prepubertal boy
    c. Prepubertal girl
    d. Teenage boy

6. Which of the following is the preferred treatment for OS disease?

    a. NSAIDs
    b. Reduction in physical activity
    c. Cast
    d. Corticosteroid injections

7. Which of the following comments by the teenager with OS disease indicates a need for further teaching?

    a. "Icing my leg will help."
    b. "I need to decrease my physical activity."
    c. "I will need to rest my knee for several months to see improvement."
    d. "Quadriceps exercises will help to strengthen my knee."

8. When is physiologic healing of OS disease usually attained?

    a. 2 weeks after reduction in physical activity
    b. When the tibial tubercle fuses to the diaphysis
    c. When excision of the ossicle occurs
    d. When the knee immobilizer is in place for 1 month

Answers and Rationales

1. *Answer:* **a** (assessment)
    Rationale: OS is an overuse syndrome that occurs in physically active males (King, 2000).

2. *Answer:* **a** (assessment)
    Rationale: OS is an overuse syndrome; the pain occurs with running, jumping, going up steps, and kneeling.

3. *Answer:* **c** (assessment)
    Rationale: OS presents with tenderness of the tibial tubercle.

4. *Answer:* **b** (analysis/diagnosis)
    Rationale: Osteochondritis is another overuse syndrome that occurs in teenage boys (King, 2000).

5. *Answer:* **d** (analysis/diagnosis)
    Rationale: Teenaged boys are more at risk to develop OS disease (King, 2000).

6. *Answer:* **b** (implementation/plan)
    Rationale: The preferred treatment for OS is reduction in physical activities. NSAIDs are not effective other than for pain relief. Corticosteroid injections can weaken the quadriceps. Casting is reserved only for severe cases.

7. *Answer:* **a** (evaluation)
    Rationale: Rest and exercises are appropriate for OS disease. Several months of rest may be required to see improvement in the pain. Ice may provide short-term relief but does not help in the condition itself (King, 2000).

8. *Answer:* **b** (evaluation)
    Rationale: Physiologically, OS is caused by cartilage detachment during a growth spurt. It is considered traction apophysitis. Healing occurs over a period of months (Wall, 1998).

OSTEOARTHRITIS *Pamela Kidd*

OVERVIEW
Definition

- Osteoarthritis (OA) is defined as a degenerative disease of the cartilage of joints with reactive formation of new bone at articular margins.
- Primary OA is the most common form. Its cause is unknown and it affects most commonly the distal interphalangeal (DIP) joints and less commonly, the proximal interphalangeal (PIP) joints, the metatarsophalangeal and carpometacarpal joints of the hip, knee, metatarsophalangeal joint of the big toe, and cervical and lumbar spine.
- Secondary OA may occur in any joint as a result of articular injury (fracture, overuse of joint, or metabolic disease) resulting from either intraarticular (including rheumatoid arthritis, congential dislocation of hip) or extraarticular causes.

Incidence

- OA is the most common form of arthritis and affects approximately 20 million Americans.
- Ninety percent of people have radiographic evidence of OA by age 40 in weight-bearing joints.

Pathophysiology

Cartilage thickens initially but then collagen starts to break down and cartilage ulcers can occur. Remodeling of bone (osteocyte formation) occurs, leading to spur formation. The joint capsule thickens, chronic synovitis develops, and periarticular muscle wasting appears.

Factors Increasing Susceptibility
- Age
- Heredity, with equal distribution across genders
- Repetitive motion/stress to a joint
- Obesity

Protective Factors
- Non–weight-bearing exercise
- Estrogen
- Ascorbic acid (may inhibit lysosomal enzymes that destroy cartilage)

ASSESSMENT: SUBJECTIVE/HISTORY
Symptoms

- Ask about duration of symptoms, morning stiffness, pain, systemic symptoms.
- Ask about insidious onset, morning stiffness of less than 30 minutes, pain on movement, limitation of movement, pain relieved by rest, nocturnal pain after vigorous exercise
- Inquire how OA affects activities of daily living (ADLs) or instrumental activities of daily living (IADLs).

Medication History

Use of antiinflammatory or analgesic agents (results, any other prescribed or OTC medications)

Family History

Inquire about family history of OA.

Dietary History

Overall nutritional assessment with emphasis on weight reduction, if necessary.

ASSESSMENT: OBJECTIVE/PHYSICAL EXAMINATION
Physical Examination

A problem-oriented physical examination should be conducted, keeping in mind potential systemic manifestations of rheumatoid arthritis (RA) (e.g., dermatologic, pleurisy, splenomegaly, ocular manifestations), which might necessitate a complete physical examination. Pay attention to the following:

- Assess vital signs, weight, B/P, pulse. Note general appearance, gait, and activity level.
- Inspect musculoskeletal system. Inspect affected joints for deformities, nodes, numbers of affected joints, symmetry of affected joints, erythema. Affects joints with the greatest load (hips, knees, and ankles). Heberden nodules may occur in females (autosomal trait) in the interphalangeal joints.
- Observe affected joints in active and passive range of motion.
- Palpate affected joints for warmth, tenderness, crepitus, and edema. Crepitus, joint instability, negative deformity, Heberden's nodes, valgus/varus deformities, negative joint effusion, quadricep atrophy.
- Assess muscle strength.
- Assess joint stability.

Diagnostic Procedures

- Obtain radiographic evidence of narrowing of joint space, soft tissue swelling, and marginal osteophytes.
- Erythrocyte sedimentation rate (ESR), complete blood count (CBC), uric acid level, and C-reactive protein may be ordered to support OA as a diagnosis of exclusion.

DIAGNOSIS

Because articular inflammation is absent or minimal and systemic manifestations are absent, OA is seldom confused; however, diagnosis is not always straightforward. In those instances, the following conditions may be included in the differential diagnoses of OA: rheumatoid arthritis, gout, pseudogout, psoriatic arthritis, septic arthritis, malignancy, osteoporosis, and tendinitis (bursitis). (See Table 3-78.)

TABLE **3-78** Differential Diagnosis of Osteoarthritis

Gout/pseudogout	Acute onset, typically nocturnal, monoarticular
	Hyperuricemia
	Asymptomatic between episodes
	Quick response to NSAIDs
	Pseudogout: acute, recurrent but not chronic, involving principally knees and wrists
Psoriatic arthritis	Psoriasis precedes arthritis in 80% of cases
	Asymmetric arthritis
	No rheumatoid factor present
	Commonly sacroiliac joint involvement
	Usual lack of osteoporosis
	May have ankylosing spondylitis
Septic arthritis	Sudden onset
	Usually monarticular, often in weight-bearing joints
	Infection with causative organisms elsewhere in body
	Large joint effusions
Osteoporosis	Spontaneous fractures
	Loss of height
	Demineralization especially of hip, spine, pelvis

THERAPEUTIC PLAN
Nonpharmacologic Treatment

- Massage
- Distraction
- Heat or cold application to affected area
- Whirlpool
- Swimming

Pharmacologic Treatment

- The objectives of therapy are to restore function, relieve pain, and maintain joint motion.
- Analgesics such as acetaminophen and aspirin are often adequate to control the pain associated with OA. Because the role of inflammation is not well-defined, the use of stronger NSAID medications should be considered as second-line. Enteric-coated aspirin to reduce GI upset is recommended.

NOTE: *Gastropathy associated with the use of NSAIDs is a major U.S. health problem. When possible, prescribe Cox2 inhibitors (Vioxx, Celebrex). Risk factors for GI hemorrhage include advanced age, previous or present peptic ulcer disease, previous GI hemorrhage, alcoholism, and use of concomitant anticoagulants or high-dose corticosteroids. Nonacetylated salicylates produce the least inhibition of platelet aggregation. See Table 3-79.*

Client Education

- Weight loss, if needed
- Exercise to maintain ROM and increase strength
- Periods of rest during the day
- Proper posture
- Use of assistive aids: canes, walkers, crutches
- Heat and cold to relieve muscle spasm and provide pain relief
- Physical therapy
- Surgery in some cases

Referral/Consultation

- Orthopedic surgeon for joint replacement or arthroscopic procedures as needed for inadequate pain relief and limitation with ADLs
- Physical therapy for flexibility and strength training

TABLE **3-79** Pharmacologic Considerations: Osteoarthritis

DRUG	CONSIDERATION
Acetaminophen	Use in mild-moderate joint pain without inflammation. Good choice for hypertensive client; no sodium retention.
NSAIDs	Promotes sodium and water retention, GI upset; new Cox2 inhibitors effects on kidneys not well established. Worse if client is taking antihypertensive medication.
Tramadol (Ultram)	Synthetic opioid agonist. No effect on blood pressure. Use with NSAID can decrease the dose of the NSAID than when using NSAID alone.
Glucosamine and Chondrotin	Nutritional supplement. Clinical improvement in symptoms is achieved, but the mechanism is not known. Safety and purity of supplement have not been assured.

GI, Gastrointestinal; *NSAIDs,* nonsteroidal antiinflammatory drugs.

Prevention

- Detection of congenital hip dislocation with proper treatment
- Non–weight-bearing exercise or decreasing high-impact activities
- Proper weight

EVALUATION/FOLLOW-UP

- Evaluate monthly with change in medication or post physical therapy referral.
- May need more frequent follow-up if client is also hypertensive and using NSAIDs.

COMPLICATIONS

- Joint failure
- Immobility
- Fractures, falls

REFERENCES

Birchfield, P. (2000). Arthritis. In D. Robinson, P. Kidd, & K. Rogers (Eds.), *Primary care across the lifespan.* St. Louis: Mosby.

Campbell, J., & Linc, L. (1999). Managing osteoarthritis pain. *ADVANCE for Nurse Practitioners, 7*(4), 57-58, 60.

Center for Health Information. (2001). *A focus on management of osteoarthritis in older adults with hypertension.* Chicago: Center for Health Information.

Puppione, A. (1999). Treatment strategies for older adults with osteoarthritis: How to promote and maintain function. *Journal of the American Academy of Nurse Practitioners, 11,* 167-171.

Review Questions

1. Which of the following statements about OA is *true?*
   a. "OA is a reversible degenerative disease."
   b. "OA is associated with exacerbations and remissions."
   c. "OA is a degenerative disease of the cartilage of the joints."
   d. "OA is an autoimmune process."

2. Joints commonly involved in OA are all of the following, *except:*
   a. Hip
   b. Neck
   c. Knee
   d. Interphalangeal joints

3. The pathologic condition of OA is caused by which of the following?
   a. Osteocyte formation
   b. Cartilage metabolism
   c. Muscle wasting
   d. Autoimmune dysfunction

4. OA is characterized by all of the following, *except:*
   a. Joint effusions
   b. Crepitus
   c. Joint pain
   d. Muscle atrophy

5. How long does joint stiffness in OA last?
   a. Less than 30 minutes
   b. All day
   c. 1 hour
   d. No stiffness

6. Diagnosis of OA is confirmed by which of the following?
   a. Physical examination
   b. Joint film
   c. C-reactive protein level
   d. ESR

7. What is first-line therapy for OA?
   a. Aspirin
   b. Ibuprofen
   c. Cox2 inhibitor (Vioxx)
   d. Tramadol (Ultram)

8. Radiographic findings in OA include all *except* which of the following?
   a. Narrowing of synovial space
   b. Effusion in the synovial space
   c. Calcific body formation
   d. Soft tissue swelling

Answers and Rationales

1. *Answer:* **c** (analysis/diagnosis)
   Rationale: Rheumatoid arthritis is an autoimmune process with exacerbations and remissions. OA is not reversible.

2. *Answer:* **b** (assessment)
   Rationale: The cervical spine is not frequently involved.

3. *Answer:* **b** (analysis/diagnosis)
   Rationale: The first step in a degenerative process is the cartilage breakdown, which leads to remodeling of bone and spur formation. Muscle wasting appears late in the disease.

4. *Answer:* **a** (assessment)
   Rationale: Effusions are associated with inflammatory processes. OA is a degenerative process.

5. *Answer:* **a** (assessment)
   Rationale: In RA, stiffness lasts longer. Mobility improves stiffness in OA instead of increasing inflammation in RA.

6. *Answer:* **b** (analysis/diagnosis)
   Rationale: C-reactive protein and ESR may be obtained to rule out autoimmune diseases (RA). Physical examination may be highly suspicious, but only radiograph films can confirm the diagnosis.

7. *Answer:* **a** (implementation/plan)
   Rationale: Because inflammation is not severe in OA, aspirin should be tried first for pain relief. Ibuprofen would be next, followed by Cox2 inhibitors then tramadol, unless the client has GI disease.

8. *Answer:* **b** (analysis/diagnosis)
   Rationale: Effusion occurs with inflammation, not with cartilage metabolism.

OSTEOPOROSIS *Cheryl Pope Kish*

OVERVIEW
Definition

Osteoporosis is a systemic skeletal disease characterized by low bone mass and microarchitectural deterioration of bone tissue, leading to enhanced bone fragility and consequent increase in fracture risk. Primary osteoporosis refers to deterioration of bone mass that is not associated with chronic illness or medication use; rather, it relates to aging and decreased gonadal function. Secondary osteoporosis is associated with chronic conditions that contribute to significant accelerated bone loss.

Incidence

Osteoporosis is considered a major health threat for 25 million U.S. citizens, 80% of whom are women. Osteoporosis accounts for 1.5 million fractures annually. American women are more likely to die from a hip fracture or its sequelae than from breast cancer.

Pathophysiology

- Throughout life, new bone is constantly being formed by osteoblasts, and older bone is being resorbed by osteoclasts. Bone loss represents a net deficit in the bone remodeling cycle. After peak bone mass is reached around the age of 30, there is a small deficit in bone formation during each cycle of bone remodeling. One cause of net deficit is the low estrogen state associated with menopause.

- Trabecular bone sites such as the spine, pelvis, distal radius, and femur are generally the first to show osteoporotic changes. These represent common sites of osteoporotic fractures. Further aging brings greater bone loss in cancellous and cortical bone that leads to hip fracture.

- Box 3-14 lists the causes of secondary osteoporosis.

Protective Factors

- Black race, obesity, early menarche
- Estrogen replacement therapy (ERT) immediately after menopause (retards menopause, related acceleration of bone loss)

Factors Increasing Susceptibility

- Increasing age
- White or Asian race
- Family history
- Small stature
- Smoking
- Physical inactivity
- Female gender
- Early menopause
- Low body weight
- Low calcium intake
- Excessive alcohol intake
- High caffeine intake

Box 3-14   Secondary Causes of Osteoporosis

ENDOCRINOPATHIES
Hypercortisolism
Hyperthyroidism
Hyperparathyroidism
Hypogonadism
Hyperprolactemia

DRUGS
Corticosteroids
L-thyroxine
Heparin
Barbiturates
Phenytoin
Methotrexate
Alcohol
Aluminum-containing antacids
Tobacco
Isoniazid

OTHER CONDITIONS
Immobilization
Diabetes mellitus
Chronic renal disease
Hepatic disease
Scurvy
Chronic obstructive lung disease
Rheumatoid arthritis
Osteomalacia
Systemic mastocytosis
Malabsorption

GENETIC CONDITIONS
Marfan's syndrome
Osteogenesis imperfecta
Klinefelter's syndrome
Turner's syndrome
Ehler's Danlos syndrome
Homocystinuria

ASSESSMENT: SUBJECTIVE/HISTORY
History of Present Illness

- Often asymptomatic
- Negative self-image because clothes do not fit right
- With vertebral fractures, acute pain with a sudden onset, localized to specific vertebrae with local tenderness and radiating bilaterally; pain that subsides within 2 to 6 weeks
- Constipation secondary to painful bowel irritation and compression
- Possible modest-to-moderate scoliosis or kyphosis, especially if fracture occurs at T2-T11
- Chronic pain in the paraspinal muscles that localizes to the lumbar area even when a fracture occurs in the thoracic area; pain in mid-back with activity
- Hip fractures associated with falls that are painful, with distortion of the leg and an inability to bear weight on the leg
- Kyphosis
- Protuberant abdomen
- Abdominal discomfort
- Back pain

Past Medical History

- Fractures
- Scoliosis
- Loss of 1.5 cm or more of height (based on maximum self-reported height)
- Age of menarche
- Late menarche
- Athletic amenorrhea
- Amenorrhea secondary to anorexia nervosa
- Hyperprolactinemia
- Gonadotropin-releasing hormone agonist therapy
- Premature or surgical menopause
- Irregular menses
- Oligomenorrhea
- Malignancies such as multiple myeloma
- Endocrinopathies such as hypogonadism if male
- Seizures (treatment with phenytoin)

Medication History

- Current and past medications
- ERT

Family History

- Osteoporosis
- Maternal hip fracture (most strongly associated with osteoporosis)

Psychosocial History

- Ask about current and lifetime physical activity patterns (include types of exercise and recreational sports).
- Calculate packs/years of cigarette smoking.
- Evaluate for alcohol use; determine whether the client drinks more than two drinks per day.
- Determine level of exercise in job and leisure activity and amount of time exposed to sunlight.

Dietary History

- Review over the lifetime anything affecting nutrition: eating disorders, gastrectomy or intestinal bypass surgery, malabsorption syndrome, diet high in protein, caffeine, sodium, and phosphorus and low in calcium.
- Use of dairy products is a good guide to evaluating calcium intake.

ASSESSMENT: OBJECTIVE/PHYSICAL EXAMINATION
Physical Examination

- Generally a complete history and physical examination is indicated to rule out other pathologic conditions.
- Observe for visible deformity of the spine (e.g., dorsal kyphosis).
- Record height and compare with self-reported maximum height.

Diagnostic Procedures
Laboratory Procedures

- Obtain laboratory data to rule out other pathologic conditions and to identify secondary causes of osteoporosis.
- CBC, ESR, serum calcium, phosphorus, alkaline phosphatase, creatinine levels, liver function tests, thyroid function tests, urine calcium, and glucose are normal in uncomplicated osteoporosis.
- Abnormalities suggest secondary pathologic conditions.
- Deoxypyridinoline and N-telopeptides are biochemical markers of bone resorption. In a client who is unable to obtain dual-energy x-ray absorptiometry (DEXA), a high level of urinary deoxypyridinoline or N-telopeptide suggests active bone turnover and high future fracture risk.

Radiographic Procedures

- Measurement of bone mass confirms the existence of osteoporosis. Low bone mass increases the risk of fracture.
- DEXA is the preferred method because of its 10-minute scan time, precision, and low radiation exposure. The spine and hip are commonly scanned. DEXA is a good technique for assessing future fracture risk.
- Dual-energy photon absorptiometry (DPA) is the next preferred method; however, the scan time is longer than with DEXA.
- Single-energy photon absorptiometry (SPA) is limited to peripheral sites.
- Quantitative computed tomography (QCT) has a higher cost and radiation exposure.

- Bone density testing: The National Osteoporosis Foundation Clinical Guidelines recommend determining bone mass measurements for the following:
  - Estrogen-deficient women
  - A vertebral abnormality that is seen on radiography
  - Initiation of glucocorticosteroid therapy
  - Presence of primary hyperparathyroidism
- Interpretation of bone density testing is based on a T score, which refers to the number of standard deviations above (+) or below (–) the average value in young adults of the same gender (the control group).
  - Normal bone density = T score greater than –1.
  - Osteopenia is low bone mass indicated by a T score between –1 and –2.5.
  - Osteoporosis is a bone density indicated by a T score less than –2.5 or the presence of fragility fractures, irrespective of the bone density test results (McClung, 1999).
- The following lists expected findings in osteoporotic women:
  - Decreased radiodensity
  - Changes in vertebral body shape
  - Generalized osteopenia
  - Fractures (particularly vertebral compression fractures)

DIAGNOSIS

For information on differential diagnosis, refer to Box 3-14.

Children

- Physical activity and dietary calcium influence the bone mass of the developing skeleton; these may each contribute up to 40% of the total variance in bone density.
- Weight-bearing recreational activities such as basketball, soccer, and tennis are associated with a modest increase in bone mass at the radius and hip and to a lesser extent in the spine.
- Participation in non–weight-bearing activities such as bicycling and swimming is associated with either no change or a reduction in bone mass.

Adolescents

Early behavioral factors such as diet, smoking, alcohol use, and exercise are major determinants of peak bone mass in later life and therefore osteoporosis.

THERAPEUTIC PLAN

- The objective is to increase bone mineral density and decrease the risk of osteoporotic fractures.
- Consult with a physician regarding suspected fractures in the presence of secondary causes or complicated cases.
- The plan depends on client problems (e.g., care of client with fracture, physical therapy for soft tissue trauma).

Pharmacologic Treatment

- ERT may be used.
- Treatment with biphosphate. Alendronate (Fosamax) may be used if not contraindicated.
  - Biphosphate decreases bone resorption and prevents bone loss.
  - Biphosphate binds to hydroxyapatite and specifically inhibits the activity of osteoclasts; inhibits osteoclastic resorption.
  - Prescribe 10 mg/day to be taken 30 minutes before breakfast with a full glass of water.
  - Instruct the client to wait at least 30 minutes in an upright position before eating or drinking anything else.
  - Instruct the client to take calcium and vitamin D supplement to increase bone mass.
  - Persons living in northern climates in winter may need to increase their vitamin D during this time.
  - Side effects of nausea and abdominal pain are common.
- Intranasal calcitonin may be used.
  - Suppresses osteoclast activity and subsequently bone resorption.
  - Has an analgesic effect on osteoporotic fracture pain.
  - Prescribe 200 IU/day; 1 puff in one nostril, alternating nostrils each day.
  - Prescribe adequate calcium and vitamin D concurrently.
  - Reserved for clients with severe osteoporotic fractures and skeletal pain.
- Calcium supplements may be used.
  - Prescribe calcium carbonate, citrate, or phosphate, usually 1000 to 1500 mg/day divided into two separate doses to be taken between or after meals or at bedtime.
  - Tums and several other brands of antacids contain calcium carbonate in varying strengths (read label). Os-Cal is a chewable tablet, but it is generally more expensive than Tums.
  - Avoid calcium tablets made from bone meal or dolomite because they contain lead, mercury, or arsenic.

Prevention

- Prevention begins in childhood and continues throughout life.
- The NP should consider teaching the following to every client of any age as appropriate:

Exercise

- Assist the client to develop a plan that allows for gradual buildup of muscle strength and endurance.
- Advise the client to avoid excessive exercise (e.g., marathon running).

O

- Encourage regular, diverse, weight-bearing exercise two to three times weekly. Treadmill, climbing a Stairmaster, tennis, using a Nordic-track apparatus, and low-impact aerobics are desirable.

Calcium Intake
- See Table 3-80 for dietary sources (preferred).
- See Table 3-81 for optimal requirements.
- Average calcium intake in diet at age 40 to 65 is 450 to 650 mg/day.
- Calcium is needed on a consistent basis.
- Only elemental calcium is absorbed. Elemental calcium by type of calcium is as follows:

  Calcium carbonate   40%
  Calcium phosphate   39%
  Calcium citrate   24%
  Calcium lactate   13%
  Calcium gluconate   9%
- Taking calcium supplements between meals increases bioavailability.
- Calcium carbonate absorption is impaired in persons who have an absence of gastric acid; these persons should take calcium carbonate with food.
- Calcium citrate does not require gastric acid for absorption and can be used in older adults who have reduced gastric acid.
- Advise the client to take 500 mg calcium hs. Take 500 mg bid if a larger dose is required.
- Advise the client to add a multivitamin with 400 mg vitamin D qd to ensure adequate absorption.
- There is a risk of ectopic calcium deposition if too much vitamin D is ingested.

Estrogen Replacement Therapy
- Counsel postmenopausal women regarding ERT; it is never too late, but immediate replacement is preferable.
- Benefits: Prevents bone loss and osteoporotic fractures; may protect some from coronary artery disease; elevates HDL levels; relieves menopausal/genitourinary symptoms.

- Risks and side effects are intermittent bleeding, breast tenderness, abdominal fullness, weight gain.
- More serious side effects are HTN, thrombosis, migraine headaches, endometrial hyperplasia. Relationship to breast cancer is undetermined.
- Progesterone is used in conjunction with estrogen if uterus is present to avoid endometrial cancer; omitted after hysterectomy.
- No difference in increase in bone mass with type or method of estrogen.

TABLE 3-81 Optimum Calcium Requirements Recommended by the National Institutes of Health Consensus Panel

AGE GROUP	OPTIMAL DAILY INTAKE OF CALCIUM (MG)
INFANTS	
Birth to 6 months	400
6 months to 1 year	600
CHILDREN	
1 to 5 years	800
6 to 10 years	800-1200
ADOLESCENTS/YOUNG ADULTS	
11 to 24 years	1200-1500
MEN	
25 to 65 years	1000
Older than 65 years	1500
WOMEN	
25 to 50 years	1000
Older than 50 years (postmenopausal)	1500
On estrogens	1000
Not on estrogens	1500
Older than 65 years	1500
Pregnant and nursing	1200-1500

From National Institutes of Health Consensus Conference. (1994). Optimal calcium intake. *Journal of the American Medical Association, 272,* 1943.

TABLE **3-80**   Calcium Content of Selected Foods

DAIRY FOODS*	CALCIUM CONTENT (MG)	NONDAIRY FOODS*	CALCIUM CONTENT (MG)
Skim milk	300	Calcium-fortified orange juice	300
Whole milk	290	Oysters, raw, 13-19	226
Yogurt (plain, no-fat)	415	Salmon, canned, 3 oz.	167
Frozen yogurt (fruit)	240	Sardines, canned with bones	372
Swiss chess, 1 oz.	270	Collard greens, cooked	357
Cheddar, mozzarella cheese, 1 oz.	205	Turnip greens, cooked	252
Part-skim ricotta cheese, 4 oz.	335	Broccoli, cooked	100
Vanilla ice cream	176	Soybeans, cooked	131
Cottage cheese (low-fat), 4 oz.	78	Tofu, 4 oz.	108
		Almonds, 1 oz.	75

*1 cup unless otherwise specified.

- Regular breast examinations, mammograms, pelvic and Pap smears are necessary.
- Tamoxifen increases bone mass but is not used for primary treatment.

Fall Prevention (Older Adults)

- Wear flat, rubber-soled shoes.
- Use cane or walker as needed.
- Use proper lifting techniques.
- Assess number and types of medications.
- Check visual acuity.
- Assist with home safety modifications, including provision of hand grips, safety mats, adequate lighting, and removal of clutter.

Screening

- Use bone density testing for clients who have several osteoporotic risk factors and as a baseline measurement before pharmacologic treatment.
- According to National Osteoporosis Foundation Clinical Guidelines, bone mass measurements should be obtained in estrogen-deficit women as part of the consideration for the use of hormone replacement or the need for other treatment modalities.
  - For women whose bone mass is 1 SD below the mean peak bone mass, hormone replacement or some other form of treatment should be recommended.
  - Women with bone mass 1 SD above the mean require no intervention.
  - Women with bone mass within 1 SD of the mean should be followed with measurements taken at 1- to 5-year intervals, depending on the initial value.

EVALUATION/FOLLOW-UP

- Prevention: Maintenance of adequate bone mass throughout life without fractures
- Screening: High-risk clients identified and therapy instituted
- Pharmacologic therapy: Resolution of client problems, decrease in advancement of osteoporosis, and/or prevention of complications such as excess disability

REFERENCES

Berarducci, A., & Lengacher, C. A. (1998). Osteoporosis in perimenopausal women: Current perspectives. *American Journal of Nurse Practitioners, 2*(9), 9-14.

Burki, R. E. (1999). Trends in osteoporosis management. *Clinical Advisor,* February, 22-29.

Crandall, C. (2001). Osteoporosis: New guidelines for screening and diagnosis. *Consultant,* February, 247-250.

Crandall, C. (2001). Osteoporosis: Update on prevention and treatment. *Consultant,* February, 259-265.

Kessenich, C. R. (2000). Osteoporosis in primary care: The role of biochemical markers and diagnostic imaging. *American Journal of Nurse Practitioners, 4*(2), 24-29.

Kish, C. P. (2002). A 49-year-old Asian woman with osteoporosis. In D. L. Robinson (Ed.), *Clinical decision making for nurse practitioners in primary care: A case study approach.* Philadelphia: Lippincott.

Lawson, M. T. (2001). Evaluating and managing osteoporosis in men. *Nurse Practitioner, 26*(5), 26-51.

Levin, R. M. (1999). Controversies in the prevention and management of osteoporosis. In *Comprehensive approach to osteoporosis: Diagnosis and management.* Lexington, MA: NPACE.

Lucata, A. (1999). Update on osteoporosis: Strategies for prevention and treatment. *Women's Health Primary Care, 2*(3), 229-244.

McClung, B. L. (1999). Using osteoporosis management to reduce fractures in elderly women. *Nurse Practitioner, 24*(3), 26-42.

National Institutes of Health Consensus Conference. (1994). Optimal calcium intake. *Journal of the American Medical Association, 272,* 1943.

Rousseau, M. E. (1998). Dietary prevention of osteoporosis. *Lippincott Primary Care Practice, 1*(5), 307-319.

Schussheim, D. H., & Siris, E. S. (1998). Osteoporosis: Update on prevention and treatment. *Women's Health Primary Care, 1*(2), 133-140.

Siris, E. S., & Schussheim, D. H. (1998). Osteoporosis: Assessing your patient's risk. *Women's Health Primary Care, 1*(1), 99-106.

South-Paul, J. E. (2001). Osteoporosis: Part I. Evaluation and assessment. *American Family Physician, 63,* 897-904, 908.

South-Paul, J. E. (2001). Osteoporosis: Part II. Nonpharmacologic and pharmacologic treatment, *American Family Physician, 63,* 1121-1128.

The continuing challenge of osteoporosis. (2000). Supplement to *The Female Patient,* September, 1-16.

Woodhead, G. A., & Moss, M. M. (1998). Osteoporosis: Diagnosis and prevention. *Nurse Practitioner, 23*(11), 18, 23-32.

Review Questions

Situation: Mrs. Jones, a 57-year-old obese white woman, has a thoracic vertebral fracture. The DEXA reveals generalized osteopenia. Past medical history includes anorexia nervosa between the ages of 14 and 20 years, cigarette smoking and coffee drinking all her life, gastrectomy for peptic ulcer disease at age 40, hysterectomy at age 40, and a seizure disorder since age 20. Medication is phenytoin (Dilantin).

1. Which of the following is *not* a risk factor for osteoporosis?
   a. Gastrectomy
   b. Smoking
   c. Anorexia nervosa
   d. Obesity

2. Which of the following would be expected on Mrs. Jones' physical examination?
   a. Dorsal kyphosis
   b. Scoliosis
   c. Lordosis
   d. No loss of height

3. Given Mrs. Jones' history, she would be classified as which of the following?
   a. Primary, type I osteoporosis
   b. Primary, type II osteoporosis
   c. Secondary osteoporosis
   d. Both primary and secondary osteoporosis

4. Assume that results from breast, pelvic, and Pap smears are normal. Considering Mrs. Jones' age and condition, which of the following should be done?

    a. Discuss starting ERT immediately.
    b. Delay ERT for 1 year.
    c. Do not recommend ERT.
    d. Prescribe only calcium citrate.

5. Mrs. Jones returns 3 weeks later for evaluation. If therapy is successful, all the following should happen, *except:*

    a. Acute pain to subside
    b. Absence of pain
    c. Increased mobility
    d. Dorsal kyphosis

Answers and Rationales

1. *Answer:* **d** (assessment)
Rationale: Obesity is a protective factor for osteoporosis.

2. *Answer:* **a** (assessment)
Rationale: Dorsal kyphosis is a likely finding with vertebral fracture at the thoracic level. One would not expect this patho-logic condition to cause scoliosis or lordosis. With vertebral fractures, there is usually some loss of height.

3. *Answer:* **d** (analysis/diagnosis)
Rationale: It is likely that both types of osteoporosis exist. Mrs. Jones' age, the absence of ERT, combined with prema-ture surgical hysterectomy predisposes her to osteoporosis, which would be accentuated by smoking and caffeine and alcohol intake. Her history of gastrectomy and phenytoin (Dilantin) use predisposes her to secondary osteoporosis.

4. *Answer:* **a** (implementation/plan)
Rationale: It is never too late to benefit from ERT, and there is no benefit in delaying treatment.

5. *Answer:* **b** (evaluation)
Rationale: Acute pain should have subsided. Absence of pain and resolution of the dorsal kyphosis are unrealistic ther-apeutic goals at 3 weeks after the fracture. The kyphosis may not disappear, and it may take several more weeks for the pain to subside.

OTITIS *Denise Robinson*

OVERVIEW
Definition

Otitis media (OM) is an inflammation of the middle ear. Acute OM is defined as the presence of fluid in the mid-dle ear associated with signs or symptoms of acute local or systemic illness. There is inflammation and bulging of the tympanic membrane (TM), along with ear pain with OM. Otitis media with effusion (OME) is defined as the pres-ence of fluid in the middle ear in the absence of signs or symptoms of acute infection.

    Classification. Acute OM lasts approximately 3 weeks. Onset is typically rapid, but may be subtle or insidious. The TM bulges and is erythematous, injected, and opaque. An effusion develops in the middle ear, causing poor tympanic membrane mobility.

    Subacute OM is defined as acute OM that lasts 4 to 8 weeks. The tympanic membrane may remain purulent or have a serous appearance. The drum may continue to bulge slightly, retract, or even return to its normal position. Tym-panic mobility is decreased as a result of effusion.

    OME presents longer than 8 weeks. TM is usually in retracted position. Effusion becomes thick and mucoid. Effusion may be clear or dark. Air bubbles signify a higher likelihood that the effusion will resolve; otherwise, referral to an ear, nose, and throat specialist for ventilation tube placement may be appropriate.

    Otitis externa (OE) is an infection of the external auditory canal, commonly known as swimmer's ear.

Incidence
OM

- Second only to upper respiratory infections (URIs) for largest number of office visits for children.
- Accounts for 24.5 million pediatric visits per year.
- Peak incidence is 6 to 36 months; it is least frequent in the 4- to 7-year-old age group.
- Risk is greater for boys, children in day care, those whose parents smoke, and children who have not been breast-fed.
- Peak occurrence is October through April, with a decline in summer.

OE

- Affects all ages.
- Occurs following swimming, aggressive cleaning of ear canal, and trauma.

Pathophysiology

    OM. OM typically follows a URI. The most accepted theory is that the eustachian tubes become blocked from chronic negative pressure. This leads to formulation of fluid or effusions in the middle ear. This fluid becomes infected and inflamed, causing bulging of the TM.

Common Organisms Causing OM

- *Streptococcus pneumonia* (31%) (Gram positive, no beta lactamase producing)
- *Haemophilus influenza* (22%) (Gram negative, 20% to 40% beta lactamase producing)

Moraxella catarrhalis (7%) (Gram negative, 90% beta lactamase producing)

OE. Trauma or excessive dryness or wetness can cause a change in the pH of the ear canal from acid to alkaline, making the external canal susceptible to superinfection. Organisms that cause external OM include the following:
- *Staphylococcus aureus*
- *Pseudomonas* (most common)
- *Streptococcus pneumococcus*
- *Candida aspergillus*

Factors Increasing Susceptibility to OM
- Anatomic anomalies of the midface
- Eskimo, Latino, or Native American ethnicity
- Sibling or parent with chronic otitis
- Allergies, such as atopic dermatitis or asthma
- Day care attendance

Protective Factor. Breastfeeding.

Factors Increasing Susceptibility to OE
- Trauma to ear canal from aggressive cleaning
- Excessive dryness of ear canal
- Excessive moisture of ear canal
- Frequent swimming/showering
- High humidity
- Underlying dermatitis

ASSESSMENT: SUBJECTIVE/HISTORY
Symptoms
OM
- Usually preceded by upper respiratory symptoms.
- Otalgia is often worse at night.
- Otorrhea usually signifies rupture of the TM.
- Hearing loss is corrected once the effusion resolves.
- Fever is absent in one third of cases.
- Diminished appetite may be present.
- The client may have restless or little sleep.
- Diarrhea or vomiting may be present.
- Tinnitus may be present.
- Infants may pull at ears, although this is not a reliable sign because it can be habitual. Often will not suck on bottle or breast.
- Toddlers can often talk about ear pain.
- For school-age children and adults, primary symptom is ear pain.
- In older adults, OM is less common, but may not exhibit fever.

OE
- Otalgia
- Pain when ear is moved
- Ear discharge

Past Medical History
- Ask about infants who drink bottle while lying down.

- Determine exposure to smoke
- Ask about allergies (including atopic dermatitis and asthma) and any craniofacial abnormalities.
- Ask about episodes of otitis, hearing loss.
- Ask about myringotomy (PE) tubes.

Medication History
Ask about recent use of antibiotics and any other medications.

Family History
- Inquire about siblings or parents with frequent otitis.
- Determine family history of allergies.
- Determine exposure to smoke.

Psychosocial History
- Ask about frequent absences from school.
- Ask about day care attendance.
- Frequent swimming or showering is a risk factor.

Dietary History
OM may be associated with food allergies.

ASSESSMENT: OBJECTIVE/PHYSICAL EXAMINATION
Physical Examination
- Obtain vital signs (weight is needed for children for drug dosing purposes).
- Perform a thorough examination of head, eyes, ears, nose, throat, heart, lungs, and skin.
- Check TM position, color, translucency, mobility (best indicator of infection).
- In acute OM, membrane usually is erythematous, no mobility, no light reflex, and the middle ear may contain fluid that is pink, red, or yellow (indicating pus). Membrane may be bulging and opaque and can perforate, leaving purulent drainage in the external canal (TM not usually visible in this case).
- In OME, membrane may appear slightly thickened but without redness. Mobility is poor and fluid is clear. Air bubbles may also be seen.
- In OE, there may be tenderness of ear when pinna is moved. Ear canal is erythematous, edematous, and inflamed with moist debris. If the canal is grossly swollen, the TM may not be visible. The whole ear canal can be filled with purulent discharge.
- Cervical lymph nodes are enlarged on the affected side.

Diagnostic Procedures
- Visual examination is the primary diagnostic tool. Pneumatic otoscopy is an extremely valuable and simple procedure (eardrum will have poor mobility).
- Tympanometry can be helpful when used as an adjunct to physical examination.
- CBC may show an increased white blood cell (WBC) count, as with any illness, but usually it is not diagnostic and does not correlate with severity of illness.

- Culture of ear drainage is not routinely done because most common organisms can be predicted and the result does not change the treatment plan. If culture comes back showing no organism but the client has symptoms and visual examination shows otitis, the client still requires treatment.

DIAGNOSIS

Differential diagnoses include the following:
- External otitis
- Cellulitis
- Malignant otitis
- Sinusitis
- Pharyngitis
- Tumor
- In older adults, problems caused by wearing hearing aid

THERAPEUTIC PLAN
Pharmacologic Treatment

OM
- Prescribe antibiotic therapy (10-day course).
- First-line therapy is amoxicillin (40 to 60 mg/kg/day) for low-risk children.
- For clients with high risk factors (attend day care with more than 6 children, antibiotics in past 3 months, frequent past OM episodes, or younger than 2 years of age), treat with 80 to 90 mg/kg/day
- Second-line therapy is amoxicillin-clavulanate, cefaclor, cefuroxime axetil, or cefixime. Indicated for resistant organisms, allergy to penicillins, treatment failure with amoxicillin, persistent otitis, and for prophylaxis when amoxicillin has been ineffective.
- If perforation is present, need systemic antibiotic plus ear drops such as Cortisporin Otic.
- For prophylaxis therapy amoxicillin or trimethoprim-sulfamethoxazole is preferred. Dose is half of therapeutic dose given in single dose hs. May be continued as long as 6 months. Because of increasing bacterial resistance, prophylaxis should be used judiciously and only in select children. Researchers have found that children taking prophylaxis antibiotics are 6 times as like to be carriers of penicillin-resistant *S. pneumonia* than those who were not on preventive medication.
- Analgesic therapy includes the following:
  - Auralgan otic suspension
  - Acetaminophen or ibuprofen
  - Acetaminophen with codeine (if severe pain)

OE
- Prescribe polymyxin, neomycin, hydrocortisone, and propylene glycol (Cortisporin Otic) or Cortisporin TC (for those with increased cerumen), 3 drops in affected ear tid or qid.
- Ciprofloxacin (Cipro Otic) or ofloxacin (Floxin) can also be given as ear drops for OE.

- If canal is occluded because of swelling and debris, a systemic antibiotic such as amoxicillin/clavulanate (Augmentin) or clarithromycin (Biaxin) may be prescribed and an ear wick should be inserted to help the ear drops get into the canal.
- Analgesics may be needed because OE can be very painful.

Client Education
OM
- Complete the full course of antibiotic.
- Side effects of medication may include upset stomach, diarrhea allergic reactions, and others.
- Especially important to educate parents of nonverbal children.
- Recheck when antibiotic course is completed if nonverbal client or verbal client is still having symptoms.
- Avoid smoke exposure.
- For infants, avoid having them drink from bottle while lying down.
- Reassure parents that episodes of otitis diminish with time (as the eustachian tubes lengthen).
- Avoid water entering the ear for 7 days if a perforated eardrum is present.

OE
- Ear canal should be kept dry for 7 days (no swimming or showering).
- Discuss with parents how to instill drops: have client lie on side, pull affected ear back and up, then instill drops without allowing dropper to touch ear; remain in lying on side for at least 5 minutes.
- Demonstrate and explain the proper technique to clean ears and minimal use of cotton swabs or instruments to clean ears (to prevent trauma).

Referral/Consultation
OM
- Children: Chronic otitis not relieved after antibiotic therapy; unresolved effusions; hearing loss; glue ear; delayed speech
- Adults: Persistent tinnitus or hearing loss; recurrent otitis

OE
- Persistent OE
- Hearing loss

Prevention
OM
- Breastfeeding helps prevent the development of OM.
- Avoid exposure to secondhand smoke.
- Reduce or eliminate day care attendance.
- Eliminate pacifier use after age 1.
- Administration of pneumococcal and influenza vaccine is recommended.

OE

- Avoidance of precipitating factors
- Prophylaxis with topical solutions:
  - Acetic acid (vinegar) or vinegar-and-alcohol (helps dry out canal and keep pH acidic): prophylactic instillation of 1 to 2 drops after contact with water
- Thorough drying of external auditory canal after washing or wearing hearing aids can be helpful.

EVALUATION/FOLLOW-UP

OM

- Antibiotic treatment failure is described as a lack of improvement in signs and symptoms after 3 days of treatment. Activity against drug-resistant strep pneumonia should guide the choice of a second antibiotic in this case. Only three meet this criteria: amoxicillin-clavulanate (Augmentin), cefuroxime axetil (Ceftin), and ceftriaxone (Rocephin).
- Recurrent otitis is defined as six episodes by 6 years of age, five episodes in 1 year, or three episodes in 6 months. Refer to ear, nose, and throat specialist for possible hearing loss and PE tube placement.
- Recheck acute/chronic OM in office every 10 days while receiving antibiotics.

OE

No follow-up is needed unless symptoms persist.

COMPLICATIONS

Factors associated with increased risk of recurrence of OM are the following:
- Young age at first ear infection (younger than 6 months)
- Male gender
- Positive family history of recurrent ear infections
- Participation in day care
- Exposure to cigarette smoke

REFERENCES

Bojab, D., Bruderly, T., & Abdulrazzak, Y. (1996). Otitis externa. *Otolaryngology Clinics of North America, 29*(5), 761-782.

Calandra, L. (1998). Otitis media with effusion. *Advance Nurse Practitioners, 6*(2), 67-70.

Dowell, S., Butler, J., & Giebink, G. (1999). Acute otitis media: Management and surveillance in an era of pneumococcal resistance-a report from the drug resistant Streptococcus pneumonia. Therapeutic working group. *Pediatric Infectious Disease Journal, 18,* 1-9.

Eden, A. N., Fireman, P., & Stook, S. E. (1996). Managing acute otitis: A fresh look at a familiar problem. *Contemporary Pediatrics, 13*(3), 64-93.

Glasziou, P. P., Del Mar, C. B., & Sanders, S. L. (2001). Antibiotics for acute otitis media in children (Cochrane Review). In *The Cochrane Library.* Oxford: Update Software.

Hanson, M. J. (1996). Acute otitis media in children. *Nurse Practitioner, 21*(5), 72-80.

Mirza, N. (1996). Otitis externa: Management in the primary care office,. *Postgraduate Medicine, 99*(5), 153-154.

Kaleida, P. (1997). The complete exam for otitis. *Contemporary Pediatrics, 14*(9), 93-101.

Robinson, D. (2000). Otitis media and otitis externa. In D. Robinson, P. Kidd, & K. Rogers (Eds.), *Primary care across the lifespan.* St. Louis: Mosby, 831-838.

Stevenson, L., & Brooke, D. S. (1995). Managing otitis media with effusion in young children. *Journal of Pediatric Health Care, 9*(1), 36-39.

Tigges, B. (2000). Acute otitis media and pneumococcal resistance: Making judicious management decisions. *Nurse Practitioner, 25*(1), 69-87.

Review Questions

1. A 6-year-old girl is brought in by her mother for treatment of an earache. The child's past medical history is negative except for one episode of streptococcal sore throat. The parents smoke in the home. Which of the following increases the likelihood that the child has OM?

- **a.** Gender of the child
- **b.** Exposure to secondhand smoke
- **c.** Age of the child
- **d.** Previous episode of streptococcal sore throat

2. Which of the following physical examination data would best help discriminate OM from OE?

- **a.** Hearing loss
- **b.** Drainage, material in ear canal
- **c.** Pain on examination of the ear
- **d.** Decreased TM motility

3. A parent asks the NP whether her child should avoid water in the ear canal after a diagnosis of OM. The best response is:

- **a.** "This is not necessary, unless your child's eardrum perforates."
- **b.** "Your child should avoid water in the ear canal for 7 days."
- **c.** "Water in the ear canal may cause the infection to last longer."
- **d.** "Use ear plugs during bathing."

4. Which of the following is the drug of choice for OM?

- **a.** Erythromycin
- **b.** Amoxicillin
- **c.** Clarithromycin (Biaxin)
- **d.** Amoxicillin/clavulanate (Augmentin)

5. Clients with which of the following should be referred?

- **a.** OM with initial effusion
- **b.** Speech delay
- **c.** Acute OE
- **d.** Prophylactic therapy for OM

6. Which of the following is correct regarding prophylactic antibiotics for OM?

- **a.** All children should be on antibiotics if they have more than one episode of OM per year.

b. Prophylactic antibiotics increases the chance of developing penicillin-resistant strep pneumonia.
c. Prophylactic antibiotics should never be prescribed.
d. Azithromycin (Zithromax) is the drug of choice for prophylactic antibiotics.

7. Max is a 3-year-old who was diagnosed with OM and placed on amoxicillin. What are the indications that treatment failure has occurred in this situation?
a. Diarrhea after every dose of amoxicillin
b. Continued fever and ear pain after 3 days
c. Child has cough, runny nose, and irritability
d. Decreased hearing and continued effusion after 5 days

8. Kristin has had multiple episodes of OE. What preventive actions could you suggest to avoid future episodes of OE?
a. Avoid swimming.
b. Clean the ear canal thoroughly every day.
c. Use vinegar and alcohol ear drops after water exposure.
d. Use a cotton-tipped swab to keep the ear canal free of cerumen.

Answers and Rationales

1. *Answer:* **b** (assessment)
Rationale: Boys have shorter eustachian tubes than girls and are at a higher risk for OM. The incidence decreases at age 4 years. A previous episode of streptococcal sore throat is not relevant unless it was recent (within 1 month) (Robinson, 2000).

2. *Answer:* **d** (assessment)
Rationale: Both conditions can result in hearing loss. If the TM ruptures in OM, material may be in the ear canal. Although pain on manipulation of the tragus is classic for OE, pain on manipulation of the ear can be present in both conditions. In OE the tympanic membrane is normal (Robinson, 2000).

3. *Answer:* **a** (implementation/plan)
Rationale: Only in OE and OM with perforation is water in the ear canal avoided for at least 7 days (Eden, Fireman, & Stook, 1996).

4. *Answer:* **b** (implementation/plan)
Rationale: Amoxicillin is the preferred drug for OM (Tigges, 2000).

5. *Answer:* **b** (implementation/plan)
Rationale: Recurrent ear infections can produce scarring and hearing loss, which leads to speech delays. The other situations do not require referral. Clients undergoing prophylactic therapy need monthly rechecks (Robinson, 2000).

6. *Answer:* **b** (implementation/plan)
Rationale: The use of prophylactic antibiotic treatment for recurrent OM should be done selectively and judiciously because of the increase in resistance of *S. pneumonia* (Tigges, 2000).

7. *Answer:* **b** (evaluation)
Rationale: Resistance is defined as a lack of improvement in signs and symptoms after 3 days of treatment (Tigges, 2000).

8. *Answer:* **c** (evaluation)
Rationale: Use of vinegar and alcohol changes the pH of the ear canal and helps keep the ear canal dry. Instilling the drops after water exposure may help prevent the development of swimmer's ear (Robinson, 2000).

OVARIAN CYSTS   *Cheryl Pope Kish*

OVERVIEW
Definition

Most ovarian cysts, fluid-filled sacs on the ovary, are functional in nature—normal and usually transient with a diameter less than 8 cm. Polycystic ovary syndrome, which involves multiple ovarian cysts, is a complex endocrine disorder of hypothalamic-pituitary dysfunction that causes hyperandrogenemia, insulin resistance, chronic anovulation, and infertility.

Incidence

Ovarian neoplasms account for approximately 289,000 hospital admissions in the United States every year. Most women, however, experience functional ovarian cysts that neither cause problems nor come to medical attention unless found on coincident pelvic examination (approximately 90%). Ovarian cysts represent one of the most common causes of adnexal mass and tenderness in women of childbearing age. Ovarian cysts generally do not occur before puberty or after menopause. Polycystic ovary syndrome (PCOS) is considered the most common endocrine disorder of reproductive age, with an incidence in that group of 6%. With some 625,000 new cases annually, PCOS is the United States' leading cause of infertility.

Pathophysiology

Cystic masses of the ovary occur as part of the normal monthly menstrual cycle. There are two types of functional ovarian cysts: follicle and corpus luteum cysts.

Follicle Cysts. Follicle cysts, physiologic structures resulting from faulty resorption of fluid from incompletely developed ovarian follicles, are the most common ovarian cysts. Their size ranges from microscopic to 8 cm. They are usually asymptomatic, disappearing spontaneously within 60 days. Follicle cysts may be associated with an abnormally long or short intermenstrual interval, thus causing irregular periods.

Corpus Luteum Cysts. A less common, transient structure resulting from failure of the corpus luteum to degenerate after ovulation is referred to as a corpus luteum cyst. This cyst causes local pain and tenderness on examination.

Multiple Inactive Ovarian Cysts. Multiple inactive ovarian cysts are associated with PCOS or Stein-Leventhal syndrome and are caused by androgen excess and anovulation. This pathology affects 15- to 30-year-olds and causes infertility. In addition to bilateral polycystic ovaries, the affected woman has insulin resistance with impaired glucose tolerance, small breasts, a large clitoris, obesity, secondary amenorrhea, enlarged muscle mass, acne, and oily skin. Fifty percent have hirsutism, with male pattern distribution. The pathophysiologic condition is not completely understood; an abnormally high ratio of luteinizing hormone (LH) to follicle-stimulating hormone (FSH) is a hallmark feature.

Differentiating functional, benign, and malignant masses is a challenge for the NP, who may not be able to diagnose the exact pathologic condition. Ovarian masses are always presumed to be cancerous until proven otherwise.

Ovarian Cancer. Ovarian cancer, a potentially lethal malignancy of ovarian tissue, is asymptomatic in early stages. Its cause is unknown. In many cases, malignancy has spread before symptoms occur. Vague GI symptoms (anorexia, early satiety, dyspepsia, bloating, and increased belching) are sometimes seen 6 months or less before the disease is discovered. The mass is irregular and adheres to surrounding tissue; firm nodules are frequently noted in the cul de sac or along the uterosacral ligaments. It is most common among women of childbearing age.

Protective Factors. Use of oral contraceptive pills (OCPs) and pregnancy protect against ovarian cysts by suppressing ovarian activity, including ovulation.

ASSESSMENT: SUBJECTIVE/HISTORY
Functional Ovarian Cysts

Presenting symptoms may include vague, local pressure, heaviness, and aching in the affected side. Follicle cysts occur in the first half of the menstrual cycle. Corpus luteum cysts occur in the last half of the menstrual cycle. Ask about the following:

- Menstrual history: last menstrual period (LMP), age at menarche or menopause
- Pregnancy history
- Type and extent of pain
- Sexual history: Use of contraception, exposure to sexually transmitted diseases (STDs)
- High-risk behaviors that might lead to pelvic inflammatory disease (PID), confusing the diagnosis
- Any other physical problems

- Dyspareunia
- Radiation exposure
- Use of talc on perineum

Polycystic Ovary Syndrome

Ask about menstrual and sexual histories and about attempts to become pregnant.

Suspicion of Torsion or Rupture of Functional Cyst

Ask about the following:

- LMP: Usually occurs 14 to 60 days after last period.
- General aching followed by sudden severe abdominal pain may be present.
- Weakness, syncope, and dizziness may occur with sudden blood loss.
- Activity that preceded sudden pain (client often reports exercise, trauma, or sexual intercourse immediately preceding).

Ovarian Cancer

Ask about the following:
- Increasing abdominal girth
- Vague GI complaints (dyspepsia, anorexia, early satiety, increased bloating and belching)
- Weight loss

Medication History

- Note use of OCPs.
- Ask about use of analgesia for discomfort.
- Ask about use of medications for indigestion, nausea, and constipation.

Family History

Ask about first-degree relatives who have had cancer. Inquire if other female relatives have PCOS.

Psychosocial History

- Ask about smoking, alcohol use, and other drug use.
- Inquire about sexually risky behavior, including multiple sexual partners, treatment for STDs or PID.
- Ask how pelvic aching affects lifestyle, including sexual relationship.

Dietary History

Determine whether high-fat diet places client at risk for ovarian cancer. Note dietary contribution to obesity, if present.

ASSESSMENT: OBJECTIVE/PHYSICAL EXAMINATION
Physical Examination

- Perform a problem-centered physical examination, with special attention to general appearance, vital signs, and abdominal and pelvic examinations.
- Determine weight and height.

- Note central obesity.
- Note acne and oily skin.
- Note masculinization (voice, breast atrophy, hair distribution).
- Palpate the thyroid gland.
- Check the heart, carotid bruits.
- Note abdominal girth, presence of ascites, and fluid wave.
- Check bowel sounds and palpate for general tenderness.
- Perform a pelvic examination gently to avoid inadvertent rupture of ovarian cyst.
- Note the size of the clitoris.
- Note the size, contour, and position of uterus.
- Note cervical motion tenderness and the presence of cervical or vaginal discharge.
- Assess the adnexa for tenderness and the presence of a mass or enlarged ovary.
- Perform rectovaginal examination to confirm size of adnexal mass and to locate in relation to uterus (usually lateral).
- Note nodularity posterior cul de sac and along uterosacral ligaments.
- If client has a history of sudden, severe abdominal pain, note position on examination table. With ruptured cyst, client usually lies quietly, with knees drawn up toward abdomen.
- Assess for acute abdomen, looking for pain, rigidity, rebound, and other peritoneal signs.

Diagnostic Procedures

Pelvic or Transvaginal Ultrasonography

- Ultrasonography differentiates between cyst and solid mass and aids in determining which clients should be followed up and which clients should be referred.
- CBC should be obtained, with special attention to WBC count and existence of shift to left.
- Urine or serum human chorionic gonadotropin (HCG) should be determined to rule out intrauterine or ectopic pregnancy.
- Calcium 125 radioimmunoassay should be performed if at risk for ovarian cancer.
- FSH, LH, testosterone level, lipids, prolactin, FBS, dehydroepiandrosterone-S (rules out virilizing tumor), 17-hydroxyprogesterone level (rules out adult-onset adrenal hyperplasia). Check level of these in clients in whom PCOS is suspected. (Findings associated with PCOS are LH to FSH ratio of 3:1; increased testosterone, increased FBS, possibly increased lipids.)

DIAGNOSIS

Rule out the following:
- Functional ovarian cyst
- Solid ovarian mass
- Ovarian cancer

- Tubal mass (ectopic pregnancy, endometrioma, leiomyoma, tuboovarian abscess)
- PCOS

When client has findings suggestive of acute abdomen associated with a ruptured cyst, rule out the following:
- Ectopic pregnancy
- Appendicitis
- Diverticulitis
- Tuboovarian abscess
- PID

THERAPEUTIC PLAN

- Functional cyst: Consider reevaluating in 2 to 3 weeks, just before ovulation.
- Unilateral cyst smaller than 8 cm in premenopausal client that is mobile: Treat conservatively and wait to resolve (4 to 6 weeks); repeat pelvic examination every 3 to 4 weeks. Repeat ultrasonography as needed to confirm size. Consider suppression with OCPs. If mass persists or enlarges, refer.
- Consider referral of postmenopausal woman with enlarged ovary or cyst.
- Treatment of PCOS includes the following:
  - Prescribe OCPs or medroxyprogesterone acetate for irregular menses.
  - For hirsutism, advise manual hair removal or anti-androgen (Spironolactone).
  - For infertility, refer to infertility specialist.
  - For obesity, provide dietary counseling, advise exercise program.
  - For insulin resistance, prescribe metformin (Glucophage) 500 to 850 mg bid. (Resolving the problem of insulin resistance has been associated with ovulation in some women.)

Pharmacologic Treatment

Use of OCPs may aid resolution in 80% of functional cysts.

Client Education

- Discuss possible cause and course of functional cysts.
- Teach what to expect if torsion or hemorrhage occurs; reassure client that these are rare complications, but prepare her to respond by notifying caregiver or going directly to emergency department.
- Advise about lifestyle changes that decrease the risk of ovarian cancer.
- Women with PCOS should be advised about the risk associated with this diagnosis and appropriate follow-up: three times greater risk of endometrial cancer, breast cancer, ovarian cancer, diabetes mellitus, coronary heart disease, and all the co-morbidities associated with obesity. If this woman becomes pregnant, she will experience the following risks in her pregnancy: pregnancy-induced hypertension (PIH), spontaneous abortion, gestational diabetes mellitus, and low birthweight.

Women using antiandrogen drugs for hirsutism should understand that it may take 6 months for the drugs to be effective. Recommend shaving, depilatories, waxing, bleaching, or electrolysis.

Referral/Consultation

- For cysts larger than 8 cm or persisting for two cycles, refer client to surgeon for evaluation and treatment. Large cysts are more subject to torsion and hemorrhage.
- If a lesion is suspected not to be a functional cyst, refer the client.
- In a postmenopausal client, if the cyst is smaller than 5 cm and the client does not have other risk factors, observe. Recheck at 6 weeks, 3 months, and 6 months. Refer the client if there is any increase in size of mass.
- Refer any child who is prepubertal and has an adnexal mass.
- Refer any postmenopausal older woman who has an enlarged ovary.
- In the event of symptoms of rupture or torsion, refer for emergency care.
- Clients with PCOS should be referred for initial diagnosis and early management; however, depending on the setting, they may be co-managed by the primary care provider.

Prevention

There is some indication that ovarian cysts are preventable with the use of OCPs.

EVALUATION/FOLLOW-UP

- Most functional cysts resolve in 8 weeks, either spontaneously or with the aid of OCPs. Clients taking OCPs should be followed up for untoward effects. Women with a history of functional ovarian cysts should continue to have annual clinical examinations. Cysts sometime recur.
- If an adnexal mass occurs during pregnancy, ectopic pregnancy must be ruled out. A fetal sac of intrauterine pregnancy should be seen on pelvic ultrasonography with an HCG level of 6500 IU and on transvaginal ultrasonography with an HCG level of 2000 IU. Physician management is warranted.
- Clients with polycystic ovaries should have an annual examination to reevaluate the appropriateness of OCPs and to determine the desire for childbearing, which would require ovulation induction. Because of their anovulatory status without treatment, these clients need to be followed up carefully for endometrial cancer related to prolonged unopposed endogenous estrogen.
- Follow-up for ovarian cancer depends on the client's situation. It is usually done by a physician and oncology team. Because of its insidious nature, most ovarian cancer has spread before diagnosis. Despite aggressive treatment, 5-year survival is only 30% or less.

COMPLICATIONS

- Rupture or torsion of large cysts
- Undiagnosed or misdiagnosed ovarian cancer

REFERENCES

Bowman, M. A., Braly, P. S., Johnson, S., et al. (1996). Who are you screening for cancer and when? *Patient Care, 30,* 54-87.

Carlson, K. J., Eisenstat, S. A., Frigoletto, F. D., & Schiff, I. (1995). *Primary care of women.* St. Louis: Mosby.

Drake, J. (1998). Diagnosis and management of the adnexal mass. *American Family Physician, 57*(10), 2471-2478.

Hunter, M. H., & Sterrett, J. J. (2000). Polycystic ovary syndrome: It's not just infertility. *American Family Physician, 62,* 1079-1088, 1090.

Lemke, D. P., Pattison, J., Marshall, L. A., & Cowley, D.S. (1995). *Primary care of women.* Norwalk, CT: Appleton & Lange.

Marantides, D. Management of polycystic ovary syndrome. *Nurse Practitioner, 22*(12), 34-41.

Markle, M. E. (2001). Polycystic ovary syndrome: Implications for the APN. *Journal of the American Academy of Nurse Practitioners, 13*(4), 160-163.

Patel, S. R., & Korytokowski, M. T. (2000). Polysyctic ovary syndrome. *Women's Health Primary Care, 3*(1), 55-69.

Robinson, D., Kidd, P., & Rogers, K. M. (Eds.). (2000). *Primary care across the lifespan.* St. Louis: Mosby.

Slowery, M. J. (2001). Polycystic ovary syndrome: New perspectives on an old problem. *Southern Medical Journal, 94*(2), 190-197.

Smith, R. P. (1997). *Gynecology in primary care.* Baltimore: Williams & Wilkins.

Star, W. L., Lommel, L. L., & Shannon, M. T. (1995). *Women's primary care: Protocols for practice.* Washington, DC: American Nurses Publishing.

Thompson, S. D. (1998). Ovarian cancer screening: A primary care guide. *Lippincott's Primary Care Practice, 2*(3), 244-250.

Tweedy, A. (2000). Polycystic ovary syndrome. *Journal of the American Academy of Nurse Practitioners, 12*(3), 101-105.

Youngkin, E. O., & Davis, M. S. (1998). *Women's health: A primary care clinical guide.* Norwalk, CT: Appleton & Lange.

Review Questions

1. Which of the following clinical manifestations is associated with a diagnosis of PCOS?
  - **a.** Infertility
  - **b.** Excessive menstrual flow
  - **c.** Reports of dry, flaking skin
  - **d.** Unexplained weight loss

2. In Miss Logan, a 26-year-old with a history suggestive of ruptured ovarian cyst, which objective finding best supports that diagnosis?
  - **a.** She is thrashing about on the examination table.
  - **b.** She is lying quietly on the examination table, with her legs drawn up toward her abdomen.
  - **c.** She has excessive dark, bloody vaginal drainage.
  - **d.** She has dry, hot skin and a high fever.

3. Which of the following is (are) appropriate differential diagnoses when an ovarian cyst ruptures?

    a. Ruptured ectopic pregnancy
    b. Appendicitis
    c. Tuboovarian abscess from salpingitis
    d. All the above

4. An enlarged left ovary is found on a prepubescent girl. What is the most appropriate action?

    a. Advise the girl and her mother that menses should be starting soon.
    b. Start low-dose OCPs for 3 months.
    c. Refer the client to a surgeon immediately.
    d. Document the presence of a cyst and plan to follow up in 2 weeks.

5. Ms. Slade, a 30-year-old woman, has a family history of ovarian cancer. In consultation with the physician, the NP orders OCPs as a protective factor for Ms. Slade. What follow-up is appropriate in these circumstances?

    a. Annual examination and ultrasonography
    b. Monthly calcium 125 radioimmunoassay
    c. Biannual endometrial biopsy
    d. Pap smear every 3 months

6. Which symptom group would make the NP suspect ovarian cancer in a 45-year-old woman?

    a. Anorexia, early satiety, and dyspepsia
    b. Pelvic pain, vaginal bleeding, and dyspareunia
    c. Weight gain, pedal edema, and hirsutism
    d. Diarrhea, breast enlargement, and abdominal tenderness

Answers and Rationales

1. *Answer:* a (assessment)
    Rationale: Infertility, acne, oily skin, weight gain, and amenorrhea are classic features of PCOS (Carlson, Eisenstat, Frigoletto, & Schiff, 1995).

2. *Answer:* b (assessment)
    Rationale: Peritoneal irritation caused by ruptured ovarian cyst causes clients to attempt to minimize pain by lying quietly, with the knees drawn up toward the chest (Smith, 1997).

3. *Answer:* d (analysis/diagnosis)
    Rationale: Ruptured ovarian cysts mimic appendicitis, ruptured ectopic pregnancy, and salpingitis (Smith, 1997).

4. *Answer:* c (implementation/plan)
    Rationale: An adnexal mass in a premenstrual girl needs immediate referral (Drake, 1998).

5. *Answer:* a (evaluation)
    Rationale: With a family history, annual clinical examination and ultrasonography is recommended (Carlson et al., 1995).

6. *Answer:* a (assessment)
    Rationale: Common signs of ovarian cancer include a 6- to 12-month history of increased belching, bloating, acid indigestion, early satiety, and anorexia (Thompson, 1998).

PANCREATITIS   *Pamela Kidd*

OVERVIEW
Definition

Inflammation of the pancreas is caused by a variety of mechanisms including alcohol abuse, cholelithiasis, trauma, or drug abuse. Classified as acute (edema and cellular infiltration) or chronic (both may lead to necrosis of cells).

Incidence

Unknown.

Pathophysiology

Pancreatitis can be caused by many conditions. Regardless of cause, the end result is the same: liberation of pancreatic enzymes into the tissues of the pancreas. In the mildest form of pancreatitis, edema results, but no changes in the structure of function of the pancreas occur. In severe pancreatitis, repeated attacks occur, leading to loss of tissue and acinar units so clients develop pancreatic insufficiency with steatorrhea or diabetes. In the most severe form, tissue destruction occurs, leading to involvement of the blood vessels, which causes hemorrhage pancreatitis. The mortality rate of hemorrhage pancreatitis ranges from 50% to 85%.

Protective Factors. None.

Factors Increasing Susceptibility
- Alcohol ingestion
- Cholelithiasis
- Medications
- Pancreatic cancer
- Abdominal trauma or surgery
- Ulcer with pancreatic involvement
- Viral infections
- Metabolic hypercalcemia, hypertriglycemia

ASSESSMENT: SUBJECTIVE/HISTORY
Symptoms

Symptoms range from mild epigastric pain to sudden, intense abdominal pain with shock and cyanosis. Clients present with the following:

- Complaints of abdominal pain, usually worse with walking and lying down, better with sitting and leaning forward; may radiate to the back
- Nausea/vomiting
- Epigastric pain
- Ask about the following:
  - Abdominal trauma

- Previous episodes of pancreatitis or gallbladder attacks
- A heavy meal immediately preceding the attack
- Bowel movements (BMs), episodes of diarrhea, last BM

Past Medical History

- Episodes of gastritis
- History of diabetes or glucose intolerance
- Cholecystitis/cholelithiasis
- Peptic ulcer disease
- Hyperlipidemia

Medication History

Ask about use of sulfonamides, thiazides, furosemide, tetracycline, valproic acid, and pentamidine.

Family History

- Ask about family history of alcohol abuse and dependence.
- Ask about family history of pancreatitis.

Dietary History

- High fat diet may precipitate attack.
- Heavy meal or alcohol ingestion may precipitate attack.

ASSESSMENT: OBJECTIVE/PHYSICAL EXAMINATION

Physical Examination

The extent of the physical examination depends on the acuteness of the client's symptoms. The main focus of the examination is the abdomen, but a more complete examination may be warranted depending on the client's complaints.

- *Vital signs:* Fever of 38.4° C to 39° C, tachycardia, or hypotension may be present.
- *General:* Observe for jaundice.
- Assess lungs.
- Assess cardiovascular system.
- Assess bowel sounds (may be absent), peristaltic waves, distention.
- Look for Cullen's sign (discoloration around umbilicus) or Grey turner (flank discoloration). Hemorrhage may occur with retroperitoneal bleeding in severe inflammation.
- Assess percussion.
- *Palpation:* Assess for tenderness, especially in the upper abdomen (usually without guarding, rigidity or rebound), masses, Murphy's sign, liver size and tenderness.
- *Rectal:* Tenderness may be present on digital rectal examination (DRE).

Diagnostic Procedures

Diagnostic procedure are outlined in Table 3-82.
- Computed tomography (CT) scan will show enlarged pancreas.
- Abdominal x-ray film may show colon cut-off sign (gas filled transverse colon abruptly ending at site of pancreatic inflammation).

DIAGNOSIS

Differential diagnoses are outlined in Table 3-83.

P

TABLE **3-82** Diagnostic Procedures for Pancreatitis

DIAGNOSTIC TEST	FINDINGS/RATIONALE
Serum amylase	The most specific aid in the diagnosis of pancreatitis, often only transiently elevated; may return to normal in 48-72 hours. As many as 20% of clients with pancreatitis have a normal or borderline amylase. Elevations of 1000 U/dL are almost always caused by pancreatitis or obstruction of the pancreatic duct. Morphine can mildly elevate an amylase levels.
Lipase, ALT, AST, alkaline phosphatase	Lipase elevated in pancreatitis. ALT and AST elevated when associated with alcoholic hepatitis or choledocholithiasis; alkaline phosphatase levels are mildly elevated.
CT/US	An enlarged pancreas on either a CT scan or ultrasound increases the likelihood that the pancreas is the cause of the acute abdominal pain. Best in diagnosing late complications, especially pseudocysts or abscess.
Bilirubin	Mildly elevated bilirubin is seen with pancreatitis (approximately 20% of clients).
Glucose	May be increased in severe pancreatitis.
Calcium	May be mildly decreased in pancreatitis. In severe pancreatitis, the calcium level may be very low, low enough to cause tetany. A decrease in serum calcium correlates well with the severity of the disease.
CBC	Elevated WBC levels are seen in acute pancreatitis.
C-reactive protein	An elevation within 48 hours indicates pancreatic necrosis.
Stool culture	Excess fecal fat in chronic pancreatitis.

ALT, Alanine transferase; *AST,* aspartame transferase; *CBC,* complete blood count; *US,* ultrasound.

THERAPEUTIC PLAN

The treatment of acute pancreatitis is supportive. Clients with the following signs should be admitted to the intensive care unit for care:

- White blood cell (WBC) count higher than 16,000
- Serum glucose higher than 200 mg/dL
- Tachycardia higher than 130 BPM
- Low urine output
- Decreasing serum calcium
- Respiratory distress

Nonpharmacologic Treatment

General measures for acute pancreatitis are the following:

P = pain control, meperidine
A = arrest shock, intravenous fluids
N = nasogastric tube for vomiting
C = calcium monitoring
R = renal evaluation
E = ensure pulmonary function
A = antibiotics
S = surgery or special procedures in selected cases

Chronic Pancreatitis

- Provide pain control, advise alcohol abstinence.
- Prescribe pancreatic enzyme supplements for maldigestion.
- For diabetes mellitus, prescribe insulin.
- Oral intake should be withheld because it stimulates release of pancreatic enzymes and therefore continued tissue damage during the acute phase. No fluid or food should be given until the client is pain free and has bowel sounds.

- A low fat diet should be followed in chronic pancreatitis.
- Recommend small meals high in protein for chronic pancreatitis.

Pharmacologic Treatment

No specific pharmacologic treatment; depends on the extent of the pancreatitis and the presence of infection.

Client Education

The importance of alcohol abstinence should be stressed.

Referral/Consultation

A surgeon or internal medicine physician should be consulted in all cases of severe acute pancreatitis during the work-up phase to make sure that, if the cause is surgically correctable, exploration is done quickly.

Prevention

Avoid alcohol.

EVALUATION/FOLLOW-UP

- Depends on symptoms.
- Follow-up of amylase level; if it remains elevated, perform ultrasound for pseudocyst.
- In most clients, acute pancreatitis is a mild disease that resolves spontaneously in a few days.
- The severity of pancreatitis can be determined by using Ranson's criteria. When three or more of the following are present, a more severe course can be predicted:
  1. Age older than 55
  2. WBC count higher than 16,000 cells/mm^3
  3. Blood glucose higher than 200 mg/dL

TABLE **3-83** Differential Diagnoses for Pancreatitis

DIAGNOSIS	DATA SUPPORT
Cholithiasis	RUQ abdominal pain, jaundice, epigastric tenderness, positive Murphy's sign; US may show gallstones; in chronic cholecystitis, pain may be present after meals, heartburn.
PUD/perforation	Severe abdominal pain, client appears toxic, abdominal guarding and rigidity.
Intestinal obstruction	Abdominal pain, distention, and vomiting are hallmark symptoms. Obstipation (inability to pass gas or stool) may also be present. Bowel sounds may be absent, high pitched or weak depending on the location of the bowel obstruction.
IBS/IBD	LLQ abdominal pain, constipation, diarrhea.
Chronic pancreatitis	90% caused by alcohol abuse, increased amylase; as the pancreatitis goes on, pancreatic function decreases. Fat malabsorption occurs, calcification may be seen on plain abdominal radiograph film in 20% of clients. DM may also be present. Abdominal CT shows characteristic changes: dilated ducts, pseudocysts, and enlargement of the pancreas.
Carcinoma of the pancreas	Pain is the most common presenting symptom. Complains of dull ache in the epigastrium with radiation depending on the location of the tumor. Client also complains of constipation and crampy lower abdominal pain. Initial diagnosis frequently is IBS. Jaundice may be seen only with tumor of head of pancreas. CT scan and endoscopy examination via ERCP will show tumor.

CT, Computed tomography; *DM,* diabetes mellitus; *ERCP,* endoscopic retrograde cholangio-pancreatography; *IBD,* irritable bowel disease; *IBS,* irritable bowel syndrome; *PUD,* peptic ulcer disease; *RUQ,* right upper quadrant; *US,* ultrasound.

4. Base deficit higher than 4 mEq/L
5. Aspartate transaminase higher than 250 units/L
6. Lactate dehydrogenase higher than 350 units/L

Complications

- Pancreatic cancer
- Sepsis
- Dehydration

REFERENCES

Friedman, L. (2001). Liver, biliary tract and pancreas. In L. Tierney, S. McPhee, M. Papadakis (Eds.), *Current medical diagnosis and treatment* (40th ed.). New York: McGraw Hill.

Skaife, P., Kingsnorth, A. (1996). Acute pancreatitis: Assessment and management. *Postgraduate Medicine 72*, 277.

Review Questions

1. Which of the following assessment data best suggests a diagnosis of pancreatitis?

- **a.** Abdominal pain improved with walking
- **b.** Sudden intense abdominal pain
- **c.** Nausea and vomiting
- **d.** Fever and chills

2. Which of the following diets may precipitate a pancreatic attack?

- **a.** High carbohydrate
- **b.** High protein
- **c.** High fat
- **d.** High volume of fluids

3. The nurse practitioner (NP) notices flank discoloration when examining a client with a history of pancreatitis. The NP interprets this sign as of which of the following?

- **a.** Indication of cholecystitis
- **b.** Indication of renal calculi
- **c.** Indication of retroperitoneal bleeding
- **d.** Cullen's sign

4. In acute attacks, the NP should do which of the following?

- **a.** Order a low fat diet.
- **b.** Instruct the client to increase oral fluids.
- **c.** Instruct the client to eliminate protein in the diet.
- **d.** Instruct the client to take nothing by mouth.

Answers and Rationales

1. *Answer:* b (assessment)
Rationale: The pain in pancreatitis is sudden and intense, and is relieved with sitting and leaning forward. Nausea and vomiting, fever, and chills are present but may also occur with cholecystitis, intestinal obstruction, appendicitis, and other abdominal conditions.

2. *Answer:* c (analysis/diagnosis)
Rationale: High-fat diet may cause an attack resulting from the need for more pancreatic enzymes for breakdown of fats.

3. *Answer:* c (analysis/diagnosis)
Rationale: In acute pancreatitis, hemorrhage may occur, creating discoloration of the flanks (Grey turner sign) and around the umbilicus (Cullen's sign). Murphy's sign (holding of breath on palpation of right subcostal margin) is present in cholecystitis.

4. *Answer:* d (implementation/plan)
Rationale: Although a high fat diet may precipitate an attack, during an attack, oral intake should be withheld because it stimulates release of pancreatic enzymes and therefore continued tissue damage during the acute phase. No fluid or food should be given until the client is pain free and has bowel sounds.

PAPANICOLAOU SMEAR   *Cheryl Pope Kish*

OVERVIEW
Definition

The Papanicolaou (Pap) smear is a cytologic screening test used to detect cancer and precancerous lesions of the uterine cervix by examination of cells collected from the exocervix and endocervix. It does not diagnose cervical cancer; colposcopy with biopsy and endocervical curettage is diagnostic. The Pap test is considered an integral component of the routine health maintenance of women in the United States; national standards suggest initiating the examination with the onset of sexual activity or at age 18, whichever is earliest.

Incidence

- More than 50 million Pap smears are done in the United States annually.
- Pap smear is considered the most effective screening test ever developed; since its introduction in the 1940s, the incidence of cervical cancer has decreased by 70%.

Pathophysiology

- Cells are sampled from transformation zone, the squamocolumnar junction (SCJ) of the cervix, which is an area of rapid cell turnover and squamous metaplasia.

- At puberty, squamous tissue slowly replaces glandular tissue on the ectocervix under the influence of estrogen. In reproductive-age women, the SCJ is usually readily visible on ectocervix; as women mature, lack of estrogen causes the SCJ to recede within the endocervical canal, making it more difficult to visualize and adequately sample.
- Human papillomavirus (HPV) is now considered the causal agent in 99.8% of cervical cancers worldwide. HPV strains 16, 18, 31, 33, 39, and 42 are strongly associated with cervical cancer (Association of Reproductive Health Professionals, 2001).
- Cervical cancer is a progressive disease with a number of histologically definable stages. Invasive cancer and its precursor lesions are detectable by cytologic examination before clinical signs appear.

Factors Increasing Susceptibility. The presence of the following risk factors for cervical cancer establish a need for Pap screening and for more aggressive management of non-reassuring results:

- First coitus at younger than 18 years old increases risk.
- Three sexual partners in lifetime increases risk.
- Multiparity increases risk.
- Low socioeconomic status (secondary to decreased preventive care) increases risk.
- Advancing age increases risk.
- Compromised immune status (i.e., immunosuppressant therapy, organ transplantation, human immunodeficiency virus [HIV]) increases risk.
- Smoking increases risk (nicotine is carcinogen and smoking decreases immune capacity).
- Male partner with history of multiple partners or sexually transmitted diseases (STDs) increases risk.
- Personal history of STDs, especially HPV, increases risk.
- Diethylstilbestrol (DES) exposure in utero increases risk.
- Cervical dysplasia: Risk of cervical cancer is 100 times greater with dysplasia history.

ASSESSMENT: SUBJECTIVE/HISTORY
History of Present Illness

In women presenting for Pap tests or those for whom the Pap smear is being recommended as part of health maintenance, the following history is important:

- Last menstrual period (LMP) should be determined. Premenopausal women are ideally scheduled for Paps in mid-cycle (epithelial cells are under highest estrogen influence and risk of menstrual bleeding is decreased).
- Determine gestational stage, if pregnant.
- Risk factors for cervical cancer should be assessed.
- Douching, antifungals, intercourse before examination with potential to interfere with adequacy of sample should be determined.

Symptoms

Signs and symptoms of cervical cancer are post-coital bleeding, intermenstrual bleeding, menorrhagia, and vaginal discharge.

Past Medical History

- Date and results of previous Pap smears; details of any Pap follow-up
- Contraception used
- Recent cancer treatment

Medication History

Medication use, especially hormone replacement therapy (HRT), oral contraceptive pills (OCPs) or other hormonal contraception.

Family History

- Family history of cervical cancer, breast or colon cancer in first-degree relatives

ASSESSMENT: OBJECTIVE/PHYSICAL EXAMINATION
Physical Examination

- On pelvic examination, note any perineal, vaginal or cervical lesions. Inspect cervix for areas of nodularity and friability.
- Characterize any vaginal discharge.
- After fully visualizing SCJ, collect sample of cells from ectocervix, then endocervix.
- Perform a complete bimanual examination.

Diagnostic Procedures

Procedure for obtaining Pap smear is as follows:

- Explain procedure thoroughly, showing models and actual equipment to facilitate understanding.
- Assist woman into comfortable lithotomy position and drape for privacy.
- Select speculum appropriate for woman's size and childbirth history. Warm speculum with water, do not use lubricant, which interferes with adequacy of sample.
- With full visualization of SCJ, carefully remove excess vaginal discharge obscuring cervix with large swab. Spotting does not preclude examination; heavy vaginal bleeding does because blood obscures squamous cells.
- Collect cells from ectocervix with spatula, using a 360-degree sweep. Wipe cells onto prelabeled glass slide.
- Collect cells from endocervix with cytobrush. Roll or twist cells from brush onto glass slide. Samples from endocervix and ectocervix do not need to be separated on the slide. Some clinicians prefer to use a cotton-tipped applicator for endocervical collections on pregnant women to minimize bleeding from a friable cervix. The cotton-tip should be moistened with saline to prevent cells from being trapped within its fibers.

- What is the nature and duration of the abuse?
- Are the violent episodes escalating?
- Are the violent episodes associated with alcohol or drug abuse?
- Is the abusive partner harming the children?
- Does he control her activities, money, or the children?
- Does she have access to family, advocacy, and support services?
- How is the abuse affecting her? Her children?
- Is there suicidal or homicidal ideation?

ASSESSMENT: OBJECTIVE/PHYSICAL EXAMINATION
Physical Examination

- Physical examination is based on the nature of the injuries or the presenting complaint.
- Observe for scratches, bite marks, contusions, lacerations, abrasions, and fractures. Note extent of injuries. Use diagrams, body maps or photographs (one with client's face) to reveal extent of injury (informed consent required for photographs).

A complete physical examination is warranted with particular attention to the following areas:

- *General:* Assess responsiveness, evidence of general well-being, affect, presence of unattended physical problems.
- *Head, eyes, ears, nose, and throat (HEENT):* Assess for head trauma, patchy hair loss, pupils; funduscopic examination revealing retinal hemorrhage; hemorrhage of sclerae; bleeding from ears or nose; blood behind tympanic membrane.
- *Skin:* Assess for bruises in different stages of healing; burns; physical marks of an object (e.g., looped cord, belt buckle); restraint marks on extremities, neck, or mouth; human bite marks; scratches; lacerations and abrasions.
- *Chest:* Assess for evidence of fractured ribs.
- *Breasts:* Assess for bite marks and soft tissue injury.
- *Abdomen:* Assess for tenderness, organomegaly, bruising, and pregnancy.
- *Musculoskeletal:* Assess for tenderness or swelling of joints, signs of spiral fractures or dislocations; generalized muscle tenderness or injury.
- *Neurologic:* Assess mental status.
- *Genitalia:* Assess genital, urethral, vaginal, or anal bruising or bleeding; swollen, red vulva or perineum; vaginal discharge, cervical or perineal lesions consistent with STD.

Diagnostic Procedures

- Obtain accurate and thorough descriptions of clinical findings suggestive of abuse (diagrams, body maps, and photographs are helpful).
- Obtain radiography and laboratory tests as warranted by history and physical.
- Obtain wet prep using KOH and saline to assess for WBC count, clue cells, or trichomonads as indicated.
- Obtain cultures for gonorrhea and chlamydia as indicated.
- Obtain blood test for syphilis, HIV if at risk.
- Test for hCG if pregnancy suspected. (In cases in which victim may be pregnant, assess before administration of medications.)

DIAGNOSIS

- Women rarely present with complaints of abuse. Unless there is an obvious injury that can be traced to an abusive cause, a diagnosis can only be made by putting together the clues that indicate abuse as a possible cause or factor for seeking care.
- Diagnosis is based on history and physical findings suggestive of partner violence.
  Differential diagnoses include the following:
  - Unintentional or accidental injury
  - Symptomatology consistent with systemic disease (e.g., bruising associated with blood dyscrasias) or co-morbidity.

THERAPEUTIC PLAN
Nonpharmacologic Treatment

- Provide supportive clinic environment that encourages disclosure. Posters about domestic violence and literature on walls or in waiting rooms or bathrooms provide the unspoken message that the topic is one of concern to clinicians in the practice. Emphasize that the woman is not to blame for her abuse and does not deserve to be hurt.
- Acknowledge seriousness of situation and concern.
- Inform about cycle of violence.
- Provide safety and privacy for disclosure. If partner comes into examination room, consider asking woman for urine specimen that will get her out of his presence and meet her at the bathroom.
- Inform her of her legal rights.
- Avoid pitfall of being a "rescuer." Caregivers cannot direct the woman's decisions or make choices about staying in the relationship, even if they are concerned about the ultimate fate of the victim, should she choose to remain. Clearly explore the options with her: notifying authorities, leaving family home and entering shelter, legal remedies, availability of social service provider, emergency assistance numbers.
- Encourage woman to consider her safety and that of her children. She is the best judge of their safety in the home.
- Encourage safety exit plan and help her consider what to pack when she is ready to leave. Encourage her to place greatest priority on safety for herself and her children. (The majority of victims are a greatest risk at or within two weeks of leaving the relationship.)

P

- Inform her of support groups and provide literature and information about community resources.
- If woman has suicidal ideation, establish verbal contract that she will seek help before hurting herself.
- Refer for job training and employment counseling.

Pharmacologic Treatment

- Provide emergency care for injury and physical pain.
- Treat for syphilis, gonorrhea, chlamydia, trichomonas, and genital herpes as appropriate. Provide prophylactic treatment if exposure is known or woman is unreliable for follow-up.
- Provide emergency contraception if unwanted coitus preceded examination by less than 72 hours.
- Treat symptomatically as indicated (e.g., for anxiety, provide antianxiety agents; for depression, provide antidepressants).

Prevention

The following represent possible preventive strategies:

- Challenge society's social stereotypes of women and partner violence and teaching nonviolent measures for conflict resolution in relationships.
- Eliminate intergenerational abuse.
- Teach self defense and assertiveness.
- Recognize control and dominance by partners early in relationships.
- Teach young women how alcohol and drug abuse decrease effective decision making in relationships.
- Educate women in early dating relationships about partner violence and cycle of violence.

EVALUATION/FOLLOW-UP

- Same-day telephone follow-up if returning to relationship.
- Confirm follow-up with referrals.
- Monitor progress of case until resolution.
- Schedule follow-up appropriate to chief complaint.
- Schedule annual physical examination.

COMPLICATIONS

- Death, disability, severe physical, emotional, or mental disorders associated with abuse, including chronic pain
- Continuation of abuse in this relationship and potentially in families of children who witness this abuse
- Increased likelihood of substance abuse
- Restricted activities, career opportunities, and decreased self-efficacy of woman
- Suicide (1:6 of abuse victims attempt) or homicide

REFERENCES

American College of Obstetricians and Gynecologists. (1995). Domestic violence. *ACOG Technical Bulletin* 209, 1-9.

Bachman, G. (1996). Domestic violence. In C. J. Johnson, B. E. Johnson, J. L. Murray, B. S. Apgar (Eds.), *Women's health care handbook* (pp. 83-191). Philadelphia:, Hanley & Belfus.

Brown, K. M. (2000). *Management guidelines for women's health nurse practitioners*. Philadelphia: FA Davis.

Chez, R. A., King, M. C., & Brown, J. (1997) Homing in on abuse: What to ask and how to listen. *Contemporary Nurse Practitioner*, Spring, 20-28.

Coeling, H., & Harmon, G. (1997). Learning to ask about domestic violence. *Women's Health Issues*, 7, 263-268.

Cromwell, S. L. (2001). Domestic abuse and violence. In D. Robinson, C. P. Kish: *Core concepts in advanced practice nursing* (pp. 547-560). St. Louis: Mosby.

Domestic violence: Ending the cycle of abuse (1998). *Clinical Review 8*(1), 55-69.

Hartman, S. J. (2000). Battered women in a small town. *AWHONN Lifelines, 4*(4), 35-39.

Hinterliter, D., Pitula, C. R., & Delaney, K. R. (1998). Partner violence. *American Journal for Nurse Practitioners 2*(3), 32-40, 1009.

Is your patient a victim of domestic violence? (2000). *Women's Health in Primary Care 3*(3), 176-178.

McClellan, A. C., & Killeen, M. R. (2000). Attachment theory and violence toward women by male intimate partners. *Journal of Nurse Scholarship, 32*(4), 353-360.

McFarlane, J. M., & Parker, B. (1994). *Abuse during pregnancy: A protocol for prevention and intervention*. White Plains, NY: March of Dimes Birth Defect Foundation.

Petter, L. M., & Whitehill, D. L. (1998). Management of female sexual assault. *American Family Physician, 58*(4), 920-928.

Poirier, L. (1997). The importance of screening for domestic violence in all women. *Nurse Practitioner, 22*(5), 105-122.

U.S. Public Health Service. (1997). Put prevention into practice. Violence. *Journal of the American Academy of Nurse Practitioners, 9*(5), 227-234.

Quillian, J. P. (1996). Screening for spousal or partner abuse in a community health setting. *Journal of the American Academy of Nurse Practitioners 8*(4), 155-160.

Ragozine, J. E. (1998). Abuse during pregnancy: The role of the nurse practitioner. *Contemporary Nurse Practitioner*, Spring, 3-10.

Smith, M. A., & Shimp, L. A. (2000). *Twenty common problems in women's health care*, New York: McGraw-Hill.

Stewart, J. (2000). Becoming advocates for battered women. *Clinical Review 10*(6), 25-28.

Valente, S. M. (2000). Evaluating and managing intimate patient violence. *Nurse Practitioner, 25*(5), 18-35.

Warshaw, C. (1996). *Improving the healthcare response to domestic violence: A resource manual for health care providers* (2nd ed.). San Francisco: Family Violence Prevention Fund.

Weis, B. D. (Ed.). (2000). *Twenty common problems in primary care*. New York: McGraw-Hill.

Review Questions

1. Which of the following behaviors on the part of a male partner is consistent with the tension-building phase of domestic abuse?

- **a.** Says he hopes he will never hit his loved one again and buys her a new blouse.
- **b.** Yells about an over-cooked egg and uses profanity.
- **c.** Hits the wall with his fists and pulls his partner's hair.
- **d.** Apologizes profusely for his bad behavior and hugs his partner.

2. Which of the following factors is consistent with an increasing risk for partner violence?

  a. Rebellion against close family relationship in childhood
  b. Strict upbringing in childhood
  c. Substance abuse
  d. Service in the military forces

3. Which of the following factors is *not* likely to be a barrier to an NP's routine assessment for partner violence?

  a. Fear of ineffectiveness in providing care if the woman discloses.
  b. Belief that the client population does not include groups commonly battered by partners.
  c. Reluctance to become involved in personal issues of clients.
  d. A personal history of victimization.

4. Which of the following remarks by the NP is most likely to facilitate disclosure of partner abuse?

  a. "Has your husband ever been violent in your presence?"
  b. "Would you like us to ask you questions about your home life and relationship?"
  c. "Tell me about your husband and how he treats you and your children."
  d. "In this practice, we are interested in client safety. How safe are you feeling in your present relationship?"

5. Which injury sites are most common when abuse occurs during pregnancy?

  a. Hands, arms, and head
  b. Abdomen, breasts, and genitals
  c. Face, back, and legs
  d. Wrists, buttocks, and feet

6. Betsy presents with injuries suspicious of domestic abuse. Which factor is consistent with such suspicions on the part of the NP?

  a. Betsy's listing of her symptoms is prolonged and rambling.
  b. Betsy has injuries in varied stages of healing inconsistent with the reported cause.
  c. Betsy's husband accompanies her to the clinic.
  d. Betsy cannot remember one of the medication dosages she takes daily.

7. A group of NPs, concerned about the numbers of battered women being seen in their practice, discuss prevention strategies. Which strategy has the greatest potential to decrease incidence of partner violence?

  a. Arrange for local law enforcement agency to teach a course in safe firearm use.
  b. Educate young women about the cycle of violence in dating relationships.
  c. Stress the importance of annual examination.
  d. Routinely assess all women seen in the practice for abuse.

8. Which of the following women victims of partner violence is at the greatest risk of homicide?

  a. Penny, who has announced her intention to leave the home
  b. Nan, a college freshman dating the campus hero
  c. Janice, a lesbian client in a long-term relationship
  d. Shawn, who recently disclosed her abuse to her priest

Answers and Rationales

1. *Answer:* **b** (evaluation)
  Rationale: Walker's theory of the dynamics of partner abuse describes the tension building behaviors as those of mounting conflict: finding fault, criticizing, threatening, and being verbally abusive.

2. *Answer:* **c** (assessment)
  Rationale: Substance abuse is highly correlated with partner violence. Childhood abuse, not a strict upbringing, is associated. There is no evidence that a close family or military service increases the risk for violent behavior in a relationship (Valente, 2000).

3. *Answer:* **d** (evaluation)
  Rationale: A personal history of victimization is not likely to stand as a barrier to assessing for partner violence; instead, someone who is or has been a victim might be more sensitive to this clinical problem (Cromwell, 2001).

4. *Answer:* **d** (implementation/plan)
  Rationale: All women should be assessed for partner violence. It is helpful to use an approach that suggests that abuse is not considered trivial, shameful, or irrelevant, and to give permission to tell by suggesting that these issues of safety are addressed with all clients (Hinterliter, Pitula, & Delaney 1998).

5. *Answer:* **b** (assessment)
  Rationale: During pregnancy, common sites of abuse are the breasts, head and face, abdomen, and genitalia (McFarlane & Parker 1994).

6. *Answer:* **b** (assessment)
  Rationale: Vague, non-specific complaints can be a clue of abuse; even nonabused clients sometimes give a long, rambling history. The fact that her husband accompanied her does not mean that she is being abused; there is no indication in the question that he remains in the examination room or answers questions asked of her (which would raise some suspicion). Many clients, when stressed, have difficulty remembering drug dosages. Injuries in varied stages of healing, especially when they are inconsistent with reports of causation, should raise suspicion of abuse (Valente, 2000).

7. *Answer:* **b** (implementation/plan)
  Rationale: Educating women about violence in relationships so that they can recognize patterns of control and dominance is a helpful preventive strategy (Stewart, 2000).

8. *Answer:* **a** (evaluation)
  Rationale: Women who are victims of partner violence are at greatest risk at or within two weeks of leave-taking from the abusive relationship (Smith & Shimp, 2000).

PEDICULOSIS PUBIS *Cheryl Pope Kish*

OVERVIEW
Definition

Pediculosis pubis is a parasitic infection of the genital region caused by the Phthirus pubis, or crab louse, which can be mechanically spread to affect other hairy areas of the body: axilla, chest, abdomen, thighs, and eyelashes.

Incidence

Pediculosis pubis infestation is more common in adolescents and young adults who are sexually active. It is highly contagious (90% to 95% acquisition rate per contact with an infected partner). Transmission occurs during intimate personal or sexual contact. Infestation can occur in children as a result of sexual abuse. This infestation affects all social, racial, and economic groups.

Pathophysiology

The pubic louse, Phthirus pubis, is an ectoparasite spread by sexual contact. It attaches to the base of the shaft of pubic hair and feeds by piercing skin. During the 25- to 30-day life cycle, this louse lays eggs (nits). Nits hatch in 5 to 10 days; adult pubic lice, blood-obligate parasites, probably survive no more than 24 hours off their human host. It is the saliva of the louse that creates pruritic symptoms through a histamine response. The louse can spread to hair in other parts of the body (axilla, trunk, abdomen, eyelashes) but likely does so by mechanical means on the client's hands rather than from crawling. The louse is also spread by contaminated bedding and clothing.

Protective Factors. Caution in selection of intimate partners lends some protection against pubic lice.

Factors Increasing Susceptibility. Sexual contact with an individual infected with pubic lice increases the probability of transmission.

ASSESSMENT: SUBJECTIVE/HISTORY
History of Present Illness

- Intense itching, often worse at night (some clients are asymptomatic initially)
- Known exposure

Symptoms

- Pruritus in pubic area
- Difficulty sleeping
- Irritability or distraction related to itching

Family History

Inquire about infestation in family members.

Psychosocial History

- Client may have had multiple sexual partners.
- Client may have lifestyle that involves shared clothing, towels, or beds.
- In children with symptoms, inquire about sexual abuse.
- Because a stigma exists concerning lice infestations, it is important to assess the client's perceptions. There are many misconceptions about infestation.

ASSESSMENT: OBJECTIVE/ PHYSICAL EXAMINATION
Physical Examination

- Strong lighting and a magnifying lens facilitate identification of lice and nits. The examiner should always wear gloves when examining for lice.
- Visualize lice or oval white nits on pubic hair (and in other hairy areas, including eyelashes). (The parasite is not always seen.)
- Pinpoint black specks (lice feces) may occasionally be noted on the skin and underwear.
- Check for lesions of secondary infection from scratching. Inguinal lymph nodes may be enlarged when secondary infection exists.
- Symptoms of other STDs may coexist with pediculosis pubis. Appropriate testing is essential.

Diagnostic Procedures

Diagnosis is made by visualization of the louse or nits. Removing the louse for visualization under a microscope aids in confirmation. A Wood's lamp may be used because lice fluoresce. This is normally not necessary for diagnosis.

DIAGNOSIS

Confirm the presence of lice and nits by carefully examining pubic hair. Differential diagnoses include scabies and seborrheic dermatitis.

THERAPEUTIC PLAN
Nonpharmacologic Treatment

Assist the client in dealing with any anxiety or embarrassment associated with this diagnosis.

Pharmacologic Treatment

- Pediculicides are required to kill lice and nits. Most are contraindicated in children younger than 2 years and in pregnant and lactating women.
- Types of pediculicides are as follows:
  - Pyrethrins (with piperonyl butoxide) 0.3% (A200, RID, Triple X): Leave shampoo on for 10 minutes, then rinse thoroughly. Reapplication may be

needed in 7 to 10 days. Products are available over the counter (OTC).

- Permethrin 1% cream rinse (Nix, Elimite): Available OTC, this drug has a 97% to 99% cure rate and minimal side effects. Apply to the area, leave on for 10 minutes, and rinse thoroughly. Reapplication is not usually necessary but may be done 7 to 10 days after initial treatment. Do not exceed two applications in 24 hours. Avoid contact with mucous membranes. May be used in pregnancy. Caution those with ragweed allergies.
- Lindane (Kwell): Prescription is required. Product comes as 1% lotion, 1% cream, and 1% shampoo. Shampoo, leave on pubic area for 4 minutes, then rinse. Repeat in 1 week if necessary. Product must be used with caution because it may cause neurotoxicity, which causes headache, dizziness, and seizures. Lindane should not be used on acutely inflamed skin nor should it be used in pregnant or lactating women or in children less than 2 years of age or in those with known seizure disorders. Avoid any contact with the eyes during application.
- Treat secondary bacterial infections as needed.
- To treat lice-infested eyelashes, apply petrolatum 3 to 4 times a day for 10 days. Remove any visible lice gently. Never use pediculicides (anti-lice medications) on the eyelashes.

Client Education

- Reassure the client that pediculosis is curable, does not cause long-term effects, and is a problem in all socioeconomic groups.
- Teach how to disinfect the personal articles and how to clean the environment, reinforcing that lice do not jump or fly but spread through crawling and direct contact.
  - Machine wash all washable clothing and bedding used within the last 48 hours with hot water and detergent (water should be hotter than 125° F).
  - Dry clothing and bedding on as high a heat as possible in a clothes dryer for at least 20 minutes.
  - Dry clean clothing and personal items that cannot be washed. Upholstered furniture and pillows that might be contaminated may be ironed with a hot iron or sprayed with products that contain pyrethrin (Black Flag and Raid).
  - Place other items that have been exposed to infestation in a plastic bag and keep it closed for 2 weeks; lice will die of starvation.
  - Recommend that sexual partners in the last month be treated.
- Absolute prevention demands sexual abstinence with exposed individuals and not sharing clothing, bedding, or towels with others.

Referral/Consultation

Referral to a physician is necessary for the following:

- Treatment failure requires referral.
- Lice in eyelashes that persist despite treatment requires referral.
- Coexisting dermatologic conditions requires referral.
- If pediculosis pubis is seen in a child, appropriate authorities should be notified regarding the potential for child sexual abuse.
- Refer client to National Pediculosis Association for more information if desired.

EVALUATION/FOLLOW-UP

- All sexual contacts for the past month should receive treatment.
- Reapplication of pediculicide may be necessary in 7 to 10 days if symptoms persist or recur.

COMPLICATIONS

- Secondary infection
- Sensitivity reactions to treatment
- Excoriations

REFERENCES

Cash, J. C., & Glass, C. A. (2000). *Family practice guidelines.* Philadelphia: Lippincott.

Crain, E. F., & Gershel, J. C. (1997). *Clinical manual of emergency pediatrics.* New York: McGraw-Hill.

Dunphy, L. M., & Winland-Brown, J. E. (2001). *Primary care: The art and science of advanced nursing practice.* Philadelphia: FA Davis.

Fenstermacher, K., & Hudson, B. T. (1997). *Practice guidelines for family nurse practitioners.* Philadelphia: WB Saunders.

Fitzpatrick, T. B., Johnson, R. A., Polano, M. K., Suurmond, D., & Wolff, K. (1997). *Color atlas and synopsis of clinical dermatology,* New York, McGraw-Hill.

Forsman, K. E. (1995). Pediculosis and scabies: What to look for in patients who are crawling with clues. *Postgraduate Medicine, 98*(6), 89-100.

Hawkins, J. W., Roberto-Nichols, D. M., & Stanley-Haney, J. L. (1997). *Protocols for nurse practitioners in gynecologic settings.* New York: Tiresias Press.

Ismail, M. A. (2000). Skin diseases: Pediculosis pubis. *Contemporary OB/GYN, 5,* 178-180.

Miller, H. S., McEvers, J., & Griffith, J. A. (1997). *Instructions for obstetric and gynecologic patients* (2nd ed.). Philadelphia: WB Saunders.

Youngkin, E. O., & Davis, M. S. (1998). *Women's health: A primary care clinical guide.* Norwalk, CN: Appleton & Lange.

Review Questions

1. Merritt, a 21-year-old college student presents to the student health clinic with complaints of intense itching in her pubic

P

area for 2 days. She says, "I'm trying to study for final exams, but this is so miserable, I can't stand it." Which information from the history is most consistent with a diagnosis of pediculosis pubis?

   a. An isolated sexual encounter over last weekend with someone she met at a party
   b. Swimming over the weekend in a dirty pond
   c. Picking strawberries in a wooded area with sorority sisters 2 days ago
   d. Trying on a dress at a "garage sale" 1 week ago.

2. Which information about the itching is consistent with a pediculosis infestation?

   a. The itching is most intense when she is sitting in class.
   b. The itching is worse at night.
   c. Warm showers before sleep relieve the itching for 6 to 8 hours.
   d. The itching intensified when she sunbathed yesterday.

3. The NP examines Meritt's pubic region carefully. What objective finding suggests the presence of pediculosis pubis?

   a. Painful, red linear vesicles across the mons pubis
   b. Honey-yellow crusted lesions scattered over the mons pubis and labia majora
   c. Flea-bite-type rash covering all the perineum, buttocks, and upper thighs
   d. Small dark specks clinging to the pubic hair

4. What symptoms other than itching are common with pediculosis pubis?

   a. Gray, homogenous vaginal discharge with a musty odor
   b. Tender inguinal lymphadenopathy
   c. Healing lesions at different stages: some fluid-filled, others scaling
   d. Distraction, irritability, difficulty sleeping

5. The NP suspects that the infestation is caused by the crab louse. How can the suspicion be confirmed?

   a. Cover the suspect area with acetic acid; silvery fluorescence denotes lice.
   b. Perform a serum Phthirus titer.
   c. Remove a louse and evaluate it under the microscope or shine a Wood's lamp onto the area in question.
   d. Ask Merrit to contact her sexual partner to determine if he has similar symptoms.

6. What conditions should be considered as differential diagnoses for Merritt?

   a. Scabies
   b. Ringworm
   c. Condyloma acuminata
   d. Pityriasis rosea

7. An 18-year-old who discloses a history of multiple sexual partners and whose menstrual period is 2 weeks overdue is suspected to have pediculosis pubis and a secondary infection in several excoriated areas on her mons. Which action should precede treatment?

   a. Pregnancy test
   b. Skin scraping viewed under microscope
   c. Wet prep to check for clue cells
   d. Patch test for permethrin allergy

8. The NP provides a woman with pediculosis pubis with comprehensive education about the infestation, prevention, treatment, and environment management. Which comment made by the woman indicates a need for further teaching?

   a. "I will wash clothes and linens in hot water and dry them in a clothes dryer."
   b. "If the medicine I use does not solve the problem, I can reapply it one time before returning for follow-up."
   c. "Only sexual partners I've had this week need to be treated."
   d. "If I get the infestation in my eyelashes, I should cover them with petroleum jelly twice daily for 10 days."

9. For which of the following clients with pediculosis pubis is lindane (Kwell) contraindicated?

   a. Joyceen, an 11-year old girl who was abused by an uncle
   b. Teresa, who is menstruating
   c. Mary Grace, who is breastfeeding her 2-month old
   d. Ann, who is allergic to iodine

10. Which follow-up is essential for Mona, a 13-year-old with pediculous pubis?

   a. "Are her menstrual periods heavier following the lindane treatment?"
   b. "Has she been sexually abused?"
   c. "Is she allergic to eggs or chickens?"
   d. "Does she use sanitary pads or tampons?"

Answers and Rationales

1. **Answer: a** (analysis/diagnosis)
   Rationale: Pediculosis pubis is spread by sexual contact (Ismail, 2000).

2. **Answer: b** (assessment)
   Rationale: Itching appears worse at night and may affect sleep (Hawkins, Roberto-Nichols, Stanley-Haney, 1997).

3. **Answer: d** (assessment)
   Rationale: Dark specks clinging to the pubic hair with the history of pruritus are suspicious of the crab louse (Hawkins, Roberto-Nichols, Stanley-Haney, 1997).

4. **Answer: d** (analysis/diagnosis)
   Rationale: Itching can cause irritability and distraction; worse symptoms at night often cause difficulty sleeping (Ismail, 2000).

5. **Answer: c** (analysis/diagnosis)
   Rationale: It is not always easy to see the crab louse, but the diagnosis can be confirmed by direct visualization of the louse under the microscope (Ismail, 2000).

6. **Answer: a** (analysis/diagnosis)
   Rationale: Scabies is always one of the differential diagnoses (Hawkins, Roberto-Nichols, Stanley-Haney, 1997).

7. **Answer: a** (implementation/plan)
   Rationale: Lindane (Kwell), one of the most effective treatments, is contraindicated in pregnant women; pregnancy must

be ruled out in this case because history indicates that the client may be pregnant (Hawkins, Roberto-Nichols, Stanley Haney, 1997).

8. *Answer:* c (evaluation)
   Rationale: Individuals with whom the affected individuals have had sexual contact within the last month should be treated (Ismail, 2000).

9. *Answer:* c (implementation/plan)
   Rationale: Lindane (Kwell), one of the most effective treatments, is contraindicated in lactating women and children younger than age 2 (Cash & Glass, 2000).

10. *Answer:* b (evaluation)
   Rationale: Children who receive a diagnosis of pediculosis pubis are followed for sexual abuse (Dunphy & Winland-Brown, 2001).

PELVIC INFLAMMATORY DISEASE   *Cheryl Pope Kish*

OVERVIEW
Definition

Pelvic inflammatory disease (PID) is a clinical syndrome that occurs when pathogens from the vagina and cervix ascend to the upper reproductive tract. It may involve inflammation of the uterus, fallopian tubes, and ovaries, most often referring to salpingitis.

Incidence

Approximately 1 in 7 women of childbearing age in the United States has been treated for PID. More than 1 million women experience PID each year; 70% are less than 25 years old and one third are younger than 19 years.

Pathophysiology

The majority of cases of PID in the United States are caused by sexually transmitted infections.

Protective Factors
- Sexual abstinence
- Consistent use of barrier contraceptives, OCPs, or progestin-only contraceptives
- Mutually monogamous relationship

Factors Increasing Susceptibility
- Age younger than 25 years
- Cigarette, alcohol, and illicit drug use
- Previous history of PID
- History of STDs in which treatment of self or partner was not assured
- Multiple or new sex partners within 30 days of symptoms
- Nulliparity
- Pelvic instrumentation
- Use of IUD
- Douching or menses within 1 week of symptoms

Common Pathogens
- Up to 60% of cases are caused by *Chlamydia trachomatis* or *Neisseria gonorrhoeae.*

- Other common organisms cultured from those with PID include *Mycoplasma hominis, Ureaplasma urealyticum, Bacteroides, Peptostreptococci, Escherichia coli,* and some endogenous aerobes and anaerobes.
- Usually more than one pathogen is present. Incubation depends on causative organisms.
- Bacterial vaginosis and trichomoniasis may also be present.

ASSESSMENT: SUBJECTIVE/HISTORY
Symptoms
- Determine onset, duration, and course of present symptoms. Characterize pain and determine its association with voiding, defecation, and coitus.
- Lower abdominal pain, fever, chills, nausea, and vomiting in are present in acute PID.
- Dysuria, postcoital bleeding may be present.
- Increased vaginal discharge may be present.
- Atypical or chronic PID features include vague symptoms, such as abnormal vaginal bleeding and dyspareunia; 25% of clients experience right upper quadrant (RUQ) pain.

Past Medical History
- Previously diagnosed STD or PID or known exposure to sexually transmitted infection
- History of endometriosis
- History of IUD use, therapeutic abortion, or dilation and curettage
- Date of LMP
- Unprotected intercourse

Medications

Inquire about recent or current antibiotic use.

Psychosocial/Sexual History
- Age
- Cigarette, alcohol, or illicit drug use
- Number of sexual partners
- Recent new partner
- Use of contraception and type used
- Use of douching

P

ASSESSMENT: OBJECTIVE/ PHYSICAL EXAMINATION

Physical Examination

A focused physical examination should be performed with special attention to the vital signs and abdomen and pelvic examinations. Particular notice should be made of the following classic examination findings:

- Lower abdominal tenderness, bilateral adnexal tenderness, and cervical motion tenderness (CMT) (Chandelier sign).
- Guarded gait, with client taking small steps while holding her lower abdomen
- Oral temperature higher than 100.4° F (38° C)
- Mucopurulent discharge
- Cervical friability

Diagnostic Procedures

Laboratory Tests

- Obtain wet prep to assess WBC count, trichomonas, and yeast.
- Do cervical cultures for *N. gonorrhoeae*. Do not wait for culture results before treating acute PID.
- Cervical culture or nonculture test (DNA probe) for *C. trachomatis*.
- Do pregnancy test; results influence treatment plan.
- Obtain complete blood count (CBC) with differential; WBC count will be elevated higher than 10,000 cells/mm^3 unless client is immunocompromised.
- Perform urinalysis
- Erythrocyte sedimentation rate (ESR) may be elevated above 15 to 20 mm/hr (not commonly performed).
- C-reactive protein level may be elevated (not commonly performed).
- Perform serologic tests for syphilis and HIV, as well as hepatitis B surface antigen (HbsAg). Results influence treatment plan.

Diagnostic Tests

- PID is diagnosed on the basis of the clinical examination. It is confirmed by wet prep and cultures.
- Laparoscopy is considered for clients not responding to treatment or to rule out another diagnosis.
- Ultrasonography may rule out other causes of symptoms (e.g., tuboovarian abscess, ectopic pregnancy, appendicitis).
- Endometrial biopsy sample shows histopathologic evidence of endometritis. Combined with transvaginal ultrasonography, biopsy may be an alternative to laparoscopy when the diagnosis is in question Endometrial biopsy is contraindicated in pregnancy.

DIAGNOSIS

The Centers for Disease Control and Prevention (CDC) has set the following criteria for diagnosing PID:

- Minimum criteria (all three must be present): lower abdominal tenderness, adnexal tenderness, CMT
- Additional routine criteria: oral temperature higher than 101° F (38.3° C); abnormal vaginal or cervical discharge; elevated ESR; elevated C-reactive protein; and laboratory evidence of chlamydia or gonorrhea
- Additional elaborate criteria (based on diagnostic procedures that are technically more complicated and costly): biopsy evidence of endometritis; ultrasonography or radiographic evidence of inflammatory mass; laparoscopic abnormalities consistent with PID

Differential diagnoses include the following:

- Ectopic pregnancy
- Appendicitis
- Ovarian torsion
- Ovarian cyst
- Tuboovarian abscess
- Endometriosis
- Pyelonephritis
- Urinary tract infection (UTI)
- Vaginitis
- Uterine fibroids
- Threatened abortion
- Diverticulitis

THERAPEUTIC PLAN

Because of the serious complications of untreated PID, most references suggest treatment even when the diagnosis is only probable, not positive.

Pharmacologic Treatment

Outpatient Care

- Regimen A: Cefoxitin sodium (Mefoxin) 2 g IM, plus probenecid (Benemid) 1 g PO in a single dose, concurrently; or ceftriaxone (Rocephin) 250 mg IM, or other parenteral third-generation cephalosporin plus doxycycline 100 mg PO bid for 14 days.
- Regimen B: Ofloxacin (Floxin) 400 mg bid, for 14 days, plus metronidazole (Flagyl) 500 mg PO bid for 14 days. Instruct client to avoid alcohol with metronidazole. Fluoroquinolones are generally contraindicated in pregnant and lactating women.

Inpatient Care

- Regimen A: Cefoxitin (Mefoxin) 2 g IV q6h, or cefotetan (Cefotan) 2 g IV q12h, plus doxycycline (Vibramycin) 100 mg PO or IV q12h. Continue this regimen for at least 48 hours after clinical improvement. Continue doxycycline 100 mg PO bid for 14 days.
- Regimen B: Clindamycin phosphate (Cleocin phosphate) 900 mg IV q8h, plus gentamicin (Garamycin) in a loading dose of 2 mg/kg IV or IM, followed by a maintenance dose of 1.5 mg/kg q8h. Continue this regimen for at least 48 hours after clinical improvement.

Continue doxycycline 100 mg PO bid, or clindamycin hydrochloride (Cleocin hydrochloride), 450 mg PO qid, for 14 days or longer.

- In the presence of tuboovarian abscess, clindamycin may be substituted for doxycycline for continued coverage because it is more efficacious against aerobic pathogens.

Referral

Hospitalization is warranted in the following cases:

- Acute surgical abdomen (appendicitis or ectopic pregnancy) cannot be ruled out.
- Pelvic abscess is suspected.
- Client is HIV-positive or is immunosuppressed.
- Severe illness with nausea and vomiting preclude oral treatment as an outpatient.
- Woman cannot tolerate outpatient treatment, is unable to follow the regimen, or is unreliable.
- Woman has failed to respond to outpatient management within 72 hours.
- The woman is pregnant. Clinical judgment is warranted in this case.

Client Education

- Abstain from sexual intercourse until treatment is completed and symptoms have resolved.
- Partner should be tested and treated for any STD.
- Complete all medication, even when feeling better.
- Return for follow-up as instructed.

Referral/Consultation

The NP is well served by consulting with a physician in any case in which there is uncertainty about the severity of the PID or when subtle symptoms make diagnosis uncertain.

Prevention

- Prevent STDs (counsel for safe sexual behaviors; screen target groups).
- Treat STDs promptly in both women and their partners with CDC-recommended regimens.
- Consider prophylactic antibiotics for insertion of IUDs.
- Advise against douching routinely.

EVALUATION/FOLLOW-UP

Client should return for follow-up 72 hours after initiation of medication, sooner if symptoms worsen. If there is no clinical improvement at 72 hours, hospitalization is required for intravenous treatment. Further studies are also warranted at this time to assess for other possible diagnoses. *C. trachomatis* continues to be excreted after treatment. Repeat cultures cannot be done until 3 to 6 weeks after the original culture to ensure accuracy.

COMPLICATIONS

- Fitz-Hugh-Curtis syndrome occurs in 5% to 30% of cases of pelvic infection. It is caused by inflammation of the capsule surrounding the liver. Affected clients have RUQ pain that is intense enough to obscure the symptoms of pelvic pain.
- Infertility as a result of tubal scarring occurs in 10% to 30% of clients after the first episode of PID, depending on the severity of the infection. Infertility rates continue to rise with each subsequent episode of PID, reaching 50% to 75% after three or more cases. Ectopic pregnancy rates also increase as a result of scarred fallopian tubes. Chronic pelvic pain of unknown cause may be a complication.
- Even women with only one episode of PID are at increased risk for long-term sequelae: chronic pelvic pain, ectopic pregnancy, dyspareunia, and infertility. PID is the most common cause of infertility worldwide.

REFERENCES

Cash, J. C., & Glass, C. A. (2000). *Family practice guidelines*. New York: Lippincott.

Centers for Disease Control and Prevention. (1998). 1998 guidelines for treatment of sexually transmitted diseases. *MMWR: Morbidity and Mortality Weekly Report, 47*(RR-1), 1-111.

Hawkins, J. W., Roberto-Nichols, D. M., Stanley-Haney, J. L. (1997). *Protocols for nurse practitioners in gynecological settings* (6th ed.). New York: Tiresias.

Hoar, S. (1998). Pelvic inflammatory disease. *Lippincott's Primary Care Practice, 2*(3), 307-311.

Ivey, J. B. (1997). The adolescent with pelvic inflammatory disease: Assessment and management. *Nurse Practitioner, 22*(2), 78-91.

MacKay, T., Soper, D., & Sweet, R. L. (1997). PID: Suspect more, treat more, hospitalize less. *Patient Care, 31*(12), 109-129.

Mott, A. M. (1998). Prevention and management of pelvic inflammatory disease by primary care providers. *American Journal of Nurse Practitioners 2*(5), 7-15.

Newkirk, G. (1996). Pelvic inflammatory disease: A contemporary approach. *American Family Physician, 53*(4), 1127-1139.

Robinson, D., Kidd, P., & Rogers, K. M. (2000). *Primary care across the lifespan*. St. Louis: Mosby.

Rome, E. S. (1999). Managing pelvic inflammatory disease in adolescents. *Women's health in primary care, 2*(10), 819-832.

Smith, R. P. (1997). *Gynecology in primary care*. Baltimore: Williams & Wilkins.

Smith, M. A., & Shimp, L. A. (2000). *Women's health care*. New York: McGraw-Hill.

Youngkin, E. Q., & Davis, M. S. (1998). *Women's health: A primary care clinical guide*. Stamford, CN: Appleton & Lange.

Review Questions

1. What are the minimum diagnostic criteria for PID?
   a. RUQ pain, fever, and vomiting
   b. CMT, left adnexal pain, and vaginal discharge
   c. Lower abdominal pain, CMT, and bilateral adnexal pain
   d. Abnormal vaginal bleeding, dyspareunia, and elevated WBC count

2. Which of the following physical findings is suggestive of PID?

- **a.** Vaginal discharge mucopurulent
- **b.** Right lower quadrant pain
- **c.** Cervical friability
- **d.** CMT

3. Which of the following regimens is appropriate for a 21-year-old client who is having her first episode of PID, is afebrile, and is in her first trimester of pregnancy?

- **a.** Ofloxacin 400 mg bid for 14 days, plus metronidazole 500 mg bid for 14 days
- **b.** Cefoxitin 2 g IV q6h, plus doxycycline 100 mg PO bid for 14 days
- **c.** Ceftriaxone 250 mg IM, and doxycycline 100 mg PO bid for 14 days
- **d.** Clindamycin 900 mg IV q8h, with gentamicin loading dose 2 mg/kg IV, and maintenance dose 1.5 mg/kg q8h.

4. Your client has been treated for 4 days with intravenous cefoxitin and intravenous doxycycline for PID with culture positive for *N. gonorrhoeae*. When should she initially return for follow-up after her discharge from the hospital?

- **a.** In 4 to 6 weeks for repeated culture
- **b.** Only if symptoms recur
- **c.** In 72 hours
- **d.** In 7 to 10 days after completion of medication

5. In atypical PID, the most probable causative organism is which of the following?

- **a.** *C. trachomatis*
- **b.** *N. gonorrhoeae*
- **c.** *Bacteroides*
- **d.** *Peptostreptococcus*

6. Your client has been taking ofloxacin 400 mg, and metronidazole 500, mg both PO bid, for 14 days. At her initial 72-hour follow-up appointment, she has minimal resolution of her symptoms. Which approach is *not* appropriate?

- **a.** Hospitalize client.
- **b.** Order abdominal ultrasonography.
- **c.** Start cefotetan 2 g, and doxycycline 100 mg IV q12h.
- **d.** Recheck on outpatient basis in 24 hours.

7. Which of the following clinical presentations is most consistent with PID?

- **a.** Pelvic pain in a 12-year-old whose menarche was 6 months ago
- **b.** Lower abdominal pain in a 19-year-old with onset one week after menses
- **c.** Increased vaginal discharge and pelvic cramps in a 47-year-old married woman
- **d.** Pain, worse with Valsalva's maneuver, in a 53-year-old divorced client

8. A group of NPs is concerned that they are seeing so many women with PID in their practice. They believe that prevention education is warranted, but their time and funding is limited. Which target group is most appropriate as their first priority?

- **a.** 25- to 30-year-old married professional women
- **b.** Teens from Amish and Quaker groups in the practice
- **c.** 15- to 24-year-olds who are known to be sexually active

- **d.** All women seen in their clinic who volunteer for the education

9. Prevention education has been offered to a target group of women at high risk for PID. Which comment made by a member of the group indicates a need for clarification?

- **a.** "When I have sex with my boyfriend, we should use a condom."
- **b.** "If I use tampons for my periods, I should wash my hands first."
- **c.** "Using a douche every month will wash out the germs that cause infection."
- **d.** "If I suspect that I have been exposed to a STD, I should come to the clinic."

10. Peggy has been treated at home with an oral regimen for PID. When should she return for follow-up, assuming her symptoms are improving?

- **a.** 24 hours
- **b.** 72 hours
- **c.** 7 days
- **d.** 10 days

Answers and Rationales

1. **Answer: c** (assessment)
Rationale: RUQ pain is a symptom of complications from PID. Unilateral pain is more indicative of appendicitis or ectopic pregnancy. Abnormal uterine bleeding, dyspareunia, and an elevated WBC count are associated with PID, but are not minimum diagnostic criteria (Newkirk, 1996).

2. **Answer: d** (assessment)
Rationale: The pain of PID originates from the cervix. The pain should be with motion of cervix. Pregnancy may accompany PID, but is not diagnostic (Mott, 1998).

3. **Answer: d** (implementation/plan)
Rationale: Hospitalization is warranted for the pregnant client. Choice d is the regimen used for hospitalized clients. Choice a, in addition to being an outpatient regimen, also contains ofloxacin, which is not for use during pregnancy. Choice c includes doxycycline, which is best avoided during pregnancy (Mott, 1998).

4. **Answer: d** (evaluation)
Rationale: A 4- to 6-week follow-up is in addition to the 7- to 10-day follow-up. The 72-hour time is from initiation of therapy. The client should not be discharged from the hospital without clinical improvement (Smith, 1997).

5. **Answer: a** (assessment)
Rationale: *C. trachomatis* is an often asymptomatic STD, including cases of PID. Choices b, c, and d are also causes of PID, but these are less likely to be asymptomatic (Robinson, Kidd, & Rogers, 2000).

6. **Answer: d** (implementation/plan)
Rationale: This client has not improved after 72 hours of treatment. She warrants hospitalization and intravenous antibiotics. Further diagnostic tests are indicated to determine if she

is simply not responding to oral medications or there is another possible diagnosis (CDC, 1998).

7. Answer: b (assessment)
Rationale: The risk of PID increases in those younger than 25 years of age and occurs almost exclusively in menstruating women (Mott, 1998).

8. Answer: c (implementation/plan)
Rationale: Women 15 to 24 years old are at the highest risk of PID, especially if they are sexually active and use inconsistent barrier contraception. This group is an appropriate first choice for prevention education (Mott, 1998).

9. Answer: c (implementation/plan)
Rationale: Douching increases the risk of PID by enabling organisms to ascend into the pelvis more easily (Mott, 1998).

10. Answer: b (evaluation)
Rationale: Clients who are treated for PID on an ambulatory basis should be reevaluated in 72 hours. If symptoms are not responding to treatment, they should return earlier (Robinson, Kidd, & Rogers, 2000).

PELVIC PAIN   *Cheryl Pope Kish*

OVERVIEW
Definition

Acute pelvic pain refers to sudden onset of pain of a gynecologic nature with duration of 3 months or less. Chronic pelvic pain is pain that occurs in any region of the pelvis and endures beyond 6 months. Pain is associated with actual or potential tissue damage or may be psychogenic in nature.

Incidence

Pelvic pain is a common complaint evaluated by those in primary care practice. Chronic pelvic pain accounts for 10% of gynecologic consults.

Pathophysiology

Four sequential phases are involved between noxious stimulus and pain: (1) nociception, the origination and detection of a neural signal caused by the noxious stimulus; (2) recognition of pain or noxious event; (3) an affective response to the pain, often referred to as suffering; and (4) pain behavior or adaptive change in response to the experience of pain. Psychosocial factors modify and compound the pain experience through a complex interaction: individual variability, expectations of pain, cultural influences, previous experiences with pain, trained responses to pain, and emotional state. Pain response is unpredictable and varies from person to person and in the same person over time. The exact pathophysiologic mechanism relates to the cause of pain. Table 3-84 identifies common causes of acute and chronic pelvic pain.

ASSESSMENT: SUBJECTIVE/HISTORY

Rapid onset of symptoms is often associated with emergent conditions that must be ruled out immediately and referred appropriately. Emergent conditions are often associated with fever, hypotension, tachycardia, decreased bowel sounds, guarding, and rigid abdomen or hemorrhage, which create situations of jeopardy.

History of Present Illness

● Obtain a comprehensive view of pain: onset, chronology and regularity, duration, radiation. Have woman

TABLE **3-84**   Common Causes of Acute and Chronic Pelvic Pain

ACUTE PELVIC PAIN	CHRONIC PELVIC PAIN
Pregnancy-related	Endometriosis
Ectopic pregnancy	Malignancy–uterine,
Abortion (spontaneous	ovarian, colon
or voluntary)	Leiomyoma
	Adhesions
Infection	Uterovaginal prolapse
PID	Interstitial cystitis
Tuboovarian abscess	Musculoskeletal
Endometritis	Psychogenic pain
Masses	Posttraumatic stress
Ovarian cysts	response—sexual abuse
Torsion fibroids	
Torsion on ovaries, tubes	
Hormonal/Cyclical	
Dysmenorrhea	
Mittelschmerz	
Gastrointestinal	
Appendicitis	
Diverticulitis	
Irritable bowel syndrome	
Inflammatory bowel disease	
Intestinal obstruction	
Urinary	
UTI	
Renal calculi	
Other Common Causes	
Adhesions	
Sexual abuse	
Musculoskeletal	

UTI, Urinary tract infection.

quantify pain on a 0 to 10 scale. Ask what factors alleviate pain and what factors exacerbate it. Ask about associated symptoms, such as nausea, fever. Determine if a relationship exists between pain and voiding, defecating, coitus, meals, activity, position, and menstrual cycle. Identify LMP. Ask about contraception being used and possibility of pregnancy. Ask about similar pain episodes in past and how treated. Determine how many doctor's visits or emergency department visits have been necessitated because of pain.

- Ask about fever, nausea, vomiting, urinary symptoms, gastrointestinal (GI) symptoms, and vaginal discharge.

Past Medical History

- Ask about mental health problems and history of sexual abuse.
- Obtain obstetrical history, sexual history, and menstrual history. Ask specifically about sexually risky behaviors, exposure to STDs, a new partner in the previous month, and past and current contraception.
- Identify chronic diseases, surgery, (especially pelvic surgery in the previous 12 to 24 months) or work-ups for infertility. Ask about last Pap smear and results, any treatment of dysplasia. Ask about significant weight gain or loss.

Medication History

Inquire about current medications and drug allergies.

Dietary History

Inquire about foods that make symptoms worse.

Psychosocial History

Inquire about work and leisure activities and how pain is affecting them. Determine the amount of support from significant others and their perceptions of the situation. Ask about current life stressors and life changes that may be compounding pain. Ask about libido and whether pain is related to coitus.

ASSESSMENT: OBJECTIVE/PHYSICAL EXAMINATION

Physical Examination

Notice whether the woman looks sick, her gait into the examination room, her mobility in climbing onto the examination table, and her position once on the table. Note affect. Perform the following components of a focused assessment:

- Vital signs
- *Abdominal examination:* bowel sounds, bruits, distention, organomegaly, masses, tenderness, surgical scars, suprapubic tenderness, guarding, rebound, peritoneal signs (psoas, McBurney's sign, obturator, Markel's test)

- *Low back examination:* costovertebral angle tenderness (CVAT), musculoskeletal tenderness, range of motion (ROM)
- *Pelvic examination:* perineal trauma, cystocele/rectocele; vaginal lesions or trauma, pain on normal palpation; cervical os open or closed, lesions, discharge, friability, CMT, changes associated with pregnancy; uterine size, shape, position, mobility, and tenderness; adnexal masses, fullness, or tenderness
- *Rectal examination:* masses, lesions, bleeding

Diagnostic Procedures

First-line tests include the following:

- Pregnancy test
- CBC and differential
- Sedimentation rate
- Urinalysis
- Wet prep and cervical cultures, if indicated
- Pelvic ultrasound, if indicated (transvaginal if suspect ectopic or spontaneous abortion)

Second-line testing depends on history and physical findings, and includes the following:

- Blood chemistry
- Urine culture
- Abdominal radiograph examination

DIAGNOSIS

- The close anatomic proximity of pelvic organs and some shared sensory innervation complicates diagnosis. See Table 3-85 for suggested differential diagnosis.

NOTE: *GI, genitourinary (GU), musculoskeletal, and malignancy-related symptoms must also be ruled out in arriving at a definitive diagnosis.*

Chronic Pelvic Pain

Chronic pain often has the additional features of depression and fatigue. Finding an organic cause can be time-consuming and complicated. Because it is prolonged, chronic pain contributes to pain-related behaviors that become integral to one's personality. Dealing with chronic pain takes an emotional toll on the individual and family. Support by the NP is of inestimable value.

Psychogenic Pelvic Pain

Women with psychogenic pain may have insignificant physical variations or minimal lesions, but no significant organic cause for their pain has been discovered. Women between 25 and 45 years of age are particularly susceptible. Psychogenic pain may be a sequela to pelvic surgery or sexual abuse. It has additional features of fatigue, depression, sexual dysfunction, somatization, and substance abuse. Some psychogenic pain is related to ignorance, fear,

TABLE **3-85**   Differential Diagnosis: Pelvic Pain

DIAGNOSIS	CLINICAL FEATURES SUPPORTING DIAGNOSIS
Endometritis	Symptoms after delivery, abortion, or instrumentation; chills, fever, vaginal discharge (possibly purulent), tender uterus
Endometriosis	Cyclic pain, worse over time; dysmenorrhea, dyspareunia; pelvic tenderness
Dysmenorrhea	Occurs premenstrually and first 1-3 days of menses; cramping
Adhesions	Localized pain, increases with activity; follows surgery 12-24 months or endometriosis; pain with mobility, thickening on examination
Ectopic pregnancy	Acute, unilateral, 6-8 weeks after LMP; light bleeding possible; hypovolemia—collapse with tubal rupture; Cullen's sign, positive hCG, positive ultrasound
PID	Fever, chills, increased WBC count and ESR, nausea, vomiting, rebound, CMT, history STD
Torsion tube/ovary	Acute, unilateral, pain with motion; adnexal mass on exam or ultrasound
Mittelschmerz	Sharp pain or dull ache, localized lower quadrant; 14 days before expected menses; absent with hormonal contraception
Abortion (spontaneous, voluntary)	Cramping, bleeding, positive hCG, cervical changes, ultrasound diagnostic
Leiomyoma (fibroid)	Pressure, fullness unless twisted or entangled with organs; tenderness on examination possible; irregular uterine contour, enlarged; abnormal uterine bleeding
Appendicitis	Sequential: periumbilical early, later to RLQ pain, nausea, anorexia, rebound, fever, increased WBC count, peritoneal signs positive
Ovarian cyst	Acute or dull pain localized to side of cyst; pelvic tenderness unilaterally; palpable thickness on adnexa; with torsion: acute pain with nausea and vomiting; CMT to that side.

CMT, Cervical motion tenderness; *ESR,* erythrocyte sedimentation rate; *hCG,* human chorionic gonadotropin; *LMP,* last menstrual period; *PID,* pelvic inflammatory disease; *RLQ,* right lower quadrant; *STD,* sexually transmitted disease; *WBC,* white blood cell.

and decreased pain threshold. The medical future for women with this kind of pain is bleak unless they accept the reality of their pain and are willing to seek psychologic help. Having an NP who refuses to abandon them is of incredible value to such clients.

THERAPEUTIC PLAN

Treatment measures for pelvic pain clearly relate to the causative factor. Prompt referral for emergent conditions; antibiotics for infectious processes; appropriate analgesia; and treatment of the underlying cause of the pain are acceptable modalities.

EVALUATION/FOLLOW-UP

The timing and nature of follow-up depends on the cause of pelvic pain and the clinical manifestations. The NP consults with a physician or refers women in the following situations:

- Diagnosis is uncertain.
- Diagnosis requires medical or surgical intervention beyond the scope of the NP.
- Signs and symptoms worsen or recur after treatment.
- There is no response to standard treatment measures.

COMPLICATIONS

Clearly, some causes of pelvic pain are life threatening and failure to respond promptly and appropriately can result in catastrophic events. Chronic unremitting pain and psychogenic pain may be associated with despondency and suicide.

REFERENCES

Brown, K. M. (2000). *Management guidelines for women's health nurse practitioners.* Philadelphia: FA Davis.

Hawkins, J. W., Roberto-Nichols, D. M., Stanley-Haney, J. L. (2000). *Protocols for nurse practitioners in gynecologic settings* (7th ed.). New York: Tiresias Press, Inc.

Robertson, C. (1998). Differential diagnosis of lower abdominal pain in women of childbearing age. *Lippincott's Primary Care Practitioner, 2*(3), 210-229.

Robinson, D., Kidd, P., Rogers, K. M. (2000). *Primary care across the lifespan.* St. Louis: Mosby.

Smith, R. P. (1997). *Gynecology in primary care.* Baltimore: Williams & Wilkins.

Tierney, L. M., McPhee, S. J., & Papadakis, M. A. (2001). *Current medical diagnosis and treatment.* New York: Lange Medical Books/McGraw-Hill.

Van Zandt, S. (2000). Pelvic pain in women: Better understanding of an elusive diagnosis. *Clinical Review 10*(9), 51-69.

Youngkin, E. Q., & Davis, S. M. (1998). *Women's health: A primary care clinical guide.* Stamford, CN: Appleton & Lange.

Review Questions

1. Bronte is a 19-year-old woman with dull ache in her lower abdomen. Which historical finding is commonly seen in women with chronic pelvic pain?

a. Obsession with a vigorous excessive program.
b. Insistence on a strict vegetarian diet and no caffeine.
c. History of childhood sexual abuse by a relative.
d. Oral sex as a substitute for intercourse to prevent pregnancy.

2. What is the major difference between acute and chronic pelvic pain?
a. Acuity of symptoms
b. Duration of symptoms
c. Intensity of pain
d. Coincident constitutional symptoms

3. Which of the following diagnostic tests is not considered first line for diagnosing pelvic pain?
a. CBC and differential
b. Urinalysis
c. Pregnancy test
d. CT of pelvis

4. Abby presents with severe cramping in her lower abdomen, chills and fever, and increased vaginal discharge. Examination reveals a tender uterus and purulent drainage from the cervical os. WBC screen reveals increased WBC count and a shift to the left. Which finding raises the index of suspicion that this is endometritis versus PID?
a. History of hospitalization for similar symptoms in the past
b. Unprotected sex with new sexual partner within last 60 days
c. Recent insertion of a progestin-IUD for contraception
d. Presence of a prosthetic heart valve since childhood

5. Meredith complains of pain in her left lower quadrant of two-week duration, worse with movement. She denies nausea, vomiting, GU symptoms, or fever. Bimanual examination shows tenderness on the left. The remainder of the examination is normal. Which finding is consistent with a diagnosis of pelvic pain related to pelvic adhesions?
a. DepoProvera for birth control
b. Life-time history of eight sexual partners
c. History of irregular periods for a few months
d. Salpingectomy for ectopic pregnancy 18 months ago

6. The NP is trying to decide if Annie's unilateral lower left quadrant (LLQ) pain that occurs midcycle is related to Mittelschmerz. Which clinical finding negates Mittelschmerz as a cause of the pain?
a. Annie has the pain only on the left.
b. Annie takes combination OCPs.
c. Annie describes the pain as 4 on a 0 to 10 scale.
d. Annie also has symptoms of premenstrual syndrome (PMS).

Answers and Rationales

1. **Answer: c** (assessment)
Rationale: Childhood sexual abuse has a strong correlation with pelvic pain after the event and in adulthood (Smith, 1997).

2. **Answer: b** (analysis/diagnosis)
Rationale: Acute pain is defined as lasting less than 3 months, whereas chronic pain is said to last longer than 6 months (Tierny, et al, 2001).

3. **Answer: d** (analysis/diagnosis)
Rationale: The CT of the pelvis is not a first-line test for diagnosing pelvic pain (Hawkins, et al, 1997).

4. **Answer: c** (analysis/diagnosis)
Rationale: Endometritis is associated with a history of childbirth, abortion, or recent pelvic instrumentation (Van Zandt, 2000).

5. **Answer: d** (analysis/diagnosis)
Rationale: Pelvic adhesions as a cause of pain should be suspected with a history of surgery within the previous 12 to 24 months or endometriosis (Smith, 1997).

6. **Answer: b** (analysis/diagnosis)
Rationale: Mittelschmerz as a cause of pelvic pain does not exist in women who use hormonal contraception that suppresses ovulation (Smith, 1997).

PEPTIC ULCER DISEASE *Denise Robinson*

OVERVIEW
Definition

- Peptic ulcer disease (PUD) is an ulcer, sore, or lesion that forms in the lining of the stomach or duodenum where acid and pepsin are present.
- Duodenal ulcer affects the proximal part of the small intestine. These ulcers follow a chronic course characterized by remissions and exacerbations.
- Gastric ulcer affects the stomach mucosa.

Incidence

- Approximately 20 million Americans develop at least one ulcer during their lifetime.

- Ulcers are rare in teenagers and even more uncommon in children.
- In young children, ulcers of the stomach and duodenum are typically secondary to systemic illnesses or drugs.
- In older children and adolescents, duodenal ulcers have a relapsing course that is increasingly thought to be related to coexisting chronic, active antral gastritis and *Helicobacter pylori* infection. Duodenal ulcers usually occur for the first time between ages 30 and 50, and occur more frequently in men than women.
- Out of all ulcers, approximately 80% are duodenal and 20% are gastric.
- Approximately 5% of all gastric ulcers are malignant.

- Each year ulcers affect approximately 4 million people; more than 40,000 people have surgery because of persistent symptoms or problems from ulcers; approximately 6,000 people die of ulcer-related complications.

Pathophysiology

PUD occurs when the mucosal barrier is impaired or overwhelmed by aggressive factors such as acid or pepsin. By definition, ulcers extend through the muscularis mucosae and are larger than 5 mm. The role of stress in the development of PUD is uncertain. Three major causes of PUD are recognized: nonsteroidal antiinflammatory drugs (NSAIDs), chronic *H. pylori* infection and acid hypersecretory states such as Zollinger-Ellison syndrome.

Protective Factors. The stomach's natural defenses are the following:
- Mucus production provides a lubricant-like coating that shields stomach tissues.
- Bicarbonate production neutralizes and breaks down digestive fluids.
- Good blood supply increases cell renewal and repair.

Factors Increasing Susceptibility
- Bacterial virulence
- Physiologic stress: surgical procedures, severe trauma, burns, shock
- Medications: corticosteroids, NSAIDs (increases risk of gastric ulcers 40 fold)
- Gender/age: men ages 30 to 50, women older than 60 years of age
- Familial predisposition
- Physiologic incompetence: bile reflux from incompetent pyloric sphincter, delayed or abnormal gastric emptying

Children
- Association with bile acid and reflux
- Association with *H. pylori*
- Secondary factors that increase susceptibility
- Stress
- Major systemic illness
- Burns
- Head trauma
- Excess acid
- G-cell hyperplasia (pseudo–Zollinger-Ellison syndrome)
- Mastocytosis
- Drugs
- NSAIDs
- Corticosteroids
- Corrosives
- Gastroduodenal Crohn's disease
- Cystic fibrosis
- Sickle cell disease
- Juvenile-onset diabetes mellitus
- Common Pathogens

ASSESSMENT: SUBJECTIVE/HISTORY
History of Present Illness
- Obtain a clear statement of the chief complaint.
- Ask about the manifestation of pain; noting the location, intensity and whether or not the pain radiates, is relieved or aggravated by food.
- Explore GI symptoms of nausea, vomiting, changes in bowel habits, dysphagia, weight loss or gain, change in appetite.
- Ask about other symptoms such as history of testicular atrophy, gynecomastia, and alopecia (may be indicative of hepatic cirrhosis).
- Determine blood type. Type O has been associated with the adherence of *H. pylori*. Assess allergies.
- In the elderly, ask about excessive belching, bloating, flatulence, nausea and vomiting, diarrhea, rectal bleeding, number of BMs per day, and dietary history.

Symptoms
Up to 20% may be asymptomatic (silent ulcers).

Duodenal Ulcers. Intermittent epigastric pain described as a gnawing or burning is present in 80 to 90% of clients; heartburn is also present. Pain often occurs between meals and in the early hours of the morning, may awaken the client at night. Nausea and vomiting may be present (significant nausea and vomiting is uncommon and suggests gastric outlet syndrome or gastric malignancy). Loss of appetite, fatigue and weakness, tarry stools, and dyspepsia may be present.

Gastric Ulcers
- Pain often aggravated or triggered by food; weight loss common.
- Older clients may be asymptomatic until disease has advanced (GI bleeding, pancreatitis).

Associated Symptoms
Associated symptoms are chest pain and diarrhea.

Past Medical History
- Ask about previous episodes of PUD.
- Ask about any other chronic illnesses, especially illnesses that might be treated with NSAIDs.
- Ask about rheumatoid arthritis (RA).

Medication History
- NSAIDs, especially acetylsalicylic acid and higher doses of other NSAIDs
- During first 3 months of NSAIDs therapy for elderly
- Concomitant steroid therapy

Family History
Ask about family history of polyps, GI cancers, alcohol consumption, smoking, and psychologic disorders.

P

Psychosocial History

In older adults, consider losses and role changes in the past year. May need to ask about death of loved ones, retirement, changes in living situations.

Diet History

- Ask about the consumption of alcohol, caffeine, foods that increase or relieve the symptoms, and patterns of consumption and elimination.
- Ask older adults to record diet for 3 days to give a more accurate pattern.

ASSESSMENT: OBJECTIVE/PHYSICAL EXAMINATION

Physical Examination

A problem-oriented physical should be conducted with particular attention to the following:

- *Vitals signs and weight:* Assess general appearance and hydration status, including turgor and orthostatic changes.
- *Cardiovascular:* Rule out cardiac insufficiency.
- *Abdomen:* Perform a complete examination, especially noting areas of tenderness, bruits, hums, or rubs. Note size of organs and CVAT. Mild localized epigastric tenderness to deep palpation may be present.
- *Genital/rectal:* Examine external genitalia for atrophy; perform a DRE.

Diagnostic Procedures

- Check hemoglobin (Hgb) and hematocrit (Hct) levels to check for anemia.
- All clients with new or recurring ulcers should be tested for *H. pylori;* once positive, antibodies are always positive, so cannot be used to check for reinfections.
- Check the upper GI system.
- Endoscopy is becoming the test of choice because it is more sensitive; ulcers can be photographed and tissue taken for biopsy.

DIAGNOSIS

Differential diagnoses include the following:

- PUD
- Gastric cancer
- Angina
- Cholecystitis
- Pancreatitis

THERAPEUTIC PLAN

The goals of treatment are to relieve pain, aid healing, prevent recurrence and prevent complications.

Nonpharmacologic Treatment

- Smoking cessation
- Discontinue the use of NSAIDs
- Discontinuation or decrease of consumption of alcohol and caffeine
- Stress management
- No specific diet; avoidance of irritating foods

Pharmacologic Treatment

There are a variety of regimens used for eradication of *H. pylori* (see Table 3-86). There is not any one "right" regimen. Some of the most common regimens used today are listed in the following. Three-times-daily regimens should be taken with meals, and four-times-daily regimens should be taken with meals and hs.

Children

- In children with primary ulcers, long-term maintenance therapy with an H₂ blocker is an option that might be considered to reduce the high rate of ulcer recurrence. However, consideration must also be give to cost and compliance with long term acid suppression. Eradication of *H. pylori* if identified is appropriate for children.
- Children with secondary ulcers are usually at low risk for recurrence once the underlying illness has been resolved.

Client Education

- Disease process, expected outcomes and possible complications
- Stress reduction
- Stop smoking
- Medications, especially NSAIDs

Referral/Consultation

- Persons who fail to respond to treatment
- Significant weight loss
- Symptoms of peritonitis (abdominal rigidity, rebound tenderness, fever)
- Suspected gastric ulcers

Prevention

- No smoking
- Avoidance of NSAIDs and corticosteroids

EVALUATION/FOLLOW-UP

- Consider rechecking *H. pylori* status if dyspepsia continues because its presence may be a weak predictor of persistent infection.
- Follow up in 2 to 4 weeks after initial visit, and 6 to 8 weeks thereafter until stable.
- Children with positive *H. pylori* need to be followed closely because they are at risk for development of gastric cancer.

COMPLICATIONS

Perforation of ulcer.

TABLE **3-86** Common Regimens Used for Eradication of *H. pylori*

DRUG	DOSAGE	COMMENTS
Bismuth (Pepto-Bismol)	2 tablets qid	Duration of regimen 1-2 weeks, omeprazole
Metronidazole (Flagyl)	250 mg tid/qid	should be continued up to 4 weeks
Tetracycline	500 mg tid	
Omeprazole (Prilosec)	20 mg bid	
Bismuth	2 tablets qid	Duration of regimen 1-2 weeks
Metronidazole	250 mg tid/qid	H_2-blocker may be continued for 4-6 weeks;
Tetracycline	500 mg qid	not recommended in children
(Helidac includes above medications)		Give with full glass of water
Positive H_2-blocker		Avoid alcohol during treatment; may antagonize OCPs; photosensitivity
Bismuth	2 tablets qid	Duration 1-2 weeks
Metronidazole	250 mg tid	
Amoxicillin	500 mg tid/qid	
Bismuth	2 tablets qid	Duration 1-2 weeks
Clarithromycin (Biaxin)	500 mg tid	
Tetracycline	500 mg qid	
Bismuth	2 tablets qid	Duration 1-2 weeks
Clarithromycin	500 mg tid	
Amoxicillin	500 mg qid	
Bismuth	2 tablets qid	Duration 8 days
Clarithromycin	500 mg bid	
Omeprazole	20 mg bid	
Metronidazole	500 mg bid	Duration 1-2 weeks
Omeprazole	20 mg bid	
Clarithromycin	500 mg bid	
Amoxicillin	1 g bid	Duration 1-2 weeks
Omeprazole	20 mg bid	
Clarithromycin	500 mg bid	
Amoxicillin	1 g bid	Duration 1-2 weeks
Omeprazole	20 mg bid	
Metronidazole	500 mg bid	
Clarithromycin	500 mg bid	Duration 2 weeks
Amoxicillin	1 g bid	Not recommended for children
Lansoprazole (Prevacid)	30 mg bid	

Adapted from Robinson, D. (2000). Peptic ulcer disease. In D. Robinson, P. Kidd, & K. Rogers (Eds.), *Primary care across the lifespan* (pp. 881-886). St. Louis: Mosby.

REFERENCES

Aronson, B. (1998). Update on peptic ulcer drugs. *American Journal of Nursing, 98*(1), 41-46.

Cave, D. R., & Hoffman, J. S. (1996). Management of *Helicobacter pylori* infection in ulcer disease. *Hospital Practice, 31*(1), 63-4, 67-9, 73-5.

Cerda, J. J. et al (1995). Peptic ulcer disease: now you can cure, *Patient Care, 29*(20), 100–109.

Cornell, S. (1997). New treatments for peptic ulcer disease. *ADVANCE for Nurse Practitioners 5*(3), 57-59.

Damianos, A. J., & McGarrity, T. J. (1997). Treatment strategies for *Helicobacter pylori* infection. *American Family Physician, 55*(8), 2765-2774.

Dohil, R., Israel, D., Hassal, E. (1997). Effective 2-week therapy for *Helicobacter pylori* disease in children. *American Journal of Gastroenterology, 92*(2), 244-247.

Heslin, J. M. (1997). Peptic ulcer disease: Making a case against the prime suspect. *Nursing 27*(1), 634-639; quiz 97, 34–40.

Johnson, D. A. (1996). New dimensions in *Helicobacter pylori* infection. *Emergency Medicine 28*(2), 74-85.

Jones, N., & Sherman, P. (1998). *Helicobacter pylori* infection in children. *Current Opinion in Pediatrics 10*(1), 19-23.

Kato, S., Takeyama, J., Ebina, K., & Naganuma, H. (1997). Omeprazole-based dual and triple regimens for *Helicobacter pylori* eradication in children. *Pediatrics, 100*(1), E3.

Lewis, J. H. (1995). Peptic ulcer disease: Update on management in the *H. pylori* era. *Consultant 35*, 91-94.

McColl, K., el-Nujumi, A., Murray, L., el-Omar, E. M., Dickson, A., Kelman, A. W., & Hilditch, T. E. (1998). Assessment of symptomatic response as predictor of *Helicobacter pylori* status following eradication therapy in patients with ulcer. *Gut 42*(5), 618-622.

National Institutes of Health. (1995). *Stomach and duodenal ulcers.* Bethesda, MD: National Digestive Diseases Information Clearing House. NIH publication No. 95-38.

Prescribers Letter. (1998). *Efficacy of peptic ulcer treatment.* Document #130804, Prescribers Letter.

Robinson, D. (2000). Peptic ulcer disease. In D. Robinson, P. Kidd, & K. Rogers. (Eds.) *Primary care across the lifespan* (pp 881-886). St. Louis: Mosby.

Rowland, M., & Drumm, B. (1998). Clinical significant of *Helicobacter* infection in children. *British Medical Bulletin, 54*(1), 95-103.

Sherman, P. M. (1994). Peptic ulcer disease in children: Diagnosis, treatment, and the implication of *H. pylori. Gastroenterology Clinics of North America 23*(4), 707-725.

Review Questions

1. Mr. T., a 55-year-old white man, seeks treatment with a sharp left upper quadrant abdominal pain associated with nausea and vomiting. The pain seems to come on as a sharp spasm or cramping discomfort, which turns into a burning sensation that goes to the chest. The pain sometimes awakens him at night. He reports that he has taken Mylanta for 7 years for indigestion. Which of the following is most likely the cause of Mr. T.'s pain?

   a. Diverticulitis
   b. Pancreatitis
   c. PUD
   d. Coronary artery insufficiency

2. Your next step in caring for Mr. T. would be which of the following?

   a. Give sublingual nitroglycerin to relieve the associated chest pain.
   b. Change his antacid.
   c. Obtain additional medical history data.
   d. Check his vital signs.

3. The fact that Mr. T.'s pain is not associated with activity and awakens him at night makes it less likely that his problem is which of the following?

   a. Coronary artery insufficiency
   b. PUD
   c. pancreatitis
   d. diverticulitis

4. For optimal effect in PUD, when should antacids be given?

   a. 1 hour before meals
   b. 1 hour after meals
   c. Immediately after meals
   d. immediately before meals

5. The NP needs to differentiate between gastric and duodenal ulcers. Unlike duodenal ulcers, gastric ulcers are associated with which of the following?

   a. Abdominal pain is not relieved by food.
   b. Anorexia, nausea, and vomiting are not usually present.
   c. Gastric ulcers heal faster than duodenal ulcers.
   d. Treatment for gastric ulcers is different than duodenal ulcers.

6. Follow-up after treatment of a gastric ulcer should consist of which of the following?

   a. No follow up is needed if no symptoms are present.
   b. Monthly hemoccult specimens are necessary.
   c. Endoscopy should be done to check healing and potential for gastric cancer.
   d. Maintenance H_2 should be continued for at least 6 months after symptoms disappear.

7. Which of the following physical findings might be present in a client you suspect has a peptic ulcer?

   a. Severe abdominal tenderness with guarding
   b. Rebound tenderness
   c. Mild localized epigastric tenderness to deep palpation
   d. Tenderness on rectal examination

8. Which comment by the client with PUD indicates a need for further instruction?

   a. "I need to quit smoking."
   b. "I need to take antacids before every meal."
   c. "Decreasing my use of NSAIDs would be helpful."
   d. "Taking my medications as prescribed will be helpful in eradicating the *H. pylori.*"

Answers and Rationales

1. Answer: c (analysis/diagnosis)
   Rationale: Manifestations of PUD include intermittent epigastric pain. Pain begins 1 to 3 hours after eating, frequently awakening the person at night. Pain is relieved by food, antacids, and dyspepsia (Robinson, 2000).

2. Answer: c (assessment)
   Rationale: More information is needed about Mr. T.'s symptoms and history before an informed decision can be made for treatment (Cornell, 1997).

3. Answer: a (analysis/diagnosis)
   Rationale: Pain associated with coronary artery insufficiency is usually precipitated by physical activity, persists no more than a few minutes, and subsides with rest (Robinson, 2000).

4. Answer: b (implementation/plan)
   Rationale: Antacids are given to reduce the total acid load in the GI tract and to elevate the gastric pH to reduce pepsin activity. Duration of activity is less than 1 hour. To be most effective, antacids must be given 1 hour after meals (Damianos, et al, 1997).

Continued

Product	Manufacturer	Description	Indication	Application	Advantages	Comments
COMPRESSION DRESSINGS						
Coban (use with Unna's boot) CircAid Profore Unna's boot	3-M Coloplast/Sween Smith & Nephew/United Biersdorf	Elastic stockings or bandages applied to the lower extremities	Venous insufficiency	Irrigate with saline or commercial noncytotoxic cleanser Change q3-7 days exudate May require use of protective cream/ointment to prevent contact dermatitis (do not apply to ulcer)	Promotes venous blood return Prevents blood pooling Decreases edema	Arterial ulcers Ulcers with mixed arterial-venous cause ABI <0.8 Contact dermatitis may develop as a result of zinc oxide impregnated wraps
ENZYMATIC DEBRIDING AGENTS						
Santyl Accuzyme	Knoll Pharmaceuticals Health Point Medical	Debriders digest necrotic tissue by differing methods	Dermal ulcers, partial- or full-thickness wounds	Irrigate with saline or commercial noncytotoxic cleanser	Daily application Nonsurgical method of debridement Does not harm healthy tissue (these two products only) Provides moist environment	Secondary dressing May require cross-hatching of eschar
FOAMS						
Allevyn LYOfoam PolyMem	Smith & Nephew/United ConvaTee Ferris Manufuacturing	Absorbs exudate May be non-adherent or have adhesive backing	Management of exuding cutaneous wounds Infected or noninfected wounds	Irrigate with saline or commercial noncytotoxic cleanser	Daily application Nonocclusive May use under compression dressing	May require secondary dressing
GAUZE						
Numerous		Nonocclusive fiber dressing with loose, open weave	Minimal to heavy exudating wounds Infected wounds Debridement	Irrigate with saline or commercial noncytotoxic cleanser Change q6-8h	Readily available Deep wound packing May use with infected wounds or with topical agents Nonocclusive Comfortable	Wound bed may dessicate Nonselective wound debridement May cause bleeding/pain on removal Secondary dressing required Frequent dressing changes Dressing may "shed"

ABI, Ankle-trachial index.

TABLE **3-88** Options in Lower Extremity Wound Management—cont'd

CATEGORY/TRADE NAME	MANUFACTURER	DESCRIPTION	INDICATIONS/ CONTRAINDICATIONS	APPLICATIONS	ADVANTAGES	DISADVANTAGES
HYDROCOLLOIDS						
Comfeel	Coloplast/Sween	A wafer dressing	Clean, granular wounds	Irrigate with saline	Forms moist gel	For noninfected wounds
Duoderm CGF	ConvTec	composed of	Minimal to moderate	or commercial	wound bed	only
Restore	Hollister	hydrophilic particles	exudating wounds	noncytotoxic	Impermeable to	Contraindicated for
Tegasorb	3-M	in an adhesive form	Venous ulcers in	cleanser	fluids/bacteria	arterial/neuropathic
		covered by a water	conjunction with	Change q3-7 days	Conformable	Impermeable to gases
		resistant film or foam	Unna's boot		Good thermal	May leave residue
			Full-thickness wounds		insulation	on skin
			without tunneling			
			or undermining			
			Noninfected wounds			
			only			
			Autolysis			
AMORPHOUS HYDROGELS						
Carrasorb	Carrington	Gel composed of	Partial- or full-thickness	Irrigate with saline	Forms moist wound	May dehydrate
	laboratories	94% water to	wounds	or commercial	Conformable	Minimal to moderate
Carrasyn Gel	Carrington	96% glycerin	Arterial and	noncytotoxic	Manages exudate	absorption
	Laboratories		neuropathic ulcers	cleanser	by swelling	Requires secondary
IntraSite Gel	Smith & Nephew/			Cover with gauze/	Autolysis	dressing
Restore	United			transparent		May require dressing
Hydrogel	Hollister			dressing to		changes if appropriate
Solosite	Smith & Nephew/			prevent		Secondary dressing not
	United			dehydration		used
				of gel		
SKIN SEALANTS						
AllKare	ConvaTec	Vapor-permeable film,	Prevents epidermal	Irrigate with saline	Protects skin from	Burns, if applied to
Protective	Hollister	nonwater soluble	stripping caused by	or commercial	epidermal stripping	denuded skin
Barrier Wipes	Smith & Nephew/		adhesive products	noncytotoxic	when adhesives	Must apply before each
Skin Gel	United			cleanser	are removed	application of adhesive
Protective	Coloplast/Sween			Apply, allow to dry		
Wipes				before placing		
Skin Prep				adhesive on skin		
Sween Prep						

TRANSPARENT DRESSINGS

Product	Manufacturer	Description	Indications	Application	Advantages	Comments
Opsite	Smith & Nephew/United	A semiocclusive translucent dressing with partial or continuous adhesive composed of polyurethane or copolymer thin film	Partial-thickness wounds; Clean, granular wounds; Minimally exudating wounds; Peripheral neuropathy ulcers; Cover dressing for hydrogels, alginates, enzymatic debriding agents	Irrigate with saline or commercial noncytotoxic cleanser; Change q3-7 days; Requires at least 24 hours wear time for effective use; Apply skin sealant to periwound skin before applying	Semi-occlusive; Gas permeable; Easy inspection of wound; Protection; Impermeable to fluids/bacteria; Comfortable; Self-adherent; Pain reduction; Moist environment; Resists shear	For noninfected wounds only; Not absorptive; May cause peritrauma on removal; Maceration may occur with large amounts of exudate
Tegaderm	3-M					

CELL PROLIFERATION

Product	Manufacturer	Description	Indications	Application	Advantages	Comments
Becaplermin (Regranex)	Ortho-McNeil	A recombinant human platelet-derived growth factor in a topical gel	Lower extremity diabetic neuropathic ulcer in conjunction with other ulcer care practices; DO NOT use in children younger than 16 years; Cover with saline-moistened dressing; Leave in place 12 hours; Remove and rinse with saline to remove residue; Cover with plain, moist dressing; Pregnancy: C	Each square inch of ulcer surface requires ⅔ inch length of gel (cm^2 of ulcer requires 0.25 cm)	Very few side effects	Wound and SQ tissue must have adequate blood supply; Complex dosing (Box 3-17)

SQ, Subcutaneous.

Peripheral Neuropathy

- Do not smoke.
- Comply with medications.
- Control diabetes.
- Avoid exposure to cold.
- Avoid friction.
- Avoid moisture between toes.
- Avoid going barefoot.
- Obtain routine professional foot care for toenails, corns, calluses.
- Use well-fitting footwear.
- Use pressure reduction for heels and other bony prominences.
- Avoid use of external heat (heating pad, hot water bottle, hydrotherapy).
- Practice daily foot care, which includes skin inspection; wash and dry well, especially between toes; keep skin moisturized; wear clean socks.
- Avoid use of OTC medications for corns and calluses.
- Avoid temperature extremes.

Referrals

- Request referral for orthotic footwear if altered gait or orthopedic deformity occurs.
- Refer to ET/WOC nurse for wound care or debridement depending on comfort level of NP.
- Refer to home health care worker if assistance needed for wound care.
- Refer for vascular surgeon if ABI is less than 0.5, if pain increases, or if ulcer fails to respond within 2 to 4 weeks.
- Refer to dietitian.
- Refer to podiatrist.
- Refer to orthotist.
- Refer to endocrinologist.
- Provide other referrals as indicated.

Prevention

- Movement
- Avoid compression of tissue (leg crossing), bedrest
- Adequate glucose control in diabetes

EVALUATION/FOLLOW-UP

NOTE: *Each client's follow-up should be individualized.*

- Venous insufficiency: Follow-up every 4 to 7 days for the first 2 weeks if compression dressing becomes saturated, because decrease in edema requires more frequent dressing changes; then every 3 to 4 weeks if followed by home health or family member instructed to change dressing daily and prn for dressing saturation; if not followed by home health or family member changing dressing, then weekly and prn for dressing changes.
- Arterial insufficiency: Follow-up weekly for the first 2 weeks, then every 4 weeks and prn for change in status of affected lower extremity.
- Peripheral neuropathy: Follow-up weekly for 4 to 6 weeks; then every 2 to 3 weeks and prn for change in status of affected lower extremity.

See Table 3-88 for options in lower extremity wound management. See Box 3-17 for calculations for Regranex gel dosing.

COMPLICATIONS

- Infection
- Osteomyelitis
- Chronic ulcer

REFERENCES

Alguire, P. C., & Mathes, B. M. (1997). Chronic venous insufficiency and venous ulceration. *Journal of General Internal Medicine, 12*(6), 374-382.

Barr, D. M. (1996). The Unna's boot as a treatment for venous ulcers. *Nurse Practitioner 21*(7), 55-56, 61-64, 71-72.

Crossland, M., Shawler, L., & Boykin, J. (1998). The chronic wound. *ADVANCE for Nurse Practitioner, 6*(8), 61-65.

DePalma, R. G. (1996). Venous ulceration: A cross-over study from nonoperative to operative treatment. *Journal of Vascular Surgery, 24*(5), 788-792.

Erickson, C. A., Lanza, D. J., Karp, D. L., Edwards, J. W., Seabrook, G. R., Cambria, R. A., Freishleg, J. A., & Towne, J. B. (1995). Healing of venous ulcers in an ambulatory care program: The roles of chronic venous insufficiency and patient compliance. *Journal of Vascular Surgery, 22*(5), 629-636.

Box 3-17 Calculations for Regranex Gel Dosing

- Measure the greatest length and the greatest width of the ulcer.
- Calculate the length of gel that should be squeezed from the 15-g tube using the following formulas:

Inches
Length × Width × 0.6
For example, if the ulcer measures 2 inches × 2 inches, a 1½-inch length of gel should be used [1 × 1 × 0.6 = 1.2].

Each square inch of ulcer surface requires approximately ⅔-inch length of gel.

Centimeters
Length × Width × 4
For example, if the ulcer measures 4 cm × 2 cm, a 2-cm length of gel should be used [(4 × 2) 4 = 2].
Each square centimeter of ulcer surface requires approximately a 0.25-cm length of gel.

From Regranex package insert, December 1997, Ortho-McNeil Pharmaceutical, Raritan, New Jersey.

Hafner, J., Bounameaux, H., Berg, G., Brunner, U. (1996). Management of venous leg ulcers. *Journal for Vascular Diseases, 25*(2), 161-167.

Hall, P., & Schumann, L. (2001). Wound care: Meeting the challenge. *Journal of the American Academy of Nurse Practitioners, 13*(6), 258-266.

Harris, A. H., Brown-Etris, M., & Troyer-Caudle, J. (1996). Managing vascular leg ulcers part I: Assessment. *American Journal of Nursing, 96*(1), 38-43.

Holloway, G. A. (1996). Arterial ulcers: Assessment and diagnosis. *Ostomy Wound Management, 42*(3), 50-51.

Kenkre, J. E., Hobbs, P. D., Carter, Y. H., Thorpe, G. H., Holder, R. L. (1996). A randomized controlled trial of electromagnetic therapy in the primary care management of venous leg ulcerations. *Family Practitioner 13*(3), 235-241.

Kowallek, D. L., & DePalma, R. G. (1997). Venous ulceration: Active approaches to treatment. *Journal of Vascular Nursing 15*(2), 50-57.

Lagua, R., Claudio, V. (1996). *Nutrition and diet therapy reference dictionary* (4th ed.). Florence, KY: International Thomas Publishing.

Lavelle, M. (2000). Lower extremity ulcers. In D. Robinson, P. Kidd, K. Rogers, (Eds.). *Primary care across the lifespan.* St. Louis: Mosby.

Maune, J., & Giordano, J. (1997). Experience with open-heeled Unna boot application technique. *Journal of Vascular Nursing, 15*(2), 63-72.

Miller, M. (2001). Managing chronic wounds: Myths and misconceptions. *Clinical Advisor, 4*(6), 72-74.

Nelzen, O., Bergquist, D., & Lindhagen, A. (1997). Long-term prognosis for patient with chronic leg ulcers: A prospective cohort study. *European Journal of Vascular and Endovascular Surgery, 13*(5), 500-508.

Regranex Package Insert, December 1997, Ortho-McNeil Pharmaceutical, Raritan, New Jersey.

Richard, L. E. (1997). Compression therapy and venous ulceration: Another point of view. *Journal of Wound Ostomy Continence Nursing 24*(3), 180.

Sanford, J. P., Gilbert, D. N., Moellering, R. C. (1997). *The Sanford guide to antimicrobial therapy.* Kansas City, MO: Hoechst Marion Roussel.

Sieggreen, M. (1997). Limb and life: Principles of leg ulcer management. *ADVANCE for Nurse Practitioners, 5*(3), 17-18, 21-22, 24, 26.

Sieggreen, M. Y., & Maklebust, J. (1996). Managing leg ulcers. *Nursing, 26*(12), 41-46.

Sieggreen, M. Y., Cohen, J. K., Kloth, L. C., Harding, K. G., Stotts, N. A. (1996). Commentaries on venous leg ulcers diagnostic and treatment draft guidelines. *Advances in Wound Care: The Journal for Prevention and Healing, 9*(4), 18-26.

Smith, P. D. (1996). The microcirculation in venous hypertension. *Cardiovascular Research 32*(4), 789-795.

Stacey, M. C., Jopp-Mckay, A. G., Rashhid, P. et al: (1997). The influence of dressings on venous ulcer healing: a randomized trial. *European Journal of Vascular and Endovascular Surgery, 13*(2), 174-179.

Review Questions

1. When the client complains of pain on movement in the extremities the NP should consider which of the following diagnoses?

   a. Vascular insufficiency
   b. Leg ulcer
   c. Arterial insufficiency
   d. Peripheral neuropathy

2. Which of the following best describes a venous stasis ulcer?

   a. Ruddy skin with surrounding erythema or brown staining
   b. Deep, pale, wound bed
   c. Thin, dry, taut wound bed
   d. Infection and necrosis usually present

3. An ABI is used to document which of the following?

   a. Circulation in a diabetic client
   b. Arterial circulation
   c. Degree of neuropathy
   d. Degree of pedal edema

4. The NP assesses a leg ulcer as exposed dermis with pink tissue. This ulcer would be classified as which of the following?

   a. Stage 1
   b. Stage 2
   c. Stage 3
   d. Stage 4

5. In what situation is compression therapy *contraindicated?*

   a. ABI less than 0.8 mm Hg
   b. Diabetic client
   c. Venous insufficiency
   d. Presence of leg ulcer

6. Which of the following statements indicates effective client education in a client with a leg ulcer produced by arterial insufficiency?

   a. "I will keep my leg elevated."
   b. "I will avoid constrictive clothing."
   c. "I will not ambulate until the ulcer has started healing."
   d. "I will apply ice as needed for pain."

7. Which of the following indicates the need for antibiotic treatment for a leg ulcer?

   a. Draining wound
   b. Colony count greater than 1×10^5
   c. Presence of fever and chills
   d. Presence of wound odor

8. Under what circumstances should topical therapy be used with caution in treating a leg ulcer?

   a. In an ulcer produced by venous insufficiency
   b. In an ulcer produced by arterial insufficiency
   c. In an ulcer produced by peripheral neuropathy
   d. When an ulcer is infected

9. Which of the following dietary supplements promotes wound healing?

   a. Carbohydrates
   b. Magnesium
   c. Vitamin C
   d. Vitamin E

P

Answers and Rationales

1. Answer: c (analysis/diagnosis)
Rationale: Vascular insufficiency produces very little pain. Peripheral neuropathy is painless. Pain may not be associated with ulcer formation.

2. Answer: a (assessment)
Rationale: Ulcers from arterial insufficiency are usually pale and deep. Skin changes in arterial insufficiency are taut, thin, dry, and loss of hair. Ulcers in peripheral neuropathy tend to be infected and necrotic because they go so long without detection.

3. Answer: b (implementation/plan)
Rationale: ABI findings are not reliable in diabetic clients. It may be used in mixed-cause ulcers, but it is used to determine degree of arterial circulation.

4. Answer: b (analysis/diagnosis)
Rationale: Stage I: involves only the epidermis
Stage II: dermis is exposed, pink with possible red tissue buds
Stage III: involves subcutaneous tissue with possible exposed fascia
Stage IV: destruction of fascia with possible exposed tendon or bone.

5. Answer: a (implementation/plan)
Rationale: An ABI of less than 0.8 mm Hg indicates inadequate circulation, which would be further compromised by compression. Compression therapy may be used in diabetic clients. Compression therapy is used to help heal leg ulcers produced by venous insufficiency.

6. Answer: b (evaluation)
Rationale: In arterial insufficiency, the leg should be maintained in a dependent or neutral position. Ambulation should be encouraged to tolerance. Exposure to cold should be avoided to prevent further vasoconstriction. Constrictive clothing should be avoided to help promote arterial flow.

7. Answer: b (implementation/plan)
Rationale: Fever and chills may indicate another health problem. Drainage and odor can be part of healthy wound healing. Only a colony count is indicative of the need for antibiotic treatment.

8. Answer: b (implementation/plan)
Rationale: Topical therapy in arterial insufficiency may cause the fragile epidermis around the ulcer to macerate. Infection may indicate the need for topical therapy. Topical therapy can be used in venous insufficiency and in peripheral neuropathy.

9. Answer: c (analysis/diagnosis)
Rationale: Vitamin C and zinc promotes wound healing. Although not listed as an option, protein also supports wound healing.

PERTUSSIS (WHOOPING COUGH, *BORDETELLA PERTUSSIS*) *Denise Robinson*

OVERVIEW
Definition

- Pertussis is an acute bacterial disease involving the respiratory tract caused by *Bordetella pertussis*. Whooping cough syndrome may also be caused by *B. parapertussis, Mycoplasma pneumoniae, Chlamydia trachomatis, C. pneumonia, B. bronchiseptica* and certain adenoviruses.
- The disease occurs in three stages, as follows:
  - Catarrhal stage involves a mild upper respiratory infection (URI) with progressive cough that lasts 1 to 2 weeks; cultures are most sensitive at this time.
  - Paroxysmal stage involves coughing spells with classic whooping sound; lasts 4 to 6 weeks. Culture zero percent after fifth week.
  - Convalescent stage involves a gradual decrease in cough and other symptoms; lasts several weeks to months.

Incidence

- Communicable for 3 weeks after the onset of paroxysmal stage in untreated patients. Five days after the onset of treatment they are communicable.
- Affects women more than men.
- Infants 1 to 2 months old are highly susceptible; disease is most severe in first year of life.
- Half of all deaths occur in infants younger than 1 year of age.
- Highest rates in occur in children younger than 5 years of age.
- Adolescents and adults have mild cases of pertussis that are not associated with whooping cough.
- Incidence rates have risen steadily in past years; although primary vaccination is effective, protection is transient. Outbreaks occur every 3 to 4 years in people who have been immunized. Infected adults and adolescents with mild disease are the reservoir for more severe infection in infants and young children (Scott, Clark, & Miser, 1997).

Pathophysiology

Caused by the gram negative bacillus *B. pertussis,* a strict anaerobe whose only reservoir is humans. Spread by respiratory secretions. Highly contagious (transmission rates can be 100% in close contacts). Incubation period is 6 to 10 days but can range from 5 to 21 days. Infected persons can transmit the disease after the first week of incubation and remain infectious until 3 weeks after onset of symptoms (Scott, et al, 1997).

ASSESSMENT: SUBJECTIVE/HISTORY
History of Present Illness

- Infants have coughing spells with hypoxemia, apnea, posttussive vomiting, and neurologic disorders such as tremor or seizures.
- Symptoms wane gradually, with 6 to 10 weeks duration.
- Adolescents and adults have mild upper respiratory symptoms that progress to severe paroxysms of cough. Fever is absent or minimal. Cough is persistent, insidious, worse at night with mild, nonspecific URI. Adults may also have sweating and sneezing attacks, hoarseness, sinus pain, and headache.

Symptoms

- Infants have paroxysms of cough, often with a characteristic respiratory whoop, followed by vomiting.
- In infants younger than 6 months symptoms may be atypical.
- Apnea is a common manifestation and the whoop is often absent.
- In adults, the cough may not have the classic whooping sound.

Past Medical History

- Immunization history
- Previous infection
- Environmental exposure (illness at home, work, school, day care)
- Travel (to area with high incidence)
- Communicable disease history

Medication History

Current medications.

Family History

Illness among family members.

Psychosocial History

School/day care exposures.

ASSESSMENT: OBJECTIVE/PHYSICAL EXAMINATION
Physical Examination

- Assess vital signs.
- Observe HEENT for symptoms of URI.
- Assess respiratory system. Observe respirations, auscultate chest.

Diagnostic Procedures

- Nasopharyngeal cultures are 80% sensitive when obtained during the first 2 weeks; negative cultures are common, especially late in the course of the disease; sensitivity is 14% after the fourth week and 0 after the fifth week.
- Direct fluorescent antibody performed on nasal smears also can be used to diagnosis pertussis.
- In CBC, leukocytosis with a predominance of lymphocytes may be noted.
- Chest radiograph may reveal perihilar infiltrates, atelectasis, or emphysema.

DIAGNOSIS

- Many cases of pertussis go unrecognized because the classic cough is uncommon.
- Pertussis should be considered in any client with symptoms of an URI followed by cough paroxysms. Also consider pertussis in client that has had an unexplained cough for longer than 14 days; a diagnosis of pertussis can be made with a sensitivity of 84% (Scott, et al, 1997).

Differential Diagnoses

- Bacterial tracheitis involves respiratory stridor, high fever, copious purulent secretions; follows streptococcus, staphylococcus, or *Haemophilus influenza* type B (Hib) infection.
- Congenital subglottis stenosis is a possibility.
- In croup, child wakens at night with barking cough, hoarseness, inspiratory stridor and possible respiratory distress. Usually afebrile. Episodes are mild to moderate and resolve quickly when exposed to humidity.

THERAPEUTIC PLAN
Nonpharmacologic Treatment

- Supportive care should be provided.
- Infants with apnea and cyanosis should be hospitalized for antibiotic therapy, observation, and supportive care. Respiratory isolation should be used until the completion of 5 days of antibiotic therapy.

Pharmacologic Treatment

- Erythromycin is the drug of choice, given for 14 days; clarithromycin (Biaxin) can also be given. Side effects include nausea, vomiting, and diarrhea; abdominal cramping; and anorexia. Trimethoprim-sulfamethoxazole (TMP/SMX, Bactrim) is an effective alternative if erythromycin is not tolerated.
- There are many drug interactions. Check before prescribing.
- Regardless of immunization status, a 14-day course of erythromycin, ethylsuccinate for household and close contacts is recommended.
- Health care workers also may need to be treated for 14 days after occupational exposure to pertussis.
- Antibiotics are appropriate during any phase of the illness. Goal late in the course of the illness is to clear the organism from the nasopharynx and limit the spread of disease rather than reduce the length of symptoms.

Client Education

- Students and school staff should not return to school until 5 days of antibiotic treatment have been completed.
- Discuss need for immunization, possible adverse events after pertussis vaccine or antipyretic prophylaxis after administration of diphtheria/tetanus/pertussis immunization.

Referral/Consultation

- Immediate referral with hospitalization of infants younger than 6 months
- Consultation with all other cases

Prevention

- Immunization per recommended schedule

EVALUATION/FOLLOW-UP

Report to local health authority.

COMPLICATIONS

- Pneumonia is the most common cause of death.
- Other complications include seizures and encephalitis.

REFERENCES

American Academy of Pediatrics. (2000). Pertussis. In G. Peter (Ed.). *2000 Red book: Report of the committee on infectious disease* (25th ed., pp. 394-407). Elk Grove Village, IL: AAP.

American Public Health Association. (2000). *Control of communicable diseases manual* (17th ed., pp. 347-351). Washington, DC: APHA.

Cooper, L. (2000). Pertussis. In D. Robinson, P. Kidd, K. Rogers, (Eds.). *Primary care across the lifespan* (pp. 895-897). St. Louis: Mosby.

He, Q., Viljanen, M. K., Arvilommi, H., et al: (1998). Whooping cough caused by *Bordetella pertussis* and *Bordetella parapertussis* in an immunized population. *Journal of the American Medical Association, 280*(7), 635-637.

Scott, P., Clark, J., & Miser, W. (1997). Pertussis: An update on primary prevention and outbreak control. *American Family Physician 56*(4), 1121-1128.

Yaari, E., Yafe-Zimerman, Y., Schwartz, S. B., et al. (1999). Clinical manifestations of *Bordetella pertussis* infection in immunized children and young adults. *Chest 115*(5), 1254-1258.

Review Questions

1. Which of the following historical data is consistent with a diagnosis of pertussis in adults?
- **a.** Mild URI followed by a persistent cough
- **b.** Whooping cough which occurs in paroxysms followed by vomiting
- **c.** Apnea and shortness of breath
- **d.** Sore throat and nasal discharge

2. In infants, what historical information will the parents most likely give related to pertussis?
- **a.** Mild URI and vomiting
- **b.** Hypoxemia with coughing spells
- **c.** Chills and loss of consciousness
- **d.** Vomiting and diarrhea

3. Pertussis presents in three stages. The description of symptoms (coughing spells, inspiratory whoop, posttussive vomiting) is characteristic of which stage of Pertussis?
- **a.** Catarrhal
- **b.** Paroxysmal
- **c.** Convalescent
- **d.** Recovery

4. Pertussis must be differentiated from croup. Compared with pertussis, croup is described as which of the following?
- **a.** Coughing with postcoughing vomiting is present.
- **b.** Cough worsens at night.
- **c.** Child wakes at night with barking cough, hoarseness, inspiratory stridor, and possible respiratory distress.
- **d.** Wheezing worse at night, sob, nasal flaring.

5. A client comes in with persistent cough. You are suspicious of pertussis. He has had the cough for approximately 5 weeks. What is the likelihood that a nasopharyngeal culture will yield any results related to pertussis at this time?
- **a.** 90%
- **b.** 50%
- **c.** 30%
- **d.** 0%

6. Which of the following clients should be evaluated for hospitalization with pertussis?
- **a.** 3-month-old infant
- **b.** 12-month-old child
- **c.** 25-year-old female
- **d.** 55-year-old male

7. What is the drug of choice for treatment of pertussis?
- **a.** Bactrim
- **b.** Penicillin
- **c.** Erythromycin
- **d.** Ciprofloxacin (Cipro)

8. Which of the follow rationales for treating a client who has had a cough for 4 weeks and is positive for pertussis by culture is true?
- **a.** Reduces length of coughing and symptoms.
- **b.** Reduces complications related to pertussis.
- **c.** Reduces the incidence of airway reactivity.
- **d.** Reduces the spread of disease.

Answers and Rationales

1. *Answer:* a (assessment)
Rationale: In adults, the characteristic whooping cough is absent; most adults have a URI preceding the development of a persistent cough (Scott, et al, 1997).

2. *Answer:* b (assessment)
Rationale: Pertussis in children presents in a much more severe fashion than in adults and adolescents. Hypoxemia with cough, apnea, and neurologic disorders are common (Scott, et al, 1997).

3. *Answer:* b (analysis/diagnosis)
Rationale: The symptoms of coughing spells, inspiratory whoop, and posttussive vomiting are consistent with the second stage of Pertussis (Scott, et al, 1997).

4. *Answer:* c (analysis/diagnosis)
Rationale: Croup consists of the following symptoms: child wakens at night with barking cough, hoarseness, inspiratory stridor, and possible respiratory distress. Nighttime cough is nonspecific and could apply to any respiratory illness. Coughing following by vomiting is also very nonspecific. It may apply to both croup and pertussis (Cooper, 2000).

5. *Answer:* d (analysis/diagnosis)
Rationale: The best time to obtain a sensitive culture for pertussis is during the first 2 weeks of the URI and coughing.

After 4 weeks, the sensitivity of a culture for pertussis drops to 14% and after 5 weeks it drops to 0% (Scott, et al, 1997).

6. *Answer:* a (evaluation)
Rationale: The most cases of death related to pertussis are in children younger than 1 year of age. Any child younger than 1 year should be evaluated carefully and hospitalization should be considered.

7. *Answer:* c (implementation/plan)
Rationale: The treatment of choice for pertussis is erythromycin (Cooper, 2000).

8. *Answer:* d (implementation/plan)
Rationale: Even though the use of erythromycin does not alter the clinical course at this point in the illness, the antibiotic does clear the organism from the nasopharynx and reduces the spread of disease (Scott, et al, 1997).

PITYRIASIS ROSEA *Denise Robinson*

OVERVIEW
Definition

Pityriasis rosea is an exanthematous, maculopapular red scaling eruption that occurs largely on the trunk.

Incidence

- Pityriasis is mainly a disorder of fair-skinned whites, and is uncommon in those with Mediterranean heritage.
- It is common in ages 10 to 35, occurring more in the spring and fall in temperate climates. It accounts for approximately 2% of outpatient dermatologic visits.
- Occurs in women more than in men.
- There is no racial predilection.

Pathophysiology

- Unknown cause
- Perhaps a viral or autoimmune disorder

  Protective Factors. None.
  Factors Increasing Susceptibility
- Climate
- Fair complexion

ASSESSMENT: SUBJECTIVE/HISTORY
History of Present Illness

- Development of skin lesion, usually on trunk; after 1 to 2 weeks, a generalized secondary eruption occurs.
- Complaints of itching are as follows:
  - Absent (25%)
  - Mild (50%)

- Severe (25%)
- Although most clients are asymptomatic except for the rash, 5% of clients complain of headaches, malaise, arthralgias, chills, nervousness, vomiting, diarrhea, or constipation before the appearance of the herald patch (Hsu, Le, & Khoshevis, 2001).

SYMPTOMS

Fever and malaise are rare.

Past Medical History

Noncontributory.

Medication History

Recent use of corticosteroids.

Family History

Less than 5% affected give positive family history (FH).

Psychosocial History

Ask about stressful situations.

ASSESSMENT: OBJECTIVE/PHYSICAL EXAMINATION
Physical Examination

- Assess height, weight, and general appearance.
- Use a problem-oriented approach with particular attention to the following:
  - General skin lesions: type, shape, arrangement, distribution
  - Hair and nail involvement

P

- Discrete erythematous small fawn colored, fine scaling lesions scattered in a characteristic pattern: the long axes of the lesions follow the lines of cleavage in a "Christmas tree" distribution. Usually confined to the trunk and proximal aspects of arms and legs; rarely involves face. Color is dull pink or tawny. "Herald patch" is 2 to 6 cm patch that precedes the rash by days to weeks. The Herald patch is an oval, slightly raised patch, bright red, with fine collarette scale at periphery.

Diagnostic Procedures

- KOH wet mount: abscence of hyphae
- Rapid plasma reagin: negative
- Lyme titer: negative

DIAGNOSIS

Differential diagnoses include the following:

- Drug eruption: consider if on captopril or barbiturates
- Secondary syphilis: maculopapular rash, especially on palms and soles
- Lyme disease: systemic symptoms, erythema migrans
- Tinea corporis: small, scaling, sharply marginated lesions, and hyphae
- guttate psoriasis: lesions occur rapidly, frequently after streptococcal pharyngitis

THERAPEUTIC PLAN

Nonpharmacologic Treatment

- Symptomatic treatment
- Colloidal bath
- Lukewarm oatmeal bath
- Ultraviolet B (UVB) phototherapy or natural sunlight exposure for itching (works best if in first week of rash)

Pharmacologic Treatment

Diphenhydramine (Benadryl) for itching (caution clients about sleepiness).

Client Education

- Reassure clients that they do not have a "blood disease" and are not contagious. Remission usually occurs spontaneously in 6 to 12 weeks.
- Recurrences are uncommon, but do occur.
- Hot water may exacerbate rash.
- Strenuous activity may aggravate rash.

Referral/Consultation

- If no improvement in expected time frame, refer.
- If rash persists for longer than 6 weeks, a skin biopsy is needed to rule out parapsoriasis.

Prevention

None.

EVALUATION/FOLLOW-UP

Return for reevaluation if lesions last 6 weeks.

COMPLICATIONS

None.

REFERENCES

Dunn, S. (1998). *Primary care consultant.* St. Louis: Mosby.

Fitzpatrick, T., Johnson, R., Wolff, K. (2000). *Color atlas and synopsis of clinical dermatology* (4th ed.). New York: McGraw-Hill.

Habif, F. (1996). *Clinical dermatology: A color guide to diagnosis and therapy.* (3rd ed.). St. Louis: Mosby.

Horio, T. (1998). Skin diseases that improve by exposure to sunlight. *Clinical Dermatology, 16*(1), 59-65.

Hsu, S., Le, E., & Khoshevis, M. (2001). Differential diagnosis of annular lesions. *American Family Physician, 64,* 289-96.

Pomeranz, A., & Fairley, J. (1998). Pityriasis. *Pediatric Clinics of North America 45*(1), 49-63.

Wyndham, M. (1997). Pityriasis. *Practitioner, 241*(1575), 358.

Review Questions

1. A 22-year-old woman comes in with a slightly pruritic, scaling, red, maculopapular rash on her trunk. The round, dome-shaped lesions are arranged along lines of skin cleavage. She recalls what she thought was a patch of ringworm that appeared before the rash. The probable diagnosis is which of the following?

    a. Tinea versicolor
    b. Acne
    c. Seborrheic dermatitis
    d. Pityriasis rosea

2. You examine a scraping from a client's lesions under the microscope with KOH. You would expect to find which of the following in pityriasis rosea?

    a. Negative hyphae
    b. Positive hyphae
    c. Cocci with central black dots
    d. Cocci with central pallor

3. A 12-year-old girl comes in with a rash on her arms and legs for the last 4 days. It does not itch, and fever and chills are not present. She has not used any new products at home. She reports that she first thought it was ringworm but then it spread. Her mother states that she helps at a day care center sometimes after school, and at least one other child has similar symptoms. Which of the following diagnoses would be most appropriate for this scenario?

    a. Tinea versicolor
    b. Lyme disease
    c. Psoriasis
    d. Rosea

4. Your plan of care for the client with rosea includes which of the following?

    a. Recommend that she stay home from work until the rash starts to disappear because it is contagious.

b. Prescribe selenium sulfide.
c. Prescribe coal tar preparations and retinoids.
d. Prescribe colloidal baths, calamine lotion, antihistamines, and topical steroids.

5. A 16-year-old girl is being treated for rosea. She returns to your office in 3 days, upset that the symptoms have not gone away and that her return appointment is not for another 2 weeks.

a. Inform the client that the 2-week appointment is appropriate to determine progress, but it will take 6 to 12 weeks for the rash to disappear.
b. Inform her that she should not get so excited; the rash does not look that bad.
c. Tell her that it is all right that she came back to the office early; lots of people get excited and return early.
d. Inform her that your schedule is full for the day and she is welcome to change her appointment to an earlier time if there are openings.

6. Which of the following clients would be more likely to contract pityriasis rosea?

a. 35-year-old Italian female
b. 15-year-old black female
c. 18-year-old white female
d. 6-year-old white male

7. The best treatment for pityriasis rosea is which of the following?

a. Hydrocortisone
b. Mupirocin (Bactroban)
c. Symptomatic treatment only
d. Clotrimazole 1% (Lotrimin)

8. Which of the following comments by the client with pityriasis rosea indicates a need for further teaching?

a. "Warm oatmeal baths will help my rash."
b. "I should stay out of the sun."
c. "Acyclovir will treat my rash."
d. "I can use hydrocortisone for itching."

Answers and Rationales

1. *Answer:* d (analysis/diagnosis)
Rationale: Rosea is usually preceded 2 to 10 days by a larger, single, red macule, the "herald patch" (Fitzpatrick, et al, 2000).

2. *Answer:* a (assessment)
Rationale: For a diagnosis of tinea, microscopic examination of skin scraping with KOH reveals black clusters of spores and hyphae. You would not expect this in pityriasis rosea (Habif, 1996).

3. *Answer:* d (analysis/diagnosis)
Rationale: Rosea is frequently misdiagnosed as ringworm. The single herald patch precedes the general rash by days to a week (Fitzpatrick, et al, 2000).

4. *Answer:* d (implementation/plan)
Rationale: Treatment usually is not necessary; however, the treatments listed in choice d may shorten the duration of the disease (Fitzpatrick, et al, 2000).

5. *Answer:* a (evaluation)
Rationale: Teaching clients about the disease process helps them to know what to expect. It takes 6 to 12 weeks for the rash to go away (Fitzpatrick, et al, 2000).

6. *Answer:* c (assessment)
Rationale: Pityriasis rosea is most common between the ages of 10 and 35 in those with light skin (Fitzpatrick, et al, 2000).

7. *Answer:* c (implementation/plan)
Rationale: Symptomatic treatment is all that is needed for pityriasis rosea (Fitzpatrick, et al, 2000).

8. *Answer:* c (evaluation)
Rationale: Symptomatic treatment such as staying out of the sun, oatmeal baths and hydrocortisone are appropriate. Acyclovir is not appropriate for this rash and will not treat it (Fitzpatrick, et al, 2000).

PNEUMONIA *Pamela Kidd*

OVERVIEW
Definition

Pneumonia is an inflammatory process of the parenchyma of the lung (bronchioles and the alveolar spaces) that is caused by infection.

Classification

- Community-acquired
- Hospital-acquired (nosocomial)

Incidence

- Pneumonia is the most common cause of death related to an infectious disease.

- Pneumonia is the sixth overall cause of death in the Unites States and the fourth leading cause of death among the elderly.
- Pneumonia occurs most often during the winter months and early spring.

Pathophysiology

- Aspirated oropharyngeal secretions
- Inhalation of infected droplets
- Lymphohematogenous spread from another site
- Direct introduction of organisms from a diagnostic or treatment procedure or trauma

Protective Factors

- Cough and gag reflexes to protect against gross aspiration
- Mucociliary lining of the tracheobronchial tree
- Immune response: leukocytes and phagocytosis

Factors Increasing Susceptibility

- Altered upper respiratory tract flora: predisposition to more virulent organisms as a result of recent antibiotic therapy, recent hospitalization, diabetes, or alcoholism
- Altered immune status: diabetes, AIDS, alcoholism, malignancy, chemotherapy, uremia, sickle cell disease
- Impaired cough and gag reflex: increased risk of aspiration with altered mental status, alcohol or drug intoxication, anesthetics, cerebrovascular accident, seizure
- Impaired function of natural defense mechanisms: mucociliary clearance damaged by smoking, inhaled environmental pollutants, chronic obstructive pulmonary disease (COPD), CHF, alcohol, viral infection
- Mechanical bypass of normal defense: tracheal intubation, chest tube
- Underlying lung pathologic condition: pulmonary embolus or contusion, foreign body, atelectasis
- Chest wall pain: postoperative pain, chest trauma, myopathy

Common Pathogens

- *Streptococcus pneumoniae* is by far the most common cause of bacterial pneumonia, accounting for 70% of cases and common on an outpatient basis (higher frequency winter months).
- *Staphylococcus aureus* and Hib may also cause bacterial pneumonia. Both are more common in hospitalized clients. *H. influenza* is more common in heavy smokers (Davis, Kane, & Plouffe, 1999).
- Influenza A is the most common cause of viral pneumonia in older children, adolescents and adults.
- Respiratory syncytial virus is the most common cause of pneumonia in infants.
- *Mycoplasma pneumoniae* is common in school age children and young adults.
- Other pathogens that cause pneumonia in infancy include *Chlamydia*, group B streptococcus, parainfluenza viruses, and *Bordetella pertussis*.
- Aspiration pneumonia may be caused by *Staphylococcus aureus, Escherichia coli, Klebsiella pneumoniae, Pseudomonas aeruginosa, Proteus,* and *Enterobacter*.
- The most common pathogens in people 65 and older are *S. pneumoniae, H. influenza,* and other gram-negative bacilli. Other possible pathogens include *M. catarrhalis, Legionella* species (more common in summer), *M. tuberculosis,* and endemic fungi.

ASSESSMENT: SUBJECTIVE/HISTORY
Symptoms

- Typically pneumonia presents with an abrupt onset of fever, chills, and productive cough, but can have an atypical presentation with an insidious onset and dry cough.
- Inquire about onset and duration of symptoms.
- Inquire about associated symptoms, including difficulty breathing, shortness of breath, wheezing, retractions, nasal flaring, difficulty sleeping, difficulty speaking or weak cry, difficulty eating, rhinorrhea, earache, sore throat, hoarseness.
- Inquire about possibility of aspiration or foreign body.
- Inquire about systemic symptoms including fever, chills, rash, malaise, muscle aches, vomiting, and seizures.
- Inquire about self-help measures and other family members who might be ill.
- Inquire about recent hospitalizations or treatments.
- Inquire about smoking and the possibility of alcohol or drug use.

Past Medical History

- For children, inquire about underlying disease such as reactive airway disease, bronchopulmonary dysplasia, cystic fibrosis, tracheomalacia, congenital heart disease, sickle cell disease, seizures, and HIV/AIDS.
- For adults, inquire about underlying disease such as COPD, diabetes, chronic renal failure, CHF, liver disease, cancer, and HIV/AIDS.

Medications

- Inquire about immunization status in both children and adults.
- Inquire about recent antibiotic use.

Family History

Noncontributory.

Dietary History

Noncontributory.

ASSESSMENT: OBJECTIVE/PHYSICAL EXAMINATION
Physical Examination

- Assess vital signs for temperature elevation, tachypnea, tachycardia, hypotension, and HTN.
- Observe for pallor or cyanosis, dyspnea, pursed lips, grunting, or nasal flaring.
- Inspect the chest for retractions and use of accessory muscles, as well as increased anterior-posterior diameter.
- Dullness to percussion may indicate lobar consolidation.
- Auscultate the chest, assessing for asymmetry and equal inspirations and expirations.
- Assess for crackles and rales, wheezing, bronchial breath sounds, increased vocal fremitus, bronchophony, egophony, and whispered pectoriloquy (signs of consolidation).

- Infants with a respiratory rate greater than 60 breaths/minute and children younger than 3 years old with a respiratory rate greater than 40 breaths/minute with chest retractions is a sensitive and specific indication of lower respiratory tract infection.

Diagnostic Procedures

See Table 3-89 for diagnostic procedures for pneumonia.

DIAGNOSIS

When the presenting features are fever and cough, consider one of the following:
- Lower respiratory tract infection such as pneumonia and bronchitis (in children, bronchiolitis is more common than bronchitis)
- Pulmonary embolus (fever, usually low grade)
- Septic pulmonary cough

When the presenting feature is dyspnea in a younger client, consider one of the following:
- Pulmonary embolus
- Pneumonia
- Pneumothorax
- Reactive airway disease/asthma
- Costochondritis/pleuritis

When the presenting feature is dyspnea in an older adult consider one of the following:
- Acute myocardial infarction
- Pulmonary embolism

- CHF
- Exacerbation of COPD
- Pneumonia
- Pulmonary abscess
- Rib fracture

THERAPEUTIC PLAN

Nonpharmacologic Treatment

- Fever care
- Increase fluids

Pharmacologic Treatment

- See Table 3-90 for pharmacologic therapy for empiric outpatient treatment of children.
- Consider administering procaine penicillin IM or ceftriaxone (Rocephin) IM to ensure initial compliance and avoid problems related to vomiting.
- Severely ill infants and children should be hospitalized and treated with intravenous antibiotic therapy.
- Indications for hospitalization are moderate to severe respiratory distress including respiratory rate higher than 70 breaths/minute, marked retractions, cyanosis, grunting, oxygen saturation less than 88% to 90%, systemic toxicity, dehydration, or mental status change.
- Infants and children at greatest risk of deterioration include those with sickle cell disease, malnutrition, immunodeficiency, cardiac or pulmonary disease, those

TABLE **3-89** Diagnostic Procedures for Pneumonia

DIAGNOSTIC PROCEDURE	FINDINGS
Chest radiograph (needed for both inpatient and outpatient; mandatory for confirmation of diagnosis, to rule out acute bronchitis and unnecessary use of antibiotics)	Bacterial pneumonia presents with lobar or segmental consolidation, abscess, pneumatocele, or pleural fluid. Mycoplasmal and viral pneumonia presents with interstitial infiltrates with possible hyperexpansion but no consolidation. Fungal, mycobacterial, staphylococcal pneumonia present with patchy distribution of granulomas with possible necrosis and cavity development.
Pulse oximetry	Determines oxygen saturation. Less than 90% indicates need for supplemental oxygen therapy.
Complete blood count (needed for inpatients)	Assess for leukocytosis which may or may not be present with bacterial pneumonia and neutrophilia which may be present with mycoplasmal or viral pneumonia.
Blood culture (needed for inpatients, two pretreatment blood cultures)	Bacteremia is present in 10% to 25% of cases and is associated with high fever.
Sputum cultures (needed for inpatient, optional for outpatient)	Assess organism identification. Adequate sampling imperative and may be hampered by dehydration and weak cough. Can be obtained by bronchoscopy or transtracheal aspiration.
Acid fast stains and culture	Assess for tuberculosis.
Arterial blood gases (optional)	PaO_2 <80 mm Hg indicates hypoxemia. Used to determine severity of the illness.
Immunofluorescent staining and ELISA	Rapid viral diagnostic techniques for RSV. Both tests are done on nasopharyngeal secretions and may identify cases which may benefit from early ribavirin treatment.

ELISA, Enzyme-linked immunosorbent assay; *RSV,* respiratory syncytial virus.

TABLE **3-90** Pharmaceutical Therapy for Empiric Outpatient Treatment of Children

For an infant younger than 6 months	Erythromycin, amoxicillin	Alternatives include TMP/SMX, erythromycin ethyl succinate (if allergic to penicillin)
0 to 7 days old	Erythromycin/sulfisoxazole (Pediazole)	
Older than 2 months	Erythromycin/sulfisoxazole	
Older children	Amoxicillin	Alternatives include erythromycin/ sulfisoxazole (Pediazole), TMP/SMX, cefaclor (Ceclor), cefixime (Suprax), or amoxicillin/clavulanate (Augmentin)

TMP/SMX, Trimethoprim-sulfamethoxazole.

who are taking immunosuppressive drugs, or who were premature.

- Infants and children whose families have no communication or means of transportation should be considered high risk.
- See Table 3-91 for drugs for older clients on an outpatient basis.
- *H. influenzae* is a common pathogen in smokers and should be treated with a macrolide.
- Most antibiotics should be prescribed for 10 to 14 days, except azithromycin which is given for 7 days because of its long half-life and significant pulmonary penetration. *Clients on corticosteroids may require more than 14 days of antibiotics.*
- Azithromycin should not be used if bacteremia is suspected because it does not yield appreciable serum levels.
- See Box 3-18 for indications for hospitalization for an adult with community-acquired pneumonia.

Client Education

- Stress the importance of rest, fluids, nutrition, antibiotics, and antipyretics.
- Teach deep breathing and cough techniques.
- Report to health care provider any change in color or characteristics of sputum, decreased activity tolerance, persistent fever, increased chest pain, or lack of overall improvement.
- Encourage smoking cessation if appropriate.

Referral/Consultation

- Consultation with a physician is indicated for severe respiratory distress or in the presence of comorbidity.
- Consult when referring for inpatient hospitalization.

Prevention

Recommend influenza and pneumococcal vaccines as appropriate.

TABLE **3-91** Drugs for Older Clients on an Outpatient Basis

For outpatient without cardiopulmonary disease, no modifying risk factors (e.g., risk factor for drug resistance, nursing home resident)	Azithromycin, clarithromycin, and erythromycin; if allergic, use doxycycline
For outpatient with cardiopulmonary disease or modifying factors	Beta-lactam antibiotic: oral cefuroxime, high dose amoxicillin, amoxicillin-clavulanate plus macrolide *or* antipneumococcal fluoroquinolone (levofloxacin, moxifloxacin)

Box 3-18 Indications for Hospitalization for an Adult with Community-Acquired Pneumonia

Age older than 60 years
Unstable vital signs (heart rate higher than 125 beats per minute, systolic blood pressure higher than 90 mm Hg)
Respiratory rate greater than 30 breaths per minute
Altered mental status
Hypoxemia (PO_2 <60 mm Hg)
Severe underlying disease (chronic obstructive pulmonary disease, diabetes mellitus, liver disease, heart failure, renal failure)
Immunocompromised (HIV infection, cancer, corticosteroid use)

Complication from pneumonia (extrapulmonary infection, meningitis, cavitation, multilobar involvement, sepsis, abscess, empyema, pleural effusion)
Severe electrolyte, hematologic, or metabolic abnormality (sodium <130 mEq/L, hematocrit <30%, absolute neutrophil count <1000/mm^3, serum creatinine >2.5 mg/dL)
No resources for self-care at home
Failure to respond to outpatient treatment within 48 to 72 hours

EVALUATION/FOLLOW-UP

Assess for response to treatment and improvement within 48 to 72 hours.

COMPLICATIONS

- Septic shock
- Respiratory failure
- Death

REFERENCES

American Thoracic Society. (2001). Guidelines for the initial management of adults with community-acquired pneumonia. *The American Review of Respiratory Disease, 163,* 1730.

Davis, A., Kane, G., & Plouffe, J. (1999). The changing care of community-acquired pneumonia. Infectious diseases special report. *Patient Care for Nurse Practitioners, 3,* 52-63.

Green, D., & San Pedro, G. (2001). Making sense of guidelines for CAP. *Clinical Advisor, 9*(suppl), 3-10.

Horowitz, H., Niederman, M., & Schaffner, W. (1999). HIV disease, persistent fever, nonresolving pneumonia, tuberculosis. *Patient Care Nurse Practitioner, 2*(3), 20-22, 25-28, 31-34, 39-40.

King, D. E., & Pippin, H. J. (1997). Community-acquired pneumonia in adults: Initial antibiotic therapy. *American Family Physician, 56*(2), 544-549.

Rogers, K. (2000). Pneumonia. In D. Robinson, P. Kidd, K. Rogers (Eds.), *Primary care across the lifespan.* St. Louis: Mosby.

Review Questions

1. An alcoholic client is at risk for pneumonia because of all the following except:
   a. Possible impaired gag reflex and aspiration
   b. Impaired immune status
   c. Underlying lung pathologic conditions
   d. Impaired mucociliary clearance

2. The organism most likely responsible for pneumonia in a middle school age child during the fall is which of the following?
   a. *Pneumocystis*
   b. *H. influenzae*
   c. *Mycoplasma*
   d. Fungus

3. Which of the following is a positive clinical sign on the physical examination indicating pneumonia?
   a. Wheezing
   b. Hyperresonance
   c. Dullness on percussion
   d. Decreased vocal fremitus

4. A client who has a diagnosis of pneumonia returns to the clinic after not responding to antibiotic treatment after 48 hours. The client has a respiratory rate of 36 breaths/minute. The NP should do which of the following?
   a. Consult with the physician about hospitalization of the client.
   b. Prescribe two oral antibiotics.
   c. Prescribe a metered-dose inhaler.
   d. Treat symptoms because the pneumonia is most likely viral in nature.

5. A client treated with azithromycin for pneumonia has improved but is not well. The NP should do which of the following?
   a. Consult with the physician about hospitalization of the client.
   b. Prescribe another antibiotic.
   c. Prescribe another round of azithromycin.
   d. Suggest the use of a vaporizer.

6. A client who is a heavy smoker is diagnosed with pneumonia. The NP should prescribe which of the following?
   a. Fluoroquinolone
   b. Beta lactam
   c. Macrolide
   d. TMP/SMX

7. Which pathogen is most common cause of outpatient bacterial pneumonia?
   a. *Streptococcus pneumoniae*
   b. *Staphylococcus aureus*
   c. *M. pneumoniae*
   d. *H. influenzae*

Answers and Rationales

1. **Answer: c** (analysis/diagnosis)
   Rationale: Altered consciousness and elevated blood alcohol levels may impair the gag reflex and decrease leukocyte production and mucociliary action.

2. **Answer: c** (analysis/diagnosis)
   Rationale: Mycoplasma organisms are more common in children and young adults and in enclosed settings during the seasons of fall and winter.

3. **Answer: c** (assessment)
   Rationale: Wheezing indicates obstruction. Hyperresonance indicates overinflation. Decreased vocal fremitus may indicate collapsed lung. Dullness indicates fluid and consolidation.

4. **Answer: a** (implementation/plan)
   Rationale: Indications for hospitalization are failure to respond to outpatient treatment after 48 to 72 hours and respiratory rate greater than 30 breaths/minute. Other criteria include altered mental status, systolic blood pressure of 90 mm Hg or less, co-morbidities, PO_2 less than 60 mm Hg.

5. **Answer: b** (evaluation)
   Rationale: There is no information suggesting the need for hospitalization. Another antibiotic may be indicated if the client remains ill after one course. Doubling the use of a single antibiotic increases drug resistance and is not effective. Vaporizers are more helpful in relieving congestion in nasal breathers (infants) or preventing URIs.

6. **Answer: c** (implementation/plan)
   Rationale: *H. influenzae* is a common pathogen in smokers and responds to macrolide therapy.

7. **Answer: a** (analysis/diagnosis)
   Rationale: *S. aureus* and *H. influenza* are frequent pathogens in hospitalized clients. Pneumonia accounts for more than 70% of cases of outpatient bacterial pneumonia.

P

POLYPHARMACY *Pamela Kidd*

OVERVIEW
Definition
Iatrogenic drug reaction from treating chronic conditions with medications in adults with physiologic and anatomic changes related to aging.

Incidence
About 60% of older adults take 5 to 15 medications daily. Up to 80% of drug-related hospitalizations are preventable (French, 1996).

Pathophysiology
Common health problems in people older than age 65 are cardiovascular disease, dementia, arthritis, diabetes, cancer, macular degeneration, auditory disorders, constipation, depression, and osteoporosis (Resnick, 2000). These health problems have multisystem affects, are chronic in nature, and are frequently treated with drugs.

Protective Factors
- No use of OTC drugs
- No use of prescribed drugs
- Use of one pharmacy and one provider

Factors Increasing Susceptibility
- Visual impairment (may not read instructions)
- Auditory impairment (may not hear instructions)
- Memory or cognitive deficit
- Decreased glomerular filtration rate
- Reduced hepatic clearance
- Increase in body fat (fat soluble drugs have longer half-lives)
- Decrease total body water (water soluble drugs become more concentrated)
- Decrease serum albumin (reduction in protein binding of drugs leaving more active [unbound] drug available)

ASSESSMENT: SUBJECTIVE/HISTORY
Symptoms
Delirium, development of new symptoms may suggest a dose-related response or drug interaction at cellular level.

Past Medical History
- Glaucoma: Oral carbonic anhydrase inhibitors can cause anorexia and weight loss; topical beta-blockers can cause bradycardia and asthma.
- Arthritis: Indomethacin produces confusion in the elderly. Regularly-dosed acetaminophen is a better alternative.
- HTN: Thiazide diuretics are first-line drugs in HTN, but the use of thiazides worsens gout (if present).
- URI: OTC cold remedies can create confusion, constipation, and urinary retention because of anticholinergic actions.

Medication History
- Antihypertensives, NSAIDs, central nervous system (CNS) depressants, and steroids may cause depression and the need for more medication to treat the depression.
- Diuretics, anticholinergics, and sedatives have the greatest number of undesirable side-effects in the elderly.

Family History
Not relevant.

Dietary History
Not relevant.

ASSESSMENT: OBJECTIVE/PHYSICAL EXAMINATION
Physical Examination
CNS changes are typical signs of drug toxicity; therefore a neurologic (including mental status) examination is appropriate.

Diagnostic Procedures
- Obtain serum drug levels for drugs with a narrow therapeutic window (phenytoin, lithium, tricyclic antidepressant [TCA]).
- Obtain renal function laboratory tests (blood urea nitrogen [BUN], creatine, basic metabolic profile).
- Obtain serum albumin level (in case of protein-bound drugs).
- Other diagnostic procedures depend on presenting symptom to rule out drug interaction or reaction as cause.

DIAGNOSIS
Differential diagnoses include the following:
- Lack of adherence to drug therapy causing symptoms related to nontreatment of a chronic condition (e.g., no money or way of getting prescriptions filled).
- Knowledge deficit regarding drug treatment (lack of understanding).
- Drug toxicity can occur in some older adults with "normal" serum therapeutic levels.
- Drug interactions are possible.

THERAPEUTIC PLAN

Nonpharmacologic Treatment

- NPs must be receptive to nonpharmacologic interventions. These include but are not limited to mental health support through counseling, avoidance of stimulants (e.g., caffeine), use of music and massage therapy, prayer, and, in some cases, helping a client to get a low-maintenance pet (Shuler, Huebscher, & Hallock, 2001).
- It may be useful to modify mobility and diet to treat a condition.
- Consider heat, cold, elevation of extremities, and manipulation of clothing (e.g., stockings, shoes) as treatment strategies.

Pharmacologic Treatment

When prescribing, follow these steps:
- Begin with less than usual adult dose.
- Increase dose slowly.
- Allow an adequate trial period before discontinuing drug (may take longer to see desired effect).
- Whenever possible, use the least number of daily doses to achieve desired effect.
- Keep number of pills needed to achieve the dose low.
- Make changes infrequently.
- Try to discontinue drug in a controlled manner (schedule frequent office visits over the trial period, do a daily-check in by phone).

Client Education

- Use variety of ways to teach the client.
- Encourage client to call office with any question about how to take drug or about new symptoms.
- Have family member come each visit for reinforcement of instructions and plan.
- Provide printed (large print) materials, videos for personal use from drug company, as well as one-on-one teaching.

Referral/Consultation

- Consult with pharmacist when choosing medication, considering addition of another drug, or discontinuing a drug if in doubt.
- Consult with geriatric medicine specialist.

Prevention

- Make changes slowly and one at a time in the drug therapy plan.
- Simplify drug treatment whenever possible.

EVALUATION/FOLLOW-UP

- Depends on drug that may be causing the interaction or toxicity. When phasing a drug in or out, evaluate at least once a week and sooner if potential therapeutic window is narrow.
- At each visit, examine current medications for possible interactions or toxicity.

COMPLICATIONS

Complications are related to the drugs involved.
- Renal failure
- Death
- Delirium
- Falls
- Tremors

REFERENCES

French, D. (1996). Avoiding adverse drug reactions in the elderly patient: Issues and strategies. *Nurse Practitioner 21*(9), 90-107.

Resnick, N. (2000). Geriatric medicine. In L. Tierney, S. McPhee, M. Papadakis, (Eds.), *Current medical diagnosis and treatment* (39th ed., pp. 47-70). New York: McGraw-Hill.

Shuler, P., Huebscher, R., & Hallock, J. (2001). Providing wholistic care for the elderly: utilization of the Shuler nurse practitioner practice model. *Journal of the Academy of Nurse Practitioners, 13*(7), 297-303.

Review Questions

1. All *except* which of the following are reasons for iatrogenic drug reactions in the elderly?
- **a.** Auditory impairment
- **b.** Visual impairment
- **c.** Decreased body fat
- **d.** Decreased serum albumin level

2. Which of the following diagnostic tests does *not* assist the NP in anticipating iatrogenic drug reactions?
- **a.** Serum drug levels
- **b.** BUN, creatine
- **c.** Serum albumin
- **d.** Urinalysis

3. Which of the following is a rule to follow when prescribing drugs in the elderly?
- **a.** Do not increase the dose.
- **b.** Begin with a child's dose.
- **c.** Use the least number of daily doses to achieve effect.
- **d.** Make changes over a period of 1 week.

4. The *least* likely diagnosis to consider when a new symptom occurs or there is no improvement of symptoms in a client receiving multiple drugs is which of the following?
- **a.** Knowledge deficit
- **b.** Drug toxicity
- **c.** Drug interaction
- **d.** Suicidal ideation

Answers and Rationales

1. *Answer:* c (analysis/diagnosis)
 Rationale: Body fat increases as one ages, allowing fat soluble drugs to have a longer half-life.

P

2. ***Answer:*** **d** (analysis/diagnosis)

Rationale: Serum drug levels help assess dosage needed for drugs with a narrow therapeutic window. Renal function is important in determining the glomerular filtration rate and elimination of drugs. Serum albumin is important in assessing the amount of free (unbound) drug in drugs that are protein bound. A urinalysis does not provide additional information.

3. ***Answer:*** **c** (implementation/plan)

Rationale: A dose can be increased, but should be increased slowly. Start with the lowest adult dose or a little less.

A child's dose may not be effective. Changes are made slowly, but there is no exact period for making a change.

Answer: **d** (evaluation)

Rationale: There is not enough information in the question to determine if the client is mentally unhealthy. The use of multiple drugs could support the other three diagnoses occurring.

PREMATURE LABOR AND BIRTH *Cheryl Pope Kish*

OVERVIEW
Definition

Premature or preterm labor refers to labor that begins before 37 completed weeks of pregnancy. Premature delivery refers to childbirth that occurs before the woman completes her 37th week of pregnancy.

Incidence

Despite technological advances and an improved standard of living in the United States, the incidence of premature birth has not declined in the past 40 years. Surprisingly, the relative magnitude of the problem has increased, now affecting 1 in 10 births. Preterm birth is the attributing factor in 83% of neonatal mortality not caused by congenital anomalies. Preterm newborns are significantly affected by complications of prematurity.

Pathophysiology

The cause of premature labor is not always known; it appears to be multifactorial.

Factors Increasing Susceptibility
- Demographic factors
  - Age younger than 18 or older than 40 years
  - Age at first pregnancy 35 years or older
  - Less than high school education
  - Black race
- Lifestyle factors
  - Unmarried
  - Smoking more than 11 cigarettes daily
  - Substance abuse, especially cocaine
  - Exposure to job-related teratogens and strenuous activity
  - High stress levels
  - Poverty, inadequate housing
  - Underweight with poor weight gain in pregnancy
  - Lack of prenatal care
- Medical risks predating pregnancy
  - Maternal illness (diabetes mellitus, renal and cardiac disease, HTN, hyperthyroidism)
- Poor obstetric history
  - Previous premature labor

- Premature birth
- History second trimester abortion
- Uterine factors
  - Multiple pregnancy
  - Polyhydramnios
  - Fibroids
  - Uterine and cervical abnormalities (e.g., incompetent cervix, bicornate uterus, DES exposure)
  - Trauma
- Infection
  - UTI or asymptomatic bacteruria
  - Group B streptococcus, bacterial vaginosis (linked to premature rupture of membranes [PROM])
  - STDs
  - Chorioamnionitis

ASSESSMENT: SUBJECTIVE/HISTORY

Establish risk of preterm labor. Many risk-scoring systems have been developed within the context of global prevention programs but have been found to have low positive predictive value. However, risk factors as outlined previously should be considered within the context of a comprehensive prenatal history.

Symptoms
- Increased uterine contractions that can be painful or painless
- Menstrual-like cramps
- Constant backache unrelieved by rest
- Diarrhea or intestinal cramping
- Constant pelvic pressure
- Urinary frequency
- Change in color, amount, or consistency of vaginal discharge

ASSESSMENT: OBJECTIVE/PHYSICAL EXAMINATION
Physical Examination
- Conduct thorough prenatal physical examination, noting systemic and uterine factors that place the woman at risk of preterm labor.
- Screen pregnant women for infection highly correlated with preterm labor.

- Based on history and assessment of risk, note uterine contractions through direct palpation of the uterine fundus or with external monitoring. Note also fetal response to uterine contractions by assessing fetal heart rate either manually or through external fetal monitoring.
- Perform sterile, gentle digital examination of the cervix if indicated by history to determine effacement and dilatation (or refer woman to physician for such examination). Because serial cervical assessments are necessary to detect progressive cervical changes, having one clinician perform these examinations minimizes subjectivity in examination findings.
- Note premature rupture of the amniotic membranes by performing Nitrazine (pH) test; amniotic fluid, which is alkaline, will turn the test paper blue. In the presence of PROM, the NP should avoid a digital cervical examination. A sterile speculum examination assists in evaluating pooling, ferning, and Nitrazine testing.

Diagnostic Procedures

- Women at risk for preterm labor and those with either history or physical findings suggestive of same are referred to an obstetrician for evaluation.
- Perform an ultrasound examination of cervical length. As ultrasound cervical length shortens to less than 30 mm at 24 and 28 weeks, there is increased risk of preterm labor (Sayres, 2001).
- Fetal fibronectin is a fetal basement membrane protein found in cervicovaginal secretions, indicating a disruption of the fetal-maternal uterine interface. In high-risk women, it is considered predictive of preterm labor.
- Cervical cultures for chlamydia and gonorrhea, perineal and perirectal culture for group B *streptococcus,* wet mount for bacterial vaginosis, and urinalysis may be done.
- Perform drug screening for high risk individuals.

DIAGNOSIS

One must differentiate Braxton-Hicks contractions from true labor. Criteria for defining preterm labor include the following:

- Gestational age between 20 and 37 weeks
- Uterine contractions evident on fetal monitor with frequency of 5 to 8 minutes and at least one of the following:
  - Rupture of the membranes
  - Cervical change
  - Positive fetal fibronectin (fFN)

THERAPEUTIC PLAN
Nonpharmacologic Treatment

- Recommend bedrest.
- Refer for surgical management of incompetent cervix, if present.
- Provide fetal surveillance.

- Ensure adequate hydration. Dehydration may precipitate uterine irritability. Have woman drink four glasses of water and reassess contractions.

Pharmacologic Treatment

- Once preterm labor has been established, fetal prognosis depends on medical intervention to delay delivery; therefore immediate referral to a physician is imperative if it has not already occurred. Pharmacologic management of the woman experiencing preterm labor generally includes tocolysis. Antibiotics may be ordered for maternal upper genital tract infection and chorioamnionitis. Glucocorticoids (Betamethasone or Dexamethasone) may be prescribed to accelerate fetal lung maturation through stimulation of surfactant release in alveoli.
- Prescribe tocolysis. Unless there is indication of fetal distress, chorioamnionitis, or maternal medical instability, tocolysis will likely be used to attempt to delay delivery. Beta-sympathomimetics (Ritodrine or Terbutaline) or magnesium sulfate are the most common drugs used in tocolysis and function by causing smooth muscle relaxation. The calcium channel blocker nifedipine is used less commonly.

Prevention

- Provide early and continuous risk assessment.
- Provide prenatal education, including how to recognize and respond to symptoms of preterm labor. Because 50% of women with preterm uterine contractions do not perceive them as painful, women must be taught how to recognize painless uterine contractions and evaluate their frequency, duration, and intensity.
- Recommend lifestyle modification to minimize risks, including not smoking, practicing safe sexual behaviors, not using illicit drugs, limiting stress and strenuous activity. Prevent dehydration.
- Modify employment as necessary to decrease risk.
- Advise adequate nutrition and prenatal vitamins. Calcium supplements should be ordered for those at risk from low socioeconomic status or with lactose intolerance.
- Educate to palpate for uterine contractions after sexual activity in high-risk women. Those with early cervical changes may be advised to abstain from coitus. Condom use (barrier to prostaglandin in semen as a cause of uterine contractions) may be recommended for those at very high risk. Nipple stimulation as a sexual activity should be avoided.
- Intervene in situations of domestic violence.

EVALUATION/FOLLOW-UP

The clinician may decide to schedule more frequent prenatal visits for the woman at risk for preterm labor. She will need to know how to recognize and respond quickly to symptoms and to have a plan in mind for timely transport to the hospital for evaluation. Ideally, women experiencing preterm labor are transferred to a tertiary care center. In the event that preterm birth is inevitable, a dialogue between the woman, her partner, and neonatology staff can be reassuring.

COMPLICATIONS

Outcomes associated with prematurity account for more than 60% of neonatal morbidity and mortality. A clinical approach that includes risk assessment, preventive strategies, early recognition of preterm labor and timely response are critical.

REFERENCES

Escher-Davis, L. (1996). Fetal fibronectin: A biochemical marker for preterm labor. *AWHONN Lifelines, 4*(3), 1, 6-7.

Maloni, J. A. (2000). Preventing preterm labor. *AWHONN Lifelines 4*(4), 26-33.

Ruiz, R. J.(1998). Mechanisms of full-term and preterm labor: Factors influencing uterine activity. *Journal of Obstetrical, Gynecological, and Neonatal Nursing 27*(6), 652-660.

Sayres, W. (2001). Preterm labor. In S. D. Ratcliffe, E. G. Baxley, J. E. Byrd, (Eds.), *Family practice obstetrics* (2nd ed., pp. 329-348). Philadelphia: Hanley & Belfus.

Star, W. L., Shannon, M. T., & Lommel, L. L. (1999). *Ambulatory obstetrics* (3rd ed.). San Francisco: University of California–San Francisco Nursing Press.

Von Der Pool, B. (1998). Preterm labor: Diagnosis and treatment. *American Family Physician, 57*(10), 2457-2464.

Weismiller, D. G. (1999). Preterm labor. *American Family Physician, 59*(1), 593-602.

Youngkin, E. Q., & Davis, M. S. (1998). *Women's health: A primary care clinical guide.* Stamford, CN: Appleton and Lange.

Review Questions

1. Which of the following factors in a woman's history places her at risk for premature labor?

   a. Oligohydramnios
   b. Sedentary life style
   c. Smoking
   d. Previous cesarean delivery

2. Rebakah, a black woman at 27 weeks' gestation, is considered at risk for preterm labor because of her race. She calls to report irregular uterine contractions of 1-hour duration. Which response by the NP is most appropriate?

   a. Assure her that these are Braxton Hicks contractions and explain how they differ from labor contractions.
   b. Advise her to lie down and increase her fluid intake.
   c. Tell her to go to the hospital immediately for evaluation.
   d. Recommend strict pelvic rest for the remainder of the pregnancy.

3. An NP teaches Beth Reardon how to recognize preterm labor. Which symptom listed by Beth indicates a need for further teaching?

   a. Pelvic pressure not relieved by lying down
   b. Intestinal cramping and diarrhea
   c. Mucoid vaginal discharge
   d. Vaginal bleeding

4. Peggy is 35 weeks pregnant and is being evaluated for premature labor. Which clinical finding is not a defining criteria for this diagnosis?

   a. Rupture of the membranes
   b. Uterine contraction approximately 5 to 8 minutes apart evident on electronic fetal monitor.
   c. Cervical dilation and effacement
   d. Blood-tinged vaginal discharge

5. Sandra says that the physician mentioned collecting a specimen for a fetal fibronectin test and asks what kind of specimen will be used. Which answer by the NP is accurate?

   a. Blood
   b. Urine
   c. Amniotic fluid
   d. Cervicovaginal fluid

6. Which of the following factors is not considered a risk factor for preterm labor?

   a. History of trichomonas
   b. History of three voluntary abortions
   c. Pyelonephritis
   d. Previous premature labor

Answers and Rationales

1. *Answer:* c (assessment)
   Rationale: Smoking, especially more than 11 cigarettes daily, is associated with higher risks of preterm labor (Sayres, 2001).

2. *Answer:* b (implementation/plan)
   Rationale: Dehydration increases uterine irritability. Having the woman lie down and increase her fluid intake may cause contractions to decrease (Ruiz, 1998).

3. *Answer:* c (assessment)
   Rationale: One of the signs of preterm labor is a change in vaginal discharge's color, amount, or consistency. Mucoid discharge is highly suggestive (Maloni, 2000).

4. *Answer:* d (assessment)
   Rationale: Although blood-tinged vaginal discharge can be a symptom of preterm labor reported by the woman, it is not a defining diagnostic sign. Definitive diagnosis is based on gestational age and uterine contractions plus rupture of membranes, documented cervical change, or fFN (Sayres, 2001).

5. *Answer:* d (assessment)
   Rationale: Fetal fibronectin is assessed in a specimen of vaginocervical secretions (Sayres, 2001).

6. *Answer:* a (assessment)
   Rationale: A history of trichomonas is not a risk of preterm labor (Sayres, 2001).

PREMENSTRUAL SYNDROME   *Cheryl Pope Kish*

OVERVIEW
Definition

Premenstrual syndrome (PMS) is a cluster of unpleasant, often distressing, physical, psychologic, and behavioral symptoms (more than 100 have been identified) that occur in the second half (premenstrual or luteal phase) of the menstrual cycle and decrease dramatically within 1 to 2 days after onset of menses. Premenstrual dysphoric disorder (PMDD) is viewed by some as a distinct clinical entity similar to PMS with more psychologic symptoms; others view PMDD as the most severe form of PMS.

Incidence

As many as 90% of all menstruating women have some recurring premenstrual symptoms. For 20% to 40% of women, symptoms are severe enough to require medical intervention; 5% suffer debilitating symptoms of PMDD. Peak incidence is during the 20s and 30s; PMS rarely occurs in teenagers.

Pathophysiology

The exact cause has not been established, but there have been numerous theories of cause over time. Currently, the two working hypotheses relate to a blunted response to serotonin and CNS-mediated interactions with sex hormones. The disorder is certainly related to the menstrual cycle; if the cycle is surgically or pharmacologically eliminated, symptoms disappear.

Protective Factors
- Regular exercise
- Current use of OCPs
- Menopause

Factors Increasing Susceptibility
- Being of reproductive age
- Increased parity
- Stressful lifestyle

ASSESSMENT: SUBJECTIVE/HISTORY
Symptoms

- Symptoms are best assessed through a prospective daily symptom diary, calendar, or checklist. Retrospective recall is less accurate.
- Assess current health status.
- Conduct obstetric history.
- Note current and past contraceptive use and any relationship to symptoms.
- Conduct detailed menstrual history: menarche; LMP; history of dysmenorrhea; when PMS symptoms were first noted; and usual frequency, duration, and flow of menstruation. Determine how menstruation is per-

ceived by client and whether it is magnified in importance to her lifestyle.
- Ask about typical day and stress level. Determine how this varies throughout cycle.
- Self-diagnosis is common. If this is the case, ask what made the client draw the conclusion that she has PMS.
- Let the client identify which symptoms she finds most distressing and which she considers a priority for intervention.

Past Medical History

- Determine history of chronic illness, noting particular effects of PMS on chronic illness.
- Ask specifically about lupus, fibrocystic disease, thyroid disease, chronic fatigue syndrome, and mood or anxiety disorders, which may mimic PMS.
- Determine history of psychiatric illness.
- Determine history of surgery.
- Determine whether the client has any drug or other allergies.

Medication History

Ask about current use of prescription or OTC medications, including those for menstrual-related symptoms.

Family History

- Ask about first-degree relatives with PMS.
- Ask about family history of psychiatric illness.

Psychosocial History

- Ask how symptoms affect work or school, leisure, and relationships.
- Ask about use of alcohol, tobacco, or illicit drugs.
- Determine how significant others have responded to diagnosis, if applicable. (Remember that PMS diagnosis is controversial and sometimes discounted by others, including health care professionals. For some, diagnosis is stigmatizing. For those reasons, syndrome should be validated and treated seriously by the NP.)
- If depression is a primary symptom, assess for suicide risk.

Dietary History

- Ask about food cravings.
- Use dietary recall to determine fat, refined sugar, caffeine, and sodium intakes.

ASSESSMENT: OBJECTIVE/PHYSICAL EXAMINATION
Physical Examination

Problem-oriented physical examination should be performed, with attention to symptom-related clusters, vital

P

signs, weight and presence of edema, skin, heart, thyroid, breasts, abdomen, and pelvis.

Diagnostic Procedures

- There is no single test diagnostic for PMS because no physiologic or biochemical factors are consistently altered. Laboratory tests may be ordered on the basis of individual symptoms or to rule out organic causes.
- Diagnosis is made on the basis of evaluation of a menstrual symptom calendar, diary, or checklist that indicates 30% increase in luteal phase symptoms 10 to 14 days before the menses when compared with those during and 10 to 14 days after. To be diagnosed as PMS, symptoms must occur in three consecutive cycles and be serious enough to require medical intervention. The hallmark feature is presence of minimum 7-day symptom-free interval in the first half of the cycle. The client should keep this record for 2 to 3 months to provide enough data for evaluation.

DIAGNOSIS

Rule out the following:
- Endocrine, metabolic, neurologic, and gynecologic disorders
- Underlying chronic illness with exacerbation related to menstrual cycle
- Acute illness with coincidental occurrence during luteal phase
- Psychiatric illness

PMDD has been associated with five or more of the following symptoms for 1 year during most of the luteal phase of the menstrual cycle. Symptoms must impair some aspect of the woman's life; other diagnoses must be excluded as a cause:
- Marked depression
- Marked anxiety
- Marked affective lability
- Persistent or marked anger, irritability, or interpersonal conflicts
- Decreased interest in usual activities
- Subjective sense of difficulty concentrating
- Lethargy, easy fatigability, or marked decreased energy
- Marked change in appetite with overeating and food cravings
- Hypersomnia or insomnia
- Subjective sense of being overwhelmed or out of control
- Other symptoms: breast tenderness, headache, joint or muscle aches, bloating, weight gain

THERAPEUTIC PLAN
Nonpharmacologic Treatment

- Recommend a risk-reduction diet such as that of American Heart Association and American Cancer Society.
- Advise moderate aerobic exercise at least three times each week (has been shown empirically to reduce symptoms).
- Consider cognitive behavioral therapy designed to reduce negative emotions through cognitive restructuring, problem-solving related to symptoms, and responsible assertiveness with a therapist skilled in this approach.
- Recommend relaxation therapy (e.g., yoga, tai chi).

Pharmacologic Treatment

- Review daily ratings to determine the most troublesome or persistent problems and select therapy most likely to affect as many of those as possible. Clients should be encouraged to try lifestyle changes before trying drugs except in the most serious cases.
- PMS is treated symptomatically. OCPs may help by suppressing ovulation. OCPs work best when symptoms are more physical than psychologic.
- Use of mild diuretics, such as spironolactone, during luteal phase may decrease edema and bloating.
- Synthetic androgens, such as danazol (Danocrine), or gonadotropin-releasing hormone (GnRH) analogs such as leuprolide (Lupron), may also be used in consultation with a physician, usually as a last resort. These drugs cause hypoestrogenic states; bone loss is a concern.
- Several drugs are effective for many women but without fully documented rationale: magnesium 200 to 400 mg/day and calcium 1200 mg/day.
- Psychotropic drugs may be necessary for anxiety or depression and anxiety. The selective serotonin reuptake inhibitors (SSRIs) seem to work best; TCAs can be useful for some depression not responsive to the SSRIs. Anxiolytics may be used for marked anxiety.

Client Education

- Teach record-keeping system with menstrual-symptom diary, checklist, or calendar. Being actively involved in management is sometimes therapeutic in itself.
- Provide understandable information about menstrual cycle and its relationship to symptoms.
- Educate client's significant others about illness to enlist their support.
- Role-play assessment of needs and dealing with difficult situations.
- Suggest scheduling difficult situations for symptom-free intervals as much as possible.
- Assist with stress reduction and management. Yoga and meditation may be helpful.
- Discourage client from placing blame for all negative circumstances on PMS to avoid perceptual victim role. Discourage menstrual magnification.
- Advise regular aerobic exercise.

- Advise frequent small meals that are low in fat and refined sugar, contain minimal sodium, and are high in complex carbohydrates and water. A low-fat vegetarian diet has been effective for many women. Foods high in tryptophan, a precursor of serotonin, may also be effective. Examples of these foods are legumes, dried peas, lentils, peanuts and peanut butter, cashews, whole wheat bread, brown rice, oatmeal, hard cheese, eggs, fish and shellfish.
- Advise reduction of caffeine and methylxanthines (coffee, tea, chocolate). This is especially helpful for breast tenderness.
- Suggest limiting alcohol intake and eliminating smoking.

Referral/Consultation
- Refer client to PMS support group, PMS clinic, or subspecialty if available.
- Refer client for psychotherapy if indicated by symptoms.
- Refer client to physician if no response to treatment or with exacerbation of chronic illness.

Prevention
Because no cause has been identified for PMS, there is no known prevention.

EVALUATION/FOLLOW-UP
Return to clinic monthly for 3 months, then annually or as needed for evaluation of symptom management. Closely monitor effectiveness of treatment and side effects.

COMPLICATIONS
No medical complications have been identified with failure to treat or undertreat PMS, although quality of life is affected by failure to treat or to treat appropriately. With untreated marked depression, it is possible that suicide risk increases.

REFERENCES

Cash, J. C., & Glass, C. A. (2000). *Family practice guidelines.* Philadelphia: Lippincott.

Daugherty, J. E. (1998). Treatment strategies for premenstrual syndrome. *American Family Physician, 58*(1), 183-194.

Evidence-based recommendations for managing premenstrual syndrome (2000). *Women's Health Primary Care 3*(10), 735-738.

Hawkins, J. W., Roberto-Nichols, E. M., Stanley-Haney, J. L. (1997). *Protocols for nurse practitioners in gynecologic settings.* New York: Tiresias.

Robinson, D., Kidd, P., & Rogers, K. M. (2000). *Primary care across the lifespan.* St. Louis: Mosby.

Smith, M. A., & Shimp, L. A. (2000). *Twenty common problems in women's health care.* New York; McGraw-Hill.

Star, W. L., Lommel, L. L., & Shannon, M. T. (1995). *Women's primary health care: Protocols for practice.* Washington, DC: American Nurses Publishing.

Taylor, D. L. (1994). Evaluating therapeutic change in symptom severity at the level of individual women experiencing severe PMS. *Image: Journal of Nursing Scholarship, 26*(1), 25-33.

Young, M. (2000). PMS and PMDD: Identification and treatment. *Patient Care, 35*(2), 29-50.

Youngkin, E. Q., & Davis, M. S. (1998). *Women's health: A primary care clinical guide.* Norwalk, CN, Appleton & Lange.

Review Questions

1. Which of the following psychologic symptoms is least indicative of a diagnosis of PMS?
- **a.** Irritability
- **b.** Anxiety
- **c.** Aggression
- **d.** Manic affect

2. Before a diagnosis of PMS may be made, the NP must determine when in the menstrual cycle symptoms occur. In which case is a diagnosis of PMS most justified?
- **a.** Symptoms consistently occur on day 14 of a 28-day cycle.
- **b.** Symptoms consistently occur in the first 5 days after menstrual flow ceases.
- **c.** Symptoms occur throughout the entire menstrual cycle every other month.
- **d.** Symptoms occur during the luteal phase of the cycle.

3. Which of the following suggestions is least appropriate for the 25-year-old client with PMS?
- **a.** Eat frequent, small meals with limited refined sugars, fats, and sodium; limit alcohol intake.
- **b.** Schedule difficult activities for symptom-free days if possible.
- **c.** Remind any significant other that conflicts and confrontations in the relationship may be blamed on her diagnosis.
- **d.** Schedule regular aerobic exercise weekly.

4. Which of the following factors most justifies more frequent follow-up of the client with PMS?
- **a.** She has become engaged to marry her college boyfriend.
- **b.** She recently changed to a part-time management position so that she can enroll in graduate school.
- **c.** She has bought a puppy.
- **d.** She joined a gym to make exercise easier to schedule.

5. Which objective measure is most suited to diagnosing PMS?
- **a.** Vital signs
- **b.** CBC and clotting profile
- **c.** Chemistry panel 20
- **d.** Menstrual symptom checklist

6. Ann Kovick is a 25-year-old who comes in for an annual examination. She mentions recent onset of symptoms suggestive of PMS. Which factor in Ann's history increases her risk for PMS?
- **a.** She works as a flight attendant.
- **b.** Both her sisters have significant premenstrual symptoms.

P

c. She jogs and swims regularly at a health club.
d. She uses OCPs for birth control.

7. Which symptom documented in Ann's menstrual diary is most diagnostic of PMS?
   a. Severe menstrual cramps and backache
   b. Premenstrual frothy, slightly malodorous vaginal discharge
   c. Leg cramps more noticeable immediately after menses
   d. Irritability and tearfulness in the four days before her period

8. The practitioner spends time counseling Ann about symptom management. Which comment made by Ann indicates her need for additional instruction?
   a. "I will start eating less fried and salty foods."
   b. "I can expect these symptoms to get progressively worse until I go through menopause."
   c. "Attending a support group with other women who experience PMS may help me to deal better with the problem."
   d. "Limiting my coffee, tea, cola, and chocolate intake may help alleviate some of the breast tenderness."

9. The NP suggests to a woman with PMS that foods high in tryptophan have proven effective in some women. Which of the following food groups are high in tryptophan?
   a. Brown rice, dried peas, and shrimp
   b. White bread, green peas, and almonds
   c. Asparagus, potatoes, and cabbage
   d. Lettuce, spinach, and parsley

10. What drug is commonly used in treatment of PMS?
    a. Amantadine
    b. Fluoxetine (Prozac)
    c. Chlordiazepoxide (Librium)
    d. Dielyclomine hydrochloride (Bentyl)

Answers and Rationales

1. Answer: d (assessment)
   Rationale: Irritability, anxiety, and aggression are common features of PMS. Depressed, not manic, affect is common (Young, 2000).

2. Answer: d (analysis/diagnosis)
   Rationale: A hallmark of the PMS diagnosis is occurrence of the symptoms during the luteal or premenstrual phase of the menstrual cycle (Young, 2000).

3. Answer: c (implementation/plan)
   Rationale: Blaming everything negative on the diagnosis of PMS causes the client to become a perpetual victim (Robinson, Kidd, & Rogers, 2000).

4. Answer: b (evaluation)
   Rationale: A stressful lifestyle that includes balancing career, family, and other commitments predisposes toward PMS (Robinson, Kidd, & Rogers, 2000).

5. Answer: d (assessment)
   Rationale: A menstrual symptom checklist, diary, or calendar is the most effective measure for assessing PMS symptoms (Hawkins, Roberto-Nichols, & Stanley-Haney, 1997).

6. Answer: b (assessment)
   Rationale: PMS in a first-degree relative is a factor that increases the probability of the client having PMS (Robinson, Kidd, & Rogers, 2000).

7. Answer: d (analysis/diagnosis)
   Rationale: PMS symptoms occur in the luteal or premenstrual phase of the menstrual cycle (Hawkins, et al., 1997).

8. Answer: b (implementation/plan)
   Rationale: Symptoms of PMS are most common in the 20s and 30s but do not necessarily progress. With appropriate intervention, most can be managed effectively (Robinson, Kidd, & Rogers, 2000).

9. Answer: a (evaluation)
   Rationale: Foods high in tryptophan, a precursor of serotonin, have been effective in some women. Choice a includes three foods high in tryptophan. Other options include no foods high in the chemical precursor to serotonin (Young, 2000; Evidence-based recommendations for managing premenstrual syndrome, 2000).

10. Answer: b (implementation/plan)
   Rationale: Prozac and the other SSRI antidepressants have been empirically shown to be effective agents for treating PMS and PMDD (Young, 2000).

PROSTATE CANCER   *Pamela Kidd*

OVERVIEW
Definition

Malignant neoplasm of the prostate gland is called prostate cancer.

Incidence

Prostate cancer has overtaken lung and colon cancers to become the most common cancer in men, accounting for 21% of all newly discovered cancers in men. The lifetime probability that a man will have prostate cancer is between 6% and 9%; the probability of death as a result of prostate cancer is approximately 2%.

Pathophysiology

Prostate cancer incidence increases with age, and blacks have a threefold higher incidence than whites; however, there is no clear cut causal relationship to environment, socioeconomic status, fertility, or endogenous androgen level. Regional differences do exist and may reflect unknown environmental factors or variation in detection methods.

Protective Factors. White race and young age are protective factors.

Factors Increasing Susceptibility
- Black race, advancing age
- Multiple sex partners

ASSESSMENT: SUBJECTIVE/HISTORY
Symptoms
- Hesitancy
- Frequency
- Nocturia
- Decreased force and caliber of stream
- Urge incontinence

Approximately 20% of individuals with prostate cancer have symptoms of metastatic cancer, such as spinal or other bone pain and gross hematuria.

Past Medical History
History of multiple STDs.

Medication History
Noncontributory.

Family History
First-degree relative with prostate cancer increases risk.

Dietary History
Noncontributory.

ASSESSMENT: OBJECTIVE/PHYSICAL EXAMINATION
Physical Examination
- A complete physical examination may be necessary to assess for signs of cancer in other organs.
- Check abdomen for distended bladder and abdominal pain.
- Check musculoskeletal system for pain in back with ROM or palpation.
- Check genital and rectal regions. Perform an examination of the external genitalia. Assess for prostate tenderness, enlargement, or nodules.
- A problem-oriented approach should be conducted, paying particular attention to vital signs, weight, general appearance, and hydration.

Diagnostic Procedures
- Always obtain a prostate-specific antigen (PSA) before rectal examination or 1 week later. Obtain postvoid urine residual to check for obstruction.
- One of the difficulties with PSA measurements is that PSA levels cannot predict if a slow growing tumor is likely to become aggressive. PSA does predict more tumors at an earlier stage than DRE (Goolsby, 2001). In men with prostate cancer, 75% have an abnormal PSA level (higher than 4 ng/mL). Norms for reading PSA levels are based on age and ethnicity.
- A prostate biopsy should be conducted by a urologist for men who have a PSA level higher than 4.0 ng/mL, rise in PSA between tests of more than .075ng/mL, or abnormal DRE.

DIAGNOSIS
The differential diagnoses include the following:
- Chronic nonbacterial prostatitis
- Prostatodynia
- STD
- Urethral stricture
- Acquired or congenital bladder neck contracture
- Chronic urethritis

THERAPEUTIC PLAN
Nonpharmacologic Treatment
- A seated position may enhance voiding with obstruction.
- Surgery (radical prostatectomy) or radiotherapy is usually used. Both procedures are associated with incontinence and sexual dysfunction.

Pharmacologic Treatment
- Anti-androgen drugs (Bicalutamide), estrogen for androgen dependent prostate cancer, leuprolide (Lupron), GnRH analogue

Client Education
- Screen all men at age 50 who have at least a 10-year life expectancy.
- Screen men with first-degree relative with known prostate cancer and Black men at age 40 to 45.

Referral/Consultation
An NP should immediately refer cases of suspected prostate cancer to a urologist.

Prevention
Prevention techniques are not known.

COMPLICATIONS
- Metastasis
- Urinary obstruction
- Renal failure
- Death

REFERENCES

Goolsby, M. J. (2001). Use of PSA measurement in practice. *Journal of the American Academy of Nurse Practitioners, 13*, 246-248.

Hostetler, R. M., Mandel, I. G., & Marshburn, J. (1996). Prostate cancer screening. *The Medical Clinics of North America, 80*(1), 83-99.

P

Liebman, B. (1996). Clues to prostate cancer. *Nutrition Action Health Letter,* March, 12-13.

Peters, S. (1997). For men only: An overview of three top health concerns. *ADVANCE for Nurse Practitioners,* April, 53-57.

Review Questions

1. Which of the following is the most common cancer in males?

   a. Lung cancer
   b. Skin cancer
   c. Prostate cancer
   d. Colon cancer

2. Of the following assessment areas, which is most important to consider in a client with possible prostate cancer?

   a. Ethnicity
   b. Age
   c. Previous STD
   d. Previous UTIs

3. Which of the following clients should have a prostate biopsy?

   a. Client with an abnormal DRE
   b. Client with a PSA rise of 0.50 ng/mL between tests
   c. Client with PSA level of 3.0 ng/mL
   d. Client with hematuria

4. Which of the following indicates adequate education of a 40-year-old black client?

   a. "I will get a PSA level drawn at age 50."
   b. "I do not need a PSA level drawn because there is no history of prostate cancer in my first-degree relatives."
   c. "I need my PSA level checked now."
   d. "PSA levels are less accurate than DRE."

Answers and Rationales

1. *Answer:* **c** (assessment)
   Rationale: Prostate cancer now occurs more frequently than lung and colon cancer.

2. *Answer:* **a** (assessment)
   Rationale: Although incidence of prostate cancer increases with age, black men have a three times higher incidence than non-black men. Multiple STDs also increase the risk, but one episode of an STD does not. UTIs have no correlation with the occurrence of prostate cancer.

3. *Answer:* **a** (implementation/plan)
   Rationale: A PSA will predict more tumors at an earlier stage than DRE but any client with an abnormal DRE should be biopsied. A rise of 0.75 ng/mL indicates the need for biopsy. A PSA level higher than 4.0 ng/mL also indicates a need for biopsy. Hematuria may indicate a UTI.

4. *Answer:* **c** (evaluation)
   Rationale: A black man should have his PSA level checked at age 40 to 45 regardless of family history of prostate cancer. A PSA predicts more tumors at an earlier stage than DRE.

PROSTATITIS *Pamela Kidd*

OVERVIEW
Definition

There are four types of prostatitis:
   1. Acute bacterial prostatitis is an infection usually caused by gram-negative rods, especially *Escherichia coli* and *Pseudomonas* species, and less commonly by gram-positive organisms, such as *Enterococcus.*
   2. Chronic bacterial prostatitis (CBP) is an infectious process that may evolve from acute bacterial prostatitis, but not always. Gram-negative rods are the most common causal agent, and only one gram-negative rod, *Enterococcus,* is associated with chronic infection.
   3. Chronic a-bacterial prostatitis/chronic pelvic pain syndrome is caused by organisms transmitted sexually (*Chlamydia, trichomonas,* and *gonorrhea*).
   4. Asymptomatic inflammatory prostatitis is the fourth type of prostatitis (Nickel, Nigro, & Hennenfent, 1999).

Incidence

Bacterial prostatitis is the most important cause of UTIs in men. Both acute and CBP can occur in men of any age but are not seen in children. Chronic abacterial prostatitis (CAP) accounts for up to 90% of all prostatitis (Lovejoy, 2001).

Pathophysiology

- Bacterial prostatitis is most likely caused by ascending urethral infection, reflux of infected urine, extension of rectal infection, or hematogenous spread. The most common pathogen is *E. coli;* others may be *Klebsiella* or *Pseudomonas* organisms.
- In CAP syndrome an inflammatory process occurs in the prostate as a complication of urethritis.

Protective Factors. Youth is the only protective factor.

Factors Increasing Susceptibility
- Advancing age
- Previous history of prostatitis
- Sexual activity

ASSESSMENT: SUBJECTIVE/HISTORY
Symptoms

For acute bacterial prostatitis, the signs and symptoms include acute onset of the following:
- Fever
- Irritative voiding symptoms (frequency, nocturia, urgency)
- Perineal or suprapubic pain
- Lower back pain
- Fatigue
- Occasional hematuria or penile tip pain
- Pain with BMs

Older adults may be asymptomatic, and fever may not be as pronounced.

Chronic Bacterial Prostatitis
- Fever
- Urgency
- Nocturia frequency
- Perineal or suprapubic discomfort that is often dull and poorly localized
- Hematospermia or painful ejaculation
  Older adults may be asymptomatic.

Chronic Abacterial Prostatitis. CAP exhibits the same symptoms as CBP.

Past Medical History
- Epididymitis
- Recurrent UTIs

Medication History
Noncontributory.

Family History
Noncontributory.

Dietary History
Noncontributory.

ASSESSMENT: OBJECTIVE/PHYSICAL EXAMINATION
Physical Examination

A complete physical examination may be necessary.
- Check abdomen for distended bladder and abdominal pain.
- Check musculoskeletal system for pain in back with ROM or palpation.
- Perform an examination of the external genitalia. Assess for prostate tenderness, enlargement, or nodules.

Diagnostic Procedures
- For acute and CBP and CAP, obtain three voided specimens (only two are needed if no signs of urethritis are present). Obtain urethral urine, midstream bladder urine, and postprostatic massage urine. Expressed prostatic secretions are usually obtained by a urologist.
- In acute bacterial prostatitis, the client will exhibit exquisitely tender prostate on physical examination, and results from culture will be positive.
- PSA may be elevated because of inflammation. Do not check PSA unless there is reason found during the examination to suspect prostate cancer (Lovejoy, 2001).

DIAGNOSIS

To differentiate bacterial from abacterial see Table 3-92. The differential diagnoses also include the following:
- Prostatodynia
- STD
- Urethral stricture
- Acquired or congenital bladder neck contracture
- Chronic urethritis
- Benign prostatic hypertension (BPH)
- Prostate cancer

THERAPEUTIC PLAN
Nonpharmacologic Treatment
- Taking sitz baths may be beneficial.
- Adding lycopenes (tomatoes, sauces containing tomatoes) to the diet is recommended.
- Spicy foods, caffeine, and alcohol should be avoided because these seem to aggravate symptoms.
- Encourage sexual activity.

Pharmacologic Treatment
- Antibiotic treatment for acute bacterial prostatitis includes quinolones or TMP/SMX for at least 2 weeks and perhaps for 30 days. CBP is treated with the same medications but for at least 4 to 16 weeks. Quinolones are the drugs of choice. Up to 4 months of treatment may be necessary.

TABLE **3-92**   Differentiating Between Bacterial and Abacterial Prostatitis

	CBP	CAP
Postprostatic massage urine	Positive bacteria, WBC count	No bacteria, positive WBC count
Midstream urine	Positive bacteria (also indicative of cystitis)	
EPS	Positive bacteria	WBC count 10-20 mm^3, no bacteria

CAP, Chronic abacterial prostatitis; *CBP,* chronic bacterial prostatitis; *EPS,* expressed prostatic secretions; *WBC,* white blood cell.

- CAP is treated with doxycycline, erythromycin, or ciprofloxacin for 7 to 10 days. Frequently, antibiotics are not helpful and treatment focuses on decreasing symptoms. Oxybutynin chloride can be used for irritative voiding.

Client Education

- A seated position may enhance voiding with obstruction.
- Increased water intake is important.
- Reduction of caffeine in diet is essential.
- Compliance with medication regimen is essential.
- Bacterial prostatitis has a chronic, relapsing nature.
- Isolated bacterial prostatitis does not cause impotency or infertility.

Referral/Consultation

- Refer men with suspected prostate cancer or chronic, relapsing cases of bacterial prostatitis to a urologist.
- Indications for urologic investigation include treatment failures with appropriate medications, chronic relapsing cases of bacterial prostatitis, or suspected prostate cancer.

PREVENTION

Condoms are preventative.

EVALUATION/FOLLOW-UP

Recheck urine and prostatic secretions after antibiotic therapy.

COMPLICATIONS

- Sexual dysfunction from chronic prostatitis
- Pyelonephritis, epididymitis from acute prostatitis

REFERENCES

Fugh-Berman, A. (1996), A better way to shrink an enlarged prostate. *Health Confidential,* January, 10.

Hostetler, R. M., Mandel, I. G., Marshburn, J. (1996). Prostate cancer screening. *Medical Clinics of North America, 80*(1), 83-99.

Liebman, B. (1996). Clues to prostate cancer. *Nutrition Action Health Letter,* March, 12-13.

Lovejoy, B. (2001). Diagnosis and management of chronic prostatitis by primary care providers. *Journal of the American Academy of Nurse Practitioners, 13,* 317-321.

Nickel, J., Nigro, M., & Hennenfent, M. (1999). Research guidelines for chronic prostates: Consensus report from the first National Institutes of Health International Prostatitis Collaborative Network. *Urology 54,* 229-233.

Peters, S. (1997). For men only: An overview of three top health concerns. *ADVANCE for Nurse Practitioners* April, 53-57.

Stoller, M., Presti, J., & Carroll, P. (2001). Urology. In L.M. Tierney, S. J. McPhee, M. A. Papadakis (Eds.), *Current medical diagnosis and treatment* (40th ed.). New York: McGraw-Hill.

Review Questions

1. Which symptom is most indicative of acute bacterial prostatitis?
   - a. Poorly localized pain
   - b. Hesitancy
   - c. Acute onset of symptomatology
   - d. Urge incontinence

2. An exquisitely tender prostate is most likely to be associated with which of the following?
   - a. Acute bacterial prostatitis
   - b. BPH
   - c. Prostate cancer
   - d. CBP

3. A 70-year-old man has nocturia, frequency, and dribbling. Which of the following diagnoses would you *not* consider as a possible diagnosis?
   - a. Prostate cancer
   - b. Acute bacterial prostatitis
   - c. BPH
   - d. UTI

4. What should the NP do for a man who has shown no response to treatment for his fourth episode of CBP in the last 5 months?
   - a. Give a prescription for medication effective against gram-positive organisms.
   - b. Refer to a urologist.
   - c. Counsel about his adherence to prescribed treatment.
   - d. Ask him to return to the clinic in 1 week.

5. Routes of prostatic infection include all *except* which of the following?
   - a. Reflux of infected urine
   - b. Ascending urethral infection
   - c. Systemic bacterial infection
   - d. Invasion of rectal bacteria

6. Which of the following is a common presenting symptom of CBP?
   - a. Pain on ejaculation
   - b. Low back pain
   - c. Suprapubic pain
   - d. Pain on urination

Answers and Rationales

1. ***Answer:* c** (assessment)
   Rationale: Perineal/suprapubic pain that is poorly localized is more indicative of CBP, whereas urge incontinence and hesitancy may be associated with BPH or prostate cancer. Acute onset of symptoms is associated with acute bacterial prostatitis.

2. ***Answer:* a** (assessment)
   Rationale: With CBP the prostate gland may or may not be tender but not exquisitely tender. With BPH, there is enlargement of the gland but it may not be tender. In prostate cancer painless nodules are most likely palpated.

3. *Answer:* b (analysis/diagnosis)

Rationale: Prostate cancer and BPH are both more common in older men; dribbling is not often seen in acute bacterial prostatitis but may be seen with UTI.

4. *Answer:* b (evaluation)

Rationale: NPs should refer clients with chronic relapsing episodes of bacterial prostatitis to a urologist.

5. *Answer:* c (analysis/diagnosis)

Rationale: Bacterial prostatitis is most likely caused by ascending urethral infection, reflux of infected urine, extension of rectal infection, or hematogenous spread.

6. *Answer:* a (assessment)

Rationale: Low back pain and pain on urination occurs in acute bacterial prostatitis. Suprapubic pain can occur in both acute bacterial prostatitis and CBP.

PSORIASIS *Pamela Kidd*

OVERVIEW
Definition

- Vulgar psoriasis is a common, plaque-type, genetically determined chronic disease of the skin. It is characterized by the presence of sharply demarcated, dull-red, scaly plaques, particularly on the extensor prominences and in the scalp.
- Flexural psoriasis appears in the groin, on the genitalia, in the axilla, at the umbilicus, and in the folds of fat around the abdomen.

Incidence

One of the most common skin disorders, psoriasis affects 1% to 2% of the population. It can begin at any age but commonly makes its first appearance in the later 20s and in the seventh decade. However, one third of clients are affected before 20 years of age, especially women. Men and women are otherwise affected equally. There is a lower incidence in West Africans, Native Americans, and Asians.

Pathophysiology

Skin lesions are caused by rapid epidermal cell proliferation. The cause of psoriasis remains a mystery. It is clear that there is a genetic component, with an estimated heritability of 90% overall. Certain human leukocyte antigen groupings are also associated with an increased likelihood of the disease.

Protective Factors. Avoid injury to nonpsoriatic areas.

Factors Increasing Susceptibility
- Multifactorial inheritance
- Minor trauma (Koebner's phenomenon)
- Endocrine factors
  Stress and obesity exacerbate existing psoriasis.

ASSESSMENT: SUBJECTIVE/HISTORY
Symptoms

- Skin: Pruritus, pustules, papules, and plaques may be present.
- Systemic: Arthritis (resembles RA), fever, and acute illness may be present.

- Nail involvement: Resembles fungal infection with striping, pitting, fraying, or separation of the distal margin and thickening discoloration and debris under the nail plate.
- Hair growth is usually unaltered.

Associated Symptoms

- Hypothermia
- Hemodynamic changes (shunting of blood to the skin)

Past Medical History

- Other skin disorders
- Trauma (surgeries, minor bumps)
- Infections
- Allergies
- Infection (HIV, streptococcal URI)
- STD and associated risk factors
- Sun overexposure

Medication History

- Corticosteroids
- Lithium
- Alcohol consumption
- Chloroquine
- Beta-blockers
- Interferon-alpha

Family History

Ask about family history of skin disorders.

Dietary History

Obtain dietary history for calorie count, especially in older adults. (Increased metabolic rate and increased calories are needed.)

ASSESSMENT: OBJECTIVE/PHYSICAL EXAMINATION
Physical Examination

A problem-oriented physical examination should be conducted, with particular attention to the following:
- General appearance of client: uncomfortable, "toxic," or well
- Vital signs

P

- Skin lesions: type, shape, arrangement, and distribution of lesions
- Auspitz's sign: pinpoint areas of bleeding when silvery scales are removed with fingernail
- Hair and nails
- Mucous membranes

Diagnostic Procedures

- Laboratory findings are inconsistent in uncomplicated psoriasis.
- Perform a serum HIV test to determine HIV serostatus in at-risk individuals with sudden onset of psoriasis.
- Perform a throat culture for streptococci: Lesions that are small and red macules that gradually become scaly are usually a result of streptococcal infection.

DIAGNOSIS

Differential diagnoses include the following:
- Seborrheic dermatitis
- Lichen simplex chronicus
- Candidiasis
- Psoriasiform drug-related eruptions
- Glucagonoma syndrome
- Secondary syphilis

THERAPEUTIC PLAN

Nonpharmacologic Treatment

Trunk
- UVB phototherapy with emollients
- Psoralen ultraviolet A-range (PUVA) photochemotherapy

Pharmacologic Treatment

Treatment is based on the location of the lesion and extent of the disease. If inflammation is present, it should be suppressed with topical steroids or antibiotics before using tar, anthralin, and calcipotriol because these agents irritate the skin. No systemic steroids should be used because they may induce pustular lesions. Treatment is stopped when induration is gone. Hyperpigmentation is common after the plaque heals.

Elbow, Knees, and Isolated Plaques
- Apply topical fluorinated corticosteroids in ointment base; cover with plastic wrap and leave on overnight.
- Apply hydrocolloid dressing; leave on 24 to 48 hours.
- When using topical anthralin preparations, avoid flexures and eyes.

Scalp
- Mild: tar shampoos followed by betamethasone valerate (Betatrex, Valisone)
- Severe: salicylic acid, 2% to 10% in mineral oil, cover with plastic cap

Trunk (Generalized)
- Refer client to dermatologist for more than 20% involvement.
- Prescribe topical corticosteroids, anthralin, vitamin D_3.
- Prescribe methotrexate given weekly.
- Prescribe combination therapy with etretinate (Tegison) or methotrexate and PUVA.

Client Education

- Instruct the client to avoid rubbing or scratching the lesions because this trauma stimulates the psoriatic process.
- Explain medication effects and side effects.
- Explain disease process.
- Avoid overexposure to the sun; psoriasis may develop in areas of sunburn.
- Cold may make psoriasis worse.

Referral/Consultation

Refer clients with the following to a dermatologist:
- Erythrodermic psoriasis
- Generalized pustular psoriasis
- Subacute psoriasis
- Extensive flexural psoriasis
- Extensive psoriasis vulgaris
- Elderly or incapacitated client
- Psoriasis that interferes with client's functioning
- Psoriasis severe enough to be distributed throughout the trunk (generalized)
- Psoriatic arthritis or inflammatory disease

Prevention

There is no known prevention. Sunshine can clear the disease.

EVALUATION/FOLLOW-UP

Initial follow-up is in 2 weeks to assess effectiveness of treatment. Follow-up is at 2-month intervals thereafter.

COMPLICATIONS

Scarring.

REFERENCES

Berger, T. (2001). Skin, hair, and nails. In L. Tierney, S. McPhee, M. Papadakis (Eds.), *Current medical diagnosis and treatment.* New York: McGraw-Hill.

Habif, T. (1996). *Clinical dermatology* (3rd ed.). St. Louis: Mosby.

Naldi, L., Parazzini, F., Peli, L., Chatenond, L., Cainelli, T. (1996). Dietary factors and the risk of psoriasis: Results of an Italian case-control study. *British Journal of Dermatology 134,* 101-106.

Young-Hughes, S. (2000). Psoriasis. In D. Robinson, P. Kidd, & K. Rogers (Eds.), *Primary care across the lifespan.* St Louis: Mosby.

Review Questions

1. The cause of psoriasis remains a mystery. It is clear that there is a genetic component, with an estimated heritability of 90% overall. The other organism associated with psoriasis is which of the following?

- **a.** *S. aureus*
- **b.** *Streptococcus*
- **c.** HIV infection
- **d.** *E. coli*

2. Which of the following physical findings is usually found in a client with psoriasis?

- **a.** Red patches with raised borders on groin and thigh, often in a butterfly pattern
- **b.** Nails thickened with debris
- **c.** "Herald patch" of 2 to 6 cm; round, erythematous, scaling plaque resembling ringworm
- **d.** Auspitz's sign: pinpoint area of bleeding when silvery scales are removed with the fingernail

3. Psoriatic lesions usually are which of the following?

- **a.** Bilateral, rarely symmetric
- **b.** Unilateral
- **c.** Bilateral, usually symmetric
- **d.** Associated with hair loss with scalp involvement

4. For a client with known psoriasis who comes in with joint inflammation, your next step should be which of the following?

- **a.** Start NSAIDs to control the pain associated with swollen joints.
- **b.** Refer client to a physician.
- **c.** Recommend physical therapy with moist heat to joints.
- **d.** Do nothing. The symptoms will resolve spontaneously.

5. Treatment for mild psoriasis is likely to start with which of the following?

- **a.** Coal tar preparations followed by topical steroids
- **b.** Debridement of necrotic plaques
- **c.** UVB phototherapy
- **d.** Methotrexate given weekly

6. The teaching plan of a client taking anthralin should include all the following *except:*

- **a.** It may cause erythema and burning of the normal skin.
- **b.** It stains clothing, sheets, and bath enamel.
- **c.** It should be used in the flexures and on plaques near the eyes.
- **d.** It will aggravate inflamed psoriasis and may induce pustulation.

7. A client with psoriasis is started on a regimen of coal tar and topical steroids. The client should be instructed to return for follow-up at what time?

- **a.** In 2 weeks
- **b.** In 6 months
- **c.** After she completes the medication
- **d.** In the winter, when her symptoms are expected to worsen

Answers and Rationales

1. Answer: b (analysis/diagnosis)
   Rationale: A history of streptococcal infection ("strep throat") 7 to 10 days before the appearance of the lesions is recognized as a precipitating factor in psoriasis.

2. Answer: d (assessment)
   Rationale: Auspitz's sign is most indicative of psoriasis; the other choices are more indicative of other skin disorders.

3. Answer: a (assessment)
   Rationale: The pattern of psoriasis is bilateral, rarely symmetric; hair loss is not a common feature even with severe scalp involvement.

4. Answer: b (implementation/plan)
   Rationale: Refer clients with extensive disease, psoriatic arthritis, or inflammatory disease to a physician.

5. Answer: a (implementation/plan)
   Rationale: Coal tar is effective in psoriasis, although its mode of action is unknown. It is used with topical steroids covered with plastic wrap at night to reverse the inflammatory process.

6. Answer: c (implementation/plan)
   Rationale: Anthralin should not be used in the flexures because burning is inevitable. It should not be used anywhere near the eyes.

7. Answer: a (evaluation)
   Rationale: Client should have follow-up in 2 weeks to evaluate the effectiveness of the treatment.

RED EYE *Denise Robinson*

OVERVIEW
Definition

Red eye refers to conjunctival blood vessel injection of eye with an unknown cause.

Incidence

- Red eye is a frequent complaint among clients seen in both the provider's office and emergency department. Approximately 5% of all clients requiring immediate care have eye complaints.
- Approximately 1300 eye injuries occur each year from the use of BB guns and air guns.
- In young clients the most common cause of visual blurring is refractive error.

Pathophysiology

Injection of the conjunctival blood vessels occurs with eyelid abnormalities and in response to inflammation, trauma, allergies, and increased pressure in the eye. The pathophysiology varies with each condition.

Factors Increasing Susceptibility

- Environmental exposure to chemicals, such as cleaning agents or superglue
- Unsupervised sports leading to increased risk of eye injury
- Errant baseballs (most common cause of ocular injury in sports)
- Non using of protective eye goggles
- Long-term use of topical steroids (longer than 4 to 6 weeks), which may produce glaucoma
- Presence of systemic disease, such as Lyme disease, Kawasaki syndrome, or juvenile rheumatoid arthritis (JRA)

ASSESSMENT: SUBJECTIVE/HISTORY
History of Present Illness

- Determine if onset is sudden or gradual.
- Determine if visual problem is present in one or both eyes.
- Determine exposure to chemicals; if chemical exposure to eye, begin flushing eye immediately with copious amounts of water.
  - Cleaning chemicals, especially those containing lye or alkaline products
  - Recent use of superglue (cyanoacrylate glue)
- Ask about cosmetic use.
- Ask about trauma to eye via thrown objects, such as rocks, balls, darts, or pencils.
- Determine if there is a foreign body (FB) in eye, such as metal, sawdust, trees/bark, or rust; ask if FB seen.

- Ask about tears overflowing onto the cheeks in newborn.
- Find out if there has been mucoid material on eyelids and, if so, when.
- Ask about light sensitivity and excessive production of tears.
- Ask about itching of eyes, conjunctival edema, and eye discharge. Determine whether these symptoms are recurrent, bilateral, or seasonal.
- Ask about symptoms of otitis media.
- Ask about vision, such as blurry vision, photophobia, pain, inability to see, "floaters" in vision, double vision, or halos around lights.
- Ask about exposure to conjunctivitis in school and home settings.
- Determine whether the client has obtained any treatment such as flushing of the eye.
- Ask about most recent eye examination.

Past Medical History

- Ask about recent upper respiratory infection.
- Determine if client has any systemic illnesses, such as the following:
  - Otitis media
  - Kawasaki syndrome
  - JRA
  - Ataxia-telangiectasia (Louis-Bar syndrome)
  - Lyme disease
  - Collagen disease (dry eyes)
  - Diabetes mellitus (ask about glucose level)
  - Hypertension
  - Glaucoma
  - Migraine headache
- Ask about previous eye problems or refractory correction.
- Ask about contact lens use.
- Ask about previous eye surgery, including condition that required surgery, date performed, and outcome.
- Ask about conditions that may cause client to be immunocompromised, such as the following:
  - Acquired immune deficiency syndrome
  - Chemotherapy
- In children, ask if the child was preterm or if he or she was resuscitated or oxygen was used as a newborn.

Medication History

- Eye drops: over-the-counter (OTC), prescription, vaso-constrictors, or artificial tears
- Oral medications:
  - Diuretics, antihistamines, or antidepressant medications for dry eyes
  - Psychotropic agents

- Digitalis products for yellow vision
- Drugs that dilate the pupil

Family History

- Family history of eye disease or other eye problems
- Retinoblastoma or cancer of retina (autosomal dominant disorder)
- Color blindness, cataracts, diabetes mellitus, glaucoma, retinitis, macular degeneration
- Refractory problems: nearsighted, farsighted, strabismus
- Skin rashes in other family members or exposure to skin rashes

Psychosocial History

- Ask about any changes in activities of daily living (ADLs) related to vision.
- Ask about activities or participation in sporting activities that may endanger eye.

Associated Symptoms

- Clear nasal discharge
- Nausea and vomiting
- Headache
- Dizziness

ASSESSMENT: OBJECTIVE/PHYSICAL EXAMINATION
Physical Examination

It is critical to examine the client in a well-lit room. It is important to follow the same routine for every client with a red eye.
- Eye: Use ophthalmic anesthetic to facilitate examination.
  - Always check visual acuity (V/A) when a client presents with a red eye. It provides information about vision and a baseline against which to compare progress.
  - Check visual fields.
  - Check extraocular muscles (Figure 3-15).
  - Check pupil response.
  - In children, do the cover/uncover test.
- Eyelids: Examine for evidence of inflammation, edema, and ptosis.
  - Inspect bulbar and palpebral conjunctiva for FB, discharge, color, lacrimal ducts, or corneal arcus.
- External eye: Examine for corneal clarity and FB, color of iris, size, shape, and reactivity.
  - Determine eye pressure using tonometer or palpation.
  - Perform funduscopic exam.
  - Check for red reflex and lens clarity.
  - Check disc margins, physiologic cup, blood vessels, retina, and macula.
  - Use slit lamp to visualize anterior structures.
- Head, eyes, ears, nose, and throat (HEENT): Check for lymphadenopathy.
  - Examine face carefully for injuries or inflammation.

Diagnostic Procedures

- Complete blood count (CBC): Rule out systemic disease.
- Thyroid: rule out hyperthyroidism, which can cause certain oculomotor palsies.
- Fasting glucose: Rule out diabetes.
- Erythrocyte sedimentation rate (ESR): Rule out arteritis.
- Fluorescein stain/blue filter light: Detect corneal abrasions/defects.
- Culture of eye discharge: Culture is not routinely done; should be checked if gonorrhea is suspected (culture both eyes, even if only one is symptomatic).

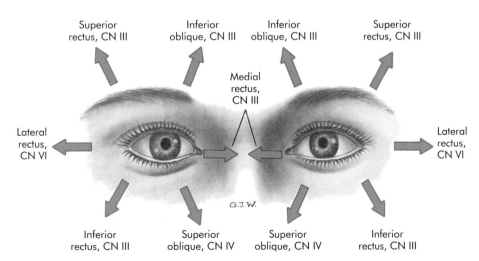

FIGURE **3-15** Cranial nerves and extraocular muscles associated with the six cardinal fields of gaze. (From Seidel H. M. [1999]. *Mosby's guide to physical examination* [4th ed.]. St. Louis: Mosby.)

DIAGNOSIS

Almost always, redness of the eye is caused by one of the conditions described as follows. Differential diagnoses are as follows:

- Bacterial conjunctivitis
- Viral conjunctivitis
- Allergic conjunctivitis
- Subconjunctival hemorrhage
- Corneal disease
- Acute narrow angle glaucoma
- Uveitis
- Eyelid swelling
  - Acute dacryocystitis
  - Blepharitis
  - Hordeolum (sty)
  - Chalazion

THERAPEUTIC PLAN

Pharmacologic Treatment

- Drug choices include ophthalmic antibiotic drops/ointments.
  - Viral topical agents
  - Topical antihistamine/decongestants
  - Mast cell stabilizer
  - Topical nonsteroidal antiinflammatory drugs (NSAIDs)
- Anesthetic agents may also be used.

Nonpharmacologic Treatment

- Cool compresses may relieve some discomfort.
- Eyelids should be washed daily with a gentle, neutral soap, such as baby shampoo, to remove crusting.
- Good handwashing and aseptic technique should be practiced.

Client Education

- Wash hands meticulously after touching the eye.
- Keep towel and washcloth separate.
- Discard any eye makeup to prevent reinfection and cross infection.

Referral

Immediately refer to ophthalmologist if any of the following are present:

- Intraocular FB or penetrating injury suspected
- Superglue in eye
- Hyphema
- Closed angle glaucoma
- Herpes dendritic keratitis
- Hyperacute bacterial conjunctivitis
- Herpes zoster of ophthalmic branch of trigeminal nerve
- Eyelid laceration if laceration crosses the eyelid margin or in the inner canthus involving the tear duct system (if fat is seen, the orbit has been entered)

- Vision loss caused by central retinal artery occlusion, retinal tears and detachments, traumatic injuries, and endophthalmitis (infection of eye usually caused by staphylococcus epidermis, which may occur after ocular surgery when client reports pain and loss of vision)

Consultation

Consult with physician if unsure of diagnosis or if V/A reveals change in vision.

Prevention

- Use good aseptic technique/handwashing.
- Wear protective eye goggles.

EVALUATION/FOLLOW-UP

- Corneal abrasions should be reevaluated in 24 hours.
- Any change or nonimprovement in V/A should be reevaluated.
- Reexamination of the eye should indicate that all tests have returned to normal baseline.
- Use of V/A can provide protection both for client and nurse practitioner (NP).
- V/A always should be measured on any client with eye problems.

COMPLICATIONS

- Loss of vision
- Blurred vision

REFERENCES

Bertolini, J., & Pelucio, M. (1995). The red eye. *Emergency Medical Clinics of North America, 13*(3), 561-579.

Davey, C. (1996). The red eye. *British Journal of Hospital Medicine, 55*(3), 89-94.

Donnefild, E., Kaufman, H. & Schwab, I. (1993). Conjunctivitis: Update on diagnosis and treatment. *Patient Care, May 30*, 22-48.

Easterbrook, M. Jonston, R., Howcroft, M. (1997). Assessment and management of ocular foreign bodies. *The Physician and Sportsmedicine, 25*(2), 77-87.

Hara, J. (1996). The red eye: Diagnosis and treatment. *American Family Physician, 54*(8), 2423-2430.

Michelson, P. E. (1997). Red eye unresponsive to treatment. *Western Journal of Medicine, 166*(2), 145-147.

Morrow, G., & Abbott, R. (1998). Conjunctivitis. *American Family Physician, 57*(4), 735-746.

Robinson, D. (2000). Red eye. In D. Robinson, P. Kidd, K. Rogers, (Eds.), *Primary care across the lifespan* (pp. 949-957). St. Louis: Mosby.

Ruppert, S. (1996). Differential diagnosis of pediatric conjunctivitis (red eye). *Nurse Practitioner, 21*(7), 12-26.

Silverman, H., Nunez, L. & Feller, D. (1992). Treatment of common eye emergencies. *American Family Physician, 45*(5), 2279-2287.

Small, R. (1991). Five steps toward a differential diagnosis. *Consultant, July*, 29-31.

Weber, C., & Eichenbaum, J. (1997). Acute red eye. *Postgraduate Medicine, 101*(5), 185-186.

Weinstock, F., & Weinstock, M. (1996). Common eye disorders: Six patients to refer. *Postgraduate Medicine, 99*(4), 107-110.

Review Questions

1. The NP provides instruction about eye drops to a mother of a child with conjunctivitis. Which comment by the mother indicates a need for further instruction?

   a. "I'm going to give these eye drops every 4 hours."
   b. "I should clean the eye before I put in the eye drops."
   c. "I can use the eye drops we already have—my son had conjunctivitis a couple months ago."
   d. "I should not touch the dropper to his eye."

2. Which of the following symptoms would *not* usually be identified by a client with a corneal abrasion?

   a. Photophobia
   b. Mild to moderate pain
   c. Mucopurulent discharge
   d. Hyperemia

3. Which of the following is the most common cause of blurring in children?

   a. Conjunctivitis
   b. Refractive error
   c. Eye trauma
   d. Chemical conjunctivitis

4. A client believes that a wood chip flew into his eye. Which of the following interventions is an appropriate first action?

   a. Apply antibiotic and an eye patch.
   b. Administer pain medication.
   c. Flush the eye with a liter of normal saline.
   d. Administer anesthetic to eye.

5. A 22-year-old female comes to the office reporting eye pain. Her eyes itch, and there is a clear discharge from both eyes. On examination the conjunctiva are diffusely injected and swollen. When everted, the eyelids show large papillae present. Which of the following diagnoses is most like in this situation?

   a. Bacterial conjunctivitis
   b. Viral conjunctivitis
   c. Allergic conjunctivitis
   d. Chemical conjunctivitis

6. Callie was playing with a mosaic kit of her mother's when she suddenly started crying. She said her eyes hurt and were burning. What is the priority action at this time?

   a. Administer anesthetic eye drops.
   b. Do a V/A test.
   c. Apply an eye patch.
   d. Begin lavage of eyes with copious amounts of normal saline.

7. Nancy comes into the office with eye pain; she feels as if there is something in her eye. Which of the following historical data is *not* consistent with a diagnosis of corneal abrasion?

   a. "I wear contacts."
   b. "My daughter poked me in the eye."
   c. "I was raking leaves."
   d. "I was applying facial cream."

8. Joanna was diagnosed with a corneal abrasion caused by an FB. When should she expect her eye to feel back to normal?

   a. 2 hours
   b. 8 hours
   c. 96 hours
   d. 24 to 36 hours

Answers and Rationales

1. *Answer:* **c** (evaluation)
   Rationale: The mother should not use a medication prescribed for someone else. She should give the eye drops every 4 hours, cleaning the eye before administration of the eye drops, and not touching the dropper to the eye (Robinson, 2000).

2. *Answer:* **c** (assessment)
   Rationale: Photophobia, mild to moderate pain, and hyperemia all are associated with corneal abrasion. Mucopurulent drainage is associated with bacterial conjunctivitis (Ruppert, 1996).

3. *Answer:* **b** (analysis/diagnosis)
   Rationale: The most common cause of blurring in young children is refractive error. Conjunctivitis does not cause blurred vision. Trauma and chemical conjunctivitis are not the most common causes of blurred vision (Robinson, 2000).

4. *Answer:* **d**
   Rationale: With wood, no amputation should be done because the wood swells. Administering an anesthetic is the first thing to do so that a complete examination can be conducted (Robinson, 2000).

5. *Answer:* **c** (analysis/diagnosis)
   Rationale: The most common complaint with allergic conjunctivitis is itchy, red eyes. There frequently is a clear discharge present (Hara, 1996).

6. *Answer:* **d** (implementation/plan)
   Rationale: If chemical exposure is suspected, immediate initiation of normal saline lavage is recommended (Robinson, 2000).

7. *Answer:* **d** (assessment)
   Rationale: A corneal abrasion typically presents with a history of an FB in the eye, scratches by contacts, or mild trauma to the eye (Hara, 1996).

8. *Answer:* **d** (evaluation)
   Rationale: A client with a corneal abrasion typically should feel better in 24 hours. The client should have follow-up if the eye is not feeling better in that time frame (Robinson, 2000).

R

RHEUMATOID ARTHRITIS *Pamela Kidd*

OVERVIEW
Definition

Rheumatoid arthritis (RA) is defined as an immunologically mediated chronic inflammatory disease of unknown cause that affects primarily joints but may have generalized manifestations.

JRA has three major presentations: (1) acute febrile form with salmon macular rash, arthritis, splenomegaly, leukocytosis, and polyserositis; (2) polyarticular (five or more joints involved) pattern that resembles adult disease, with chronic pain and swelling of many joints; and (3) pauciarticular (less than five joints involved) disease characterized by chronic arthritis of a few joints, often the large weightbearing joints, in asymmetric distribution. Up to 30% of children (1 to 16 years old) with this form of disease develop iridocyclitis, which can cause blindness if untreated.

Incidence

RA affects approximately 7 million Americans; women are affected more than men, based on diagnostic criteria. The incidence increases with age and peaks in the fourth decade. There is increased risk during the first 3 months postpregnancy. The onset of JRA is between 2 and 4 years of age; the rate of JRA in girls is almost twice that of boys.

Pathophysiology

An unknown mechanism triggers the immune system to attack the synovium of various joints, leading to synovitis (Browning, 2001). Rheumatoid factor (RF) antibodies develop against antibody immunoglobulin G, which is transformed into an antigen to be destroyed. The immune complexes deposit in the synovium and erode soft tissue, cartilage, and bone.

Factors Increasing Susceptibility
- Heredity
- Positive family history
- Female gender

Protective Factors
- Intact immune system
- Male gender

ASSESSMENT: SUBJECTIVE/HISTORY
Symptoms

Ask about duration of symptoms, morning stiffness, pain, and systemic symptoms.
- With RA, prodromal systemic symptoms of malaise, fever, weight loss, and morning stiffness lasting 30 to 60 minutes may occur. Joints usually affected are the proximal interphalangeal (PIP) and metacarpophalangeal but *not* the distal interphalangeal joints of the hands and metatarsophalangeal joints of the foot, shoulders, elbows, knees, ankles, and wrists.
- In children, the disease affects one or more joints with nonmigratory arthropathy; tends to involve larger joints or PIPs and lasts longer than 3 months with systemic manifestations of fever, rash, nodules, or leukocytosis.
  - Onset of JRA is related to age of child with systemic involvement and is more likely in younger children.

Associated Symptoms

- RA is articular inflammation with swelling, pain, erythema, and warmth. Progression of joint involvement is centripetal and symmetric. Tenosynovitis and rheumatoid nodules may occur. Be alert for systemic manifestations, such as vision loss, conjunctivitis, pain associated with pleural effusion, carpal tunnel syndrome, cutaneous lesions, rashes, neuropathies, and vasculitis.
- In JRA a characteristic salmon-colored, maculopapular rash is seen in 25% to 50% of children. The rash may be intermittent and associated with fever spikes and increased splenomegaly. May precede joint symptoms by 3 years.
- In adults and older adults inquire how RA affects ADLs or instrumental activities of daily living.
- In children consider how RA may affect their daily life and school performance.

Past Medical History

- History of metabolic, endocrine, autoimmune, or other musculoskeletal diseases (postural or developmental defects, joint instability, past meniscectomy) are common.
- In children, past medical history may be unremarkable.

Medication History

Note use of antiinflammatory or analgesic agents (indicate results and any other prescribed or OTC medications).

Family History

Inquire about family history of RA or musculoskeletal, endocrine, autoimmune, or metabolic diseases.

Dietary History

Perform an overall nutritional assessment with emphasis on weight reduction, if necessary.

ASSESSMENT: OBJECTIVE/PHYSICAL EXAMINATION

Physical Examination

A problem-oriented physical examination should be conducted, keeping in mind potential systemic manifestations of RA (e.g., dermatologic problems, pleurisy, splenomegaly, ocular manifestations) that might necessitate a complete physical examination. Assess the following:

- Assess vital signs, weight, blood pressure, and pulse. Note general appearance, gait, and activity level.
- Musculoskeletal system: Inspect affected joints for deformities, nodes, numbers of affected joints, symmetry of affected joints, and erythema.
- Observe affected joints in active and passive range of motion (ROM).
- Palpate affected joints for warmth, tenderness, crepitus, and edema.
- Assess muscle strength.
- Assess joint stability.
- Assess skin for soft-tissue nodules.
- Assess popliteal area for cysts (Baker's cysts).

Diagnostic Procedures

There are no definitive tests for RA or JRA; however, the following diagnostic tests may help to include or exclude the diagnoses:

- RA: ESR (Westergren method) provides useful but nonspecific information in confirming inflammatory disease. An ESR greater than 60 mm/h indicates severe inflammation. The ESR, useful in following response to treatment, is not useful when inflammatory disease is in remission.
- RF is not pathognomonic of RA but is present in 70% to 80% of people meeting the criteria for RA. A significant titer is a finding of 1:80 or greater, although it may be negative in early disease.
- Antinuclear antibodies (ANAs) are present in 20% to 30% of people with RA; ANAs are more common in those with extraarticular manifestations of RA and in those with a high titer of RF.
- A CBC will show the white blood cell count as normal or slightly elevated; it may reveal normocytic, hypochromic anemia (the anemia of chronic disease). The platelet count often is elevated also. Anemia may be present due to gastric blood loss from use of NSAIDs.
- In children, positive RF by latex fixation occurs in about 15% of cases; ANAs may be present in pauciarticular disease and the client may have a normal ESR in the presence of active disease. Platelet count may be elevated.
- Radiographs may reveal soft-tissue swelling, joint space narrowing, or bony erosions.

DIAGNOSIS

- For diagnosis of RA, four of the following criteria must be present: for at least 6 weeks, client must have morning stiffness, symmetric arthritis of three or more joints or arthritis of hand joints, or rheumatoid nodules, positive RF, and radiographic changes.
- Other differential diagnoses are osteoarthritis (OA), polymyalgia rheumatica, systemic lupus erythematosus (SLE), Sjögren's syndrome, vasculitis, gout, pseudogout, scleroderma, septic arthritis, psoriatic arthritis, Lyme disease, malignancy, and polymyositis. (See Table 3-93.)
- For JRA, differential diagnoses include rheumatic fever, Osgood-Schlatter disease, fracture, slipped capital femoral epiphysis, Henoch-Schönlein purpura, infections, SLE, Lyme disease, neoplasms (leukemia, lymphoma, neuroblastoma), and syndromes of psycho-organic origin.

THERAPEUTIC PLAN

Nonpharmacologic Treatment

- Exercise to maintain ROM and increase strength.
- Rest during the day.
- Selectively rest affected joints to prevent contractures (e.g., splinting at night).
- Apply heat and cold to relieve muscle spasm and provide pain relief.
- Engage in physical therapy.

Pharmacologic Treatment

- The objectives of therapy are to restore function, relieve pain, and maintain joint motion (Table 3-94).
- With RA and JRA, aspirin is effective and inexpensive, and it may be the first NSAID used. (Try Cox 2 inhibitors, such as Vioxx, Celebrex, or Mobic, to decrease gastrointestinal [GI] side effects.) If NSAIDs fail to provide relief quickly, try disease-modifying antirheumatic drugs (DMARDs).
- DMARDs, such as antimalarials, corticosteroids, cytotoxic drugs, and gold salts, may be effective. DMARDs are used in people with RA who show evidence of progressive joint involvement, persistent inflammation, elevated ESR/RF, and radiographic changes. The use of DMARDs early in the course of the disease in these people may prevent disability and morbidity because 90% of erosive changes can occur within 2 years. Use of DMARDs almost always accompanies the use of NSAIDs, should be used in consultation with the collaborating physician, and may necessitate a referral to a specialist.

NOTE: *Gastropathy associated with the use of NSAIDs is a major health problem in the United States. Risk factors for GI*

R

TABLE **3-93** Differential Diagnoses

DIAGNOSIS	DATA SUPPORT
Osteoarthritis	Asymmetric joint pain, worse after activity, no systemic symptoms
Polymyalgia rheumatica	Age >50 usually Pain and stiffness in shoulder and pelvic girdle Frequently accompanied by fever Anemia and increased ESR
Systemic lupus erythematosus	Young women primarily Rash over areas exposed to sunlight 90% experience joint symptoms Positive ANA Decreased Hgb, WBCs, platelets
Osgood-Schlatter disease	Young athletes Prepatellar bursa swelling Anterior tibial tuberosity tenderness
Lyme disease	Headache/stiff neck Arthralgias, arthritis, myalgias often chronic and recurrent Flat or slightly raised red lesion that expands with central clearing

ANA, Antinuclear antibodies; *ESR*, erythrocyte sedimentation rate; *Hgb*, hemoglobin; *WBCs*, white blood cells.

TABLE **3-94** Pharmaceutical Treatment

GENERIC NAME	USE	CONSIDERATIONS
Etanercept (biologic response modifier)*	Used when DMARD is not effective	Approved for JRA also; slows degree progression on radiographs; inhibits tumor necrosis factor
Methotrexate DMARD	Used in conjunction with NSAID	Takes 1-2 months for relief of symptoms
Sulfasalazine (Azulfidine) DMARD	Used frequently in conjunction with methotrexate	Takes 1-2 months for benefit; readjust dose after 2 weeks of use
Steroids	May be used for flare ups or for intraarticular use	Beware of inducing osteoporosis; taper quickly

* Restricted access in the United States.
JRA, Juvenile rheumatoid arthritis.

hemorrhage include advanced age, previous or present peptic ulcer disease, previous GI hemorrhage, alcoholism, and use of concomitant anticoagulants or high-dose corticosteroids. Nonacetylated salicylates produce the least inhibition of platelet aggregation.

- In children, NSAIDs have replaced salicylates in liquid form. NSAIDs have a decreased dosage frequency and diminished side effects, which enhance compliance. Take naproxen 7.5 mg/kg bid; ibuprofen 10 mg/kg qid; or tolmetin sodium 10 mg/kg tid. Aspirin 75 to 100 mg/kg in 3 divided doses is equally effective (do not give aspirin if the client has been exposed to chickenpox or Asian flu). For those children who fail to respond to NSAIDs, methotrexate is a second-line medication (5 to 10 mg/m²/wk). Injectable gold salts are an alternative.

- Older adults have an increased risk of NSAID-induced gastropathy as well as other serious side effects from chronic NSAID use (e.g., renal failure, fluid retention). As with other pharmaceutical treatments, it may be necessary to start with lower dosages and titrate upward until symptoms are controlled.

Client Education

- Encourage weight loss to desirable weight, if needed.
- Promote use of assistive devices, such as canes, walkers, crutches, or splints, if needed.
- Inform children and parents that disease activity progressively diminishes with age and, in 95% of cases, ceases by puberty. In a few cases, the disease will persist into adulthood. Problems after puberty relate to joint damage, but RA presenting in adolescence may precede adult disease.

Referral

- For JRA, consult with pediatric rheumatologist at onset of diagnosis.
- For children and adults who do not respond to therapy or have severe disease, treatment is a team approach and should include referrals for nutritional counseling, physical and/or occupational therapy, and surgery when necessary.
- Children with ophthalmic involvements should be referred to an ophthalmologist.

Prevention

No preventive measures are known.

EVALUATION/FOLLOW-UP

- Follow-up depends on the severity of the disease. If medications are to be advanced weekly, laboratory evaluations should be performed and clients should be seen on a weekly basis until symptoms are controlled. At the follow-up visits reinforce client education measures and assess for psychosocial adaptation to and coping with the disease.
- Children: If JRA is stable, children may be seen on a routine basis that meets both the family's and the provider's needs. Laboratory studies, such as CBC, appropriate for medication regimen and disease process should be obtained to follow progress of the disease and to observe for side effects of medications.
- Adults: Once the disease is stable, adults also may be evaluated on a routine basis.

COMPLICATIONS

- Deformity
- Disability

REFERENCES

Browning, M. A. (2001). Rheumatoid arthritis: A primary care approach. Journal of the American Academy of Nurse Practitioners. 13, 399-408.

Bynum, D. T. (1997). Clinical snapshot: Gout. American Journal of Nursing, 97(7), 36-37.

Cornell, S. (1997, March). New directions in rheumatoid arthritis. *Advance*, 61-64.

Halin, J. (2001). Treatment of rheumatoid arthritis: Etanercept a recent advance. *Journal of the American Academy of Nurse Practitioners. 12*, 433-441.

Hery, W. W., Groothius, J. R., Hayward, A. R., & Leven, M. J. (Eds.). (1997). *Current pediatric diagnosis and treatment.* Stamford, CT: Appleton & Lange.

Hooker, R. S. (1996, January). Osteoarthritis of the hip and knee: Managing a common joint disease. *Clinicians Review*, 54-67.

Hurst, J. W. (1996). *Medicine for the practicing physician.* Stamford, CT: Appleton & Lange.

Peck, B. (1998). Rheumatoid arthritis: Early interventions can change outcomes. *ADVANCE for Nurse Practitioners, 6(7):* 35-38, 41.

Ross, C. (1997). A comparison of osteoarthritis and rheumatoid arthritis: Diagnosis and treatment. *The Nurse Practitioner, 22,* 20-41.

Review Questions

1. JRA is characterized by all *except* which of the following?
   - **a.** Polyarticular
   - **b.** Acute febrile form
   - **c.** Occurs as a result of articular injury
   - **d.** Pauciarticular

2. How long does morning stiffness in RA last?
   - **a.** 30 to 60 minutes or longer
   - **b.** Less than 30 minutes
   - **c.** Throughout the day
   - **d.** An indefinite period

3. Which of the following is a characteristic of a typical client with RA?
   - **a.** Man
   - **b.** 40 years or older
   - **c.** Overweight
   - **d.** Older than 65 years of age

4. Which of the following applies to the anemia often associated with RA?
   - **a.** Microcytic, hypochromic
   - **b.** Macrocytic, normochromic
   - **c.** Normocytic, hypochromic
   - **d.** Microcytic, normochromic

5. The differential diagnosis of RA includes all the following *except*:
   - **a.** Gout
   - **b.** OA
   - **c.** Tendinitis
   - **d.** Polymyalgia rheumatica

6. Which of the following drugs may be the first drug to use in treating RA?
   - **a.** Enteric coated aspirin
   - **b.** Ibuprofen
   - **c.** Celebrex
   - **d.** Etanercept

7. After treatment with sulfasalazine is initiated, when should the client next be seen?
   - **a.** 1 month
   - **b.** 1 to 2 weeks
   - **c.** 1 to 2 days
   - **d.** 3 to 5 days

Answers and Rationales

1. ***Answer:* c** (assessment)
   Rationale: JRA has three major presentations: (1) acute febrile form with salmon-colored maculopapular rash, arthritis, splenomegaly, leukocytosis, and polyserositis; (2) polyarticular

R

(five or more joints) pattern with swelling and chronic pain; (3) pauciarticular (fewer than five joints) disease with chronic arthritis of a few joints, often weightbearing joints, in an asymmetric distribution.

2. **Answer: a** (assessment)
Rationale: RA typically has a history of morning stiffness lasting 30 to 60 minutes or even longer, whereas with OA morning stiffness lasts 15 to 30 minutes.

3. **Answer: b** (assessment)
Rationale: The typical client with RA is female, with the incidence peaking in the fourth decade of life.

4. **Answer: c** (implementation/plan)
Rationale: Clients with RA often exhibit anemia that is referred to as "anemia of chronic disease." This anemia is a normocytic, hypochromic anemia with reduced red blood cell mass.

5. **Answer: c** (analysis/diagnosis)
Rationale: Because of joint involvement or inflammatory characteristics, OA, gout, and polymyalgia should be considered in the diagnosis of RA.

6. **Answer: a** (implementation/plan)
Rationale: Aspirin is effective and inexpensive. Ibuprofen may cause GI upset. Cox 2 inhibitors may be used to decrease GI side effects, but they are not first-line drugs. Etanercept is a biologic response modifier and is used when DMARDs are not helpful.

7. **Answer: b** (evaluation)
Rationale: The usual time frame for follow-up after initiation of treatment with sulfasalazine is 1 to 2 weeks to consider raising the dosage. This time frame allows for adequate blood levels and a trial for symptomatic relief.

ROSEOLA *(ROSEOLA INFANTUM, EXANTHEM SUBITUM)* Denise Robinson

OVERVIEW
Definition

Roseola is an acute viral illness caused by an infection of the *Herpes viride* family, with most cases caused by human herpes virus (HHV)-6 (80% to 92% of cases). Some cases may be due to HHV-7.

Incidence

- Infection occurs throughout the year and as often in males as in females.
- The mean incubation period is 9 to 10 days. It is contagious before and during the febrile period.
- It is rare before age 3 months and after 4 years and peaks at 6 to 12 months of age. There is a 90% occurrence in children before age 2. One-third of children experience clinical symptoms.
- The condition is most common in spring. Outbreaks rarely are recognized. Infection may occur without symptoms.

Pathophysiology

- Oral viral shedding is the theory of how the virus is spread.
- Mode of transmission is unknown, but the HHV-6 genome may be persistent in lymphocytes and in salivary glands.
- There are antibodies to HHV-6 in cord blood. More than 90% of children have antibodies to HHV-6 by age 3.
- Adults frequently have high levels of antibody for HHV-6, suggesting a long-lived state of viral latency.

ASSESSMENT: SUBJECTIVE/HISTORY
History of Present Illness

- Roseola is associated with abrupt onset of fever as high as 41° C (106° F) that lasts 3 to 5 days.
- Child may be mildly lethargic and irritable.
- The child frequently looks well despite the fever.

Past Medical History

- Immunization history
- Communicable disease history

Medication History

Determine current or new medications.

Family History

- Illness among family members
- Age of siblings

Psychosocial History

Inquire about environmental exposure (e.g., day care).

Common Symptoms

An erythematous, maculopapular rash appears on the trunk following the fever and spreads to the extremities, neck, and face. The rash fades within 24 hours.

Associated Symptoms

Occasionally pharynx, tonsils, and tympanic membranes (TMs) are injected. In immunocompromised hosts, HHV-6 infection has been associated with pneumonitis.

Seizures may occur, usually in the preeruptive stage of roseola.

ASSESSMENT: OBJECTIVE/PHYSICAL EXAMINATION

Physical Examination

- *HEENT:* Observe pharynx, tonsils, and TMs for injection.
- *Extremities:* Observe trunk, arms, neck, face, and legs for erythematous, maculopapular, pinpoint, nonpruritic rash.

Diagnostic Procedures

Diagnostic procedures are not usually necessary.

DIAGNOSIS

Differential diagnoses include the following:

- Fifth disease (warm, red, nontender, "slapped cheeks" rash that spreads in 1 to 2 days to trunk, neck, and buttocks, and then fades with central clearing leaving a lacy, reticulated rash that lasts 2 to 40 days)
- Impetigo
- Rubeola (erythematous, maculopapular rash that begins on face and becomes generalized, sometimes ending in branny desquamation)
- Prodromal fever
- Conjunctivitis
- Coryza
- Cough
- Koplik's spots on buccal mucosa
- Scabies
- Meningitis
- Scarlet fever (a fine erythematous rash that blanches on pressure; often felt more easily than seen [sand papery]; most often on the neck, chest folds of the axilla, the elbow, groin, and inner thighs; cheeks may appear flushed and pale around the mouth; follows a strep infection, usually strep pharyngitis)

THERAPEUTIC PLAN

Pharmacologic Treatment

Control fever for children at risk of febrile seizures by using acetaminophen or ibuprofen (ages 6 months to 2 to 3 years or previous history of febrile seizures).

Nonpharmacologic Treatment

- Provide supportive care as needed.
- Keep child home.
- Ensure the child gets adequate rest until the fever ends.

Client Education

- Roseola is a self-limiting disease.
- High fever can cause seizures.
- Child should be well hydrated.

Referral

Refer if client exhibits any of the following:

- Prolonged high fever
- Febrile seizures
- Signs of meningeal irritation

Consultation

Obtain consultation for immunocompromised individuals.

Prevention

None.

EVALUATION/FOLLOW-UP

None.

COMPLICATIONS

Complications are rare but may occur in a client with hyperpyrexia, persistent seizures, severe encephalitis, or fatal hepatitis.

REFERENCES

American Academy of Pediatrics. (2000). Human Herpesvirus 6 (including Roseola). In G. Peter, (Ed.), *2000 Red Book: Report of the Committee on Infectious Disease* (25th ed.). Elk Grove Village, IL: American Academy of Pediatrics.

American Public Health Association. (2000). *Control of Communicable Diseases Manual* (17th ed.). Washington, DC: American Public Health Association.

Review Questions

1. The rash of roseola differs from that of measles in which of the following ways?

- **a.** Roseola rash starts on the trunk.
- **b.** Measles is a maculopapular rash.
- **c.** Roseola is pink.
- **d.** Measles is a nonpruritic rash.

2. Which of the following historical data is consistent with a diagnosis of roseola?

- **a.** "I have a stuffy nose."
- **b.** "My neck is stiff."
- **c.** "I have a high fever."
- **d.** "I have diarrhea."

3. The time sequence of the fever and rash in roseola is best described by which of the following?

- **a.** Cold symptoms, rash, and then fever
- **b.** High fever that then resolves followed by a rash starting on the trunk
- **c.** Rash starting on the face, spreading to trunk, followed by a fever
- **d.** Fever and rash occur together

4. The best treatment for roseola is which of the following?

- **a.** Treatment for fever with acetaminophen or ibuprofen and rest

R

b. Viral medications such as acyclovir, fluids, and rest

c. Antibiotics such as amoxicillin, antipyretic medications, and rest

d. Lumbar puncture, hospitalization, and symptomatic care

5. Which of the following is the causative agent for roseola?

a. Herpes viride family

b. Herpes zoster family

c. Human parvovirus

d. Group A beta hemolytic streptococci

Answers and Rationales

1. **Answer: a** (assessment)
   Rationale: Both measles and roseola are pink to red, maculopapular, nonpruritic rashes. Roseola starts on the trunk, whereas measles usually starts on the face (American Academy of Pediatrics, 2000).

2. **Answer: c** (assessment)
   Rationale: The first typical sign of roseola is a high fever (102° F-105° F). Neck stiffness, diarrhea, and cold symptoms are not typical of roseola (American Academy of Pediatrics, 2000).

3. **Answer: b** (analysis/diagnosis)
   Rationale: The initial symptom in roseola is a high fever that resolves, followed by a rash that starts on the trunk (American Academy of Pediatrics, 2000).

4. **Answer: a** (implementation/plan)
   Rationale: Treatment for roseola is supportive: fever reduction, fluids, rest, and reassurance. Antiviral agents, antibiotics, and hospitalization are not needed (American Academy of Pediatrics, 2000).

5. **Answer: a** (analysis/diagnosis)
   Rationale: Roseola is caused most frequently by HHV-6, a member of the herpes viride family (American Academy of Pediatrics, 2000).

RUBELLA (GERMAN MEASLES, 3-DAY MEASLES) *Denise Robinson*

OVERVIEW
Definition
Rubella is a mild viral communicable disease.

Incidence
- Rubella most often occurs in late winter or early spring and has a 14 to 21 day incubation period.
- The condition is contagious a few days before the rash appears and 5 to 7 days after the rash appears.
- Cases have decreased 99% from the prevaccine era.
- Congenital rubella syndrome (CRS) occurs in up to 90% of infants born to females who acquire rubella during the first trimester of pregnancy. The risk falls to 10% to 20% by the sixteenth week, and CRS occurs rarely after the twentieth week.

Pathophysiology
- Rubella is caused by a virus and is present in nasopharyngeal secretions, blood, feces, and urine during the clinical illness.
- It is spread by direct contact with infected people by their nasopharyngeal secretions and respiratory droplets or transplacentally.
- It replicates in the nasopharynx and regional lymph nodes.
- The condition usually is self-limiting and does not manifest complications.
- Infants with CRS can shed the virus in their urine and nasopharyngeal fluids for 1 year.

- Active immunity is acquired by natural infection (permanent) or immunization (thought to be life-long). Infants born to immune mothers are protected for 6 to 9 months.
- Of young adults, 10% are susceptible primarily because of lack of vaccination.

ASSESSMENT: SUBJECTIVE/HISTORY
History of Present Illness
- Young children may experience mild coryza and diarrhea.
- Older children and adults may have a sore throat.
- Prodromal symptoms last 1 to 5 days, followed by a rash that begins on the face and spreads downward to the trunk and extremities.
- Lesions remain pink and discrete.

Past Medical History
- Immunization history
- Communicable disease history

Medication History
Determine use of any current or new medications.

Family History
- Rash or illness among household contacts
- Family immunization history
- Pregnancy of family members/close contacts

Psychosocial History
Ask about known exposures.

TABLE **3-95** Prevention of Rubella

DRUG	DOSE	COMMENTS
MMR	Adults : 0.5 ml SQ Children: 0.5 ml SQ First dose at 12-18 months, Second dose at 4-6 years or 11-12 years	All nonimmunized persons should receive MMR (live virus). Ask about egg allergies or reaction to neomycin. Do not give to pregnant women. Inform women of reproductive age not to become pregnant for 3 months after vaccine. Ensure plan for reliable contraception is in place.

Adapted from Cooper, L. (2000). Rubella. In D. Robinson, P. Kidd, K. M. Rogers, (Eds.), *Primary care across the lifespan.* St. Louis: Mosby.
MMR, Measles-mumps-rubella.

Common Symptoms

- Exanthem is a pink, maculopapular eruption.
- It begins on the face and spreads down to trunk and extremities.
- The facial rash clears as extremity rash erupts.
- The rash usually clears in 3 to 5 days.
- Lesions remain pink and discrete.
- Anorexia, headache, and malaise are *not* common.

Associated Symptoms

Postauricular and suboccipital lymphadenopathy are symptoms associated with rubella.

ASSESSMENT: OBJECTIVE/PHYSICAL EXAMINATION
Physical Examination

- Inspect skin, noting characteristics of exanthem.
- To rule out other exanthems, inspect the following:
  - HEENT: Assess mouth for discrete rose spots on soft palate (Koplik's spots are not present).
  - Check for nuchal rigidity.
  - Check for retroauricular, posterior cervical, and postoccipital adenopathy (no other disease causes tender enlargement of the nodes to the extent of rubella).
- Chest: Auscultate heart.
- Abdomen: Check for splenomegaly.
- Joints: Check for polyarthritis (in older girls and women); most likely in hands.

Diagnostic Procedures

Clinical diagnosis is often inaccurate. The following laboratory tests are important.
  - CBC: Look for mild leukopenia with lymphocytosis.
  - Rubella antibody: Draw titer during the acute phase.

DIAGNOSIS

Differential diagnoses include Kawasaki syndrome, roseola, rubeola, scarlet fever, infectious mononucleosis, and drug rash.

THERAPEUTIC PLAN
Pharmacologic Treatment

Symptomatic care includes the following:
  - Acetaminophen
  - Ibuprofen suspension

Nonpharmacologic Treatment

Exclude from school, work, or day care for at least 7 days after onset of rash.

Client Education

- Discuss need for preventive immunization.
- Inform patient to identify pregnant female acquaintances and avoid contact with them (explain why).

Referral/Consultation

Refer pregnant females, especially in the first trimester.

Prevention

- Passive protection can be afforded by immune serum globulin given in a large dose within the first 7 to 8 days of exposure.
- Encourage active immunization with measles-mumps-rubella (MMR) vaccine (Table 3-95).

EVALUATION/FOLLOW-UP

- Return to have convalescent titer drawn.
- Report to local health authority.
- Make phone contact in 72 hours.

COMPLICATIONS

Possible complications include encephalitis, thrombocytopenic purpura, and congenital rubella.

REFERENCES

American Academy of Pediatrics. (2000). Rubella. In: G. Peter. (Ed.). *1997 Red Book: Report of the Committee on Infectious Disease* (25th ed., pp. 456-462). Elk Grove Village, IL: American Academy of Pediatrics.

American Public Health Association. (2000). *Control of Communicable Diseases Manual.* (17th ed., pp. 405-410). Washington, DC: American Public Health Association.

Cooper, L. (2000). Rubella. In D. Robinson, P. Kidd, K. Rogers (Eds.), *Primary care across the lifespan* (pp. 969-971). St. Louis: Mosby.

Review Questions

1. Which of the following historical data is consistent with a diagnosis of rubella?

R

a. Fever, muscular pain (especially in the neck), headache, and malaise
b. Fever, hacking cough, Koplik's spots
c. Exudative pharyngitis, enlarged posterior lymph nodes
d. Facial exanthem, posterior cervical, postoccipital lymphadenopathy

2. Which of the following symptoms is the most characteristic sign of rubella?

a. Retroauricular, posterior cervical, postoccipital lymphadenopathy
b. Discrete rose spots on soft palate
c. Facial rash
d. Slight inflammation of pharynx

3. It is important to differentiate between rubella and rubeola (measles). Compared with rubella, measles is associated with which of the following?

a. Low-grade fever
b. Lymphadenopathy
c. Splenomegaly
d. Koplik's spots

4. The most effective prevention for rubella includes which of the following strategies?

a. Passive immunity (immune serum globulin)
b. Active immunity (MMR)
c. Good handwashing
d. Avoidance of people with URIs

5. Trudy is 6 weeks' pregnant. She went on a business trip to Mexico and is now afraid that she was exposed to rubella. Which of the following strategies is appropriate in this situation?

a. Begin active immunization with MMR.
b. Administer passive immunization with immune serum globulin.
c. Begin symptomatic treatment.
d. Administer dead virus.

Answers and Rationales

1. *Answer:* **d** (assessment)
Rationale: Rubella has a rash that starts on the face and posterior cervical and postoccipital lymphadenopathy (American Academy of Pediatrics, 2000).

2. *Answer:* **a** (assessment)
Rationale: The most characteristic sign of rubella is the lymphadenopathy. All other symptoms described are present, but lymphadenopathy is the most characteristic (American Academy of Pediatrics, 2000).

3. *Answer:* **d** (assessment)
Rationale: Koplik's spots are pathognomonic for measles (American Academy of Pediatrics, 2000).

4. *Answer:* **b** (implementation/plan)
Rationale: Active immunization is the most effective way to prevent measles.

5. *Answer:* **b** (implementation/plan)
Rationale: Passive immunization is only appropriate for nonimmune pregnant women.

RUBEOLA (MEASLES, HARD MEASLES, RED MEASLES) *Denise Robinson*

OVERVIEW
Definition

Rubeola is an acute, highly communicable viral disease caused by morbilli virus in the paramyxovirus family.

- Prodromal phase lasts 3 to 5 days, and the following symptoms precede Koplik's spots by 2 to 3 days:
  - Low-grade to moderate fever
  - Hacking cough
  - Coryza and conjunctivitis
- Rash: Temperature rises (up to 104° F to 105° F) as the rash appears. The rash starts on the neck, along the hairline and cheek. The rash spreads to include the chest, trunk, arms, and face within 24 hours. As it reaches the feet, it begins to fade on the face. The rash may become confluent in severe cases, and the rash is often slightly hemorrhagic.

Incidence

- It occurs late winter and early spring.
- There is an 8 to 12 day incubation period.

- It is contagious 1 to 2 days before any symptoms occur until 4 days after the rash appears. Since 1992, incidence in the United States has been low, at less than 1000 reported cases per year.
- Cases occur in nonimmunized populations (previously vaccinated adolescents and young adults in secondary schools and colleges), and cases are the result of vaccine failure (failure to seroconvert after 1 dose).
- The condition occurs equally among males and females.

Pathophysiology

The disease is spread by direct contact with nasal and throat secretions of an infected person or contact with articles soiled with nose/throat secretions. Immunization at 15 months of age produces immunity in 95% to 98% of recipients. A second dose may increase immunity levels to 99%. Acquired immunity after the illness is permanent.

ASSESSMENT: SUBJECTIVE/HISTORY
History of Present Illness

- Fever (as high as 105° F) with conjunctivitis and photophobia may occur.
- Dry hacking or barking cough and cold symptoms are followed by a deep-red, blotchy rash beginning on the face; The rash becomes generalized, confluent, and sometimes ends in branny desquamation.
- Koplik's spots (gray and white, sand grain-sized dots on red base on buccal mucosa opposite lower molars) appear approximately 2 days before rash appears (pathognomonic for measles).

Past Medical History

- Immunization history including number of doses of vaccine and age at time of administration
- Communicable disease history

Medication History

Inquire about current or new medications.

Family History

- Illness or rashes among household members
- Immunization history of household members

Psychosocial History

Ask about environmental exposures.

ASSESSMENT: OBJECTIVE/PHYSICAL EXAMINATION
Physical Examination

- *Skin:* Inspect skin; note characteristics of exanthem and occasionally jaundice in adults.
- *HEENT:* Note conjunctivitis, photophobia, Koplik's spots, and enlarged lymph nodes at the angle of the jaw and posterior cervical region.
- *Chest:* Auscultate heart and lungs.
- *Abdomen:* Check for slight splenomegaly and abdominal pain in adults.
- *Neurologic:* Evaluate mental status and neurologic system to rule out complications such as encephalitis.

Diagnostic Procedures

- Usually no diagnostic procedures are needed.
- Draw antibody titers at appearance of rash and 3 to 4 weeks later or measles specific immunoglobulin M antibodies 10 days after rash appears.

DIAGNOSIS

Differential diagnoses include Kawasaki syndrome, roseola, rubella, scarlet fever, and drug rashes.

THERAPEUTIC PLAN
Pharmacologic Treatment

- Give acetaminophen.
- Vitamin A should be considered for clients age 6 months to 2 years undergoing hospitalization with measles and complications or clients older than 6 months with ophthalmologic or nutritional disorders or recent immigrants.
- Given to vitamin A levels, which are reduced early in disease
- Pregnancy category X
- Postexposure prophylaxis is immune globulin: prevents or modifies disease in person exposed to measles less than 6 days before administration.

Nonpharmacologic Treatment

- Provide supportive care; cool baths are helpful for fever control.
- Rest in semi-darkened room.
- Exclude from school and day care until 4 days after rash appears.
- Maintain diet as tolerated. Encourage fluids to prevent dehydration.

Client Education

- Teach family to observe changes in level of consciousness and to monitor temperature and respirations daily.
- Practice good handwashing, disposal of tissues, and covering mouth when coughing.
- Encourage immunization.
  - MMR: all nonimmunized persons should receive MMR (live virus).
  - Ask about egg allergies or reaction to neomycin. Do not give MMR vaccine to pregnant women.
  - Give first dose of MMR vaccine at 12 to 18 months.
  - Give second dose of MMR vaccine at 4 to 6 years or 11 to 12 years.

Referral

Refer exposed pregnant females.

Consultation

Consultation should occur before administering vitamin A or if complications develop.

Prevention

- Active immunization with MMR
- Passive immunization with immune serum globulin

EVALUATION/FOLLOW-UP

- Examine daily during acute phase and 3 to 4 days after onset of exanthem to monitor development of complications.
- Report cases to local health authority.

COMPLICATIONS

Complications include otitis media, bronchopneumonia, croup, diarrhea, encephalitis (1 in 1000 cases), and death (1 to 2 in 1000 cases).

REFERENCES

American Academy of Pediatrics. (2000). Measles. In: G. Peter. (Ed.), *2000 Red Book: Report of the Committee on Infectious Disease* (25th ed.). Elk Grove Village, IL: American Academy of Pediatrics.

American Public Health Association. (2000). *Control of communicable diseases manual* (17th ed.). Washington, DC: American Public Health Association.

Cooper, L. (2000). Rubeola. In D. Robinson, P. Kidd, K. Rogers (Eds.), *Primary care across the lifespan* (pp. 972-974). St. Louis: Mosby.

Review Questions

1. Which of the following historical data are consistent with a diagnosis of rubeola?

    a. Fever, muscular pain (especially in the neck), headache, and malaise

    b. Fever, hacking cough, Koplik's spots

    c. Exudative pharyngitis, enlarged posterior lymph nodes

    d. Facial exanthem, posterior cervical, postoccipital lymphadenopathy

2. Which of the following symptoms is the most characteristic sign of rubeola?

    a. Retroauricular, posterior cervical, postoccipital lymphadenopathy

    b. Discrete rose spots on soft palate

    c. Koplik's spots

    d. Slight inflammation of pharynx

3. It is important to differentiate between rubella and rubeola (measles). Compared with rubella, measles is associated with which of the following?

    a. Low-grade fever

    b. Lymphadenopathy

    c. Splenomegaly

    d. Koplik's spots

4. The most effective prevention for rubeola includes which of the following strategies?

    a. Passive immunity (immune serum globulin)

    b. Active immunity (MMR)

    c. Good handwashing

    d. Avoidance of people with URIs

5. Trudy has leukemia and may have been exposed to rubeola. Which of the following strategies is appropriate in this situation?

    a. Begin active immunization with MMR.

    b. Administer passive immunization with immune serum globulin.

    c. Begin symptomatic treatment.

    d. Administer dead virus.

Answers and Rationales

1. *Answer:* **b** (assessment)
Rationale: Rubeola has a rash that starts on the face and Koplik's spots (American Academy of Pediatrics, 2000).

2. *Answer:* **c** (assessment)
Rationale: Koplik's spots are the most characteristic sign of rubeola (American Academy of Pediatrics, 2000).

3. *Answer:* **d** (assessment)
Rationale: Koplik's spots are pathognomonic for measles (American Academy of Pediatrics, 2000).

4. *Answer:* **b** (implementation/plan)
Rationale: Active immunization is the most effective way to prevent measles.

5. *Answer:* **b** (implementation/plan)
Rationale: Passive immunization is appropriate for pregnant women, children with untreated tuberculosis, or children with leukemia or those taking immunosuppressive drugs.

SCABIES *Denise Robinson*

OVERVIEW
Definition

Infestation of the skin with an obligate parasite, the human skin itch mite, *Sarcoptes scabiei var hominis*.

Incidence

- Most commonly seen in children, young adults, institutionalized persons of all ages, and persons with acquired immune deficiency syndrome.
- A persistently high incidence is found in developing countries and in housing where overcrowding occurs.

Pathophysiology

The impregnated female mite burrows into the skin using chemical factors in the saliva to dissolve keratin on the skin surface. Once in the burrow, the female remains there her entire life, approximately 30 days, laying two to three eggs per day. The eggs hatch in 3 to 4 days and the mites

Factors Increasing Susceptibility
- Space-occupying central nervous system (CNS) lesion
- Lack of immunization
- Premature birth
- Birth trauma
- Perinatal intracranial infection
- Positive family history of epilepsy, neurocutaneous disease, sickle cell, febrile seizures, breath-holding spells
- Developmental delay
- Chromosomal disorders
- Illicit drug use
- Chronic illness
- Meningitis and encephalitis
- Cardiac disease
- History of severe head trauma

Etiology
- Neonatal seizures are often related to birth trauma or congenital malformation.
- Seizures in infancy to early childhood (younger than 6 years) are likely caused by metabolic disorders, CNS infections, or febrile seizures.
- In children (age 6 to 10 years) seizures are most often caused by CNS infection, idiopathic epilepsy, or CNS degeneration.
- In childhood to adolescence (10 to 18 years) idiopathic epilepsy, trauma, and alcohol and drug abuse are likely causes.
- Seizures in older persons are often related to trauma, neoplasm, or stroke.

Classification of Seizures

One of the major developments in epileptology of the last few decades has been the adoption of the International Classification of Epileptic Seizures (ICES). Much of the basis for this classification, as illustrated in Box 3-20, is the recognition that the brain is highly organized, with specific functions represented in discrete anatomic regions.

ASSESSMENT: SUBJECTIVE/HISTORY
Clinical Presentation
Partial Seizures
- Simple partial seizure
  - Simple partial seizures (auras) usually last 20 to 180 seconds and are not associated with impairment of consciousness.
  - There are usually no postictal symptoms, but lethargy may occur.
- Complex partial seizures
  - Associated with impairment, but no loss of consciousness.
  - Clients typically stare but do not respond to questions or commands.
  - Usual duration is 30 to 180 seconds.
  - Auras are common.
  - Postictal symptoms are common, but usually brief (less than 20 minutes).
  - Lethargy and confusion
- Partial seizures evolving to secondarily generalized seizures
  - Clients may not recall aura, but witnesses may report that client described an aura or may observe focal movements or automatisms before the convulsion.

Generalized Seizures
- Absence (petit mal) seizure
  - Onset is usually 4 to 11 years.
  - Paroxysmal onset and offset occurs.
  - Impairment of consciousness is usually brief (less than 15 seconds).
  - Precipitated by hyperventilation.

S

Box 3-20 Epileptic Seizures: Classification and Characteristics (Proposed by the International Classification of Epileptic Seizures)

PARTIAL SEIZURES (FOCAL SEIZURES)
Simple partial seizures
Complex partial seizures
   Simple partial onset followed by impairment of consciousness
   With impairment of consciousness at the onset
Partial seizures evolving to generalized seizures

GENERALIZED SEIZURES (CONVULSIVE OR NONCONVULSIVE)
Absence seizures
Typical absence seizures (petit mal)
Myoclonic seizures

Clonic seizures
Tonic seizures
Tonic-clonic seizures
Atonic seizures
Infantile spasms

UNCLASSIFIED EPILEPTIC SEIZURES
Includes all those seizures that cannot be classified because of incomplete data or because they defy classification into the above categories; for example, neonatal seizures with swimming movements.
Status Epilepticus

From Baker, D. (2000). Seizures. In D. Robinson, P. Kidd, & K. Rogers (Eds.), *Primary care across the lifespan* (p. 990). St. Louis: Mosby.

- Aura, postictal confusion, or lethargy are not present.
- May be frequent (more than 100 per day).
- Myoclonic Seizure
  - Brief, shock-like jerk of muscles or group of muscles are present.
  - Two types, as follows:
  Nonepileptic: often unilateral
  Epileptic myoclonus: usually bilateral, symmetrical movements
- Tonic seizure
  - Brief episode with sudden increase in tone in trunk or extremities are present.
  - Seizures usually last less than 20 seconds.
- Tonic-clonic (grand mal) seizure
  - May be partial (beginning focally) or primary generalized (bilateral/symmetrical onset).
  - There is an initial brief tonic phase lasting 2 to 10 seconds with loss of consciousness, extensor rigidity, fall, often a cry; superior deviation of eyes and pupil dilation.
  - Secondary clonic phase with bilateral jerking lasts 30 to 180 seconds; rate of jerking usually slows; often a large jerk is followed by flaccidity and coma.
  - There may be hypersalivation, tongue biting, and urinary incontinence.
  - Postictal period lasts minutes to hours with lethargy, confusion, decreased attention, and depression.
- Atonic seizure
  - Brief episodes with sudden decrease in tone in trunk or extremities are present.
  - Onset usually in childhood.
  - Seizures last less than 15 seconds.
  - There is a sudden loss of postural tone, from head nod to fall with major trauma.
  - May be accompanied by tonic seizures.
  - Injury is common, and these clients often require helmets.
  - Primarily seen in Lennox-Gastaut syndrome.

Unclassified Seizures
- Lennox-Gastaut syndrome
  - Begins at age 1 to 7 years.
  - Often coexists with atonic seizures.
  - Client falls are common.
  - Symmetrical jerking of proximal arms with twitching of facial muscles (mouth and eyes).
- West syndrome (infantile spasms)
  - Presents at 2 months of age to 1 year.
  - There is sudden flexion of extremities, head, and trunk for limited time.
  - Untreated, infantile spasms subside within 1 to 4 years but often are replaced by other forms of seizures; prognosis is poor.
- Febrile seizures

- Usually occur between 6 months and 5 years, and most commonly occur before 13 months of age.
- They are brief, generalized, short, and nonfocal.
- Client is febrile before seizure and has no evidence of CNS infection.
- Prognosis is excellent because fewer than 3 percent of children with simple febrile seizures will have nonfebrile seizures subsequently.

Status Epilepticus
- Characterized by a seizure that continues longer than 30 minutes or by repeated seizures associated with impaired awareness for more than 30 minutes.
- They are medical emergencies that can cause brain damage and death.
- Thus any tonic-clonic seizure lasting longer than 5 to 10 minutes should be treated.

History of Present Illness
- Determine what type of seizure occurred by asking client, family members, and witnesses.
- Obtain a good description of the seizure.
- Determine whether it was focal (involving only the face, or one extremity, or one side of the body); immediately generalized (involving all extremities); or started as a focal seizure and then generalized to involve the extremities; and how long it occurred.
- Ask whether the client lost consciousness.
- When client is aroused, determine if there was any evidence of an aura.
- Did the client lose control of bowel or bladder?
- Was there a period of postictal lethargy, and how long it occurred?
- Describe how the client acted after the seizure.
- Is there any associated illness or fever or any sleep deprivation?
- Determine the relationship of seizure to the time of day, meals, fatigue, emotional stress, excitement, menses, discontinuing medication, activity before attack, and frequency of occurrence.
- Inquire about history of trauma, drug withdrawal, particularly alcohol, barbiturates, or benzodiazepines, and any exposure to toxins.

Past Medical History
- Obtain birth history.
- Obtain prenatal history for children: infection, substance abuse, bleeding, preterm labor, diabetes, hypertension (HTN).
- Assess labor and delivery, whether there were complications, whether oxygen was needed.
- In neonates, assess gestation, infections, apnea, major complications, or congenital anomalies.
- Determine whether there is a history of cardiac arrhythmias, valve disease, stroke, and malignancies.
- Determine the presence of any diabetes or renal disease.

- Obtain history of head trauma with loss of consciousness, febrile seizures.
- If the client has had seizures before, determine the following:
    - Precipitating factors
    - Whether the seizure is the same as those in the past
    - Medication compliance
    - More frequent occurrence

Medication History

Determine what medications the client is taking.

Family History

Determine if there is a family history of seizures or neurologic disorders.

Psychosocial History

Determine the following:
- Any recent travel
- Occupation
- Alcohol consumption and amount
- Drug abuse with type and amount of drug or drugs
- Type and age of dwelling; lead screen
- Description of attainment of development milestones/school performance

Dietary History

Determine the type of foods client has eaten in the recent past.

ASSESSMENT: OBJECTIVE/PHYSICAL EXAMINATION

Physical Examination

- Observe for an injury pattern.
- Determine vital signs, head circumference in children, height, weight.
- Perform a complete neurologic examination: mental status, speech, cranial nerves, eye fundus, strength, tone, reflexes, cerebellar.
- Perform a complete cardiovascular examination: bruits, murmurs, abnormalities of rhythm.
- Observe the skin for any abnormalities (often associated with congenital disorders).
- Assess café-au-lait spots: neurofibromatosis.
- Assess adenoma sebaceum (reddish nodules over the nose, cheeks, and, occasionally, the chin or shagreen patch [like untanned leather] over the dorsum of the trunk): tuberous sclerosis.
- Assess hemangioma involving one side of face or involving one side of body: Sturge Weber.
- Assess abdomen: liver size.

Diagnostic Procedures

- Obtain electrolytes glucose levels, and renal and liver function tests.
- Assess lead level.

- Obtain a drug screen.
- EEG is the most helpful test in terms of diagnosing and classifying seizures disorders.
- Computed tomography (CT) and magnetic resonance imaging (MRI) are indicated in first-time seizures, or with intractable seizures or focal neurologic abnormalities.
- Obtain lumbar puncture.
- Perform genetic studies.

DIAGNOSIS

Differential Diagnosis

- Syncope
- Vasovagal attack
- Cardiac disorder
- Nonepileptic seizures
- Breath-holding spells
- Paroxysmal rapid eye movement (REM) sleep behavior
- Panic attack

THERAPEUTIC PLAN

Immediate Management

- Maintain clear airway by turning client on side with head down; remove vomitus or dentures.
- Do not try to pry tight jaws open to place an object between the teeth.
- Protect client from injuries.
- Administer oxygen if cyanotic.
- Status epilepticus (seizure longer than 10 minutes' duration) necessitates transportation to an emergency department and immediate consultation with a physician.

Principles of Treatment

- Consult physician for all first-time seizures.
- The decision to treat a first-time seizure is difficult and should be based on the interpretation of the subtle clinical, historical, and laboratory findings.
- The final decision about treatment must be made individually for each client, and should consider the potential psychological, vocational, and physical consequences of further seizures.
- A provoked seizure is one for which the factors that precipitated the episode can be identified and remedied, such as physical injury and drug overdose.
- In febrile seizures, the initial treatment is lowering the temperature with acetaminophen, ibuprofen, or cool baths. (Generally, febrile seizures do not require anticonvulsant therapy; however, frequent recurrent febrile seizures may require prophylactic treatment with oral phenobarbital.)

Pharmacolgic Treatment

- Generally 80% of seizures can be controlled with anticonvulsants.

- Antiepileptic drug (AED) selection is based on the preference of the health care provider. The NP may actively participate in the process of selecting the AED, monitoring its administration, and assessing the client's response, including side effects.
- If AED treatment is chosen, then consider the following:
  - The goal of AEDs is to prevent the recurrence or lessen seizures while avoiding side effects from the drugs.
  - Choose an agent appropriate to the seizure type.
  - Initiate treatment with a single drug; consider cost and toxicity.
  - When dosing, consider the half-life of the drug in terms of how often the drug should be given and how long it takes to achieve a steady-state level.
  - When you have to add additional drugs, add one at a time.
  - When you want to stop one or all drugs, taper them off; do not stop abruptly.
  - Hematologic and hepatic monitoring should be done at initiation of therapy, once during the first few months, whenever clinical symptoms occur, and annually or less often.
  - Individualize treatment to seizure type, response to medication, and maintenance of appropriate blood levels.
  - Clients at high risk for recurrence should be treated for a 2-year period.

See Table 3-97 for choosing the correct AED for the type of seizure.

Special Considerations

Reproductive Health and Pregnancy

NOTE: *Preconception counseling is imperative: If seizure free for 2 years, consider an attempt at drug withdrawal before conception.*

- Fertility rates may be lower in women with localization-related epilepsy.

- Family planning may be affected by the high failure rate of oral contraceptives and AEDs.
- Changes in hormones over the menstrual cycle may influence the frequency of seizures.
- Pregnancy causes a large increase in circulating serum proteins; because most drugs are protein bound, there may be a decrease in free or active blood levels, especially during the first trimester. Free drug levels should be measured rather than total serum drug level.
- Pregnant women with epilepsy have more frequent seizures (30% to 50%) and pregnancy complications (blunt abdominal trauma caused by falls or motor vehicle accidents [MVAs]).
- The probability of teratogenesis in fetuses of epileptic women treated with AEDs is higher than that in fetuses of untreated epileptic women (rates of stillbirth, neonatal death and perinatal death are 3 times greater) (200 to 300 times risk of stillbirth, prematurity, developmental delay).

Other problems associated with epilepsy in pregnancy include the following:
- Increased risk of bleeding
- Decreased fetal growth
- Decreased childhood intelligence

Elderly Population

- Common causes of epilepsy in older adults are cerebrovascular disease and neoplasms, as well as metabolic derangements and head trauma.
- A slower metabolic rate often requires a decrease in dosage of AEDs.
- The possibility of drug interactions is increased mainly because many elderly take numerous medications.
- The cost of AEDs may be of great concern to those on a fixed income.
- Failing memory can make compliance difficult, especially when the drug requires multiple daily doses.

TABLE **3-97**   Choosing the Correct AED for the Type of Seizure

TYPE OF SEIZURE	AED DRUGS TO CONSIDER
Simplex and complex, partial	Preferred: carbamazepine, phenytoin, divalproex sodium, valproic acid; acceptable: gabapentin, lamotrigine, topiramate
Absence	Preferred: ethosuximide, valproic acid, divalproex sodium; acceptable: methsuximide (Celontin Kapseals: no information available)
Tonic-clonic	Phenytoin, valproic acid, carbamazepine, divalproex sodium
Myoclonic and atonic	Clonazepam
Special considerations	Felbamate for treatment of Lennox-Gastaut syndrome; gabapentin for use as add-on therapy in refractory simple and complex partial seizures; lamotrigine for treatment of partial seizures and possibly also tonic-clonic, absence, and atonic seizures; vigabatrin for childhood forms of epilepsy

From Baker, D. (2000). Seizures. In D. Robinson, P. Kidd, & K. Rogers (Eds.), *Primary care across the lifespan* (p. 995). St. Louis: Mosby.
AED, Antiepileptic drug.

Nonpharmacologic Treatment

- The degree to which activities should be restricted is individualized for each person and depends on the type, frequency, and severity of the seizures, the response to therapy, and the length of time the seizures have been controlled.
- The client should be encouraged to follow a regular and moderate routine in lifestyle, diet, exercise, and rest. (Sleep deprivation may lower the client's threshold to seizures.)
- Normal, healthy activities are encouraged for children, and participation in competitive sports is determined on an individual basis. Contact sports such as football, karate, or wrestling are avoided, but basketball, baseball, and tennis are allowed.
- A variety of special diets are recommended for the treatment of seizures. One of the recommendations includes eating a healthy, well-balanced diet. Also, the ketogenic diet that stimulates the ketosis and acidosis of starvation has been advocated as therapy for epilepsy.
- Avoid excessive amounts of caffeine and alcohol.

Client Education

- Make sure that the client and/or parent understands the goals and time frame of treatment and that they have been provided with information and support about seizures.
- Teach families what to do in the emergency management of seizures. To avoid unnecessary medical intervention and to ensure that observers respond appropriately to seizures, the client may want to wear an identification bracelet that notes the condition and the phone number of a contact person.
- Counseling in children is especially important, emphasizing the significance of seizures, that they can live a normal life within some limits, and that they must learn to cope with some of the attitudes of the public regarding seizures.
- Areas of psychosocial difficulty should be identified early in the course of treatment so that disabilities related to epilepsy can be minimized by using the necessary social, educational, vocational, and psychological support services.
- Review each state law concerning driving an automobile.
- If the client has good control of seizures, minimum restrictions are needed, such as swimming with a buddy or wearing a helmet with some sports.
- Stress the importance of drug compliance and instruct the client about the actions and side effects of medications, including the following:
  - AEDs reduce effectiveness of oral contraceptives.
  - AEDs are teratogenic.
  - AEDs and other drugs may display numerous interactions.

- Review with the client that many factors tend to precipitate seizures in some clients and should be avoided, including the following:
  - Sleep deprivation
  - Fever
  - Strobe lights
  - Psychologic stress
  - Excessive alcohol
- A client who is not well-controlled should not have pertussis vaccine.
- It is important to encourage a healthy attitude toward the child and his or her disease and to help the parents feel competent in their ability to meet their responsibilities to the child. Many parents refrain from correcting or punishing the child, especially if they have had the experience of such an emotional stress precipitating an attack. The child should not be made to feel that he or she is different.
- The child needs to learn about the disease and the role that medication plays in contributing to his or her well-being. As soon as he or she is old enough, the child should assume responsibility for taking medication.

Referral/Consultation

- Consult a specialist for treatment of clients with West syndrome and Lennox-Gastaut syndrome.
- Consultation with a neurologist is recommended before pregnancy in those women contemplating pregnancy to ascertain that an AED is indicated and to consider alteration of the current regimen to one that has a lower risk to the fetus.
- New options are available for refractory seizures.
  - Vagus nerve stimulator are available.
  - Anterior lobe resection is the most common surgery for seizure.
- Consult physician on all first-time seizures.
- Consult physician about clients who have complicating factors such as persistent seizures, change in seizure pattern, and serious infection.
- Consult physician regarding clients who may require hospitalization, such as children with a complex febrile seizure.

Prevention

- Prevention of high fevers and infection
- Use of seat belts and bike helmets to prevent closed head injuries

EVALUATION/FOLLOW-UP

- Follow-up is indicated according to the chosen AED.
- In general, follow up every 3 to 6 months to evaluate seizure control and side effects of drugs.
- Follow-up for clients on AEDs are the following:
  - Draw blood level of drug.
  - Consult with physician.

S

- Follow-up is indicated according to the chosen AED for blood work related to liver function and serum drug concentrations.
- Always ascertain any untoward side effects that the client may be experiencing.
- Reinforce education as described previously.
- Clients who are seizure free for 2 years can be considered for medication withdrawal.
- Focal motor seizures are more likely to recur than generalized seizures, and those with a history of neonatal seizures have a greater risk of seizure recurrence.

COMPLICATIONS

Inability to function on a day-to-day basis because of frequent and debilitating seizures.

REFERENCES

Baker, D. (2001). Seizures. In D. Robinson, P. Kidd, & K. Rogers (Eds.), *Primary care across the lifespan* (pp. 989-999). St. Louis: Mosby.

Celano, R. (1998). Diagnosing pediatric epilepsy: An update for the primary care clinician. *Nurse Practitioner, 23*(3), 69-96.

Curry, W., & Kulling, D. (1998). Newer antiepileptic drugs: Gabapentin, lamotrigine, felbamate, topiramate and fosphenytoin. *American Family Physician, 57*(3), 513-520.

Henneman, P. L., DeRoos, F., & Lewis, R. J. (1994). Determining the need for admission in patients with new-onset seizures. *Annals of Emergency Medicine, 12*(6), 1108-1113.

Kaplan, P. W. (1999). Seizure disorders. In L. R. Barker, J. R. Burton, & P. D. Zieve (Eds.), *Principles of ambulatory medicine* (5th ed., pp. 1230-1251). Baltimore: Williams & Wilkins.

Kuhn, B. R., Allen, K. D., & Shriver, M. D. (1995). Behavioral management of children's seizure activity: Intervention guidelines for primary care providers. *Clinical Pediatrics, 34*(11), 570-575.

Leppik, I. E. (1996). *Contemporary diagnosis and management of the patient with epilepsy* (2nd ed.). Newtown, PA: Handbooks in Health Care.

Marks, W., & Garcia, P. (1998). Management of seizures and epilepsy. *American Family Physician, 57*(7), 1589-1604.

McLachlan, R. S. (1993). Managing the first seizure. *Canadian Family Physician, 39*, 885-888, 891-893.

Moore-Sledge, C. M. (1997). Evaluation and management of first seizures in adults. *American Family Physician, 56*(4), 1113-1120.

Morrell, M. J. (1994). XII Epilepsy. In D. C. Dale (Ed.), *Scientific American medicine* (pp. 1-19). New York: Scientific American.

Rochester, J. (1997). Epilepsy in pregnancy. *American Family Physician, 56*(6), 1631-1638.

Review Questions

1. M. J. comes to the emergency department today with his 74-year-old wife, stating that he thinks his wife has had a seizure. What presenting symptoms would lead you to believe that a tonic-clonic seizure may have taken place?

   a. Headache, fever, and general malaise
   b. Eyes rolled back in head while lying rigid, then jerking for 30 seconds
   c. Fall on the floor
   d. Unable to speak after waking this morning

2. What is the most important test in classifying and diagnosing epilepsy?

   a. Brain scan
   b. Electrocardiogram (ECG)
   c. EEG
   d. Complete blood count (CBC)

3. What differential diagnosis would be included with a 3-week-old baby girl who turns very red in the face and then passes out after crying?

   a. Panic attack
   b. Nonepileptic seizures of psychogenic origin
   c. Breath-holding spells
   d. Partial seizure evolving to secondarily generalized seizure

4. Once it has been determined that a seizure has taken place, it is then important to determine whether the seizure was provoked to determine treatment. Which of the following options does not indicate a provoked seizure?

   a. Occurs without cause
   b. Occurs with sustained head injury after a motor vehicle crash
   c. Occurs with a high fever
   d. Associated with acute alcohol withdrawal

5. P. S., a 31-year-old woman, has been treated many years with several AEDs for her seizures and comes to see you because she wants to get pregnant. What would be an appropriate decision to make in her case?

   a. Take her off all AEDs right away to prevent any harm to the fetus in case pregnancy occurs.
   b. Refer her to a neurologist.
   c. Inform her that pregnancy will cause a decrease in seizures.
   d. Inform her that the fertility rate in women with localization-related epilepsy is the same as that of women without epilepsy.

6. Which of the following physical findings suggests a congenital reason for seizures?

   a. Café au lait spots
   b. Tender temporal artery
   c. Tense trapezius muscles bilaterally
   d. Soft fontanelle

7. Sara is having a tonic-clonic seizure. Which of the following needs is the greatest priority at this time?

   a. Determine if she has a temperature.
   b. Pry her jaws open to place a tongue blade inside.
   c. Administer diazepam (Valium).
   d. Turn her on her side with her head down.

8. Which of the following comments by the client regarding seizure management indicates a need for more teaching?

a. "I can drive my car when I have good days."
b. "I need to be aware of all the drugs I take and their side effects."
c. "Antibiotics can affect the blood level of my seizure medications."
d. "I should avoid stress and strobe lights."

Answers and Rationales

1. Answer: b (assessment)
Rationale: Tonic-clonic (grand mal) seizures have an initial brief tonic phase with extensor rigidity and superior deviation of the eyes and a secondary clonic phase with bilateral jerking lasting 30 to 180 seconds. Often a large jerk is followed by flaccidity and coma. There may be hypersalivation, tongue biting, and incontinence. The postictal period lasts minutes to hours with lethargy and confusion (Devinsky & Sloviter, 1993).

2. Answer: c (analysis/diagnosis)
Rationale: The EEG is the single most important diagnostic test in the diagnosis and classification of seizures, although it is not uncommon for a standard 30-minute recording to show no definite interictal activity in the presence of diagnosed epilepsy (Scheuer & Pedley, 1990).

3. Answer: c (analysis/diagnosis)
Rationale: Often infants cry so hard while holding their breath that they pass out temporarily (Mikati & Browne, 1993). The other choices of panic attack and pseudoseizures are not indicated in an infant. The last choice of partial seizure evolving to secondarily generalized seizure also is not indicated because there may be focal movement or automatisms seen before the convulsion that were not seen in this infant.

4. Answer: a (analysis/diagnosis)
Rationale: A provoked seizure is one in which the factors that precipitated the episode can be identified and remedied, such as those mentioned other than the first choice. An unprovoked seizure is one without an outside influence (Uphold & Graham, 1994).

5. Answer: b (evaluation)
Rationale: Consultation with a neurologist is recommended before pregnancy in those women contemplating pregnancy to ascertain that an AED is indicated and to consider alteration of the current regimen to one that would have a lower risk to the fetus (Messenheimer, 1996). The other choices are inappropriate.

6. Answer: a (assessment)
Rationale: Certain skin abnormalities are indicative or associated with congenital seizures (Baker, 2000).

7. Answer: d (analysis/diagnosis)
Rationale: Immediate management of a seizure includes making sure the airway is open by placing the client on his or her side, and then removing vomitus or dentures. The teeth should not be pried apart to insert a tongue blade. Valium is not appropriate unless it is a case of status epilepticus (Baker, 2000).

8. Answer: a (evaluation)
Rationale: Each state has different requirements regarding driving and seizures. Usually there must be a period in which the person is seizure free before obtaining the right to drive (Baker, 2000).

SICKLE CELL ANEMIA *Denise Robinson*

OVERVIEW
Definition

Sickle cell anemia is a condition in which there is an abnormality of the globin genes (i.e., a hemoglobin disorder). (Both parents must have sickle hemoglobin [Hb S] for the child to have sickle cell anemia; only one S is present for the sickle cell trait). A better term than anemia might be hemoglobinopathy because hemoglobin has a structural change in the amino acid sequences of the globin chains. Sickle cell anemia is characterized by severe chronic hemolytic disease resulting from premature destruction of the brittle, poorly deformable erythrocytes.

Incidence

- Sickle cell anemia affects more than 70,000 blacks, with one third between 2 and 16 years old. It is the most common single gene disorder in blacks (Wethers, 2000a).
- Sickle cell anemia occurs in 1 out of 400 black infants.
- Eight percent of blacks are heterozygous carriers of the sickle gene and have the trait.

- The sickle cell trait and anemia affect persons from many parts of Africa, the Mediterranean area, and parts of Turkey, the Middle East, and India.

Pathophysiology

Hb S differs from normal adult hemoglobin by a substitution of a glutamic acid at the sixth position of its amino acid chains by valine. In the oxygenated state, the Hb S functions normally. When this hemoglobin is deoxygenated, an interaction occurs that causes the formation of polymers; these elongate to form rigid, crystal-like rods. This polymerization is responsible for the spiny, brittle character of sickle erythrocytes under conditions of decreased oxygen. Other symptoms of sickle cell anemia are caused by the ischemic changes resulting from vascular occlusion caused by high numbers of sickled cells. These are referred to as "crises."

Manifestation of sickle cell by age are as follows:
- Newborn: No clinical features of sickle cell are exhibited; hemolytic gradually develops over 2 to 4 months as the fetal hemoglobin is replaced by Hb S.

S

Other signs and symptoms are uncommon before age 5 to 6 months.

- First indication of sickle cell might be hand-and-foot syndrome: acute sickle dactylitis. This may be first sign that sickle cell disease is present in the child; it occurs in up to 50% of children before the age of 3. Symptoms include painful, symmetrical swelling of hands and feet. The underlying abnormality is necrosis of the small bones, which is thought to be caused by the decreased blood supply caused by the rapidly expanding bone marrow.
- Painful vasoocclusive episodes characterize the symptoms in other age groups. Most clients have some pain on a daily basis. Illness such as fever, hypoxia, and acidosis may precipitate the crises and pain, but the pain can occur without an apparent precipitant event.
- Young children: Pain often involves extremities.
- Older children: Head, chest, abdominal and back pain are more common.
  - Acute pain episodes may evolve to infarction of bone marrow or bone. Splenic infarcts are common in children from 6 to 60 mos.
  - Cerebrovascular accidents (CVAs) are common; up to 10% of preadolescent and older clients demonstrate symptoms consistent with cerebral occlusion.
  - Renal function is progressively impaired; most clients older than age 5 exhibit renal problems.
  - Because of the altered splenic function, sickle cell anemia clients are more susceptible to meningitis, sepsis, and other serious infections.
  - Chronic leg ulcers occur in late adolescence and beyond.
- Adults: Common manifestations include the following:
  - Bacterial sepsis
  - Aplastic crises
  - Bone infarction
  - Stroke
  - Priapism
  - Acute multiorgan failure
  - Chronic problems include leg ulcers, avascular necrosis of the hip, cholecystitis, and chronic organ failure of the liver, kidney, and lung.

ASSESSMENT: SUBJECTIVE/HISTORY
History of Present Illness and Past Medical History

History of symptoms related to sickle cell include the following:

- Irritability
- Dyspnea
- Fatigue
- Palpitations
- Headache
- Edema
- Jaundice
- Bleeding
- Pallor
- Infection
- Heart murmur
- Chronic illness
- Drug use
- Bone pain
- Past viral infections
- Number of hospitalizations

Medication History

Ask about use of anticonvulsants.

Family and Psychosocial History

- Determine ethnic origin.
- Ask about other children in family with sickle cell anemia.
- Ask about prior testing for sickle cell trait or disease.

ASSESSMENT: OBJECTIVE/PHYSICAL EXAMINATION
Physical Examination

Perform a complete physical examination with increased attention to the following:

- Vital signs, weight, height (children typically have delayed growth and development)
- General: Sensitivity to cold, weight loss, lethargy
- Skin: Jaundice, bleeding, pallor, petechiae, purpura
- Mouth: glossitis, angular stomatitis
- Eyes: Eyelid edema, retinal hemorrhage
- Respiratory: Tachypnea
- Cardiovascular: Tachycardia, murmur, or gallop; angina; myocardial infarction (MI); congestive heart failure
- Abdominal: Hepatosplenomegaly or other masses, lymphadenopathy, anorexia (spleen size should be noted every exam)
- Musculoskeletal/extremities: Bone pain, leg ulcers
- Neurologic: Headache, vertigo, irritability, depression, impaired thought processes

Diagnostic Procedures

- In 41 states and the District of Columbia, newborns are required to be screened for sickle cell anemia (Wethers, 2000a).
- Obtain CBC, including all indexes, mean corpuscular volume (MCV), mean corpuscular hemoglobin (MCH), mean corpuscular hemoglobin concentration (MCHC). White blood cell (WBC) count frequently is elevated to 12,000 to 20,000/mm^3 with a predominance of neutrophils. Platelet count is usually increased. Hemoglobin may typically be between 7 and 10 g/dL.

- Blood smear: Typically reveals target cells, poikilocytes, and irreversibly sickled cells. These findings permit differentiation from sickle cell trait. Reticulocyte counts range from 5% to 15%, and nucleated red cells and Howell-Jolly bodies are often present; reflects state of erythroid activity of bone marrow (normal 0.5% to 1.5%).
- Erythrocyte sedimentation rate (ESR) is slow.
- Liver function tests are abnormal.
- Bilirubin levels are elevated.
- Bone marrow may be hyperplastic with erythroid predominance.
- Obtain hemoglobin studies, electrophoresis; sickle cell: hemoglobin (Hb) SS; sickle cell trait: Hb AS; solubility tests such as Sickledex and Sicklequik are not recommended because they do not identify other genetic variants. They are also inaccurate in the newborn (Wethers, 2000a).

DIAGNOSIS

- Assess presence of Hb SS or Hb AS on electrophoresis studies.
- Differential diagnoses include the following: Symptoms of occlusion may lead the diagnoses to diseases such as rheumatic fever, rheumatoid arthritis (RA), osteomyelitis, and leukemia.

THERAPEUTIC PLAN

- The goal of treatment is to provide early diagnosis, comprehensive medical care, and prophylactic care to reduce episodes of infection and complications.
- Recommend referral to hematologist for multidisciplinary approach and pain management for sickle cell anemia.

Nonpharmacologic Treatment

- Any illness with fever of 38.5° C should be evaluated with blood cultures, IV broad-spectrum antibiotics, and careful observation.
- Red cell transfusions improve oxygen-carrying capacity during crises; the most common indication for transfusion is stroke.

Pharmacologic Treatment

- Folic acid to ensure adequate amounts for the high erythrocyte turnover
- Prophylactic penicillin starting by the age of 2 months until at least 6 years of age
- Pneumococcal vaccination
- Yearly influenza vaccine

Client Education

- Identify causes of sickle cell crisis and disease process.
- Be aware of precipitating factors, including the following:
  - Cold exposure
  - Decreased fluid intake
  - Exercise at high altitude
  - Overexertion, emotional or physical stress
  - Increased blood viscosity
  - Viral or bacterial infections
  - Surgery, blood loss
- Emphasize need for routine health care.
- Provide psychosocial support.

Prevention

- Identification of sickle cell traits in parents before pregnancy
- Complications associated with treatment failure
- Tissue ischemia and infarction causes damage to virtually every organ system.

EVALUATION/FOLLOW-UP

- Children should be followed every 3 months until they are 2 years old, then every 6 months until the age of 5. After age 5, visits should occur yearly.
- Periodic urinalysis should be done to check for early signs of renal disease.
- Retinal examinations should occur after the age of 10 to rule out retinal disease.
- Right upper quadrant pain may indicate gallbladder disease, and an ultrasound should be done.
- Adolescents can participate in sports but must avoid overexertion, dehydration, and extremes of temperature. They should stop at the first sign of fatigue.
- Adolescents will have catch-up growth.
- Genetic counseling should be offered to all adolescents, as well as family planning and contraception information.

REFERENCES

Bates, B. (1995). *Physical exam and history taking* (6th ed.). Philadelphia: J. B. Lippincott.

Cunningham, F., Gant, N., Kenneth, J., Laveno, M., Clark, S., Hauth, J., & Wenstrom, K. (2001). Hematological disorders. In F. G. Cunningham, (Ed.), *Williams obstetrics* (21st ed.). Norwalk, CT: Appleton & Lange, 1307-1338.

Kalinyak, K. (1997). Anemias. In R. Arceci (Ed.), *Hematology/oncology/stem cell transplant handbook* (2nd ed., pp. 87-116). Cincinnati: Hematology Oncology Division of Children's Hospital Medical Center.

Lane, P., Nuss, R., & Ambruso, D. (2001). Hematologic disorders. In W. Hay, A. Hayward, M. Levin, & J. Sondheimer (Eds.), *Current pediatric diagnosis and treatment.* Norwalk, CT: Appleton & Lange.

Mitus, A., & Rosenthal, D. (1995). History and physical examination of relevance to the hematologist. In R. Handlin, S. Lux, & T. Stossel (Eds.), *Blood: Principles and practice of hematology* (pp. 3-19). Philadelphia: J. B. Lippincott.

Wethers, D. (2000a). Sickle cell disease in childhood, part I: Laboratory diagnosis, pathophysiology and health maintenance. *American Family Physician, 62,* 1013-1020, 1027-1028.

Wethers, D. (2000b). Sickle cell disease in childhood, part II: Diagnosis and treatment of major complications and recent advances in treatment. *American Family Physician, 62,* 1309-1314a, 1027-1028.

Review Questions

1. Which of the following historical information is typical in clients with sickle cell anemia?

   a. Pain
   b. Hematuria
   c. Weight gain
   d. Alopecia

2. Which of the following should be noted during the physical examination?

   a. Skin color
   b. Enlarged spleen
   c. Rash
   d. Height and weight

3. Which of the following is likely to be found in adolescents during their examination?

   a. Weight gain
   b. Alopecia
   c. Delayed growth and development
   d. Increased lead level

4. Which of the following has made a dramatic impact on morbidity and mortality of sickle cell disease in children?

   a. Early recognition of the disease
   b. Prophylactic treatment with penicillin
   c. Folic acid replacement
   d. Avoiding dehydration

5. Which of the following comments by the mother of a child with sickle cell indicates a need for further teaching?

   a. "I need to monitor Sara's temperature."
   b. "Swelling of the hands and feet needs to be addressed immediately."
   c. "A low-grade fever can be treated with Tylenol."
   d. "Sam can play tennis if he wants to."

Answers and Rationales

1. *Answer:* **a** (assessment)
   Rationale: Every sickle cell client, whether in crisis or not, is likely to have pain (Wethers, 2000a).

2. *Answer:* **b** (assessment)
   Rationale: It is important to note spleen size on every examination; it can indicate a splenomegaly caused by infarction or an enlarged spleen resulting from infection crisis.

3. *Answer:* **c** (assessment)
   Rationale: Most teens have delayed growth and development; they usually are approximately 2 years behind. Teens can be reassured that they will attain average height (Wethers, 2000a).

4. *Answer:* **b** (implementation/plan)
   Rationale: Prophylactic penicillin has made a big difference in terms of morbidity and mortality for children diagnosed with sickle cell disease (Wethers, 2000a).

5. *Answer:* **c** (evaluation)
   Rationale: Parents need to understand that any fever elevation needs to be treated aggressively and warrants medical attention (Wethers, 2000a).

SINUSITIS: ACUTE AND CHRONIC *Pamela Kidd*

OVERVIEW
Definition

- Sinusitis is defined as inflammation of the mucous lining of the paranasal sinuses.
- Acute sinusitis is a symptomatic sinus infection lasting up to 4 weeks. Subacute sinusitis lasts 4 to 12 weeks. Recurrent acute sinusitis is four or more episodes annually with resolution between episodes. Chronic sinusitis is a symptomatic sinus infection that persists for longer than 12 weeks, despite adequate treatment (Casiano, 2000).

Incidence

Sinusitis is one of the most common complaints leading to office visits. This common health problem is prevalent in all ages and is equally prevalent in both sexes. In fall, winter, and spring, it usually follows a viral upper respiratory infection (URI); in summer, it is often associated with swimming and diving or allergic rhinitis.

Pathophysiology

- Maxillary and ethmoid sinuses are present from birth.
- Frontal sinus develops after age 2.
- Sphenoid sinus develops after age 7.
  Causes include the following:
  - Response to a virus, bacterium, or allergen
  - Fungal infestation
  - Mechanical obstruction
  - Trauma
  - Air pollution, tobacco smoke, or low humidity
  Similar pathogens that occur in adults and children are the following:
- *Streptococcus pneumoniae* (35%) and *Haemophilus influenzae* (35%)
- *Moraxella catarrhalis* (5%), a common cause in children
- *Streptococcus pyogenes* and β-hemolytic streptococcus (10%)
- Viruses (9%)
- Chronic: mixture of aerobic and anaerobic bacteria; *S. aureus;* pathogens often opportunistic

Protective Factors

- A protective mucous blanket traps bacteria and other irritants, covers the respiratory cilia, and is most consistent along predetermined pathways to the sinus ostia.

Factors Increasing Susceptibility. Any interference with the normal cleansing of the mucosal cilia increases susceptibility. Chemotherapy and immunosuppression can interfere with the functioning of cilia.

ASSESSMENT: SUBJECTIVE/HISTORY
Symptoms

Persistent symptoms of URI for more than 10 days that have not begun to abate, including the following:

1. Acute symptoms: Nasal discharge (serous, mucous mucopurulent*), cough (in children*/in adults†), nasal obstruction/congestion*, tooth or facial pain,† pain with chewing/dental pain,† sore throat, decreased or loss of sense of smell, a metallic taste in the mouth, and headaches often worse at night and early in the morning.
2. Chronic symptoms are the same as acute sinusitis, but last longer than 30 days.
3. Children often have more nonspecific complaints than adults. Suspect sinusitis if URI symptoms persist beyond 10 days without improvement, especially with persistent cough; the child with URI seems sicker than usual with high fever and has purulent nasal drainage and periorbital swelling; the allergic child has an acute exacerbation of respiratory symptoms.

Associated Symptoms

- Early morning periorbital edema; fever;† malaise/fatigue;† increased pain while coughing, bending forward, and making sudden head movement*

NOTE: *Diagnosis of bacterial rhinosinusitis requires two or more major criteria*; or one major and two minor criteria†; or purulent rhinorrhea.*

Past Medical History

Ask about history of diabetes, asthma, or immunosuppression; a seasonal relationship with symptoms; allergies; recent nose trauma, dental work, or URI; and past sinusitis episodes and treatments.

Medication History

Inquire about recent use of antibiotics (very important in chronic sinusitis related to increased incidence of drug resistance), steroids, decongestants, nasal sprays, or antihistamines.

Family History

- Ask about a family history of asthma, allergies, and chronic sinusitis.
- For children, inquire whether a smoker resides in the household; ask about household pets.
- For adults, ask whether the client is a smoker or whether a smoker resides in the household; ask about household pets.

Dietary History

Not relevant.

ASSESSMENT: OBJECTIVE/PHYSICAL EXAMINATION
Physical Examination

A problem-oriented physical examination should be conducted, with particular attention to the following:

- Vital signs: Include temperature.
- Eyes: Look for allergic shiners or periorbital edema.
- Nasal mucosa: Assess for color, edema, and mucopurulent discharge. Look for polyps and patency of both nares. Examine structures of the nasal septum. Unilateral pain and intranasal bleeding are associated with neoplasm (Casiano, 2001).
- Ears, throat, and mouth: Look for signs of inflammation.
- Frontal and maxillary sinuses: Look for pain on percussion and inability to transilluminate. Palpate for tender, doughy swelling over forehead (subperiosteal abscess).
- Maxillary teeth: Percuss to check for a dental source of maxillary sinusitis.
- Neck and jaw: Assess for lymphadenopathy, neck rigidity.
- Neurologic: Assess for headache (possible symptom of intracranial complication).
- Heart and lungs: Auscultate.

Diagnostic Procedures

No diagnostic procedures are indicated for typical presentation. The following may be indicated in some cases:

- Sinus radiographs may be needed for refractory cases. Obtain a Waters plain radiographic view; air-fluid level or complete opacification of the sinuses and thickening of the mucosal lining are most diagnostic.
- CT scan or MRI is indicated for chronic sinusitis or symptoms of intracranial complication.
- Allergy testing may be indicated.

DIAGNOSIS

Differential diagnoses include the following:

- Rhinitis: Allergic, vasomotor, or viral
- Dental abnormality, abscesses, or periodontitis
- URI
- Cluster or migraine headaches

---

*Major criteria; †minor criteria

- Nasal polyps
- Foreign body (especially children)
- Tumor
- Temporal arteritis

THERAPEUTIC PLAN

Goals are management of infection, establishment of drainage, and relief of pain.

Nonpharmacologic Treatment

- Steam inhalation promotes nasal vasoconstriction and drainage.
- Use saline nasal washes.
- Humidify the air. Increase fluid intake.
- Apply warm compresses to the face.

Pharmacologic Treatment

- Antimicrobial agents (minimum of 2 weeks' therapy for acute sinusitis); *do not use* until symptoms have worsened and lasted more than 5 days, or have been present (without worsening) 10 or more days or if bacterial source is suspected (see Symptoms section).
- First-line antibiotics are amoxicillin-clavulanate, erythromycin-sulfisoxazole, cefuroxime, cefpodoxime proxetil, trimethoprim-sulfamethoxazole (TMP/SMX), and loracarbef.
- Second-line treatment (for use in clients who already were treated for sinusitis using first-line agents) are respiratory quinolones (moxifloxacin, levofloxacin), and macrolides for children.
- For chronic sinusitis, use the same antibiotics but extend the therapy for 3 to 4 weeks. If drug resistance is suspected, use TMP/SMX, clindamycin, ciprofloxacin, and consider combination therapy.
- Topical decongestants (Afrin or Neo-Synephrine spray) should not be used for more than 7 days (Casiano, 2001).
- Oral decongestants are used in combination with mucolytics (e.g., Humibid, Zephrex, Entex).
- Analgesics and antipyretics

Client Education

- Avoid swimming and diving during the acute phase.
- Encourage smoking cessation.
- Avoid allergens.

Referral

Ear, nose, and throat referral is indicated for recurrent sinusitis or complications of acute sinusitis.

Prevention

Do not smoke.

EVALUATION/FOLLOW-UP

- Instruct client to return if no improvement within 48 hours or swelling develops in the periorbital area.
- Schedule a return visit in 10 to 14 days.

COMPLICATIONS

- Orbital cellulitis
- Frontal subperiosteal abscess
- Epidural abscess
- Meningitis

REFERENCES

Baker, R. (1996). *Handbook of pediatric primary care.* Boston: Little, Brown.

Casiano, R. R. (2000). Treatment of acute and chronic rhinosinusitis. *Seminars in Respiratory Infection, 15,* 216.

Casiano, R. R. (2001). A rational approach to treating rhinosinusitis. *Supplement to the Clinical Advisor,* September, 17-24.

Wilder, B. (1996). Management of sinusitis. *Journal of the American Academy of Nurse Practitioner, 8*(11), 525-529.

Review Questions

1. Risk factors for the development of acute rhinosinusitis include which of the following?

   a. Family history of diabetes
   b. Recent antibiotic therapy
   c. Allergic rhinitis
   d. History of migraine headaches

Situation: A 20-year-old male college student reports having had a "cold" for 3 weeks. His symptoms are yellow nasal discharge, facial pain increased with bending over, and a low-grade fever. He has no known allergies. Family history shows a sister with asthma and a father with chronic sinusitis. Vital signs and ears are normal. Nasal mucosa are erythematous with yellow discharge. Pharynx appears benign. Sinuses are tender to percussion.

2. The NP makes a tentative diagnosis of acute sinusitis. What additional information would be helpful in confirming the diagnosis?

   a. Considering the time of the year
   b. Client's eating habits
   c. Client's smoking history
   d. Impaired light transmission of maxillary sinuses

3. Major signs and symptoms for a diagnosis of rhinosinusitis include all of the following, *except:*

   a. Purulent nasal discharge
   b. Facial pain
   c. URI symptoms lasting longer than 10 days
   d. Teary eyes

4. In addition to antibiotics, which other medications are necessary for the treatment of acute rhinosinusitis?

   a. Antifungals
   b. Antihistamines
   c. Decongestants
   d. Antihistamine-decongestant combinations

5. A client returns 1 week after being seen for sinusitis with complications of acute sinusitis. Her treatment should include which of the following?

a. Antifungal medication
b. Antihistamines
c. Eyes, ears, nose, and throat (EENT) referral
d. Nasal irrigation

6. Which of the following symptoms are more indicative of acute rhinosinusitis?

a. Maxillary sinus pain, vomiting, and diarrhea
b. Cluster headaches, clear nasal discharge, and diffuse wheezes
c. Periorbital edema, purulent nasal discharge, and cough
d. Productive cough, chest congestion, and rhonchi

7. To confirm the suspicion of rhinosinusitis in a refractory case, which of the following tests is most reliable?

a. CBC with differential
b. Sinus radiograph, Waters view
c. Sedimentation rate
d. Serum complement

8. Client education for a client with acute rhinosinusitis should include all *except* which of the following.

a. Smoking cessation
b. Warm compresses to the face
c. Humidifying the air
d. Antihistamines

Answers and Rationales

1. *Answer:* **c** (assessment)
Rationale: Allergic rhinitis is a risk factor for the development of sinusitis because it interferes with the normal cleansing of the mucosal cilia. Diabetes, recent antibiotic therapy, and migraine headaches do not affect this process.

2. *Answer:* **d** (assessment)
Rationale: Impaired light transmission of maxillary sinuses is diagnostic for maxillary sinusitis; the other choices are not.

3. *Answer:* **d** (analysis/diagnosis)
Rationale: Teary eyes are associated with allergic rhinitis.

4. *Answer:* **c** (implementation/plan)
Rationale: Decongestants are considered a necessary part of the treatment plan because they thin secretions; thus sinus drainage is enhanced. Antihistamines dry the mucous membranes and thicken the secretions, making drainage more difficult.

5. *Answer:* **c** (evaluation)
Rationale: EENT referral is indicated for complications of acute rhinosinusitis.

6. *Answer:* **c** (assessment)
Rationale: Periorbital edema, purulent nasal discharge, and cough are frequently seen in both acute and chronic sinusitis. Vomiting, diarrhea, diffuse wheezes, and rhonchi may or may not be present.

7. *Answer:* **b** (analysis/diagnosis)
Rationale: Sinus radiographs in the Waters view are specific for sinusitis.

8. *Answer:* **d** (implementation/plan)
Rationale: All are client education recommendations except for antihistamines, which dry out the mucous membranes, making secretions thicker and more difficult to drain.

SKIN CANCER AND OTHER SUN-RELATED CONDITIONS   *Pamela Kidd*

OVERVIEW
Definition

Benign or Premalignant Lesions
- Seborrheic keratosis is the proliferation of immature keratinocytes and melanocytes. They are beige, brown, or black plaques with a velvety or warty surface.
- Actinic keratosis is damage to keratinocytes caused by sunlight's ultraviolet energy. Affects dorsum of hands, forehead, scalp, nose, and ears. Lesions are rough, adherent crusts on erythematous base. One in 1000 lesions progress to become squamous cell carcinoma.
- Nevi is hyperplasia and proliferation of melanocytes located in the epidermis, dermis, and occasionally subcutaneous tissue. It may be present from birth.

Incidence
- Seborrheic keratosis affects mainly men 30 years and older.
- Actinic keratosis is common in fair-skinned persons in middle to old age.

- Nevi is more common in whites with a family history of nevi.
- Half of all new cancers are skin cancers. Both basal cell and squamous cell carcinoma have a better than 95% cure rate if detected and treated early. Melanoma is more common than any nonskin cancer among people between 25 and 29 years old. The three most common cancerous lesions are reviewed in Table 3-98.

Pathophysiology

It is not known exactly what circumstances trigger conversion of a precancerous lesion to a cancerous lesion.

Protective Factors
- Dark skin
- Youth

Factors Increasing Susceptibility for All Skin Lesions
- Working outdoors
- Frequent sun exposure without sunscreen

S

TABLE **3-98** Comparison of Cancerous Skin Lesions

TYPE	OBJECTIVE DATA
BASAL CELL CARCINOMA	
Nodule-ulcerative	Small, firm, waxy papule often with telangiectasis, may ulcerate
Superficial	Erythematous, sharply circumscribed, scaly macule or thin plaque
Morpheaform	Scarlike lesion, whitish/yellow, smooth and shiny
Pigmented	Blue, brown, or black, waxy papule
SQUAMOUS CELL CARCINOMA	
Common	Firm to hard, erythematous, scaly or ulcerated nodule
Bowen's disease/in situ	Erythematous, sharply circumscribed, scaly macule or thin plaque
MELANOMA	
Superficial, spreading	Usually brown but can be brown, black, blue, red, or white or any combination of those colors; flat papule, plaque, or macule, usually greater than 6 mm in diameter
Nodular	Symmetric, uniform papule or nodule in the colors noted immediately above
Lentigo maligna	Tan or brown with focal surface elevation usually on sun-exposed surface
Acral lentiginous	May be pigmented band in the nail fold (Hutchinson's sign) tan or brown macule similar to lentigo maligna

- History of sunburn
- High altitude (atmosphere provides less protection)

Factors Increasing Susceptibility for Skin Cancer
- Smoking
- Immunosuppression
- Industrial carcinogen exposure
- Intense, intermittent, sun exposure
- Light hair and blue eyes
- Inability to tan
- Radiation treatment

ASSESSMENT: SUBJECTIVE/HISTORY
Symptoms

Ask about duration of lesions. Lesions present since birth are usually nonmalignant. Ask about recreational hobbies that involve the outdoors and occupation with sun exposure. Ask about systemic symptoms such as fatigue and weight loss.

Noncancerous Lesions
- Clients with seborrheic keratosis: Complain of "stuck-on" brown spots over trunk that may bleed when irritated by clothing or picking.
- Clients with actinic keratosis: May seek treatment because there are multiple lesions and they are cosmetically displeasing.
- Clients with nevi: Usually seek treatment because of increasing number of nevi or change in appearance of a nevi.

Cancerous Lesions
- Clients with basal cell carcinoma: Report that lesion gets red, peels, or bleeds, then improves, only to repeat the cycle again.

- Clients with squamous cell carcinoma may complain of firm, hard, nodule.
- Clients with melanoma: Usually report change in color, size, or border of a preexisting lesion.

Past Medical History

Chronic illness or immunosuppression are relevant.

Medication History
- Use of corticosteroids
- Use of sunscreen

Family History
- Family history of melanoma is relevant.
- Familial atypical mole and melanoma syndrome (family history of melanoma in a first- or second-degree relative), multiple nevi (greater than 50), and atypical moles are relevant. These persons have a lifetime risk nearing 100% for the development of melanoma.

Dietary History

Noncontributory.

ASSESSMENT: OBJECTIVE/PHYSICAL EXAMINATION
Physical Examination
- Have client undress and inspect entire body for lesions.
- Use the ABCD approach to skin inspection:
  A = asymmetry
  B = border irregularity
  C = color varies (usually brown, tan, blue, red, black, or white)
  D = Diameter larger than 6 mm (pencil eraser)
- Use epiluminescence microscopy to magnify and illuminate lesions.

Noncancerous Lesions

- In seborrheic keratosis, size varies from 1 to 3 cm. May be skin-colored, tan, brown, or black. Usually oval with a warty, greasy feel. Distributed on face, neck, scalp, back, and upper chest.
- In actinic keratosis, there are multiple lesions, which are flat or slightly elevated, brownish or tan, scaly lesions with stuck-on appearance. May be up to 1.5 cm. Feel like sandpaper.
- Nevi are usually flat and symmetrical; brown or black in color.

Cancerous Lesions

- Basal cell carcinoma can be nodular, ulcerative, pigmented, or superficial. Usually whitish, brown, or black with ill-defined borders. Seen on face and other exposed areas. Very slow growing.
- Squamous cell carcinoma are isolated, keratotic, eroded, ulcerated lesions (papule, plaque, or nodule). Grow rapidly, with a central ulcer and an indurated, raised border on a red base.
- Melanoma is a pigmented lesion (usually brown, tan, blue, red, black, or white) that is asymmetrical with irregular borders. Frequently greater than 6 mm. There are many forms of melanoma. One form in persons of African descent results in Hutchinson's sign. This is pigment extending onto nail fold with subungual pigmented lesion. It is highly predictive of melanoma.

Diagnostic Procedures

Skin biopsy (usually performed by dermatologist) is indicated for the following symptoms:

- Asymmetry in lesions
- Appearance of a new pigmented lesion
- Irregular or notched borders
- Bleeding
- Irregular color or variegated shades
- Change in surface or elevation
- Expanding diameter
- Lesion sensitive
- When in doubt, biopsy

DIAGNOSIS

Differential diagnoses are all presented in this chapter except for warts. See previous content for discriminating information.

Warts

Warts are most common in children and young adults. Lesions disrupt normal skin lines and have a pinpoint black dot. They appear most commonly at sites of irritation and are usually skin-colored or pink and 1 mm in size.

THERAPEUTIC PLAN

Nonpharmacologic Treatment

Remove noncancerous lesions with electrocautery or liquid nitrogen. Refer all clients with cancerous lesions for removal. Photograph all lesions before they are removed. Record the date, location, name, and size of lesion and place in client record.

Pharmacologic Treatment

Sunscreens reduce local immunosuppression induced by ultraviolet radiation. People of all ages and ethnicity benefit from their use. Use sun protection factor (SPF) of at least 15 that protects against both ultraviolet A and ultraviolet B rays. Apply every hour.

Client Education

- After removal of lesions, area may be hypopigmented.
- Perform skin self-examination every month and report changes to health care provider. Encourage family member to perform inspection.
- Use sun-blocking agents with P-aminobenzoic acid.
- Wear hats.

Teach what to look for in skin lesions that indicates need to see health care provider. Client should contact the health care provider if any of the following are seen:

- Change in color
- Change in size
- Change in shape
- Change in elevation
- Change in surface
- Change in surrounding skin
- Change in sensation (itching, tenderness, pain)
- Change in consistency (softening, friability)

Referral/Consultation

Referral to dermatologist for removal of lesions and for biopsy.

Prevention

- Decrease sun exposure.
- Change clothing apparel. Cover body with cotton clothing.
- Do not tan.

EVALUATION/FOLLOW-UP

For actinic keratosis, have skin checked by provider every 6 months because new lesions frequently occur.

COMPLICATIONS

- Development of skin cancer
- Metastasis and death

REFERENCES

Berger, T. (2001). Skin, hair, and nails. In L. Tierney, S. McPhee, & M. Papadakis (Eds.), *Current medical diagnosis and treatment* (40th ed.). New York: McGraw-Hill.

Boynton, R., Dunn, E., & Stephens, G. (1998). *Manual of ambulatory pediatrics* (4th ed.). Philadelphia: Lippincott.

Butler, J. (1997). Playing detective: Assessing skin lesions in primary care. *Advanced Nurse Practitioner, 5*(8), 41-43.

S

Epstein, J., Kaplan, L., & Levine, N. (2000). The value of sunscreens. *Patient Care Nurse Practitioner, 3*(6), 17-18, 24, 28-30.

Kidd, P. (2000). Skin cancer and other sun-related conditions. In D. Robinson, P. Kidd, & K. Rogers (Eds.), *Primary care across the lifespan.* St. Louis: Mosby.

Review Questions

1. Which of the following in a client's history places the client most at risk for melanoma?

   a. Gender
   b. Age
   c. White ethnicity
   d. Intense intermittent sun exposure

2. When removing a lesion for biopsy purposes, which technique should be used?

   a. Electrocautery
   b. Liquid nitrogen
   c. Laser
   d. Knife or scalpel excision

3. When distinguishing between basal cell and squamous cell carcinoma, the NP should focus on which of the following?

   a. Texture of the lesion
   b. Color of the lesion
   c. Borders of the lesion
   d. Location of the lesion

4. A client who had an actinic keratosis lesion removed returns with hypopigmentation at the site. The NP recognizes this as which of the following?

   a. Normal
   b. Fungal infection
   c. Precancerous area
   d. Secondary bacterial infection

Answers and Rationales

1. *Answer:* **d** (assessment)
   Rationale: Males in the 30- to 50-year-old range are most at risk for all sun-related skin conditions. Whites are also at higher risk. However, intense intermittent sun exposure is associated with melanoma.

2. *Answer:* **d** (assessment)
   Rationale: Accompanying skin should be included with excision for biopsy purposes. The other techniques destroy the histologic composition of the tissue.

3. *Answer:* **c** (analysis/diagnosis)
   Rationale: Both may be firm nodules and vary in color. Both may develop anywhere on the body. However, basal cell lesions tend to have a cycle of bleeding, peeling, and improvement with the borders ill defined. Squamous cell lesions have an indurated, raised border on a red base.

4. *Answer:* **a** (evaluation)
   Rationale: Hypopigmentation occurs frequently after removal.

SLEEP DISORDERS   *Pamela Kidd*

OVERVIEW
Definition

- Sleep disorders include a variety of disorders that interfere with the quality and quantity of sleep. Common sleep problems include insomnia (restless legs syndrome [RLS], periodic leg movements in sleep [PLMS], chronobiologic disorders); hypersomnias (narcolepsy, sleep apnea); and parasomnias (sleepwalking, nightmares). The average adult needs 6 to 9 hours of sleep per night.
- Insomnia is defined as "involuntary sleeplessness severe enough to interfere with daytime alertness and energy level." Insomnia is classified as primary (no apparent cause) or secondary (identifiable cause). It may also be classified as transient (only a few nights), short term (lasting up to 3 weeks), and long term (lasting longer than 3 weeks).

Incidence

One of three Americans has difficulty sleeping over the course of a year, and more than 50 million people have some type of sleeping disorder. Approximately one half of all elderly persons aged 65 and older experience insomnia. Insomnia is the most frequent sleep complaint. Women older than age 40 are more likely to complain of difficulty sleeping.

Pathophysiology

- The average newborn sleeps 18 hours a day, with a high proportion of REM sleep. Circadian patterns do not develop for at least several weeks or months. Sleep continues to be polyphasic, with daytime naps, until the child is 5 or 6. The amount of sleep decreases with age; the quality and quantity of sleep drops sharply with puberty. The elderly tend to sleep less, usually an average of 6.5 hours. The sleep tends to be lighter, with more arousals and near disappearance of slow wave sleep. Sleep onset and final awakening come earlier. Severe insomnia also increases with age, and excessive daytime sleepiness is also increased. Sleep apnea and PLMS occur frequently in the elderly, disturbing nighttime sleep.
- The sleep-wake cycle is controlled by the circadian rhythm located in the hypothalamus. Two of the neurotransmitters associated with sleep are serotonin and gamma-aminobutyric acid.

- A normal sleep cycle is a complex electrophysiologic process consisting of alternating periods of wakefulness, REM sleep, and non–rapid eye movement (NREM) sleep. A sleep cycle consists of two different types of sleep:
  - REM sleep
  - NREM sleep
- Growth hormone is secreted during NREM sleep.
- The immune system is more active during NREM sleep.

Protective Factors. Regular exercise.

Factors Increasing Susceptibility
- Previous history of sleep disorders
- Diagnosis of psychiatric disorder
- Anxiety
- Depression
- Alcohol and drug use
- Tobacco use
- Pain and discomfort
- Orthopnea
- Nocturia
- Gastroesophageal reflux disease (GERD)
- Asthma
- Fibromyalgia

ASSESSMENT: SUBJECTIVE/HISTORY
Symptoms
Clients may complaint of the following:
- Difficulty falling asleep
- Awakening in the middle of the night
- Awakening early in the morning
- Symptoms associated with sleepiness
- Fatigue
- Irritability
- Decreased concentration
- Anxiety
- Depression

Ask about the following:
- How long has the insomnia been happening?
- How long does it take you to fall asleep once you go to bed?
- Do you remain asleep all night?
- How much sleep do you get?
- How sleepy are you during the day?
- Do you feel well-rested in the morning?
- What type of bedtime routine do you have?
- Do you exercise before bedtime?
- Do you use tobacco?
- Ask about substance abuse or dependence.

Ask about recent stressors that may interfere with sleep, including the following:
- Cold, noise, new baby, pain
- Travel across time zones
- Occupation: shift work

Past Medical History
Ask about the following:
- History of psychiatric disorders: anxiety, depression
- Thyroid disorders
- Renal disorders
- GERD
- Orthopnea
- Nocturia
- Fibromyalgia
- Chronic obstructive pulmonary disease
- Arthritic disorders
- Neurologic disorders: Parkinson's disease, past head trauma, CVA

Medication History
Ask about the use of the following:
- Melatonin
- Sleep aids
- Cold and allergy medications
- Nicotine
- Prescription drugs that may cause insomnia
- Anti-Parkinson's: amantadine, diphenhydramine, pergolide
- Cardiovascular: beta-blockers, calcium channel blocking agents
- Conjugated estrogens
- Nonsteroidal antiinflammatory drugs (NSAIDs)
- Psychotropics: alprazolam (Xanax), clozapine (Klonopin), fluoxetine (Prozac)
- Muscle relaxants: cyclobenzaprine (Flexeril)
- Beta-adrenergics: aminophylline, theophylline, metaproterenol sulfate (Alupent)
- Diuretics: if they cause nocturia

Family History
- Ask about family history of sleep disorders.
- Ask about family history of RLS or PLMS.

Dietary History
- Caffeine (3- to 7-hour half-life)
- Alcohol use

ASSESSMENT: OBJECTIVE/PHYSICAL EXAMINATION
Physical Examination
- Rule out physical or organic causes of insomnia.
- Assess vital signs.
- Assess general appearance.
- Assess head, eyes, ears, nose, and throat (HEENT), including presence of nasal stuffiness and post nasal drip.
- Assess lungs for wheezing and shortness of breath.
- Do a baseline assessment of the cardiovascular system.
- Assess abdomen for urinary tract infection (UTI); assess for costovertebral angle tenderness and suprapubic tenderness.

Diagnostic Procedures

- CBC, arterial blood gases, comprehensive metabolic panel, urinalysis, thyroid-stimulating hormone levels, iron levels, B_{12} levels, and Holter ECG can help rule out endocrine, renal, or cardiac disorders that may precipitate sleeping disorders.
- See Table 3-99 for sleep related diagnostic procedures.

DIAGNOSIS

See Table 3-100 for differential diagnosis.

THERAPEUTIC PLAN

Nonpharmacologic Treatment

- The plan should identify specific short-term goals, such as the following:
  - Shorter sleep latency
  - Delayed morning wake-up
  - Fewer nocturnal awakenings
- Advise the following sleep hygiene measures:
  - Maintain a regular wake/sleep schedule.
  - Bedtime routine (e.g., bathing, storytelling, and rocking) can facilitate a winding down process.
  - Exercise daily but not within 3 hours of bedtime.
  - Do not nap during the day.
  - Do not use the bed for anything other than sleep and sex.
  - No caffeine (after 12 noon), and limit to two cups per day, no alcohol (in the evening), or nicotine (before bedtime) (Elliott, 2001).
- Cognitive therapy involves teaching techniques to reduce anxiety and initiate behavioral changes to improve sleep hygiene. Examples include the following:
  - Talking about the frustration of not falling asleep: Bed restriction (out of bed if awake for more than 30 minutes). No reading, eating, or watching TV in bed.
  - Education about sleep and daytime napping (okay if midday and less than 1 hour); no caffeine, alcohol, or nicotine late in the day.
  - Reframe concept of poor sleep in a positive manner: bright light exposure (especially in morning),

and exercise in the afternoon (Singer & Sack, 1997).
  - Biofeedback, muscle relaxation techniques, and breathing exercises may be helpful as an adjunct to treatment.
- Chronobiologic treatment: Use of bright natural or artificial light should be carefully timed so the circadian rhythm is phase shifted to move sleep propensity to a later time. The client needs to rise early to receive light therapy.
- Stimulus-control therapy is based on the premise that there is a conditioned response to environmental cues.
  - Get out of bed if unable to go to sleep within 30 minutes. Do not go or return to bed until sleepy.
  - Get out of bed at the same time each day.
  - Do not watch TV, read, work, or eat in bed.
- Relaxation therapy is based on using meditation, imagery, and progressive muscle relaxation.
- Sleep restriction therapy focuses on decreasing the amount of time spent in bed.
  - Go to bed much later than usual.
  - Stay in bed only as long as you are sleeping.
  - Rise at the same time each day.
  - Increase the time spent in bed by 15 minutes a week at the start of bedtime.
  - A sleep debt occurs to encourage falling and staying asleep.
- Snoring: Losing weight, avoiding sedating medications or alcohol, and using appliances to avoid sleeping on back (e.g., sew tennis ball to the back of the nightshirt) may decrease snoring. Surgery may be considered as an option. Polysomnographic evaluation should be done before surgery.
- Sleep terrors: Reassure the parents. In persistent sleep terrors, medication may be justified.

Pharmacologic Treatment

- Barbiturates are not recommended because they decrease REM sleep and may cause an REM rebound effect.

TABLE **3-99** Sleep-Related Diagnostic Procedures

DIAGNOSTIC TEST	FINDING/RATIONALE
Sleep diary	Keep a sleep diary for 2 weeks: document sleep onset and wake times, rating sleep quality and daytime fatigue and sleepiness.
EEG	Identifies the changes specific to psychiatric problems, as well as identification of the stages of sleep.
EMG	Test that records the state of the muscle contraction when the muscle is stimulated.
EOG	Helps correlate brain waves with eye movements.
PSG	All-night sleep study: Test that includes EEG, EOG, EMG of submental and anterior tibialis muscles, respiratory muscles, nasal airflow, ear oximetry, and ECG. Not helpful in most cases, except for refractory insomnia.
Sleep study	Records respiratory effort, heart rate, ECG, O_2 saturation.

ECG, Electrocardiogram; *EEG,* electroencephalogram; *EMG,* electromyogram; *EOG,* electrooculogram; *PSG,* polysomnograph.

TABLE **3-100** Differential Diagnoses of Sleep Disorders

DIAGNOSIS	DATA SUPPORT
Anxiety	25% of people with chronic insomnia have an anxiety disorder. The client complains of difficulty falling asleep and staying asleep.
Depression	90% of all clients who have depression complain of insomnia. EEG reflects a sleep disturbance.
Chronic insomnia	Diagnosis of exclusion; it may develop after a period of sleep disruption. Sometimes it continues after the cause disappears. Long-term sedatives may cause chronic insomnia.
RLS	An irresistible need to move, stretch, or rub the lower extremities. Creepy-crawly sensations are sometime described. Periodic limb movements are also present, which can lead to further sleep disturbances. This syndrome affects approximately 5% of the population. It sometimes appears in females during pregnancy, but can run in families, and tends to worsen with age.
PLMS	These are repetitive myoclonic movements of the lower extremities that come in bursts lasting from a few seconds to minutes; they usually occur in the first half of the night. These movements are associated with brief arousals, leading to nonrestorative sleep and daytime sleepiness. The prevalence increases with age: 5% in those age 30 to 50, and up to 44% in those older than age 65. These are not the same as nocturnal leg cramps. Best documented by PSG. A PLMS index of more than five muscle jerks an hour is considered positive.
Alcohol and drugs	Alcohol causes decreased alertness, but it also suppresses slow-wave sleep, making sleep lighter. Alcohol also tends to produce a rebound arousal effect in the second half of the night, thus producing less sleep overall. Amphetamines and cocaine also cause a decrease in sleep.
Medical disorders	Pain, rheumatic disorders, neuromuscular disease, cardiac disease, pulmonary disease, dyspepsia, IBD, and nocturia are all causes of insomnia. Fibromyalgia is another disorder that interferes with normal sleep patterns.
Neurodegenerative diseases	AD and PD cause an interference with day/night differences. Akinesia in PD may cause physical discomfort, and the medication can cause arousal.
Snoring	Snoring may signify obstruction of the airway. Occurs in males more than females, although more snoring is seen in postmenopausal females. Obesity, supine positions, alcohol, smoking, and possibly genetic factors may increase snoring.
Sleep apnea	OSA is a major cause of CV morbidity and daytime sleepiness. OSA includes a wide range of upper airway narrowing. Approximately 2% of women and 4% of men have OSA in midlife. Symptoms include loud snoring that gets worse with age and increased weight, snorting and gagging sounds, night sweats, abrupt awakenings with a feeling of choking, and profound sleep disruption (Singer & Sack, 1997). PSG confirms the diagnosis. Surgical uvuloplasty, tracheostomy, CPAP, and dental appliances are options for treatment.
Sleep terrors	These occur in children, usually ages 3 to 6, when they awaken with a scream, appear terrified, heart racing, sweating. They may last from a few minutes to 30 minutes. Attempts to comfort the child usually do not work and finally the child goes back to a quiet sleep. In the morning, the child does not remember the episode. Sleep terrors involve a partial arousal from Stage IV (deep sleep).
Nightmares	True nightmares occur in REM sleep. They are usually transient problems, generally triggered by personal events. Persistent nightmares may indicate a mental health problem and warrant referral to a mental health specialist.
Sleepwalking	Occurs during stage IV (deep sleep). Occasional sleep walking is common in children and may follow a personal stressor.

AD, Alzheimer's disease; *CPAP,* continuous positive airway pressure; *CV,* cardiovascular; *EEG,* electroencephalogram; *IBD,* irritable bowel disease; *OSA,* obstructive sleep apnea; *PD,* Parkinson's disease; *PLMS,* periodic leg movements in sleep; *PSG,* polysomnograph; *RLS,* restless leg syndrome.

- In short-term insomnia, short-term therapy with benzodiazepines should be used in conjunction with a sleep-hygiene program. See Table 3-101.
- For RLS, stretching before bedtime, opioids, L-dopa, and sedative-hypnotics may be helpful. There is a national support group for this disorder.
- For PLMS, benzodiazepines may be helpful in increasing the sleep continuity but do not reduce the number of leg movements. Opioids work well but should be reserved for those with severe symptoms.

Client Education

- The concern in sleepwalking is accidental injury. Protective measures should be taken, including installing gates in front of stairwells, keeping windows shut and locked, and so on.

- Flexibility and compromise is necessary with teenagers. Advise about adding naps, avoiding driving while sleepy, and avoiding working late at night while in school.
- Avoid caffeine, alcohol, and excessive time in bed while awake.
- Use of a "white noise" machine may help block out environmental noises.
- For those with delayed sleep phase, avoid late-night activity.
- Any foods or drinks that seem to intensify insomnia or interfere with sleep should be avoided.
- Sugary snacks and heavy meals late in the evening may stimulate metabolism, making it difficult to fall asleep or sleep restfully.
- Caution client about drinking alcohol with benzodiazepines. Mixing them can cause death.

TABLE **3-101**   Pharmacologic Treatment of Sleep Disorders

DRUG	DOSE	COMMENTS
BENZODIAZEPINES		Alter sleep structure, reducing REM and slow-wave sleep. Generally safe for younger adults. Use for short-term treatment of insomnia. **Clients with sleep apnea, severe respiratory problems, or alcohol abuse should not be given these drugs.** Pregnancy: X
Temazepam (Restoril)	7.5 mg to 30 mg at bedtime Elderly 7.5 mg	
Estazolam (ProSom)	Maximum treatment of 1 month Initially 1 mg at bedtime May increase to 2 mg at bedtime	Side Effects: abuse potential, CNS depression, somnolence, dizziness, confusion, anxiety, paradoxical excitement
Zolpidem (Ambien)	5 to 10 mg hs	Short half-life (1.4 to 3.8 hours). Preserves normal sleep architecture. Recommend getting into bed quickly because of swift onset. Pregnancy: B Side Effects: dizziness, daytime fatigue, diarrhea, drugged feelings, amnesia
Zaleplon	10 mg adult, 5 mg elderly hs	Best for difficulty falling asleep because of short half-life
SEDATING ANTIDEPRESSANTS		Some feel that these drugs are better choices for long-term treatment, although this has not been studied. Less impairment of nighttime breathing and slow-wave sleep. Use special care in elderly.
Trazodone (Desyrel)	50 to 150 mg hs	
Nefazodone (Serzone)	200 mg in divided doses	
Doxepin (Sinequan)	75 mg at hs	
Amitriptyline (Elavil)	50 to 100 mg at hs	Pregnancy: C Side Effects: nausea, insomnia, dizziness, constipation, blurred vision confusion
Diphendydramine (Benadryl)	25 to 50 mg hs	Generally safe and effective for short-term use. Tolerance develops quickly. Caution: anticholinergic effects.
Valerian root	400 to 900 mg 30 to 60 minutes before going to bed	Efficacy and safety not established.
Melatonin	0.5 mg is a reasonable starting dose	Has sleep-promoting effects in many people. Considered an experimental drug. Greater than 0.5 mg produces plasma levels greater than occurs naturally. Avoid "pineal extracts." Use synthetic melatonin. This may be helpful in cases of chronobiological disorders (e.g., jet lag). A person with delayed sleep phase may take melatonin early in the evening (8 to 9 P.M.) hours before endogenous melatonin is secreted, to reset the body clock to an earlier time.

CNS, Central nervous system; *REM,* rapid eye movement.

Referral/Consultation

- Any client with refractory insomnia should be referred to a sleep disorder center.
- Physician consultation may be appropriate before ordering expensive sleep tests or to order controlled substances.

Prevention

Eating a small protein meal 1 hour before bedtime may assist sleep in elderly (Shuler, Huebscher, & Hallock, 2001).

EVALUATION/FOLLOW-UP

- Re-evaluate clients who have been taking benzodiazepines for 2 to 3 weeks.
- Re-evaluate the client if insomnia continues for more than 3 weeks.

COMPLICATIONS

- Depression or anxiety
- Mood disorder
- Alcohol abuse
- Motor vehicle crash secondary to sleepiness

REFERENCES

Cupp, M. (1997). Melatonin. *American Family Physician, 56*(5), 1421-1425.

Elliott, A. C. (2001). Primary care assessment and management of sleep disorders. *Journal of the American Academy of Nurse Practitioners, 13*(9), 409-417.

Ellsworth, A., Witt, D., Dugdale, D., Oliver, L. (1998). *Mosby's 1998 medical drug reference.* St. Louis: Mosby.

Healthcare Consultants of America. (1998). *1998 physicians fee and coding guide.* Augusta, GA: HCA.

Insomnia: What to do when you can't get a good night's sleep. *Mayo Clinic Health Letter, 16*(4), 1-3.

Kirkwood, C. K. (2001). *Treatment of insomnia. Continuing education program # 424-000-01-010-H01.* New York: Power-Pak C.E. (1998).

Mosier, W., Nelson, S., & Walgren, K. (1998). Wanted: A good night's sleep. *Advanced Nurse Practitioner, 6*(5), 30-35.

Phillips, B., Amstead, M., & Gottlieb, D. (1998). Monitoring sleep and breathing: Part I, monitoring breathing. *Clinical Chest Medicine, 19*(1), 203-212.

Riedel, B., & Lichstein, K. (1998). Objective sleep measures and subjective sleep satisfaction: How do older adults with insomnia define a good night's sleep? *Psychology of Aging,* 13(1), 159-163.

Sack, R., Lewy, A., & Hughes, R. (1998). Use of melatonin for sleep and circadian rhythm disorders. *Annals of Medicine, 30*(1), 115-121.

Sahelian, R. (1998). Use of melatonin for insomnia. *American Family Physician, 57*(8), 1783.

Shuler, P., Huebscher, R., & Hallock, J. (2001). Providing wholistic care for the elderly: Utilization of the Shuler Nurse Practitioner Practice Model. *Journal of the American Academy of Nurse Practitioners, 13*(7), 297-303.

Singer, C., & Sack, R. (1997). Sleep disorders. In M. Feldman & J. Christensen (Eds.), *Behavioral medicine in primary care.* Stamford, CT: Appleton & Lange, 237-246.

Wilson, K., Watson, S., & Currie, S. (1998). Daily diary and ambulatory activity monitoring of sleep in patients with insomnia associated with chronic musculoskeletal pain. *Pain, 75*(1), 75-84.

Review Questions

1. Symptoms of sleepiness may include all *except* which of the following?
- **a.** Weakness
- **b.** Irritability
- **c.** Depression
- **d.** Anxiety

2. Which of the following differential diagnoses would be appropriate for a client whose chief compliant is difficulty staying asleep?
- **a.** Primary insomnia
- **b.** Hypothyroidism
- **c.** Chronic fatigue
- **d.** Narcolepsy

3. All of the following differential diagnoses would be considered in a client who has fatigue and sleepiness during the day, *except:*
- **a.** Primary insomnia
- **b.** Hyperthyroidism
- **c.** Secondary insomnia
- **d.** Chronic fatigue

4. Which of the following indicates adequate education of a client with a sleep disorder?
- **a.** "I will not drink coffee after 12 noon."
- **b.** "I will not drink coffee after 5 P.M."
- **c.** "I will limit my coffee intake to three cups per day."
- **d.** "I will drink coffee in bed."

5. Which of the following applies to short-acting barbiturates?
- **a.** Used to treat PLMS.
- **b.** May cause REM rebound effect.
- **c.** Cause major daytime drowsiness.
- **d.** Contraindicated in sleep disorders.

6. Which of the following is *not* true of behavioral sleep therapies?
- **a.** Cognitive therapy uses relaxation techniques.
- **b.** Stimulus control therapy is based on the idea that sleep disorders may be a conditioned response to an environmental cue.
- **c.** Relaxation therapy uses meditation and imagery to promote rest.
- **d.** Sleep restriction therapy decreases the amount of time spent in bed.

Answers and Rationales

1. ***Answer:*** a (assessment)
 Rationale: Weakness is a neuromuscular-related symptom that is not related to sleep disorders.

S

2. *Answer:* **a** (analysis/diagnosis)
Rationale: Hypothyroidism, chronic fatigue, and narcolepsy are associated with excessive sleep.

3. *Answer:* **b** (analysis/diagnosis)
Rationale: Hyperthyroidism produces hyperactivity and lack of sleepiness.

4. *Answer:* **a** (evaluation)
Rationale: Coffee has a half-life of 3 to 7 hours, so it should not be drunk after 12 noon. Drinking any beverage in bed promotes poor sleep hygiene.

5. *Answer:* **b** (implementation/plan)
Rationale: Barbiturates are short acting and do not cause daytime sleepiness. Benzodiazepines increase sleep continuity and are used in treating PLMS.

6. *Answer:* **a** (analysis/diagnosis)
Rationale: Cognitive therapies reduce anxiety and help initiate behavior change through talking about the condition, learning more about treatment of the problem, and reframing the problem in a positive manner.

SPRAINS, STRAINS, AND FRACTURES *Denise Robinson*

OVERVIEW
Definition

An injury to one of the ligamentous structures of the body is termed a *sprain*. A *strain* is trauma to a muscle or musculoskeletal unit of the body from an excessive forcible stretch. Loss in continuity in the substance of the bone is called a *fracture*.

Pathophysiology

- Fractures are classified as either open or closed. Open fractures are exposed to the external environment and are highly prone to serious infection. Description of a fracture includes the anatomic location and degree of displacement, rotation, translation, or shortening. Fractures into the joint are called *intraarticular fractures*. Fracture patterns are described as transverse, oblique, spiral, comminuted, or greenstick. The Salter-Harris classification is commonly used to describe growth plate fractures in children.
- Sprains involve ligaments, which connect bones together and can sustain injuries. Ligamentous injuries are classified as first degree, second degree, or third degree, depending on the extent of injury. A completely torn ligament is classified as a third-degree sprain, whereas a mildly stretched ligament is classified as a first-degree sprain.

Common Injuries/Fractures

- Elbow: Radial head subluxation (nursemaid's elbow) is a dislocation of the radial head in which the head becomes caught beneath the annular ligament. Lateral epicondylitis (tennis elbow) is a tendinitis at origins of the wrist extensors that originate at the lateral epicondyle of the humerus.
- Wrist: Colles' fracture is a fracture of the distal radius and is the most common type of adult wrist fracture. Scaphoid fractures are common carpal bone fractures because of the scaphoid bone's anatomic location spanning both rows of carpal bones.

- Hand: Ulnar collateral ligament injury of the metacarpophalangeal (MCP) joint (gamekeeper's thumb or skier's thumb) is caused by a forced hyperabduction of the thumb. Boxer's fracture is a fifth metacarpal fracture.
- Fingers: Mallet finger is a flexion deformity of the distal interphalangeal joint of the finger. Distal phalanx fractures are fractures of the distal tip of the fingers.
- Knee: See "Knee Injuries."
- Ankle: Ankle sprains are most commonly caused by inversion of the ankle, resulting in injury to one or more of the lateral ankle ligaments (anterior talofibular ligament, calcaneofibular ligament, and posterior talofibular ligament). Eversion ankle injuries commonly injure the deltoid ligament of the medial ankle. Ankle fractures involve either the medial malleolus, the lateral malleolus, or both.
- Foot: A fracture of the fifth metatarsal (Jones fracture) frequently occurs with ankle sprains.
- Toes: Toe fractures occur from direct trauma.

ASSESSMENT: SUBJECTIVE/HISTORY
History of Present Illness

- Exact mechanism of injury
- Timing of injury
- Description/location of pain
- Radiation
- Quality
- Timing
- Severity
- Aggravation and relief
- Previous treatment

Symptoms

- Swelling
- Deformity
- Masses
- Paralysis
- Gait changes

Past Medical History

- Previous injuries
- Surgery
- Exercise
- Allergies

Medication History

Ask about recent or present use of pain medications, NSAIDs, and other medications.

Family History

Inquire about orthopedic problems.

Psychosocial History

- Occupational job description
- Smoking
- Alcohol intake
- Conditioning

History of Common Injuries and Fractures

- Elbow: Nursemaid's elbow commonly occurs in children 1 to 3 years of age as they are being pulled up by an extended arm. Tennis elbow results after repetitive wrist and elbow activity in persons with limited conditioning.
- Wrist: Colles' fracture is associated with a fall on an outstretched hand. Scaphoid fractures are usually seen in young adults who have sustained a fall on an outstretched hand.
- Hand: Gamekeeper's thumb or skier's thumb includes a history of forced hyperabduction of the thumb, such as when skiers fall while holding onto ski poles. Boxer's fracture is associated with a forceful punch with a closed fist.
- Fingers: Mallet finger is usually caused by a jamming injury of the finger or a forced flexion of the distal phalanx. Distal phalanx fractures are frequently associated with crush injuries.
- Knee: Meniscus injuries occur in all age groups and are often associated with athletic activity in which a hyperextension, hyperflexion, or rotational injury occurs. Collateral ligament injuries occur as a result of varus or valgus stress to the knee. Anterior cruciate ligament (ACL) injuries occur with twisting motion, a quick stop, or a hyperextension. ACL injuries are also associated with an audible pop. Posterior cruciate ligament (PCL) injuries are associated with a direct blow to the anterior portion of the tibia (see "Knee Injuries" for more detail).
- Ankle: Ankle sprains usually result from an inversion injury in which the lateral ligaments of the ankle are damaged. Ankle fractures may occur as a result of inversion or eversion injuries.
- Foot: Jones fracture usually occurs as a result of an inversion injury of the foot and often accompanies an ankle sprain.

- Toes: Toe fractures usually occur from direct trauma such as stubbing or secondary to an object striking the toe.

ASSESSMENT: OBJECTIVE/PHYSICAL EXAMINATION
Physical Examination

- A problem-oriented physical examination should be conducted, with particular attention to vital signs, general assessment, musculoskeletal area of complaint, adjacent musculoskeletal areas, and neurovascular status distal to the injury.
- Vital signs should be relatively normal with common, non-life-threatening injuries.
- General assessment should note the client's response to pain, gait, and how the client holds the injured extremity.
- Musculoskeletal assessment should include observation for swelling and effusion, palpation of adjacent and actual areas of injury, evaluation of ROM, and special physical testing to diagnose specific conditions.
- Neurovascular assessment should be performed distal to the injury. Check pulses, sensation, and capillary refill.

Specific Physical Findings of Common Injuries and Fractures

- Elbow: Nursemaid's elbow is characterized by a child holding the affected arm limply in adduction, pain elicited with palpation of the radial head, and resistance to ROM. Tennis elbow is characterized by pain over the lateral epicondyle aggravated with resisted finger and wrist extension.
- Wrist: Colles' fracture is characterized by the classic "dinner fork" appearance, with considerable pain and resistance to ROM with palpation. Concomitant median nerve injury commonly occurs with Colles' fracture; numbness and tingling of the thumb, index and long fingers, and radial half of the ring fingers should be noted. Scaphoid fractures are characterized by wrist pain localized to the snuffbox area with palpation.
- Hand: Gamekeeper's thumb or skier's thumb is characterized by a painful ulnar aspect of the MCP joint of the thumb, with a possible abnormal opening of the MCP joint with stress. Boxer's fractures demonstrate swelling along the dorsum of the hand, with pain elicited on palpation of the fifth metatarsal. Commonly, a malrotation of the involved digit also exists.
- Fingers: Mallet finger is a flexion deformity of the distal phalanx and inability to actively extend the distal interphalangeal joint. Distal phalanx fractures are often associated with crush injuries and therefore are associated with lacerations, contusions, and subungual hematoma.

- Knee: Meniscus injuries are characterized by mild swelling, joint line tenderness, and positive results from a McMurray's test. Medial collateral ligament (MCL) injuries are associated with joint line pain, mild swelling, joint effusion, pain, or laxity with valgus stress. Lateral cruciate ligament (LCL) injuries include joint line pain, swelling or effusion, and pain or laxity with varus stress. ACL injuries frequently include a joint effusion with a positive anterior drawer sign or positive Lachman's sign. PCL injuries are associated with minimal swelling but a positive posterior drawer sign or a positive sag sign of Godfrey.
- Ankle: Ankle sprains include mild-to-severe swelling over the area involved, with mild-to-severe pain over the lateral ligaments and lateral malleolus. Inversion ankle sprains are often difficult to differentiate from distal fibular avulsion fractures because both have similar physical findings. Include palpation of the distal tibia, fibula, all ankle ligaments, and the fifth metatarsal base. Joint laxity reveals a positive anterior drawer sign and indicates a significant ligamentous injury.
- Foot: Jones fracture is associated with a painful, swollen lateral foot with pain elicited on palpation of the fifth metatarsal.
- Toes: Toe fractures are swollen, contused, and painful with palpation.

Diagnostic Procedures

Consider x-ray examinations with significant pain, swelling, effusion, or contusion.

Radiographic Findings of Common Injuries and Fractures

- Elbow: Nursemaid's elbow and tennis elbow show no specific radiographic findings.
- Wrist: Colles' fractures reveal a fractured distal radius with a dorsally angulated distal fragment. Scaphoid fractures typically do not show up on initial x-ray examination but may be evident on follow-up x-ray examination 7 to 10 days after injury.
- Hand: Gamekeeper's thumb or skier's thumb usually demonstrates normal findings on radiograph, but occasionally an avulsion fracture of the ulnar aspect of the distal thumb metacarpal exists. Boxer's fractures reveal a fracture of the fifth metatarsal, which frequently is medially angulated.
- Fingers: Finger fractures may reveal crush injuries to the distal phalanx; transverse or spiral fractures of the phalanges may be present. Intraarticular fractures must be referred to an orthopedic surgeon.
- Knee: Soft tissue injuries (ACL, MCL, PCL, LCL, and meniscus injuries) usually reveal normal findings on radiographs, with the exception of a visible joint effusion or soft tissue swelling. Occasionally a ligament rupture reveals a small avulsion fracture.
- Ankle: Ankle sprains usually reveal normal findings on radiographs with soft tissue swelling, but can include avulsion fractures of the distal fibula or tibia. Ankle fractures may reveal malleolar fractures of the tibia or fibula or bimalleolar fracture of both the tibia and fibula. Trimalleolar fractures reveal a bimalleolar fracture and a fracture of the posterior tibial malleolus.
- Foot: Jones fractures reveal a fracture to the fifth metatarsal.
- Toes: Toe fractures are usually obvious on x-ray film.

DIAGNOSIS

The differential diagnoses include the following:

- Sprain
- Strain
- Fracture
- Tendinitis
- Osteoarthritis
- RA
- Cellulitis
- Gout
- Gonococcal arthritis
- Tumors
- Degenerative changes
- Congenital disorders
- Overuse syndromes
- Infections
- Bursitis
- Plantar fascitis

THERAPEUTIC PLAN

Nonpharmacologic Treatment

RICE

- **R**est any injured part of the musculoskeletal system. Rest time varies according to the seriousness of the injury.
- **I**ce all musculoskeletal injuries in an attempt to control swelling. Continue ice application as long as swelling exists. Ice can be applied for 15 minutes at a time.
- **C**ompression controls edema and provides comfort and support. Compression can be accomplished with elastic bandages, neoprene braces, custom-made splints, and commercially made splints.
- **E**levate all injured extremities. Upper extremities should be elevated with a sling.

Joint Protection/Immobilization

- The injured joint should be protected with application of a splint.
- Splinting allows for postinjury swelling.
- Never apply a circumferential cast to an acutely injured extremity.
- Use crutches for lower extremity injuries.
- Many splints are commercially made; easy-to-apply custom-made splinting material includes plaster and fiberglass.
- Immobilization also assists in pain control.

Splints for Particular Injuries

- Volar cock-up: wrist sprains, Colles' fractures
- Sugar tong upper extremity: Colles' fracture, forearm fractures
- Posterior splint upper extremity: radial head fractures, fractures about the elbow and forearm
- Thumb spica: gamekeeper's thumb or skier's thumb, scaphoid fractures
- Ulnar gutter: boxer's fractures
- Metal finger splint: finger sprains
- Stax splint: mallet finger
- Knee immobilizer: knee injuries
- Bimalleolar splint: ankle sprains
- Posterior splint lower extremity: ankle sprains, Jones fracture, foot fractures, fractures of the lateral or medial malleolus
- Posterior splint with stirrups: severe ankle sprains, malleolus fractures, foot fractures

Pharmacologic Treatment

- Antiinflammatory drugs and muscle relaxants are the drugs of choice for musculoskeletal injury.
- NSAIDs are indicated for musculoskeletal injury. NSAIDs inhibit prostaglandin synthesis, which decreases pain. Common NSAIDs include ibuprofen (Motrin), naproxen (Naprosyn), etodolac (Lodine), and diclofenac (Voltaren). Do not prescribe NSAIDs to clients with peptic ulcer disease, allergy to NSAIDs or aspirin, renal dysfunction, or pregnancy.
- Myorelaxants are indicated for pain related to muscle spasm. Common muscle relaxants include cyclobenzaprine (Flexeril) and chlorzoxazone (Parafon Forte). Muscle relaxants should be prescribed for short periods of time (3 to 5 days).
- Over-the-counter (OTC) analgesics such as acetaminophen are for less severe pain and for clients who are unable to take NSAIDs.
- Narcotic analgesics are indicated only for fractures with severe pain and should be given for several days only.

Client Education

- RICE: Emphasize the importance of rest, ice application, use of splints or elastic bandage wraps, and elevation. These measures tend to decrease swelling and help control pain.
- Pathophysiologic condition: Explain injury pathophysiologic condition with expected outcomes.
- Cast and splint care: Give detailed information concerning splint care, including bathing instructions, removal and application instructions if indicated, and tips for observation of signs of neurovascular compromise.
- Medications: Include potential medication side effects and instructions for administration. Advise the client to take NSAIDs with food to avoid abdominal discomfort. Muscle relaxants and narcotic analgesics may cause drowsiness; advise the client not to operate machinery or work above ground level.

Referral

- Immediate referral to an orthopedic surgeon for long bone fractures, displaced fractures, intraarticular fractures, all fractures with neurovascular compromise, and knee injuries with significant effusion or instability
- Referral to an orthopedic surgeon within 3 to 5 days for simple nondisplaced fractures and grade II to III ankle sprains of the ankle and knee after appropriate splinting and client education
- Referral to an orthopedic surgeon for all minor injuries that do not respond to conservative management

Prevention

- Warm up before exercise.
- Complications associated with treatment failure
- Neurovascular damage associated with swelling and misdiagnosis
- Weak ligaments if not treated

EVALUATION/FOLLOW-UP

- Recheck all minor injuries and sprains in 1 week. For those that do not show improvement, consider a referral to an orthopedic surgeon.
- Begin rehabilitation for minor injuries and sprains as soon as possible to prevent contractures and loss of conditioning.
- Continue prescribing NSAIDs with food.

REFERENCES

Alonso, J. (1996). Ankle fractures. In V. Masear (Ed.), *Primary care orthopedics* (pp. 122-127). Philadelphia: W. B. Saunders.

Anderson, B. (1996). *Office orthopedics for primary care.* Philadelphia: W. B. Saunders.

Balano, K. (1996). Anti-inflammatory drugs and myorelaxants: Pharmacology and clinical use in musculoskeletal disease. *Primary Care, 23*(2), 329-334.

Connolly, J. (1996). Acute ankle sprains: Getting and keeping patients back up on their feet. *Consultant,* August, 1631-1639.

DiChristina, D. (1996). Fractures and ligamentous injuries of the ankle. In V. Masear (Ed.), *Primary care orthopedics* (pp. 117-122). Philadelphia: W. B. Saunders.

Dvorkin, M. (1993). *Office orthopedics.* Norwalk, CT: Appleton & Lange.

Garth, W. (1996). Knee injuries in sports. In V. Masear (Ed.), *Primary care orthopedics* (pp. 88-101). Philadelphia: W. B. Saunders.

Lillegard, W. A. (1996). Common upper extremity injuries. *Archives of Family Medicine, 5,* 159-168.

Martin, J. (1996). Initial assessment and management of common fractures. *Primary Care, 23*(2), 405-409.

Meislin, R. (1996). Managing collateral ligament tears of the knee. *Physician Sports Medicine, 24*(3), 67-80.

Robinson, D., Kidd, P., & Rogers, K. (Eds.). (2000). *Primary care across the lifespan*. St. Louis: Mosby.

Savage, P. L. (1996). Casting and splinting techniques. In V. Maeser (Ed.), *Primary care orthopedics* (pp. 337-346). Philadelphia: W. B. Saunders.

Swenson, E. J. (1995). Diagnosing and managing meniscal injuries in athletes. *Journal of Musculoskeletal Medicine*, June, 35-45.

Thordarson, D. B. (1996). Detecting and treating common foot and ankle fractures. *Physician Sports Medicine, 24*(9), 29-38.

Torburn, L. (1996). Principles of rehabilitation. *Primary Care, 23*(2), 335-343.

Review Questions

1. Which of the following fractures is characterized by the classic "dinner fork" appearance?

   a. Jones fractures of the foot
   b. Mallet finger deformity
   c. Boxer's fracture of the hand
   d. Colles' fracture of the wrist

2. Ankle injuries are most commonly associated with which one of the following?

   a. Inversion injuries in which the lateral ligaments are damaged
   b. Eversion injuries in which the deltoid ligament is injured
   c. Fractures of the first metatarsal
   d. Proximal fibula fractures

3. Radiographic findings consistent with a Colles' fracture include which one of the following?

   a. Fractured distal radius with a dorsally angulated fragment
   b. Fractured distal radius with a volar displaced fragment
   c. Avulsion fracture of the lateral fibula
   d. Fractured midshaft radius

4. Nursemaid's elbow is associated with which one of the following mechanisms of action?

   a. Repetitive wrist motion
   b. Pulling up a young child by an extended arm
   c. Repetitive forearm motion as seen with golf and tennis
   d. A fall on an outstretched hand in young children

5. Which one of the following is the most common type of adult wrist fracture?

   a. Boxer's fracture
   b. Scaphoid fracture
   c. Colles' fracture
   d. Mallet finger

6. Which one of the following best describes the mechanism of action for NSAIDs?

   a. NSAIDs inhibit H_2 receptors in the gastric mucosa.
   b. NSAIDs alter pain receptors in the brain by altering serotonin release.
   c. NSAIDs inhibit prostaglandin synthesis, thereby decreasing I pain.

   d. NSAIDs relax the skeletal muscle by decreasing stimulation along the axons.

7. Which one of the following describes appropriate follow-up time for minor injuries or sprains?

   a. Recheck all injuries in 24 hours.
   b. No follow-up is needed for minor injuries.
   c. Recheck minor sprains and injuries in 1 week.
   d. Recheck common injuries in 4 to 6 weeks.

8. Sylvia fell down the steps leading to her house. She is complains of pain on the outside of her ankle and that it hurts to bear weight. On examination she has ecchymosis and swelling on the lateral side of her ankle. There is no actual bone tenderness and no ligamentous laxity. The injury in this client is most likely which of the following?

   a. Grade 1 sprain of the lateral side of the right ankle
   b. Grade 2 sprain of the lateral side of the right ankle
   c. Grade 3 sprain of the lateral side of the right ankle
   d. Most likely an ankle fracture

Answers and Rationales

1. Answer: d (assessment)
   Rationale: When viewed from the side, the wrist with a displaced Colles' fracture resembles a dinner fork, with the tines resembling the fingers.

2. Answer: a (assessment)
   Rationale: Lateral ankle ligaments are weaker than medial ankle ligaments and are injured with common inversion of the ankle (DiChristina, 1996).

3. Answer: a (assessment)
   Rationale: In a Colles' fracture, the distal radius is fractured. The fragment is dorsally angulated, with shortening at the fracture site (Dvorkin, 1993).

4. Answer: b (assessment)
   Rationale: Nursemaid's elbow typically is characterized by a history of a jerk on the upper extremity of a young child who has an extended elbow (Lillegard, 1996).

5. Answer: c (assessment)
   Rationale: Colles' fracture is the most common adult wrist fracture and is associated with a fall on an outstretched hand (Dvorkin, 1993).

6. Answer: c (implementation/plan)
   Rationale: NSAIDs decrease prostaglandin synthesis via inhibition of cyclooxygenase. Prostaglandins are associated with the development of pain after trauma (Balano, 1996).

7. Answer: c (evaluation)
   Rationale: Most athletes with grade I ankle sprains are able to return to full activity in 1 to 2 weeks (DiChristina, 1996). Therefore, follow-up is indicated at about 1 week after injury.

8. Answer: a (analysis/diagnosis)
   Rationale: Because there is no bone point tenderness, it is unlikely that the ankle is fractured. With no ligamentous laxity, this is a grade 1 sprain (Robinson et al., 2000).

STRABISMUS *Denise Robinson*

OVERVIEW
Definition

Strabismus is a deviation of one or both of the eyes. The eyes fail to stay in alignment. Strabismus may be manifest (occurs under binocular conditions) or latent (occurs only under monocular conditions). Manifest deviations can be intermittent, constant, alternating, or unilateral. Strabismus is categorized as medial deviation (esotropia, most common type, 50%), lateral deviation (exotropia, 25%), or vertical deviation (hyperopia, least common type, 10%, accompanied by head tilt to minimize diplopia usually caused by fourth cranial nerve paresis).

Incidence

Approximately 5% of children have strabismus.

Pathophysiology

- Healthy neonates often have intermittent or alternating strabismus. Proper alignment is not established until approximately the first month of age. An intermittent exotropia ("walleye") can be normal until 6 months of age. Esotropia ("cross-eye") is more often a sign of a pathologic condition and is significant if noted after 2 months of age. If the condition persists, a loss of vision (amblyopia) can result from suppression of the image in the deviating eye.
- Binocular vision is the result of coordinated and simultaneous use of both eyes so that the images perceived by the brain are combined to appear as one single image. Strabismus may interfere with the ability of the eyes to work together in unison as they focus on an object. As a result, the brain receives different messages. Deviation of the eye causes the focus of the image to occur outside the macula of the retina, resulting in a blurred image. The brain attempts to correct this by focusing on the clearer image. The brain then suppresses the blurred image of the deviated eye and relies more on the vision of the unaffected eye.
- Strabismus can result from an altered reflex arc in the CNS, or it can also result from cranial nerve palsies, neuromuscular disorders, or craniofacial abnormalities.

ASSESSMENT: SUBJECTIVE/HISTORY
History of Present Illness

- Parents report deviation of the eye.
- Complain of squinting.
- Complain of visual difficulties.
- Parents report school problems.
- Ask parents if their child's eyes work together. Do the eyes appear crossed when focusing on an object up close or when the child is tired?
- Ask the parent about a constant assumed head position such as tilting of the head.

Past Medical History

Strabismus may be associated with cerebral palsy, hydrocephalus, congenital cataracts, colobomas, retinoblastomas, and prematurity associated with intraventricular hemorrhage or regressed retinopathy.

Family History

Inquire about a family history of eye problems, including strabismus, amblyopia, patching therapy, glasses, and eye muscle surgery.

ASSESSMENT: OBJECTIVE/PHYSICAL EXAMINATION
Physical Examination

- Screening for visual problems is essential at every well-child visit (see Table 3-6).
- Ideally the infant or child should be awake and alert.
- Observe for assumed head tilt.
- Observe the eyes, including the eyelids, for size, shape, symmetry, and general appearance.
- Observe as to whether the infant or child follows an object or the examiner's face.
- Assess the red reflex for color, brightness, and symmetry. The room should be slightly darkened, and the ophthalmoscope should be set on +1 diopter.
- Assess for pupillary reflex (infants older than 2 months). The pupils should constrict and remain constricted as a light is moved from one pupil to another.
- Assess the Hirschberg or corneal light reflex (tests for ocular alignment). The reflection of light from each cornea should be symmetrical and in the center of each pupil. In the presence of strabismus, the reflected light appears off-center in the affected eye.
- Assess for extraocular movements.
- Assess an older infant or child with the cover/uncover test at a distance and at close range (also tests for ocular alignment). One eye is covered by the examiner, who looks for movement in the contralateral eye. The covered eye is then uncovered, assessing for movement in that eye. Repeat the same sequence on the other eye. The cover/uncover test differentiates phoria from tropias.
- Assess for visual acuity of each eye and both eyes together.
- If either esotropia or exotropia is found on examination, note whether it is intermittent, constant, or alternating (i.e., asymmetrical light reflex).
- The Hirshberg corneal reflex test is performed by projecting a light source onto the cornea of both eyes while the child looks straight ahead. The positions of

S

the light reflex in each eye are compared. If the eyes are in proper alignment, the light reflex is in the same location on the cornea of each eye. If they are not, the test result is positive for strabismus.

- The cover/uncover test is the only test for latent strabismus. To perform the cover/uncover test, have the child look at a distant object. Cover one eye and watch for movement of the uncovered eye (movement of the uncovered eye when alternate eye is covered). If no movement occurs, there is no apparent misalignment of that eye. Repeat the test with the other eye.
- Record abnormal result of Snellen or other visual acuity test.

Diagnostic Procedures

The diagnosis of strabismus is made by clinical inspection and eye examination. No lab testing is needed.

DIAGNOSIS

Differential diagnoses include the following:
- *Pseudostrabismus* has the appearance of strabismus secondary to the presence of epicanthal folds and a wide, flat nasal bridge with more of the white of the eye being exposed temporally than nasally. Cover/uncover tests and corneal light reflexes are symmetrical (can be ruled out by the Hirschberg test).
- *Nonparalytic strabismus* is secondary to an imbalance in ocular tone. The deviation is constant in all directions of the gaze and is classified by the direction of the deviation.
- *Paralytic strabismus* is secondary to weakness or paralysis of the ocular muscles. The deviation varies by the direction of the gaze.

THERAPEUTIC PLAN

- Three principles of therapy are the following:
  1. Correction of the visual image clarity on the retina
  2. Alignment of bilateral vision
  3. Augmented development of the amblyopic visual cortex by intermittent occlusion of the preferred eye (Broderick, 1998)
- The order in which these therapies take place depends on the clinical presentation, the degree of amblyopia, and the age of the child.
- Treatment of the amblyopia is the most time-critical aspect of therapy (see "Amblyopia").

Nonpharmacologic Treatment

- Force the use of the suppressed eye by patching the preferred eye.
- Surgery may be considered to align the eyes. Children who attain proper alignment of the eyes by age 2 have the best chance of developing binocular vision.

Pharmacologic Treatment

- A mydriatic, such as atropine, can be used to blur the vision in the "good" eye of the child if a patch is not tolerated.
- Ocutinune is a rarely used medical alternative to surgery. It works by preventing the release of acetylcholine from nerve terminals, which functionally paralyzes the muscle. This drug is meant to temporarily overcorrect the deviated eye. The hope is that, when the drug wears off in approximately 2 months, the eye will not revert to its original position. The success rate is approximately 50%. The most common side effect is drooping of the eyelid.

Client Education/Prevention

- The child must wear the patch until vision is normalized.
- The treatment is age-dependent. The younger the child, the faster the normalization of vision is seen.
- Parents should know that noncompliance is the most frequent reason for failure of amblyopia therapy. Other factors such as age at time of treatment, severity of amblyopia, and other eye conditions can affect success of therapy.
- Children should have eye screening incorporated into all well-child visits.
- Provide reassurance to parents when infants less than 6 months of age have pseudostrabismus. This eye crossing disappears as the child grows. It is not a true strabismus.

Referral

Immediate referral to an ophthalmologist is necessary for the following:
- A child of any age with a constant or fixed deviation
- A child 6 months of age or older with intermittent exotropia
- A child 2 months of age or older with intermittent esotropia

Treatment by the ophthalmologist depends on the cause of the strabismus but may involve patching, corrective lens, or surgery. Speed of intervention helps increase changes of an optimal outcome with full restoration of vision.

EVALUATION/FOLLOW-UP

- Assess parent's and child's compliance and understanding of treatment and follow-up treatment recommended by the ophthalmologist.
- Frequent vision and observation will be needed in clients who have occlusion therapy to monitor treatment. It is important to monitor the "good" eye so it does not also develop amblyopia.

- The child needs to continue therapy until vision in the affected eye is normalized or until no further improvement is seen.
- The child with pseudostrabismus less than 6 months of age should be reevaluated in 1 month. For an older child with pseudostrabismus, reevaluate for strabismus in 3 months.

COMPLICATIONS

- By the end of 10 years, it is not known if amblyopia treatment can affect the eyes, so there is a window for which therapy is effective. It is currently believed that the sensitive period for amblyopia is 10 years of age.
- Strabismus is detrimental to childhood development, educational achievement, and self esteem.
- Vision loss may occur in affected eye: monocular vision loss.
- Strabismus also causes impairment of depth perception, peripheral vision, and contrast sensitivity.
- The most common reason for failure of amblyopia therapy is noncompliance.

REFERENCES

Bane, M., & Beauchamp, G. (2001). Update on vision screening. *Review of Ophthalmology* [online journal] *8*, 3.

Broderick, P. (1998). Pediatric vision screening for the family physician. *American Family Physician, 58*(3), 691-700, 703-704.

Eisenbaum, A. (2001). Eye. In W. Hay, A. Hayward, M. Levin, & J. Sondheimer (Eds.), *Current pediatric diagnosis and treatment.* Stamford, CT: Appleton & Lange.

Essman, S., & Essman, T. (1992). Screening for pediatric eye disease. *American Family Physician, 46*(4), 1243-1252.

Lempert, P. (2001). Prevention may be the best way to deal with amblyopia. *Ophthalmology Times, 26*(7), 60.

Mills, M. (1999). The eye in childhood. *American Family Physician, 60*, 907-918.

Moseley, M., & Fielder, A. (2001). Improvement in amblyopic eye function and contralateral eye disease: Evidence of residual plasticity. *Lancet, 357*, 902-904.

Nelson, W. (1996). *Textbook of pediatrics.* Philadelphia: W. B. Saunders.

Rogers, K. (2000). Strabismus. In D. Robinson, P. Kidd, & K. Rogers (Eds.), *Primary care across the lifespan.* St. Louis: Mosby, 1032-1034.

Talsma, J., & Donahue, S. (2001). Screening urged for kids 2 and older. *Ophthalmology Times, 26*(4), 1.

Review Questions

1. A deviation of one or both of the eyes in which the eyes fail to stay in alignment is which of the following?
- **a.** Myopia
- **b.** Conjunctivitis
- **c.** Strabismus
- **d.** Ptosis

2. What is another way to check for ocular alignment besides the Hirschberg test?
- **a.** Red reflex
- **b.** Cover/uncover test
- **c.** Visual acuity with tumbling Es
- **d.** Funduscopy examination

3. Eyes deviated outward is known as which of the following?
- **a.** Hyperopia
- **b.** Exotropia
- **c.** Esotropia
- **d.** Myopia

4. Consider strabismus if the parents report which of the following?
- **a.** A droopy eyelid
- **b.** A lazy eye or wandering eye
- **c.** A cloudy lens
- **d.** Staring spells

5. To screen for latent strabismus, perform which of the following tests?
- **a.** Hirschberg test
- **b.** Snellen test
- **c.** Cover/uncover test
- **d.** Bruckner test

6. To rule out pseudostrabismus, perform which of the following tests?
- **a.** Hirschberg test
- **b.** Snellen test
- **c.** Cover/uncover test
- **d.** Bruckner test

7. Immediate referral to an ophthalmologist is necessary for which of the following children?
- **a.** Child of any age with a constant or fixed deviation
- **b.** Child younger than 6 months with intermittent exotropia
- **c.** Child younger than 2 months with intermittent esotropia
- **d.** Child of any age with alternating deviation

8. How should a child 3 months of age with intermittent esotropia should be managed?
- **a.** Continue to observe until 6 months of age.
- **b.** Immediate referral is necessary.
- **c.** Ask parents to call if it becomes fixed.
- **d.** Reassure the parents that this is normal.

Answers and Rationales

1. *Answer:* c (diagnosis/analysis)
Rationale: The definition of strabismus is a deviation of one or both eyes in which the eyes fail to stay in alignment (Rogers, 2000).

2. *Answer:* b (assessment)
Rationale: Both the Hirschberg corneal reflex test and cover/uncover test check for alignment. The red reflex test checks for opacity of the cornea, cataract, and others.

S

A funduscopic examination looks at the retina, optic disc, and the macula (Mills, 1999).

3. *Answer:* b (assessment)
Rationale: Eyes deviating outward (walleye) is exotropia.

4. *Answer:* b (assessment)
Rationale: The report of a lazy or wandering eye is often an indication of strabismus (Mills, 1999).

5. *Answer:* c (assessment)
Rationale: The cover/uncover test is one of the few tests for strabismus that reveals latent strabismus (Nelson, 1996).

6. *Answer:* a (assessment)
Rationale: Pseudostrabismus can be ruled out with the Hirschberg test. With pseudostrabismus, the light reflex is in the same location on the cornea of each eye (Nelson, 1996).

7. *Answer:* a (plan/implementation)
Rationale: A child of any age with fixed or constant strabismus needs immediate referral to an ophthalmologist. This indicates a more problematic form of strabismus (Essman & Essman, 1992).

8. *Answer:* b (plan/implementation)
Rationale: A child who is 3 months old with intermittent esotropia should receive an immediate referral to an ophthalmologist because of the increased complication rate with esotropia (Essman & Essman, 1992).

SUBSTANCE ABUSE *Denise Robinson*

OVERVIEW
Definition
- Substance: drug of abuse, a medication or toxin
- Substance abuse: recurrent use results in the following:
  - Failure to fulfill obligations
  - Use in hazardous situations
  - Legal problems
- Substance dependence: recurrent use over 12 months leads to three or more of the following:
  - Tolerance: need more of substance for same effect, or less effect with same amount
  - Withdrawal: symptoms typical for the substance when the substance is stopped
  - Unsuccessful efforts to cut back in use
  - Much time spent obtaining or recovering from effects of substance
  - Continued use despite adverse physical or psychological effects
- *Meeting the definition of substance dependence supersedes the definition of substance abuse* (American Psychiatric Association [APA], 1994).

Incidence
- Approximately 8% to 20% of primary care clients (adults and adolescents) have problem drinking (abuse or dependence).
- There is a 5:1 male/female ratio.
- Highest incidence occurs in ages 18 to 24 years (17% to 24% of males, 4% to 10% of females), with decreased incidence for older clients.
- Approximately 3% to 40% of pregnant women who are alcohol dependent give birth to infants with fetal alcohol syndrome.
- In adolescents ages 12 to 17, 18% used alcohol in the past month, 35% in the past year.
- In the elderly with problem drinking, 70% have a chronic, long-standing problem, 30% have a late-onset problem.

- Alcohol abuse costs $85.8 billion per year.
- Other drugs of abuse (besides alcohol) are more commonly used by teens and young adults, by men, the unemployed, those living in urban areas, and those who have not completed high school. The estimated cost of substance abuse is $47 billion per year.
- Of pregnant women, 5.5% used illicit drugs at least once during pregnancy; 1.1% used cocaine.

Pathophysiology
See Table 3-102.

Factors Increasing Susceptibility
- Positive family history
- Genetics
- Cultural attitudes
- Availability of substances
- Personal experience with the substance
- Stress (APA, 1994)

Pregnant Women
- Alcohol use
- Cigarettes
- Poverty
- Poor nutrition
- Inadequate prenatal care

ASSESSMENT: SUBJECTIVE/HISTORY
History of Present Illness
- May need to confirm or get an additional perspective from another family member if possible.
- Ask about quantity, frequency of use.
- Consider that client might under-report (common).
- May present with vague complaints.
- Frequently seen for gastrointestinal (GI) complaints.
- If client admits to substance abuse or dependence, find out the following:
  - Age substance use began

TABLE **3-102** Pathophysiology of Substance Abuse

DRUG	INTOXICATING EFFECTS	HEALTH CONSEQUENCES
Alcohol	CNS depression, sedation, lack of coordination, altered mood Blood alcohol 150 to 200 mg/dL Legal driving level less than 100 mg/dL in most states (some have changed limit to less than 80 mg/dL) 12 to 24 hours after use stops: weakness, sweating, hyperreflexia, GI symptoms, seizures, hallucinations, delirium tremens	Consequences are cirrhosis, peripheral neuropathy, dementia, cardiomyopathy, CHF, arrhythmia, pancreatitis, gastritis, thiamine deficiency. **Women:** Adverse health effects develop sooner with less consumption than men. **Pregnant women:** FAS with 7 to 14 drinks per week. More risk early in pregnancy or with binge drinking. FAS: fetal growth retardation, facial deformities, CNS dysfunction (microcephaly, mental retardation, behavior problems). Any alcohol may cause risk. **Adolescents and young adults:** Contributes to leading cause of death (MVA) and other problems (injuries, homicides, suicides, unsafe sex, legal problems). **Elderly:** Slowed metabolism: elevated alcohol with less drinking. Isolation, falls, malnutrition, dementia, self-neglect, suicide
Marijuana	Euphoria, increased taste perceptions, relaxation, drowsiness	Consequences are asthma, bronchitis, memory impairment, pharyngitis.
Cocaine, amphetamine	Stimulates CNS: euphoria, hyperactivity, alertness, grandiosity, anger, impaired judgment, altered pulse, blood pressure Other symptoms: perspiration, chills, paranoia, seizures, chest pain, MI, arrhythmia Acute withdrawal: depression, suicidal ideation Withdrawal: fatigue, unpleasant dreams, psychomotor retardation or agitation, increased appetite	Consequences of chronic use are fatigue, social withdrawal, weight loss. Consequences of snorting are nasal mucosal irritation, perforated nasal septum. Cocaine and amphetamines are short acting, producing rapid dependence. Consequences of dependence are large amounts of money for repetitive use, prostitution. Increased incidence of STDs. Consequences of amphetamine use are diaphoresis, flushing, hyperreflexia, insomnia, irritability, restlessness, tachycardia. Consequences of chronic use are confusion, depression, headache, paranoia.
Opioids	CNS depressant: drowsiness, decreased vital signs, dry mouth, constipation, euphoria, flushing, itchy skin	Tolerance is achieved within 2 to 3 days after prescribed use. Withdrawal occurs within 4 to 6 hours, resulting in CNS hyperactivity, anxiety, increased respirations, yawning, perspiration, lacrimation, rhinorrhea. Dependence associated with high death rate from overdose, injuries, violence. Men may experience erectile dysfunction. Women may experience irregular menses. Pregnant women risk withdrawal in newborn.
PCP	Ataxia, disinhibition, euphoria	Consequences are panic attacks, sweating, sensitivity to sensation.
Hallucinogens	Altered visual perception	Consequences are hallucinations, flashbacks, panic attacks, psychosis. IDU may involve shared needles, leading to hepatitis B, hepatitis C, hepatitis D, HIV, septicemia, bacterial endocarditis, localized cellulitis.

From Renfrow, V. (2000). Substance abuse. In D. Robinson, P. Kidd, & K. Rogers (Eds.), *Primary care across the lifespan* (p. 1038). St. Louis: Mosby.
CHF, Congestive heart failure; *CNS,* central nervous system; *FAS,* fetal alcohol syndrome; *HIV,* human immunodeficiency virus; *IDU,* injection drug use; *MI,* myocardial infarction; *MVA,* motor vehicle accident; *PCP,* phencyclidine hydrochloride.

- Amount and pattern of use, including binges
- Method used to support habit (e.g., stealing, prostitution, employment)
- History of injected drug use or needle sharing
- Presence of withdrawal symptoms, including the following:
  - Alcohol: morning shakes, seizures, hallucinations
  - Opioids: nausea, vomiting, diarrhea, abdominal pain or cramps, chills, runny nose and eyes, sweating, bone or muscle pain
  - Cocaine: depression, suicidal thoughts
- Determine whether any treatment has been sought.
- Determine length of substance-free periods and remissions.
- Determine circumstance of remission (e.g., incarceration, inpatient unit).
- Assess legal history (e.g., convictions for driving under the influence).
- Assess work history.

Most Frequent Presenting Symptoms

- Anxiety
- Depression
- Fatigue
- Headache
- Weight loss
- Rhinorrhea
- Dysphagia
- Cough
- Shortness of breath
- Dysuria
- Chest pain
- Edema
- Genital discharge
- Rectal bleeding
- Constipation
- Rash
- Paresthesia

Past Medical History

Ask about substance-related illnesses and hospitalizations related to the following:

- History of head injury
- MVA
- Other injuries or fractures
- Seizures
- Learning disorders
- HTN
- Cardiovascular disease
- Pneumonia
- Emphysema
- Pancreatitis
- Hepatitis (alcoholic or viral)
- HIV status
- Cirrhosis
- Cancer

- Sexual dysfunction
- Frequent sexually transmitted diseases (STDs)
- Abuse: physical, emotional, sexual
- Psychiatric disorders: depression, suicide, anxiety (alcohol, sedative/hypnotics, cocaine, opioids), bipolar disorder (alcohol, sedative/hypnotics, cocaine, opioids), paranoia (alcohol, cocaine, stimulants) hyperactivity or attention deficit hyperactivity disorder (alcohol, cocaine, stimulants), sleep disorders (alcohol, sedative/hypnotic, cocaine, stimulants, opioids), dementia (alcohol, sedative/hypnotics), amnesiac disorders (alcohol)
- Gynecologic history: last menstrual period (LMP), birth control method, gravity, parity, abortions, ectopic pregnancies, complications during pregnancy, source of prenatal care, history of drug use during pregnancy, health of newborns

Medication History

- Current medications
- Psychotropics
- Prescription drugs of abuse (opioids, benzodiazepines, barbiturates, stimulants)

Family History

- Determine history as far back as at least two generations and include current close relatives.
- Assess substance abuse or dependence in the family.
- Assess effect of substance problem on family.

Psychosocial History

Ask about the following (concentrate on losses related to substance abuse):

- Losses: jobs, property, relationships, children, self-respect, health
- Marital history
- Number and ages of children
- Occupation (frequent absences from work)
- Financial status
- Legal problems
- Adequacy of housing (consider homelessness)
- Sexual preferences and practices
- Cigarette smoking
- Alcohol use: If a nondrinker ask why, whether they ever drank in the past, and when drinking stopped.

See Table 3-103 for drug abuse screening.

ASSESSMENT: OBJECTIVE/PHYSICAL EXAMINATION

Physical Assessment

- Problem oriented, guided by substance of abuse, symptoms, risk behaviors
- See Table 3-104.

Diagnostic Procedures

See Table 3-105.

TABLE **3-103** Substance Abuse Screening

SCREENING TEST	SCREENING QUESTIONS	FINDINGS
CAGE Questionnaire*	Ask first if the client uses alcohol. If yes, ask the following: Have you ever felt you ought to **cut** down on drinking? Have people ever **annoyed** you by criticizing your drinking? Have you ever felt bad or **guilty** about your drinking? Have you ever had a drink first thing in the morning to steady your nerves or get rid of a hangover? **(eye opener)** Address other drug use after giving the CAGE.	One "yes" response should raise suspicions of alcohol abuse. More than one "yes" response should be considered a strong indication that alcohol abuse exists. 100% specificity for those without alcohol abuse or dependence, 37% sensitivity of true cases with one "yes" answer, 66% sensitivity with three "yes" answers, 82% sensitivity with two "yes" answers, and 90% sensitivity with one "yes" answer.
DAST†	Ask the following: Have you ever used drugs other than those required for medical reasons? Have you abused prescription drugs? Do you abuse more than one drug at a time? Can you get through the week without using drugs? Are you always able to stop using drugs when you want to? Do you abuse drugs on a continuous basis? Do you try to limit your drug use to certain situations? Have you had 'black outs' or 'flashbacks' as a result of drug use? Do you ever feel bad about your drug use? Does your spouse (or parents) ever complain about your involvement with drugs? Do your friends or relatives know or suspect you abuse drugs? Has your drug use ever created problems between you and your partner? Has any family member ever sought help for problems related to your drug use? Have you ever lost friends because of your use of drugs? Have you ever neglected your family or missed work or school because of drug use? Have you ever been in trouble at work or school because of drug use?	

Continued

TABLE **3-103** Substance Abuse Screening—*cont'd*

SCREENING TEST	SCREENING QUESTIONS	FINDINGS
	Have you ever lost a job because of drug abuse?	
	Have you ever gotten into fights when under the influence of drugs?	
	Have you ever been arrested because of unusual behavior while under the influence of drugs?	
	Have you ever been arrested for driving while under the influence of drugs?	
	Have you engaged in illegal actions to obtain drugs?	
	Have you ever been arrested for possession of illegal drugs?	
	Have you ever experienced withdrawal symptoms as a result of heavy drug intake?	
	Have you had any medical problems as a result of your drug use (memory loss, hepatitis, convulsions, bleeding)?	
	Have you ever gone to anyone for help for a drug problem?	
	Have you ever been in a hospital for medical problems related to your drug use?	
	Have you ever been involved in a treatment program for drug use?	
	Have you ever been treated as an outpatient for problems related to drug use?	
Screening Follow-Up Questions‡	HALT BUMP mnemonic:	Helps determine preoccupation with substance abuse.
	Do you usually use drugs or drink to get **high?**	
	Do you sometimes drink or use drugs **alone?**	
	Have you found yourself **looking** forward to using drugs or drinking?	
	Have you noticed an increased **tolerance?**	
	Do you have memory lapses or **blackouts** that occur while drinking?	
	Do you find yourself using or drinking in **unplanned** ways?	
	Do you use drugs or drink when you feel anxious, stressed, or depressed for **medical reasons?**	
	Do you work at **protecting** your supply, having drugs or alcohol at all times?	
	FATAL DT mnemonic:	Used to identify important information, including negative consequences that have resulted from substance abuse.
	Family history of alcohol or substance abuse problems?	
	Alcoholics anonymous or other 12-step program attendance?	
	Thoughts of having alcoholism or being drug dependent?	
	Attempts or thoughts of suicide?	
	Legal problems?	
	Driving while intoxicated or using drugs?	
	Tranquilizer or disulfiram (Antabuse) use?	

POPULATION TO SCREEN	SCREENING QUESTIONS	FINDINGS
Pregnant women: All pregnant women should be screened for drugs and alcohol.	Include questions of tolerance, for example, "How many drinks can you hold?" Also ask about other substances or drugs.	Tolerance: Three or more drinks to feel high or ability to drink five drinks at a time. Two or more drinks per day or binge drinking may result in FAS.
Adolescents: All adolescents should be screened for tobacco, alcohol, and drug use.	Ask about school, extracurricular activities, friends, nighttime activities, neighborhood, and family life. Then screen for alcohol and drug use, asking the following questions: Do you know anyone who smokes, drinks alcohol, or uses drugs? Does anyone in your family smoke, drink, or use drugs? Have you ever used tobacco, alcohol, or drugs in the past? Now? Ask directly about drug and alcohol use, specific substances, and frequency and duration of use. Ask if there is a problem and if the client is interested in getting help.	If the client admits to substance abuse, gather information about the following: Tobacco dependence in clients younger than 17 years of age Poor grades (more than two Ds or Fs on two consecutive report cards) Experiences of rape, incest, or physical abuse Frequent drunkenness in early adolescence Chronic deceptiveness, aggression, hostility or resentment Staying away from home for 48 hours or longer without parental permission Sexual promiscuity
Older adults§	Alcohol is the most likely abused substance for the elderly at 2% to 10% of the population. Screen client with recent stresses in life and his or her ability to cope with stress. Then ask the client, "Have you drunk any alcohol in the past year? Have you used any drugs in the past year?" If the client's answer is "yes," use the CHARM screen, as follows: Have you ever thought about **cutting** down? **How** do you use? Do you have rules about drinking or drug use? Has your pattern of drinking or drug use changed recently? Has **anyone** expressed concern about your alcohol or drug use? What **role** do alcohol and drugs play in your life? Have you ever used alcohol or drugs **more** than you intended? Have you ever had problems with your **medications** or taken more than prescribed?	

From Renfrow, V. (2000). Substance abuse. In D. Robinson, P. Kidd, & K. Rogers (Eds.), *Primary care across the lifespan* (pp. 1038-1041). St. Louis: Mosby.

*Ewing, J. (1984). Detecting alcoholism: The CAGE questionnaire. *Journal of the American Medical Association, 252*(14), 1905-1907.

†Skinner, H. (1982). The drug abuse screening test. *Addictive Behavior, 7*(4), 363-371.

‡Clark, W. (1985). The medical interview: Focus on alcohol problems. *Hospital Practice, 20*(11), 59-65.

§Summicht, G. (1991). *Sailing with horses: Adventures with older substance abusers.* Madison, WI: PICADA.

DAST, Drug abuse screening test; *FAS,* fetal alcohol syndrome.

TABLE **3-104**   Physical Assessment for Substance Abuse

SYSTEM	FOCUS AREA/FINDINGS
General	Vital signs, temperature if infection suspected Hygiene, weight loss (stimulants, cocaine, opioids)
Mental status	Affect (full, flat, blunted, inappropriate, labile, restricted), alertness, orientation, mood (dysphoric, elevated, euthymic, restricted)
Skin	Lesions, scars, tracks, jaundice (alcohol, IV opioids), contusions and bruises (alcohol, sedative/hypnotic), petechiae, diaphoresis (sedative hypnotics), spider angiomas (alcohol, stimulants), burns, especially on fingers (alcohol), needle marks (opioids), homemade tattoos (cocaine, IV opioids), increased vascularity of face (alcohol), piloerection (opioid withdrawal)
HEENT	Eyes: Pupillary response (pinpoint: opioid intoxication, dilated: opioid withdrawal), accommodation EOM, nystagmus (vertical: PCP, lateral: alcohol, sedative/hypnotics), sclera (jaundice), funduscopy if blood pressure high Nose: condition of mucosa and septum (perforated: cocaine), rhinorrhea (cocaine, opioids) Mouth and pharynx: dentition (periodontal disease: alcohol), lesions, increased gag reflex (alcohol), excessive yawning (alcohol, opioid withdrawal) Neck: thyroid size, asymmetry, mass, carotid bruit (increased head/neck cancer with alcohol use)
Chest	Chest diameter, breath sounds, hoarseness (cocaine, opioids, nicotine), chest trauma (especially rib fracture: alcohol, sedative/hypnotics), adventitious sounds: wheezing (nicotine, cocaine), gynecomastia (alcohol)
Cardiovascular	Rate, rhythm, murmurs, rubs, gallops, arrhythmias (alcohol, cocaine, stimulants), HTN (alcohol), cardiomyopathy (alcohol), subacute endocarditis (IV opioids, cocaine), thrombophlebitis (cocaine, opioids)
Abdomen	Bowel sounds, bruit, hepatosplenomegaly (alcohol), tenderness, esophagitis, gastritis, epigastric and RUQ tenderness (alcohol)
Neurologic	Tremors (alcohol, sedative hypnotics), sensation/symptoms of neuropathy (alcohol, sedatives/hypnotics), reflex sympathetic dystrophy (alcohol, sedative/hypnotics, opioids) coordination, gait, reflexes (hyperactive: alcohol, cocaine, opioids intoxication)
Genital/rectal	Examine if symptomatic, or if high-risk behavior vaginitis (opioids, alcohol, cocaine)
GU	Penile scars or tracks (IV opioid), atrophic testes (alcohol)
Extremities	Check peripheral pulses, look for palmar erythema, compression syndromes ("Saturday night palsy"), peripheral edema, myopathies (alcohol)

From Caulkner-Burnett, I. (1994). Primary care screening for substance abuse. *Nurse Practitioner, 19*(6), 42-48.
EOM, Extraocular muscles; *GU,* genitourinary; *HEENT,* head, eyes, ears, nose, and throat; *HTN,* hypertension; *PCP,* phencyclidine hydrochloride; *RUQ,* right upper quadrant.

DIAGNOSIS

- Substance intoxication (specify substance): excessive use of substance, with expected symptoms of behavioral and physical manifestations based on the substance used
- Substance withdrawal (specify substance): development of a substance-specific syndrome because of discontinuation or reduction in substance use that has been heavy and prolonged
- Substance abuse: Maladaptive pattern of substance use leading to clinically significant impairment (during 12-month period); failure to fulfill major role obligations at work, school, home; recurrent use in situations in which it is physically hazardous (e.g., driving car); arrests for substance-related activities; continued use despite these problems (does not meet criteria for substance dependence)

- Substance dependence: tolerance; withdrawal; inability to cut down on use of substance; great amount of time spent procuring substance; social, occupational, or recreational activities given up or reduced because of substance use; substance use continued despite physical or psychological problems likely caused by the substance (during preceding 12 months)

Consider substance abuse or dependence when the following criteria are present:

- Frequently missed appointments
- Frequent excuses for missed work
- Report of lost prescriptions or request for frequent refills
- Frequent emergency department visits for headache, stomach pain, tooth problems, fights, MVA

TABLE **3-105** Diagnostic Testing for Substance Abuse

DIAGNOSTIC TEST	FINDING/RATIONALE
GGT*, AST*, ALT*, LDH, Alkaline phosphatase, total bilirubin, cholesterol, triglycerides, uric acid, MCV	Increased in chronic excessive alcohol intake Also sensitive: AST/ALT ratio greater than 1 Other causes of elevated GGT: drugs (anticonvulsants, tranquilizers) or metabolic diseases (DM, hyperlipidemia)
Blood alcohol level	Provides level of intoxication. The following are indicators of abuse: 300 mg/100 mL at any time, 100 mg/100 mL during routine physical examination, 150 mg/100 mL without evidence of intoxication.
CBC	Screen for low Hgb/Hct from alcoholic gastritis and elevated MCV. Consider advanced disease with low WBC and low platelets (bone marrow depression).
HIV screen	If high-risk behaviors
Hepatitis panel	
RPR	
TSH, T4	Screening
Chest radiograph	Screen for adult smokers
Toxicology tests	Excretion rates vary. Positive results occur for 1 to 4 days after use (several weeks for long-term marijuana use). Prevent false-positive result with confirmatory tests on same sample (per routine laboratory procedure). Record list of current medications in case of cross-reactivity. Consider direct observation of urine collection (prevent sample tampering). Newborn meconium toxicology confirms recent maternal use. Consider screening for those involved in serious MVA, a suicide attempt, unexplained seizure, violent outbursts of temper, antisocial acts, promiscuity, syncope, or unexplained cardiac arrhythmia
Screening for drugs of abuse: Color or spot tests	Easy to use, low cost, immediate results, but specific compounds difficult to identify. High concentration of drug required to achieve a color reaction

Adapted from American Medical Association. (1987). Scientific issues in testing. *Journal of the American Medical Association, 257,* 3110-3114, and *Patient Care,* December 15, 1989, from Renfrow, V. (2000). Substance abuse. In D. Robinson, P. Kidd, & K. Rogers (Eds.), *Primary care across the lifespan* (p. 1043). St. Louis: Mosby.
*Most sensitive.
ALT, Alanine transaminase; *AST,* aspartate aminotransferase; *CBC,* complete blood count; *DM,* diabetes mellitus; *GGT,* gamma-glutamyltransferase; *Hct,* hematocrit; *Hgb;* hemoglobin; *HIV,* human immunodeficiency virus; *LDH,* lactate dehydrogenase; *MCV,* mean corpuscular volume; *MVA,* motor vehicle accident; *RPR,* rapid plasma reagin; *T4,* thyroxine; *TSH,* thyroid-stimulating hormone; *WBC,* white blood cell.

- Family history of substance use
- Social history of financial or marital problems, or loss of custody of children

THERAPEUTIC PLAN

- The primary treatment approach is the use of brief intervention techniques that last approximately 5 to 10 minutes.
- Discuss diagnosis with client; discuss findings in a nonjudgmental, caring manner. State the negative consequences of the client's substance use and express concern that the client may be developing a problem with drugs or alcohol. Elicit the client's reaction. When clients are ready to change their substance use behavior, a quit date can be negotiated and a behavior contract developed. Follow-up calls to provide support have been found to be helpful. Referral to a person or program specific for substance abuse or dependence may be another option. The following algorithm identifies the initial management of a client thought to have a substance problem.

Nonpharmacologic Treatment

- Client should commit to and participate in a treatment plan.
- A well-balanced diet is important to anyone who has nutritional deficits caused by substance abuse or dependence.

Pharmacologic Treatment

Consider inpatient detoxification if any of the following apply:

- History of alcohol withdrawal seizures
- No stable home environment
- High potential for withdrawal problems, determined according to the following characteristics:
  - Age older than 40 years
  - Male gender

S

- Daily consumption of more than one-fifth of liquor
- Drinking around the clock to maintain a steady blood level
- Excessive drinking for longer than 10 years
- Development of tremulousness and anxiety within 6 to 8 hours of cessation
- History of seizures, hallucinations, delusions with alcohol withdrawal
- Presence of an acute medical problem such as pneumonia
- Alcohol level higher than 250 mg/dL
- Acute intoxication: See Table 3-106.

Client Education

- Discuss with all clients the risks of driving while intoxicated by drugs or alcohol.
- All pregnant women should be encouraged to abstain from alcohol and drugs during pregnancy.
- Explain the need for repeated attempts to achieve goals.
- Have client identify anxiety-provoking situations.
- Develop strategies for resisting temptations.
- Explain the disease process.
- Discuss prevention strategies.
- Role of family members can be very important during treatment. A sober and responsible family member or friend is an integral part of outpatient medical detoxification. Family and friends can encourage the client to do the following:
  - Encourage client to attend Alcoholics Anonymous or Narcotics Anonymous meetings.
  - Provide a safe, loving environment.
  - Watch for serious withdrawal symptoms.
  - Assist with medications.
  - Drive the client to appointments.
  - Provide for massages and hot baths for muscle cramps and anxiety.
  - Minimize the risk of relapse by keeping the client away from situations that may lead to relapse.
  - Dispose drugs/alcohol in the home environment.
  - Facilitate participation in a treatment program.

Referral/Consultation

- Federal law protects the confidentiality of persons receiving alcohol and drug abuse prevention and treatment services. A signed consent form must be completed for release of information.
- Minors: Check state laws. Referral may be required in the presence of medical emergencies, court orders, client crime against staff or program, approved research, initial child abuse reports.
- Level of treatment: Match personality, background, mental condition, duration, and extent of substance use and type of substance with level of treatment.
- Refer to psychiatrist or addiction specialist for inpatient treatment care. For outpatient care, use of support groups, employee assistance programs, and individual or family counseling may be appropriate.

EVALUATION/FOLLOW-UP

- Monitor the client closely.
- If referred to an addiction specialist, be aware of progress and the need to be consistent with interventions used.
- Do not refill prescriptions if client claims they have been lost, stolen, or otherwise unable to be filled.
- Convey a clear message regarding your thoughts and policies concerning substance use. Development of an office policy regarding controlled substances is recommended.

REFERENCES

American Medical Association. (1987). Scientific issues in testing. *Journal of the American Medical Association, 257,* 3110-3114

American Psychiatric Association. (1994). *Diagnostic and statistical manual of mental disorders* (4th ed.). Washington, DC: APA.

Ash, K., Schikis, M., & Schwartz, M. (1989). Helping the teenage drug user. *Patient Care,* 614-627.

TABLE **3-106**   Therapeutic Treatment for Substance Abusers

SUBSTANCE	TREATMENT
Alcohol and barbiturate intoxication	Supportive care is the rule.
Benzodiazepine intoxication	The antagonist flumazenil (Mazicon, 0.1-0.2 mg/min. IV up to 1 mg) can be used to reverse toxic effects.
Opiate intoxication	If the client is unconscious and respiration is depressed, the opiate antagonist naloxone (Narcan, 0.4-2.0 mg IV q3 min) can be used to revive the client. Narcan causes physical withdrawal in dependent clients. If a total dose of 10 mg is given with no response, a drug other than an opiate is involved.
Stimulant intoxication	Treated only if client is overtly psychotic and agitated. Lorazepam (Ativan) 2-4 mg IM q30 min up to 6 hours prn for agitation. Monitor cardiac function.
Hallucinogens, marijuana, inhalants	Reassurance or talk-down therapy may be helpful. If not, use lorazepam as described above.
PCP	Minimize sensory input; talk-down therapy is not recommended. More unpredictable; leave client alone in dimly lit room. Lorazepam may be needed.

From Renfrow, V. (2000). Substance abuse. In D. Robinson, P. Kidd, & K. Rogers (Eds.), *Primary care across the lifespan* (p. 1046). St. Louis: Mosby.

Brown, R. L. (1992). Identification and office management of alcohol and drug disorders. In M. Fleming & K. Barry (Eds.), *Disorders* (p. 40). St. Louis: Mosby.

Caulkner-Burnett, I. (1994). Primary care screening for substance abuse. *Nurse Practitioner, 19*(6), 42-48.

Clark, W. (1985). The medical interview: Focus on alcohol problems. *Hospital Practice, 20*(11), 59-65.

Ewing, J. (1984). Detecting alcoholism: The CAGE questionnaire. *Journal of the American Medical Association, 252,* 1905-1907.

Grinspoon, L. (1995). Treatment of drug abuse and addiction: part I. *Harvard Medical Letters, 12*(2).

Hoksema, H., & deBock, M. (1993). The value of laboratory tests for the screening and recognition of alcohol abuse in primary care patients. *Journal of Family Practice, 37*(3), 268-275.

National Institute on Alcohol Abuse and Alcoholism. (1990). *Seventh special report to the U.S. Congress on alcohol and health.* Rockville, MD: U.S. Department of Health and Human Services, USDHHS Publication ADM 90-1656.

Renfrow, V. (2000). Substance abuse. In D. Robinson, P. Kidd, & K. Rogers (Eds.), *Primary Care Across the Lifespan.* St. Louis, Mosby.

Saunders, J., Aasland, O., Babor, T., de la Fuente, J. R., & Grant, M. (1993) Development of the alcohol use disorders identification test (AUDIT): WHO collaborative project on early detection of persons with harmful alcohol consumption–II. *Addiction, 88*(6), 791-804.

Schonberg, S. (1998). *Substance abuse: A guide for health professionals.* Elk Grove Village, IL: The American Academy of Pediatrics/Pacific Institute for Research and Evaluation.

Schulz, J., & Barry, K. (1992). Alcohol and drug treatment and role of 12-step programs. In M. Fleming & K. Barry (Eds.), *Addictive disorders* (p. 84). St. Louis: Mosby.

Skinner, H. (1982). The drug abuse screening test. *Addictive Behavior, 7*(4), 363-371.

Substance Abuse and Mental Health Services Administration. (1994). *Treatment for alcohol and other drug abuse: Opportunities for coordination.* Rockville, MD: U.S. Government Printing Office, Technical Assistance Publication Series: 11 (DHHS Publication No. (SMA) 94-2075).

Sumnicht, G. (1991). *Sailing with horses: Adventures with older substance abusers.* Madison, WI: Prevention and Intervention Center for Alcohol and Other Drug Abuse (PICADA).

U.S. Department of Health and Human Services, Public Health Service. (1994). *Clinician's handbook of preventive services: Put prevention into practice.* Washington, DC: U.S. Government Printing Office.

U.S. Preventive Services Task Force. (1996). *Guide to clinical preventive services* (2nd ed.). Baltimore: Williams & Wilkins.

Warner, A. (1996). *Drug testing: Practices and pitfalls.* Cincinnati, OH: University of Cincinnati Medical Center, Division of Toxicology. Unpublished handout.

West, D., & Kinney, J. (1996). An overview of substance use and abuse. In J. Kinney (Ed.), *Clinical manual of substance abuse* (2nd ed., p. 31). St. Louis: Mosby.

Review Questions

1. Which of the screening techniques is most sensitive for risky drinking practices in pregnant women?

   a. CAGE screening
   b. Items about alcohol use on a questionnaire
   c. Questions about tolerance in history
   d. Direct questions about amount of alcohol consumed

2. Careful routine screening for drug use other than alcohol is especially indicated for which of the following clients?

   a. Women
   b. Clients older than 65
   c. Adolescents and pregnant women
   d. Clients younger than 65

3. Which test results are highly suggestive of alcohol abuse?

   a. Elevated gamma-glutamyltransferase (GGT), elevated MCV, and alanine transaminase (ALT)/aspartate aminotransferase (AST) ratio of less than 1
   b. Elevated GGT, decreased MCV, and elevated sodium
   c. High-density lipoprotein, elevated WBC, and elevated total bilirubin
   d. Decreased MCHC, elevated GGT, elevated potassium

4. What is the best way to prevent false-positive urine drug tests?

   a. Have a trained laboratory technician collect the specimen.
   b. Send the report to the primary provider.
   c. Run confirmatory tests on a positive sample.
   d. Send a list of the prescribed drugs with the specimen.

5. Meeting the definition of substance dependence does not include which of the following?

   a. Headaches
   b. Tolerance
   c. Much time spent obtaining or recovering from the substance
   d. Withdrawal

6. Pregnant women who are opioid dependent have improved outcomes with which of the following?

   a. Detoxification with benzodiazepine
   b. Direct confrontation at each visit about the harmful effects of drugs on the fetus
   c. Examination for needle marks (tracks) at each visit
   d. Methadone maintenance

7. A 44-year-old man with elevated GGT and other serum liver test results normal agrees to discontinue alcohol use. When should he be told to return for a follow-up GGT to determine if his alcohol consumption is affecting his liver?

   a. 1 month
   b. 2 to 3 months
   c. 1 week
   d. Every 4 months for 1 year

8. How often should a pregnant 25-year-old diagnosed with cocaine dependence should be instructed to return for follow-up prenatal visits?

   a. According to the number of weeks' gestation (standard schedule) as long as she agrees to enter a treatment program
   b. More frequently than the standard schedule

c. With regular psychiatric evaluations scheduled throughout pregnancy

d. Determined by an alcohol use disorders identification test questionnaire administered at each visit

---

Answers and Rationales

1. *Answer:* **c** (assessment)
Rationale: Light drinking in pregnant women is hazardous and may not be uncovered by direct questioning or screening questionnaires. Questions about tolerance are more revealing. Two drinks per day or binge drinking is most risky during pregnancy. Women who drink three or more drinks to feel high or who can drink five drinks at a time demonstrate tolerance (U.S. Preventive Services Task Force, 1996).

2. *Answer:* **c** (assessment)
Rationale: Drug abuse has increased among adolescents. Drug use during pregnancy is associated with adverse outcomes, with the potential for developmental delay (U.S. Preventive Services Task Force, 1996).

3. *Answer:* **a** (analysis/diagnosis)
Rationale: Alcohol use causes elevated GGT by microsomal enzyme induction, elevated MCV from red blood cells destroyed by hypersplenism, and ALT/AST ratio of less than 1 with suppressed ALT from nonviral hepatitis.

4. *Answer:* **c** (analysis/diagnosis)
Rationale: False-positive results can be reduced by performing a second, more specific confirmatory test (U.S. Preventive Services Task Force, 1996).

5. *Answer:* **a** (analysis/diagnosis)
Rationale: The definition of substance dependence includes three of the following in the same 12 months: tolerance, withdrawal, inability to cut down use, much time spent obtaining the substance or recovering from its effects, and continued use despite adverse effects (APA, 1994).

6. *Answer:* **d** (implementation/plan)
Rationale: Methadone maintenance improves outcomes in pregnant, opioid-dependent women. Opiate withdrawal is dangerous during pregnancy. Regular contact to obtain methadone can improve prenatal care (U.S. Preventive Services Task Force, 1996).

7. *Answer:* **b** (evaluation)
Rationale: GGT should return to normal within 2 to 3 months after cessation of alcohol use.

8. *Answer:* **b** (evaluation)
Rationale: Outcomes are improved in substance-dependent pregnant women with more frequent prenatal visits (U.S. Preventive Services Task Force, 1996).

SYNCOPE *Pamela Kidd*

OVERVIEW
Definition

Syncope is defined as a transient loss of consciousness accompanied by unresponsiveness and loss of postural tone with spontaneous recovery. It is associated with bradycardia and hypotension.

Incidence

Syncope is most likely to occur in the older adult; prevalence increases with age from 2% in ages 65 to 69 years to 12% in those older than 85 years.

Pathophysiology

Vasomotor syncope is caused by excessive vagal tone or impaired reflex control of the peripheral circulation (Massie & Amidon, 2001). Orthostatic hypotension is caused by autonomic neuropathy (diabetes), hypovolemia, and drugs. Cardiogenic syncope occurs in response to mechanical problems of the heart (e.g., aortic stenosis, cardiomyopathy) or automaticity (e.g., sick sinus syndrome) and conduction disorders. Another cause of syncope is carotid sinus hypersensitivity. Syncope usually occurs with tight collars or neck turning, such as with shaving.

Factors Increasing Susceptibility
- Pregnant women, as a result of a change in blood flow, particularly when changing position
- Smoking
- Increased stress
- Obstructed venous return to the heart
- Acute pain
- Fluid loss

ASSESSMENT: SUBJECTIVE/HISTORY
Symptoms
- Prodromal period consists of nausea, headache, diaphoresis, pallor, sense of impending loss of consciousness.
- Recovery is rapid, with a postevent period of headache, fatigue, and nausea.
- Ask about the circumstances around the syncopal episode: what the client was doing, where he or she was, and a subjective description of the event. For women of childbearing age, ask for date of LMP and about contraceptive use.
- Timing of the syncopal episode is critical: Does it occur after micturition, defecation, coughing, or swallowing? These events may lead to a transient hypotension that

results in syncope. If after exercise, consider cardio-genic source of syncope.

- Chest pain
- Shortness of breath
- Pleuritic chest pain

Past Medical History

- Hypotension
- Cardiovascular or peripheral vascular disease
- Atrial fibrillation
- Ventricular aneurysms
- Aortic stenosis
- Hypoglycemia
- Seizures
- Pulmonary disease
- Carotid artery disease

Medication History

- Medications can provoke carotid sinus hypersensitiv-ity (e.g., digitalis, beta-blockers, alpha-methyldopa, and calcium-channel blockers).
- In older adults, the medications most likely to cause syncope are phenothiazine, tricyclic antidepressants, adrenergic blocking drugs, diuretics, and antihyperten-sive medications.

Family History

- History of cardiovascular disease
- History of CVA

Dietary History

Syncope can be precipitated by swallowing, so the timing in relationship to meals is important. Also, if the client is taking antihypertensive medications with a meal or just before, hypotension can develop, causing a syncopal episode. Poor nutrition can also cause dehydration and hypotension, leading to syncope.

ASSESSMENT: OBJECTIVE/PHYSICAL EXAMINATION
Physical Examination

- A complete physical examination is indicated with a chief complaint of syncope. Special attention should be paid to the cardiovascular examination. Orthostatic vital signs should be taken, and hydration status should be assessed.
- A decrease in blood pressure of 20 mm Hg or greater upon arising from the supine to standing position oc-curs in orthostatic hypotension. Tachycardia may also occur, providing the autonomic nervous system is functioning.

Diagnostic Procedures
Laboratory Tests
- CBC
- Electrolytes

- Glucose
- Creatine kinase
- Possibly troponin I if MI is a possibility.

Radiologic Tests
- Obtain echocardiogram if history of heart disease.
- If trauma to head during syncopal episode, consider CT scan of head.
- Consider carotid artery Doppler study if any indication of CNS problem.

Other Tests
- An ECG may reveal arrhythmias.
- Consider doing 3-day Holter monitoring.
- Consider tilt table.
- Consider other electrophysiologic testing if all other test results are negative.

DIAGNOSIS

Seizure is often confused with syncope. In syncope, motor activity is less common and incontinence rarely occurs. However, differential diagnoses include all of the follow-ing:

- Pulmonary embolus
- MI
- Vasovagal syncope
- Situational syncope
- Drug-induced syncope
- Orthostatic hypotension
- Postprandial hypotension
- Aortic stenosis
- Pulmonary HTN
- Idiopathic hypertrophic subaortic stenosis
- Carotid sinus syncope
- Subclavian steal
- Coronary artery disease
- Transient ischemic attack
- Seizure
- Psychogenic syncope
- Left atrial myxoma
- Tetralogy of Fallot
- Arrhythmias
- Hypoglycemia
- Pregnancy

THERAPEUTIC PLAN
Nonpharmacologic Treatment

- Sleep in a semi-erect position.
- Wear waist-high elastic hosiery.
- Add salt supplementation to diet.
- Postprandial hypotension is improved with caffeine.

Pharmacologic Treatment

- The therapeutic plan depends on the diagnosis. Con-sider using aspirin 81 mg/day for platelet inhibition.
- Vasoconstrictor agents may be used.

- Midodrine 2.5 to 10 mg tid may be prescribed.
- Ephedrine 15 to 30 mg tid may be prescribed.

Client Education

Clients should be educated to change positions slowly, waiting before actually moving after a position change has been made.

Referral/Consultation

Referral should be made to an appropriate specialist based on initial diagnostic test findings. In most cases, this is a cardiologist or a neurologist.

Prevention

- Avoid periods of prolonged recumbency.
- Avoid abrupt postural changes.

EVALUATION/FOLLOW-UP

Clients should be followed closely until a cause for the syncopal episode is known.

COMPLICATIONS

- Head injury
- Death

REFERENCES

Aminoff, M. (2001). Nervous system. In L. Tierney, S. McPhee, & M. Papadakis (Eds.), *Current medical diagnosis and treatment* (40th ed.). New York: McGraw-Hill.

Larson, L. (2000). Syncope. In D. Robinson, P. Kidd, & K. Rogers (Eds.), *Primary care across the lifespan.* St. Louis: Mosby.

Massie, B., & Amidon, T. (2001) Heart. In L. Tierney, S. McPhee, & M. Papadakis (Eds.), *Current medical diagnosis and treatment* (40th ed.). New York: McGraw-Hill.

Review Questions

1. All *except* which of the following can lead to a syncopal event?
   a. Micturition
   b. Swallowing
   c. Neck turning with shaving
   d. Sleeping

2. Which of the following is a medication that can cause carotid sinus hypersensitivity?
   a. Beta-blockers
   b. Aspirin
   c. Acetaminophen
   d. NSAIDs

3. Although a full physical examination is important when assessing a client with syncope, to what part of the examination should special attention be paid?
   a. Pulmonary systems
   b. GI systems
   c. Cardiovascular systems
   d. Ears, nose, and throat

4. Clients receiving antihypertensive medications should be taught which of the following?
   a. Take medications just before meals.
   b. Change positions slowly (from lying to standing, waiting a few minutes in sitting position before standing, and standing a few minutes before beginning to walk).
   c. Put the head between the knees before standing up.
   d. Skip medications if feeling light-headed.

5. Clients with a diagnosis of carotid sinus hypersensitivity should be taught which of the following?
   a. Avoid changing positions quickly.
   b. Avoid high-calorie meals.
   c. Avoid tight collars.
   d. Avoid sweets.

6. Which symptom or clinical sign differentiates syncope from generalized seizure?
   a. Headache before event
   b. Incontinence
   c. Impending loss of consciousness
   d. Actual loss of consciousness

Answers and Rationales

1. **Answer: d** (analysis/diagnosis)
   Rationale: Choices a and b are situational causes of syncope, and choice c refers to carotid sinus hypersensitivity; therefore choice d is the correct answer.

2. **Answer: a** (analysis/diagnosis)
   Rationale: Beta-blockers provoke carotid sinus hypersensitivity by their dilatory effect as well as slowing the electrical impulse.

3. **Answer: c** (assessment)
   Rationale: Although the cause of syncope is often undetermined, the most likely cause is cardiovascular.

4. **Answer: b** (implementation/plan)
   Rationale: Because of the effect of antihypertensive medications on the vascular tree, if clients are taught to change position slowly, the vascular tree is given a chance to adjust to the change so that the brain continues to be perfused adequately.

5. **Answer: c** (implementation/plan)
   Rationale: Tight collars may stimulate carotid sinus hypersensitivity by putting pressure on the carotid sinus and partially obstructing flow, particularly if the head is turned.

6. **Answer: b** (evaluation)
   Rationale: In syncope, motor activity is not common and incontinence rarely occurs. Loss of consciousness may occur in both conditions. Both conditions may be preceded by headache and a sense of impending unconsciousness.

SYPHILIS *Cheryl Pope Kish*

OVERVIEW
Definition

Syphilis is a complex multisystem disease caused by the spirochete *Treponema pallidum*. Historically, syphilis has been known as the "great imitator" because its symptoms mimic so many other illnesses.

Incidence

The incidence of syphilis varies greatly from country to country. Developing countries have a higher incidence. The World Health Organization reports 4 million cases worldwide. In the United States, prevalence is declining steadily because of federal and state programs. Incidence is highest in the southern states. There is a 60% occurrence rate in those 15 to 25 years old.

Pathology

- Pathogenesis: Exposure to the spirochete *T. pallidum* results in its rapid penetration through intact mucous membranes or abraded skin to the blood and lymphatics, where it causes a systemic infection. The median incubation period in humans is 21 days. A primary lesion develops at the site of inoculation. This lesion remains for 2 to 6 weeks and heals spontaneously.
- The generalized lesions, lymphadenopathy, and malaise of secondary syphilis usually appear 6 to 8 weeks after the primary lesion (chancre) heals. These lesions subside spontaneously in 2 to 6 weeks, and the affected person then enters the latent phase.
- The latent phase may be undetectable except by serologic examination. One third of untreated cases progress to tertiary syphilis, with manifestations such as cardiovascular syphilis, neurovascular syphilis, and gummas (granulomatous tumors involving various organs).
- Classification: Syphilis is classified into groups primarily on the basis of presenting clinical manifestations of the disease.
- Primary syphilis: After exposure to an infected individual, a primary lesion (chancre) develops at the site of inoculation in approximately 3 weeks (range is 3 to 90 days). This is a painless, indurated, clean-based lesion that may not be noticed, depending on its location. Common sites of this primary lesion, known as a chancre, include the penis, anus, cervix, vulva, and vagina. Without treatment, the chancre resolves in 3 to 6 weeks.
- Secondary syphilis: If untreated, primary syphilis progresses to a secondary stage between 2 weeks and 2 months. The secondary stage is characterized by a generalized, hyperpigmented, maculopapular rash that includes the palmar and plantar surfaces. Concomitant

symptoms include sore throat, fever, malaise, generalized nontender lymphadenopathy, and patchy alopecia, including scalp hair, eyebrows, and beard. Rarely, hepatitis and meningitis may also be seen. The secondary lesions of syphilis resolve within 2 to 10 weeks with or without treatment. Systemic involvement can occur in this stage or thereafter.
- Latency: The period of untreated resolution of symptoms of secondary syphilis, an asymptomatic stage, is called *latency* and is subdivided into early and late latency. Early latency is within 1 year of the initial infection. Late latency is longer than 1 year after the initial infection.
- Tertiary stage: Tertiary syphilis develops in up to 40% of untreated or undertreated persons. This stage is characterized by further involvement of multiple systems. It most commonly presents as neurosyphilis. CNS effects can include meningitis, cranial nerve involvement, focal lesions or stroke, paresis, dementia, ataxia, and tabes dorsalis (wide-based "steppage" gait). An eye abnormality, Argyll-Robertson pupils, are small, irregular pupils bilaterally that react to accommodation but not to light.
- Cardiovascular manifestations of tertiary syphilis are rare and include aortic damage, aneurysms, and valve insufficiency. Gummatous syphilis, also uncommon, is characterized by soft tissue, tumor-like lesions called gummas, in the skin, bone, liver, brain, or other organs. They are painless but progressively destructive lesions.
- Congenital syphilis refers to the form of syphilis transmitted from an infected mother to her unborn child through transplacental spread of the spirochete. The classic manifestations of congenital syphilis include maculopapular rash, snuffles, mucous patches, hepatosplenomegaly, jaundice, osteochondritis, chorioretinitis, and iritis.

Factors Increasing Susceptibility
- Unprotected sexual intercourse increases risk.
- Multiple sexual partners increases risk.
- Exchange of sex for drugs, especially crack cocaine, increases risk.
- History of other sexually transmitted illnesses increases risk.
- Infectivity: Approximately 50% of named contacts of primary and secondary syphilis become infected. The actual risk from a single exposure is probably lower.

ASSESSMENT: SUBJECTIVE/HISTORY
Symptoms

Primary Syphilis
- Chancre: painless ulcer at the site of inoculation, usually genital
- Lymphadenopathy, usually in the groin

S

Secondary Syphilis

- Rash, especially on palms of hands and soles of feet: nonpruritic, copper-colored
- Painless lymphadenopathy
- Fever, sore throat, and malaise
- Patchy hair loss
- Painless white mucous patches on mucous membranes
- Symptoms of meningitis or hepatitis

Tertiary Syphilis

- Subjective symptoms depend on the organ system or systems involved.
- Tertiary syphilis is usually found during an extensive workup on an inpatient basis.

Congenital Syphilis

- Snuffles (rhinitis)
- Maculopapular rash with desquamation and sloughing of the epithelium, particularly on the palms and soles
- Vesicular rash and bullae
- Congenital syphilis may be seen as saddle nose or anterior bowing of lower extremities.
- Abdominal organomegaly
- Anemia, thrombocytopenia

History of Present Illness

Ask about contact with an infected individual (specify what sort of contact, be specific).

Symptoms

- Determine when symptoms began, whether onset was acute or gradual, how many days, weeks, or months symptoms have persisted (be specific).
- Ask about associated symptoms, including discharge, odor, dysuria, lesion, genital itch, abdominal rash, or scrotal pain.
- Determine presence of precipitating factors, whether the client has had unprotected sex.
- Ask about any relieving factors.
- Determine what kinds of treatments have been used so far.

Past Medical History

- Previous STDs: When they occurred, type, course, and treatment, compliance with treatment, test of cure
- Sexual history: Number of partners, sexual preference, last exposure, type of exposure, use of barrier contraception or other birth control, use of sex acts to obtain money or drugs
- Gynecologic history: LMP/normal, pregnancy status (gravida, para, abortus), last Pap smear and results

Medication History

- Present medications: prescription, OTC, illicit
- Drug allergies
- Note particularly antibiotics used in preceding 2 weeks

Psychosocial History

- Assess economic factors, including whether the client can afford medications and whether the client has access to follow-up care.
- Assess alcohol or drug history.
- Determine whether client uses intravenous or intramuscular drugs.
- Travel: Yaws, endemic syphilis, and pinta are three nonvenereal *Treponematoses*. These must be considered in clients who have traveled to developing countries.

ASSESSMENT: OBJECTIVE/PHYSICAL EXAMINATION

Physical Examination

- Check vital signs.
- Inspect skin and hair (note patchy alopecia in a pattern opposite to that of male pattern baldness: progresses from occiput to temples, with loss of eyelashes and lateral third of eyebrows).
- Examine mouth, noting ulcers, exudate, patches, and pharyngitis.
- Palpate lymph nodes (neck, supraclavicular, axillary, epitrochlear, inguinal).
- Auscultate the heart and lungs.
- Perform a neurologic examination.
- Assess the genital and perianal areas for lesions and rashes.

Diagnostic Procedures

- Consider testing for multiple STDs.
- Screen for pregnancy to enable early treatment: Congenital syphilis is preventable if maternal syphilis is treated in early pregnancy. Nontreponemal tests should be used for screening, and positive results should be confirmed with treponemal testing.
- Darkfield microscopy is a definitive test for syphilis. Allows identification of *T. pallidum* from serous exudate from lesion examined under a microscope in a properly equipped lab by specially trained personnel.
- Serology tests are the following:
  - Nontreponemal tests: Results are either reactive (positive) or nonreactive (negative). Titers correlate with disease activity. Reactive results need confirmation with treponemal tests.
    - Venereal Disease Research Laboratory (VDRL) test
    - Rapid plasma reagin (RPR) test
  - Treponemal tests
    - Fluorescent treponemal antibody absorption (FTA-ABS) test
    - Microhemagglutination assay for antibody to *T. pallidum* (MHA-TP) test
  - Once positive, the FTA-ABS, VDRL, and RPR usually remain reactive indefinitely regardless of treatment or disease activity.

- Culture of cerebrospinal fluid to detect neurosyphilis.

DIAGNOSIS

Differential diagnoses include the following:
- Primary syphilis
- Secondary syphilis
- Tertiary or late syphilis
- Congenital syphilis
- Other: herpes simplex virus

THERAPEUTIC PLAN
Nonpharmacologic Treatment

The nonpharmacologic treatment focuses on client education and prevention of transmission to sexual partners and the fetus in an infected mother.

Pharmacologic Treatment

- Primary and secondary syphilis of less than 1 year duration (adult)
  - Benzathine penicillin G 2.4 million units IM
  - Only use alternative if client is allergic to penicillin and not pregnant (may refer for desensitization).
  - Doxycycline, 100 mg PO bid for 14 days
  - Tetracycline, 500 mg qid for 14 days
  - Erythromycin, 500 mg PO qid for 14 days
- Primary and secondary syphilis of less than 1 year duration (child): Give benzathine penicillin G 50,000 units/kg IM, total 2.4 million units or less.
- Late latent and tertiary syphilis: Give benzathine penicillin G 2.4 million units IM every week for 3 weeks.
- Syphilis in Pregnancy
  - Penicillin, 2.4 million units IM (dosage and type of penicillin are debatable)
  - No alternative is available in pregnancy. All the traditional alternatives have unacceptable side effects.

Client Education

- Jarisch-Herxheimer reaction is thought to be a reaction to lysis of treponemes. It occurs in approximately 30% of clients treated for primary syphilis and 70% of those treated for secondary syphilis within 24 hours of treatment. Usually, presenting symptoms are fever, chills, myalgia, headache, palpations, flushing, and so on, but it can be severe enough to cause hypotension. Mild forms can be treated with aspirin. More severe forms require emergency care to prevent end-organ damage. The reaction in pregnant women may trigger labor or cause fetal distress; pregnant women should be advised to seek care immediately if contractions or decreased fetal movement occur.
- Explain importance of compliance with medication if one of the multidose, multiday therapies is initiated.
- Explain importance of barrier protection, including correct use of condoms.
- Encourage client to inform partner of STDs.

- Advise abstinence during treatment and until symptoms resolve.
- Identify of chancre and other signs of STDs in partners.
- Encourage client to limit partners; use barrier protection.
- Explain the risk of other STDs.
- Advise HIV testing and counseling as appropriate.

Prevention

- Screen new sex partners.
- Use condoms.
- Abstain while lesions are present.
- Undergo treatment in early pregnancy to prevent congenital disease.

Referral/Consultation

- Pregnancy
- Penicillin allergy
- HIV positivity
- Persistent elevation of titer
- Late latent syphilis
- Gummas
- Neurosyphilis
- Cardiovascular syphilis
- Congenital syphilis

EVALUATION/FOLLOW-UP

- Nontreponemal tests at 1 month after treatment and then every 3 months for at least 1 year are required for evaluation. Adequate treatment of primary or secondary syphilis is indicated by a fourfold decrease in the titer by 3 months and by 6 months in latent syphilis. Some clients have a VDRL result that remains unchanged on subsequent testing after treatment. These clients are considered "serofast" or "seroresistant." For most clients, the titer continues to decrease until it is nonreactive. A fourfold increase in the titer indicates a reinfection that requires further treatment.
- A VDRL result obtained from cord blood of a neonate may be reactive as a result of the passive transfer of antibodies from the mother. A VDRL should be performed every month for 3 or 4 months to determine whether the titer is rising or falling. If the titer falls or becomes nonreactive, then the infant had maternal transfer and not congenital syphilis.
- Syphilis is a reportable disease.

COMPLICATIONS

- With untreated syphilis during pregnancy, up to 40% of infants die, and those who survive have the congenital form of the illness.
- Tertiary syphilis is associated with long-term complications impacting the quality of life. Twenty-eight percent of those with tertiary syphilis die from the illness.
- Untreated disease or undertreatment is a public health concern because of the risk of transmission of a long-

term progressive disease, which can ultimately cause dementia and death.

REFERENCES

Birnbaum, N. R., Goldschmidt, R. H., & Buffett, W. O. (1999). Resolving the common clinical dilemmas of syphilis. *American Family Physician, 59*(8), 2233-2242.

Cash, J. C., & Glass, C. A. (2000). *Family practice guidelines.* Philadelphia: Lippincott.

Gerrig, J. N. (1998). Preventing and recognizing STDs in the adolescent. *Lippincott's Primary Care Practice, 2*(3), 312-314.

Hawkins, J. W., Roberto-Nichols, D. M., & Stanley-Haney, J. L. (1997). *Protocols for nurse practitioners in gynecologic settings.* New York: Tiresias Press.

Rawlins, S. (2001). Nonviral sexually transmitted infections. *Journal of Obstetric and Gynecologic Neonatal Nursing, 30*(3), 324-331.

Robinson, D., Kidd, P., & Rogers, K. M. (2000). *Primary care across the lifespan.* St. Louis: Mosby.

Shaffa, S. D. (1998). Vaginitis and sexually transmitted diseases. In E. Q. Youngkin & M. S. Davis (Eds.), *Women's health care: A primary care clinical guide* (2nd ed., pp. 265-300). Stamford, CT: Appleton & Lange.

Smith, M. A., & Shimp, L. A. (2000). *20 common problems in women's health care.* New York: McGraw-Hill.

Star, W. L., Lommel, L. L., & Shannon, M. T. (1995). *Women's primary health care: Protocols for practice.* Washington, DC: American Nurses Publishing.

Trotto, N. E. (1999). Are you up to date? *Patient Care,* May 30, 74-76, 81, 85-103.

Uphold, C. R., & Graham, M. V. (1998). *Clinical guidelines in family practice.* Gainesville, FL: Armarrae Books.

Review Questions

1. Tia is a 20-year-old woman who comes to your clinic with a generalized maculopapular rash that includes her palmar and plantar surfaces. She has been living in a metropolitan area, has no regular source of income, and has a history of crack cocaine use. She has syphilis diagnosed. What stage of syphilis does she have?

  a. Primary
  b. Secondary
  c. Tertiary
  d. Late latent

2. Mark is a 25-year-old marketing executive. He is married and has two children. Mark has made an appointment to discuss a penile lesion. Several weeks ago on a business trip, he had unprotected intercourse with a woman he met at the hotel bar. Since returning home, he has had unprotected intercourse with his wife. If this is syphilis, which of the following would apply to the lesion?

  a. The lesion would be a painful erosion associated with tender inguinal lymph nodes.
  b. The lesion would be a painless, indurated lesion associated with rubbery inguinal lymph nodes.
  c. The lesion would be an indication of an early stage that is too early to be transmitted to his wife.

  d. The lesion would be a sign of irreversible damage associated with syphilis.

3. To determine the efficacy of treatment for syphilis, which of the following quantitative tests should be done?

  a. Microscopic examination
  b. Dark-field examination
  c. VDRL
  d. Scraping of the lesion

4. One diagnostic test for syphilis is examination of a scraping from a suspected chancre under a dark-field microscope. A positive test result would show which of the following?

  a. A Gram-positive diplococcus
  b. Clue cells and many WBCs
  c. Giant cells
  d. A corkscrew-shaped organism

5. A 15-year-old anonymous female client arrives at the STD clinic after being told by her boyfriend that she needs to go to the clinic because he had syphilis. She is anxious, hostile, and angry. The best way to treat her exposure to syphilis and to ensure compliance is to treat her with which of the following?

  a. Treat with ceftriaxone (Rocephin), 250 mg IM 1.
  b. Treat with benzathine penicillin G, 2.4 million units IM.
  c. Nothing, wait until serology returns before treatment.
  d. Treat with erythromycin, 500 mg PO qid for 14 days.

6. Mr. Craig is a middle-aged man who presents for a job-required RPR. Results are positive. His history is indicative of some risk for exposure to STDs. What action by the NP is appropriate?

  a. Swab urethra to obtain fluid for dark-field microscopy.
  b. Order FTA-ABS to determine diagnosis of syphilis.
  c. Treat him with procaine penicillin.
  d. Order VDRL to confirm RPR findings.

7. A woman at 30 weeks' gestation is treated for primary syphilis. The NP provides anticipatory guidance related to the Jarisch-Herxheimer reaction. Which statement by the client indicates a need for further instruction?

  a. "I may have fever, headache, and muscle aches in the next 24 hours as the treatment begins to break down the infection."
  b. "If I have this reaction to treatment, Tylenol should make me feel better."
  c. "This reaction you described means I have a serious allergy to penicillin and should go to the emergency department."
  d. "If the reaction you described causes labor contractions or changes in fetal movement, I should seek care immediately."

8. When should a person treated for syphilis have an initial follow-up visit?

  a. 3 months
  b. 6 months
  c. 9 months
  d. 12 months

9. Which of the following drugs is appropriate for treating primary syphilis in a client with an allergy to penicillin?

TENDONITIS/BURSITIS *Denise Robinson*

OVERVIEW
Definition
Inflammation of tendons and bursae of involved joints

Incidence
- After low back pain, shoulder pain is a common problem in middle-aged adults.
- Stages of impingement syndrome occur in the shoulder (Table 3-108).
  - Bursitis (subacromial, subdeltoid)
  - Tendinitis (rotator cuff, biceps tendon, calcific tendinitis)
  - Rotator cuff tears

Pathophysiology
- A bursa is a thin-walled sac lined with synovial tissue located where tendons rub against tendons. Its purpose is to act as a shock absorber and to reduce friction. Bursitis is an inflammation of the synovium. Common locations include the following:
  - Subacromial bursa (located superior to the glenohumeral joint, above the supraspinatus muscle and below the acromion)
  - Olecranon bursa (facilitates smooth movement of the skin over the olecranon during elbow flexion and extension)
  - Ischial bursa
  - Trochanteric
  - Prepatellar bursa
- A tendon is a cord that attaches a muscle to a bone. Repetitive overuse causes micro-tears of the tendons, which become inflamed and painful. Common locations include the following:
  - Epicondyle (tennis elbow or golf elbow)
  - Rotator cuff, consisting of four muscles: subscapularis, supraspinatus, infraspinatus, and teres minor (subacromial bursa provides lubrication for rotator cuff; rotator cuff is stabilizer of glenohumeral joint)

Factors Increasing Susceptibility
- Age
- Overuse
- Instability of glenohumeral joint
- Poorly vascularized tendons
- Rotary motions of forearm
- Diabetes mellitus

ASSESSMENT: SUBJECTIVE/HISTORY
History Associated with Present Illness
Ask about the following:
- Dominant hand
- Frequent lifting overhead (e.g., painting)
- Frequent elbow flexing (e.g., swimming, gymnastics, weight lifting)
- Direct trauma to the elbow
- Repeated rotary movements of the elbow
- Pain: onset, location, radiation, interference with sleep
- Cause of pain: lifting, fall, motor vehicle accident, injury at work, pulling, sports injury, no apparent cause
- Pain with movements of putting on coat, combing hair, washing back
- Sleeping on side
- Swelling
- Fever
- Weak, stiff, or loose joint
- Limitations in range of motion (ROM) of affected joint
- Current ability to work

Relieving/Aggravating Factors
- Treatments that have been tried and associated results
- History of bursitis or tendonitis (any tests or injections)

Symptoms
- Erythema
- Pain with ROM

TABLE **3-108** Impingement Syndrome in the Shoulder

STAGE	CLIENTS MOST LIKELY AFFECTED	SYMPTOMS
I: Bursitis	Athletes younger than 25 years (swimmers, throwers)	Pain after exercise or activity Mild, dull ache
II: Tendonitis	Occurs most commonly in laborers who reach overhead, ages 25-40 years	Pain occurs during activity as well as after Pain is vague but increases in intensity, usually during sleep
III: Rotator cuff tear	Laborers younger than 40 years with long history of shoulder problems	Sudden severe episode of pain Pain occurs during activity, after activity, and during sleep Stiffness and weakness

From Robinson, D. (2000). Bursitis. In D. Robinson, P. Kidd, & K. Rogers (Eds.), *Primary care across the lifespan* (p. 1077). St. Louis: Mosby.

T

- Swelling
- Pain on palpation

Past Medical History

- Previous joint surgery of affected part
- Arthritis

Medication History

- Use of nonsteroidal antiinflammatory drugs (NSAIDs) or other analgesics for pain
- Other medications

Family History

Determine whether family members have arthritis.

Psychosocial History

- History of alcohol use
- History of smoking
- Occupation that require lifting or repetitive movements (e.g., mining, painting)

ASSESSMENT: OBJECTIVE/PHYSICAL EXAMINATION

Physical Examination

Focused physical examination is conducted with particular attention to the following:

- General: Check the client's overall appearance and response to pain.
- Observe for swelling, erythema, atrophy, or asymmetry.
- Palpate for tenderness or swelling.
- Conduct a head compression test.
- Screen for cervical spine pathologic abnormality. Have the client sit. Gently but firmly apply pressure to the client's head. Pain localized to the neck indicates disk degeneration. Burning pain or pain down the shoulder or arm implies nerve root involvement, in which case a detailed neurologic examination should be performed.
- Check ROM.
- Perform Apley's scratch test: Have the client place his or her arm and hand behind the back to try to touch opposite scapula.
- Check the impingement sign.
- Check for a point of tenderness at the greater tuberosity of the humerus.
- Check for a painful arc of abduction.
- Neer impingement sign: Bring the client's arm into full flexion and note whether the pain increases.
- Hawkins impingement sign: Flex the client's arm to 90 degrees, bend the elbow internally so as to rotate the shoulder, and note whether pain increases.
See Table 3-109.

DIAGNOSIS

Differential diagnoses include the following:

- Arthritis or autoimmune disorders
- Septic bursitis or arthritis
- Crystal deposition
- Reflex sympathetic dystrophy
- Osteoarthritis
- Fibromyalgia
- Tumor

Most likely diagnoses related to shoulder pain are the following:

- Impingement syndrome
  - Bursitis: subacromial, subdeltoid
  - Tendonitis: rotator cuff, biceps tendon, calcific tendonitis
  - Rotator cuff tear
- Shoulder instability
- Adhesive capsulitis (frozen shoulder)
- Inflammation of the acromioclavicular joint

THERAPEUTIC PLAN

The treatment plan should address both pain management and facilitation of healing through rehabilitation. Use of the following PRICEMM mnemonic may be helpful (Salzman, 1997):

- **P**rotection: Use padding, braces, and changes in technique to avoid future injury.
- **R**est: Avoid activities that exacerbate pain.
- **I**ce: Apply to affected site for 20 minutes, 3 times a day.
- **C**ompression: Apply elastic bandage over swollen bursae (olecranon).
- **E**levation: Elevate affected limb above heart.
- **M**odalities: Physical modalities are ultrasound, electric stimulation, and heat.
- **M**edications: Prescribe NSAIDs, acetaminophen, or injectable corticosteroids.

Pharmacologic Treatment

NSAIDs are indicated for musculoskeletal injury. NSAIDs inhibit prostaglandin synthesis and decrease pain. *Do not* prescribe NSAIDs to those with peptic ulcer disease, allergy to NSAIDs or aminosalicylic acid (ASA), renal dysfunction, or pregnant women.

Nonpharmacologic Treatment

- Activity should be modified to prevent further injury.
- Pain should be the guide regarding extent of activity.
- ROM should be continued to prevent loss of function, especially in the shoulder.
- Physical therapy should be initiated.
  - Specific exercises to strengthen the rotator cuff
  - Flexibility exercises
  - Ultrasound to reduce inflammation by molecular vibration
- Use elbow cushion for olecranon bursitis.
- Splinting of elbow in 90 degrees of flexion for epicondylitis for 3 to 5 days may be helpful.

TABLE **3-109** Physical Examination Findings Based on Cause of Pain

CAUSE	CHARACTERISTICS	KEY PHYSICAL EXAMINATION TESTS
Subacromial/ subdeltoid bursitis	Shoulder pain with insidious onset worse at night; no specific injury recalled	ROM with elevation, internal rotation, and abduction
	Overhead lifting is uncomfortable	Most painful motion between 70 and 120 degrees of abduction Impingement sign: forcibly forward flexing the internally rotated arm more than 90 degrees if pain produced
Rotator cuff injury	Pain, weakness, and loss of motion Pain is with overhead or above-the-shoulder activities Pain worse at night (wakes from sleep) and when lying on shoulder	Anterior/lateral tenderness Assess for signs of impingement: moving shoulder through passive ROM (forward flexion, internal and external rotation with arm abducted 90 degrees with 5 to 10 lb of force directed inferiorly on acromion, narrowing subacromial space
Adhesive capsulitis (frozen shoulder)	Pain when putting on coat or washing back Decreased ability to go to sleep	Putting on coat or washing back (external rotation of shoulder) Pain implies adhesive capsulitis
Little League shoulder	Pain with throwing motion	Injury to proximal humeral physis of an adolescent resulting from repetitive stress of throwing Later presents as tendonitis in adult
Olecranon bursitis	Tender, swollen area of redness on back of elbow 40% have history of trauma to bursa	Goose egg swelling at tip of elbow
Epicondylitis: medial (golf)	Pain on medial or lateral aspect of elbow, made worse by grasping	Pain is most noticed 1 to 2 cm distal to epicondyle Resisted dorsiflexion or volar flexion may cause pain
Lateral (tennis)	Pain may radiate into arm or distally into forearm	Normal ROM, no swelling, normal radiograph results
Trochanteric bursitis	More common in women than in men Pain in lateral hip and proximal thigh Worsened when sitting in chair or car	Tenderness over greater trochanter Pain with hip flexion and external rotation Leg length discrepancies may exist ROM usually normal and painless
Prepatellar bursitis	Pain, swelling, and redness over knee Trigger is usually minor trauma (kneeling on floors)	Swelling over patella No distention of knee joint
Baker cyst	Swelling behind knee May have sense of fullness behind knee	Cystic swelling in popliteal space If bursa ruptures: acute swelling of lower leg, mimicking deep vein thrombosis

From Robinson, D., Kidd, P., & Rogers, K. (2000). *Primary care across the lifespan.* St. Louis: Mosby.
ROM, Range of motion.

- Apply a compression band for chronic epicondylitis.
- Leg length discrepancies may be part of the cause of trochanteric bursitis, and shoe lifts may be helpful to reduce pain.

Client Education

- Emphasize the importance of active rest (keep doing ROM exercises).

- A sling may be helpful initially (emphasize the need to continue ROM exercises to prevent frozen shoulder).
- Explain the benefits of NSAIDs.
- Teach exercises that restore normal function, including the following:
  - Begin with ROM exercises.
  - Work up to resistance exercises using rubber bands or light weights.

- Continue with resistance training with weight machines or free weights.
- Aerobic exercises help by increasing blood flow to site.
- Stop smoking.
- Surgery may be needed for tears to tendons when pain continues or if there is weakness.

Referral

- Corticosteroid injection
  - If conservative measures do not work in 3 to 4 weeks, consider referring for injection.
  - Administer no more than three injections during a 12-week period.
  - Do not repeat series in less than 12 months from previous injection.
- Surgery
  - Consider referral for surgery if no improvement is achieved after 3 months of therapy.
  - Perform arthroscopy to debride subacromial space.
- Rehabilitation exercises

Consultation

Discuss options of steroid injection.

Prevention

- Adequate warmup before commencing activities
- Good level of conditioning before new activities attempted
- Complications associated with treatment failure are the following:
  - Limited ROM
  - Pain

EVALUATION/FOLLOW-UP

Return as close as possible to normal ROM and pain-free status.

REFERENCES

Benjamin, J. (1993) Hip pain. In H. Green, W. Johnson, & M. Maricic (Eds.), *Decision making in medicine* (pp. 398-399). St. Louis: Mosby.

Brunet, M., Norwood, L., & Sykes, T. (1997). What to do for the painful shoulder. *Patient Care*, 56-83.

Burckhardt, C., Jones, K., & Clark, S. (1998). Soft tissue problems associated with rheumatic disease. *Lippincott's Primary Care Practitioner, 2*(1), 20-29.

Fongemie, A., Buss, D., & Rolnick, S. (1998). Management of shoulder impingement syndrome and rotator cuff tears. *American Family Physician, 57*(4), 667-678.

Genovese, M. (1998). Joint and soft-tissue injection: A useful adjuvant to systemic and local treatment. *Postgraduate Medicine, 103*(2), 125-134.

Reveille, J. (1997). Soft tissue rheumatism: Diagnosis and treatment. *The American Journal of Medicine, 102*(suppl. 1A), 24S-29S.

Robinson, D. (2000). Tendinitis/bursitis. In D. Robinson, P. Kidd, & K. Rogers (Eds.), *Primary care across the lifespan.* St. Louis: Mosby.

Rotator cuff injuries: When your shoulder throws you a curve. (1998). *Mayo Clinic Health Letter, 16*(2), 1-3.

Salzman, K., Lillegard, W., & Butcher, J. (1996). Lower extremity bursitis. *American Family Physician, 53*(7), 2317-2324.

Salzman, K., Lillegard, W., & Butcher, J. (1997). Upper extremity bursitis. *American Family Physician, 56*(7), 1797-1812.

Review Questions

1. Which of the following historical indications is consistent with a diagnosis of subacromial bursitis?
  - **a.** Pain at night when sleeping
  - **b.** Pain when arm abducted to shoulder height
  - **c.** Pain when weight carried in arm only
  - **d.** Pain when shoulder touched

2. Which of the following signs noted at the time of physical examination is consistent with subacromial bursitis?
  - **a.** Positive impingement sign
  - **b.** Positive Tinel's sign
  - **c.** Positive Phalen's maneuver
  - **d.** Positive Patrick's sign

3. Missy has been diagnosed with tennis elbow. This implies pain at what location?
  - **a.** Medial epicondyle
  - **b.** Lateral epicondyle
  - **c.** Olecranon
  - **d.** Epicondyle and olecranon

4. Which of the following is the treatment of choice for subacromial bursitis?
  - **a.** Surgery
  - **b.** Splint
  - **c.** NSAIDs
  - **d.** Sling

5. Which of the following comments by a client with tendonitis indicates a need for further teaching?
  - **a.** "I should do gentle exercises if the pain is not bad."
  - **b.** "NSAIDs should be taken with food."
  - **c.** "Ice to the affected area is helpful."
  - **d.** "I can continue with my swimming."

Answers and Rationales

1. *Answer:* b (assessment)
  Rationale: Clients with subacromial bursitis complain of pain when the arm is lifted and when lifting overhead (Robinson, 2000).

2. *Answer:* a (assessment)
  Rationale: Positive results of an impingement test are indicative of subacromial bursitis (Robinson, 2000).

3. *Answer:* b (analysis/diagnosis)
   Rationale: Tennis elbow refers to pain in the lateral epicondyle. Golf elbow refers to pain in the medial epicondyle (Robinson, 2000).

4. *Answer:* c (implementation/plan)
   Rationale: The treatment for bursitis and tendonitis is rest, ice, compression, and elevation (RICE) or PRICEMM. Both advocate the use of antiinflammatory medications (Robinson, 2000).

5. *Answer:* d (evaluation)
   Rationale: The client should avoid activities that worsen the pain. Gentle exercises, ice, and NSAIDs are all appropriate. Once the pain is gone, the client can continue swimming (Robinson, 2000).

TESTICULAR/SCROTAL MASS   *Pamela Kidd*

OVERVIEW
Definition

A hydrocele is a result of the collection of fluid between the two layers of the tunica vaginalis in the scrotum. A varicocele is the result of dilation of the veins in the spermatic cord. Testicular cancer is a tumor of the testicles.

Incidence

- Although most common in infants, hydroceles can form as a result of testicular pathologic abnormality in adult men.
- Varicoceles are most common in older boys and adolescents and are rare before puberty. They are present in up to 20% of all males.
- A varicocele is a result of dilated veins in the spermatic cord. It can be associated with infertility in adulthood.
- Testicular cancer is tumor of the testis and is most common in young men, with an average age of 32 years. It represents 1% of all cancers in males.

Pathophysiology

- Hydroceles are described as communicating and non-communicating. In a communicating hydrocele, the processus vaginalis is patent between the peritoneal cavity and the tunica vaginalis, allowing the peritoneal fluid to shift back and forth through this opening. In a noncommunicating hydrocele, the processus vaginalis has closed, but there is residual fluid in the tunica vaginalis.
- Communicating hydroceles can be associated with inguinal hernias and usually occur at birth or during the neonatal period.
- Hydroceles in adulthood are usually associated with testicular pathologic abnormality.
- Varicoceles are caused by incompetent valves of the internal spermatic venous system. Left-sided varicoceles are most common; their cause is unknown. Right-sided varicoceles may represent acute venous obstruction from tumor or intraabdominal pathologic abnormality.
- Varicoceles are associated with male infertility. The exact cause is unknown but is speculated to be a result of alteration of scrotal temperature secondary to increased blood flow, which affects spermatogenesis and sperm motility.
- Approximately 97% of testicular tumors are germinal in origin. Seminoma is the most common, with embryonal cell carcinoma, teratoma, and choriocarcinoma being the next most common. Testicular tumors spread along the lymphatic system in predictable and preferential pathways.
- There is a significant increase in the incidence of testicular cancer in clients with cryptorchidism. Cancer can develop in both the undescended and the contralateral descended testis.

Factors Increasing Susceptibility. The exact exposure is not known, but miners, oil and gas workers, food and beverage processors, and janitors have increased risk of testicular cancer.

Protective Factors. Testicular self-examination is important.

ASSESSMENT: SUBJECTIVE/HISTORY
Symptoms

Hydrocele
- Inquire about onset and duration, constant or intermittent pattern of scrotal swelling, pain, and color change.
- Inquire about associated swelling or mass in the inguinal area.
- A communicating hydrocele in an infant often presents with progressive swelling throughout the day and resolves overnight.
- New onset of a hydrocele in an adult or scrotal hemorrhage after minor trauma may be a sign of testicular cancer.

Varicocele
- Inquire about onset and duration, pattern of swelling (including intermittent or constant, left-sided or right-sided), and pain (including heaviness).
- Varicoceles are often described as a "bag of worms."
- Most varicoceles are asymptomatic.
- Inquire about associated infertility, if appropriate.

T

Testicular Cancer

- Inquire about onset and duration, increasing size of mass, and presence of pain.
- Inquire about associated symptoms of a hydrocele or hemorrhage from trauma.
- Inquire about the practice of testicular self-examination.

Past Medical History

- Inquire about past genitourinary surgery or history of an undescended testis.
- History of human immunodeficiency virus (HIV) increases risk.
- Determine whether the client has previously been treated for testicular cancer.

Medication History

Noncontributory.

Family History

Family history of testicular cancer increases risk.

Dietary History

Noncontributory.

ASSESSMENT: OBJECTIVE/PHYSICAL EXAMINATION
Physical Examination

- Assess for gynecomastia. A client with a suspicious testicular mass may or may not have associated gynecomastia.
- Perform an abdominal examination.
- Palpate the inguinal area for swelling, masses, or pain. Assess for lymphadenopathy.
- Inspect scrotum and testes for size, shape, symmetry, swelling, masses, lesions, and color in both a supine and a standing position.
- Palpate each testis specifically for the epididymis and vas deferens.
- Assess swelling or masses by transillumination. Hydroceles produce brilliant transillumination.
- New onset of a hydrocele in an adult is often associated with testicular pathologic abnormality.
- Testicular cancer does not transilluminate and is free of fixation from the scrotum.
- Tumor often replaces the testicle, making the testicle difficult to discern on examination.
- Ultrasound is indicated to help define suspicious masses.

Diagnostic Procedures

- Ultrasonography differentiates fluid from solid masses and intratesticular from extratesticular masses.
- The following tumor marker screenings differentiate origin of testicular tumors:
  - Serum alpha fetoprotein (AFP)

- Human chorionic gonadotropin (HCG)
- Lactic dehydrogenase
- Semen analysis is indicated when a client has a varicocele and infertility is questioned.

DIAGNOSIS

- Inguinal hernia is commonly associated with scrotal mass.
- Testicular torsion is a sudden onset of severe scrotal pain caused by twisting of testicular appendages.
- Epididymitis is the most common cause of painful scrotal swelling in postpubertal males; associated with fever, urethral discharge, and urinary symptoms, including pyuria.
- Acute orchitis is a red, warm, painful, sudden swelling of the testes associated with viral parotitis (mumps).
- Spermatocele is a cyst that contains sperm and is well circumscribed, does not transilluminate, and persists when client is supine.
- Cryptorchidism is the failure of testes to descend into scrotum.

THERAPEUTIC PLAN
Nonpharmacologic Treatment

Hydrocele

- In infancy, a hydrocele usually resolves spontaneously during the first year of life and requires no specific therapy.
- If the hydrocele is associated with an inguinal hernia, referral to a surgeon is indicated at any age.
- An adult with a hydrocele needs further evaluation to rule out testicular pathologic abnormality. Ultrasonography may be indicated.

Varicocele

- Most varicoceles are asymptomatic and do not require treatment.
- If pain is present, causing a dull ache or heavy sensation, refer the client for surgical evaluation.
- A right-sided varicocele warrants evaluation of an intraabdominal obstruction at any age.
- A left-sided varicocele with sudden onset in an older man warrants evaluation for a possible renal tumor with resultant occlusion of the spermatic vein.
- If infertility is a concern and the client has an abnormal semen evaluation, refer the client for surgical correction.

Testicular Cancer

- Computed tomography (CT) of the abdomen may be indicated for staging of disease.
- Radiography of the chest and CT of the lungs may also be indicated to assess for metastatic disease.
- Surgical management of testicular cancer consists of radical orchiectomy with high ligation of the spermatic

cord via an inguinal approach. Bone marrow transplant and radiation therapy are also considered.

- Serum AFP and HCG levels, if previously elevated, can be monitored to determine recurrence of disease.
- Five-year survival rate exceeds 90% in most cases.

Pharmacologic Treatment

Chemotherapy.

Client Education

- Educate parents about the benign nature of hydroceles.
- Educate parents and adolescents about varicoceles and the possible association of infertility. Caution adolescents about the importance of appropriate birth control.
- Educate all adolescent and adult males about the importance of testicular self-examination.

Referral

Obtain surgical consult if indicated.

Prevention

Testicular self-examination beginning at puberty provides early detection. There are no preventative measures at this time.

EVALUATION/FOLLOW-UP

Fertility may need to be assessed after treatment.

COMPLICATIONS

- Metastasis
- Death
- Infertility

REFERENCES

Hagan, C., & White, J. (1999). Common but curable: Responding to symptoms of testicular cancer. *ADVANCE for Nurse Practitioners, 7*(4), 25-26, 28, 30.

Hoekelman, R. A. (1997). *Primary pediatric care* (3rd ed., pp. 1103-1104). St. Louis: Mosby.

Junnila, J., & Lassen, P. (1998). Testicular masses. *American Family Physician, 57*(4), 685-692.

Rogers, K. (2000). Testicular mass. In D. Robinson, P. Kidd, & K. Rogers (Eds.), *Primary care across the lifespan.* St. Louis: Mosby.

Review Questions

1. A client is diagnosed with a variocele. How should the nurse practitioner (NP) proceed with the client?
   a. Assess whether the client has experienced any sexual dysfunction.
   b. Determine whether the client wants to start a family.
   c. Warn the client that he is at higher risk for sexually transmitted diseases (STDs).
   d. Instruct the client that he must perform monthly testicular self-examinations because he is at higher risk for testicular cancer.

2. Which of the following increases the likelihood of testicular cancer?
   a. Repeated bicycle riding
   b. Saddle injury
   c. Vocation as a janitor
   d. 40 years of age

3. Which of the following is true of hydroceles?
   a. They may occur acutely.
   b. They result from dilated veins in the spermatic cord.
   c. They do not transilluminate.
   d. They are associated with cryptorchidism (failure of the testes to descend).

4. A client diagnosed with testicular cancer asks about his plan of care. What is the NP's answer?
   a. The survival rate is approximately 50%.
   b. Serum hormone levels will be monitored to determine recurrence after treatment.
   c. Management will be with radiation.
   d. Testicular self-examinations should *not* be performed right now.

Answers and Rationales

1. ***Answer:* b** (implementation/plan)
   Rationale: Varicoceles are associated with male infertility. Referral for fertility assessment and counseling may be needed. There are no associations between variocele and testicular cancer, sexual dysfunction, or STDs.

2. ***Answer:* c** (assessment)
   Rationale: Testicular cancer is most prevalent around age 32 years. Injury and repetitive motion are not associated with testicular cancer. Occupational exposure seems to be associated with testicular cancer, although the exact relationship is not known. Janitors are at higher risk, as are gas and oil workers, food and beverage workers, and miners.

3. ***Answer:* a** (analysis/diagnosis)
   Rationale: Hydroceles in an adult occur acutely and are associated with testicular cancer. They transilluminate well. Dilated veins in a spermatic cord are varicoceles. Hydroceles are not associated with cryptorchidism, but cryptorchidism is also associated with testicular cancer.

4. ***Answer:* b** (implementation/plan)
   Rationale: Testicular self-examinations should be performed because cancer could occur in the unaffected testicle. Serum AFP and HCG levels are monitored longitudinally to determine recurrence of the disease. Surgery is usually indicated, with radiation as an additional therapy. There is an approximate 90% survival rate.

T

THYROID DISEASE *Cheryl Pope Kish*

OVERVIEW
Definition

Hypothyroidism is the undersecretion of the thyroid hormones triiodothyronine (T3) and thyroxine (T4). It is termed *cretinism* when it causes brain damage as a congenital condition and *myxedema* when it is a life complication of hypothyroidism in adults. Hyperthyroidism is the oversecretion of a thyroid hormone. Thyroid nodules refer to tumors that occur in a thyroid gland that is otherwise normal.

Incidence

Hypothyroidism and hyperthyroidism have a prevalence of 0.5% in the general population, but have a higher prevalence in selected groups. Adults have an incidence of approximately 11% to 15% of hypothyroidism. Postmenopausal women are more at risk for developing hypothyroidism. Approximately one in 500 children is treated for hypothyroidism in the United States. Approximately 2% of the adult population has hyperthyroidism, most often young women, although it can occur in men and at any age.

Thyroid nodules occur in 2% to 3% of adults, usually three to four times more often in women than in men. Overall, altered thyroid function is the most common endocrine problem observed during primary care.

Pathophysiology

Two thyroid hormones, T3 and T4, are produced by the body. Production and release of T4 by the thyroid gland is regulated by the anterior pituitary gland by means of a thyroid-stimulating hormone (TSH). Increases in T4 or T3 result in decreased production of TSH, whereas decreases in T4 or T3 result in increased TSH production. TSH production is primarily regulated by thyrotropin-releasing hormone, which is produced by the hypothalamus. These mechanisms produce a negative feedback loop maintaining T4 and T3 within therapeutic ranges.

Primary Hypothyroidism. Primary hypothyroidism is an insufficient quantity of thyroid tissue or loss of functional thyroid tissue because of iatrogenic causes such as thyroidectomy or autoimmune responses (Hashimoto's disease). Hypothyroidism also often follows treatment of hyperthyroidism with radioactive iodine.

Secondary Hypothyroidism. Secondary hypothyroidism is less common. It usually occurs along with other anterior pituitary deficiencies and is most often caused by a pituitary tumor.

Hyperthyroidism. Hyperthyroidism is an increased level of thyroid secretion, usually as a result of an autoimmune disorder in which the body produces thyroid-stimulating antibodies against TSH receptors on the thyroid cells, pathologically stimulating the thyroid cells (Graves disease). Graves disease is the cause of hyperthyroidism in approximately 90% of cases. Various types of thyroiditis cause the other 10% of hyperthyroidism.

Thyroid Nodules. Nodules on the thyroid gland are usually thyroid adenoma, thyroid cyst, or thyroid carcinoma. Of these, only thyroid cancer poses a risk to the client.

Factors Increasing Susceptibility
- Newborn
- Strong familial history of thyroid disease
- Postpartum period
- History of autoimmune disorders
- Iatrogenic, surgical, or radiation treatments
- Medications
- Thyroid carcinoma: men, young age, history of neck irradiation, positive family history
- Obesity

ASSESSMENT: SUBJECTIVE/HISTORY
Symptoms
Hypothyroidism
- Congenital abnormalities
- Infrequent crying
- Hypoactivity
- Poor feeding
- Inconsistent bowel habits
- Lethargy
- Temperature instability

Adult: Early Signs
- Fatigue
- Dry skin
- Weight gain
- Cold intolerance
- Constipation
- Heavy menstrual flow

Adult: Later Signs
- Excessively dry skin
- Coarse hair texture
- Alopecia
- Increased weight gain
- Decrease in mental awareness
- Depression
- Pain or swelling in neck
- Mask-like face
- Myxedema
- Thick, dry, scaly skin
- Enlarged tongue

- Muscle weakness
- Joint pain

Hyperthyroidism

- Nervousness, irritability, decreased concentration, restlessness, tremor
- Weight loss despite increased appetite; anorexia in older adults
- Heat intolerance, sweating
- Skin changes: silky, hyperpigmentation over joints
- Hair loss
- Neck mass
- Eyes: bulging (exophthalmos)
- Shortness of breath
- Symptoms of heart failure: palpitations, angina
- Menstrual irregularities: amenorrhea, oligomenorrhea

Thyroid Nodules

- Neck mass
- Neck discomfort
- Hoarseness
- Dysphagia

Past Medical History

- Allergies
- Last menstrual period and characteristics
- Past neck irradiation

Medication History

Inquire about any iodine-containing or antithyroid medication.

Family History

Ask about other family members with endocrine disorders.

Dietary History

Inquire about the type of diet the client usually eats.

ASSESSMENT: OBJECTIVE/PHYSICAL EXAMINATION

Physical Examination

A problem-oriented physical examination should be conducted with particular attention to the following:
- Vital signs, weight, and general appearance
- Hypothyroidism
  - Slow movements, lethargy, and irritability
  - HEENT: hair texture coarse, inspect neck/thyroid, dull facies
  - Cardiovascular: cardiomegaly, slow heart rate
  - Abdomen: decreased bowel sounds
  - Neurologic examination: deep tendon reflexes, persistently opened posterior fontanelle; brisk reaction and prolonged reaction, large anterior fontanelle

- Skin: plaques with sharp raised margin, with complaints of pruritus
  - Infant: sometimes symptomatic as early as 2 weeks; sometimes asymptomatic for up to 1 month; irreversible mental changes occurring before symptoms sometimes become evident
- Hyperthyroidism
  - Eyes: forward protrusion of globe, lid lag, stare, limitation in ability to converge
  - Thyroid: enlargement or asymmetric, enlargement in the young, may not find enlargement in older adults, bruit
  - Cardiovascular: sinus tachycardia, atrial fibrillation, systolic flow murmurs, cardiac failure
- Thyroid nodules
  - Thyroid: enlargement, consistency

Diagnostic Procedures

- Hypothyroidism
  - T4 screen of all newborns in the United States; TSH measured if T4 is low
  - Increased TSH and decreased T4
  - Additional laboratory data: Lytes, blood urea nitrogen, creatinine, glucose, calcium, lipids
- Hyperthyroidism
  - TSH undetectable or below normal
  - T4 elevated
- Thyroid nodule
  - Radioiodine scanning and ultrasonography: no discrimination between benign and malignant lesions
  - Fine-needle aspiration (FNA): most reliable and useful method of identifying malignancy

DIAGNOSIS

Differential diagnoses include the following:
- Hypothyroidism
  - Ischemic heart disease
  - Depression
  - Nephrotic syndrome
  - Liver disease
- Hyperthyroidism
  - Cancer
  - Cardiac: congestive heart failure, atrial fibrillation
  - Psychologic problems: anxiety
  - Tremors: neurologic problems
  - Fibromyalgia
- Thyroid nodule
  - Benign adenoma
  - Thyroid cancer

THERAPEUTIC PLAN

Pharmacologic Treatment

Hypothyroidism

- Levothyroxine: Lifelong replacement is required. Both generic and brand name products are equally bioavail-

T

able. However, preparations should not be interchanged; rather the same product should be ordered to ensure consistent blood levels. Dosage may be increased depending on symptoms and laboratory results.

- Caution should be used with older adults with heart disease. A lower initial dose is recommended.
- Thyroid hormone replacement should be taken daily at approximately the same time each day, ideally before breakfast. Iron, antacids, and cholesterol-lowering agents should be taken at least 4 hours before or after the thyroid drug. Symptoms should begin to improve within 2 weeks.

Hyperthyroidism
- Medications are administered for 12 to 24 months and include Lugol iodine solution, propylthiouracil (preferred for pregnant women), and methimazole (Tapazole), antithyroid drugs.
- A major side effect of thyroid-suppressant drugs is agranulocytosis.
- Treatment with levothyroxine must be administered after the client's condition becomes hypothyroid.
- Radioactive iodine works by destroying overactive thyroid tissue. A disadvantage is the high rate of post-treatment hypothyroidism requiring lifelong replacement therapy. This treatment is contraindicated during pregnancy and lactation. Antithyroid medication must be discontinued 2 weeks before administration of radioactive iodine; however, propranolol for symptom relief may be continued. Women should not become pregnant for at least 6 months after treatment.
- Surgery, called thyroidectomy, can be performed but is less commonly used than in the past.
- Beta-adrenergic blockers (propranolol) can be used for symptomatic relief of palpitations, tachycardia, tremors, and nervousness.

Nonpharmacologic Treatment
Thyroid Nodule. Refer the client to a physician or surgeon for FNA. A smooth, soft, mobile nodule that is tender is likely to be benign, whereas a firm or hard, irregular, fixed and non-tender nodule is more likely to be malignant.

Client Education
Congenital Hypothyroidism
- Educate the family about the disease process and the importance of early treatment to prevent brain damage and to ensure normal physical growth.
- Emphasize the importance of follow-up to obtain a euthyroid level.

Adult Hypothyroidism
- Educate the family about the side effects of medication and the signs and symptoms of hyperthyroidism.

- Alert families to the genetic component of thyroid disorders.
- Thyroid storm is a complication of hyperthyroidism.
- Thyroid storm is a medical emergency, with symptoms of fever, sinus tachycardia, nervousness, cardiovascular collapse, and shock.

Referral
- For congenital hypothyroidism, refer the client to a physician and pediatric endocrinologist.
- For an adult with myxedema, cardiac disease, hypothyroidism caused by pituitary gland or hypothalamus dysfunction, or hyperthyroidism, refer the client to an endocrinologist.
- For congenital hyperthyroidism, refer the client to a pediatric endocrinologist.

Prevention
Thyroid disorders are not considered preventable diseases.

EVALUATION/FOLLOW-UP
- For congenital hypothyroidism, monitor T4 and TSH every 2 to 4 weeks after therapy is begun, then monthly until the client is 1 year old, and then bimonthly until the client is 3 years old.
- For adult hypothyroidism, reassess thyroid levels 4 to 6 weeks after treatment and monitor thyroid levels every 6 to 12 months.

COMPLICATIONS
Failure to treat hypothyroidism appropriately can potentially result in life-threatening myxedema, whereas failure to treat hyperthyroidism may result in life-threatening thyroid crisis. Failure to identify and promptly refer a client with a thyroid nodule might result in a missed diagnosis of cancer.

REFERENCES

Bishnoi, A., & Sachmechi, I. (1996). Thyroid disease during pregnancy. *American Family Physician, 53*(1), 215-220.

Burman, K. D. (2001). Diagnosing Graves' disease. *Women's Health in Primary Care, 4*(4), 318.

Demester, N. (2001). Diseases of the thyroid. *Clinician Reviews, 11*(7), 59-64.

Elliott, B. (2000). Diagnosing and treating hypothyroidism. *The Nurse Practitioner, 25*(3), 92-105.

Falsetti, D. (2001). The lifelong lurker. *ADVANCE for Nurse Practitioners,* April, 63-68.

Keating, H. J. (2000). A wanderer with an enlarged thyroid. *The Clinical Advisor,* March, 58-68.

Kuritzky, L. (2001). Hypothyroidism. *American Journal for Nurse Practitioners, 5*(5), 26-41.

Larson, J., Anderson, E. H., & Koslawy, M. (2000). Thyroid disease: A review for primary care. *Journal of the American Academy of Nurse Practitioners, 12*(6), 226-232.

Madison, L. D. (1998a). Today's approach to managing hyperthyroidism. *Women's Health in Primary Care, 1*(5), 452-465.

Madison, L. D. (1998b). The work-up for solitary thyroid nodules: A logical approach. *Women's Health in Primary Care, 1*(8), 641-644.

Robinson, D., Kidd, P., & Rogers, K. M. (2000). *Primary care across the lifespan.* St. Louis: Mosby.

Slatosky, J., Shipton, B., & Wahba, H. (2000). Thyroiditis: Differential diagnosis and management. *American Family Physician, 61*(4), 1047-1052.

Trotto, N. E. (1999). Hypothyroidism, hyperthyroidism, hyperparathyroidism. *Patient Care,* September 15, 186-218.

Youngkin, E. Q., & Davis, M. S. (1998). *Women's health: A primary care clinical guide.* Norwalk: Appleton & Lange.

Review Questions

1. Which factor in a woman's history is considered a positive sign for thyroid nodules?
   a. Menopause
   b. Head or neck irradiation
   c. Young age
   d. Normal body weight

2. Which physical finding is most suggestive of hyperthyroidism?
   a. Dull hair
   b. Flat affect
   c. Weight gain
   d. Anxious speech

3. Which of the following laboratory test results are indicative of hypothyroidism?
   a. Increased TSH and decreased T4
   b. Normal TSH
   c. Decreased TSH and increased T4
   d. Normal T4

4. A thyroid biopsy is considered mandatory with which of the following findings?
   a. Increased TSH and decreased T4
   b. Thyroid nodule
   c. Thyrotoxicosis
   d. Decreased TSH and increased T4

5. Ellie is a 34-year-old client being treated with levothyroxine for hypothyroidism. Which of the following does not indicate that her medication needs to be adjusted?
   a. Tremor
   b. Fatigue
   c. Increased energy
   d. Chest pain

6. For which of the following clients is radioactive iodine treatment an appropriate therapy?
   a. Susan, who is breastfeeding her daughter
   b. Sam, a middle-aged smoker
   c. Ellen, a 26-year-old primigravida
   d. Andrea, who is currently taking Tapazole

7. Mrs. O'Brien, a 52-year-old woman who has received a prescription for Synthroid, is provided with education about the drug. Which comment by Mrs. O'Brien, indicates a need for *further* instruction?

   a. "I'm glad I will have to take this pill for only a few months; I don't like taking medicine."
   b. "I need to take this pill everyday; before breakfast will be fine."
   c. "With this medicine, I should begin to feel better within the next 2 weeks or so."
   d. "I should take my iron tablet at least 4 hours apart from this medicine."

8. In examining the thyroid gland of a middle-aged woman, the NP discovers a solitary nodule. Which action is most appropriate?
   a. Begin thyroid hormone replacement therapy immediately.
   b. Order antithyroid antibody levels.
   c. Refer the client for FNA.
   d. Schedule radiography of the chest.

9. Which of the following medications may be helpful in reducing the tremors, nervousness, and palpitations of a client with hyperthyroidism?
   a. Dicyclomine (Bentyl)
   b. Propranolol (Inderal)
   c. Phenobarbital
   d. Levodopa

10. Once an adequate replacement dose has been established for a client taking thyroid replacement hormone, how often will her serum TSH and T4 levels need to be evaluated?
    a. Monthly
    b. Every 3 months
    c. Every 6 months
    d. Annually

Answers and Rationales

1. *Answer:* b (assessment)
   Rationale: Head and neck irradiation is considered a risk factor for developing thyroid malignancies (Youngkin & Davis, 1998).

2. *Answer:* d (assessment)
   Rationale: Clients with hyperthyroidism may have anxious and pressured speech. Flat affect, weight gain, and dull hair are more characteristic of hypothyroidism (Youngkin & Davis, 1998).

3. *Answer:* a (analysis/diagnosis)
   Rationale: Hypothyroidism is confirmed by a high TSH and a low T4 level (Elliott, 2000).

4. *Answer:* b (implementation/plan)
   Rationale: A thyroid biopsy is necessary for a client with a thyroid nodule (Demester, 2001).

5. *Answer:* c (evaluation)
   Rationale: A tremor and chest pain may indicate increased levels of thyroid secretion, whereas fatigue may indicate decreased levels of thyroid secretion. Increased energy is the desired response (Youngkin & Davis, 1998; Larson, et al., 2000).

6. *Answer:* b (implementation/plan)

Rationale: Radioactive iodine is contraindicated in pregnant and lactating women and in those who have recently breast-fed. Antithyroid medications, such as methimazole (Tapazole), should be discontinued 2 weeks before beginning radioactive iodine therapy (Madison, 1998a).

7. *Answer:* a (evaluation)

Rationale: Thyroid hormone replacement is generally administered as a lifelong replacement therapy (Elliott, 2000).

8. *Answer:* c (implementation/plan)

Rationale: A solitary thyroid nodule should be referred for FNA to rule out thyroid cancer (Madison, 1998b).

9. *Answer:* b (implementation/plan)

Rationale: Beta-adrenergic blockers, such as propranolol (Inderal), control tremors, nervousness, tachycardia, and palpitations in clients with hyperthyroidism (Trotto, 1999).

10. *Answer:* c (evaluation)

Rationale: Once the thyroid dose is stabilized, clients should have TSH and T4 levels measured every 6 months for evaluation of their condition (Elliott, 2000).

TINEA INFECTION   *Denise Robinson*

OVERVIEW
Definition

Tinea is a fungal infection caused by an organism known as a *dermatophyte*, which is capable of colonizing keratinized tissues such as the epidermis, nails, hair, tissues of various animals, and feathers of birds. The dermatophytes rarely affect deep layers of tissue or cause systemic infections.

Incidence

- **Tinea capitis/ringworm** of the scalp is a fungal infection of the hair follicles and the surrounding skin.
- **Tinea barbae/ringworm** of the beard is similar to tinea capitis but affects the beard and mustache.
- **Tinea corporis/ringworm** of the glabrous skin affects the trunk and extremities, with the exclusion of the palms of the hands, soles of the feet, and the groin.
- **Tinea versicolor** typically appears on the trunk, neck, and proximal extremities.
- **Tinea pedis/athletes foot** is a fungal infection of the feet and is the most common infection.
- **Tinea manuum** is a fungal infection of the palmar and interdigital areas of the hand.
- **Tinea cruris/"jock itch"** is a fungal infection of the groin areas, including genitalia, pubic area, and perineal and perianal skin.
- **Tinea unguium/onychomycosis** is ringworm of the nails, more commonly affecting the toenails than the fingernails.
- The estimated cost of treatment of fungal infections in 1994 was 400 million dollars.

Pathophysiology

Infection begins when a fungal spore adheres to the skin under suitable conditions (trauma to tissue and moist, occlusive environment). Within 4 to 6 hours, the spore germinates. The germinating spores develop hyphae and complete the life cycle by producing more spores. As the dermatophyte grows on the skin, there may be no clinical signs of infection. Some persons may be symptomatic carriers. Dermatophyte colonizations are not highly infectious. Inflammation associated with the fungal growth is usually an allergic response to fungal antigens that have affected the epidermal layer composed of living cells.

Common Pathogens
- *Epidermophyton*
- *Microsporum*
- *Trichophyton rubrum*

ASSESSMENT: SUBJECTIVE/HISTORY
History of Present Illness

- Duration of occurrence
- Location of occurrence
- Associated symptoms, including the following:
  - Itching
  - Burning
  - Pain
  - Excessive sweating
- Current treatments
- Contact with infected animals or persons
- History of shared combs, towels, or clothing
- Recent travel
- Use of communal showers or swimming areas
- Environmental exposures, such as contact sports and use of sports facilities
- Swimming
- Gardening

Past Medical History

- General medical condition, especially hepatic, renal, status of endocrine systems, and immunosuppressive disorders
- History of previous occurrence and past treatments
- History of other skin disorders or allergies

Medication History

Current medications.

Family History

- History of tinea infections
- History of other skin disorders
- Other family members with skin disorders

Psychosocial History

Assess living conditions.

ASSESSMENT: OBJECTIVE/PHYSICAL EXAMINATION
Physical Examination

General physical examination of involved area includes the following:
- Conducting careful evaluation of the skin, using good lighting source
- Checking all body surfaces with clothes removed
- Checking for lymph node enlargement

Diagnostic Procedures

- KOH preparation: Obtain several hair roots. The area within 5 to 6 cm of the infection is the most important area. Scalp scrapings from the active margin of the suspected infection may be used. Place the scrapings on a slide and add 10% aqueous KOH. Let the specimen sit for 5 to 10 minutes to clear the keratinous material. A drop of ink may be added to highlight the hyphae. Hyphae appear as long, translucent, branching filaments of uniform width. Septa may be visible as lines of separation at irregular intervals. Visualization of hyphae and spores under a standard light microscope should be suitable for diagnostic purposes.
- Wood's lamp: Dermatophytes fluoresce a yellowish color. Not all strains causing tinea fluoresce.
- Fungal culture: Several hairs or scrapings from an infected area may be obtained and placed on the appropriate test medium. Dermatophyte test media have a color indicator, which changes the medium from yellow to pink or red in the presence of a dermatophyte. Although this yields a more precise diagnosis, the results take longer. Such precision is not usually necessary. For most clinical purposes, classification of fungal infection by anatomic site is preferred.

DIAGNOSIS

Differential diagnoses are addressed in Table 3-110.

THERAPEUTIC PLAN
Pharmacologic Treatment

Topical creams are the treatment of choice for all forms of tinea except tinea capitis and tinea barbae, which require topical and oral medications. Oral agents penetrate the hair shaft, and topical agents limit the spread of spores.

Oral antifungal medications are used for tinea capitis and resistant infections. Common side effects are GI complaints and headache.

Tinea Capitis/Tinea Barbae
Children

🔥**CAUTION:** *Need to specify* microsize *or* ultramicrosize *because formulations and dosages are different.*

- Griseofulvin, ultramicrosize (14 to 23 kg: 31.25 to 82.5 mg q12h or 62.5 to 165 mg qd; heavier than 23 kg: 125 to 330 mg qd)
- Lamisil (3 to 6mg/kg/day for 1 to 4 weeks)
- Ketoconazole not recommended for children

Adults
- Griseofulvin (250 to 373 mg qd)
- Ketoconazole (3.3 to 6.6 mg/kg/day, up to 200 mg qd for 6 to 8 weeks)
- Lamisil (250 mg qd for 2 weeks)

Topical Therapy/Adjunctive Therapy
- Prescribe 2.5% selenium sulfide shampoo to prevent spread of infection (available by prescription only).
- Advise use of 1% Selsun Blue shampoo (can be purchased over-the-counter [OTC]).
- Prescribe prednisone 1 to 2 mg/kg qd for 5 to 10 days in *adults* with inflammatory tinea capitis.
- There are many drug interactions; check before prescribing.
- Side effects, in increasing order, are terbinafine < itraconazole < ketoconazole < griseofulvin (Fitzpatrick, Johnson, Wolff, & Suurmond, 2001).

Tinea Corporis
- Topicals are usually effective.
- Miconazole nitrate l% (Monistat) can be used.
- Clotrimazole 2% (Lotrimin) can be used.
- Econazole 1% (Spectazole) can be used.
- Ketoconazole 2% (Nizoral) can be administered qd, as noted previously.
- Terbinafine 1% (Lamisil) can be administered qd for 7 days.
- Butenafine 1% (Mentax) can be administered qd for 2 weeks.
- Apply bid for 2 weeks after clinical signs and symptoms have disappeared.
- Oral agents are for widespread, inflammatory, or resistant infections.
- Griseofulvin (500 to 1000 mg) can be administered qd.

Tinea Versicolor: Topical
- Selenium sulfide lotion 2.5% (Selsun) can be applied.
- Miconazole cream 2.5% can be applied.
- Clotrimazole 1% can be applied.
- Thiosulfate 25% can be applied.
- Apply beyond the borders of the affected areas for 5 to 10 minutes every day for 2 weeks.

T

TABLE **3-110** Tinea Infections

TYPE	RISK FACTORS	CLASSIC LESIONS	DIFFERENTIAL DIAGNOSIS
Tinea capitis/ tinea barbae	Children 2 to 10 years old; males; blacks; contact with infected persons and animals; confined/crowded living quarters; sharing of combs, brushes, hats; attending daycare; poor hygiene; immunosuppression; occlusive pomades; tight braiding; family history	Scalp, beard, mustache Noninflammatory areas of alopecia with characteristic black dots caused by breaking of hair shaft at level of follicle; patchy, round areas of hair loss; single or multiple erythematous plaques with follicular papules, nodules, crusting Inflammatory: swollen hairless purulent area develops, accompanied by suppurative folliculitis; pus may be present at site; scarring and permanent hair loss can occur; often associated with cervical adenopathy, important finding to differentiate from other alopecias	Seborrhea dermatitis Atopic dermatitis Psoriasis Alopecia areata Impetigo Bacterial folliculitis
Tinea corporis	Children, occlusive clothing, attending daycare, pets, immunosuppression	Trunk and extremities, excluding palms of hands and soles of feet Anular plaque with scaling, vesicle formations, and papules seen in an advancing border with hypopigmented or light brown center; may occur singly or in groups of three to four	Nummular eczema Granuloma anular Psoriasis Lichen planus Seborrhea dermatitis Pityriasis rosea
Tinea versicolor	Humidity, warm temperatures, occlusive clothing, excessive sweating, sharing of footwear, tropical climates	Trunk, neck, proximal extremities Presents as small oval or round hyperpigmented or hypopigmented sharply marginated macule; fine scales appear with scratching of the skin surface; colors range from white to red-brown; opportunistic infection caused by normal flora on the skin; chance of periodic recurrence	Pityriasis alba Seborrhea dermatitis Secondary syphilis Pityriasis rosea Vitiligo
Tinea pedis and tinea manuum	Communal showers and pools, occlusive footwear, excessive sweating, sharing of footwear, tropical climates	Surface of feet Mild to moderate erythema between toes, macerated and scaly skin between toes, and plantar and lateral surfaces of feet; vesicles and pustules in severe cases; foot odor Tinea manuum associated with tinea pedis, unilateral in nature	Contact dermatitis Interdigital psoriasis Eczema
Tinea cruris	Occlusive and tight clothing, athletic supporters, obesity, wet swimsuits, diagnosis of tinea pedis or tinea unguium, immuno-suppression, men	Genitalia, pubic area, perineal area, and perianal skin Anular formation of erythematous, raised, well-marginated border; area within border is often pigmented redbrown; lesions rarely extend beyond genitocrural crease and medial upper thigh; lateral or bilateral; first site involved usually left medial thigh adjacent to scrotum	Candidiasis Erythrasma Psoriasis Seborrhea Dermatitis Lichen simplex chronicus Benign familial chronic pemphigus Intertrigo
Tinea unguium	Tinea pedis, immuno-suppression, diabetes, elderly with venous insufficiency, trauma to nails	Nails Lose luster and become opaque yellow in color, thicken, lifting up nail bed, distal edge becomes brittle and crumbles	Candidiasis Psoriasis

From Bushong, K. (2000). Tinea. In D. Robinson, P. Kidd, & K. Rogers (Eds.), *Primary care across the lifespan* (p. 1099). St. Louis: Mosby.

- Oral medications usually are not needed to treat tinea versicolor but may be used in resistant cases or for prophylaxis.

Tinea Pedis and Tinea Manuum
- Apply clotrimazole, miconazole, tolnaftate, or Terbinafine HCl creams bid to the feet, and apply for 2 weeks after the condition has cleared.
- Apply butenafine 1% qd after bathing for 4 weeks.
- Talcum powder or antifungal powders (OTC) can be used.
- In severe cases, use Burrows solution for lesions that are oozing.
- For tinea cruris, apply clotrimazole or miconazole topical cream bid for 3 to 4 weeks.
- For children, 1% terbinafine can be applied qd for 7 days.
- Butenafine 1% can be applied qd after bathing for 2 weeks.
- Oral treatment can be administered in resistant cases.

Onychomycosis. Topical medications are usually not effective.
Oral
- Itraconazole (Sporanox) (200 mg daily for 90 days or pulse therapy of 1 week on and 3 weeks off for three to six rounds of therapy for 3 to 6 months)
- Griseofulvin (1000 mg/day in divided doses for 4 to 6 months for fingernails and 12 to 18 months for toenails; not usually recommended because itraconazole and terbinafine are available
- Terbinafine HCl (250 mg qd for 6 weeks for fingernails and 12 weeks for toenails; pulse therapy also used)
- Side effects: nausea, monitor liver function
- Antacids avoided within 2 hours

Nonpharmacologic Treatment
- Children in a day care setting do not need to be isolated once treatment has begun.
- Children may return to school after beginning oral therapy.

Client Education
- Side effects and drug interactions associated with oral antifungal medications are possible.
- Clean the environment and fomites to remove fungal scales.
- Avoid sharing brushes, combs, hats, towels, and other items that can transmit fungal scales.
- Search out infected animals, including pets, and treat appropriately.
- Do not use oils on the hair or scalp.
- Avoid braiding hair.
- Apply creams after bathing and reapply after swimming or exercising.

- The recurrence rate is high, and treatment may be needed each spring before tanning season.
- Wear leather shoes or nonocclusive shoes.
- Remove wet swimsuits as soon as possible.
- Use drying powders on the feet.
- Wear sandals or rubber shoes in communal areas.
- Keep skin dry.
- It may be necessary to culture and treat other family members. All family members can use selenium sulfide shampoo to prevent recurrence by asymptomatic carriers.

Referral/Consultation
- Collaborate with physician regarding any clients requiring oral antifungal medications.
- Collaborate with physician regarding any client not showing improvement within 2 weeks.

Prevention
- Dryness
- Loose fitting clothes and nonocclusive footwear
- Cotton undergarments and socks
- Good hygiene; benzol peroxide wash
- Wearing footwear in communal areas
- Not sharing personal care items, such as combs, brushes, mats, or towels

EVALUATION/FOLLOW-UP
- Reevaluate all cases of tinea in 2 weeks for response to therapy.
- Resistant infections and tinea capitis may require follow-up visits every 2 to 4 weeks until clear.
- Monitor hepatic, renal, and hematopoietic functions monthly while receiving oral antifungals.
- Monitor for superimposed bacterial infections at the follow-up visit. Cultures and gram stains may be needed to determine appropriate antibiotic therapy. Monitor the client for side effects and drug interactions associated with oral antifungals.
- Check for resolution of lesions.

COMPLICATIONS
- Tinea tends to be chronic; it may provide a portal for lymphangitis or cellulitis, especially in clients whose leg veins have been used for open heart surgery.
- Chronic untreated kerions result in scarring alopecia.

REFERENCES

Abdel-Ranman, S. M., & Nahata, M. C. (1997). Oral terbinafine: A new antifungal agent. *The Annals of Pharmacotherapy, 31*(4), 445-456.

Bakos, L., Brito, A. C., Castro, L. C., Gontijo, B., Lowy, G., Reis, C. M., Ribeiro, A. M., Sonza, F. H., Villar Mdo, L., & Zaitz, C. (1997). Open clinical study of the efficacy and safety of terbinafine cream 1% in children with tinea corporis and

T

tinea cruris. *The Pediatric Infectious Disease Journal, 16*(6), 545-548.

Bergus, G. R., & Johnson, J. S. (1993). Superficial tinea infections. *American Family Physician, 48*(2), 259-267.

Bushong, K. (2002). Tinea. In D. Robinson, P. Kidd, & K. Rogers (Eds.), *Primary care across the lifespan* (p. 1099). St Louis: Mosby.

Degreef, H. J., & DeDoncker, P. R. (1994). Current therapy of dermatophytosis. *Journal of the American Academy of Dermatology, 31*(3), S25-S29.

Drake, L. A., Dinehart, S. M., Farmer, E. R., et al. (1996) Guidelines of care for superficial mycotic infections of the skin: tinea capitis and tinea barbae. *Journal of the American Academy of Dermatology, 34*(2), 2909-293.

Faergemann, J., Mork, N. J., Haglund, A., & Odegard, T. (1997) A multicentre (double-blind) comparative study to assess the safety and efficacy of fluconazole and griseofulvin in the treatment of tinea corporis and tinea cruris. *British Journal of Dermatology, 136*(4), 575-577.

Fitzpatrick, T., Johnson, R. A., Wolff, K., & Suurmond, K. (2001). *Color atlas and synopsis of clinical dermatology.* New York: McGraw Hill.

Frieden, I. J., & Howard, R. (1994). Tinea capitis: Epidemiology, diagnosis, treatment, and control. *Journal of the American Academy of Dermatology, 31*(3 Pt 2), S42-S46.

Greer, D. L., Weiss, J., Rodriguez, D. A., Hebert, A. A., & Swinehart, J. M. (1997). A randomized trial to assess once-daily topical treatment of tinea corporis with butenafine, a new antifungal agent. *Journal of the American Academy of Dermatology, 37*(2), 231-235.

Hoffmann, T. J., & Schelkum, P. H. (1995). How I manage athlete's foot. *The Physician and Sports Medicine, 23*(4), 29-32.

Lesher, J., Levine, N., & Treadwell, P. (1994). Fungal skin infections: Common but stubborn. *Patient Care, 28*(2), 16-30.

Lesher, J. L., Babel, D. E., Stewart, D. M., Jones, T. M., Kaminester, L., Goldman, M., & Weintraub, J. S. (1997). Butenafine 1% cream in the treatment of tinea cruris: a multicenter, vehiclecontrolled, double-blind trial. *Journal of the American Academy of Dermatology, 36*(2), S20-S24.

Martin, A. G., & Kobayashi, G. S. (1999). Superficial fungal infection: dermatophytosis, tinea, nigra, piedra. In T. B. Fitzpatrick, I. Freedberg, A. Eisen, K. Woeff, & S. Katz. (Eds.), *Dermatology in general medicine.* New York: McGraw Hill, 2421-2451.

Martin, A. G., & Kobayashi, G. S. (1993). Yeast infections: Candidiasis, pityriasis (tinea) versicolor. In T. B. Fitzpatrick, I. Freedberg, A. Eisen, K. Woeff, & S. Katz (Eds.), *Dermatology in general medicine.* (5th ed.). New York: McGraw Hill, 2452-2467.

Pierard, G. E., Arrese, J. E., & Pierard-Franchimont, C. (1996). Treatment and prophylaxis of tinea infections. *Disease Management, 52*(2), 209-224.

Reilly, K. (1996). Tinea versicolor. In M. D'Ambro (Ed.), *Griffith's 5-minute clinical consult* (pp. 1062-1063). Baltimore: Williams & Wilkins.

Stevenson, L., & Brooke, D. S. (1994). Tinea capitis. *Journal of Pediatric Care, 8*(4), 189-190.

Tschen, E., Elewski, B., Gorsulowsky, D. C., Pariser, D. M. (1997). Treatment of interdigital tinea pedis with a 4-week once daily regimen of butenafine hydrochloride 1% cream. *Journal of American Academy of Dermatology, 36*(2), S9-S14.

Review Questions

1. James is an 8-year-old black boy who comes to the clinic with a report of hair loss. You examine his head and observe a lesion that you know to be characteristic of tinea capitis. What are the characteristics of the lesion?

    a. Round, erythematous plaque with black dots

    b. Erythematous macule with pustules in the center

    c. Red, raised area with white crusting and yellow exudate

    d. Circular area without hair, of normal skin color

2. Which of the following is the treatment of choice for tinea capitis?

    a. Corticosteroid topical gel, qd

    b. OTC 1% selenium shampoo

    c. Detoconazole, 5 to 10 mg/kg/day, and 2.5% selenium sulfide shampoo

    d. Griseofulvin, 10 to 20 mg/kg/day, and 2.5% selenium shampoo

3. Which of the following is most likely to cause a client to seek treatment for tinea versicolor?

    a. Intense pruritus

    b. Pain and tenderness, with ROM to shoulder joints

    c. Cosmetic appearance

    d. Oozing of serous fluid from the pustule

4. Which of the following is an appropriate treatment for tinea pedis?

    a. Apply clotrimazole cream bid for 2 weeks.

    b. Apply clotrimazole cream bid until the feet remain free of lesions for 2 weeks.

    c. Administer griseofulvin, 1g qd in divided doses, for 4 weeks.

    d. Apply soaks of hydrogen peroxide and vinegar bid for 2 weeks.

5. Which of the following represents an accurate statement concerning tinea?

    a. Client should be reevaluated when treatment is complete.

    b. A follow-up appointment is not necessary unless there is a secondary bacterial infection.

    c. All cases of tinea should be evaluated 2 weeks after therapy has been initiated.

    d. All cases of tinea should be evaluated every 2 weeks until lesions have cleared.

6. You see a client with recurring rash in the groin area. You decide that the client has tinea cruris on the basis of the classic location of the lesions. Where are the lesions located?

    a. Scrotum

    b. Glans penis

    c. Scrotum, glans penis, and around the rectum

    d. Medial aspect of the thigh bilaterally

7. To avoid recurrence of tinea pedis, you instruct Mark, a 19-year-old college student, to do all except which of the following?

    a. Avoid leather shoes.
    b. Wear rubber sandals in communal areas.
    c. Dry carefully between his toes.
    d. Wear absorbent cotton socks.

8. Which of the following historical indications is consistent with the diagnosis of tinea pedis?

    a. Itching and burning between the toes
    b. Bleeding and ecchymosis between the toes
    c. Purulent discharge
    d. White patch noted on the distal or lateral underside of the nail

Answers and Rationales

1. *Answer:* **a** (assessment)
Rationale: Examination of the scalp reveals areas of alopecia with characteristic black dots, caused by breaking of the hair shaft at the level of the follicle, leaving a spore filled remnant of hair (Lesher, Levine, & Treadwell, 1994).

2. *Answer:* **d** (implementation/plan)
Rationale: Griseofulvin is the drug of choice to treat tinea capitis in pediatric clients. In addition, the client should use a shampoo with 2.5% selenium sulfide to help prevent the spread of infection (Lesher et al. 1994).

3. *Answer:* **c** (assessment)
Rationale: The presenting complaint is usually cosmetic, because lesions often fail to tan with sun exposure. Pruritus is often mild or absent (Fitzpatrick et al. 1996).

4. *Answer:* **b** (implementation/plan)
Rationale: Use clotrimazole cream until the infection clears and then for a few weeks afterward (Hoffmann & Schelkum, 1995).

5. *Answer:* **c** (evaluation)
Rationale: Clients should be seen in 2 weeks to evaluate the effectiveness of treatment (Fitzpatrick, et al. 2001).

6. *Answer:* **d** (analysis/diagnosis)
Rationale: Infection involves the medial aspect of the upper thigh on one or both legs (Lesher et al. 1994; Bergus & Johnson, 1993).

7. *Answer:* **a** (implementation/plan)
Rationale: Treatment of tinea pedis begins by emphasizing hygiene, specifically thorough drying of the feet after bathing. Absorbent cotton socks may help to maintain dryness, and shoes should be made of leather to allow the feet to breathe. It would be prudent to wear sandals or other protective footwear in the locker room (Lesher et al. 1994; Hoffmann & Schelkum, 1995).

8. *Answer:* **a** (assessment)
Rationale: The lesions of tinea pedis are dry, scaling, maceration, peeling, and fissuring of toe webs. It is most common between the fourth and fifth toes (Fitzpatrick, et al. 2001).

TINNITUS   *Denise Robinson*

OVERVIEW
Definition

Tinnitus is the perception of abnormal ear or head noises.

Incidence

- Most people suffer from occasional intermittent tinnitus, which lasts for several minutes; this occurs even in persons with normal hearing.
- Continuing tinnitus usually means the person has suffered sensory hearing loss.
- Approximately 1% of the population in the United States suffers from chronic tinnitus that causes severe distress and requires some kind of management intervention.
- The overall prevalence of unexplained tinnitus is 11%.
- Tinnitus seems to be clearly associated with somatization disorders (42%) or hypochondriacal disorder (27%).

Pathophysiology

Some forms of tinnitus may be caused by loss of the normal masking effect of ambient noise, with the emergence of otherwise subaudible tympanic, vascular, or muscular noises.

ASSESSMENT: SUBJECTIVE/HISTORY
History of Present Illness

- Ringing or buzzing in ears
- Ask about the following:
  - Involvement of one ear or both ears
  - Ringing or buzzing associated with movement or rotation
- Decreased hearing (90% of clients with decreased hearing also experience tinnitus)
  - Hearing loss was gradual or sudden
  - Hearing acuity fluctuation
- Associated symptoms such as vertigo, otalgia, or otorrhea
  - Ear pain
  - Discharge from ear
  - Being nervous or depressed
  - Inability to sleep or concentrate because of noises
- Temporomandibular symptoms
  - Facial muscle pain
  - Preauricular pain
  - TMJ sounds: jaw clicking, popping, catching, locking
  - Limited mouth opening

T

- Increased pain while chewing
- Difficulty talking or singing
- History of recent trauma or injury to neck, jaw, or mouth
  - Previous treatment for unexplained facial or jaw pain
  - Told by dentist that client grinds teeth
  - Treatment for grinding teeth
  - Last dental visit
- Screening questions for clients with TMJ disorder are the following:
  - Difficulty, pain, or both when opening your mouth (e.g., when yawning)
  - Jaw become stuck, locked, or "go out"
  - Difficulty, pain, or both when chewing, talking, or using jaws
  - Aware of noises in the jaw joints
  - Jaws regularly feel stiff, tight, or tired
  - Pain in or about the ears, temples, or cheeks
  - Frequent headaches, neck aches, or toothaches

Past Medical History

- Ask about history of ear problems or disease.
- Ask about history of anxiety or depression.
- Ask about history of migraines.
- Ask about history of syphilis, diabetes, hypothyroidism, or head trauma as a possible cause of hearing loss.

Medication History

- Ask about use of ASA or other ototoxic drugs.
- Ask about aminoglycosides, diuretics, quinine, or furosemide.

Family History

- Ask about a family history of hearing loss.
- Ask about a family history of migraines.

Psychosocial History

- Ask about exposure to excessive noise and use of ear plugs.
- Ask about coping strategies used to date to adjust to tinnitus.

ASSESSMENT: OBJECTIVE/PHYSICAL EXAMINATION
Physical Examination

The examination should concentrate on the head and neck.

- HEENT: Evaluate for upper respiratory infection.
- Ear: Evaluate TM and external canal.
  - Complete pneumatic otoscopy: Check for TMJ movement.
  - Obtain tympanogram.
- Face: Assess masseter and temporal muscles and preauricular area for pain or tenderness. Inspect the face, jaw, and dental arches for symmetry.

- Ask the client to open and close the mouth, keeping your fingers over the preauricular areas; be alert for joint sounds.
- Mouth: To measure the mouth opening, use a millimeter rule on the teeth and have the client open as wide as possible. The distance between the maxillary and mandibular teeth should be measured. Less than 40 mm is considered a restricted mouth opening.
- Inspect the teeth for significant wear, mobility, or decay. Look at the buccal mucosa for riding and the lateral edges of the tongue for scalloping. These are signs of clenching and bruxism.
- Neurologic examination: Check sensation of the face, and note whether facial movement is symmetrical and whether there are rapid alternating movements.
- Hearing: Have the client repeat aloud words presented in a soft whisper, normal speaking voice, or shout. Have the opposite ear occluded and repeat on the other side.
  - Child 0 to 3 months responds to noise.
  - Child 3 to 5 months turns to sound.
  - Child 6 to 10 months responds to name.
  - Child 10 to 15 months imitates simple words.
  - To conduct the Weber test, place the tuning fork on the forehead or front teeth. Have the client indicate where sound is best heard.
  - To conduct the Rinne test, place the tuning fork alternately on the mastoid bone and in front of the ear canal.

Diagnostic Procedures

- For audiometric studies, a hearing test is conducted in a sound-proof room. Pure-tone thresholds in decibels are obtained over the ranges of 250 to 8000 Hz for both air and bone conduction. All clients with hearing loss should be referred for audiometric testing unless the cause is easily remediable (e.g., impacted cerumen).
- Speech discrimination testing evaluates the clarity of hearing. Results are reported as percentage correct.
- Tympanogram used to detect fluid in the middle ear and to determine the mobility of the TM. An electroacoustic device is used to measure the compliance of the TM. Results are shown in a graphic form. It is most reliable in children younger than 6 months.
- Audiogram: Small handheld audioscopes can provide an approximate indication of hearing impairment. Usually four pure tones are emitted in sequence. This test can be affected by background noise, so the examination room must be quiet.
- The tinnitus handicap inventory (THI) consists of a self-perceived rating scale to determine the effect of tinnitus on the activities of daily living (ADLs) and the severity of the tinnitus handicap (Newman et al. 1997).

DIAGNOSIS

Differential diagnoses include the following:

- Pulsatile tinnitus is caused by conductive hearing loss; carotid pulsations are more apparent. This condition may indicate a vascular abnormality, such as glomus tumor, carotid vasoocclusive disease, arteriovenous malformation, or aneurysm.
- Sensory hearing loss is caused by conditions affecting the eighth cranial nerve leading to sensorineural hearing loss. The tinnitus can be caused by hyperirritability of the acoustic nerve.
- Acoustic neuroma can cause unilateral tinnitus or hearing loss, mild positional vertigo, or sense of imbalance. Audiometry demonstrates significant sensorineural hearing loss with poor discrimination.

THERAPEUTIC PLAN
Pharmacologic Treatment

- Nortriptyline (Pamelor): Treatment seems to be effective in reducing tinnitus, possibly because of treatment of underlying depression. Side effects include drowsiness and anticholinergic effects.
- Fluoxetine (Prozac): Side effects include CNS stimulation, fatigue, headaches, somnolence, and sexual dysfunction.
- Misoprostol (Cytotec): Side effects include diarrhea, abdominal pain, flatulence, and headaches.
- Melatonin: Melatonin seems to improve tinnitus according to the THI, although the improvement is not statistically significant. Sleeping also seems to improve tinnitus. Clients with THI scores are most likely to benefit. Side effects and a safety profile have not been established, and approval has not been received from the Food and Drug Administration for use with tinnitus.

Nonpharmacologic Treatment

- The sound of a radio may help a person with tinnitus to go to sleep (FM radio delivers a broader spectrum of frequencies and is preferred).
- Use of "white noise" may be helpful to mask sounds.
- Bedtime sedation can be helpful to ensure adequate sleep.
- Some people with tinnitus recommend the following:
  - Avoid stress.
  - Get adequate rest.
  - Do not drink alcohol.
  - Take ginkgo biloba at meals.
  - Use a splint for TMJ disorders.

Diet. Avoid caffeine.

Client Education

- Give the client reassurance that the sounds are not caused by a serious intracranial condition.

- Tinnitus clinics and support groups are available.
- Tinnitus management training includes using white noise, biofeedback, and relaxation therapies. With these methods, tinnitus was found to be less annoying, but the loudness of the tinnitus did not change nor did the tinnitus awareness.

Referral/Consultation

- Noises that originate from the region of the client's ear and are audible to the examiner should be referred to an otolaryngologist.
- Clients that have tinnitus that lateralizes to one ear should also be referred to an otolaryngologist.
- Clients with temporomandibular disorders with coexisting tinnitus should be referred to a dentist. Improvement in TMJ disorder also improves tinnitus.
- Clients with severe tinnitus may benefit from surgery; cochlear resection and microvascular decompression are available, but clear-cut efficacy has not been shown.

Prevention

None.

EVALUATION/FOLLOW-UP

- Conduct a follow-up examination in 2 weeks to evaluate the effectiveness of the anti-depressant.
- Evaluation should determine how well the client is sleeping.
- Determine the effectiveness of masking tinnitus using biofeedback, relaxation, or white noise.

COMPLICATIONS

Decreased ability to sleep and interference with ADLs is possible.

REFERENCES

Denk, D. M., Heinzl, H., Franz, P., & Ehrenberger, K. (1997). Caroverine in tinnitus treatment: A placebo-controlled blind study. *Acta Otolaryngology, 117*(6), 825-830.

Dineen, R., Doyle, J., & Bench, J. (1997). Managing tinnitus: A comparison of different approaches to tinnitus management training. *British Journal of Audiology, 31*(5), 331-344.

Ellsworth, A., Witl, D., Drydale, D., & Oliver, L. (2002). *Mosby's 2003 medical drug reference.* St. Louis: Mosby.

Gelb, H., Gelb, M., & Wagner, M. (1997). The relationship of tinnitus and craniocervical mandibular disorders. *Cranio: The Journal of Craniomandibular Practice, 15*(2), 136-143.

Hiller, W., Janca, A., & Burke, K. (1997). Association between tinnitus and somatoform disorders. *Journal of Psychosomatic Research, 43*(6), 613-624.

Meikle, M. (1997). Electronic access to tinnitus data: The Oregon tinnitus data archive. *Otolaryngology Head and Neck Surgery, 117*(6), 698-700.

Newman, C., Sandridge, S., & Jacobsea, G. (1997). Psychometric adequacy of the tinnitus handicap inventory (THI) for evaluating treatment outcomes. *Journal of the American Academy of Audiology, 9*(2), 153-160.

Parnes, S. (1997). Current concepts in the clinical management of patients with tinnitus. *European Archives of Otorhinolaryngology, 254*(9-10), 406-409.

Rizzardo, R., Savastano, M., Maron, M. B., Mangialaio, M., Salvadori, L. (1998). Psychological distress in patients with tinnitus. *Journal of Otolaryngology, 27*(1), 21-25.

Robinson, D. (2000). Tinnitus. In D. Robinson, P. Kidd, & K. Rogers (Eds.), *Primary care across the lifespan* (pp. 1104-1107). St. Louis: Mosby.

Rosenberg, S., Silverstein, H., Rowan, P. T., Olds, M. J. (1998). Effect of melatonin on tinnitus. *Laryngoscope, 108*(3), 305-310.

Shemin, L. (1998). Fluoxetine for treatment of tinnitus. *Otolaryngology and Head and Neck Surgery, 118*(3 Pt 1), 421.

Tyler, R. (1997). Perspective on tinnitus. *British Journal of Audiology, 31*(6), 381-386.

Wright, E., & Bifano, S. (1997). Tinnitus improvement through TMD therapy. *Journal of the American Dental Association, 128*(10), 1424-1432.

Review Questions

1. Steve complains of ear noise. Which of the following historical indications is consistent with tinnitus?

   a. Jaw popping and locking
   b. Decreased hearing
   c. Bruxism
   d. Frequent headaches

2. What other information is important to determine in relation to tinnitus?

   a. Use of ASA
   b. Loudness of noises heard
   c. History of dental decay
   d. History of frequent sinusitis

3. Which of the following descriptions is consistent with a Weber test?

   a. Place the tuning fork on the mastoid bone; when unable to hear the sound, place in front of the ear canal.
   b. Place the tuning fork on the forehead; have the client indicate where it is heard best

   c. Conduct a pencil and paper test to determine the effect of tinnitus on the ADLs.
   d. Conduct a hearing test in a sound-proof room.

4. Which of the following diagnostic tests is first line in cases of tinnitus?

   a. Rinne test
   b. Weber test
   c. Audiometric studies
   d. Audiogram

5. Which of the following interventions can be used before definitive diagnosis to help decrease tinnitus?

   a. Hypnotics and sedatives
   b. White noise machine
   c. Relaxation therapy
   d. NSAIDs

Answers and Rationales

1. **Answer: b** (assessment)
   Rationale: Decreased hearing is present in 90% of those with tinnitus (Parnes, 1997).

2. **Answer: a** (assessment)
   Rationale: It is important to determine whether the client has a history of taking ototoxic drugs such as ASA, aminoglycosides, diuretics, quinine, or furosemide (Parnes, 1997).

3. **Answer: b** (assessment)
   Rationale: The Weber and Rinne tests should be conducted during the physical examination. A Weber test compares bone conduction; the tuning fork is placed on the forehead. A Rinne test compares bone and air conduction; the tuning fork is placed on the mastoid bone (Robinson, 2000).

4. **Answer: c** (analysis/diagnosis)
   Rationale: The first-line test for tinnitus is audiometric studies because 90% of clients with tinnitus have hearing loss. The other tests are adequate for screening purposes but are not diagnostic (Parnes, 1997).

5. **Answer: b** (implementation/plan)
   Rationale: A white-noise machine makes a steady consistent noise, which helps to block out the tinnitus noise (Parnes, 1997).

TRANSIENT ISCHEMIC ATTACKS *Pamela Kidd*

OVERVIEW

Definition

Defined as cerebral ischemia that is transient or reversible in nature, a transient ischemic attack (TIA) presents with acute focal neurologic deficit, usually lasting less than 20 minutes but sometimes lasting up to 24 hours. Signs of cerebral ischemia lasting longer than 24 hours and less than 7 days is defined as reversible ischemic neurologic deficit (RIND).

Incidence

The incidence of cerebral ischemia has declined for clients younger than 70 years, probably as a result of aggressive hypertension and cardiovascular management. TIAs precede 50% to 75% of strokes caused by carotid artery thrombosis. However, among all stroke types, TIAs precede only approximately 10%. Approximately one third of clients who experience TIAs will experience cerebral infarction within 5 years.

Pathophysiology

Atherosclerosis and inflammatory disease processes damage arterial walls, leading to the development of cerebral thrombosis. TIAs represent thrombotic particles causing an intermittent blockage of circulation. There is increased risk of vascular damage with prolonged hypertension, degeneration of the endothelial wall of vessels, and adherence of platelets and fibrin.

Factors Increasing Susceptibility
- Smoking
- Increased stress levels

Protective Factors. Aspirin use.

ASSESSMENT: SUBJECTIVE/HISTORY
Symptoms
- Sudden onset of paralysis or paresis of one extremity or extremities on one side of the body
- Numbness, tingling, clumsiness of an extremity or both extremities on one side of the body
- Aphasia
- Visual disturbances
- Sensation of spinning
- Facial paralysis or drooping
- Headache, drooling, slurred speech

Past Medical History
- Hypertension
- Diabetes
- Hyperlipidemia
- Cardiovascular or peripheral vascular disease
- Gout
- Atrial fibrillation (increases stroke risk by almost 18% per year if two additional risk factors are present)
- Ventricular aneurysms
- Heart valve replacement

Medication History
Use of oral contraceptives.

Family History
- History of cardiovascular disease
- History of cerebral vascular accidents

Dietary History
Excessive intake of salt, carbohydrates, and fats.

ASSESSMENT: OBJECTIVE/PHYSICAL EXAMINATION
Physical Examination
- General appearance: confusion, facial drooping
- Vital signs: hydration status (dehydration can lead to hypovolemia and orthostatic hypotension), orthostatic changes (systolic blood pressure of 110 in normally hypertensive client may in fact be hypotensive), hypertension (should not be based on an isolated blood pressure, but rather trending of the blood pressure unless it is higher than 210 systolic or 120 diastolic)
- HEENT:
  - Eyes: Check the reactivity of the pupils (remember that in the elderly, the eyes may not have a brisk response), and check for visual field deficit.
  - Throat: Check the client's ability to swallow.
  - Neck: Check whether the neck is supple, listen to carotid arteries for bruits, and check for diminished or absent carotid pulsations.
  - Cardiovascular: Listen for irregular rhythms, murmurs, and artificial heart valves (clicks).
  - Check extremities for possible signs of deep vein thrombosis.
- Neurologic: cranial nerve deficits, especially facial paresis or paralysis, possible abnormalities of the gag reflex, tongue, extraocular movements
- Deep tendon reflexes normal or hyperactive in upper extremities
- Level of consciousness, memory, speech, walking, balance (Romberg), sensory perception, and motor ability (e.g, hand grips, lifting leg off the table and holding against pressure, etc.)

Diagnostic Procedures
- Diagnostic tests should include electrocardiogram (ECG) and CT of the head (results should be normal). Lumbar puncture is used if there is likelihood of septic embolism from bacterial endocarditis.
- Laboratory tests are complete blood count (CBC) and comprehensive metabolic profile.
- Other radiologic tests that may be considered include duplex Doppler study to determine the patency of the carotid arteries. If there is significant stenosis of the carotid arteries (greater than 70%), arteriography should be performed.

DIAGNOSIS
Differential diagnoses include TIA, RIND, and stroke (brain attack) (Table 3-111).

Underlying causes include atrial fibrillation, infective endocarditis, meningitis, recent anteroseptal myocardial infarction, valvular heart disease or heart valve replacement, carotid stenosis, polycythemia, blood dyscrasias (especially those resulting in hypercoagulable states), connective tissue diseases, hypertension, and chemical imbalances (particularly glucose and sodium).

THERAPEUTIC PLAN
The therapeutic plan depends on whether an underlying condition, such as carotid artery stenosis or uncontrolled hypertension, was determined. Treatment of the underlying condition is imperative.

T

TABLE **3-111** TIA Diagnosis, Findings, and Evaluation

DIAGNOSIS	FINDINGS	EVALUATION
Stroke (brain attack)	Neurologic deficit	None, other than physical examination; need to be admitted for further evaluation and initiation of tissue plasminogen activator; consult physician
RIND	Neurologic deficit	None, other than physical examination; need admission to hospital to determine whether RIND or brain attack
TIA	History of unilateral weakness, confusion, clumsiness of arm or leg, visual disturbance, facial paralysis, aphasia, headache, slurred speech; Normal results of physical examination and no neurologic deficits May indicate carotid bruit	12-Lead ECG; consider CT or magnetic resonance imaging of head, CBC, comprehensive metabolic profile; may want to consider duplex Doppler study of carotid arteries to evaluate for stenosis; arteriography is reserved for stenoses greater than 70% as revealed by Doppler study

CBC, Complete blood count; *CT,* computed tomography; *ECG,* electrocardiogram; *RIND,* reversible ischemic neurologic deficit; *TIA,* transient ischemic attack.

Nonpharmacologic Treatment

None.

Pharmacologic Treatment

Choices for inhibiting platelet aggregation are the following:

- Aspirin (81 mg daily): Enteric coated is best for the elderly. Use 325 mg/day if atrial fibrillation is present and the client is younger than 60 years of age with no other stroke risk factors.
- Ticlopidine (250 mg bid) is reserved for clients with aspirin intolerance and requires close monitoring of the CBC.
- Warfarin (5 mg/day; 2.5 mg/day for clients 75 years of age or older): The goal is to obtain an international normalized ratio (INR) between 2 and 3 during 1 to 2 weeks. Check the INR three times during the first week, twice during the next week, and weekly thereafter. The risk of bleeding increases with an INR higher than 4.5. Warfarin interacts with most antibiotics (antibiotic potentiates the drug).
- Surgical: If carotid artery stenosis is significant, carotid endarterectomy may be indicated.

Client Education

Assess for bleeding (stools, urine, unusual bruising, bleeding gums) if the client is receiving an anticoagulant.

Referral

- All clients with TIA should be referred to a physician/neurologist.
- Work with a pharmacist to identify other possible medication interactions with warfarin.

Prevention

- Low fat diet
- Regular aerobic exercise
- No smoking

EVALUATION/FOLLOW-UP

Clients with TIAs should be followed at least weekly and instructed to call if any neurologic symptoms occur or depending on the symptoms of the underlying risk conditions. If unidentified, frequency of check-ups vary from clinic to clinic. However, clients should be evaluated every 4 to 6 months or immediately if symptoms recur.

COMPLICATIONS

- Stroke/brain attack
- Death

REFERENCES

Blank, F. (2000). Thrombolytic therapy for clients with acute stroke in the ED setting. *Emergency Nursing, 26*(1), 24-30.

Larson, L. (2000). Transient ischemic attacks. In D. Robinson, P. Kidd, & K. Rogers (Eds.), *Primary care across the lifespan.* St. Louis: Mosby.

Turpie, A., Weart, C., & White, R. (1998). Anticoagulation: Promises and pitfalls. *Patient Care for Nurse Practitioners, 1*(2), 44-55.

Review Questions

1. TIAs represent which of the following?
   a. Total, permanent occlusion of circulation to a small area of the brain
   b. Hemorrhage of a small vessel in the brain
   c. Intermittent occlusion of circulation in the brain
   d. Permanent occlusion of circulation to a large area of the brain

2. Diseases associated with TIAs include all *except* which of the following?
   a. Atrial fibrillation
   b. Hyperlipidemia
   c. Cardiovascular or peripheral vascular disease
   d. Arthritis

3. Which of the following objective findings may be related to TIA?

    a. Heberden nodes
    b. Carotid bruit
    c. Tenderness in both wrists
    d. Increased grip in both hands

4. Which of the following reasons accounts for why polycythemia can result in a TIA?

    a. The blood is too thin, resulting in decreased perfusion
    b. The blood is too thick, resulting in clotting
    c. The tissue is resistant to insulin
    d. The platelets are inhibited

5. Ticlopidine may be used for inhibition of platelets in clients with TIA who have which of the following?

    a. Allergy to aspirin
    b. Allergy to acetaminophen
    c. Allergy to eggs
    d. Allergy to warfarin

6. The treatment for significant carotid stenosis (greater than 70%) is which of the following?

    a. Heart catheterization
    b. Cardiac arterial bypass surgery
    c. Carotid endarterectomy
    d. Vagotomy

7. Once the INR is between 2 and 3, how often should the client be followed?

    a. Monthly
    b. Every 6 months
    c. Yearly
    d. As symptoms occur

Answers and Rationales

1. *Answer:* **c** (analysis/diagnosis)
Rationale: By definition, the occlusion is intermittent.

2. *Answer:* **d** (assessment)
Rationale: The other diseases are associated with the potential for emboli formation and resultant TIA.

3. *Answer:* **b** (assessment)
Rationale: Carotid bruits indicate turbulence of blood flow in the carotid artery that may be stenosis or ulceration in the carotid artery, from which emboli can detach.

4. *Answer:* **b** (analysis/diagnosis)
Rationale: Polycythemia is an increase in the number of red blood cells that makes the blood have a higher viscosity and may result in abnormal clotting.

5. *Answer:* **a** (implementation/plan)
Rationale: If the client is allergic to aspirin, the platelets can still be inhibited with ticlopidine.

6. *Answer:* **c** (implementation/plan)
Rationale: Carotid endarterectomy cleans up the carotid artery such that if there are tiny emboli being sent to the brain from the carotid artery, resulting in TIA, this will be stopped and the possibility of stroke will be decreased.

7. *Answer:* **a** (implementation/plan)
Rationale: The client needs to be followed up monthly to ensure anticoagulation and to prevent stroke.

TRIGEMINAL NEURALGIA   *Pamela Kidd*

OVERVIEW
Definition

Trigeminal neuralgia (tic douloureux) is a recurrent unilateral facial pain syndrome. It most often affects the maxillary division of the trigeminal nerve. The attacks of pain may last several seconds and may be repeated one after the other. They may come and go throughout the day and may last for days, weeks, or months at a time and then disappear for the same length of time. It has no known cause.

Incidence

- There are 15,000 to 25,000 new cases in the United States each year. This may be a low estimate because of difficulty of diagnosis during the early stage and misdiagnosis as a dental disease.
- Trigeminal neuralgia is more common in women than in men.
- It occurs most often during late middle age.
- It is associated with multiple sclerosis if younger in age and occurring bilaterally.

Pathophysiology

Although there is no known cause, there is a compression hypothesis that attempts to explain the clinical findings. The pain may be caused by electrical activity generated by compression of the trigeminal nerve. Demyelinated nerve fibers, hyperexcitability, and damaged axons combined with the discharge of nearby pain fibers may cause intense pain.

Factors Increasing Susceptibility
- Gender
- Age

Protective Factors. None.

ASSESSMENT: SUBJECTIVE/HISTORY
Symptoms

- Assess for duration, frequency, and intensity of pain.
- Identify what triggers the episode of pain.
- Ask about associated headaches.
- Ask about stabbing pains or clusters of stabbing pains that are restricted to one or more divisions of the

T

trigeminal nerve. Clients describe "electric-like shocks" of pain on one side of the face. These pains may last 20 to 30 seconds. Pain varies from mild to intense. Episodes may be brief and followed by long periods of remission. Trigger zones on the face or in the mouth are characteristic of this disorder. Activities involving the face, shaving, combing the hair, eating, drinking, and brushing the teeth may trigger the pain. The affected areas may be very sensitive to hot and cold. Clients are usually anxious when examined and may have a small degree of numbness in the affected area. Some clients experience atypical forms of trigeminal neuralgia, which has a less well-defined syndrome of pain. They may experience burning or aching over longer periods on one side of the face or forehead. There are usually no other neurologic abnormalities.

Past Medical History

- Ask about the most recent dental visit and any dental problems.
- Ask about headaches and their treatment in past.
- Trigeminal neuralgia is associated with multiple sclerosis and brainstem neoplasm.

Medication History

- Ask about current medications.
- Ask about medications that the client has tried to decrease pain.

Family History

Family history of headache, facial pain, and neurologic problems.

Dietary History

Noncontributory, although eating may trigger an attack.

ASSESSMENT: OBJECTIVE/PHYSICAL EXAMINATION
Physical Examination

Complete physical and neurologic examinations should be performed. Usually no abnormal physical findings are present. Usually no evidence of sensory loss in the nerve distribution is found.

Diagnostic Procedures

- There are no specific diagnostic tests.
- Perform magnetic resonance imaging of the head to rule out multiple sclerosis and compression tumor (rare to find).

DIAGNOSIS

For differential diagnoses, see Table 3-112.

THERAPEUTIC PLAN
Nonpharmacologic Treatment

- Radiofrequency rhizotomy
- Gamma radiosurgery to trigeminal nerve root

Pharmacologic Treatment

- Medications take effect from 4 to 24 hours after initiation of therapy.
- See Table 3-113.
- When the medical therapy is ineffective, subcutaneous injection of the ganglion with glycerol can provide relief and may be repeated if necessary.

TABLE **3-112** Differential Diagnoses

DIAGNOSIS	DATA SUPPORT
Trigeminal neuralgia	Characteristic facial pain beginning near one side of mouth then shooting toward ear, eye, or nose; physical examination and CT or MRI results are usually normal
Herpes zoster/post-herpetic neuralgia	Vesicular, painful lesions involving trigeminal nerve; approximately 10% of clients suffer from post-herpetic neuralgia
Dental disease	TMJ disorder may cause facial pain, as does a dental abscess
Trigeminal neuroma/acoustic and neuroma/aneurism/multiple sclerosis/meningioma (these are secondary trigeminal neuralgias)	Pain radiates from lesion to periphery of affected nerve and is usually intermittent but may become continuous and severe; should be considered, particularly if client is older than 40 years and has pain predominately in upper division (forehead and eye) or has bilateral pain or evidence of bilateral sensory loss or associated motor weakness
Multiple sclerosis	Should be considered as contributing disease when young person presents with trigeminal neuralgia
Cluster headaches	Ipsilateral nasal congestion, rhinorrhea, lacrimation, redness of eyes, Horner syndrome; episodes usually occur at night, most often in men
Facial migraine	Pain about eyes, nausea and vomiting, diplopia
Sinus problems	History of upper respiratory infection, fever, tenderness to sinus palpation

CT, Computed tomography; *MRI,* magnetic resonance imaging; *TMJ,* temporomandibular joint.

TABLE **3-113**   Pharmacologic Treatment

DRUG	DOSAGE	COMMENTS
Carbamazepine (Tegretol)	50 mg qid, then increase to 200 mg/day until pain relieved Maintenance: 800-1200 mg/day ER: 100-200 mg/day or bid with meals; increase to 800-1200 mg/day	Pregnancy: C Side effects: aplastic anemia, bone marrow depression, photosensitivity, drowsiness Interacts with CYP3A4 inhibitors and CYP3A4 inducers Monitor CBC, Fe level, BUN level, U/A, carbamazepine levels, ECG, electrolyte level, Ca level, and LFTs Once pain is controlled, dosage may be reduced to minimum effective dosage
Phenytoin (Dilantin)	250 mg tid; adjust dose every 7-10 days Children: 5 mg/kg/day in two to three doses; maximum dose is 300 mg/day	Pregnancy: X Side effects: nystagmus, drowsiness, GI disturbances, gingival hyperplasia, hepatic disease Chewable and suspension not intended for once-a-day dosing Many drug interactions because of P450 enzyme Monitor phenytoin and thyroid levels
Baclofen (Lioresal)	5 mg tid initially, then increase by 5 mg/dose every 3 days until desired response achieved; maximum dose is 80 mg/day	Pregnancy: C Side effects: drowsiness, dizziness, weakness, fatigue, increased urinary frequency
Neurontin (Gabapentin)	300 mg tid	Pregnancy: C Do not administer within 2 hours of antacids Side effects: somnolence, dizziness, ataxia, fatigue, nystagmus

BUN, Blood urea nitrogen; *Ca,* calcium; *CBC,* complete blood count; *ECG,* electrocardiogram; *ER,* extended release; *Fe,* iron; *GI,* gastrointestinal; *LFTs,* liver function tests; *U/A,* urinalysis.

Client Education

- Reassure the client that trigeminal neuralgia is not fatal.
- Connect the client with a support group or national foundation.
- The client may require treatment from 3 months to longer than 1 year.
- Trigeminal neuralgia may remit spontaneously.

Referral

Any client experiencing atypical facial pain should be referred to a neurologist.

Prevention

Avoid activities that trigger painful episodes (usually touch and drafts).

EVALUATION/FOLLOW-UP

- A client with a typical or classic presentation may be treated and followed by the primary care provider unless response to medical management is ineffective.
- Monitor appropriate laboratory values based on medication used.
- Follow every 2 to 3 weeks for response to treatment.

- Complete resolution of the pain is the goal. Surgery is a last resort.

COMPLICATIONS

Pain.

REFERENCES

Aminoff, M. (2001). Nervous system. In L. Tierney, S. McPhee, & M. Papadakis (Eds.), *Current medical diagnosis and treatment* (40th ed.). New York: McGraw Hill.

Bowsher, D. (1997). Trigeminal neuralgia: an anatomically oriented review. *Clinical Anatomy, 10*(6), 409-415.

Bushong, K. (2000). Trigeminal neuralgia. In D. Robinson, P. Kidd, & K. Rogers (Eds.), *Primary care across the lifespan.* St. Louis: Mosby.

Fields, H. L. (1996). Treatment of trigeminal neuralgia. *The New England Journal of Medicine, 334*(17) 1125-1126.

Howard, J. (1997). Tic douloureux, Parkinson's disease and the herpes connection. *Integrated Physical Behavioral Science, 32*(3), 257-264.

Lincoff, N., Rath, P. & Herano, M. (1998). The treatment of periocular and facial pain with topical capsaicin. *Journal of Neuroophthalmology, 18*(1), 17-20.

Mabara, G. (1996). Trigeminal neuralgia: A review of current therapeutic strategies. *Journal of Phillipines Dental Association, 47*(4), 33.

T

Sist, T., Filadora, V., Miner, M., Lema, M. (1997). Gabapentin for idiopathic trigeminal neuralgia: report of two cases. *Neurology, 48*, 1467-1471.

Zakrzewska, J., Chaundry, Z., Nurmikko, T. J., Patton, D. W., Mullens, E. L. (1997). Lamotrigine (Lamictal) in refractory trigeminal neuralgia: Results from a double-blind placebo controlled crossover trial. *Pain, 73*(2), 223-230.

Review Questions

1. The client with trigeminal neuralgia complains of what type of pain?

a. Pressure-like
b. Radiating to the neck
c. Burning
d. Stabbing

2. When performing a neurologic examination of a client with trigeminal neuralgia, the NP expects to find which of the following?

a. Difficulty clenching the jaw
b. Hypersensitivity of the face to a cotton ball
c. No abnormalities
d. A problem with cranial nerve VII

3. What is the best information to provide the client regarding medications used to treat trigeminal neuralgia?

a. Relief should occur within 24 hours after the initiation of therapy.
b. The medications are always effective in relieving symptoms but the timing of the relief is not predictable.
c. The medications require a month of use before therapeutic blood levels are reached.
d. The medications may produce seizures.

4. Which of the following statements indicates effective teaching of a client with trigeminal neuralgia?

a. "If I do not go into remission, I will have permanent deformity."
b. "Treatment may require up to a year."
c. "Attacks cannot be prevented."
d. "This condition is fatal."

Answers and Rationales

1. *Answer:* **c** (assessment)
   Rationale: The pain may be described as electric shocks. If it radiates, the pain radiates to the forehead.

2. *Answer:* **c** (assessment)
   Rationale: No evidence of sensory loss in the nerve is usually found. However, if the client is having an acute attack, paresthesia of the face may occur. There is no change in motor (jaw clenching) abilities. Cranial nerve VII (facial) is not affected.

3. *Answer:* **a** (implementation/plan)
   Rationale: The medications usually provide relief in 4 to 24 hours, but local injection of the ganglion may be necessary in some cases. The drugs used are also used to prevent seizures.

4. *Answer:* **b** (evaluation)
   Rationale: Treatment usually requires 3 to 12 months. Deformity and death are not associated with trigeminal neuralgia. Attacks can be prevented by avoiding triggers (usually drafts, touching the face).

TUBERCULOSIS *Pamela Kidd*

OVERVIEW
Definition

Tuberculosis (TB) is a chronic, infectious, inflammatory, reportable disease. Clients infected with the bacillus are distinguished from those who have the disease. TB usually infects the lungs but may occur in other tissues and organs in the body (extrapulmonary).

Incidence

The World Health Organization estimates that one third of the world population is infected with *Mycobacterium tuberculosis*. The occurrence rate of TB cases in the United States in 1996 was 8 per 100,000. Those older than 65 years have the highest case rate (16 per 100,000). The number of pediatric cases has increased by 51%, compared with an increase of 19% for all ages combined. The reasons for the increased incidence are the following:

- HIV epidemic

- Immigration into the United States from countries where TB is common
- Inadequate public health efforts because of decreased funding
- Resistance to antibiotics because of misuse and noncompliance with therapy

Pathophysiology

TB is caused by the bacteria *M. tuberculosis* and is transmitted by airborne droplets. The infected person does not develop the disease unless the immune system is compromised. The disease can be pulmonary or extrapulmonary. Extrapulmonary disease includes meningitis and lymphadenitis and renal, bone, and joint involvement. The disease has the two following stages:

- Infection (primary), which means exposure but no active disease, no symptoms but positive results of tuberculin test
- Disease (symptoms present)

Factors Increasing Susceptibility

- Contact with infected persons, HIV-positive persons, or persons from Latin America, the Caribbean, Africa, and Asia (except Japan)
- Living in homeless shelters, migrant farm camps, prisons, nursing homes, or with health care workers
- Alcoholism and drug abuse
- Impaired immunity from chronic illness
- Foreign travel

Protective Factors

- Living in uncrowded conditions with good ventilation
- Avoiding exposure to infected persons and at-risk populations
- Intact immune system

ASSESSMENT: SUBJECTIVE/HISTORY
Symptoms

- Chronic cough (usually with hemoptysis) lasting longer than 2 weeks
- Night sweats
- Unexplained weight loss
- Children are less likely to have obvious symptoms
  - Chest pain
  - Fatigue
  - Fever and chills
  - Anorexia

Past Medical History

- Substance abuse
- Diabetes
- Silicosis
- Cancer
- Renal failure
- Corticosteroid treatment or immunotherapy (e.g., transplant recipient)

Medication History

Corticosteroid use of long duration may produce immunosuppression and raise likelihood of TB infection.

Family History

- Children do not transmit the disease to other children. Infection is generally transmitted by adults. A detailed family history should be obtained.
- Ask about any chronic illness among family members because immunosuppression may allow the family member to have active TB disease.

ASSESSMENT: OBJECTIVE/PHYSICAL EXAMINATION
Physical Examination

- General appearance, including vital signs (fever)
  - Examination results may be negative, including results of the chest radiograph.
- *Chest:* rales or crackles in upper posterior chest

- Assess for bronchovesicular breathing.
- Assess for whispered pectoriloquy.
- Assess for supra- and infraclavicular retraction.
- *Lymph:* lymphadenopathy

Diagnostic Procedures
Laboratory Tests

- *CBC:* Check for low hematocrit, normocytic anemia, and normochromic anemia.
- *Urinalysis:* Sterile pyuria suggests renal TB.
- *Liver enzymes:* If disseminated disease is present, these enzymes are elevated.
- *Sputum for culture and smear (acid-fast bacteria) times 3:* A positive smear is highly suggestive of TB, but only the culture is diagnostic. Cultures allow for testing for drug sensitivity to standard TB drugs.
- *TB skin test:* A 5-tuberculin unit dose of purified protein derivative should be used (Mantoux test).
  The following persons should be tested:
  - Any person who has spent time with a person who has infectious TB
  - A client with a chronic illness that puts the client at high risk for TB (e.g., HIV)
  - A client from a country with a high rate of TB
  The test should be performed at the following times:
  - If a person has been in contact with another person with active TB disease, it may take 10 to 12 weeks after exposure for the test to produce positive results. If the test is performed earlier than 10 weeks after possible exposure, retest later.
  - Children should be tested based on the incidence of TB in their community. Guidelines recommend testing when the child is between 4 and 6 years of age and again when the child is between 11 and 16 years of age.
  Read the results as follows:
  - If a person has received a bacille Calmette-Guérin (BCG) vaccination for TB, a positive tuberculin test result may occur. The size of the reaction indicates the likelihood of active disease. Reactions from BCG get smaller over time.
  - Results should be read between 48 and 72 hours after injection.
  - The basis of the reading is the presence or absence of induration determined from inspection and palpation, recorded in millimeters.
  - If a multiple puncture test instead of a Mantoux test has been performed, a positive result is vesicular in nature. If papules form, the test should be repeated using the Mantoux method (intradermal).
  Postive findings are the following:
  - More than 5 mm is a positive finding for HIV-infected persons, persons who have had close contact with someone with active TB and persons who have healed TB as evidenced by chest x-ray examination.

T

- More than 10 mm is a positive finding for persons who are from countries with high incidence and for high-risk populations (including thus with possible immunosuppression from chronic illness), including health care workers.
- More than 15 mm is a positive finding for all persons. Two-step testing involves the following:
- Used for the elderly or the immunosuppressed, this test is repeated 1 to 3 weeks after the first administration. A 6-mm increase in induration from tuberculin test 1 to tuberculin test 2 in conjunction with chronic obstructive pulmonary disease, undernutrition, diabetes, end-stage renal disease, immunosuppression, malignancy, gastrectomy, or jejunoileal bypass is also considered a positive finding (Bergman-Evans, 1998). In older clients, the second test may be positive although the first test was negative.

Tuberculin test conversion is an increase of 10 mm or more within a 2-year period (Franco-Paredes & Blumberg, 2001).

Persons previously vaccinated with BCG are as noted previously. If positive and no symptoms are present, assume latent TB. Active TB is confirmed by diagnostic testing.

Radiographic Tests
- Perform chest x-ray examination, obtaining posteroanterior and lateral views.
- Apical scarring, hilar adenopathy with peripheral infiltrate, and upper lobe cavitation may be present. Negative results of chest radiograph rule out pulmonary TB.

DIAGNOSIS
Differential diagnoses are located in Table 3-114.
- Latent TB infection: negative radiographic results, no clinical signs or symptoms, positive results of Mantoux test
- Active TB infection: positive cultures, positive radiographic results, positive results of tuberculin test, signs and symptoms are present

THERAPEUTIC PLAN
Nonpharmacologic Treatment
If weight loss is present, a high-calorie diet should be instituted.

Pharmacologic Treatment
Drug therapy plan is presented in Table 3-115.
- Rifater combines isoniazid (INH) with rifampin and pyrazinamide.
- Liver enzyme (alanine transferase [ALT], aspartame transferase [AST]) tests are necessary when administering INH with rifampin and pyrazinamide. They are performed at baseline, at 2, 4, and 6 weeks of therapy, and at the week 8 for the 2-month rifampin-pyrazinamide regimen. If the client is receiving INH, AST and ALT, he or she is assessed three times per month and then once every 3 months. If a 2.5- to 3-fold increase occurs in active disease, discontinue or switch drug therapy.
- TB of the lungs and throat is infectious. The client should stay home from work or school for at least 2 weeks after starting treatment.
- If it is difficult for the client to remember to take the drugs, consider enrolling the client in a directly observed therapy (DOT) program at the health department. If the client still has positive cultures after the required treatment, enrollment in a DOT program is recommended because this is an indicator of nonadherence.

Client Education
- Explain the difference between TB infection and TB disease. Explain that with TB infection, the person has no symptoms and cannot spread the disease to another person, but can develop active disease if not treated.
- Warn the client about the side effects of the medications, including the following:
  - No appetite
  - Nausea and vomiting
  - Yellowish skin or eyes
  - Fever longer than 3 days
  - Abdominal pain
  - Tingling in fingers and toes
  - Change in vision
  - Rash
- Emphasize the need to complete the drug therapy plan. Suggest a reminder system, such as taking the medication at the same time each day around a routine activity (e.g., brushing teeth) and using a pill dispenser.

TABLE **3-114** Differential Diagnoses

DIAGNOSIS	DATA SUPPORT
Community-acquired pneumonia (fungal)	Fever, headache, sore throat, myalgia, nonproductive hacking cough, substernal chest pain
Chronic bronchitis	Productive cough lasting longer than 3 months in at least 2 consecutive years, smoker, shortness of breath with activity, digital clubbing, hyperinflation on chest radiograph if emphysema is present

TABLE **3-115**   Pharmaceutical Treatment for Active TB

DRUG	DOSE	COMMENTS
INH	5-10 mg/kg PO qd, up to 300 mg	Side effects include peripheral neuritis and hepatitis; warn client *not* to drink alcoholic beverages; must be taken on an empty stomach every morning
RIF	10 mg/kg PO qd up to 600 mg	Side effects include hepatitis and purpura; reduces effect of OCPs and implants; use alternative contraceptive method; can turn saliva, tears, and urine orange; do not use soft contact lenses; must be taken on an empty stomach every morning
Streptomycin	15-20 mg/kg PO qd, up to 1 g	Nephrotoxic, may damage hearing
PZA	15-30 mg/kg PO qd up to 2 g	Causes hyperuricemia
Rifater	Do not administer to client younger than 15 years of age. Give client weighing less than 44 kg four tabs; 44-54 kg, five tabs; more than 55 kg, 6 tabs administered PO qd	Used in initial phase of 2-month treatment of pulmonary tuberculosis; continue treatment for 4 additional months with RIF and INH
ETB	15-25 mg/kg PO qd	Can cause optic neuritis; check visual acuity often

Note: All of these drugs can be administered two or three times weekly to promote adherence. Check an additional drug reference for proper dosage.
Note: Drug treatment for a client with latent TB infection is for a 2-month period for adults (RIF and PZA daily). If the results of the chest radiograph are abnormal, the treatment period is 12 months. Pregnant women with active TB infection, children, and persons with HIV infection need 9 months of treatment with INH.
ETB, Ethambutol; *INH,* isoniazid; *OCPs,* oral contraceptive pills; *PZA,* pyrazinamide; *RIF,* rifampin; *TB,* tuberculosis.

Referral

- In cases of systemic disease, the client should be referred to an infectious disease physician or internal medicine specialist. A pulmonologist may also be consulted.
- All cases of TB must be reported to the public health department.

Prevention

- Sleep alone until 2 weeks of treatment have been completed.
- Make sure of adequate ventilation.
- Wear masks when active disease is present or when around someone with active disease.

EVALUATION/FOLLOW-UP

- Conduct follow-up every 2 weeks for treatment with rifampin and pyrazinamide.
- Conduct follow-up monthly with INH treatment.
- Monitor visual acuity.
- Monitor renal function.
- Monitor liver enzymes.

COMPLICATIONS

- Neurologic impairment
- Renal failure

REFERENCES

Bergman-Evans, B. (1998). Tuberculosis in long-term care settings. *ADVANCE for Nurse Practitioners, 6*(12), 67-69.

Cornell, S. (1998). Back from the dead: Emerging and re-emerging infectious diseases. *ADVANCE for Nurse Practitioners, 6*(5), 67-68.

Cornell, S. (1998). Pediatric infectious disease: Updates on three top offenders. *ADVANCE for Nurse Practitioners, 6*(5), 70-72.

Franco-Paredes, C., & Blumberg, H. (2001). Latent tuberculosis infection: When to screen, when to treat. *Consultant, 41*(8), 1113-1118, 1120-1121.

Horwitz, H., Niederman, M., & Schaffner, W. (1999). HIV disease, persistent fever, nonresolving pneumonia, and tuberculosis. *Patient Care for the Nurse Practitioner,* 20-22, 25-28, 31-34, 39-40.

Kidd, P. (2000). Tuberculosis. In D. Robinson, P. Kidd, & K. Rogers (Eds.), *Primary care across the lifespan.* St. Louis: Mosby.

Review Questions

1. Which of the following applies to a client with a positive tuberculin skin test result?

- **a.** Client is ill with TB.
- **b.** Client is infected with the organism.
- **c.** Client is contagious.
- **d.** Client is allergic to the vaccine.

2. Which of the following symptoms is most indicative of TB?

- **a.** Night sweats
- **b.** Weight loss
- **c.** Fever
- **d.** Chronic cough

T

3. Pneumonia may be mistaken for TB. Which of the following should help confirm which of the two is the correct diagnosis?

a. Housing situation
b. Pulmonary examination
c. Cough characteristics
d. Chest x-ray examination

4. Treatment for TB requires which of the following?

a. Isolation
b. At least 2 months of drug therapy
c. Penicillin plus INH
d. Desensitization

5. A client who has been under your care for 12 months for treatment of TB still has positive cultures. Which of the following is the best option?

a. Consider the client a carrier and stop treatment.
b. Refer the client to a DOT program.
c. Increase the drug dosage.
d. Refer the client to a pulmonologist.

6. A client who has diabetes has a 5-mm induration with Mantoux testing. The NP interprets this as which of the following?

a. Indicative of latent infection
b. Negative
c. Two-step testing necessary
d. A Tuberculin test conversion

7. A client with active TB who is receiving rifampin and pyrazinamide has a threefold increase in liver enzymes. The NP should do which of the following?

a. Stop the medication.
b. Switch the medication.
c. Add INH.
d. Decrease the dose.

Answers and Rationales

1. *Answer:* **b** (analysis/diagnosis)
Rationale: The only positive finding is that the person has the organism. Active disease (and therefore contagious status) may not be present and is confirmed by obtaining a chest radiograph or sputum cultures.

2. *Answer:* **d** (assessment)
Rationale: All four symptoms may occur with TB. However, of these, only cough is associated with TB versus other systemic chronic diseases that compromise the immune system.

3. *Answer:* **b** (analysis/diagnosis)
Rationale: Overcrowding may cause both conditions. Cough may be associated with both conditions. Consolidation may occur with either disease. There are no significant findings of the pulmonary examination of a person with TB. In cases of pneumonia, increased vocal fremitus, dullness to percussion, crackles, and decreased breath sounds may occur.

4. *Answer:* **b** (implementation/plan)
Rationale: Isolation is not required if the person can and will control droplet spread. Treatment may consist of INH, rifampin, pyrazinamide, and, in adults, ethambutol. No one can be desensitized to TB.

5. *Answer:* **b** (evaluation)
Rationale: Clients with positive culture results must receive continued treatment. The positive culture result is usually a sign of nonadherence with treatment, and referral to a DOT program is indicated for public health. Increased dosage is not necessary and contributes to resistance.

6. *Answer:* **b** (analysis/diagnosis)
Rationale: A 5-mm induration indicates active or latent TB (depending on results of other tests and the presence or absence of signs and symptoms) in persons with HIV or persons from countries where TB is endemic. A 10-mm induration is positive for a person with diabetes. Two-step testing is used for the elderly or immunosuppressed, but only if the results of the first test are negative. Tuberculin test conversion is an increase of 10 mm or more within a 2-year period. There are not enough data in the question to assume this fact.

7. *Answer:* **b** (evaluation)
Rationale: Liver enzyme (ALT, AST) tests are necessary when administering INH with rifampin and pyrazinamide. They are performed at baseline, at 2, 4, and 6 weeks of therapy, and at week 8 for the 2-month rifampin-pyrazinamide regimen. If the client is receiving INH, AST and ALT liver enzyme are assessed three times per month and then once every 3 months. If a 2.5- to 3-fold increase occurs in active disease, discontinue the current drug and switch to another agent.

URINARY INCONTINENCE   *Cheryl Pope Kish*

OVERVIEW
Definition

Urinary incontinence is defined by the Agency for Health Care Policy and Research as "involuntary loss of urine which is sufficient to be a problem." Urinary incontinence produces a significant threat to one's quality of life; clients often experience diminished self-esteem, concerns about hygiene and skin integrity, and social isolation.

Incidence

- Exact statistics are unavailable because many persons with urinary incontinence fail to mention this condition to their health care providers because of embarrassment, belief that incontinence is a normal expectation of aging, or lack of opportunity.
- It is thought that more than 13 million Americans suffer with urinary incontinence. Women are twice as likely as men to have this problem.
- The condition is more common among aging clients, with 15% of community dwellers and 50% of those in long-term care facilities affected.

Pathophysiology

Continence depends on a compliant reservoir for urine storage and sphincter control that has two components: involuntary smooth muscle of the bladder neck and voluntary skeletal muscle of the external sphincter. There are four major categories of reversible urinary incontinence: stress incontinence, urge incontinence (detrusor instability), overflow incontinence, and functional incontinence. A fifth category (mixed) is a combination of stress and urge incontinence and is particularly common among women.

Stress Incontinence

- Accounts for 80% of urinary incontinence in women younger than 60 years.
- Associated with activities that result in increased intraabdominal pressure, such as coughing, sneezing, laughing, lifting, and exercising.
- Urine does not leak in the supine position.
- Associated with urethral sphincter insufficiency and laxity of pelvic floor muscles related to multiparity, pelvic surgery, chronic constipation, obesity, trophic changes to genital tissue from hypoestrogen state, and injuries in childbirth.

Urge Incontinence

- Urge incontinence is a less common cause of incontinence but accounts for 70% of urinary incontinence in older adults, especially men.

- Associated with involuntary bladder contractions that stimulate urge to void that cannot be overcome.
- Unrelated to position or activity.
- Causes swift leakage of moderate to large amounts of urine.
- Often caused by bladder irritation or neurogenic problems (e.g., Alzheimer disease, cerebrovascular accidents, chronic cystitis, Parkinson's disease).

Overflow Incontinence

- Overflow incontinence is a less common cause of urinary incontinence.
- Associated with chronic urinary retention; distended bladder receives additional increment of urine from kidney so that intravesical pressure just exceeds outlet resistance, allowing small amounts of urine to dribble out.
- Causes include neurologic effects of diabetes mellitus, vitamin B_6 deficiency, obstructions related to benign prostatic hypertension (BPH), strictures, or tumors, and side effect of certain medications

Functional Incontinence. This condition occurs in clients who have cognitive problems or severe restrictions to mobility that interfere with timely urination.

ASSESSMENT: SUBJECTIVE/HISTORY
History of Present Illness

- Pattern of voiding: frequency, timing, amount, causes attributed to leakage, character of urinary stream, and characteristics of urine (voiding diary can be used to provide many of these details); need to void so urgently cannot make it to toilet
- Fluid intake: time, type, and amount
- Signs and symptoms of urinary tract infection (UTI)
- Signs and symptoms of chronic illness (neurologic, diabetes)
- Symptoms of menopause (hot flashes, vaginal dryness, irritability)
- Nocturia
- Need to use absorbent pads to protect clothing from urine leakage

Past Medical History

- Obstetric history: parity, type of deliveries, operative delivery (forceps, vacuum extraction, episiotomy)
- Contraception used
- History of genital prolapse and surgery
- Last menstrual period
- Use of hormone replacement
- History of renal or urinary tract disease, including frequent UTIs

U

- History of chronic respiratory disease with cough
- History of neurologic disease or radiculopathy
- History of sexual abuse
- History of BPH

Medication History

- Sedative hypnotics, central nervous system depressants, and antipsychotics cause retention, sedation.
- Anticholinergics cause retention.
- Alpha-adrenergics relax the urinary sphincter.
- Diuretics cause frequency, urgency, and polyuria.
- Determine use of hormone replacement therapy.
- Antihistamines cause retention.
- Calcium channel blockers cause retention.
- Alpha-antagonists (e.g., doxazosin mesylate, terazosin hydrochloride, and prazosin hydrochloride) lower urethral pressure.

Psychosocial History

- Alcohol use causes frequency, urgency.
- Caffeine use causes irritation to bladder.
- Smoking is detrimental.

ASSESSMENT: OBJECTIVE/PHYSICAL EXAMINATION
Physical Examination

- The physical examination is intended to assess for systemic disease with the potential to affect continence and to evaluate the particulars of urinary incontinence.
- Obtain vital signs.
- Evaluate mental status; look for evidence of delirium or dementia.
- Assess respiratory system for acute or chronic disease associated with cough.
- Assess cardiac system for cardiac disease, including congestive heart failure.
- Check abdomen for distention, suprapubic tenderness, and masses.
- Perform pelvic examination. Note normalcy of urethral meatus. Determine whether skin of perineal area is intact. Note vaginal mucosa for evidence of estrogen deficiency. Assess vaginal tone. Observe for cystocele and rectocele (use half of speculum to facilitate this assessment). Ask woman to strain down to see whether loss of urine occurs. Test tone of levator ani muscle and ability to contract. Look for fistulae.
- Perform rectal examination. Palpate for rectocele, enlarged prostate, fecal impaction. Evaluate normal anal tone.
- Perform neurologic assessment. Check strength and sensation of lower extremities to assess pudendal nerve function reflexes, including Babinski sign, light touch, and deep tendon reflex.
- Assess musculoskeletal system. Note mobility.

Diagnostic Tests

Tests conducted by many primary care providers include the following:

- Perform urinalysis.
- Obtain urine culture and sensitivity with suspicion of UTI.
- Obtain chemistry profile with blood urea nitrogen (BUN), creatinine, calcium, and glucose to rule out systemic or renal problem as contributory.
- Ask client to keep a voiding diary.
- Consider "Q-tip" test. Cleanse area as for urinary catheterization. Insert sterile cotton swab lubricated with anesthetic gel into bladder; use goniometer to determine angle between swab and horizontal plane while resting compared with angle during Valsalva maneuver. If angle changes more than 30 degrees, urethral hypermobility (positive result for stress incontinence) is suggested.
- Refer for specialized urodynamic testing, which includes the following:
  - Postvoid measurement of residual urine.
  - Cystometry to test for detrusor instability, bladder capacity, and stress.
  - Uroflowmeter testing to measure voiding duration, amount, and rate graphically.
  - Pad test. (After dose of phenazopyridine hydrochloride [Pyridium], woman notes color of urine staining.)
  - Sphincter assessment: urethral profilometry, electromyography, combined video studies.

DIAGNOSIS

Differentiate between types of urinary incontinence: stress, urge, overflow, functional, or mixed. Determine whether the problem is transient and related to a systemic problem, medication use, or environmental factors that can be easily remedied.

THERAPEUTIC PLAN
Nonpharmacologic Treatment

Stress Incontinence

- Kegel (pelvic floor) exercises: Hold contraction for 10 seconds. Do 10 to 20 repetitions three to four times a day. Initial instructions and reminders are essential.
- For women who have incontinence only with exercise, taking an alpha agonist 30 minutes in advance and using a large or super size tampon for pelvic support may help.
- Use progressively weighted (20 to 100 g) vaginal cones held in the vagina twice daily. Correct use requires the woman to contract her pelvic musculature effectively.
- Pelvic floor electrical stimulation can be applied bid.
- Individually fitted pessaries may be useful. Teach the client to remove the appliance at night and reinsert it

in the morning after cleaning with soap and water. The two primary types are the Continence Ring and the Introl Device.

- Occlusive devices to occlude urethral meatus include the Reliance Catheter, Fem-Assist, and Impress Softpatch. The use of such devices is contraindicated in women with high pressure detrusor overactivity.
- Surgeries such as bladder neck suspension and urethral sling procedures can be performed (Burch, Marshall-Marchetti test).

Urge Incontinence

- Bladder retraining with gradual lengthening of time between voiding
- Timed voiding: opportunities at regular intervals prompted by caretakers for those with mobility or cognitive impairment
- Absorbent products to allow clients to conduct normal activities of daily life while decreasing embarrassment, discomfort, and inconvenience
- Fluid management
- Kegel exercises
- Surgery: rarely used; denervation procedures and cytoplasty reserved for nonresponsive cases

Overflow Incontinence

- Crede or Valsalva maneuver to facilitate bladder emptying
- Intermittent or indwelling or suprapubic catheterization
- Transurethral resection of the prostate: procedure of choice for men with overflow problem related to BPH; newer procedures: transurethral incision of prostate and transurethral ultrasound-guided laser-induced prostatectomy

Functional Incontinence

- Provide clear paths to toilet and good lightening in environment.
- Recommend assistive devices (e.g., canes, walkers, grab bars) to facilitate easier access to toilets.

Pharmacologic Treatment

- Stress incontinence: estrogen (systemic or vaginal topical), pseudoephedrine (Sudafed), imipramine (Tofranil)
- Urge incontinence: oxybutynin (Ditropan), imipramine (Tofranil), Flavoxate (Urispas), tolterodine (Detrik), propantheline bromide (Pro-Banthine), and dicyclomine (Bentyl); detrusor hyperactivity: oxybutynin
- Overflow incontinence: Prazosin (Minipress), bethanechol chloride (Urecholine)
  See Table 3-116 for key information about drugs.

Client Education

- Teach the client how to maintain a voiding diary for assessment. The client should note the following: time voided or leaked, time and amount of oral intake, amount of voided urine, activity at time of leakage, quantification of leak (0 = few drops, 1 = damp, 2 = wet, and 3 = soaked), and urge with or before voiding or leakage.
- Advise adequate fluid intake (four to eight glasses a day) to prevent UTI and bowel problems. More fluids may be necessary in times of hot weather or high activity. It is important to quench thirst. Note that the elderly may not feel thirst and that dehydration is possible.
- Have the client avoid fluids containing irritants (e.g., coffee, tea, carbonated drinks, alcohol). High acid beverages like orange juice, grapefruit juice, cranberry juice, and lemonade are problems for some. High sugar intake and hot spicy foods may irritate some clients.

TABLE **3-116** Key Information About Drugs for Urinary Incontinence

DRUG	EFFECTS
STRESS INCONTINENCE	
Pseudoephedrine (Sudafed) 15-30 mg PO tid	Anticholinergic effects, GI upset, insomnia, palpitations, and anxiety
Estrogen (systemic, estrogen ring, vaginal cream)	Alleviates problem of vaginal or urethral atrophy related to hypoestrogenemia. Estrogen ring and cream do not offer same protection from osteoporosis. With systemic estrogen and intact uterus, progesterone should be added.
OVERACTIVE BLADDER/URGE INCONTINENCE	
Oxybutynin (Ditropan) 2.5-10 mg bid-qid or Ditropan XL 5-15 mg daily	First-line drug. Anticholinergic effects cause blurred vision, dry mouth, and constipation. Need clearance from ophthalmologist if glaucoma is suspected. Pregnancy category B.
Tolterodine (Detrol) 1-2 mg bid	Antimuscarinic agent helpful with incontinence and has less anticholinergic effects than oxybutynin. Contraindicated in cases of urinary retention. Pregnancy category C.
Imipramine (Tofranil) 10-75 mg hs	May cause nausea and insomnia.
Dicyclomine (Bentyl) 10-20 mg qid	May cause nausea, vertigo, headache, and tachycardia.

GI, Gastrointestinal.

- Instruct the client not to postpone urination when urge is felt.
- Teach the client to try to avoid frequent urination by using distraction, working up to 2 to 4 hours between voidings. Clients with urge incontinence will likely need medication to accomplish this goal.
- Kegel exercises: Verbal and written instructions and reminder stickers can be helpful. Help the client to locate the pubococcygeal muscle through starting and stopping the urine stream. Advise the client to squeeze the muscle for 2 seconds and to relax the muscle for 10 seconds, increasing the squeezing time by 1-second increments until the client can hold the contraction for 10 seconds.
- Teach aging clients that incontinence is not an expectation of aging and should be reported so that corrective remedies can be offered.
- Prevent constipation/fecal impaction.

Referral/Consultation

- Clients who need urodynamic testing for diagnosis
- Clients who are nonresponsive to treatment
- Men with prostate nodules or asymmetry
- Clients who want to explore surgical options
- Women with cystoceles or rectoceles
- Clients with recurring UTI or hematuria with urinary infection
- Clients with neurologic disorders

Prevention

There are no recognized preventive strategies. Helpful strategies include the following:

- Estrogen replacement therapy
- Kegel exercises
- Avoiding obesity

EVALUATION/FOLLOW-UP

Monthly follow-up during initial treatment enables evaluation of strategies used. Follow-up should then be performed as needed.

COMPLICATIONS

Complications of urinary incontinence relate to effects on the quality of life regarding family, work, and leisure activities. Depression and social isolation are common. Incontinence also increases the risk of institutionalization of the elderly, falls and fractures, and increased caregiver burden.

REFERENCES

Culligan, P. J., & Heit, M. (2000). Urinary incontinence in women: Evaluation and management. *American Family Physician, 62*(11), 2433-2444, 2447, 2452.

Culligan, P. J., & Sand, P. K. (1998). Involuntary urine loss in women: Help for a hidden problem. *Patient Care,* December 15, 141-161.

Czarapata, B. J. (1999). Managing urinary incontinence. *Patient Care Nurse Practitioner, 2* (4), 37-48, 2433-2444, 2447, 2452.

Hoffman, E. (2000). Overactive bladder: Diagnosis of a hidden disorder. *Contemporary Ob/Gyn,* Summer (Suppl.), 15-21.

Miller, J. A. (2000). Urinary incontinence: A classification system and treatment protocols for primary care providers. *Journal of American Academy of Nurse Practitioners, 12*(9), 374-379.

Roberts, R. G. (2000). Current management strategies for overactive bladder. *Contemporary Ob/Gyn,* Summer (Suppl.), 22-30.

Robinson, D., Kidd, P., & Rogers, K. M. (2000). *Primary care across the lifespan.* St. Louis: Mosby.

Rovner, E. S., & Wein, A. J. (2000). Overactive bladder and urge incontinence: Establishing the diagnosis. *Women's Health and Primary Care, 3*(2), 117-126.

Shimp L. A., & Peggs, J. F. (2000). *20 common problems in women's health care.* New York: McGraw-Hill.

Shinopulos, N. (2000). Bedside urodynamic studies: Simple testing for urinary incontinence. *Nurse Practitioner, 25*(6), 18-39.

Thom, D. H. (2000). Overactive bladder: Epidemiology and impact on quality of life. *Contemporary Ob/Gyn,* Summer (Suppl.), 6-14.

Tierney, L. M., McPhee, S. J., & Papadakis, M. A. (2001). *Current medical diagnosis and treatment.*, New York: Lange Medical Books/McGraw-Hill.

Weir, A. J. (2000). Putting overactive bladder into clinical perspective. *Contemporary Ob/Gyn,* Summer (Suppl.), 1-5.

Winkler, H. A., & Sand, P. K. (1998). Stress incontinence: Options for conservative treatment. *Women's Health and Primary Care, 1*(3), 279-294.

Review Questions

1. Mrs. Connor is a 56-year-old woman experiencing incontinence. Which comment she makes about her symptoms is consistent with a diagnosis of stress incontinence?

  a. "I couldn't hold my urine twice this week; we are moving and boxes blocked my trip to the bathroom."
  b. "Recently I have had an overwhelming urge to urinate and cannot hold my urine; I can be working or just reading."
  c. "I've had multiple sclerosis for years but I hadn't started to be incontinent until the last few weeks."
  d. "I do pretty well until I laugh or lift something heavy; then I'm likely to leak urine."

2. Which factor in Mrs. Connor's history predisposes to stress incontinence?

  a. Heavy smoking with chronic cough
  b. Cesarean childbirth with both pregnancies
  c. Sedentary lifestyle
  d. Retired Air Force colonel

3. Which of the following clients is most likely to have a diagnosis of overflow incontinence?

  a. 42-year-old who occasionally leaks urine while jogging
  b. 66-year-old man with BPH
  c. 27-year-old man with renal calculi
  d. 37-year-old woman during an anxiety attack

4. Which of the following diagnostic tests is considered first-line for diagnosing urinary incontinence?

    a. Intravenous pyelogram
    b. Voiding cystogram
    c. Urine culture
    d. Renal ultrasonography

5. In which of the following situations is a referral for urodynamic testing appropriate?

    a. Postpartum client voiding frequent small amounts despite urinary distention
    b. Client with first episode of incontinence during rehabilitation after hip replacement
    c. Woman with symptoms indicative of both stress incontinence and urge incontinence
    d. Older man with residual volume of 60 ml after voiding 280 ml

6. A middle-aged woman who is experiencing leakage of urine has been provided with detailed instructions for keeping a voiding diary to facilitate diagnosis. Which notation in the diary is most helpful to diagnosis?

    a. 9:45 A.M.: damp panty liner; voided on toilet
    b. 10:00 A.M.: soaked panties and pad; urge present
    c. 4:20 P.M.: bladder contractions; unable to delay
    d. 5:50 P.M.: dry 3 hours; wearing adult diapers today

7. The nurse practitioner (NP) orders conjugated equine estrogen for a postmenopausal woman with urinary incontinence. The woman had a hysterectomy many years ago. What is the rationale for using estrogen for urinary incontinence?

    a. Estrogen increases bladder capacity.
    b. Estrogen therapy inhibits bladder contractions.
    c. Estrogen alkalinizes urine.
    d. Estrogen alleviates atrophic effects on bladder tissue.

Answers and Rationales

1. **Answer: d** (Fanalysis/diagnosis)
    Rationale: Stress incontinence is associated with activities that result in increased abdominal pressure (e.g., coughing, sneezing, laughing, lifting, and exercising) (Winkler & Sand, 1998).

2. **Answer: a** (assessment)
    Rationale: The presence of a chronic cough is associated with stress incontinence because it causes increased intraabdominal pressure (Winkler & Sand, 1998).

3. **Answer: b** (analysis/diagnosis)
    Rationale: Overflow incontinence is associated with outlet obstruction or underactivity of the detrusor (Robinson et al., 2000).

4. **Answer: c** (analysis/diagnosis)
    Rationale: Urinalysis and urine culture are considered first-line diagnostic tests in a work-up for urinary incontinence (Tierney et al. 2001).

5. **Answer: c** (analysis/diagnosis)
    Rationale: Clients with symptoms of both stress and urge incontinence should be referred for urodynamic testing to make an appropriate diagnosis (Rovner & Wein, 2000).

6. **Answer: b** (assessment)
    Rationale: Choice b is most helpful because it provides enough detail for the NP to judge the amount of urine lost and whether this amount was preceded by an urge to void. Other diary entries lack specificity or detail to be helpful (Winkler & Sand, 1998).

7. **Answer: d** (implementation/plan)
    Rationale: Estrogen receptors are present within the bladder and urethral epithelium; decreases in estrogen levels cause atrophic changes. The urethral mucosa becomes thinner, leading to lowered urethral closing pressures. Estrogen therapy remedies this problem (Czarapata, 1999).

URINARY TRACT INFECTION   *Cheryl Pope Kish*

OVERVIEW
Definition

- Cystitis is the presence of bacteria in urine, causing a change in urinary patterns. It is considered a lower UTI.
- Pyelonephritis is an infection of the renal pelvis or parenchyma. It is considered an upper UTI.
- Two infections that occur within 6 months or three infections that occur within 1 year constitute recurrent UTI.

Incidence

- UTI is the second most common infection (respiratory infection is the most common). It accounts for 7 million visits to health care providers each year.

- Every year, 20% of women complain of UTI symptoms; occurrence of UTI becomes more common with increasing age. Women have a 40% to 50% lifetime risk of UTI.
- Newborn boys have UTIs more frequently than do newborn girls, especially uncircumcised boys, but after the newborn period, most UTIs occur in girls.
- Approximately 20% of UTIs are recurrent.

Pathophysiology

UTI usually occurs as a consequence of colonization of the periurethral area by virulent organisms that subsequently gain access to the bladder.

U

Protective Factors

- Urinary acidity and osmolality
- Antimicrobial properties of the mucosa
- "Flushing" effect of urination, especially when adequately hydrated
- Cervical immunoglobulins

Factors Increasing Susceptibility

- Female gender: shorter urethra and close proximity of urethra to anus
- Bacterial virulence
- Behavioral factors: poor hygiene, wiping back to front, nonresponse to urge to void
- Abnormal urinary flow: stones, BPH, vesicoureteral reflux (structural abnormalities)
- Other host factors: decreased immunity, pregnancy, alcoholism, indwelling catheter, increased sexual activity, urinary instrumentation, bubble baths (females only), perfumed feminine hygiene products, diaphragm use, spermicides, diabetes mellitus, loss of protective lactobacilli from antibiotics and spermicide use

Common Pathogens

- *Escherichia coli* (70% to 85% of cystitis, 90% of pyelonephritis)
- *Staphylococcus saprophyticus* (10% to 20%)
- *Enterococcus* species

ASSESSMENT: SUBJECTIVE/HISTORY
Most Common Symptoms

Cystitis

- Adults: Typical symptoms include dysuria, urinary frequency, urinary urgency, hematuria, urine odor, suprapubic discomfort, small-volume voidings despite constant sensation to void, pressure, and acute onset.
- Infants: Typical symptoms include irritability, failure to thrive, systemic illness (fever), vomiting and diarrhea, abdominal pain and distention, decreased urination, change in urination pattern (enuresis), and foul odor. UTI is the most common cause of fever of undetermined origin in infants. The younger the infant, the more likely sepsis and structural abnormalities will be found.
- Toddlers: Typical symptoms include abdominal discomfort, fever, altered voiding patterns, and malodorous urine.
- Preschool: Typical symptoms include voiding discomfort and enuresis.
- School-age children and teenagers: Typical signs and symptoms are the same as for adults.
- Older adults: This group may be asymptomatic, and fever is uncommon.

Pyelonephritis

- Adults, school-age children, and older children: Fever, malaise, prostration, nausea, anorexia, and back pain can be present, and more gradual onset and toxic appearance can occur.
- Children younger than 6 years old: Nonspecific symptoms, similar to those associated with cystitis, can occur.
- Older adults: Generalized symptoms are common; in 50% of women older than 65 years, it is possible that no fever will be present until later in the course.

Associated Symptoms

- Back or flank pain
- Nausea and vomiting
- Incontinence in children (who were previously toilet trained) or older adults
- Fever
- Decreased force of urine stream
- Nocturia
- Diarrhea
- Constipation
- Vaginal discharge
- Urethral discharge
- Perianal itching

Past Medical History

- Kidney stones; UTIs; kidney, bladder, or prostate disease
- Diabetes, hypertension, multiple sclerosis
- Last menstrual period, use of barrier birth control methods, spermicides
- Allergies, date of last sexual contact, new sexual partner within preceding 6 months
- Pregnant female: recent group A beta-streptococcus infection

Medication History

Inquire about recent use of antibiotics or any other medications.

Family History

Ask about family history of kidney problems.

Psychosocial History

In children, consider possible sexual abuse. Do not ask the child about possible sexual abuse until a comfortable nurse-client relationship has been established.

Dietary History

- Increased ingestion of caffeine or carbonated drinks
- Abnormal water intake

ASSESSMENT: OBJECTIVE/PHYSICAL EXAMINATION
Physical Examination

- A problem-oriented physical examination should be conducted with particular attention to vital signs and weight, general appearance, and general hydration status, including orthostatic changes.

- Abdominal examination: Perform a full abdominal examination, and check for costovertebral angle (CVA) tenderness (common in cases of pyelonephritis). Some suggest deep palpation of the upper abdomen to confirm CVA tenderness.
- Genital examination: For women, perform a complete pelvic examination if abdominal or laboratory results do not provide data for a diagnosis of UTI. For men, perform a complete examination of external genitalia and assess for prostate tenderness or enlargement.
- Children: Assess for dehydration and activity level. Physical examination results may be essentially within normal limits.

Diagnostic Procedures

The choice of procedure is based on the documented presence of pyuria or bacteriuria in a clean-catch urine sample. Children may require catheterization to obtain a specimen.

Urine Dipstick
- Presence of leukocyte esterase
- Presence of nitrites (infection must incubate in bladder approximately 6 hours for nitrates to convert to nitrites; not all pathogens produce nitrites)

Microscopic Urinalysis
- More than 2 to 5 leukocytes/field
- More than 2 to 5 red blood cells/field
- More than 1 positive bacterial organism

A urinalysis with more than 0 to 5 epithelial cells should be considered contaminated and should be redone.

The following are indications for urine culture:
- Symptoms without pyuria or bacteriuria
- Complicated UTIs (see the following list)
- Suspected pyelonephritis
- Female clients for whom previous treatment failed

The standard definition of positive results from urine culture is 10^5 colony-forming units (CFU)/ml of uropathogen. In current practice, the criterion is CFU of 10^2 in symptomatic female clients and 10^3 in symptomatic male clients.

NOTE: *About 15% to 20% of symptomatic women have negative culture results.*

Wet Mount of Vaginal Secretions/Penile Discharge
- This test is needed only if sexually transmitted disease (STD) is suspected. Trichomoniasis may be noted on wet mount. Send culture for chlamydia and gonorrhea screening.
- Consider obtaining wet mount and vaginal cultures if a woman client has had a new sexual partner within the last 3 months.

- Obtain a complete blood count with differential, electrolytes, BUN, and creatinine measurements. This is needed only if the client is severely ill or has systemic illness or if pyelonephritis is suspected.

DIAGNOSIS

The differential diagnoses include the following:
- Nephrolithiasis
- Pyelonephritis
- Trauma
- Prostatitis
- Diabetes
- STD
- Acute urethral syndrome
- Tumor
- Pelvic inflammatory disease
- Vulvovaginitis
- Cervicitis
- Epididymitis
- BPH
- Renal tuberculosis
- Poststreptococcal glomerular nephritis
- Children: sexual abuse, constipation, appendicitis
- Older adults: menopause

THERAPEUTIC PLAN
Pharmacologic Treatment

Antibiotic treatment for UTI is based on how involved or complicated the condition is.

Uncomplicated UTI
- Prescribe 3 day course of antibiotics.
- Choice of antibiotics, first considerations: second-generation cephalosporins can be used throughout pregnancy; sulfonamides in last trimester may be associated with increased neonatal bilirubin levels; fluoroquinolones for resistant pathogens are contraindicated during pregnancy.
- Consider use of phenazopyridine (Pyridium) as urinary tract analgesic.

Complicated UTI
- Symptoms longer than 6 days' duration
- Men, children, and pregnant women
- Nosocomial infections
- Postinstrumentation infection
- Abnormal urinary flow
- Compromised host
- Diabetes mellitus
- Progressive renal deterioration

The following describes antibiotic treatment for complicated UTIs:
- For diabetic clients and pregnant women, prescribe 7- to 10-day course.
- For children, prescribe a 10-day course.

U

- For client with pyelonephritis, prescribe a 10- to 14-day course.
- For client with frequent postvoid urine residual, treat symptoms only.
- For client with a permanent Foley catheter, treat symptoms only.
- See Table 3-117 for common drug choices for treating UTI.
- Other drugs are amoxicillin and ciprofloxacin for resistant organisms.
- Consider phenazopyridine (Pyridium) as a urinary analgesic for dysuria. Adult dose is 100 mg tid for 3 days. For children older than 12 years is 12 mg/kg/day tid. Phenazopyridine is a pregnancy category B drug. Side effects include coloring all body fluids orange; possibly permanently staining soft contact lens. Warn about discoloration in clothing.

Pyelonephritis. Clients who are healthy and at low risk for complications with no nausea or vomiting can be treated on an outpatient basis. Clients who are more ill, children, and pregnant women (increased chance of premature labor) at risk for complications must be treated with IV administered antibiotics with broad activity against gram-negative bacteria. Possible drug choices include trimethoprim-sulfamethoxazole (TMP-SMX) (Bactrim) or an aminoglycoside. Referral to a urologist is required.

Interstitial Cystitis. Nine times more frequent in women, this phenomenon is often associated with allergy, fibromyalgia, vulvodynia, and irritable bowel syndrome. It is identified through exclusion of other causes of bladder pain, including bacterial cystitis. Risk factors include white race and Jewish ancestry. Pathogenesis is unclear, but there are distinct pathologic tissue changes in the bladder. Frequent urination (more than eight times during waking hours), urgency, hesitancy, and postvoid fullness are common. Pain occurs as the bladder becomes full and decreases with voiding. A voiding diary can be helpful in determining the diagnosis. Referral for urodynamic testing and treatment is appropriate.

Client Education

- Use of correct postvoiding wiping technique
- Use of barrier methods of birth control and spermicides
- Avoid use of tampons, deodorants, douches
- Need to void before and after intercourse
- Local trauma (e.g., certain sexual positions, horseback riding)
- Adequate fluid intake: increase when symptoms are noted, but avoid overhydration
- Self-administered treatment at first symptoms of UTI
- Need for good perineal hygiene
- Effect of estrogen depletion on vaginal tissues
- Use of phenazopyridine (Pyridium): orange discoloration of urine and all body fluids that may stain contact lenses and clothes
- Avoidance of sex during symptom stage
- Acidification of urine with cranberry juice during symptom stage
- Return to clinic if no improvement in 48 hours
- Suppression treatment with single postcoital medication for women with frequent recurrences related to sexual activity

TABLE **3-117** Common Drug Choice for Treating Urinary Tract Infection

DRUG	DOSAGE	IMPLICATIONS
TMP-SMZ (Bactrim DS)	Adult: 1 tablet bid For prophylaxis: ½ regular tablet hs	Pregnancy category C Cautious use in first month of life because of risk of jaundice Side effects: nausea, vomiting, abdominal pain, photosensitivity Skin rash following drug: Rule out Stevens Johnson syndrome
Nitrofurantoin microcrystals (Macrodantin)	Adult: 100 mg qid For prophylaxis: 100 mg hs qod Children: 1.25-1.75 mg/kg q6h For prophylaxis: 1-2 mg/kg bid	Pregnancy category B Side effects: nausea, vomiting, abdominal pain, amber urine GI distress: Take with food to minimize
Nitrofurantoin (Macrobid)	Adult: 100 mg bid Not for children	For children older than 2 months
Cephalexin (Keflex)	Adult: 500 mg bid Children: 10-15 mg/kg qid	Pregnancy category B Side effect: diarrhea

GI, Gastrointestinal; *TMP-SMX,* trimethoprim sulfamethoxazole.

Children

- Teach children to avoid a full bladder. Children who are toilet training require a regular schedule.
- Teach children not to delay urination. Advise children to avoid taking bubble baths and sitting in soapy bath water. Teach girls front-to-back wiping and teach uncircumcised boys how to properly clean the penis.
- Stress the implications of UTI. Ensure that parents understand that most infection causing renal scarring occurs in infancy and childhood. The consequences of UTI in children is not the same as the "annoyance" experienced by adults.

Referral/Consultation

- Hospitalize children with symptomatic pyelonephritis or sepsis.
- Refer men with UTI to a urologist.
- Refer pregnant women to an obstetrician/gynecologist or urologist. Pregnant women may need to take maintenance antibiotics during pregnancy.

Prevention

Prevention may be possible with adequate hydration and behaviors that do not introduce contaminants into the bladder.

EVALUATION/FOLLOW-UP

The following are indications for urologic investigation (intravenous pyelogram or ultrasonography of kidneys, ureters, and bladder):

- All male clients
- Children younger than 8 years (ultrasound less invasive)
- Clients with renal colic
- Clients with gross or persistent hematuria
- Persistent UTI
- Recurrent UTI/relapses
- Voiding cystourethrogram
- Clients with evidence of renal scarring

Cystitis. Simple UTIs do not require follow-up unless symptoms persist.

Children

- Obtain a second culture 2 to 3 days after treatment is begun to check for sterile urine.
- Schedule routine follow-up cultures in 1 month, then every 3 months for 1 year, then yearly for 2 to 3 years.

Pregnant Women

- Schedule monthly urine cultures during pregnancy after initial UTI is treated.
- Because of a higher incidence of asymptomatic bacteriuria, schedule monthly screenings for pregnant women with sickle cell trait.

Complicated UTI

- For all UTIs confirmed by urine culture, reassess by urinalysis 2 weeks after treatment.
- For complicated UTIs, schedule a follow-up urine culture after treatment.

For men older than 50 years, follow-up after 4 to 6 weeks is recommended.

Pyelonephritis

- Monitor urinary output.
- Follow up for evaluation of symptom assessment and directed physical examination in 24 to 48 hours.
- Schedule a test of cure 1 to 4 weeks after completion of antibiotic therapy.
- Special diagnostic studies are needed in men and children after an episode of pyelonephritis.
- Referral to a urologist is warranted.

COMPLICATIONS

- Failure to treat cystitis appropriately can lead to ascending pyelonephritis and ultimate renal damage.
- Failure to treat appropriately during pregnancy may contribute to premature delivery and related sequelae. Some drugs used to treat UTI are teratogenic during pregnancy or associated with neonatal risks.

REFERENCES

Ahmed, S. M., & Swedlund, S. K. (1998). Evaluation and treatment of urinary tract infections in children. *American Family Physician, 57*(7), 1573-1580.

Bromberg, W. D. (1998). UTIs: Part II: Treating specific populations. *Clinical Advisor,* Sept, 61-65.

Cash, J. C., & Glass, C. A. (2000). *Family practice guidelines.* Philadelphia: Lippincott.

Current management of UTI in women. *Primary Care Nurse Practitioner,* Fall, 3-22.

Hellerstein, S. (1998). Urinary tract infections in children: Why they occur and how to prevent them. *American Family Physician, 57*(1), 2440-2446.

Kurowski, K. (2000). Bacterial cystitis in women: A primary care approach. *Women's Health and Primary Care, 3*(8), 554-565.

Maloney, C. (1997). Tips for a healthy bladder. *Lippincott's Primary Care Practice, 1*(4), 447.

Myers, D. L., & Arya, L. A. (2001). Diagnosing interstitial cystitis in women. *Women's Health and Primary Care, 3*(12), 867-875.

Nygaard, I., & Johnson, M. (1996). UTI in elderly women. *American Family Practice, 53*(1), 175-182.

Orenstein, R., & Wong, E. S. (1999). Urinary tract infections in adults. *American Family Physician, 59*(5), 1225-1234.

Ringel, M. (1999). Best approaches to recurrent UTI. *Patient Care, 15,* 38-79.

Robinson, D., Kidd, P., & Rogers, K. M. (2000). *Primary care across the lifespan.* St. Louis:, Mosby.

Ryals, J. K., Vetrosky, D., & White, G. L. (1997). Urinary tract infection. *Lippincott's Primary Care Practice, 1*(4), 442-445.

Sant, G. R. (1999). Treating interstitial cystitis safely. *Patient Care, 33*(4), 32-44.

U

Towers, P. M. (2000). Urinary tract infection. *Journal of American Academy of Nurse Practitioners, 12*(4), 149-154.

Uphold, C., & Graham, M. (1998). *Clinical guidelines in family practice.* Gainesville: Barmarrae Books.

Review Questions

1. Which of the following physical findings is not consistent with cystitis?

  a. CVA tenderness
  b. Urethral discharge
  c. Mild abdominal pain
  d. Suprapubic tenderness

2. You suspect that 23-year-old Marcy has pyelonephritis. Which of the following symptoms do you expect to find?

  a. Spasmodic flank pain and hematuria
  b. Urethral discharge and dysuria
  c. Flank pain, CVA tenderness, nausea, and vomiting
  d. Urinary urgency, frequency, and suprapubic pain

3. A 38-year-old man complains of flank pain, fever, nausea, and vomiting. Which of the following diagnoses is not appropriate for this client?

  a. Bacterial cystitis
  b. Acute bacterial prostatitis
  c. Interstitial cystitis
  d. Pyelonephritis

4. Treatment for a pregnant female with cystitis includes which of the following?

  a. Tetracycline
  b. Amoxicillin
  c. Ciprofloxacin
  d. TMP-SMX (Bactrim)

5. Which of the following actions indicates that Tracy, a 19-year-old woman with frequent UTIs, understands the teaching she has received regarding her care?

  a. Tracy stops taking her antibiotic as soon as her symptoms are gone.
  b. Tracy drinks 10 quarts of water a day during the treatment.
  c. Because her roommate has similar symptoms, Tracy gives some of her pills to her roommate.
  d. Tracy returns to the office in 2 weeks for a urine culture.

6. Mrs. McGuire continues to have bladder pain despite several courses of antibiotics during the past several years. The NP considers the possibility of interstitial cystitis as a cause of the client's pain. Which question best differentiates between bacterial cystitis and interstitial cystitis?

  a. Is the pain worse during voiding or when the bladder is full?
  b. Is the pain associated with menstruation?
  c. Does she have a vaginal discharge as well as pain?
  d. Does she also have joint pain?

7. Which of the following factors is *not* associated with increased risk of UTI?

  a. Drinking bottled water
  b. Using a diaphragm for contraception
  c. Wiping back to front after toileting
  d. Female gender

8. Kathy is a 10-year-old girl with symptoms of UTI who was brought in by her mother. Which historical information is consistent with a diagnosis of cystitis?

  a. Swimming in a plastic pool
  b. Taking bubble baths
  c. Having a poor appetite
  d. Wearing cotton panties while sleeping

9. Kathy's mother asks whether it is true that girls have more UTIs than boys. What is the NP's response?

  a. This is a common misunderstanding; there is no difference in incidence in boys and girls.
  b. In fact, boys have more UTIs; girls are just more likely to complain of symptoms.
  c. The statement is true and is because of the female's short urethra and its proximity to the rectum.
  d. The incidence is greater in females, but only after menopause.

10. Gail is a college student with cystitis that the NP plans to treat with TMP-SMX and phenazopyridine hydrochloride (Pyridium). Which information is the most important to know before prescribing these medications?

  a. Does Gail wear soft contract lenses?
  b. Does Gail smoke cigarettes?
  c. Does Gail have an allergy to iodine?
  d. Does Gail eat yogurt?

Answers and Rationales

1. *Answer:* a (assessment)
  Rationale: CVA tenderness is most indicative of pyelonephritis. Urethral discharge, mild abdominal pain, and suprapubic tenderness may be found during the examination of a client with cystitis (Uphold & Graham, 1998).

2. *Answer:* c (assessment)
  Rationale: Spasmodic flank pain and hematuria may occur in association with a kidney stone. Urethral discharge and dysuria are more commonly associated with an STD. Urinary urgency, frequency, and suprapubic pain are most commonly associated with cystitis (Current Management of UTI in Women, 2000).

3. *Answer:* c (analysis/diagnosis)
  Rationale: Bacterial cystitis, acute bacterial prostatitis, and pyelonephritis must be considered in a man with flank pain, fever, nausea, and vomiting. Although interstitial cystitis is a possibility in a 38-year-old client, the other diagnoses must be considered first because symptoms do not support that diagnosis and because it is much less common in males (Uphold & Graham, 1998; Myers & Arya, 2000).

4. *Answer:* b (implementation/plan)
  Rationale: TMP-SMX (Bactrim) and ciprofloxacin are pregnancy category C drugs. Tetracycline is not appropriate for generic treatment of UTIs and is not being recommended for pregnant females or for children because of teeth staining (Bromberg, 1998).

5. *Answer:* d (evaluation)

Rationale: The client should complete the whole course of antibiotic therapy for a UTI. Although having an adequate fluid intake is recommended, 10 quarts is too much because the urinary antibiotics depend on the concentration of drug in the bladder to achieve their maximum effect. Women with frequent UTIs are considered to have complicated UTIs and should return for follow-up urine cultures (Robinson et al. 2000).

6. *Answer:* a (assessment)

Rationale: The classic symptom of interstitial cystitis is pain when the bladder is full that is relieved by voiding, whereas bacterial cystitis causes pain during voiding (Sant, 1999).

7. *Answer:* a (analysis/diagnosis)

Rationale: Bottled water does not increase the risk of UTI. Diaphragm use, wiping back to front, and being female all increase risk. (Cash & Glass, 2000).

8. *Answer:* b (assessment)

Rationale: Bubble baths increase the risk of UTI in females because of their short urethras. Bubble bath changes the surface tension of the water and organisms ascend more easily (Robinson et al. 2000).

9. *Answer:* c (analysis/diagnosis)

Rationale: The incidence of UTI is greater in females. They are predisposed because of a shorter urethra and proximity of the urinary meatus to the rectum, where contamination is more likely (Common Management of UTIs in Women, 2000).

10. *Answer:* a (assessment)

Rationale: Pyridium colors urine and all body fluids orange; a soft contact lens will become discolored as a result of orange tearing and cannot be cleaned (Robinson et al. 2000).

URTICARIA AND ANAPHYLAXIS *Denise Robinson*

OVERVIEW
Definition

- Urticaria is composed of wheals (transient edematous papules, usually pruritic and caused by edema of the papillary body). Angioedema is a larger edematous area that involves the dermis and subcutaneous tissue (Fitzpatrick, Johnson, Wolff, & Suurmond 2001).
- There are two types of generalized allergic reactions:
  - Urticaria/angioedema (usually not life threatening)
  - Anaphylaxis (life threatening)
- Urticaria/angioedema consists of lesions (extravascular accumulation of fluid in the dermis) resulting from exposure to an inciting substance.
- Anaphylaxis is an acute systemic reaction manifested by sudden onset of pruritus, generalized flush, urticaria, respiratory distress, and vascular collapse (Dambro, 1998). It results from an antigen exposure in a sensitized person.

Incidence

- Urticaria occurs at some time in 15% to 23% of the population.
- Anaphylaxis occurs in 1 of 2700 hospitalized clients.
- Hymenoptera (stinging insects) causes allergic reactions in 0.4% of the population in the United States.
- Males and females are affected equally; allergic reactions occur in all age groups.
- Food allergies are much more common in children younger than 3 years of age (8%).
- Milk allergies occur in children (2%) and in older children and adults (1% to 2%).

Pathophysiology

The underlying mechanism for both urticaria and anaphylaxis is a classic immunoglobulin (Ig)E-mediated allergy, causing an immune response in which chemical mediators (histamine and kinins) are released. Allergy-prone individuals produce more specific IgE-specific antibodies, and they have a tendency to become allergic when subjected to repeated exposures.

Causative Types

- Immunologic IgE mediated: People often have atopic background, including food, therapeutic agents, drugs.
- Complement-induced: Immune complexes activating complement and releasing anaphylatoxins that induce mast cell degranulation may be present; includes serum sickness, administration of whole blood, and immunoglobulins.
- Physical: Urticaria dermographism is present in 4.2% of population; linear urticarial lesions occur after stroking or scratching skin; itches and fades in 30 minutes.
- Cold: Urticarial lesions occur when exposed to cold; ice cube test confirms diagnosis.
- Solar: Urticaria occurs after sun exposure.
- Cholinergic: Urticaria occurs after exercise.
- Pressure angioedema is swelling induced by pressure (e.g., buttock swelling when seated, hand swelling after hammering).
- Hereditary angioedema is an autosomal dominant disorder involving angioedema of face and extremities and episodes of laryngeal edema and acute abdominal pain caused by angioedema of bowel wall; episodes can be life threatening.
- Angioedema-urticaria-eosinophilia syndrome is severe angioedema involving face, neck, extremities, and trunk and lasting 7 to 10 days; no family history is present.

U

Factors Increasing Susceptibility

- Family history of allergies
- History of allergic reaction
- History of asthma, hay fever, or other allergic disorders

Common Causes of Allergic Reactions

- Drugs with high probability of reaction (3% to 5%): penicillin, carbamazepine (Tegretol), allopurinol, gold salts (10% to 20%); medium probability: sulfonamides (bacteriostatic, antidiabetic, diuretic), nonsteroidal antiinflammatory drugs (NSAIDs), hydantoin derivatives, isoniazid (INH), erythromycin, streptomycin; low probability: (less than 1%) barbiturates, benzodiazepines, phenothiazines, tetracyclines
- Insect stings: honeybees/wasps
- Foreign serum
- Vaccines
- Blood products
- Hormones: adrenocorticotropic hormone, insulin, estradiol
- Diagnostic chemicals: iodine
- Foods: peanuts, eggs, legumes, popcorn, seafood; in children, vitamin C milk, chocolate
- NSAIDs, aspirin
- Snake venom
- Animal dander
- Latex
- Exercise

ASSESSMENT: SUBJECTIVE/HISTORY

History of Present Illness

- Determine type of bite, sting, or antigen.
- Determine location of antigen.
- Inquire about time of occurrence.

Most Common Symptoms

- Compromised respirations (may need to treat quickly, given signs and symptoms and past history)
- Urticaria: itching, transient hives on any part of the body, exposure preceding symptoms, dysphagia; edema
- Anaphylaxis: generalized itching, erythema of skin followed by sense of warmth and then generalized hives; rapidly progressive respiratory distress; edema

Associated Symptoms

- Presence of systemic symptoms, such as fever, chills, nausea, vomiting, and weakness
- Shortness of breath, chest tightness, facial swelling, or throat tightness

Past Medical History

- Hives/urticaria/anaphylaxis
- Hay fever or asthma

Medication History

- Ask about medications: Angiotensin-converting enzyme inhibitors, such as benazepril, captopril, enalapril, fosinopril, lisinopril, moexipril, quinapril, ramipril, and trandolapril, are frequently combined with other antihypertensive drugs and can cause a reaction with the first dose or after prolonged treatment as a result of a kinin-mediated reaction.
- Ask specifically about NSAIDs because many people do not think of them as medications.
- Ask about antibiotics taken recently.

Family History

Ask about allergies or allergic reactions.

Psychosocial History

- Environmental exposures: animals, chemicals in the home or workplace
- Physical agents: light, exercise, heat, and others

ASSESSMENT: OBJECTIVE/PHYSICAL EXAMINATION

Physical Examination

A problem-oriented physical examination should be conducted with particular attention to the following:

- Vital signs: hypotension
- Skin: urticaria (transient skin colored papules), pruritus, cutaneous erythema; drug reactions: macules/papules, bright red; lesions confluent after time; symmetric distribution: almost always on trunk and extremities but may spare face, nipple, periareolar area, surgical scar
- Head, eyes, ears, nose, and throat: eyelid edema, facial edema, throat swelling; rhinitis, conjunctivitis
- Respiratory status: dyspnea, wheezing, shallow respirations, increased secretions
- Cardiovascular status: tachycardia, circulatory collapse
- Neurologic assessment: confusion, coma
- General assessment: abdominal colic, nausea, vomiting, diarrhea
- Hematologic assessment: disseminated intravascular coagulation

Diagnostic Procedures

- Epicutaneous immediate reacting IgE skin test: Use food extract to determine the presence of food-specific IgE antibodies (this is a good screening method for allergies). A positive result indicates the likelihood of allergy.
- In vitro test for allergen-specific IgE antibodies: This is an appropriate test for life-threatening allergies (a negative result rules out allergy).
- Food challenge is the only method capable of confirming the suspicion of food reaction, regardless of

mechanism (a double-blind, placebo-controlled food challenge is the gold standard).

- Food diary and home challenges may possibly be helpful when reactions are not life threatening.

DIAGNOSIS

- A detailed history is of utmost importance.
- Mild reaction is characterized by urticaria that involves the superficial dermis, pruritus, and well-circumscribed wheals that may coalesce.
- Moderate reaction is characterized by bronchospasm and angioedema, which is well-demarcated localized edema that involves the entire dermis and subcutaneous tissue; common sites are the skin, gastrointestinal (GI) tract, and upper airway (GI angioedema can produce cramping abdominal pain, nausea, vomiting, and diarrhea).
- Severe reaction is anaphylaxis, a severe systemic reaction of multiple organ systems to IgE-driven mediator release in previously sensitized persons (hypotension, bronchoconstriction, and upper airway obstruction are common).

  The differential diagnoses include the following:
  - Urticaria versus anaphylactoid reactions
  - Vasovagal reaction
  - Hyperventilation episode
  - Insect bites
  - Adverse drug reactions

THERAPEUTIC PLAN

Treatment depends on the severity of the reaction. If a life-threatening systemic reaction has occurred, assess and treat the ABCs: airway, breathing, and circulation.

Life-Threatening Situation

- Initiate emergency transport service (call 9-1-1).
- Administer oxygen; assess the need for intubation.
- Administer epinephrine (1:1000 solution), 0.5 mg SC or IV, repeated every 5 to 10 minutes when necessary. It can also be administered via endotracheal tube.
- IV fluids: Administer normal saline or lactated Ringer's solution.
- Aminophylline: For bronchospasm, administer 6 mg/kg IV during a period of 10 to 20 minutes.

Non–Life-Threatening Situation

- Administer epinephrine (1:1000 solution; 0.01 ml/kg) 0.3 to 0.5 ml SC every 20 to 30 minutes, up to three doses.
- After the administration of epinephrine, administer a long-acting agent (epinephrine [SusPhrine] as a single dose, 0.150 to 0.250 ml SC).
- Administer diphenhydramine (Benadryl) 25 to 50 mg; it may help shorten the duration of the reaction.
- If extensive swelling is present at the site of a local reaction, consider adding a short course of prednisone.

- H_2 blockers: Cimetidine (Tagamet) may also help treat an allergic response. It is administered in many emergency departments concurrently with the above mentioned agents.

Client Education

- Emphasize the need to have antihistamine or epinephrine (Epi-jet or Epi-pen [spring-loaded automatic injector of epinephrine] or Ana-Kit [contains a preloaded syringe of epinephrine and a chewable antihistamine]) on hand for self-treatment for all people at risk for anaphylaxis from stings.
- Caution the client to avoid insects, food, and drugs that cause reaction.
- Advise the client to wear a medical alert tag identifying the allergy.
- Alert the client to beware of taking medications (especially over-the-counter [OTC] medications) if he or she has a history of allergic disorders, hay fever, or asthma.
- Warn the client that an acute generalized reaction means there is a potential for a life-threatening reaction in the future.
- Instruct the client that wearing shoes at all times is the single most important safeguard.
- Do not wear perfume or brightly colored clothes when outside if allergic to hymenoptera; consider pretreatment with antihistamines and corticosteroids.

Referral/Consultation

- Refer for allergy testing to identify the sensitizing agent if it is unknown.
- Immunotherapy reduces the likelihood of a similar reaction from 50% to 5%.

EVALUATION/FOLLOW-UP

- For clients who experience a moderate local reaction or a mild allergic reaction, follow up via phone in 24 hours.
- For clients who experience an anaphylactic reaction, closely monitor for 12 to 24 hours afterward.

REFERENCES

Anderson, J. (1997). Milk, eggs and peanuts: Food allergies in children. *American Family Physician, 56*(5), 1365-1374.

Dambro, M. (1998). *Griffith's 5-minute clinical consult* (6th ed.). Philadelphia: Williams & Wilkins.

Fitzpatrick, T., Johnson, R., Wolff, K., & Suurmond, D. (2001). *Color atlas and synopsis of clinical dermatology* (4th ed.). New York: McGraw-Hill.

Kidd, P., & Stuart, P. (1996). *Mosby's emergency nursing reference.* St. Louis: Mosby.

O'Brien, J. (1998). Allergic reactions: 10 questions physicians often ask., *Consultant, 38*(4), 851-866.

Robinson, D. (2000). Allergic reactions. In D. Robinson, P. Kidd, & K. Rogers (Eds.), *Primary care across the lifespan* (pp. 32-35). St. Louis: Mosby.

U

Review Questions

1. Which of the following allergies are more common in children?

- **a.** Medicine
- **b.** Pet
- **c.** Food
- **d.** Environmental

2. Which of the following children is most likely to have an allergic reaction to a first-time penicillin injection?

- **a.** An asthmatic child
- **b.** A child with an allergy to sulfa
- **c.** A boy
- **d.** A child being treated for a rash

3. Which of the following should an NP do when assessing a client for a life-threatening allergic reaction?

- **a.** Determine the distribution of hives.
- **b.** Assess the severity of itching.
- **c.** Ask about shortness of breath.
- **d.** Check for the presence of edema.

4. What should the NP's first action be when treating a client with anaphylaxis?

- **a.** Call 911.
- **b.** Administer oxygen.
- **c.** Administer epinephrine.
- **d.** Start an IV line.

5. When treating a client with a non–life-threatening allergic reaction, which of the following drugs may be used?

- **a.** Aminophylline
- **b.** Diphenhydramine (Benadryl)
- **c.** Ibuprofen
- **d.** Metaproterenol (Alupent)

6. Which of the following descriptions is consistent with a moderate allergic reaction?

- **a.** Urticaria that affect the superficial dermis, pruritus
- **b.** Bronchospasm and angioedema
- **c.** Hypotension, bronchoconstriction, wheezing
- **d.** Unconsciousness, respiratory arrest

7. Which of the following comments by the client with allergies indicates a need for further instruction?

- **a.** "I should avoid being outside when it is 'bee season.'"
- **b.** "I should always have my Epi-pen with me."
- **c.** "I wear an alert bracelet identifying my allergy."
- **d.** "If I get hurt, I will take ibuprofen or aspirin."

8. A client should be aware of which of the following side effects if he or she uses an Epi-pen?

- **a.** Hypotension
- **b.** Palpitations

- **c.** Nausea, vomiting, diarrhea
- **d.** Abdominal pain

Answers and Rationales

1. *Answer:* **c** (assessment)
Rationale: Food allergies are much more common in children. There are no age distinctions among the other three (Anderson, 1997).

2. *Answer:* **a** (assessment)
Rationale: Children with an allergic disorder or atopy (such as asthma) have an increased susceptibility for an allergic reaction. An allergy to sulfa does not indicate that the child has an allergy disorder. Boys and girls are equally affected with allergic reactions. A rash may be related to a contagious disease or a nonallergenic source (Robinson, 2000).

3. *Answer:* **c** (assessment)
Rationale: Itching, hives, and edema may be present in both anaphylaxis and urticaria/local allergic reaction. Respiratory distress is associated with anaphylaxis (Robinson, 2000).

4. *Answer:* **c** (implementation/plan)
Rationale: Although the client needs emergency transport and follow-up, the client initially needs epinephrine to counteract the effects of histamine release. Oxygen is necessary, but it will not help alone. Epinephrine can be administered SC. After the epinephrine is administered, the emergency service can be called (Robinson, 2000).

5. *Answer:* **b** (implementation/plan)
Rationale: A life-threatening reaction may be treated with aminophylline, but it would not be the first-line drug. Ibuprofen and metaproterenol (Alupent) are not used. A non–life-threatening reaction is usually treated with epinephrine, antihistamine, and, in cases of extensive swelling, prednisone.

6. *Answer:* **b** (evaluation)
Rationale: A moderate allergic reaction consists of bronchospasm and angioedema. Choice a refers to a mild reaction, whereas choices c and d describe a severe allergic reaction (Robinson, 2000).

7. *Answer:* **d** (evaluation)
Rationale: A person who has a history of allergic reactions should be very careful about taking any medications, even OTC medications, and especially aspirin or ibuprofen because they are moderate allergen causers (Fitzpatrick, et al. 2001).

8. *Answer:* **b** (evaluation)
Rationale: Use of an Epi-pen produces the "fight or flight" response. Palpitations, nervousness, and headache are common. Hypotension is not caused by epinephrine; epinephrine is more likely to cause hypertension (Robinson, 2000).

VASCULAR INSUFFICIENCY (THROMBOPHLEBITIS/DEEP VEIN THROMBOSIS) *Pamela Kidd*

OVERVIEW
Definition

Superficial thrombophlebitis (SVT) is the presence of thrombus and inflammation of the superficial veins. Deep vein thrombosis (DVT) is the presence of thrombus and inflammation in the deep venous system.

Incidence

- Occurs more commonly in women.
- All races affected equally.
- Incidence increases with advancing age.
- Occurs in children, but incidence is low.

Pathophysiology

- Thrombus prevents blood flow and oxygenation of distal tissue. Eventually, necrosis and infection occur. The thrombus may travel to the pulmonary circulation, producing infarction and death.
- SVT: The greater or lesser saphenous veins or their tributaries are most often involved.
- DVT: The calf veins are most frequently affected, but the popliteal, femoral, and ileofemoral veins are also commonly affected.

Protective Factors
- Ambulation
- Adequate fluid intake

Factors Increasing Susceptibility
- Stasis of blood flow
- Endothelial injury
- Hypercoagulability

Conditions Associated with Increased Risk
- Trauma
- Old age
- Varicosities
- Previous thrombophlebitis
- Immobility
- Cancer
- Congestive heart failure
- Myocardial infarction (MI)
- Abdominal condition
- Pelvic and lower extremity surgery
- Obesity
- Pregnancy
- Oral contraceptive pills (OCPs) and hormone replacement therapy

ASSESSMENT: SUBJECTIVE/HISTORY
Symptoms

- SVT: Symptoms include the sudden onset of pain localized to the site of the thrombus, a tender palpable cord, erythema, and warmth without generalized edema. Low-grade fever may be present.
- DVT: The physical signs for diagnosing DVT are unreliable. Calf pain, tenderness, unilateral swelling, low-grade fever, warmth, erythema, engorged, prominent superficial veins, and pain during dorsiflexion (Homans' sign) may occur but are nonspecific.

Past Medical History

- Ask about conditions that predispose toward immobility, such as recent trauma, surgery, sedentary lifestyle, MI, or stroke. Inquire concerning previous SVT or DVT, pregnancy, recent childbirth, or coagulopathies.
- DVT frequently occurs in the flaccid extremity after stroke.

Medication History

- Recent use of OCPs
- Hormone replacement therapy
- Aspirin or nonsteroidal antiinflammatory drugs (NSAIDs)

Family History

Ask about family history of blood clotting disorders, varicose veins, or DVTs.

Dietary History

Diet is noncontributory.

ASSESSMENT: OBJECTIVE/PHYSICAL EXAMINATION
Physical Examination

- A problem-oriented physical examination should be conducted with particular attention to vital signs, including temperature.
- Examine for thigh or calf tenderness on palpation, warmth, erythema, swelling, and palpable cord.
- Palpate femoral, popliteal, posterior tibial, and pedal pulses.
- Feel for enlarged, tender inguinal lymph nodes.
- Test of Homans' sign is considered unreliable by some sources. Classic signs are found in only 25% of cases of DVT.

- Pulmonary embolism may be the first clinical indication of thrombosis.

Diagnostic Procedures

- SVT is readily diagnosed by physical examination.
- For DVT, venous Doppler ultrasonography (compression ultrasonography) with duplex or color flow imaging studies to measure blood flow and detect venous obstruction should be performed. Venography is considered one of the most accurate means for diagnosis of DVT.

DIAGNOSIS

Differential diagnoses include the following:

Superficial Thrombophlebitis

- Ruptured calf muscle
- Cellulitis
- Severe muscle cramp
- Trauma

Deep Vein Thrombophlebitis

- Ruptured calf muscle
- Baker's cyst
- Trauma
- Cellulitis
- Lymphedema

THERAPEUTIC PLAN

Nonpharmacologic Treatment

Superficial Thrombophlebitis

- Discontinue OCPs or hormone replacement therapy.
- Elevate the extremity, apply heat locally, compress with elastic stockings, and cease smoking.

Pharmacologic Treatment

- Aspirin or other NSAIDs can be administered.
- DVT *usually* requires referral and hospitalization for initiation of antithrombotic therapy. However, some clients may be treated at home with low-molecular-weight heparin (LMWH). The advantage of LMWH is that there is no need to monitor the INR. Dalteparin/Fragmin (100 U/kg bid) and enoxaparin (1 mg/kg bid) are used to treat DVT.
- Warfarin (5 mg/day) can be used and overlapped with heparin treatment (for at least 5 days).
- For a first episode of DVT in a client who has had no recent surgery, trauma, or malignancy, use warfarin for 6 months.
- Warfarin can be used "chronically" for clients with recurrent DVT.

Client Education

- Proper use of compression stockings
- Avoidance of leg crossing at knees and prolonged inactivity, including sitting and standing

- Need for balance of exercise and rest
- Effects of OCPs and hormone replacement therapy on blood clotting
- Hazards of smoking
- Refraining from massaging calf to reduce pain

Referral/Consultation

- SVT: Phlebitis of a varicose vein is generally an indication for surgical removal. Refer the client to a vascular surgeon.
- DVT: DVT requires a physician referral and may require hospitalization.
- Pregnant women should be followed up by an obstetrician/gynecologist.

Prevention

Use LMWH (e.g., enoxaparin [Lovenox] for prevention of DVT after hip and knee replacement surgery or ardeparin [Normiflo] for prevention of DVT after knee replacement surgery).

EVALUATION/FOLLOW-UP

- SVT: Follow-up should include symptom assessment and directed physical examination. Migrating SVT may be a marker for carcinoma and requires investigation.
- DVT: Client should be managed in consultation with a physician.
- Complications of untreated SVT and DVT include necrosis and skin ulcer formation (SVT) and pulmonary embolus and death (DVT).

REFERENCES

Eftychiou, V. (1996). Clinical diagnosis and management of the patient with deep venous thromboembolism and acute pulmonary embolism. *Nurse Practitioner,* March, 50-69.

Stone, A. (2000). Thrombophlebitis. In D. Robinson, P. Kidd, K. Rogers (Eds.), *Primary care across the lifespan.* St. Louis: Mosby.

Turpie, A., Weart, C., & White, R. (1998). Anticoagulation: Promises and pitfalls. *Patient Care Nurse Practitioner, 1*(2), 44-55.

Review Questions

1. Risk factors for the development of DVT include which of the following?

    a. Abdominal, pelvic, and lower extremity surgery
    b. Middle-class Asian female
    c. Jogging more than 3 miles a day
    d. Pernicious anemia

2. Twenty-nine-year-old Betty Harris works as an operating room nurse. She seeks treatment for sudden onset of left calf pain, a tender palpable cord, erythema, and warmth to palpation. She is afebrile. Which of the following is the most likely diagnosis?

    a. Ruptured Achilles tendon

b. Baker's cyst
c. Ruptured calf muscle
d. SVT

3. Diagnostic studies that are useful in confirming a diagnosis of SVT include which of the following?

a. Prothrombin time
b. Complete blood count (CBC) with differential
c. Doppler studies
d. Physical findings, which usually confirm the diagnosis

4. Which of the following statements regarding the treatment of DVT is true?

a. A low-dose antibiotic should be used.
b. Only clients with symptoms should be treated.
c. Anticoagulant therapy should be started immediately.
d. Begin aspirin therapy.

5. Which of the following applies to clients with DVT?

a. Hospitalization always required.
b. Must have varicose veins stripped.
c. Should be managed in consultation with a physician.
d. Can continue hormone replacement therapy.

6. What of the following factors reported by the client is most helpful in making a diagnosis of DVT?

a. "I am in an exercise class."
b. "I do not smoke."
c. "I am 4 weeks postpartum."
d. "I stand a lot at work."

7. What is the primary emphasis in the treatment of DVT?

a. Early ambulation
b. Prevention of pulmonary emboli
c. Hypercoagulability
d. Prevention of secondary infections

8. Which of the following applies to DVT?

a. It can easily be diagnosed by physical findings.
b. It causes hypocoagulability.
c. It may not be clinically apparent.
d. It is unusual in people older than 85 years.

9. Client education for Ms. Howard, a 30-year-old postpartum woman with SVT, includes which of the following?

a. Side effects of antithrombotic medication
b. Avoidance of prolonged limb dependency
c. Need for complete bed rest
d. Need for vena cava umbrella

Answers and Rationales

1. **Answer: a** (assessment)
   Rationale: Having undergone abdominal, pelvic, or lower extremity surgery is associated with increased risk for development of thrombophlebitis. Pernicious anemia, jogging, and Asian ethnicity are not risk factors.

2. **Answer: d** (analysis/diagnosis)
   Rationale: Tender, palpable cord, erythema, and warmth to palpation are more indicative of SVT. Ruptured Achilles tendon, Baker's cyst, and ruptured calf muscle do not feature the classic symptoms listed.

3. **Answer: d** (analysis/diagnosis)
   Rationale: The physical signs of SVT are extremely reliable in diagnosing the disease. Prothrombin time and CBC with differential are nonspecific tests. Doppler studies are used to diagnose DVT.

4. **Answer: c** (implementation/plan)
   Rationale: Client requires the initiation of anticoagulation therapy. Antibiotics are not used in the treatment of thrombophlebitis, and all clients with DVT are treated because the primary goal of treatment is prevention of pulmonary embolism.

5. **Answer: c** (implementation/plan)
   Rationale: Clients with DVT are managed in consultation with a physician to regulate their antithrombotic medications.

6. **Answer: c** (analysis/diagnosis)
   Rationale: Women are more susceptible to development of thrombophlebitis within the first 6 weeks postpartum. Standing (depending on length of time) may or may not be a risk factor. Exercise helps prevent clot formation, and not smoking is also a positive finding.

7. **Answer: b** (implementation/plan)
   Rationale: The primary emphasis for treatment of DVT is prevention of pulmonary embolism.

8. **Answer: c** (analysis/diagnosis)
   Rationale: The physical signs for diagnosing DVT may not be apparent. Hypocoagulability may cause bleeding, not clotting.

9. **Answer: b** (implementation/plan)
   Rationale: Prolonged limb dependency is a risk factor for development of thrombophlebitis. Antithrombotic medication is not prescribed for SVT, nor is complete bed rest.

VISION LOSS *Pamela Kidd*

OVERVIEW

Definition

Vision loss is the decreased ability to see objects. Hyperopia is the inability to see near objects clearly because of failure to accommodate. Myopia is the inability to see distant objects. Presbyopia is the natural loss of accommodation that is caused by aging.

Incidence

Exact incidence is not known.

Pathophysiology

Visual perception begins with light entering the cornea and culminates in neural stimulation of the brain.

Protective Factors. Use of eye protection at work and play is recommended.

Factors Increasing Susceptibility. Aging can increase susceptibility.

ASSESSMENT: SUBJECTIVE/HISTORY
Symptoms

- Gradual or sudden onset of vision loss (acute onset in closed angle glaucoma and central retinal artery occlusion, gradual onset in corneal ulcer and macular degeneration)
- Partial or complete loss of vision
- Flashing lights (suspect retinal detachment)
- Monocular or binocular loss of vision (suspect hyphema or central retinal artery occlusion if monocular; suspect cerebrovascular accident or macular degeneration if binocular with partial loss)
- Pain (PQRST–**P**rovokes, **Q**uality, **R**adiates, **S**everity, **T**ime)
- Headache, scalp tenderness, jaw claudication, myalgia, fatigue (consider giant cell arteritis and ischemic optic neuropathy)
- Severe headache, nausea and vomiting, painful eye (consider closed angle glaucoma)

Past Medical History

- Hypertension
- Previous eye trauma
- Multiple sclerosis
- Diabetes
- Cataracts
- Glaucoma

Medication History

Medications are noncontributory.

Family History

- Cataracts
- Macular degeneration
- Glaucoma

ASSESSMENT: OBJECTIVE/PHYSICAL EXAMINATION
Physical Examination

Fundoscopic
- Retinal hemorrhages, soft exudates (cotton-wool patches) indicates diabetic retinopathy.
- Edema of the optic disc indicates ischemic optic neuropathy.
- Red eye indicates acute closed-angle glaucoma.
- Blood in anterior chamber indicates hyphema.
- Opacity of cornea indicates cataract.

Pupillary Reaction
- Amaurotic pupil: Pupil of one eye does not respond to light but does respond to light shone in other eye (ischemic optic neuropathy).
- Fixed, mid-dilated pupil indicates acute closed angle glaucoma.

Visual Acuity. Visual acuity should be assessed for each eye using a Snellen chart. Results are recorded as a fraction, with the test distance used as the numerator and the client's score as the denominator. A corrected acuity of less than 20/30 is abnormal (Riordan-Eva & Vaughan, 2001).

Diagnostic Procedures

- Erythrocyte sedimentation rate may be very elevated in cases of ischemic optic neuropathy.
- Temporal artery biopsy denotes presence of giant cell arteritis and ischemic optic neuropathy.
- Perform echocardiography to rule out embolization of retinal artery from cardiac valves.

DIAGNOSIS

If a client can see clearly through a pin hole on a sheet of white paper, refractive errors are not producing the vision loss. Differential diagnoses are discussed previously.

THERAPEUTIC PLAN
Nonpharmacologic Treatment

- Refer for laser surgery of vessels before hemorrhaging.
- Refer for ophthalmologic surgery to repair retinal detachment, closed angle glaucoma.
- Refer to cataract chapter for specific surgical treatment.
- In some cases of corneal abrasion, patching of the eye may be used.

Pharmacologic Treatment

Refer to the glaucoma and corneal abrasion chapters for specific treatment.

Client Education

- Seek health care with any change in vision.
- Properly use and maintain assistive devices (e.g., glasses, contact lens).

Referral/Consultation

All clients with a change in vision should be referred to an ophthalmologist.

Prevention

Vision screening should be performed every 2 years with a dilated eye examination and more frequently (yearly) if hypertension or diabetes is present.

EVALUATION AND FOLLOW-UP

- Reevaluation of visual acuity after treatment

COMPLICATIONS

Complication of untreated vision loss is blindness.

REFERENCES

Riordan-Eva, P., & Vaughan, D. (2001). Eye. In L. Tierney, S. McPhee, & M. Papadakis (Eds.), *Current medical diagnosis and treatment* (40th ed.). New York: McGraw-Hill.

Yagoda, A., & Gorman, D. (2001). Sudden monocular visual loss. *Clinical Advisor, 4*(10), 30-34.

Review Questions

1. Which of the following is true regarding symptomatology of the eyes?
   a. The older the client is, the greater the likelihood that decreased vision is caused by cataracts.
   b. Ischemic optic neuropathy often results in flashes of light in the visual fields.
   c. Blood in the anterior chamber of the eye is a benign finding that typically resolves on its own.
   d. Macular degeneration tends to occur abruptly.

2. A 20-year-old client who is unable to see objects closely because of failure to accommodate would be diagnosed with which of the following?
   a. Myopia
   b. Presbyopic
   c. Cataracts
   d. Hyperopia

3. What type of symptom is associated with the greatest risk of blindness?
   a. Binocular vision loss
   b. Sudden onset of vision loss
   c. Decreased visual acuity
   d. Painless vision loss

4. In documenting visual acuity, which of the following is true?
   a. The test distance is the denominator.
   b. A corrected acuity of 20/30 is abnormal.
   c. The figure assigned to the lowest line is the numerator.
   d. Visual acuity is assessed before and after treatment.

Answers and Rationales

1. **Answer: a** (analysis/diagnosis)
   Rationale: Cataracts tend to occur in older adults as a result of buildup of eye fibers and because of cumulative trauma from such sources as the sun and foreign bodies.

2. **Answer: d** (analysis/diagnosis)
   Rationale: Myopia is the inability to see distant objects. Presbyopia is the natural loss of accommodation caused by aging. Cataract formation may produce the inability to clearly see distant and near objects.

3. **Answer: b** (assessment)
   Rationale: True optic emergencies (ischemic optic neuropathy, acute closed angle glaucoma, temporal arteritis) produce sudden loss of vision, usually with pain and monocular in nature.

4. **Answer: d** (implementation/plan)
   Rationale: Results are recorded as a fraction with the test distance assigned to the numerator and the client's score assigned to the lowest line as the denominator. A corrected acuity of less than 20/30 is abnormal. Visual acuity is assessed before and after treatment.

VULVOVAGINITIS *Cheryl Pope Kish*

OVERVIEW
Definition

Vulvovaginitis is an infection of the vagina and vulvar tissues that occurs because the vaginal ecosystem becomes altered, either by an infectious organism or by an imbalance of normal vaginal flora.

Incidence

- More than one million health care visits annually in the United States are related to vaginal signs and symptoms. The three most common causes are bacterial vaginosis (BV), vulvovaginal candidiasis (VVC), also known as *moniliasis*, and *Trichomonas*. BV accounts for 40% to 50% of cases, VVC accounts for 20% to 25%, and *Trichomonas* accounts for 13% to 20% of cases. BV rarely occurs in monogamous couples or virgins.

- Candidiasis is incorrectly self-diagnosed and treated with over-the-counter (OTC) preparations by many women.

Pathophysiology

- BV is associated with a change in the normal vaginal ecosystem wherein vaginal flora become imbalanced; the normal flora decrease, and anaerobes predominate. The number of organisms may reach 1000 times normal, and the pH value increases. Although women with BV are symptomatic, the disorder does not cause inflammation; hence the term *vaginosis* instead of *vaginitis*.

- Vulvovaginal candidiasis is a fungal infection. In 90% of cases, the cause is *Candida albicans*, but other species can also be causative, including *C. tropicalis*, *Torulopsis glabrata* (10%), *C. parapsilosis*, and *C. krusei*. *C. albicans*, *C. tropicalis*, and *T. glabrata* are part of the normal flora of the gastrointestinal tract and vagina that can become pathogenic with changes in the vaginal pH.

- The causative organism of trichomoniasis is *Trichomonas vaginalis*, a single-cell anaerobic protozoan that is sexually transmitted.

Factors Increasing Susceptibility to Bacterial Vaginosis

- Multiple sexual partners (not considered a sexually transmitted disease [STD] but rather sexually associated disorder)
- New sexual partner within last 30 days
- Presence of intrauterine device (IUD)
- History of douching, tampon use
- Changes in normal vaginal flora associated with menses, pregnancy, OCPs, systemic antibiotics

Factors Increasing Susceptibility to *Trichomonas*

- Multiple sexual partners
- History of infected partner who does not receive treatment

Factors Increasing Susceptibility to Vulvovaginal Candidiasis

- Diabetes mellitus, especially when poorly controlled
- History of systemic antibiotics, OCPs, steroids
- Pregnancy
- Obesity
- Immunocompromise (e.g., human immunodeficiency virus [HIV], transplant)
- Wearing tight, restrictive clothing
- Douching, using perfumed feminine hygiene products and sprays, panty liners

ASSESSMENT: SUBJECTIVE/HISTORY
Typical Symptoms of Bacterial Vaginosis

- Increase in vaginal discharge with sensation of almost constant wetness; discharge is usually thin, white
- Fishy odor that improves little with bathing and is worse after intercourse and during menstruation

Typical Symptoms of *Trichomoniasis*

- Malodorous vaginal discharge (frothy yellow to green color) may be present.
- Vulvovaginal itching and irritation may be present.
- Dyspareunia may be present.
- Dysuria may be present.
- Postcoital spotting or bleeding may occur.
- Of all clients with *Trichomoniasis*, 20% to 25% are asymptomatic.
- Men may be asymptomatic or may complain of mild itching and moisture noted at the top of the penis on awakening.

Typical Symptoms of Vulvovaginal Candidiasis

- Vulvovaginal itching and burning

- Sensation of vaginal dryness despite cheesy white discharge
- Dyspareunia

History of Present Illness

- Obtain description of vaginal discharge: amount, color, odor, whether associated with itching, burning, or irritation.
- Determine whether there has been a change in symptoms with menstruation, sexual intercourse.
- Ask about onset of symptoms, duration, and course.
- Ask about remedies tried.
- Determine aggravating and relieving factors.
- Ask whether sexual partner is symptomatic.
- Ask about last menstrual period.
- Determine estrogen-status. Determine whether the woman is pregnant, lactating, or menopausal.
- Ask whether the woman is experiencing dyspareunia. (If she is, determine whether the pain is on entry or deep thrust.)

Past Medical History

- Previous sexually transmitted illness
- Chronic illness, particularly diabetes, seizure disorders, HIV or other condition that causes immunocompromised status
- Previous vulvovaginitis
- Date and results of last Pap smear

Medication History

- Recent antibiotic use
- Anticoagulants
- Birth control method, especially IUD, spermicides, OCPs
- Estrogen replacement or antiestrogen drugs such as tamoxifen (Nolvadex)

Psychosocial History

- Sexual practices, new partner
- Last intercourse (semen changes vaginal pH)
- Use of vaginal deodorants, vaginal sprays, scented tissue, bath oils, tampons, pads, panty liners, douches, changes in soaps, detergents, or fabric softeners
- Type of clothing (restrictive versus loose, synthetic fibers; type of panties, sleep without panties)

ASSESSMENT: OBJECTIVE/PHYSICAL EXAMINATION
Physical Examination

- A problem-oriented physical examination is performed with particular attention to the abdominal and pelvic areas. Visual inspection of the external genitalia, speculum examination, bimanual examination, and assessment of the abdomen and inguinal nodes are appropriate. The objective clinical findings that are commonly observed during the physical examination are noted in Table 3-118.

- The Fem Exam is a credit-card-like pH and amine test card used in some settings. Whether the pH value is being tested with this product or with regular pH paper, the sample should be obtained from the vaginal walls because the pH value of cervical mucus is normally higher.

Diagnostic Procedures

- Diagnosis can generally be made on the basis of clinical findings and the results of pH testing of vaginal secretions and microscopic analysis of a wet prep prepared with a suspension sample of vaginal discharge in normal saline solution (for BV and *Trichomonas*) and 10% KOH (for VVC).
- A whiff test for the presence of the fishy odor that is associated with the release of volatile amines when exposed to KOH is also helpful in making a diagnosis. Table 3-119 summarizes the typical findings of wet prep and pH testing.

DIAGNOSIS

The following differential diagnoses must be considered when assessing for vulvovaginitis:

- Chemical irritant exposure, contact dermatitis, or hypersensitivity reaction
- BV
- *Candidiasis*
- *Trichomoniasis*
- STD, gonorrhea, or chlamydia
- Atrophic vaginitis
- Presence of foreign body in vagina
- Cytologic vaginosis (worse during luteal phase of menstrual cycle, improves with menses, causes pruritus, dyspareunia, dysuria, and an irritating discharge); possible cause: overgrowth of lactobacilli and increased acidity; diagnosis: acid pH, increased lactobacilli, no clue cells, *candida*, or *trichomonads* evident on wet prep; treatment includes decreasing acidity with baking soda douche or sitz baths)

TABLE **3-118** Common Objective Clinical Findings of Vulvovaginitis

	BACTERIAL VAGINOSIS	VULVOVAGINAL CANDIDIASIS	TRICHOMONAS
External genitalia/vulva	Normal	Erythema, edema, excoriation Evidence of scratching	Erythema, edema, excoriation Evidence of scratching
Vaginal mucosa	Normal	Erythematous White patches along vaginal sidewalls	Erythema May have grandular appearance or thin gray pseudomenbrane that cannot be wiped off
Cervix	Normal	Normal	Punctate hemorrhages giving strawberry-like appearance (2% to 3%) Friable
Discharge	Homogenous, thin white milky to gray in color, adherent to mucosa Musty or fishy odor	Thick, cottage-cheese–like curdy white Odorless	Frothy yellow or greenish color Malodorous

TABLE **3-119** Typical Findings of Wet Prep, Whiff, and pH Testing of Vaginal Discharge

	BACTERIAL VAGINOSIS	VULVOVAGINAL CANDIDIASIS	TRICHOMONAS
pH	>4.5	<4.5	>4.5
Whiff test	Positive	Negative	Positive or negative
Wet prep	Clue Cells Rare WBC Loss of lactobacilli	Budding yeast and/or hyphae	Motile trichomonads WBCs

WBC, White blood cell.

THEREPEUTIC PLAN
Pharmacologic Treatment

Vulvovaginal *Candidiasis*

- The first-line drugs for treatment of candidiasis are the topical azoles administered intravaginally at night (e.g., Monistat, Mycelex). The topical drug may also be used externally to provide relief from pruritus and burning. These topical agents provide relief in 90% of cases. Only the topical azoles are indicated in cases of pregnancy and lactation. Oil-based topicals can weaken latex in condoms and diaphragms. Side effects tend to be vaginal burning and genital pain, itching, and rash. Table 3-120 summarizes information about prescription medications for candidiasis. Recurrent infection should be confirmed by culture.

- Recurrent VVC refers to four or more episodes of symptoms occurring within 1 year. Uncontrolled diabetes mellitus, corticosteroid use, and immunosuppression increase the risk of recurrent infection. A fasting blood glucose test should be conducted to rule out diabetes; for those at risk, HIV testing may be appropriate. If the blood glucose is normal, confirmation of recurrent candidiasis should precede maintenance therapy. Recurrence necessitates an intensive treatment regimen for 10 to 14 days with oral therapy to induce clinical remission and a negative fungal culture followed by a 6-month maintenance program.

- The pharmacologic treatment of BV and *Trichomonas* is summarized in Table 3-121.

Nonpharmacologic Treatment

Clients prone to vaginal candidiasis should consider a diet low in refined sugars.

Client Education

- Explain the vaginal ecosystem and how it is altered. Discuss how alterations contribute to vulvovaginitis.

- Advise the client not to engage in sexual intercourse until treatment is complete and symptoms subside.

- Stress the importance of completing the medication regimen even if menses begins.

- Advise against use of tampons during treatment.

- Stress perineal hygiene, cotton underwear, loose clothing, wiping front to back, not to wear panties while sleeping. Advise against feminine hygiene sprays or deodorants, scented sanitary products, douching. Soap can be drying on the perineum. Unscented mineral oil is a good cleanser and does not dry out the tissues.

- For those with *trichomoniasis,* advise treatment of sexual partners. Advise no sexual activity until both client and partner have been treated.

- For those receiving metronidazole as a treatment for BV and *Trichomonas,* advise refraining from any intake of alcohol, including mouth wash and cough medicine, for 24 hours before treatment begins and for at least 48 hours after completing treatment.

- For those prone to *candidiasis* infections, recommend a diet low in refined sugars.

- Explain that treatment of sexual partners is not required for those with *candidiasis* or BV.

- Inform the client that several alternative treatments for vaginal *candidiasis* have received anecdotal support, although they have not been substantiated by empirical study: (1) vaginal application of yogurt (plain with active cultures) to balance vaginal ecosystem once or twice daily for 1 week using a vaginal tampon; (2) gentian violet (1%) painted onto vaginal mucosa once a week for 4 or more weeks or monthly after menses for several months (remind client that gentian violet stains clothing and linens); (3) vitamin C 500 mg PO bid-qid to increase acidity of vaginal secretions; and (4) acidophilus tablets 40 million to 1 billion IU daily.

- Remind clients that OTC yeast treatments are less effective for nonalbicans species and that inappropri-

TABLE **3-120** Second-line Pharmacologic Treatment for Vulvovaginal Candidiasis

DRUG AND DOSAGE INFORMATION	IMPLICATIONS FOR CLIENT EDUCATION
INTRAVAGINAL AGENTS	
Terconazole 0.4% cream (Terazol 7) 5 g intravaginally for 7 days hs	Effective for both *Candida albicans* and nonalbicans species.
	May weaken condoms and diaphragms.
Or	Pregnancy category C
Terconazole 0.8% cream (Terazol 3) 5 g intravaginally for 3 days	Not recommended for children.
	Side effects: vaginal burning, itching, genital pain, and fever.
Or	Pregnancy category C
Terconazole 80 mg vaginal suppository hs for 3 days	Not recommended for children.
	Less effective against *Candida globrata.*
ORAL AGENT	
Fluconazole (Diflucan) 150 mg PO as single dose	Side effects: headache, nausea, GI upset, abdominal pain, and dizziness.
	Pregnancy category C

GI, Gastrointestinal.

TABLE **3-121** Pharmacologic Treatment for Vaginitis

DIAGNOSIS	DRUG AND DOSAGE	IMPLICATIONS FOR CLIENT EDUCATION
Bacterial vaginosis	Nonpregnant clients, drug of choice: Metronidazole Metronidazole (Flagyl) 2 g PO as single dose. Or Metronidazole (Flagyl) 500 mg PO bid for 7 days Or Metronidazole gel 0.75% intravaginally bid for 5 days Or Clindamycin (Cleocin) cream 2% intravaginally daily for 7 days with previous premature delivery For pregnant women: Clindamycin (Cleocin) 300 mg PO bid for 7 days Metronidazole 250 mg bid for 7 days Metronidazole 2 g PO as single dose If at low risk for preterm labor, may also use metronidazole gel For lactating women: Metronidazole can be used but breastfeeding must be discontinued 24 hours	Advise no alcohol during treatment and for 48 hours after completing medication to avoid severe Antabuse-like reaction associated with drug: abdominal pain, nausea, vomiting, and headache. Side effects: unpleasant metallic taste, furry tongue, GI upset, anorexia, constipation, headache, seizures, candida overgrowth. Not recommended for persons on phenytoin and phenobarb for seizures. Not recommended in children. Contraindicated: Chronic home disease. Clindamycin cream weakens latex condoms. Advise abstinence during treatment and for 2-3 days afterwards. Side effects: diarrhea, rash, blood dyscrasias, colitis, GI upset. Clindamycin is not recommended for children.
Trichomonas	Metronidazole (Flagyl) 2 g PO as single dose or 500 mg PO bid for 7 days	See above. Sexual partner should be treated concurrently.

GI, Gastrointestinal.

ate treatment may delay proper management. Discuss the benefits, risks, and advisability of self-diagnosis and self-treatment.

Referral/Consultation

- Referral may be necessary in cases of vulvovaginitis that is not responsive to treatment. Rule out noncompliance and reexposure before referring the client.
- A diagnosis of *trichomoniasis* in a child necessitates evaluation for sexual abuse.

Prevention

- Maintaining the normal flora of the vagina helps to prevent candidiasis and BV; however, this is not always possible. Eating yogurt that contains active culture and drinking buttermilk may help prevent candidiasis associated with antibiotic use. Refraining from behaviors such as douching that alter the vaginal ecosystem may aid in prevention of vulvovaginitis.
- *Trichomoniasis* may be prevented by limiting the number of sexual partners, screening any new partners, and consistently using condoms with each act of intercourse.

EVALUATION/FOLLOW-UP

- In general, follow-up is necessary only if symptoms persist. Women treated during pregnancy should be asked about symptoms at their next prenatal visit. Pregnant women treated for BV should be scheduled for follow-up in 1 month because BV is associated with complications of pregnancy.
- Clients who continue to have vulvar itching after treatment for candidiasis or trichomoniasis should probably undergo vulvar biopsy.
- Women who self-treat yeast infections with OTC drugs should understand that they are less effective against the nonalbicans species; anyone who self-treats should return to a provider if she has more than two recurrences during a 6-month interval.

COMPLICATIONS

- Failure to treat *candidiasis* appropriately leads to persistence of unpleasant symptoms. *Candidiasis,* especially recurrent *candidiasis,* may be associated with immune system abnormalities or undiagnosed diabetes mellitus. With OTC treatment by the client, there is no opportunity for a provider to rule out systemic disease.
- Failure to treat the woman with *trichomoniasis* and her sexual partner results in persistent symptoms that are distressing and reinfection.
- Failure to appropriately treat BV in a pregnant woman may result in chorioamnionitis, premature rupture of the amniotic membranes, premature labor, or postpartum endometritis.

- Current studies are addressing the role of vaginal flora in the transmission of viral STDs such as HIV.

REFERENCES

Cash, J. C., & Glass, C. A. (1999). *Family practice guidelines.* New York: Lippincott.

Cullins, V. E., Dominquez, L., Guberski, T., Secor, R.M., & Wysocki, S.J. (1999). Treating vaginitis. *Nurse Practitioner, 24*(10), 46-45.

Diagnosing and managing vaginal infections. (1999). *Women's Health and Primary Care, 2*(1), 63-64.

Freeman, S. B. (2000). Vaginitis: Advice for women who self-treat. *Conversations Counsel,* Spring, 6-8.

Hawkins, J. W., Robert-Nichols, D. M., & Stanley-Haney, J. L. (1997). Protocols for nurse practitioners in gynecologic settings (6th ed.). New York: Tiresias.

Hutti, M. H., & Hoffman, C. (2000). Cytologic vaginosis: An overlooked cause of cyclic vaginal itching and burning, *Journal of the American Academy of Nurse Practitioners, 12*(2), 55-57.

Mayeaux, E. J. (2001). Work-up of bacterial vaginosis: The role of pH testing. *Female Patient, 26,* 21-25.

Mead, P. B., Eisenbach, D. A., & Sobel, J. D. (1999). Update on management of vaginitis. *Contemporary Ob/Gyn, 44*(11), 26-32, 34-38.

Migeon, M. B., Desneck, L., & Elvore, J. G. (1999). Management of vaginal infections. *Clinical Advisor,* May, 26-31.

Nyirjesy, P. (2001). Chronic vulvovaginal candidiasis. *American Family Physician,* Retrieved February 15, 2001, from www.aafp.org/afp/20010215/687.html.

Robinson, D., Kidd, P., Rogers, K. (2000). *Primary care across the lifespan.* St. Louis: Mosby.

Smith, M. A., & Shimp, L. A. (2000). *20 common problems in women's health care.* New York: McGraw-Hill.

Street, R. L. (2001). Recurrent BV: An update. *Vaginitis Report,* 1:4.

Street, R. L. (2001). Tests for BV: Overlooked and underused. *Vaginitis Report,* 2:4.

Talarico, L. D. (1999). Vaginitis: Solid diagnosis means effective treatment. *Patient Care,* January 30, 86-106.

Witkin, S. S., Gidoldo, P. C., & Gregory. T. (2000). The quandary of recurrent vaginal candidiasis. *Patient Care, 34*(2), 123-129.

Review Questions

1. Betsy, a 19-year-old college student, presents to the clinic complaining of vaginal itching and burning. Which factor in Betsy's history is most consistent with a diagnosis of vaginal candidiasis?

- **a.** She prefers unscented sanitary napkins to tampons during menstruation.
- **b.** She recently completed a course of antibiotics for a respiratory infection.
- **c.** She occasionally swims laps in the college's indoor pool.
- **d.** She has seasonal allergies and takes cetirizine HCl (Zyrtec) daily.

2. Which of the following most accurately describes the classic vaginal discharge of vaginal candidiasis?

- **a.** Milky white, homogenous, and foul smelling
- **b.** Frothy green, "fishy smelling," and pruritic
- **c.** Curdy white, nonodorous, and associated with itching
- **d.** Yellow with a musty odor and associated with dysuria

3. Which microscopic finding is most consistent with a diagnosis of vaginal candidiasis?

- **a.** Clue cells
- **b.** Motile trichomonads
- **c.** Excess white blood cells
- **d.** Hyphae

4. A client with recurrent yeast infections, despite treatment, should be evaluated for which of the following?

- **a.** Diabetes mellitus
- **b.** Gonorrhea
- **c.** Graves disease
- **d.** *Shigella*

5. Which of the following diagnostic measures is appropriate for diagnosing trichomoniasis?

- **a.** Normal saline wet prep
- **b.** Rapid plasma reagent test
- **c.** KOH wet prep
- **d.** Culture of discharge

6. The nurse practitioner (NP) has provided comprehensive teaching to a woman who has just been diagnosed with *trichomoniasis.* Which comment by the client indicates that she needs further instructions?

- **a.** " I should not drink any alcohol during treatment or for 48 hours after completing the medicine."
- **b.** "I need to have my boyfriend come in to receive treatment."
- **c.** "I should abstain from sexual intercourse during treatment."
- **d.** "I need to limit my intake of dairy products during treatment."

7. Which of the following findings is inconsistent with a diagnosis of BV?

- **a.** Clue cells on wet prep
- **b.** pH value of vaginal discharge higher than 4.5
- **c.** Vulvar itching and erythema
- **d.** Positive whiff with KOH

8. Which of the following medications is appropriate for treating BV?

- **a.** Terconazole 80 mg vaginal suppository hs for 3 days
- **b.** Providone iodine douche bid for 4 days
- **c.** Metronidazole 500 mg PO bid for 7 days
- **d.** Fluconazole (Diflucan) 150 mg PO as a single dose

9. Mary Ellen is 23 weeks' pregnant when it is determined that she has BV. Because of that diagnosis, she will need to be monitored closely for which of the following?

- **a.** Premature rupture of the membranes
- **b.** Lactic acidosis
- **c.** Endometrial hypertrophy
- **d.** Placenta accreta

10. An NP teaches a group of women college students about vaginal health and prevention of vaginitis. Which statement by one of the students indicates a need for further teaching on the topic?

a. "Douching disturbs the vaginal environment and contributes to vaginal infections."

b. "I can no longer use tampons during my periods or I risk vaginitis."

c. "Wearing tight pants and nylon panties can increase the risk of vaginal infections."

d. "It is a good idea to sleep without panties to allow air to circulate to the vaginal area."

Answers and Rationales

1. *Answer:* b (assessment)
Rationale: Antibiotics contribute to vaginitis by destroying the normal flora in the vagina (Robinson et al. 2000).

2. *Answer:* c (evaluation)
Rationale: The typical vaginal discharge of candidiasis is cheesy white discharge resembling the curds of cottage cheese. It is nonodorous and causes vulvar erythema and itching (Talarico, 1999).

3. *Answer:* d (analysis/diagnosis)
Rationale: Budding yeast and hyphae are findings of a wet prep microscopic examination that are indicative of a diagnosis of candidiasis vaginal infection (Talarico, 1999).

4. *Answer:* a (implementation/plan)
Rationale: A client with recurrent yeast vaginitis needs to be assessed for diabetes mellitus and HIV infection, both of which are systemic illnesses associated with frequent candidiasis (Robinson et al. 2000).

5. *Answer:* a (analysis/diagnosis)
Rationale: A normal saline wet prep aids in diagnosing *trichomoniasis*. Trichomonads can be visualized in a wet prep viewed under the microscope. KOH destroys trichomonads (Cash & Glass, 1999).

6. *Answer:* d (evaluation)
Rationale: Persons being treated for *trichomoniasis* should be taught not to drink alcohol in any form during treatment with metronidazole (Flagyl); their sexual partners will need treatment, and they should abstain from intercourse during treatment. Dairy products are not contraindicated (Cullins et al., 1999).

7. *Answer:* c (analysis/diagnosis)
Rationale: BV does not present with itching and vulvar irritation (Cash & Glass, 1999).

8. *Answer:* c (implementation/plan)
Rationale: Metronidazole is the appropriate drug choice for BV (Mayeaux, 2001).

9. *Answer:* a (evaluation)
Rationale: BV in pregnancy increases the risk of several obstetrical complications, one of which is premature rupture of the amniotic membranes (Mayeaux, 2001).

10. *Answer:* b (evaluation)
Rationale: Tampons themselves do not seem to contribute to vaginitis; however, scented sanitary products do increase the risk because they alter the vaginal ecosystem (Freeman, 2000).

WARTS: COMMON *Denise Robinson*

OVERVIEW
Definition

Warts are virus-induced epidermal tumors caused by human papillomavirus (HPV). More than 70 genotypes of HPV have been identified. There are three types of HPV infections that occur among the general population: common wart, plantar wart, and flat wart. Warts can last from many months to several years.

Incidence

- The common wart constitutes approximately 70% of all cutaneous warts, with 20% occurring in school age children.
- Plantar warts occur in older children and young adults, representing approximately 30% of cutaneous warts.
- Flat warts also occur in children and adults, representing 4% of cutaneous warts.

Pathophysiology

- HPV is a double-stranded DNA virus of the papovavirus class. Minor trauma with breaks in the stratum corneum facilitates epidermal infection.
- Transmission occurs through the following:

- Skin-to-skin contact can transmit HPV.
- Minor trauma to the skin facilitates infection. Medical personnel may be exposed to the virus from the plume of warts treated by laser or electrosurgery, resulting in a nosocomial infection. Heredity is a factor in epidermodysplasia verruciformis, most often an autosomal recessive gene.

Factors Increasing Susceptibility. A person who is immunocompromised by human immunodeficiency virus or who has undergone organ transplantation is at increased risk of widespread cutaneous warts. There is an occupational risk associated with butchers and meat packers.

ASSESSMENT: SUBJECTIVE/HISTORY
History of Present Illness

Ask about location, onset, duration, and symptoms.

Symptoms

- Bleeding after shaving
- Cosmetic disfigurement
- Foot pain

Past Medical History

Ask about previous warts, treatments, and results.

Medication History

If the client has received previous treatment for HPV, determine what treatment was used, how often treatment was used, and whether the treatment was completed.

Family History

Ask about history of epidermodysplasia verruciformis.

ASSESSMENT: OBJECTIVE/PHYSICAL EXAMINATION

Physical Examination

- Examine the lesion, looking for characteristic lesions.
- Use a hand lens to assist in visualizing surface characteristics.
- See Table 3-122 for types of skin lesions.

Diagnostic Procedures

Decisions regarding which diagnostic procedures to use are usually based on the clinical findings.

DIAGNOSIS

Differential diagnoses include the following:
- Molluscum contagiosum
- Condyloma latum
- Lipomas, fibroma, adenoma
- Squamous cell carcinoma
- Seborrheic keratoses
- Psoriatic plaques

THERAPEUTIC PLAN

Warts may resolve spontaneously in 12 to 24 months without treatment. Approximately 50% do resolve spontaneously.

Nonpharmacologic Treatment

Soaking warts in hot water for 10 to 30 minutes every day for 6 weeks may be effective for immunocompromised clients.

Pharmacologic Treatment

- Salicylic acid, 17% (Duofilm, Occlusal-HP, Compound W): Apply a thin coat to the area, one or two times a day for a maximum of 12 weeks. Duofilm patch for children: Apply one patch, and repeat q48h for a maximum of 12 weeks. Soak the wart in warm water for 5 minutes, remove loose tissue, and dry.
- Liquid nitrogen: Apply to achieve a thaw time of 20 to 45 seconds. Two freeze-thaw times are administered every 2 to 4 weeks for several visits. Face, dorsal hands, and legs are more sensitive than palms. This treatment is useful on dry penile warts and filiform warts involving the face and body.
- Resorcinol (RA lotion) (over the counter [OTC]): Apply per package directions.
  - Apply to affected areas and rub gently. For clients who are pregnant, keep in mind that treatment can be systemically absorbed.
  - Wash hands immediately after applying. Avoid contact with eyes.
  - Do not use other topical acne preparations or other products containing peeling agents.
  - Medication may darken light colored hair.
  - Side effects are diarrhea, nausea, stomach pain, methemoglobinemia, and redness or peeling of skin.

TABLE **3-122**   Skin Lesions

VERRUCA VULGARIS (COMMON WARTS)	VERRUCA PLANTARIS (PLANTAR WARTS)	VERRUCA PLANA (FLAT WARTS)	EPIDERMODYSPLASIA VERRUCIFORMIS
Firm papules; 1 to 10 mm; skin color; round isolated or scattered discrete lesions; typically at site of trauma on hands, fingers, or knees	Early stages are small shiny papules that later develop plaque with rough surface; skin colored; may have marked tenderness; confluence of many small warts, resulting in mosaic wart; lesions may also occur on the two facing surfaces of toes; usually occur on pressure points, such as heads of metatarsal, heels, or toes	Flat papules, 1 to 5 mm on surface and 1 to 2 mm in thickness; skin colored or light brown; round, oval, polygonal, or linear if caused by traumatic inoculation; many discrete lesions, closely set; commonly on face, beard, dorsa of hand, shins	Flat wart-like lesions; may be large, numerous, and confluent; skin colored, light brown, pink, or hypopigmented; occurs on face, trunk, extremities; premalignant and malignant occur most often on face

From Robinson, D. (2000). Nongenital warts. In D. Robinson, P. Kidd, & K. Rogers (Eds.), *Primary care across the lifespan* (p. 1173). St. Louis: Mosby.

TABLE **3-123** Treatment for Types of Warts

TYPE OF WART	TREATMENT
Common	Topical salicylic preparations or cryotherapy: Cryotherapy is painful and may require continued treatments every 4 weeks until the wart is gone.
Filiform	Refer for removal by curette.
Flat	Refer for removal. These warts are resistant to treatment and are usually located in cosmetically important areas.
Plantar	Use 40% salicylic acid plasters (Mediplast). Plaster is cut to size, applied to wart, removed in 48 to 72 hours, and repeated every 24 to 48 hours. Any dead white keratin can be removed with pumice stone. This process can be continued up to 4 to 6 weeks until the wart is removed. Pain relief results during the first few days because a large part of the wart can be removed during that time. Aggressive therapies may be painful and can result in scarring. Surgical removal, cryosurgery, electrosurgery (tends to cause more scarring than cryosurgery), or laser may be considered.

From Robinson, D. (2000). Nongenital warts. In D. Robinson, P. Kidd, & K. Rogers (Eds.), *Primary care across the lifespan* (p. 1174). St. Louis: Mosby.

See Table 3-123 for treatments for various types of warts.

Client Education

Reassure the client that frequently warts go away.

Referral/Consultation

Refer the client to a dermatologist for excision of the wart.

Prevention

Good hand washing can help prevent warts.

EVALUATION/FOLLOW-UP

- Follow-up may not be indicated.
- Evaluation is determined by clinical observations of the resolving lesion.
- If the lesions are on the fingertips, return of fingerprint indicates resolution of wart.

COMPLICATIONS.

Warts not removed and still present.

REFERENCES

Feldman, S., Fleischer, A., & McConnell, R. (1998). Most common dermatological problems identified by internists. *Archives of Internal Medicine, 158*(7), 726-730.

Fitzpatrick, T., Johnson, R., Wolff, K., & Suurmond, D. (2001). *Color atlas and synopsis of clinical dermatology* (4th ed.). New York: McGraw-Hill.

Glass, A., & Solomon, B. (1996). Cimetidine therapy for recalcitrant warts in adults. *Archives of Dermatology, 32,* 680-682.

Landow, K. Y. (1996). Non-genital warts: When is treatment warranted? *Postgraduate Medicine, 99,* 245-249.

Miller, D., & Brodell, R. (1996). Human papillomavirus: Treatment options for warts. *American Family Physician, 53,* 135-143, 148-150.

Robinson, D. (2000). Nongenital warts. In D. Robinson, P. Kidd, & K. Rogers (Eds.), *Primary care across the lifespan.* St. Louis: Mosby

Sterling, J. (1995). Treating the troublesome wart. *Practitioner, 239,* 44-47.

Review Questions

1. Which of the following occupations does *not* put the workers at risk of acquiring warts on the job?
   a. Butchers
   b. Meat packers
   c. Fish handlers
   d. Teachers

2. Which of the following is the type of cutaneous wart that is often painful?
   a. Common
   b. Flat
   c. Plantar
   d. Filiform

3. Which of the following findings of a physical examination are consistent with verruca plantaris (plantar warts)?
   a. Firm papules, 1 to 10 mm, hyperkeratotic, with vegetations
   b. Small, sharp, sharply marginated papule with rough hyperkeratotic surface, studded with brown-black dots
   c. Sharply defined, flat papules, skin colored or light brown
   d. Papules, pearly white or skin colored with central keratotic plug, giving lesion a central dimple

4. Which of the following lesions are most characteristic of warts?
   a. Firm, skin-color papules
   b. Vesicles painful to touch
   c. Oval, erythematous lesion with fine, coliform edges
   d. Round, pearly white papules that are umbilicated

5. Which of the following is not an appropriate treatment for common warts?
   a. Do nothing; the warts may disappear on their own.
   b. Be aggressive with therapy; otherwise, the warts will become painful.
   c. Use salicylic acid applications.
   d. Perform cryosurgery.

6. Which of the following methods describes the transmission of warts?
   a. Respiratory droplets

b. Blood and body fluids
c. Skin-to-skin contact
d. Touching frogs

7. Which of the following warts most frequently occur in school age children?

a. Common warts
b. Plantar warts
c. Flat warts
d. Genital warts

8. Which of the following would you teach regarding preparation for removal of warts by cryosurgery (liquid nitrogen)?

a. The lesion will go away as soon as it is touched with the liquid nitrogen.
b. This procedure may cause scarring.
c. The procedure is painful and may need to be repeated.
d. The procedure is painless.

Answers and Rationales

1. *Answer:* **d** (analysis/diagnosis)
Rationale: All of those listed except teachers are at risk of coming in contact with the viruses that cause warts (Fitzpatrick, Johnson, Wolff, Suurmond, 2001).

2. *Answer:* **c** (assessment)
Rationale: Tenderness may occur with plantar warts, especially in area of pressure, such as over the metatarsal head (Fitzpatrick, et al. 2001).

3. *Answer:* **b** (assessment)
Rationale: Plantar warts are described as sharply marginated papules with brown-black dots. They are frequently painful. Choice a describes common warts, choice c describes flat warts, and choice d describes molluscum contagiosum (Fitzpatrick et al. 2001).

4. *Answer:* **a** (assessment)
Rationale: Warts are commonly firm, skin-color papules. Vesicles painful to touch are common in herpes; oval, erythematous lesions are characteristic of pityriasis; round, pearly papules are molluscum contagiosum (Fitzpatrick et al. 2001).

5. *Answer:* **b** (implementation/plan)
Rationale: Most warts spontaneously resolve. Aggressive therapies can cause scarring and pain (Fitzpatrick et al. 2001).

6. *Answer:* **c** (analysis/diagnosis)
Rationale: Warts are caused by viruses and are spread by skin-to-skin contact (Fitzpatrick et al. 2001).

7. *Answer:* **a** (analysis/diagnosis)
Rationale: Common warts represent approximately 70% of all warts, occurring in up to 20% of all school age children (Fitzpatrick et al. 2001).

8. *Answer:* **c** (implementation/plan)
Rationale: Liquid nitrogen cryosurgery to remove warts is usually painful and may require several treatments if the wart is large. Electrosurgery tends to cause more scarring than cryosurgery (Fitzpatrick et al. 2001).

WORMS (HELMINTHIASIS) *Denise Robinson*

OVERVIEW
Definition

Helminthiasis is the condition of being infected with parasitic worms.

Incidence

- Helminthic infections endemic to the United States include hookworm (uncinariasis), pinworm (enterobiasis), roundworm (ascariasis), and whipworm (trichuriasis). Humans are the only vectors of these particular helminths.
- Approximately 4 million individuals in North America have roundworm.
- Pinworm infections are ubiquitous; however, they occur more commonly in the southeastern United States where the warm, moist climate is conducive to ova incubation or larva maturation in fecally contaminated soil.
- There is also a higher incidence in immigrants/travelers from warm, tropical regions.

Pathophysiology

- Hookworms: Larvae in the soil penetrate the skin, migrate via the circulatory system to the cardiopulmonary bed where they penetrate the alveoli, migrate up the bronchial tree, and are coughed into the pharynx and swallowed. In the gastrointestinal (GI) tract, larvae mature into adults and attach themselves to the intestinal mucosa and can suck up to 0.5 mL of blood daily per worm. Hookworms also secrete an anticoagulant that contributes to additional blood loss.
- Pinworms: Ingested eggs mature and live imbedded in the wall of the cecum. Gravid females migrate to the anus to deposit eggs, which causes intense pruritus. Scratching often contaminates the fingers and enables reinfection of the host or other contacts. Chronic urinary tract infections in girls are infrequently attributed to adult worms migrating up the urethra.
- Roundworms: Larvae from ingested eggs penetrate the intestinal wall into the mesenteric venous system, migrate to the cardiopulmonary bed where they penetrate the alveoli, migrate up the bronchial tree, are coughed into the pharynx and swallowed, and mature into adult worms. Adult roundworms live in the upper small intestine and infections are often asymptomatic. Malnourishment and weight loss occur in cases of more severe infections. Infrequently, worms penetrate and

block the common bile duct or masses may cause intestinal obstruction.

- Whipworms: Ingested eggs mature and then migrate to the cecum and colon, where they imbed themselves in the intestinal mucosa. If infections are severe, the worms can consume enough blood to cause anemia and weight loss. In cases of massive infestation, obstruction of the appendiceal lumen, bloody diarrhea, and secondary infections of the colon may occur.

Factors Increasing Susceptibility
- Children and those who are institutionalized or disabled
- Lower socioeconomic groups
- Overcrowding
- Poor hygiene practices or unsanitary conditions
- Situations that contribute to soil contamination with human feces (e.g., flooding, open and untreated sewage)

ASSESSMENT: SUBJECTIVE/HISTORY

Many persons with helminthiasis remain asymptomatic unless the infection becomes severe. Onset is usually insidious, and symptoms are usually vague.

History of Present Illness

Ask about the following:
- Pruritus of feet (hookworm) or anus and vagina (pinworm)
- Transitory fever, cough, sore throat (hookworm, roundworm)
- Abdominal discomfort, distention, nausea, vomiting, diarrhea (hookworm, roundworm, whipworm)

Past Medical History

Assess for pica, institutionalization, and disability.

Family History

Signs and symptoms of helminthic infection in other family members depend on the age and degree of infestation.

Environment

Inquire about the client's living situation relative to crowding, sanitation, and hygiene (washing of hands and food). Inquire about exposure to raw sewage or human waste fertilizer.

Activity and Lifestyle

Assess for fatigue and unexplained weight loss, changes in elimination patterns, and travel to susceptible regions.

Symptoms

See Table 3-124 for a description of the most common symptoms.

Associated Symptoms

- Possible symptoms of urinary tract infection or vaginitis can occur in extensive pinworm infections.
- Rectal prolapse can result from severe whipworm infections; adult worms may be visible in the prolapsed rectum.

ASSESSMENT: OBJECTIVE/PHYSICAL EXAMINATION
Physical Examination

- Clients often do not appear symptomatic; may appear pale and anemic, underweight, malnourished; children may demonstrate retarded growth.
- Skin: Papulovesicular entry lesions are apparent in hookworm infestation; check for pallor; clubbing will be present if progressive anemia has occurred.
- Lungs: Wheeze, cough, and blood-tinged sputum may be present if larvae are in pulmonary migratory phase (roundworm, hookworm).
- Heart: Increased force and lateral displacement of point of maximal impulse (PMI) will be present if anemia-induced hypertrophy has occurred.
- Rectal area may show excoriation and erythema from scratching; pinworms may be visualized.

TABLE **3-124** Description of Most Common Symptoms

TYPE OF WORM	MOST COMMON SYMPTOMS
Hookworms	Erythema and intense itching at site of entry (usually feet); papulovesicular lesion at entry site; fever, sore throat, cough, blood-tinged sputum associated with larvae in lungs; fatigue, weight loss, nausea, vomiting, uncontrolled diarrhea, melena
Pinworms	Intense anal pruritus, restlessness (especially at night); parents may report seeing adult worms on child's anal region
Roundworms	Fever, sore throat, cough, blood-tinged sputum associated with larvae in lungs; abdominal cramps and discomfort, weight loss, nausea, vomiting, diarrhea; presence of large white or reddish round worm(s) in feces or vomit
Whipworms	Heavy worm load (more than 30,000 ova/g of feces) associated with abdominal cramps and discomfort, flatulence, weight loss, bloody mucoid diarrhea

From Niemer, L. (2000). Worms. In D. Robinson, P. Kidd, & K. Rogers (Eds.), *Primary care across the lifespan* (p. 1184). St. Louis: Mosby.

Diagnostic Procedures

- If a worm has been visualized, diagnostic tests are unnecessary.
- If a worm has not been visualized, conduct a cellophane tape test (used primarily for pinworms). Loop a piece of cellophane tape with the adhesive side out to the end of a tongue depressor. Spread the buttocks and apply the adhesive side of the tape (on depressor) to the perianal area. Rotate the tape so that it touches all of the perianal area. Apply a slide to the adhesive area and then cut the tongue depressor from the remaining tape (Robinson & McKenzie, 2000). These specimens are best obtained in the morning and before bathing.
- Collect a stool sample to test for ova and parasites.

DIAGNOSIS

Visualization of a worm in the feces or vomit (roundworm), confirmation of ova in the feces (hookworm, roundworm, and whipworm), or nocturnal anal pruritus and presence of ova on transparent tape (pinworm) constitutes diagnosis. Differential diagnoses for worms include the following:

- Asthma, pneumonia
- Duodenal ulcer, hiatal hernia, gallbladder, or pancreatic disease
- Nonspecific urinary or vaginal irritation or fungal infection, hemorrhoids, localized allergic response

THERAPEUTIC PLAN

- Unless symptomatic, clients with light hookworm (fewer than 1000 ova/g of feces) or whipworm (fewer than 10,000 ova/g of feces) infections do not require treatment. However, these infections are often accompanied by roundworm infections.

- The potential complications from wandering roundworms require that they be treated, especially before elective surgery (anesthesia stimulates hypermotility) and after the third trimester of pregnancy.
- Although annoying, pinworm infections are benign. Clients who are symptomatic for pinworms are treated. All members of the household and household contacts are generally infected and should also be treated to reduce the risk of reinfection.

Pharmacologic Treatment

See Tables 3-125 and 3-126 for pharmacologic treatment of worms.

Nonpharmacologic Treatment

- Careful hand washing after defecation and before meals is important.
- Keep fingernails short and clean.
- Avoid scratching the perianal area.
- Wash bedding, towels, and clothes of infected person.
- Snug fitting underwear may be helpful for children.

Client Education

- Helminthic infections occur from the ingestion of ova or the penetration of larvae through the skin.
- Explain the cause of the worms and teach the importance of hand washing after defecation and before eating.
- Hygiene practices, such as washing fruits and vegetables, changing underwear and linens daily (especially in cases of pinworm infections), and regular housecleaning, help prevent reinfection.
- In cases of hookworm infection, stress the importance of wearing shoes in endemic areas.

TABLE **3-125** Pharmacologic Treatment of Worms

DRUG/DOSE	COMMENTS
Pyrantel pamoate (Antiminth)	May be taken without regard to food; available as suspension 50 mg/ml; not recommended for children younger than 2 years; Side effects: vomiting, diarrhea, headache, drowsiness Mild symptoms in up to 20%
Mebendazole (Vermox)	Administer before or after meals For hookworm, administer bid for 3 days Not recommended for children younger than 2 years Chew tablet for best effect Contraindicated during pregnancy For heavy whipworm infections, continue up to 6 days or repeat course if necessary
Thiabendazole (Mintezol) tablets, 500 mg/susp, 500 mg/5 mL	Chewable tablets, take with food Safety not established for children weighing less than 30 lb Monitor hepatic or renal dysfunction carefully Side effects: dizziness, drowsiness, headache, anorexia, nausea, vomiting, diarrhea, pruritus, tinnitus

TABLE **3-126** Drugs of Choice for Various Types of Worm Infestations

INFECTING ORGANISM	DRUG OF CHOICE
Pinworm	Albendazole 400 mg PO (one dose) or Pyrantel pamoate 11 mg/kg PO (single dose) or Mebendazole 100 mg PO (single dose, repeat after 2 weeks)
Hookworm	Albendazole 400 mg PO (single dose) or Mebendazole 100 mg PO bid for 3 days or Pyrantel pamoate 11 mg/kg PO qd for 3 days
Whipworm	Albendazole 400 mg PO (single dose) or Mebendazole 100 mg PO bid for 3 days
Roundworms	Albendazole 400 mg PO (single dose) or Mebendazole 100 mg PO bid for 3 days or Pyrantel pamoate 11 mg/kg PO (single dose) (maximum, 1 g) or Thiabendazole 10 mg/kg/dose bid for 2 days PO (in clients weighing less than 150 lb) or Thiabendazole 1.5 g/dose PO (in clients weighing more than 150 lb) or Diethylcarbamazine 13 mg/kg qd for 7 days PO (children: 6 to 10 mg/kg tid for 7 to 10 days)
Larva migrans	Diethylcarbamazine 2 mg/kg PO tid for 10 days (considered superior) or Albendazole 400 mg PO bid for 5 days or Mebendazole 100 to 200 mg PO bid for 5 days

- In cases of pinworm infection, children should bathe daily (showers are preferable to baths). The nails should be kept short and nail biting discouraged.
- A social stigma is often associated with helminthiasis. Infections may have occurred while traveling. Children may have ingested eggs while playing outdoors or with contaminated objects. Families may need support.

Referral/Consultation

- Referral is not necessary unless the condition is refractory to treatment.
- For a pregnant woman with worms, consult with an obstetrician (treat ascariasis after first trimester).

Prevention

- Good hand washing, especially after using the bathroom
- No walking barefoot outside

EVALUATION/FOLLOW-UP

- Roundworm: Recheck stool in 2 weeks, continue to retreat until worms are eradicated.
- Eradicate helminths.

COMPLICATIONS

Rectal excoriation from itching is a complication associated with worms.

REFERENCES

Goldsmith, R. (1997). Infectious diseases: Protozoal and helminthic. In L.M. Tierney, S. McPhee, & M. Papadakis (Eds.), *Current medical diagnosis and treatment* (13th ed.). Stamford, CN: Appleton & Lange.

Juckett, G. (1997). Pets and parasites. *American Family Physician, 56*(7), 1763-1774.

Niemer, L. (2000). Worms. In D. Robinson, P. Kidd, & K. Rogers (Eds.), *Primary care across the life span*. St. Louis: Mosby.

Robinson, D., & McKenzie, C. (2000). *Procedures for primary care providers*. Philadelphia: Lippincott.

Roos, M. (1997). The use of drugs in the control of parasitic nematode infections: Must we do without? *Parasitology, 114*(suppl), S137-S144.

Salata, R. (2000). Infections diseases of travelers: Protozoal and helminthic infections. In T. Adreoli & C. Carpenter (Eds.), *Essentials of Medicine* (5th ed., pp. 868-874). Philadelphia: Squnders.

Sarinas, P., & Chitkara, R. (1997). Ascariasis and hookworm. *Seminars in Respiratory Infection, 12*(2), 137.

Weinberg, A., & Levin, M. (1999). Infections: Parasitic and mycotic. In W.W. Hay, M. Levin, A.R. Hayward, & J. Sondheimer (Eds.), *Current pediatric diagnosis and treatment* (14th ed.). Stamford, CN: Appleton & Lange.

Review Questions

1. Which of the following historical data is consistent with a diagnosis of pinworms?
  a. Difficulty sleeping
  b. Coughing and sneezing
  c. Nausea and vomiting
  d. Abdominal pain

2. Which of the following symptom descriptions stated by a client, in addition to rectal itching, is typical of pinworms?
  a. "I have nausea and vomiting."
  b. "My abdomen really hurts."
  c. "My rectal area is really rubbed raw."
  d. "I have had diarrhea."

3. Which of the following is a first-line test for pinworms?

a. Lower GI series
b. Stool specimen
c. Cellophane tape test
d. Sputum specimen

4. You are scheduling an appointment for a child who has rectal itching at night. When is the best time for an appointment?

a. In the morning
b. After the child has showered and eaten breakfast
c. In the afternoon
d. When the child is hungry

5. Pinworms must be differentiated from other helminths. Compared with pinworms, hookworms are associated with all except which of the following?

a. Erythema and intense itching at the site of entry
b. Systemic symptoms (fever, fatigue)
c. Intense anal pruritus
d. Blood-tinged sputum

6. Which of the following drug choices is most appropriate for treatment of pinworms in a 2-year-old child?

a. Dicyclomine (Bentyl), 25 mg pc and hs
b. Diphenoxylate with atropine (Lomotil), 1 tablet after bowel movement
c. Mebendazole (Vermox), 100 mg, 1 tablet now, repeat in 2 weeks
d. Ivermectin (Stromectol), 1 6-mg table now, repeat in 2 weeks

7. Which of the following comments by a mother of a child with pinworms indicates the need for further teaching?

a. "Washing hands after going to the bathroom is important."
b. "Wearing snug fitting underwear helps decrease the chance of spreading the disease."
c. "The other children should be treated prophylactically."
d. "Adults are immune to pinworms."

8. What other control measures should the nurse practitioner (NP) discuss with a mother of a child with pinworms?

a. Ironing the child's clothes ensures that the ova is killed.
b. A nutritious diet with fruits and vegetables helps contain the pinworms.
c. Watch for the presence of head itching; frequently, lice and pinworms are found together.
d. Wash all the linens, clothes, and towels in hot water after treating the child with the medication.

Answers and Rationales

1. *Answer:* **a** (assessment)
Rationale: Clients with pinworms usually present with difficulty sleeping because of rectal itching. The pinworms exit the rectum to lay their eggs in the perianal area, which causes itching (Niemer, 2000).

2. *Answer:* **c** (assessment)
Rationale: Perianal excoriation is common, particularly in children. They scratch the perianal area because of all the itching (Niemer, 2000).

3. *Answer:* **c** (analysis/diagnosis)
Rationale: A cellophane tape test is a first-line test because it can be performed in the office and confirms the presence of ova and pinworms (Robinson & McKenzie, 2000).

4. *Answer:* **a** (analysis/diagnosis)
Rationale: It is best to schedule the appointment for the morning, before the child has bathed, so that there is more chance of visualizing the pinworm and of having better success with the cellophane tape test. Meals have no bearing on the likelihood of the examination to visualize the ova (Robinson & McKenzie, 2000).

5. *Answer:* **c** (analysis/diagnosis)
Rationale: Hookworms do not cause intense anal pruritus. That is a classic symptom of pinworms. Symptoms of hookworm infestation include intense itching, usually at the site of entry (feet), fever, sore throat, cough, blood-tinged sputum, fatigue, weight loss, nausea, vomiting, and diarrhea (Niemer, 2000).

6. *Answer:* **c** (implementation/plan)
Rationale: Vermox is an appropriate drug for the treatment of pinworms. It is administered as a chewable tablet and then repeated one time in 2 weeks (Niemer, 2000).

7. *Answer:* **d** (evaluation)
Rationale: Adults are not immune to pinworms and may be infected by their children. It is recommended that all household members be treated for pinworms if one member is diagnosed (Niemer, 2000).

8. *Answer:* **d** (implementation/plan)
Rationale: Housecleaning activities can help decrease the transmission of pinworms back to the client and other household members (Niemer, 2000).

WOUND MANAGEMENT   *Pamela Kidd*

OVERVIEW
Definition
A wound is a structural alteration that results when energy is imparted during an interaction with a physical or chemical agent.

Incidence
Nearly 10 million wounds are treated each year in the United States.

Pathophysiology
Alteration in skin integrity produces a portal for infection and a need for granulation of new tissue.

Protective Factors
- Helmet use
- Good nutrition

Factors Increasing Susceptibility
- Chronic use of steroids, which decreases skin density
- Failure to use protective equipment at work

ASSESSMENT: SUBJECTIVE/HISTORY
Symptoms
- Bleeding (minimal to extensive)
- Pain, swelling
- Decreased range of motion at site of injury, possibly because of tendon or ligament injury
- Change in sensation at site of injury or distal to site of injury caused by nerve injury

History of Injury Event
Mechanism of Injury: Puncture Wound. Knowing the following information aids in determining what underlying tissues, organs, bones, nerves, or other elements may also be involved in the injury:
- What was the instrument that caused the puncture wound?
- How long and wide was the instrument that caused the puncture wound?
- What position was the body in when the puncture wound occurred?

Also determine the following:
- Time of injury: Wounds older than 10 hours are more prone to infection and require special attention, such as antibiotic treatment, excessive irrigation, or delayed closure (Behr, 1999).
- Determine whether first aid was administered before client's arrival at health care provider's office or emergency department.

Past Medical History
- Tetanus status
- Allergies, especially to lidocaine, iodine (Betadine), tetanus, and antibiotics
- Previous experiences with sutures
- Immunity disorders
- Diabetes
- Last menstrual period (be sure client is not pregnant before conducting radiographic studies or giving antibiotic therapy, or tetanus injections)

Medication History
Ask about current medications, especially cardiovascular and asthma medications that may cause potential harmful side effects with the use of lidocaine with or without epinephrine (elevation of heart rate or blood pressure).

Family History
Noncontributory.

Dietary History
Noncontributory.

ASSESSMENT: OBJECTIVE/PHYSICAL EXAMINATION
Physical Examination
A problem-oriented examination should be conducted with particular attention to the following:
- Vital signs
- Heart rate
  - Increase may be caused by infection.
  - Decrease may be caused by cardiac dysrhythmia.
- Blood pressure (indication of potential shock)
- Temperature (indication of infection)
- Type of wound
- Signs of infection
- Sensory, motor (including range of motion of joints above and below wound), and vascular assessment distal to injury
- Presence of foreign bodies
- Palpation of bony areas below and adjacent to injuries

Diagnostic Procedures
Radiology
- X-ray studies of the site of injury may be needed to rule out foreign bodies or bone involvement.
- Be aware that glass is be visible on radiographs only if it contains lead. Wood is not visible on x-ray films.
- If an infection is involved, an x-ray examination may help determine the depth and extent of the infection.

Wound Culture
If the wound appears infected, a wound culture should be obtained before any debridement or cleansing is performed.

DIAGNOSIS
Types of Wounds

- Lacerations
- Shearing
  - Eighty percent of soft-tissue injuries are caused by shearing injuries.
  - A sharp force is applied to the tissue by glass, metal, or knife. This results in a linear wound. The wound may be superficial, extending through the dermis, or deep, extending through the subcutaneous tissue. This type of wound is the most resistant to infection.
- Stellate
  - Caused by compression between tissues that overlay bone, and an applied force to the tissue. This injury is highly susceptible to infection and is the most common type of scalp injury.
- Compression
  - Caused by collision of two bodies applying compression to soft tissue supported by bone. Often associated with a hematoma and is most commonly associated with chin and eyebrow lacerations.
- Abrasion
  - The rubbing away of the dermal layer of skin against a firm surface may or may not include embedded material. This injury is similar to second degree burn.
  - Avulsion (tearing away or forcible separation)
  - Full thickness tearing away of the skin exposes the underlying fat.
  - Avulsion is the most common tissue injury among the elderly.
- Puncture
  - Penetration of the skin by a sharp or pointed object. This wound involves minimal bleeding and can cause serious injury to underlying tissues and structures.
- Bites
  - Include puncture and possible tearing wounds of the skin; can be of human or animal origin.

THERAPEUTIC PLAN
Nonpharmacologic Treatment

Wound Cleansing
- Irrigation under high pressure with normal saline is the most effective way to cleanse a wound. (An inexpensive and easy method is the use of a 35-cc syringe and a 19-gauge needle to create high-flow irrigation.)
- If iodine (Betadine) solution is used to cleanse the wound, it must be irrigated completely to avoid causing tissue damage.

Hair Removal
- Hair should be clipped with scissors from around the wound. Hair in the wound acts like a foreign body and may delay the healing process and potentiate the infectious process. Shaving the hair may cause injury to the hair follicle and increases the risk of infection.
- Eyebrows should never be shaved. Shaving alters the landmarks, leading to possible misalignment of the wound edges. Eyebrows grow back very slowly, causing alteration in cosmetic looks.

Wound Closure. Suturing is used for irregular and deep lacerations and for lacerations of the face, over joints, and on the hands and feet. The types of sutures are the following:
- Absorbable sutures
  - Biodegradable sutures last 2 to 6 weeks and are used for internal sutures.
  - Gut sutures are made from sheep submucosa or beef serosa; degrade rapidly.
  - Plain sutures may cause inflammatory reaction in the wound; last approximately 2 weeks.
  - Chromic sutures create less tissue reactivity but may potentiate wound infections; last approximately 4 weeks.
  - Synthetic sutures include Dexon, Vicryl, and PDS sutures. These create minimal tissue reaction and are used for closures of dermal and subcutaneous layers and for the ligation of blood vessels.
- Nonabsorbable sutures
  - Will not degrade or may degrade very slowly; generally used for external closure.
  - Silk sutures are made of natural fiber. They cause high tissue reactivity and are slow-absorbing.
  - Dacron sutures are synthetic, polyester. They are less reactive than silk; difficult to handle because of high friction.
  - Nylon sutures are synthetic. They are less reactive than Dacron. Nylon sutures create a decreased risk of infection when used for contaminated wounds.
  - Monofilament sutures are difficult to tie.
  - Multifilament sutures are easy to tie.

The following are methods of wound closure using polypropylene and polyester:
- Synthetic: Least tissue reactivity of all suture materials; presents least chance of infection when used in contaminated wounds. Hold knots better than nylon.
- Staples: Made of stainless steel and are cumbersome; cannot be used over moveable joints. Staples are excellent for linear lacerations of the scalp, trunk, and extremities. They cause increased infection rates when used in contaminated wounds.
- Steri-Strips: Used for superficial lacerations (except those over joints) that are easily approximated; reinforce facial lacerations after removing sutures.

Wound Care

- The wound should remain covered with a clean, dry dressing for 24 to 48 hours. It takes approximately 48 hours for a wound to become impermeable to bacteria.
- The suture line should then be cleaned with soap and water two to three times a day to remove exudate and crusted blood from the site. This aids in reducing scarring.
- An antibiotic ointment may be applied to the suture line. Note that neomycin may cause local reactions.
- Wounds that are likely to become contaminated should remain covered for 1 week.
- A joint should be immobilized in the position of function if movement of that joint will compromise the suture line integrity.

Suture Removal

- Face: 3 to 5 days
- Scalp: 5 to 7 days
- Neck: 4 to 6 days
- Hand and foot: 7 to 14 days
- Arm and leg: 7 to 14 days
- Chest, abdomen, and back: 6 to 12 days
- Nail bed: absorbable sutures

Pharmacologic Treatment

See Table 3-127 for tetanus immunization information.

Children

- If child is younger than 7 years, administer diphtheria-pertussis-tetanus (DPT) vaccine or diphtheria and tetanus toxoids (Td) vaccine if pertussis is contraindicated.
- Tetanus-prone wounds include wounds with the following characteristics:
  - More than 6 hours old
  - Stellate wound configuration
  - Caused by missile, crush, burn, or frostbite
  - More than 1 cm in depth
  - Contaminated by debris (e.g., soil, feces, saliva)
  - Devitalized or ischemic tissue

Analgesia

- Local anesthetic agents prevent the influx of sodium across the nerve membrane. This, in turn, decreases the rate and amplitude of depolarization of the nerve membrane. When depolarization is decreased, an action potential cannot be formed. This results in the inability to transmit an impulse. A conduction blockade is achieved, resulting in local anesthesia.
- Topical analgesia is an excellent choice for treating wounds of small children and anxious adults. These preparations are generally used on small, superficial lacerations.
- Topical mixture of tetracaine 1%, adrenaline (epinephrine) 1:4000, and cocaine hydrochloride (HCl) 4% (TAC): A cotton ball is soaked with 10 mL of the solution and then applied to the wound. Anesthesia is achieved in approximately 10 to 15 minutes. TAC should never be used on mucous membranes or areas with poor perfusion. The person holding the TAC to the wound should wear an examining glove to avoid absorption of the mixture into the skin.
- Topical mixture of lidocaine 2% to 4%, epinephrine 1:4000, and tetracaine 1% (LET) is used in the same manner as TAC. Anesthesia is achieved within 20 to 25 minutes.
- For infiltrative analgesia, see Table 3-128.
- Epinephrine 1:1000 can be added to lidocaine and bupivacaine. It aids in hemostasis of the wound and prolongs the effects of the anesthetic. It should never be used on fingers, toes, noses, tip of the ear, nipples, penis, or tarsal plate of the eye.
- Sodium bicarbonate can be added to lidocaine in a 1:10 ratio to neutralize the pH of the lidocaine. This reduces the burning sensation felt during the infiltration of the lidocaine. The shelf-life of the mixture is 1 week. Note the following:
  - 0.5% = 5 mg/cc
  - 1% = 10 mg/cc
  - 2% = 10 mg/cc
- See Table 3-129 for anesthesia options.
- See Table 3-130 for antibiotics used in wound management.
- Rabies prophylaxis should be administered if the client has been bitten by a wild animal or a domestic animal if the animal is unhealthy or is unavailable to be observed for 10 days. The local public health department should have information on the incidence of rabies in your area.

TABLE **3-127**   Tetanus Immunization

HISTORY OF ABSORBED TETANUS TOXOID	TETANUS-PRONE		NONTETANUS-PRONE	
	TD	TIG	TD	TIG
Uncertain or less than three	Yes	Yes	Yes	No
Three or more (last dose within 5 years)	No	No	No	No
Three or more (last dose within 6 to 10 years)	Yes	No	No (yes if longer than 10 years)	No

Td, Tetanus and diphtheria absorbed; *TIG*, tetanus immune globulin.

TABLE **3-128**   Local Anesthesia

AGENT	CONCENTRATION	MAXIMUM ADULT DOSE	MAXIMUM PEDIATRIC DOSE	ONSET	DURATION
Lidocaine	0.5% (5 mg/cc)	300 mg (60 cc)	4 mg/kg (0.8 cc/kg)	3 to 5 minutes	30 to 60 minutes
	1% (10 mg/cc)	300 mg (30 cc)	4 mg/kg (0.4 cc/kg)		
	2% (20 mg/cc)	300 mg (15 cc)	4 mg/kg (0.2 cc/kg)		
Lidocaine with epinephrine	0.5% (5 mg/cc)	500 mg (100 cc)	7 mg/kg (1.4 cc/kg)	2 to 5 minutes	60 to 120 minutes
	1% (10 mg/cc)	500 mg (50 cc)	7 mg/kg (0.7 cc/kg)		
	2% (20 mg/cc)	500 mg (25 cc)	7 mg/kg (0.35 cc/kg)		
Bupivacaine (Marcaine)	0.25% (2.5 mg/cc)	175 mg (70 cc)	Not recommended	5 to 10 minutes	90 to 120 minutes
Bupivacaine with epinephrine	0.25% (2.5 mg/cc)	225 mg (90 cc)	Not recommended	2 to 5 minutes	4 to 8 hours
Mepivacaine (Carbocaine)	0.5% (5 mg/cc)	400 mg (80 cc)	5 mg/kg (1 cc/kg)	5 to 10 minutes	75 to 150 minutes
Procaine	0.5% (5 mg/cc)	500 mg (100 cc)	7 mg/kg (1.4 cc/kg)	2 to 5 minutes	15 to 45 minutes
	1% (10 mg/cc)	500 mg (50 cc)	7 mg/kg (0.7 cc/kg)		
Procaine with epinephrine	0.5% (5 mg/cc)	600 mg (120 cc)	9 mg/kg (1.8 cc/kg)	2 to 5 minutes	15 to 45 minutes
	1% (10 mg/cc)	600 mg (60 cc)	9 mg/kg (0.9 cc/kg)		

TABLE **3-129**   Anesthesia Options

TYPE OF ANESTHESIA	INDICATIONS	CONTRAINDICATIONS	ADVANTAGES	DISADVANTAGES
Topical	1. Young children 2. Lacerations less than 0.5 cm	1. Not to be used on fingers, toes, nose, ear, or penis	1. Painless 2. No distortion of wound edges 3. Hemostasis	1. Must be held in place for at least 10 to 20 minutes 2. Less effective on trunk and extremities
Infiltration	1. All age groups 2. Laceration repair 3. Excision of skin lesions 4. Incision of an abscess	1. Where large toxic amounts of anesthesia are required	1. Quick 2. Generally considered safe 3. Reliable	1. Distorts wound edges 2. Requires a larger amount of medication 3. Painful
Nerve Block	1. Large wounds 2. If distortion from infiltration compromises blood flow or hampers wound closure	1. Client who is taking MAO inhibitors should not receive anesthesia with epinephrine (may lead to an exaggerated cardiac response)	1. Provides anesthesia to a larger area with less medication and fewer injections	1. May need to use local infiltrates if complete anesthesia is not obtained 2. Potential to inject into a nerve bundle or blood vessel 3. Painful

MAO, Monoamine oxidase.

Client Education

Provide the following wound care instructions to the client:

- Keep the wound clean and dry.
- Keep the dressing in place for 24 to 48 hours.
- Clean suture lines with soap and water daily. Removing crusted material from the suture line ensures proper healing.
- Antibiotic ointment can be applied if desired.
- Keep the wound elevated above the heart to decrease swelling.
- Watch for signs of infection, including redness, red streaks, swelling, pus, and fever.

Referral/Consultation

- Depending on the extent and site of the wound (e.g., multilayer or large area), client may need to be referred to surgeon or plastic surgeon.
- If infection occurs, may need to refer client to infectious disease physician.
- Refer clients with eyelid lacerations to an ophthalmologist.

TABLE **3-130**   Antibiotics Used in Wound Management

TYPE OF WOUND	MOST COMMON ORGANISM	ANTIBIOTIC	ADULT DOSE	CHILDREN'S DOSE*
Laceration (grossly contaminated wounds)	*Staphylococcus aureus*	Augmentin (amoxicillin/ clavulanate) Pregnancy category B	875/125 mg PO bid or 500/125 mg PO tid	*45 mg/kg/day in two divided doses or 20 to 40 mg/kg/day in three divided doses
		Ceftin (Cefuroxime) Pregnancy category B	250 to 500 mg PO bid	125 mg PO bid
		Keflex (Cephalexin) Pregnancy category B	250 to 500 mg PO tid	25 to 50 mg/kg/day in three divided doses
Puncture wounds	*S. aureus* and *Pseudomonas aeruginosa*	Ceftin (Cefuroxime) Pregnancy category B	250 to 500 mg PO bid	125 mg PO bid
		Augmentin (amoxicillin/ clavulanate) Pregnancy category B	875/125 mg PO bid or 500/125 mg PO tid	*45 mg/kg/day in two divided doses or 20 to 40 mg/kg/day in three divided doses
Human and animal bites	Multiple aerobic and anaerobic organisms (human, cat, dog, raccoon, bat, skunk)	Ceftin (Cefuroxime) Pregnancy category B Augmentin (amoxicillin/ clavulanate) Pregnancy category B	250 to 500 mg PO bid 875/125 mg PO bid or 500/125 mg PO tid	125 mg PO bid *45 mg/kg/day in two divided doses or 20 to 40 mg/kg/day in three divided doses
		Unasyn (ampicillin/ sulbactam) Pregnancy category B	1.5 to 3.0 g IV q6h	Doses of 200 to 400 mg/kg of ampicillin plus 100 to 200 mg/kg of sulbactam qd in divided doses have been used
		Zinacef (Cefuroxime) Pregnancy category B	750 mg to 1.5 g IV q8h	50 to 100 mg/kg/day in three divided doses
		Penicillin G Pregnancy category B	2.5 million IU IV q4h	400,000 IU/kg/day in four divided doses

*Dosage has not yet been established for children younger than 12 years of age.

- Refer clients with facial injuries to a plastic surgeon.
- Refer clients with hand injuries to an orthopaedist, hand surgeon, or plastic surgeon.
- Clients with human bites to the hand are usually admitted to the hospital for IV antibiotic therapy.

Prevention

- Home safety assessment
- Use of appropriate safety equipment

EVALUATION/FOLLOW-UP

- All suture lines should be evaluated within 2 to 3 days to ensure proper healing without complication of infection.
- Evaluate any wound that becomes infected.

- All puncture wounds should be reevaluated within 48 hours (Behr, 1999).
- Any loss of function, change of sensation, or change in color at or distal to the wound should be evaluated.
- Development of fever requires follow-up.

COMPLICATIONS

- Scarring
- Infection
- Loss of limb or digit

REFERENCES

Behr, J. (1999). Repairing lacerations in children: suture, staple, or secure? *ADVANCE for Nurse Practitioners, 7*(1), 35-39.

Dean, E., & Orlinsky, M. (1998). Nerve blocks of the thorax and extremities. In J. R. Roberts & J. R. Hedges (Eds.), *Clinical procedures in emergency medicine* (3rd ed., pp. 473-496). Philadelphia: W. B. Saunders.

Dello-Stritto, R. (2000). Wound management. In D. Robinson, P. Kidd, & K. Rogers (Eds.), *Primary care across the lifespan*. St. Louis: Mosby.

Martin, D. R. (1996). Soft-tissue injuries and lacerations. In D. A. Rund, R. M. Barkin, P. Rosen, & G.L. Sternbach. (Eds.), *Essentials of emergency medicine* (2nd ed., pp. 283-293). St. Louis: Mosby.

Orlinsky, M., & Dean, E. (1998). Anesthetic and analgesic techniques. In J. R. Roberts & J. R. Hedges (Eds.), *Clinical procedures in emergency medicine* (3rd ed., pp. 454-473). Philadelphia: W. B. Saunders.

Roberts, J. R. (1996). Pain control in the emergency department. In J. R. Roberts (Ed.), *Robert's practical guide to common medical emergencies* (pp. 119-175). Philadelphia: Lippincott.

Review Questions

1. P. J. states that she dropped a sharp knife on her foot while removing it from the dishwasher. She now has a laceration to her foot that requires stitches. P. J. states that her last Td immunization was 7 years ago. Which of the following applies to P. J.?

   a. P. J. requires Td immunization because it has been longer than 5 years since her last immunization.
   b. P. J. does not require Td immunization because the wound is considered a clean wound and her last immunization was less than 10 years ago.
   c. P. J. requires Td immunization because all wounds to the foot should be considered dirty and must be protected with prophylactic immunization.
   d. P. J. does not require Td immunization because the wound is a clean wound.

2. Tommy comes to your clinic with a long, linear laceration to his scalp. It is a clean, superficial wound without contamination. His medical history is noncontributory. He is extremely anxious and impatient. What is the best way to close this wound?

   a. Chromic gut sutures
   b. Silk sutures
   c. Staples
   d. Dacron sutures

3. J. W.'s puncture wound is at high risk for infection. The NP decides to send him home with an antibiotic. He has no known allergies. Which of the following antibiotics would the NP use to treat this adult?

   a. Amoxicillin-clavulanate
   b. Cefuroxime (Ceftin)
   c. Trimethoprim-sulfamethoxazole
   d. Bacitracin zinc–polymyxin B sulfate (Polysporin)

4. B. C. has undergone repair of a laceration to the lower leg. Discharge instructions for this client should include all *except* which of the following?

   a. The wound should be reevaluated in 2 days for possible signs of infection and to ensure that it is healing well.
   b. A topical antibiotic ointment can be applied to the suture line after cleaning.
   c. The sutures need to be removed in 5 to 7 days.
   d. The client should be seen immediately if the area becomes painful, if red streaks develop, or if drainage from the wound is noted.

5. D. K. states that he fell from his motorcycle earlier in the day. He is now reporting lacerations to his left outer thigh and left upper arm. The NP evaluates the wounds and determines that he has sustained multiple abrasions. The NP explains to D. K. that an abrasion is caused by which of the following?

   a. Shearing forces that tear away the full thickness of the skin and fat layers
   b. Shearing forces that tear away the epidermis and the upper layer of the dermis, with dirt often embedded in the wound
   c. Shearing or tearing forces that result in a linear wound that expands through the dermis
   d. Compression of soft tissue

6. A child has a laceration of his thumb that is deep and regular. Which of the following should the NP use for analgesia?

   a. Local infiltration
   b. LET
   c. TAC
   d. Nerve block

7. Effective client education is indicated by which of the following statements?

   a. "I will not remove any crusted material from the wound."
   b. "I will clean it after the sutures are removed."
   c. "I will watch for red streaks."
   d. "I will remove the dressing when I get home."

Answers and Rationales

1. *Answer:* **b** (analysis/diagnosis)
   Rationale: The wound is not considered a tetanus-prone wound, and the immunization status is up to date within the past 10 years. If a wound is tetanus prone, then the immunization status should be within the past 5 years.

2. *Answer:* **c** (implementation/plan)
   Rationale: Staples are indicated for use on the scalp, trunk, and extremities. They are especially useful when time is a factor. Chromic gut is an absorbable suture and is not indicated for skin closure. Silk and Dacron are associated with increased skin reactions.

3. *Answer:* **a** (implementation/plan)
   Rationale: The first choice of antibiotic is penicillinase-resistant penicillin or a first-generation cephalosporin. Amoxicillin-clavulanate (Augmentin) is effective in the treatment of *Staphylococcus aureus* and *Pseudomonas aeruginosa*, both of which are common organisms associated with puncture wounds. Choice b, cefuroxime (Ceftin), is an intravenously administered antibiotic and is not needed for this client. Choice c, trimethoprim-sulfamethoxazole (Bactrim), is not effective

against *P. aeruginosa*. Choice d, bacitracin-polymyxin B (Poly-sporin), is a topical antibiotic ointment and is inappropriate for use with this type of wound.

4. *Answer:* c (implementation/plan)
Rationale: Sutures to the leg should remain in place for 10 to 14 days to ensure adequate scar formation. The remaining choices are important discharge instructions that should be given to all clients who have received wound care.

5. *Answer:* b (analysis/diagnosis)
Rationale: Abrasions are often treated like burn injuries. The wound must undergo debridement to remove the dirt embed-ded in it to avoid tattooing. Choice a describes an avulsion in-jury. Choice c describes a laceration. Choice d describes a crush injury, which is usually associated with a hematoma.

6. *Answer:* a (implementation/plan)
Rationale: Topical anesthetics should not be used on fin-gers or toes because of their vasoconstrictive qualities. A nerve block would be used for a larger wound.

7. *Answer:* c (evaluation)
Rationale: Crusted material should be removed from the wound. The dressing is left in place for 24 to 48 hours. The wound should be cleaned daily. Infection may be noted by red streaks.

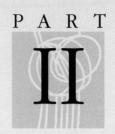

CLIENT WELLNESS

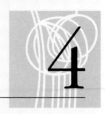

Wellness across the Lifespan

The purpose of well care is to provide individualized care to healthy clients. Identification of risks for preventable illnesses, injuries, and deaths should be incorporated into wellness care. Evidence is abundant that the majority of deaths among Americans younger than age 65 years are preventable, often through interventions introduced in the primary care office. Primary care providers have a key role in screening for many of these preventable problems. Equally important is the role of the provider in counseling clients to improve lifestyle behaviors, such as diet, smoking, alcohol use, exercise, injuries, and sexually transmitted diseases (STDs).

Although immunizations and screening tests are important, the most promising arena for prevention lies in changing the personal health behaviors of clients long before a clinical disease develops. Smoking contributes to one of every five deaths in the United States, including coronary artery disease (CAD), chronic obstructive pulmonary disease, and cerebrovascular disease. Motor vehicle crashes and injuries are compounded by failure to use seat belts and by the use of alcohol. Physical activity and dietary factors contribute to atherosclerosis, cancer, diabetes, and osteoporosis. High-risk sexual behaviors result in unintended pregnancy and various STDs, including acquired immune deficiency syndrome (AIDS). Approximately one half of all deaths in the United States can be attributed to these factors and have the potential for reduction through changes in personal behaviors (McGinnis & Foege, 1993).

Clinical preventive care can be defined as "an integral part of preventive health care concerned with the maintenance and promotion of health and the reduction of risk factors which result in injury and disease" (American College of Preventive Medicine News, 1989). Components of clinical preventive care include the following:

- Assessment of client's risk for disease
- Implementation of interventions to modify or eliminate risk for disease and injury
- Integration and monitoring of personal prevention behaviors

Barriers to preventive care include the following:

- Failure of clinician to provide recommended clinical preventive services
- Inadequate reimbursement for preventive care
- Fragmentation of health care delivery
- Insufficient time during appointment
- Recommendations from multiple sources, sometimes contradictory
- Uncertainty regarding effectiveness of preventive services

The United States Preventive Services Task Force was established in 1984 to address the issues of preventive care. This panel was charged with the task of developing preventive recommendations based on systemic review of evidence of clinical effectiveness. Its findings include the following:

- Interventions that address personal health practices are vitally important.
- The provider and the client should share decision making.
- Clinicians should be selective in ordering tests and providing preventive services.
- Every opportunity must be taken to deliver preventive services, especially for those clients with limited access to care.
- For some health problems, community-level interventions may be more effective than clinical preventive services (United States Preventive Services Task Force, 1996).
- The recommendations for health prevention and health promotion for all age groups follow.

WELL-CHILD CARE, AGES 0 TO 10 YEARS   *Denise Robinson*

GROWTH AND DEVELOPMENT

The growth and developmental guidelines and milestones for children are outlined in Tables 4-1 through 4-5.

TABLE **4-1** Growth and Development 0-12 Months

SYSTEM	0-3 MONTHS	4-6 MONTHS	7-12 MONTHS
Neurologic	Turns head side to side by 1 month. Then prone head to chest. Head lag when pulled from supine to sitting until 2-3 months. Upright head control should be obtained. Landau (ventral suspension): flexion position. Reaching/grasping; palmar grasp at birth until about 2 mo. By 3 mo growing hand-eye coordination and attempts contact with objects and can hold them briefly.	Raises head and chest with arms extended. Raises head on vertical axis and turns head from side to side. Pulled from supine to sitting with no head lag. In a sitting position, head may tilt a little forward, but no head bobbing. Head erect by 5 mo. By 5-6 mo infant is purposefully rolling over, first front to back and then back to front. By 4 mo infant loses tonic neck reflex and head stays midline with extensors in a more symmetrical position. Infant regards hands, brings them to midline and mouth (symmetrotonic posture). The infant bears the weight of an erect head and enjoys being supported in an upright position. At 4 mo infant has increased attention for various objects. By 6 mo, infant reaches out, retrieves, and transfers the object from hand to hand. After discovering hands, discovers the rest of body: face, head, trunk, lower extremeties and genitals. At 4 mo enjoy standing erect. By 5-6 mo can pull from sitting to a standing position and can bear weight by holding hands. By 6½ mo they can do this and then flex their knees momentarily. They sit alone with head erect.	By 7 mo, able to pivot in pursuit of an object. By 8-9 mo many infants stand for a few seconds independently, cruising by 9 mo. By 9-10 mo takes a few steps with hands held. Between 6-9 mo the radial-palmar grasp moves to a thumb and forefinger (pincher) grasp, by 12 mo the pincher grasp is used without the ulnar surface. At 9 mo uses finger to poke at objects. By 9 mo is able to release an object on request; looks for objects (object permanency) and finds hidden objects if in sight. By 12 mo able to release object into hand.
Vision	Newborns fixate and track an object to midline. By 2 mo objects are followed past midline. By 3 mo objects are tracked 180 degrees; peripheral vision is 180 degrees by 2 mo. By 6 wk binocular vision begins and is well established by 4 mo. Acuity at birth is 200/200-200/400. By 3-4 mo it is 20/200-20/300.	Visual accommodation equals that of adults; follows objects 180 degrees; perceives the color spectrum similar to adults; visual acuity 20/200 to 20/300. Prefers moving objects. By 5-6 mo visual acuity is 20/40-20/60. EOMI, cover-uncover test WNL.	Equal tracking; EOMI, improving eye hand coordination.
Hearing	Responds to human voice; positive startle reflex with loud noises. By 2 mo turns head to side when sound is made at ear level. By 3 mo makes initiative to look toward sounds; can discriminate between pitch sounds.	Turns to sound; responds to human voice; discriminates, between pitch sounds.	Infant can locate sounds, recognize his or her own name, and understand commands but usually doesn't obey. By 12 mo follows some simple commands.

Dental	Increase in salivation at 3 mo. May begin teething as early as 3-4 mo.	May begin teething; teeth eruption.	Lower and upper incisors usually present, lateral incisors should be erupting or present.
Nutrition	110 kcal/kg/day needed.	110 kcal/kg/day, feeding 4-6 times per day, 4-6 oz every 4-6 hours (24-32 oz).	Eating time is a socialization process for 9-12 mo old. They want to be part of family meal times. Shows interest in drinking from a cup, attempts to feed self. By 12 mo drinks from a cup; feeds self. Needs approximately 12-16 oz milk/day. By 12 mo self feeder, decrease in growth demands therefore decrease in appetite. May see picky eater.
Breast feeding	Newborn: Feed every 1-2 h. 2 wk to 1 mo: feed every 2-4 h. 1-2 mos: feed every 4-6 h.	By 4 mo tongue thrusting diminishes and infants turn their heads if full.	
Formula	Newborn: feed 2-3 oz every 2-3 h. 2 wk-1 mo: feed 3-4 oz every 3-4 h. 2-3 mo: feed 4-6 oz every 4-6 h.	Continue formula/breast. At 6 mo begin cereal.	
Sleep	Newborns alert 1/10 h. Infants are awake 3-4 h/24. By 2 mo may be awake as long as 10 h/day. Usually sleeps 4-6 h at night. By 3 mo should be sleeping 3-8 hr at night	Own bed: own room; sleeps 6-8 h; by 5-6 mo sleeps 8-10 h; 1-2 naps, begins to resist separation; begins to experience night awakening (does not need nighttime bottle) by 5-6 mo	Infants may have decreased naps to 1/day. They have more wakeful periods at night. A bedtime routine should be established.
Elimination	Stools begin as loose and watery; as the infant matures, stools become more formed. **Breastfed infants:** Stools with every feeding, UOP 6-8 wet diapers. **Formula fed infant:** Stools 1/day, 1 every other day or 1 every third day. UOP 6-8 wet diapers.	Stools more formed; color changes related to solids, bladder capacity increasing, urination decreasing.	Stools formed, 1-2/day. UOP same as 4-6 mo.
Speech/ language	By 4 wk of age makes throaty noises. Focuses on significant other and imitates. By 2 mo makes vowel sounds/cooing. By 3 mo attempts to make sounds in relation to socialization.	Continues to imitate; coos, babbles, squeals, laughs, vocalizes to mirror.	6½ mo: repetitive vowel sounds. 9 mo: enjoy imitating sounds like "Mama" and "Dada" with babbling. Recognize words said by others like mom, dog, etc. By 8-9 mo responds to own name. By 1 yr says 1-3 words related to object.
Psychosocial	Fully developed social smile develops by 3-5 wk. (Infants that do not develop social smile by 3 mo may be an early identification of problems). Newborn makes eye-to-eye contact and focuses on faces. By 3 mo can recognize familiar faces.	Infants 4 mo old begin to laugh, squeal, or blow bubbles as part of social exchange; they are able to show displeasure by facial expressions. By 4-7 mo responds to emotional tones of social contacts. By 6 mo demonstrated social preference to care givers; when mom is around can display stranger anxiety. Development of separation anxieties may depend on the infant's comfort with communication and emotional exchange.	Developing into very social being; plays games, enjoys books and being read to for very short periods. Tries to figure out how things work; likes to manipulate objects. Imitates activities of caregiver; interacts with others; parallel play; separation anxiety; stranger anxiety.

EOMI, Extraocular movements; *UOP*, urinary output; *WNL*, within normal limits.

TABLE **4-2** Well-Child (0–12 Months) Care

	0–3 MONTHS	4–6 MONTHS	7–12 MONTHS
Strategies on conducting examination	Approach slowly Conduct much of examination with infant on parent's lap Provide security object: blanket, pacifier Do noninvasive examination first (heart/lungs); examine ears and mouth last	Same	Same
S	**History:** Determine any problems/changes since last seen. Ask about sleeping, elimination, immunizations, concern of parents, birth history if has never been seen **Nutrition:** How often, how much formula/breast, feeding problems **Development:** Cuddles, follows to midline, responds to sound, smiles, parent-child interaction, moves arms/legs, can sleep 3-4 hr at a time (1 mo) can be consoled if held or spoken to; 2 mo: coos and vocalizes, pays attention to voices, on stomach, lifts head, neck and upper chest with support on forearms, some head control in upright position **Family:** Mom's health/rest, family adjustment to baby, child care issues, Dad's involvement, support system, parents getting out/rest	**History:** Determine any problems/changes since last seen. Ask about sleeping through night, elimination, immunization reaction and what immunizations completed, birth history if never seen, parents' concerns **Nutrition:** How often, how much formula/breast, feeding problems, solids **Development:** Follows 180°, responding to voice, grasps rattle, rolls over one way, lifts head to 90°, babbles, reaches for object, coos, reaches for object; 6 mo: sits up with minimal support, laughs, squeals, transfers from hand to hand, may have first tooth, no head lag, "Dada," "Mama" **Family:** Mom's health, Dad's involvement, sibling adjustment	**History:** Determine any problems/changes since last seen. Ask about sleeping, elimination, immunization reaction and what immunizations completed, birth history if never seen before, parents' concerns **Nutrition:** How often, how much formula/breast, feeding problems, solids, feeds self with finger foods, fluoride **Development:** Plays peek-a-boo, looks for fallen object, pincher grasp, "Mama," "Dada," crawls, sits without support, stands holding on, pat-a-cake, bangs two blocks together, imitates sounds, understands "no," cruises, stands alone 2-3 seconds, feeds self **Family:** Family schedule, outside supports
O	**Physical Examination:** (child is usually not fearful of strangers) Ht., Wt., HC **2 week:** Infant gains 15-30 g, back to birth weight Ht., Wt., HC Skin: Look for "Stork bite" or jaundice HEENT: Nodes, head (cranial molding in newborn: cephalohematoma or caput succedaneum), fontanelles: flat, soft, anterior: <4-5 cm, Posterior: closes by 2 mo Eye: Red reflex, ability to fix and follow human face (lack of red reflex may indicate cataracts, white spot may indicate	**Physical Examination:** (child is usually fearful of strangers) Ht., Wt., HC Skin, nodes, head (good head control at 4 mo) 6 mo: no head lag, fontanelles: flat, soft, anterior: 4-5 cm; eye: red reflex, visual tracking (cover/uncover at 6 mo), ears, nose, oropharynx, teeth and gums, neck, chest/breast, lungs, heart, abdomen, genitalia: testes descended, femoral pulse, musculoskeletal, hips: clicks/clunks, Moro and tonic neck reflexes (disappear by 6 mo), plantar grasp remains	**Physical Examination:** (child is usually fearful of strangers) Ht., Wt., HC Skin, nodes, head, fontanelles: flat, soft, eye: cover/uncover, ears, nose, oropharynx, neck, chest/breast, lungs, heart, abdomen, genitalia: testes descended, femoral pulse, musculoskeletal, plantar grasp (disappears by 8 mo), positive pincher, positive parachute reflex

retinoblastoma); ears, nose, oropharynx, neck, chest/breast (enlarged breasts in newborn), lungs, heart, abdomen, umbilicus: cord off, genitalia: testes descended, urinary stream femoral pulse, musculoskeletal, hips: clicks/clunks, neuro: Moro reflex, Palmar reflex, plantar grasp, spine, symmetrical movements

2 month: wt gain 15-30 g (1 oz/day), 1 inch/mo; skin, nodes, head, fontanelles: posterior fused, eye: red reflex, ears, nose, oropharynx, neck, chest/breast, lungs, heart, abdomen, umbilicus: cord off, genitalia: testes descended, femoral pulse, musculoskeletal, hips: clicks/clunks, Moro reflex, plantar grasp (less intense)

Dx

WCC

Possible medical problems: metabolic disorders, intestinal obstruction, cardiac anomalies, congenital defects, apnea, GER, FTT, STD: congenital syphilis, HIV, chlamydia, abuse, cradle cap, diaper rash, fever

WCC

Possible problems: FTT, URI, OM, viral exanthem, diaper dermatitis, candidias diaper rash, atopic dermatitis, gastroenteritis, dacryostenosis, conjunctivitis, abuse, constipation, teething

WCC

Possible problems: OM, diaper dermatitis, URI, amblyopia, tibial torsion, genu varum; developmental delay, trained night feeders, undescended testicles, hypospadias, abuse

P

Immunizations: DPaT # 1, Hib #1, HBV #1 (can give together as Comvax), IPV # 1, Prevnar #1 at 2 mos
Check newborn screening results at 2 wk or repeat if needed

Immunizations:
4 mo: DPaT # 2, Hib #2, HBV #2 (Comvax if not received in hospital) IPV # 2, Prevnar #2
6 mo: DPaT # 3, Prevnar #3
Sickle prep if indicated

Immunizations:
9 mo: up to date
12 mo: Hib #3, HBV #3 (Comvax), MMR #1, can offer varicella
Screen for lead level and CBC (or HCT)
TB if indicated

E

Follow-up: 2 mo; next visit at 4 mo

Follow-up: 6 mo, 9 mo

Follow-up: 12 mo, 15-18 mo

Guidance

Assess parental ability to learn, prior experience as parent, educational level
Development: Review expected developmental changes, basic trust vs mistrust
Nutrition: Continue formula/breast, (25 oz formula/day at 4-6 oz/time), 6-8 wet diapers a day, no bottle in bed or warmed in microwave, burping, avoid honey, no cereal in bottle
Safety: Car seat, crib, falls—keep hand on baby, smoke alarm, water temperature, sleep on back, sun exposure
Parenting: Cuddling, talking to baby, music,

Assess parental ability to learn, prior experience as parent, educational level
Development: Review expected developmental changes, basic trust vs mistrust
Nutrition: Continue formula/breast, (5 feedings 6-8 oz/time), can offer water espcially during hot weather. At 6 mo: Add one new food at a time/week: allergies. Can begin cereal with iron (1-2 tbsp/day) increasing up to $1/3$-$1/2$ cup 2×/day), then add vegetables (1 tsp at time) and then fruits (offer nonsweet food first), no honey, start cup

Assess parental ability to learn, prior experience as parent, educational level
Development: Review expected developmental changes, basic trust vs mistrust
Nutrition: Decrease in formula to 12-16 oz day (8 mo), introduce cup, tolerance and acceptance of new foods, meat, breads, rice, macaroni, soft cheese and egg yolks should be introduced, decrease calorie intake, child will eat if hungry. Balanced diet, uses cup, finger foods, whole milk at 1 yr
Safety: Check lead risks, gates on stairs, electrical outlets capped, car seat, playpen or

Continued

TABLE **4-2** Well-Child Care (0-12 Months)—*cont'd*

0-3 MONTHS	4-6 MONTHS	7-12 MONTHS
maternal care (rest, nipple care, eating properly, follow-up support), sibling reaction, time for partner **Potential problems:** Possible diaper rash, spitting up, colic/crying **Infant care:** Cord, circumcision care, vaginal, elimination: transition from meconium, layers of clothing	**Safety:** Car, crib, falls, smoke alarm, baby proof house, all objects go into mouth, choking, bathing, poison control number, syrup of ipecac, no baby walkers, CPR, first aid **Parenting:** Call child by name, soft music, touching games "little piggy," bedtime routine, comfort objects, distraction as discipline **Potential problems:** Possible diaper rash, teething, susceptible to infections, sleep patterns: night awakening, dental hygiene (no bottle in bed)	crib for safe place, constant watching, falls and burns, poison: ipecac, smoke free environment, lower crib mattress **Parenting:** Reinforce positive behavior, stimulation: toy phone, name body parts, blowing games, noisy push/pulls, hugs/kisses; discipline: limit but enforce rules, bedtime routine, separation and stranger anxiety, reading, dental care (no toothpaste) **Prevention:** Dental hygiene, weaning from bottle, pacifer

CBC, Complete blood count; *CPR,* cardiopulmonary resuscitation; *DPaT,* diphtheria, acellular pertussis, tetanus; *FTT,* failure to thrive; *GER,* gastroesophageal reflux; *HBV,* hepatitis B vaccine; *HC,* head circumference; *HCT,* hematocrit; *HEENT,* head, eyes, ears, nose, and throat; *Hib, Haemophilus influenza* B; *HIV,* humane immunodeficiency virus; *IPV,* inactivated poliovirus vaccine; *MMR,* measles-mumps-rubella; *OM,* otitis media; *STD,* sexually transmitted disease; *TB,* tuberculosis; *URI,* upper respiratory infection; *WCC,* well-child check.

TABLE **4-3**   Growth and Development 1-10 Years

SYSTEM	12-24 MONTHS	24-36 MONTHS	3-5 YEARS	5-10 YEARS
Neurologic	By 12 mo, the infant moves to an upright stance; takes a few independent steps or should be walking; walking should be accomplished no later than 15-18 mo. By 15 mo, gait is ataxic but symmetrical stoops and recovers; by 18 mo, walks up stairs holding on; runs; walks backwards, by 20 mo goes down stairs; at 24 mo able to run about; kicks ball. By 12 mo can release object into hand; at 15 mo can place raisin into bottle, by 18 mo can remove raisin by dumping it out. Can make a tower of blocks of two cubes at 15 mo; 18 mo can make a tower of four cubes; by 24 mo makes a tower of six cubes. Jumps up and down by 24-28 mo.	At 2 years is able to kick a ball without falling. Progresses to able to kick a ball 10 feet by 3 years. Runs and jumps with both feet, jumps from chair or step; rides a push toy to pedaling a tricycle at 3 years. By 3 years fine and gross motor skills are becoming more refined, smooth, and more coordinated. Enjoys physical play. Able to walk up and downstairs holding on to railing with 2 feet on step. Begins to scribble at 2 yr. Draws a circle, matches colors; crosses midline; can use scissors by age 3. By 3 yr can make a tower of eight blocks; makes a bridge after demonstration. Walks on tiptoe.	Preschooler is slender but sturdy, graceful, and agile, with erect posture. Hopping, skipping, and climbing. Advancing with fine motor skills; copies figures and draws recognizable pictures.	At 6-8 yr, gross and fine motor skills become more controlled; improved eye-hand coordination; prints, colors in lines, ties bow; rides bike, hops, jumps. By 10 yr, gross and fine motor skills are more precise; tricks with bicycle, cursive writing, makes crafts, organized sports.
Vision	Smooth ocular movements; depth perception, good eye-hand coordination; intense interest in bright colors and different shapes.	Visual acuity 20/80; depth perception, copies a vertical line; color recognition not until 3½ to 4 yr.	Visual capabilities continue to undergo refinement during preschool period. Color vision and depth perception are fully established. Visual acuity: 3: 20/50 4: 20/40 5: 20/30 Hyperopic	At 6-8 yr, visual acuity is 20/20, no color blindness.
Hearing	Reactive to whispering; localizes sounds well, understands most commands, recognizes name readily; recognizes familiar words.	By 3 yr acuity is at an adult level; aware of pitch and tone.	Hearing develops to an adult level; able to make fine discriminations among similar speech sounds, such as the difference between "f," "th," and "s."	Normal.
Dental	May have as many as 6 teeth; during second year, 8 more teeth should erupt. First year molars, cuspids, then second-year molars. Brushing teeth 2×/day with a washcloth until able to spit. Off bottle by 15-18 mo.	Between 24-36 mo dentition is completed.	20 deciduous teeth. Primary teeth are important for chewing, speech, and to hold spaces for secondary teeth. Older preschoolers can be responsible for brushing with gentle reminding from parents.	Permanent teeth continue to erupt; continue brushing and flossing with regular dental visits.
Nutrition	By 1 yr, change to whole milk until 2 yr. Soft table foods with more	Average 2-3 yr old needs 100 kcal/kg/day. Fat should be approximately	Average preschooler needs 95 kcal/kg/day. Has definite food	At 5-8 yr, needs approximately 80 kcal/kg/day. Increased appetite, 3

Continued

TABLE 4-3   Growth and Development 1-10 Years—cont'd

SYSTEM	12-24 MONTHS	24-36 MONTHS	3-5 YEARS	5-10 YEARS
	texture foods by 15-18 mo. Usually eat one balanced meal with decreased food intake related to decreased growth rate.	30% or less. Calcium needs to be approximately 700 mg/day.	preferences. Likely to refuse new foods.	meals/day plus 1-2 snacks. At 8-10 yr, nutrition still under primary control of parent, but eating away from home more and more and influenced by peers and television. Likes a variety of foods, especially fast foods and snacks.
Sleep	Fitful sleep at night; more REM periods. Increased tension may have fits or energy bursts at night; rock crib, bang head. Usually on nap/day. Sleeps 10-12 hr/day	Usually sleeps 10-12 hours; may still take afternoon naps; sleeps all night; enjoys sleeping with favorite toy or blanket; begins to be afraid of the dark; bed should have side rails.	Average sleep is 8-12 hr/night. Bedtime rituals still important. Nightmares and night terrors can be common in this age group because of active imaginations.	Average sleep is 8-10 hr/night. Usually resists bedtime, develops stall tactics. Parents should set limits.
Elimination	Stools formed, urine more concentrated; may show interest in "potty."	Maturation of cortex layers; sensory development for bladder/bowel control; elimination, especially BMs, is expression of pleasure in what a 2-3 yr old has to produce. Nighttime wetting is not expected to end until 5-7 years.	Should have established daytime bowel and bladder control; nighttime bladder control usually accomplished by 3-6 years. Around age 5, child should be able to manage toileting independently.	Normal patterns established
Speech/ language	At 15 mo, points to body parts. By 18 mo, vocabulary is approximately 10 words. It is not unusual for child not to have words at up to 18 mo. Usually by 18-20 mo there is rapid learning of words and meanings usually develop by this time.	By 2 years more than 50 words is common; two-word sentences, knows five to six body parts; dysfluencies are common, uses plurals, present verb tense, recognizes three colors. By 3 years speaks in three- to four-word sentences; speech is clear, uses pronouns, negatives, past tense, understands some adjectives, (e.g., big or little).	Sophisticated and complex; 3-4 yr three- and four-word sentences. At 4-5 yr, can speak four- to five-word sentences; lots of "why" questions. Speech often with hesitations, repetitions, and revisions. Stuttering and stammering should be ignored. Quality and quantity of language in home is the most important impact on the child's language development.	Understands "if," "because," and "when."
Psychosocial	Toddlers develop a sense of control over their bodies and expressively demonstrate this: temper tantrums, breath holding spells, and biting. Developing a sense of self separate from others; striving for independence by taking initiative in making choices about behaviors.	Egocentric: better sense of time, anticipates consequences from parents to form more careful actions; pretends; magical thinking, dramatic-imitation play. Moves from a sensory to intuitive learning, development of memory, symbolic play; global organization.	Separates with some apprehension at age 3. By 4-5 yr, relates to unfamiliar people easily; tolerates periods of separation. Enjoys playing and interacting with other children. Recommend preschool. Progresses from associative play to cooperative play. Egocentric behaviors still present; role play; make believe or fantasy play.	Very sociable, group play increases, becomes competitive, learns to share, cooperates in organized manner. By 8-10 yr enjoys team sports, parties, sleep-overs. Needs time for free play, do not overschedule.

BM, Bowel movement; *REM,* rapid eye movement.

TABLE **4-4** Strategies for Communication with Children and Parents by Age Group

GENERAL INTERVIEWING APPROACHES	YOUNGER THAN 6 YEARS	YOUNGER SCHOOL AGE CHILDREN	OLDER SCHOOL AGE CHILDREN
Determine who will be present for interview.	Talk to child at eye level.	Communicate with parent if child is shy.	Conduct interview with parent present.
Provide privacy.	Use play to enhance comfort.	Use concrete terminology.	For older, more mature children, parent may leave the room for the examination.
Maintain good eye contact.	Use nonthreatening words.	Allow time for child to respond.	Start with nonthreatening questions, let child know some questions may be
Gather history with child clothed.	Take time for child to respond.		uncomfortable, but are important for you to
Start with open ended questions: "How is Gretchen doing?"	Use distracting techniques: "Do you have a puppy dog in your ear?" Quiet barking will make child		know.
Ask specific questions to get specific data.	listen and cooperate.		Let child know that all children his or her age are asked these questions.
Do not use leading questions.			Information is confidential unless threat to self
Use language parents and child understand.			or others.
Be aware of cultural differences.			

TABLE **4-5**   Well-Child (1-10 Years) Care

	12-24 MONTHS	24-36 MONTHS	3-5 YEARS	5-10 YEARS
Strategies to conduct examination	Use of distraction helpful; allow child to touch and hold equipment before examination. Have parent or sibling demonstrate examination. Tell child what you are going to do instead of asking permission. Conduct much of examination on parent's lap; do noninvasive examination first (heart/lung), do ears and mouth last.	Same	Tell child what you are going to do and ask them to help. Let child role play with doll first. Allow choices when possible. Teach child about body during examination. Praise child for helping and being big boy or girl.	Modesty emerges with older school age child. Answer questions matter-of-factly. Explain use of equipment. Ensure privacy for older school age. Give choices when possible. Cover parts of body when possible. Recognize modesty over breast, pelvic, and testicular examination.
S	**History:** Determine any problems since last seen, parents' concerns. Ask about sleeping, elimination, illnesses, accidents, immunizations, birth history if never seen before. Assess lead risk. **Nutrition:** Number of meals/day, varied diet, balanced diet, fluoride, mealtime problems. **Development:** Drinks from cup, crawls up stairs, throws ball, walks well, removes clothes, stacks two or three blocks, walks up steps with help, knows body parts, speaks two- or three-word sentences, handles spoon well **Family:** Parents agree on discipline, child care, sibling rivalry.	**History:** Determine any problems since last seen, parents' concerns. Ask about sleeping, elimination, illnesses, accidents, immunizations, birth history if never seen before. **Nutrition:** Number of meals/day, varied diet, balanced diet, fluoride, mealtime problems. **Development:** Follows simple directions, knows full name, sex, knows one color, uses plurals, rides tricycle. **Family:** Discipline, child care, sibling rivalry, playmates, family activities, family history of early MI, high cholesterol.	**History:** Determine any problems since last seen, parents' concerns. Ask about sleeping, elimination, illnesses, accidents, immunizations, birth history if never seen before. **Nutrition:** Number of meals/day, varied diet, balanced diet, fluoride, mealtime problems. **Development:** Puts toys away, knows prepositions, knows three or four colors, uses verbs and full sentences, hops on one foot, dresses alone, understands opposites, copies square, triangle, draws man (with three to six parts), heel-to-toe walk, assess school readiness. **Family:** Mom and Dad's work, family happy, discipline, any new family members, smokers, alcohol, or drug use.	**History:** Determine any problems since last seen, parents' concerns. Ask about sleeping, elimination, illnesses, accidents, immunizations, birth history if never seen before. Ask about menses for girl, sexual activity. **Nutrition:** Number of meals/day, varied diet, balanced diet, fluoride, mealtime problems. **Developmental:** Behavior, chores, outside activities, reads for pleasure, knows days of week, skips rope, tells time, peer interaction, organized sports. **Family:** Family schedule, family activities, discipline, new family members, any smokers or alcohol or drug use, after school care, firearms at home, sibling problems or rivalry.

O	**Physical Examination:** (fear of strangers) Height, weight, HC Skin: nodes, head, fontanelles Eye: cover/uncover Ears, nose, oropharynx, teeth and gums, neck, chest/ breast, lungs, heart, abdomen, genitalia, musculoskeletal: gait, neurologic	**Physical Examination:** (fear of strangers) Height, weight, HC (gain 3 in/ height/yr and 5 lb/weight/yr) Skin, nodes, head, Eye: fundi, cover/uncover Ears, nose, oropharynx, teeth and gums, neck, chest/ breast, lungs, heart, abdomen, genitalia	**Physical Examination:** (may be cooperative with parents close) Height, weight, vital signs, vision screening, hearing (±3 in/yr) HTN: BP higher than 112/74 Skin, nodes, head Eye: fundi cover/uncover Ears, nose, oropharynx, teeth and gums, neck, chest/breast, lungs, heart, abdomen, genitalia	**Physical Examination:** (usually cooperative) Older child may want privacy Height, weight, vital signs (gains 5 lb and 2½ in/yr) HTN: BP higher than 116-126/76-82 Vision/hearing screening Skin, nodes, head Eye: fundi cover/uncover Ears, nose, oropharynx, teeth and gums, neck, chest/breast, lungs, heart, abdomen, genitalia, Tanner staging, scoliosis screening
Dx	WCC Possible problems: dental caries, developmental delays, intoeing, chronic OM, conductive hearing loss, croup, pica, impetigo	WCC Possible problems: speech delays, tibial torsion, nursemaid elbow, encopresis, sexual abuse, stomatitis, pinworms, septic arthritis	WCC Possible problems: HTN, primary enuresis, masturbation, night terrors, coxsackie virus, varicella, osteomyelitis, dental caries	WCC Possible problems: enuresis, poor school performance, sibling rivalry, abuse, dental caries, vision/ hearing problems, eating disorders
P	15 mo: DTaP 4, IPV 3, MMR 2 either now or at 18 mo, Prevnar 4 Screen for TB exposure Lead screen if not already done	Screen for TB exposure Offer varicella if has not had chickenpox	Offer varicella if has not had chickenpox Immunizations (5 yr) DTaP 5 IPV 4 MMR 2 (If not given at 15 or 18 mo)	Offer varicella if has not had Assess for TB, assess HBV
E	Follow-up: 15-18 mo, 2 years	Follow-up: 3 years	Follow-up: yearly check	Follow-up: yearly check
Guidance	Assess parental ability to learn, prior experience as parent, educational level. **Development:** Review expected developmental changes, autonomy vs shame. **Nutrition:** Need for balanced diet, milk intake 12-16 oz/day, decreased growth so decreased intake, avoid soda: give fruit juice, not fruit drinks, discontinue bottle, decrease junk food, limit sugar **Safety:** Discuss aspiration,	Assess parental ability to learn, prior experience as parent, educational level. **Development:** Review expected developmental changes, autonomy vs shame. **Nutrition:** Need for balanced diet, milk intake 12-16 oz/day, decreased growth so decreased intake, avoid soda: give fruit juice, not fruit drinks, discontinue bottle, decrease junk food; no potato chips, coconut, nuts, whole kernel corn, hot dogs,	Assess parental ability to learn, prior experience as parent, educational level. **Development:** Review expected developmental changes, initiative vs guilt. **Nutrition:** Need for balanced diet, milk intake 12-16 oz/day, offer raw vegetables during day, avoid soda: give fruit juice, not fruit drinks, discontinue bottle, decrease junk food **Safety:** Discuss pets, plastic bags, outdoors, poison—	Assess parental ability to learn, prior experience as parent, educational level. **Development:** Review expected developmental changes, industry vs inferiority; goes from learning through intuition to learning through concrete experiences, discuss expected pubertal changes, body odor (~10) unless going through early puberty. **Nutrition:** Need for balanced diet, avoid soda: give fruit juice, not

Continued

TABLE **4-5** Well-Child (1-10 Years) Care—*cont'd*

12-24 MONTHS	24-36 MONTHS	3-5 YEARS	5-10 YEARS
pets, plastic bags, outdoors, climbing out of crib, poison—ipecac or water, toddler car seat, close supervision, lower crib mattress, pets, window guards, lawn mower, street. **Parenting:** Provide consistent discipline, reinforce positive behavior, set limits, let child problem solve, play, read to child, thumb sucking, dental care, naps. Discuss hitting, biting, aggressive behavior, self-care, self-quieting. Do not attempt to toilet train until older than 2, limit number of caregivers, limit television, curiosity about genitalia. At 18 mo, child shares toys, help toddler express fear and frustration.	raw carrots because of risk of aspiration. **Safety:** Discuss aspiration, pets, plastic bags, outdoors, climbing out of crib, poison—ipecac, playground safety, safe after-school environment. **Parenting:** Discuss toilet training, dental care (sealants), play, reading books, television limits, one long nap/day, needs large-muscle use/activity, anticipating consequences, dramatic play, discipline: limit setting, provide positive role model, use correct terms for sex, body parts, strategies for nightmares, teeth brushing, sucking habits, praise child, family rules, respect, right from wrong, chores, handle anger, conflict resolution.	ipecac, strangers, tricycle/bike (helmets), water, matches, medications, guns. **Parenting:** Ignore stuttering, provide positive role model for speech, provide a listener to allow child to express ideas and feelings, set television limits, choices, limits, consistent schedule, positive reinforcement, family rules developed and enforced, chores, (5 yr) should learn and know telephone number and address **Preventive:** Encourage dental appointment, brushing minimum of 2×/day	fruit drinks, discontinue bottle, decrease junk food. **Safety:** Discuss the outdoors, bike helmet, strangers, car, water, guns. **Parenting:** Provide consistent schedule, positive reinforcement, family rules developed and enforced, chores, positive role model, participation in school activities, reasonable expectations, limit television, give time to talk with child, new responsibilities given with appropriate supervision, allowance, respect, communication, discuss sex education, promote abstinence, music. **Preventive:** Encourage dental appointment, brushes teeth minimum of 2×day, emergency plan developed, discuss drugs, alcohol, and smoking.

BP, Blood pressure; *DTaP,* diphtheria, acellular pertussis, tetanus; *HBV,* hepatitis B vaccine; *HC,* head circumference; *HTN,* hypertension; *IPV,* inactivated poliovirus vaccine; *MI,* myocardial infarction; *MMR,* measles-mumps-rubella; *OM,* otitis media; *TB,* tuberculosis; *WCC,* well-child care.

REFERENCES

American College of Preventive Medicine News. (1989). *The Newsletter of the American College of Preventive Medicine, 1*, 3.

American Academy of Pediatrics. (2000). Active and passive immunizations. In G. Peter (Ed.), *2000 Red book: Report of the Committee on Infectious Disease* (25th ed., pp. 1-71). Elk Grove Village, IL: American Academy of Pediatrics.

Baker, R. (1996). *Handbook of pediatric primary care.* Boston: Little Brown.

Behrman, R.E., & Kliegman, R. (1996). *Nelson: Essentials of pediatrics* (15th ed.). Philadelphia: W. B. Saunders.

Brady, M. (1994). Patient management exchange: Educating youths and their parents about the prevention of firearm injury. *Journal of Pediatric Health Care, 8*(3), 127-129.

Bright Futures. Retrieved August 20, 2002, from http://www.brightfutures.org.

Grossman, D., Cummings, P., Koepsell, T., Marshall, J., D'Amrosio, L., Thompson, R., & Mack, C. (2000). Firearm safety counseling in primary care pediatrics: A randomized, controlled trial. *Pediatrics, 106*(1 pt 1), 22-26.

Hoekelman, R. A., (2001). *Primary pediatric care* (4th ed.). St. Louis: Mosby.

McGinnis, J., & Foege, W. (1993). Actual cases of death in the US. *Journal of the American Medical Association, 270*, 2207-2212.

Phillips, D., Longlett, S., Mulrine, C., Kruse, J., & Kewney, R. (1999). School problems and the family physician. *American Family Physician, 59*(10):2816-2824.

Ramos, A. G., & Tuchman, D. N. (1994). Persistent vomiting. *Pediatrics in Review, 5*(1), 24-31.

Schmitt, B. (1987). *Your child's health.* New York: Bantam.

Thiedke, C. (2001). Sleep disorders and sleep problems in childhood. *American Family Physician, 63*, 277-284.

United States Preventive Services Task Force (1996). *Guide to clinical preventive services* (2nd ed.). Baltimore: Williams & Wilkins.

Wilson-Adkins, M., & Adkins, C. (2001). A new conjugate vaccine against pneumococcal disease. *Nurse Practitioner, 26*(5), 52, 55-56, 59-62.

Woolf, S., Jonas, S., & Lawrence, R. (1996). *Health promotion and disease prevention in clinical practice.* Baltimore: Williams & Wilkins.

Review Questions

1. A 1-month-old infant is at your clinic for a well-child examination. You will assess all except which one of the following factors?

a. Fontanelles
b. Hips
c. Weight gain between 15 and 30 g/kg/day
d. Fundi

2. A 4-year-old is in your office for a well-child examination. You will give anticipatory guidance about all except which one of the following factors?

a. Masturbation
b. Bicycle safety
c. Stranger anxiety
d. Dental hygiene and dental referral

3. An infant is seen in your office to rule out failure to thrive. His weight is less than the fifth percentile on his growth curve, but he appears healthy. The parent reports that the child spits up formula frequently. On his nutritional history, the mother reports that his intake of formula is approximately 24 to 26 ounces per day. What is the most likely diagnosis?

a. Pyloric stenosis
b. Metabolic disorder
c. Milk allergy
d. Rumination

4. The nurse practitioner (NP) performs a Denver Developmental Screening Test (DDST) for a 5-year-old. What part of the examination is this?

a. Health history
b. Treatment plan
c. Provision of anticipatory guidance
d. Assessment

5. A newborn infant does not have a red reflex. What could the lack of red reflex indicate?

a. Retinoblastoma
b. Cataracts
c. Brain damage
d. Use of narcotic substance

6. In what order would you examine a toddler?

a. Start with least invasive, proceeding to most invasive, with some parts of the examination performed with the child on the parent's lap.
b. Get the most invasive done first, then do the least invasive, performing the whole examination on the table.
c. Perform the whole examination with the child on the parent's lap.
d. Perform the whole examination while the parent holds the child down.

7. By what age has the posterior fontanel usually closed?

a. 2 months
b. 6 months
c. 8 months
d. 1 year

8. Maleka brings in her newborn for a well-child check at 1 month. The baby seems healthy; however, the NP notes that the anterior fontanel seems large. What is considered the normal size for the anterior fontanel?

a. 1 to 2 cm
b. 6 to 8 cm
c. 4 to 5 cm
d. 9 to 10 cm

9. At what age would you expect a child to be able to hop on one leg?

a. 2 years
b. 4 years
c. 6 years
d. 8 years

10. When would you discuss anticipatory guidance regarding toilet training with a parent?

a. 15 months
b. 24 months
c. 18 months
d. 30 months

11. At what age would the NP expect to see a child use his or her pincher grasp?

a. 6 months
b. 3 months
c. 9 months
d. 11 months

12. At what age would the NP generally recommend that the parents start using a time-out system for discipline?

a. 12 months
b. 18 months
c. 24 months
d. 30 months

13. You have been teaching the mother of a 12-month-old child about discontinuing the bottle. What comment by the mother indicates a need for more teaching?

a. "I should start having Morgan use a sippy cup now as much as possible."
b. "Heavenly can use a cup during the day and can have a bottle before bedtime."
c. "Discontinuing the bottle can happen overnight."
d. "Morgan doesn't really like the bottle anymore. This will be a good time to stop it."

14. At what point can a child move from a car seat to a booster seat?

a. 3 years
b. 4 years or 40 lb
c. 6 years
d. When his or her head is above the lower edge of the window

15. When should the NP discuss puberty, body changes, and body odor with a school age girl?

a. Age 8
b. Age 10
c. Age 12
d. Age 13

Answers and Rationales

1. Answer: d (assessment)
Rationale: A funduscopic examination is not routinely performed on children younger than 3 years, although it is possible to perform a funduscopic examination on a child as young as 6 to 7 months (Baker, 1996).

2. Answer: c (assessment)
Rationale: Stranger anxiety usually first occurs at approximately 9 to 18 months of age and then reoccurs at approximately 2.5 years of age. It is likely to occur when the child loses sight of the mother or is left with a sitter. These fears are often heightened at night (Schmitt, 1987).

3. Answer: d (analysis/diagnosis)
Rationale: Rumination is behavioral in nature. Ruminators often experience failure to thrive despite an otherwise healthy appearance (Ramos & Tuchman, 1994).

4. Answer: d (assessment)
Rationale: Previous DDST results may be elicited as part of the history, but current information obtained through the NP's skills is considered assessment (Bright Futures, 2002).

5. Answer: b (assessment)
Rationale: The lack of a red reflex can indicate cataracts. A white reflex may be indicative of retinoblastoma. Substance use may be indicated by small pupils (Bright Futures, 2001).

6. Answer: a (assessment)
Rationale: Perform the least invasive parts of the examination, usually heart and lungs, while the child is on the parent's lap. Then proceed to the more invasive parts, ending with mouth and ears (Baker, 1996).

7. Answer: a (evaluation)
Rationale: The posterior fontanel closes by age 2 months; it may be difficult to palpate, even before closure (Baker, 1996).

8. Answer: c (analysis/diagnosis)
Rationale: The anterior fontanel usually is approximately 4 to 5 cm. A large fontanel may indicate increased intercranial pressure, hypothyroidism, or osteogenesis imperfecta (Baker, 1996).

9. Answer: b (assessment)
Rationale: A child can generally hop on one foot at the age of 4 years (Baker, 1996).

10. Answer: c (implementation/plan)
Rationale: Generally, anticipatory guidance is provided before the expected age of completion. In this case, toilet training should not be started before 2 years, but the anticipatory guidance should be provided to the parent before the 24-month birthday.

11. Answer: c (assessment)
Rationale: A child normally uses a pincher grasp around the age of 9 months (Bright Futures, 2001).

12. Answer: c (implementation/plan)
Rationale: Time-out forms of discipline are best started when the child is 2 years old (Bright Futures, 2001).

13. Answer: b (implementation/plan)
Rationale: When stopping the bottle, it is best to do so with no withdrawal. Children at age 12 months are able to get adequate fluid from a cup. Keeping a bottle at night prolongs the difficulty of bottle separation.

14. Answer: b (implementation/plan)
Rationale: Most safety experts recommend that children should remain in a car seat until they are 4 years old or weigh 40 lb. A booster car seat is recommended for children weighing more than 40 lb (Baker, 1997).

15. *Answer:* b (implementation/plan)
   Rationale: Ten years is a good time to start discussing pubertal changes and body odor with school age girls. The NP needs to be aware that some girls may develop earlier and the timetable may need to be adjusted downward (Baker, 1997).

WELL-ADOLESCENT CARE   *Denise Robinson*

Adolescence is a period of accelerated growth, encompassing both physical and psychologic development that results in the ability of the teen to become an independent and responsible member of society.

GROWTH AND DEVELOPMENT

Pubertal changes occur in a predictable sequence for all adolescents. The age at which changes begin varies based on genetic, socioeconomic, and nutritional factors. The rate at which the changes occur is known as the *tempo*. There may be individual variances in tempo. The most prominent changes are in terms of the secondary sexual characteristics; however, changes in the endocrine glands, lymphatic system, brain, and body fat composition occur as well. See Tables 4-6 through 4-10 and Figure 4-1.

GUIDELINES FOR ADOLESCENT PREVENTIVE

The guidelines for adolescent preventative services (GAPS), according to the American Medical Association (1995), are the following:
- To deter adolescents from participating in behaviors that jeopardize health
- To detect physical, emotional, and behavioral problems early and to intervene immediately
- To reinforce and encourage behaviors that promote healthful living
- To provide immunizations against infectious disease
Recommendations for care include the following:
- Yearly visits between ages 11 and 21 years to identify those who have begun high-risk behaviors and to provide information supporting healthful habits
- Should be age-developmental appropriate and socioculturally sensitive
- NP and adolescent should have time alone without parent to discuss issues that otherwise might not be addressed
Recommendations for communication with adolescent include the following (Levenberg, 1998):
- Remind the adolescent that the information discussed will be confidential unless he or she is engaged in at-risk behaviors.
- Use non-threatening, open-ended questions to establish rapport.
- Be matter-of-fact.
- Do not lecture; instead, involve the adolescent in health education and development of a plan of action.
- Acknowledge that it is uncomfortable talking about sensitive subjects but emphasize that learning to talk about difficult subjects is an important part of growing up.
- Ask sensitive questions using the third person: "Many teenagers go to parties where alcohol is served. Do you?"
- Mnemonics to help recall information to obtain from teens:
  - HEADS
Home, habits
Education, employment, exercise
Accidents, ambition, activities, abuse
Drugs (tobacco, alcohol, others), diet, depression
Sex, suicide
  - SAFE TEENS
Sexuality
Accident, abuse
Firearms (suicide)
Emotions (suicide/depression)
Toxins (tobacco, alcohol, others)
Environment (school, home, friends)
Exercise
Nutrition
Shots, school performance (Monalto, 1998)
  - Use of a History and Physical Examination form helps maintain consistency of approach and makes sure all components are included in each examination.

Early Adolescence (11, 12, 13, and 14 Years of Age)
Subjective Data (S)
- Lifestyle: relationships, including family, peer, and school; peer group activities, including tobacco, drug, and alcohol usage; television watching
- Sexual involvement, legal history, pressure from friends to do things that the adolescent does not want to do
- Family: clearly stated rules about how teen is to act; discussion about puberty, drugs, and other health topics
- HEADS:
  - **H**ome setting: who lives with client, whether client has own room, relationships at home, what parents do for a living, recent moves, running away, new people in home
  - **E**ducation/employment: school grade performance and changes, favorite and worst subjects, repeated classes, suspension, dropping out, future education plans, relations with teachers, employers, attendance

TABLE **4-6** Growth and Development in Adolescence

MAJOR EVENTS OF PUBERTY	SKELETAL GROWTH	SECONDARY SEX CHARACTERISTICS	SEQUENCE OF EVENTS: MALE	SEQUENCE OF EVENTS: FEMALE
Typical age to begin puberty: Boys, 11 to 12 years; normal range, 9 to 14 years; Girls, 10 to 11 years; normal range, 8 to 13 years	The body attains one fourth of the total adult height, with growth occurring in the distal portions of the limbs before the proximal portions and the trunk.	Girls enter puberty earlier than boys and take longer to complete the process. The average length of pubertal events for boys is 3 to 4 years and for girls is 4 to 5 years.	Growth of testicles Pubic hair appears Growth of penis and scrotum Axillary hair First ejaculations (average age, 13 to 14 years) Growth spurt Facial hair Adult height	Ovaries increase in size Breast buds and pubic hair appear Growth spurt Pubic hair matures Breasts mature Axillary hair Menarche (age range at onset, 10 to 16 years) Adult height

TABLE **4-7** Female Tanner Stages

TANNER 1	TANNER 2	TANNER 3	TANNER 4	TANNER 5
Prepubertal; there is no observable change.	Shows small raised breast buds and sparse growth of fine, downy hair, usually along the sides of the labia.	General enlargement of the breast with elevation of the entire breast and areola from the general chest contour occurs. Breast development is best assessed from a side view. Pubic hair becomes darker, coarser, and curlier, and extends over the middle of the pubic bone. Usually the period of most rapid growth.	Areola and papilla form a contour, which is separate from the rest of the breast. Pubic hair has adult characteristics but does not extend to the medial thigh. Menarche generally occurs during this stage.	Areola has the same contour as the rest of the breast, with an increase in overall size of the breast. Pubic hair extends from thigh to thigh, and some females may have additional growth at the midline to form the shape of a triangle.

TABLE **4-8** Male Tanner Stages

TANNER 1	TANNER 2	TANNER 3	TANNER 4	TANNER 5
There is no pubic hair growth. Appearance is prepubertal. Testes are 1 cm.	Sparse growth of fine, downy hair occurs along the base of the penis. Slight enlargement, increased texture of scrotum. Testes are 2 to 3.2 cm.	Pubic hair becomes darker, coarser, and curlier, and spreads over the middle of the pubic bone. Further growth and enlargement or scrotum. Testes are 3.3 to 4 cm.	Pubic hair takes on adult-like characteristics but does not extend to the thighs. *Penis significantly enlarged in length and circumference. Increased size of testes (4.0 to 4.9 cm), and darkening of scrotal skin occur.	Pubic hair is distributed from thigh to thigh and may extend up to the navel. Genitalia are adult size (testes are approximately 5 cm).

TABLE **4-9** Coping Mechanisms of Adolescents

COPING MECHANISM	STRATEGY
Cognitive mastery	Teen attempts to learn as much as possible about situation or stressor.
Conformity	Teen attempts to be image of peers: this includes language, dress, attitude and actions.
Controlling behaviors	Teen needs to be in control of some aspect of his or her life.
Fantasy	Used more frequently by younger teens to deal with unpleasant situations.
Motor activity	Serves as safe, tension-releasing strategy through release of energy.

From Robinson, D. (2000). Well adolescent. In D. Robinson, P. Kidd, & K. Rogers (Eds.), *Primary care across the lifespan* (p. 1300). St. Louis: Mosby.

TABLE **4-10** Major Morbidities and Leading Causes of Death for Teenagers

	EARLY ADOLESCENCE (11 TO 14 YEARS)	MIDDLE ADOLESCENCE (15 TO 17 YEARS)	LATE ADOLESCENCE (18 TO 21 YEARS)
Major Morbidities	Consequence of sexual behavior (STDs, pregnancy), drugs, alcohol, smoking, and effects of adolescent mental illness	Same	Same
Leading Causes of Death	Accidents (boys more often than girls), homicides (boys more than girls), suicides (boys more than girls), cancers (boys more than girls), and heart disease (boys more than girls)	Increase of homicides by 400% and 600%; increase in suicide rates compared with 10- to 14-year-olds; alcohol involved in 50%	Same

From Robinson, D. (2000). Well adolescent. In D. Robinson, P. Kidd, & K. Rogers (Eds.), *Primary care across the lifespan* (p. 1304). St. Louis: Mosby.
STDs, Sexually transmitted diseases.

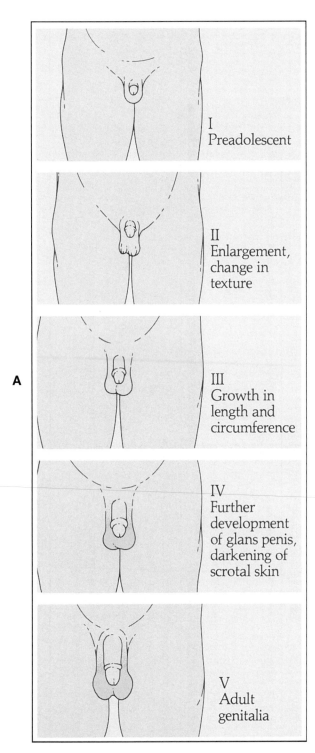

FIGURE **4-1** Schematic drawings of male and female Tanner stages. **A,** Male genital development.

- **A**ctivities: for fun, with whom, when, where, sports, church attendance, clubs, hobbies, television, car, seat belts, history of arrests, acting out
- **D**rugs: use by client, peers, family members; amounts, frequency, patterns; car driving while using; source (how paid for)
- **S**exuality: menarche, spermarche, orientation, degree and type of sexual experience, number of partners, masturbation (normalize), history of pregnancy, abortion, STD, contraception, comfort with sexual activity, history of sexual/physical abuse
- Nutrition: body image, screen for eating disorders, typical daily intake
- Mental health: suicide assessment, coping skills assessment

Objective Data (O)
- One complete physical examination during early adolescence
- Blood pressure, body mass index (BMI)
- Skin: acne
- Vision and hearing screen
- Dental screen
- Scoliosis screen
- Assess pubertal development; Tanner stage
- Screening for STDs if sexually experienced; Pap smear
  - Condyloma/lesions (female adolescents)
  - Instruction in breast self-examination (BSE) (female adolescents)
  - Gynecomastia (male adolescents)
  - Hernias, condyloma lesions (male adolescents)
  - Instruction in testicular self-examination (male adolescents)

Assessment (A)
- Well adolescent
- Possible findings: gynecomastia, irregular menses, decreased school performance in junior high, myopia

Plan (P)
- Immunizations
  - Tuberculosis (TB) screen (once between ages 14 and 16 years)
  - Tetanus and diphtheria (Td)
  - Hepatitis B vaccine (HBV) series, if not administered during childhood
  - Varicella, if no reliable history of chickenpox or if not administered during routine childhood schedule
  - Measles, mumps, and rubella (MMR), if two vaccinations are not documented as having been administered earlier during childhood
- Gynecomastia: reassurance
- Irregular menses: education regarding anovulatory cycles, reassurance, hormonal treatment if disruptive
- Anticipatory guidance
  - Education approach for a concrete thinker
  - Development: review of normal physical changes, timing of menarche for females, peer pressure
  - Injury prevention: bike helmet use, protective equipment with sports, seat belt use, sunscreen, guns locked away
  - Diet and physical activity: calcium, iron sources in diet, food choices (vegetables, fruits, milk), discuss

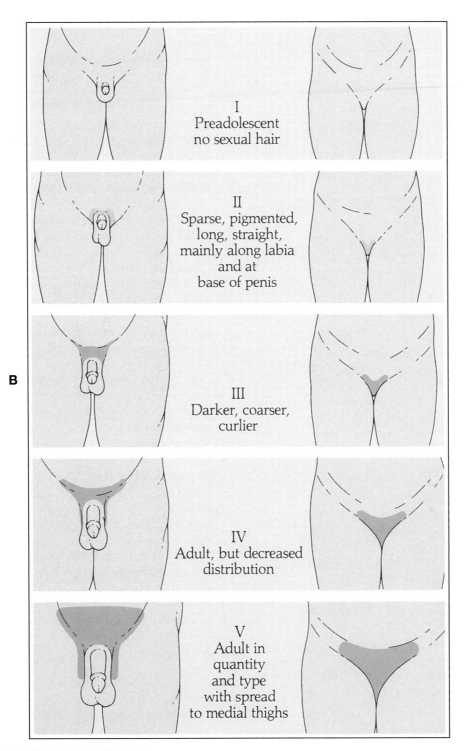

I
Preadolescent
no sexual hair

II
Sparse, pigmented,
long, straight,
mainly along labia
and at
base of penis

B

III
Darker, coarser,
curlier

IV
Adult, but decreased
distribution

V
Adult in
quantity
and type
with spread
to medial thighs

FIGURE **4-1**—cont'd **B,** Pubic hair development.

sugar, high-fat foods, exercise three times per week, athletic conditioning and fluids
- Healthy lifestyle: postponing sexual involvement; abstinence, contraception, and condoms if sexually experienced; substance use risks (more than 75% of adolescents have tried alcohol by age 14 years), dental care, adequate sleep, limit television watching

- Emotional: challenges, self-confidence, listen to friends or adults, stress, nervousness, sadness
- Normal sexual feelings, peer counseling
- Social competence: family time, respect parents' limits and consequences, social activities, groups, sports
- Peers, sibling relationships, peer pressure, peer refusal
- Responsibility: respect others, ethical role model, rules, chores, responsibilities, new skills, talents, interests

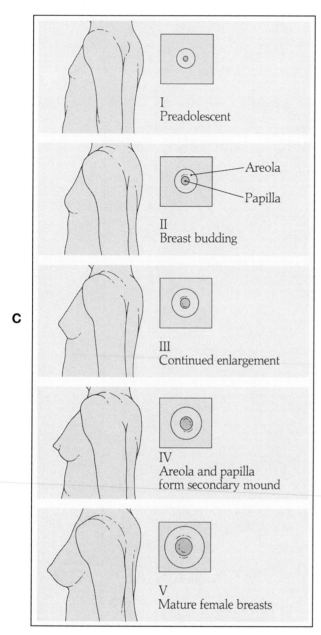

C

I
Preadolescent

II
Breast budding

Areola

Papilla

III
Continued enlargement

IV
Areola and papilla
form secondary mound

V
Mature female breasts

FIGURE **4-1**—cont'd **C,** Breast development. (Modified from Johnson, T. R., Moore, W. M., & Jefferies, J. E. [1978]. *Children are different: Developmental physiology* [2nd ed., pp. 26-22]. Columbus, OH: Ross Laboratories).

- School achievement: school transitions, attendance, homework, frustrations, dropping out, school activities, future plans, college, career
- Community interaction: religious, cultural, volunteer activities
- Suggestions for client's parents: normative adolescent development, both physical and emotional; role modeling health-related behaviors, monitoring social activities; providing opportunities to make independent decisions
- Follow-up
  - Follow-up at 3 months if menses remain irregular
  - Follow-up at 1 month for HBV 2

Middle Adolescence (15, 16, and 17 Years of Age)

Subjective (S). Information obtained from clients in early adolescence should also be elicited from those in middle adolescence. In addition, specific questions for the older teen include the following:

- What do you do for fun? Is it easy or hard to make friends?
- Do you ever feel really down and depressed? To whom do you talk about these feelings?
- How do you feel about the way you look? About your weight? What kind of exercise do you get?
- Do you work? How many hours a week?
- Do you date? Do you have a steady partner? Are you happy? Have you begun having sex? Do you use birth control? What kind?
- Are the rules in your family clear and reasonable?
- Do you smoke cigarettes, drink alcohol, or use drugs? How often?
- How is school? Is it difficult for you? What activities and sports are you involved in?

Objective (O). Objective assessment for clients in middle adolescence is the same as for those in early adolescence.

Assessment (A)
- Well adolescent
- Possible findings: acne, dysmenorrhea, sports injuries, increased conflict at home

Plan (P)
- Immunizations: none, if updated at early adolescent visit
- Acne treatment, begin with topical medications
- Dysmenorrhea: nonsteroidal antiinflammatory drugs (NSAIDs) before onset of menses and every 6 to 8 hours for the first 2 days of menses
- Eating disorder: referral for dietary assessment if BMI is lower than 5th percentile
- Rehabilitation from all sports injuries before return to play
- Anticipatory guidance: education approach for early abstract thinking style; under stress, this ability may be lost; adolescents feel invulnerable (i.e., as though things happen to others but never to them)
- Development: skin care for acne, menstrual calendar, begin career planning
- Injury prevention: stretching before physical activity, seat belts, no driving while intoxicated or riding with intoxicated driver, violence prevention and conflict resolution, job safety, emergencies, weapon safety, self-protection
- Diet and physical activity: calcium sources, fast food choices, adequate exercise levels
- Healthy lifestyle: postponing sexual involvement, contraception and condoms if sexually experienced, meth-

ods to avoid substance use, birth control, safer sex, limitation of sex partners, correct condom use, instruction in BSE, instruction in testicular self-examination, dental care, adequate sleep
- Emotional: self-confidence, strengths, trust feelings, listen to friends or adults, stress, depression, hopelessness, goals should be challenging and reasonable, handle anger, conflict resolution, support friends, peer counseling
- Social competence, responsibilities, school achievement, and community interaction same as for younger teen
- Suggestions for client's parents: communication, signs of emotional distress, monitoring use of motor vehicles, avoid weapons in home, monitor social activities
- Follow-up at 2 months for dysmenorrhea resolution (consider oral contraceptive pills [OCPs] if dysmenorrhea continues)
- Follow-up in 2 months for acne (begin combination treatment if necessary)

Late Adolescence (18, 19, 20, and 21 Years of Age)

Subjective (S). Information obtained from clients in early and middle adolescence should also be elicited from those in late adolescence. In addition, specific questions for the clients in late adolescence include the following:
- Drugs: use by client, peers, or family members; amounts, frequency, and patterns; use while driving car; source (how paid for)
- Sexuality: orientation, degree and type of sexual experience, number of partners, masturbation (normalize), history of pregnancy, abortion, STD, contraception, comfort with sexual activity, history of sexual or physical abuse, violence in dating relationships
- Nutrition screen for eating disorders, especially bulimia, body image, typical daily intake
- Mental health: depression, suicide assessment, coping skills assessment
- How client and parents deal with client's living away from home or preparing to do so

Objective (O). Objective assessment for clients in late adolescence is the same as for younger and middle adolescents. In addition, perform a Pap smear for all women regardless of sexual experience.

Assessment (A)
- Well adolescent
- Possible findings: acne, *Chlamydia*, obesity

Plan (P)
- Immunizations: none if updated at early adolescent visit
- Hyperlipidemia risk assessed; screening at age 20 years
- Acne treatment: combination therapies considered
- *Chlamydia*: single-dose therapy, partner notification

- Obesity: low-fat diet, increased exercise; referral for dietary counseling if BMI higher than 95th percentile for age and gender
- Anticipatory guidance (most of younger teen anticipatory guidance still applies to this age group): education approach for abstract thinking; abstract thoughts and increased ability to set limits and understand consequences established by late adolescence
- Development: skin care, job/school/college search, leaving "nest"
- Injury prevention: occupational safety, seat belts, no driving while intoxicated or riding with intoxicated driver, conflict resolution
- Diet and physical health: folic acid before planned pregnancy, calcium requirements, low-fat high-fiber diet, exercise
- Healthy lifestyle: contraception and condom usage, recommend one partner for sexual activity to decrease risk, moderation with alcohol, smoking cessation, substance use avoidance
  - BSE
  - Testicular self-examination
  - Dental care
  - Gay/lesbian issues
- Suggestions for client's parents: separation from adult child, role model for health-related behavior
- Follow-up at 3 months to rescreen for STDs and reevaluate acne
- Follow-up at 1 month for further nutrition education; referral to dietitian if client is interested

REFERENCES

American Medical Association. (1995). *Guidelines for adolescent preventive services (GAPS) recommendations monograph.* Chicago: American Medical Association.

American Psychiatric Association. (1994). *Diagnostic and statistical manual of mental disorders* (4th ed.). Washington, DC: American Psychiatric Association.

Barker, Burton, & Zieve (2002). *Ambulatory Medicine.* Philadelphia: Lippincott Williams & Wilkins.

Biro, F., Rosenthal, S., Rymarquis, L., & Hillard, P. (1997). Adolescent girls' understanding of Papanicolaou smear results. *Journal of Pediatric Adolescent Gynecology, 10*(4), 209-212.

Bright Futures. (2001). *Guidelines for health supervision of infants, children and adolescents.* Retrieved August 22, 2002, from http://www.brightfutures.gov.

Campbell, M., & McGrath, P. (1997). Use of medication by adolescents for the management of menstrual discomfort. *Archives of Pediatric Adolescent Medicine, 151*(9), 905-913.

Draelos, Z. K. (1995). Patient compliance: Enhancing clinician abilities and strategies. *Journal of the American Academy of Dermatology, 32,* S42-S48.

Dull, P., & Blythe, M. (1998). Preventing teenage pregnancy. *Primary Care, 25*(1), 111-122.

Elster, A., & Kuznets, N. (1994). *AMA guidelines for adolescent preventive services (GAPS): Recommendations and rationale.* Baltimore: Williams & Wilkins.

Glass, A. P. (1994) Gynecomastia. *Endocrinology and Metabolism Clinics of North America. 23*(4), 825-837.

Hurwitz, S. (1995). Acne treatment for the '90s. *Contemporary Pediatrics, 12*(8), 19-32.

Levenberg, P. (1998). GAPS: An opportunity for nurse practitioners to promote the health of adolescents through clinical preventive services. *Journal of Pediatric Health Care, 12*(1), 2-9.

Malat, B. (1998). Reducing teen health risks. *Advance for Nurse Practitioners, 6*(3), 47-50.

Monalto, N. (1998). Implementing the guidelines for adolescent preventive services. *American Family Physician, 57*(9), 2181-2190.

Moore, P., Adler, N., & Kegeles, S. (1996). Adolescents and the contraceptive pill: The impact of beliefs on intentions and use. *Obstetric and Gynecology, 88*(Suppl. 3), 48S-56S.

Neinstein, L. S. (1996). *Adolescent health care: A practical guide* (3rd ed.). Baltimore: Urban & Schwarzenberg.

Robinson, D. (2000). Well adolescent. In D. Robinson, P. Kidd, & K. Rogers (eds.), *Primary care across the lifespan* (p. 1303). St. Louis: Mosby.

Tanner, J. M. (1987). Issues and advance in adolescent growth and development. *Journal of Adolescent Health Care, 8*, 470-478.

Wheeler, M. D. (1991). Physical changes of puberty. *Endocrinology and Metabolism Clinics of North America, 20*, 1-14.

Review Questions

1. Which of the following best represents a normal sequence of pubertal events for a girl?

   a. Breast buds, axillary hair, ovaries enlarged, menarche
   b. Menarche, axillary hair, breast buds
   c. Growth spurt, breast buds, menarche
   d. Breast buds, pubic hair development, menarche

2. Acne lesions most commonly erupt on which of the following areas of the body?

   a. Face, upper arms, and abdomen
   b. Cheeks, forehead, chin, chest, and back
   c. Face, buttocks, chest, and back
   d. Cheeks, forehead, and chin

3. Which of the following is most consistent with a diagnosis of anorexia nervosa in a 15-year-old female?

   a. BMI 5%, refusal to gain weight, perception of being overweight, amenorrhea
   b. BMI 15%, concerns about gaining weight, normal menstrual cycles
   c. BMI 10%, concern with weight, active in sports, oligomenorrhea
   d. BMI 15%, satisfaction with weight, normal menstrual cycles, vegetarian diet

4. Which of the following is the correct schedule for Td vaccination?

   a. Td booster during adolescence 10 years after last diphtheria and tetanus toxoids and pertussis (DTP), diphtheria and tetanus toxoids and acellular pertussis (DTaP), or diphtheria and tetanus toxoids (DT) vaccine
   b. Td booster during early, middle, and late adolescence
   c. Td booster at age 11 to 12 years if 5 years have elapsed since last DTP, DTaP, or DT vaccine and subsequently, every 10 years
   d. Td booster at age 11 to 12 years if 5 years have elapsed since last DTP, DTaP, or DT vaccine and subsequently, every 5 years

5. A 15-year-old adolescent continues to have monthly dysmenorrhea after 3 months of receiving NSAIDs and OCPs. This adolescent should be referred for evaluation of which of the following?

   a. Secondary dysmenorrhea
   b. Primary dysmenorrhea
   c. Psychogenic pain syndrome
   d. Premenstrual syndrome

6. When performing a well-child examination on a 13-year-old, the NP discovers that the client is planning to try out for football. The client's father used to play professional football, but he died at age 51 years as the result of a heart attack. To assess the client's potential for CAD, the NP should do which of the following?

   a. Perform a careful funduscopic examination.
   b. Order a cholesterol level.
   c. Assess for hepatomegaly.
   d. Order a triglyceride level.

7. Which of the following comments by a teenager would make the NP delve more deeply into his emotional state?

   a. "I hate drinking milk."
   b. "I am getting a B in most subjects, but I am failing math."
   c. "None of my friends want to spend any time with me."
   d. "I don't get along well with my father."

8. Which of the following historical data is most important when conducting a sports physical?

   a. "Have you ever been hospitalized when playing sports?"
   b. "Have you fractured or sprained any extremities?"
   c. "Have you undergone any surgeries?"
   d. "Have you ever fainted or lost consciousness when exercising?"

9. When should a teenage girl get a Pap smear?

   a. When her mother suspects she is having sex
   b. When she becomes pregnant
   c. If she suspects she has an STD
   d. If she is sexually active

10. Appropriate anticipatory guidance for parents of an 11-year-old boy should include which of the following?

   a. Preparation for pubertal changes
   b. Explanation that their son will begin actively revolting against them
   c. Importance of letting the son make his own choices regardless of consequences
   d. Encouraging them to get dental care for the teen so that his teeth will not become rotten like theirs

11. Stacy is a 15-year-old who is concerned about her weight. Which of the following historical data is *not* helpful in finding out why she is gaining weight?

a. Sports or exercise done on a regular basis
b. Amount of TV watched
c. Whether whole milk is drunk every day
d. Participation in gym at school

12. Shateela is concerned because her menstrual period is irregular; she has had only one period since her period started 4 months ago. What information would you give her regarding the menstrual cycle?

a. Reassure her that the first periods are anovulatory and tend to be irregular.
b. Encourage her to go on OCPs to help regulate her period.
c. Tell her that irregular periods indicate that she is sexually active and she should practice abstinence.
d. Encourage her to begin Depo-Provera to help prevent pregnancy.

13. Which of the following educational approaches is most appropriate for an 18-year-old college student?

a. Presenting ideas in a concrete manner
b. Using abstract ideas as appropriate based on topic
c. Using scare tactics to frighten the student out of smoking
d. Threatening to share information with his or her parent

14. Sheila complains of having acne on her face. She indicates that it makes her feel unattractive. Sheila has papules and pustules on her chin and forehead. What is the most appropriate action to take at this time?

a. Begin antibiotics by mouth.
b. Encourage her to stop eating chocolate and high-fat foods.
c. Have her wash her face three to four times a day.
d. Begin topical preparations, such as benzol peroxide or erythromycin gel.

15. Based on the most common cause of death among 12- to 15-year-olds, the NP should discuss which of the following topics with clients in this age group?

a. Wearing seat belts
b. Safe sex
c. Screening for skin cancer
d. Being alert for heart palpitations

Answers and Rationales

1. *Answer:* d (assessment)
Rationale: Menarche generally begins within 2 to 3 years after the onset of breast development. The average age of menarche for girls in the United States is 12 to 13 years. Menarche signals the end of the rapid-growth stage (Tanner, 1987).

2. *Answer:* b (assessment)
Rationale: Acne most commonly occurs on the face (especially the forehead, chin, and cheeks), the chest, and the back. There are nearly 900 sebaceous glands/cm² in these areas, as compared with 100 glands/cm² on other skin surfaces (Hurwitz, 1995).

3. *Answer:* a (analysis/diagnosis)
Rationale: Diagnostic criteria include a refusal or inability to maintain body weight, fear of gaining weight or becoming fat despite being underweight, distorted body image, and absence of three consecutive menstrual cycles (American Psychiatric Association, 1994).

4. *Answer:* c (implementation/plan)
Rationale: The age range for administration of a Td booster has been lowered from 14 to 16 years to 11 to 12 years to ensure long-lasting immunity against tetanus. Immunity to tetanus varies with age; 28% of children vaccinated 6 to 10 years before serologic testing lacked immunity, as compared with 14% of those vaccinated 1 to 5 years before testing. The Td booster administered at age 11 to 12 years is the only exception to the administration of routine boosters every 10 years (Bright Futures, 2001).

5. *Answer:* a (implementation/plan)
Rationale: The differential diagnoses of secondary dysmenorrhea include endometriosis, pelvic inflammatory disease, uterine polyps or fibroids, and anatomic disorders. A diagnostic laparoscopy should be considered (Campbell & McGrath, 1997).

6. *Answer:* b (assessment)
Rationale: Arcus senilis may be present before the age of 50 years in someone with hyperlipidemia, but this can be noted without a funduscopic examination and is still rare in children. An enlarged liver is not associated with CAD. A triglyceride level must be obtained from a fasting specimen. A cholesterol level can be drawn the day of the examination (Barker, Burton, & Zieve, 2002).

7. *Answer:* c (assessment)
Rationale: The comment about not having any friends should serve as a "red flag" to investigate further regarding possible depression (Robinson, 2000).

8. *Answer:* d (assessment)
Rationale: Obtaining a history is the most important part of conducting a sports physical. Asking about loss of consciousness during exercise provides data regarding potential cardiac problems (Robinson, 2000).

9. *Answer:* d (evaluation)
Rationale: A girl should begin getting an annual Pap smear when she becomes sexually active or at the age of 18 years (Robinson, 2000).

10. *Answer:* a (implementation/plan)
Rationale: At age 11, upcoming pubertal changes should be discussed with parents (Robinson, 2000).

11. *Answer:* d (assessment)
Rationale: Finding out whether Stacy is involved in sports, how much TV she watches, and whether she drinks whole milk all provide data regarding why she is gaining weight. Although participating in gym class at school may help contribute to a healthful lifestyle, it is important for Stacy to exercise at least 3 times a week, drink skim milk, and decrease the amount of TV watching, if her weight high (Bright Futures, 2001).

12. *Answer:* a (implementation/plan)
Rationale: Anovulatory periods are common during the first few months after a girl's period starts. Reassurance is needed at this point (Robinson, 2000).

13. *Answer:* b (implementation/plan)

Rationale: Teens 18 and older are able to handle abstract ideas. Threatening behavior and scare tactics do not work. A concrete thinking approach is more appropriate for a younger teen (Robinson, 2000).

14. *Answer:* d (implementation/plan)

Rationale: A topical agent is the appropriate choice at this point for beginning treatment of acne (Robinson, 2000).

15. *Answer:* a (implementation/plan)

Rationale: Accidents are the most common cause of death in teens, so it is important to discuss safety related to wearing seat belts. Other causes of death include congenital heart disease, human immunodeficiency virus (HIV), and cancer (Bright Futures, 2001).

WELL-MAN CARE *Pamela Kidd*

Well-man care encompasses comprehensive care across the lifespan for men based on knowledge of men's diverse lives (Table 4-11).

PRACTICE GUIDELINES FOR PREVENTIVE CARE
Indications for Screening

- Hearing: Presbycusis is the most frequent type of hearing loss among the elderly (Scheitel et al., 1996). Annual hearing tests should be conducted after age 65 years. Hearing loss can affect social, religious, and personal aspects.
- Vision: Cataracts are common among the elderly. Counseling regarding what to look for assists the client in early detection. Vision screening every 2 years with a Snellen chart is appropriate. A funduscopic examination with eyes dilated is appropriate every 5 years until age 40 years for blacks and age 65 years for others (see glaucoma screening, following) then annually.
- Blood pressure: For persons 75 years old and older, heart disease and cerebrovascular disease are among the top five causes of death. Although the United States Preventive Services Task Force (1996) recommends a blood pressure check only every 2 years for clients with normal readings, it is a quick, effective measurement to obtain at an office visit.
- Skin: An annual skin examination is recommended for early detection of cancer, especially for those clients who are exposed to sun.
- Purified protein derivative (PPD) test is recommended for close contacts of persons with known or suspected TB, health care workers, persons with medical risk factors associated with TB, immigrants from countries with high TB prevalence, the medically under-served, low-income populations (including the homeless), alcoholics, those who are intravenous drug users (IVDUs), and residents of long-term care facilities.
- HIV: Screening for HIV is recommended for men who have had sex with men after 1975, who are or have been IV drug users (IVDUs), persons who exchange sex for money or drugs and their sex partners, those who have had bisexual or HIV-positive sex partners, those who received blood transfusion between 1978 and 1985, and persons seeking treatment for STDs.
- Rapid plasma reagin (RPR) test is recommended for persons who exchange sex for money or drugs and their sex partners, persons with other STDs (including HIV), and sexual contacts of persons with active syphilis.
- Total cholesterol should be assessed every 5 years starting at age 20 years.
- Glucose level should be assessed every 3 years beginning at age 45 years for asymptomatic persons. Screening may need to begin earlier for those who are obese, have a first-degree relative with diabetes mellitus (DM), are members of a high-risk ethnic population (black, Hispanic, Native American, Asian), are hypertensive, have had a high cholesterol or triglyceride level, or on previous testing had impaired glucose tolerance (IGT) or impaired fasting glucose (IFG).
- Digital rectal examination (DRE) should be performed annually to check for prostate and colorectal cancer starting at age 50 years.
- Prostate-specific antigen (PSA) test should be performed annually starting at age 40 years for blacks and those with a family history (first-degree relative) of prostate cancer and starting at age 50 years for all others. After age 75 years, the screening needs to be individualized based on level of activity (general life expectancy of 10 years) because it is theorized that the disease is less virulent. Treatment of prostate cancer versus cautious observation has to be weighed with morbidity and/or mortality outcomes.
- Perform fecal occult blood (FOB) test annually.
- Perform sigmoidoscopy every 5 years.
- Glaucoma screening should be performed by an eye specialist for blacks 40 years old and whites 65 years old, those with a positive family history, and those with severe myopia.
- Oral cavity: Persons who smoke or drink alcohol regularly should have dental hygiene visits every 6 months.
- Family violence: An NP must be alert to signs and symptoms of adult abuse. NPs must find a comfort level in interview techniques that can assist in identifying family violence. Explore how things are going at home, work, and in other areas of the client's life. Identify changes, both good and bad. Is the client anxious? How does the client feel about work and home in general? Be empathetic. Support the feelings of the

TABLE **4-11** Well-Man Care: 18 Years through Adulthood

SOAP	18 TO 24 YEARS	25 TO 64 YEARS	OLDER THAN 65 YEARS
S (subjective data)	**History:** medical history, surgical history, family history, medications, allergies; genogram to identify risk factors for CAD, DM, cancer, asthma, psychiatric illnesses **Lifestyle:** healthful diet and exercise, dental care, fluoridated water, risk for STDs; risk taking **Habits:** alcohol, tobacco, illicit drug, and IV drug use **Safety:** lap and shoulder seat belts; bike and motorcycle helmets; smoke detector; safe storage of firearms; use of alcohol while driving, swimming, and boating; hot water and heater settings; use of space heaters; safety with hobbies; blood transfusion between 1978 and 1985 **Ethnic Background:** Native American or Alaska Native, black **Health Maintenance:** last vision, hearing, and dental examination; Pneumovax or influenza vaccine **Social:** family relationships, employment, living arrangements, significant other **Developmental Task:** Identity versus role confusion (adolescence)	**History:** medical history, surgical history, family history, medications, allergies; genogram to identify risk factors for CAD, DM, cancer, asthma, psychiatric illnesses **Lifestyle:** healthful diet and exercise, dental care, fluoridated water, risk for STDs **Habits:** alcohol, tobacco, illicit drug, and IV drug use **Safety:** lap and shoulder seat belts; bike and motorcycle helmets; smoke detector; safe storage of firearms; use of alcohol while driving, swimming, boating; hot water and heater settings; use of space heaters; safety with hobbies; blood transfusion between 1978 and 1985 **Ethnic Background:** Native American or Alaska Native, black **Health Maintenance:** last vision, hearing, and dental examination; Pneumovax or influenza vaccine **Social:** family relationships, children, employment, living arrangements, health of parents **Developmental Tasks:** intimacy versus isolation (early adulthood), generativity versus stagnation (middle adulthood)	**History:** medical history, surgical history, family history, medications, allergies; genogram to identify risk factors for CAD, DM, cancer, asthma, psychiatric illnesses **Lifestyle:** healthful diet and exercise, dental care, fluoridated water, risk for STDs **Habits:** alcohol, tobacco, illicit drug, and IV drug use **Safety:** lap and shoulder seat belts; bike and motorcycle helmets; smoke detector; safe storage of firearms; use of alcohol while driving, swimming, boating; hot water and heater settings; use of space heaters; safety with hobbies; blood transfusion between 1978 and 1985 **Ethnic Background:** Native American or Alaska Native, black **Health Maintenance:** last vision, hearing, and dental examination; Pneumovax or influenza vaccine **Social:** loss issues, family relationships, social activities **Developmental Task:** ego integrity versus despair
O (objective data)	Height, weight, vital signs Skin Oral cavity Adenopathy Hearing Snellen Heart/lung DRE Testes Other systems dependent on risk factors and history	Height, weight, vital signs Skin Oral cavity Adenopathy Hearing Snellen Heart/lung DRE Testes Other systems dependent on risk factors and history	Height, weight, vital signs Skin Oral cavity Adenopathy Hearing Snellen Heart/lung DRE Testes Other systems dependent on risk factors and history

Continued

TABLE **4-11** Well-Man Care: 18 Years through Adulthood—*cont'd*

SOAP	18 TO 24	25 TO 64	OLDER THAN 65
A (assessment)	**Leading Causes of Death:** MVC or other unintentional injuries, homicide, suicide, malignant neoplasms, heart disease, HIV	**Leading Causes of Death:** malignant neoplasms, heart disease, MVC or other unintentional injuries, HIV, suicide, homicide	**Leading Causes of Death:** heart disease, malignant neoplasms (lung, colorectal, prostate), cerebrovascular disease, COPD, pneumonia, influenza
P (plan)	**Screening:** lipid, HIV, PPD, RPR, GC, *Chlamydia* **Immunizations:** Td, hepatitis B, hepatitis A, influenza, MMR, varicella **Counseling:** problem drinking, illicit drug use, smoking cessation, alcohol/drug cessation, no drinking/drugs while driving, healthful diet and exercise, seat belts, bike helmets, firearm safety, STD prevention and protection, contraception, regular dental and vision care, skin cancer prevention	**Screening:** lipid, HIV, PPD, RPR, GC, PSA, FOB, sigmoidoscopy, glaucoma **Immunizations:** Td, hepatitis B, hepatitis A, influenza, MMR, varicella **Counseling:** problem drinking, illicit drug use, smoking cessation, alcohol/drug cessation, no drinking/drugs while driving, healthful diet and exercise, seat belts, bike helmets, firearm safety, STD prevention and protection, contraception, regular dental and vision care, skin cancer prevention	**Screening:** lipid, FOB, HIV, PPD, RPR, PSA, sigmoidoscopy, glaucoma, hearing, mini-mental status **Immunizations:** Td, hepatitis B, hepatitis A, influenza, MMR, varicella, pneumococcal **Counseling:** problem drinking, illicit drug use, polypharmacy, smoking cessation, healthful diet and exercise, seat belts, bike helmets, firearm safety, STD prevention, regular dental and vision care, skin cancer prevention **Safety:** hot water heater set lower than 120° F, CPR training for household members, emergency phone numbers available, fall prevention

CAD, Coronary artery disease; *COPD,* chronic obstructive pulmonary disease; *CPR,* cardiopulmonary resuscitation; *DM,* diabetes mellitus; *DRE,* digital rectal examination; *FOB,* fecal occult blood; *GC, HIV,* human immunodeficiency virus; *MMC,* measles-mumps-rubella; *MVC,* motor vehicle crash; *PPD,* purified protein derivative; *PSA,* prostate-specific antigen; *RPR,* rapid plasma reagin; *STD,* sexually transmitted disease; *Td,* tetanus and diphtheria.

TABLE **4-12** Immunization Guidelines

IMMUNIZATIONS	HIGH-RISK GROUPS
Influenza	Annual vaccination of residents of chronic-care facilities; persons with chronic cardiopulmonary disorders, metabolic diseases, hemoglobinopathies, renal dysfunction, or immunosuppression; and health care providers who work with high-risk individuals
Pneumococcal	Immunocompromised institutionalized persons; immunocompromised persons with disorders such as chronic cardiac or pulmonary disease, DM, or anatomic asplenia; immunocompromised persons who live in high-risk environments or social settings (e.g., certain Native American and Alaska Native populations); and all persons older than 65 years
Tetanus	Every 10 years and in cases of severe or contaminated wounds
Hepatitis A	Persons living in, working in, or traveling to areas where the disease is endemic and where periodic outbreaks occur (certain Alaska Native, Pacific Island, Native American, and religious communities); men who have sex with men; IVDUs/street drug users. Consider for institutionalized persons and workers in these institutions; military personnel; and day-care, hospital, and laboratory workers
Hepatitis B	Blood product recipients (including hemodialysis clients), persons with frequent occupational exposure to blood or blood products, men who have sex with men, IVDU and their sex partners, persons with multiple recent sexual partners, persons with other STDs, travelers to countries with endemic hepatitis B
Varicella	Healthy adults without a history of chickenpox or previous immunization. Consider serologic testing for presumed susceptible adults

DM, Diabetes mellitus; *IVDU*, intravenous drug user; *STD*, sexually transmitted disease.

TABLE **4-13** Lifestyle Assessment

ISSUE	RECOMMENDATION
Exercise/ nutrition	Recommendations are based on individual, but periodic evaluation of weight gain or loss and counseling of dietary intake is appropriate. Disease processes that can alter appetite or ability to consume nutrition or exercise include strokes, Parkinson's disease, dementia, depression, immobility, constipation, alcoholism, dental problems, medications, and impaired taste.
Medications	There should be a periodic review of all medications taken, including those taken OTC, which can interact with prescription medications.
Smoking/tobacco	Recommend smoking/tobacco cessation to all clients.
Burns	Hot water heaters should be turned down to 48.9° C (120° F). Counsel regarding not smoking in bed. The main types of burns among the elderly are flame and scald injuries. Counsel regarding fire extinguishers and fire alarms (see note under Home Safety Issues).
MVCs	Persons older than 70 years are at an increased risk for MVCs, especially if wearing bilateral hearing aides. Polydisease entities, subsequent polypharmacologic management, and normal aging processes put the older adults at higher risk when operating a motor vehicle. Slowing of reflexes and a decrease in motor strength make the elderly more susceptible to crashes in situations that require rapid thinking and decision making, such as at intersections. Decreased hepatic mass, blood flow, and enzyme activity, as well as increased receptor site sensitivity, make the elderly more susceptible to side effects of medications. Even if they are not at risk for causing the crash, older adults tend to have more severe injuries and require hospitalizations more frequently. The heart and lungs become less pliant with age. Osteoporosis renders the elderly more vulnerable to fractures in what may seem to be a minor injury event.
Driving assessment	A periodic review of driving history, including near misses, is appropriate. Referral for formal, behind-the-wheel evaluation may be appropriate. There are some community resources that test driving skills without going through the state's department of transportation. These programs bill based on "on-road" time and "class" time, with a typical fee of $300 to $600. Some insurance companies offer reduced rates for those who go through formal programs/testing. Some automobile and other associations offer refresher courses specifically designed for the older adult driver (some at minimal or no cost). Get input from family members who have ridden in the vehicle with the older adult. A mini-mental status examination gives an indication of the elder's cognitive function. Complete hearing and vision examinations and range-of-motion and strength assessment as part of the physical examination. Review medications and alcohol use to assess for potential or actual side effects that the elder may be experiencing.

MVC, Motor vehicle crash; *OTC*, over the counter.

involved parties by identifying that other people are struggling with the same issues. Remain objective.

- Use statements such as the following:
  - "That sounds as though it can be a very difficult situation."
  - "Is there anything you may want to change?"
  - "What kinds of worries are most bothersome to you?"
  - "How do you manage this problem?"
  - "How have you managed similar problems in the past?"
  - "Who supports you?"

Immunizations

See Table 4-12.

Lifestyle and Activities

See Table 4-13.

Home Safety Issues

Assess the following:
- Security systems
- Use of throw rugs, extension cords, or appliances with frayed cords
- Use of space heaters or wood burning stoves
- Torn or frayed carpeting on stairways
- Presence of pets, which could get in the way of ambulation
- Presence of adequate lighting, both inside and outside
- Whether client parks car outside or in a garage; if client parks in street, what time client arrives home

Recommendations. In general, there should be an ABC fire extinguisher and smoke detector for each level of the home. The fire extinguisher should be a 5# extinguisher to allow for some error in usage. If there is a high-hazard area, there should be an additional fire extinguisher and smoke detector.

REFERENCES

Branch, W., & Jacobson, T. (1996). Routine preventive studies: What to include and how often. *Consultant, 36*(11), 2401-2410.

Leading causes of death. (1998). *Women's Health in Primary Care, 1*(1), 38.

Murray, S. L. (1997). What's happening: Driving and the elderly. *Journal of the American Academy of Nurse Practitioners, 9*(3), 133-136.

Nichol, K., Margolis, K., Wouremna, J., & von Sternberg, T., (1996). Effectiveness of influenza vaccine in the elderly. *Gerontology, 42*(5), 274-279.

Robinson, D. (2000). Well male. In D. Robinson, P. Kidd, & K. Rogers (Eds.), *Primary care across the lifespan.* St. Louis: Mosby.

Scheitel, S., Fleming, K., Churka, S., & Evans, J. (1996). Geriatric health maintenance. *Mayo Clinic Proceedings, 71*(3), 289-302.

United States Preventive Services Task Force. (1996). *Guide to clinical preventive services* (2nd ed.). Baltimore: Williams & Wilkins.

Review Questions

1. Which of the following differentiates the history taking that is appropriate for a well examination of a 25-year-old man as compared with a 40-year-old man?
- **a.** Health maintenance
- **b.** Lifestyle
- **c.** Safety
- **d.** Social history

2. When making a diagnosis during a well examination of a male, what factor should be considered in relation to the age of the client?
- **a.** Leading cause of death
- **b.** Co-morbidities
- **c.** Current medications
- **d.** Physical examination results

3. Which of the following immunizations should be screened for receipt in a 65-year-old client as compared with a 30-year-old client?
- **a.** Flu
- **b.** MMR
- **c.** Varicella
- **d.** Pneumococcal

4. A 45-year-old man without a positive family history for heart disease asks about cholesterol screening. How often should the NP tell the client to have his cholesterol checked?
- **a.** Every year
- **b.** Every 2 years
- **c.** Every 5 years
- **d.** Every 10 years

5. A 77-year-old client who is being treated for lung cancer should do which of the following?
- **a.** Have a PSA test performed.
- **b.** Wait for a PSA test until after treatment is finished.
- **c.** Should not undergo PSA testing.
- **d.** Depend on the results of the DRE and the PSA test.

Answers and Rationales

1. Answer: d (assessment)
Rationale: The questions asked about health maintenance, lifestyle, and safety do not differ across the lifespan. Only the areas of social history and developmental tasks achievement vary across age groups.

2. Answer: a (analysis/diagnosis)
Rationale: The leading causes of death vary by age and should be kept in mind when making a diagnosis. Co-morbidities, current medications, and physical examination results should all be considered regardless of the age of the client.

3. Answer: d (assessment)

Rationale: Pneumococcal vaccine is recommended for all clients 65 years or older regardless of risk status. MMR, varicella, and flu vaccines are recommended for everyone.

4. Answer: c (assessment)

Rationale: All adults should have cholesterol levels checked every 5 years beginning at age 25 years.

5. Answer: c (assessment)

Rationale: A PSA test is not recommended after age 75 years unless life expectancy is longer than 10 years.

WELL-WOMAN CARE   *Cheryl Pope Kish*

See Table 4-14 for a summary of well-woman care across the lifespan.

SCREENING AND IMMUNIZATIONS
Indications and Frequencies for Screening

- Blood glucose level baseline measurement is obtained at 18 to 39 years, and blood glucose is then measured every 2 years.
- Bone density test is performed in perimenopausal women, in women with high risk of osteoporosis, or after low-impact fracture.
- *Cholesterol:* Baseline measurement is obtained at 18 to 39 years, and cholesterol is then measured every 5 years. After age 40 years, measure cholesterol every 3 to 5 years.
- Dental examination should be obtained every year.
- *Eye examination with tonometry:* Get baseline measurements at 18 to 39 years and then measure every 3 to 5 years or more frequently if risk factors are present.
- Conduct gonococcus and *Chlamydia* screening if the client engages in or has any partner who engages in high-risk sexual behavior or if the client has contact with a person who has been diagnosed as having *Chlamydia.* Screen anyone in a nonmonogamous relationship.
- *Hearing:* Screen clients with regular exposure to excessive noise; establish baseline measurement at 40 years and repeat screening at age 50 years. After age 60 years, screen annually.
- *Hematocrit/hemoglobin:* Check every 2 years from age 18 to 50 years and then every 5 years.
- *HIV:* Screen if the client engages in or has any partner who engages in high-risk sexual behavior or if the client has contact with an HIV-seropositive person. Screen clients who are IVDUs. Screen women who have male partners who have had sex with men, who are IVDUs, who have long-term residence or were born in an area with high prevalence of HIV infection, or who received blood transfusion between 1978 and 1985.
- *Mammography:* Obtain baseline measurements at 35 to 40 years and then repeat every 1 to 2 years from ages 40 to 50 years and every year after age 50 years. Women with a family history of breast cancer should undergo mammography 5 years earlier than the age at which breast cancer was diagnosed in a first-degree relative.
- Perform pelvic examination and Pap smear every year from age 18 years or at the beginning of sexual activity until age 60 years and then every 1 to 2 years. In low-risk women with three consecutive normal Pap results, every 2 years is sufficient. After hysterectomy for benign disorder, a Pap smear should be obtained every other year or less often with three consecutive normal results and low-risk status.
- *Proctoscopy and sigmoidoscopy:* Screen those with a family history of familial polyposis coli or cancer familial syndrome; screen those without a family history starting at age 40 years. Repeat every 3 to 5 years. Obtain two consecutive yearly negative examination results before switching to intervals of every 3 to 5 years.
- *PPD:* Screen household members of persons with diagnosis of TB and those with other close contacts with known or suspected TB. Screen health care workers. Screen those with risk factors associated with TB (HIV seropositivity), immigrants from countries with high TB prevalence, clients from medically underserved low-income populations, those with history of alcoholism, who are IVDUs, and residents of long-term care facilities.
- *RPR test:* Screen clients who engage in or have any partner who engages in high-risk sexual behavior. Screen clients with contact with any person with a diagnosis of active syphilis.
- Perform rectal examination every year after age 40 years.
- *Rubella antibodies:* Screen anyone without evidence of immunity.
- *FOB:* Check every year after age 50 years.
- *Thyroid function:* Check every 3 to 5 years, starting at age 60 years.

Indications for Immunizations

- Influenza: Annually vaccinate residents of chronic-care facilities; persons with chronic cardiopulmonary disorders, metabolic diseases, hemoglobinopathies, immunosuppression, or renal dysfunction; and health care providers who work with high-risk clients.
- Hepatitis A: Vaccinate those who reside in, travel to, or work in areas where the disease is endemic and where periodic outbreaks occur (e.g., countries with high or intermediate endemicity, certain Native

TABLE 4-14   Well-Woman (18 to 64 Years) Care

	18 TO 39 YEARS	40 TO 64 YEARS
S (subjective data)	**History:** family history; medical history, surgical history; menstrual, gynecologic, obstetric, and contraceptive histories; immunization and infectious disease history; allergies; blood transfusion between 1978 and 1985, IVDU, occupational blood and body fluid exposure; dental care **Current:** medications, herbals, dietary intake, physical activity, contraception, sexual practices (high risk for STDs) **Safety:** abuse, smoke detectors, seat belt use, safety gear for hobbies, domestic violence **Habits:** alcohol, tobacco, or illicit drug use **Erikson's Developmental Task:** intimacy versus isolation or self-absorption	**History:** family history; medical history, surgical history; menstrual, gynecologic, obstetric, and contraceptive histories; immunization and infectious disease history; allergies; blood transfusion between 1978 and 1985, IVDU, occupational blood and body fluid exposure; dental care **Current:** medications, herbals, dietary intake, physical activity, contraception, sexual practices (high risk for STDs) **Safety:** abuse, smoke detectors, seat belt use, safety gear for hobbies, domestic violence **Habits:** alcohol, tobacco, or illicit drug use **Erikson's Developmental Task:** generativity versus stagnation
O (objective data)	**Physical Examination:** height, weight, blood pressure, adenopathy, skin, thyroid, lungs, heart, abdomen, breast, pelvic, DRE **High-Risk Groups:** oral cavity, thyroid, skin, osteoporosis screen **Laboratory and Diagnostic Procedures:** **Screening:** Pap smear; cholesterol, domestic violence **High-Risk Groups:** PPD, FPG, rubella antibodies, urinalysis for bacteriuria, HIV, RPR, gonococcus/*Chlamydia*, hearing, mammogram, colonoscopy	**Physical Examination:** height, weight, blood pressure, adenopathy, skin, thyroid, lungs, heart, abdomen, breast, pelvic, DRE **High-Risk Groups:** skin, oral cavity, thyroid, carotid bruits, osteoporosis screen **Laboratory and Diagnostic Procedures:** **Screening:** Pap smear, mammogram, cholesterol **High-Risk Groups:** PPD, FPG, rubella antibodies, urinalysis for bacteriuria, HIV, RPR, gonococcus/*Chlamydia*, hearing, FOB and sigmoidoscopy, colonoscopy, bone density test
A (assessment)	**Leading Medical Problems:** nose, throat, and upper respiratory tract infections; injuries; viral, bacterial, and parasitic infections; acute urinary tract infections; eating disorders; violence, rape; substance abuse	**Leading Medical Problems:** osteoporosis and arthritis; nose, throat, and upper respiratory tract infections; orthopedic deformities and impairments of back, arms, and legs; cardiovascular diseases; hearing and vision impairments
P (plan)	**Immunizations:** Td booster **High-Risk Groups:** HBV, influenza, MMR, pneumococcus **Counseling:** diet related to fat, cholesterol, complex carbohydrate, fiber, sodium, iron, folate, and calcium intake; exercise program; smoking cessation; limited alcohol consumption, treatment for abuse; contraceptive options and safer sex practices; BSE, skin protection from ultraviolet light, seat belt use	**Immunizations:** Td booster **High-Risk Groups:** HBV, influenza, pneumococcus **Counseling:** diet related to fat, cholesterol, complex carbohydrate, fiber, sodium, and calcium intake; brushing, flossing, and regular dental checkups; exercise program; smoking cessation; limited alcohol consumption; treatment for abuse; contraceptive options and safer sex practices; BSE; HRT; skin protection; seat belt use
E (evaluation)	**Follow-Up:** depends on risk factors and illness **Leading Causes of Death:** MVA; cardiovascular diseases; homicide; CAD; AIDS; breast cancer; cerebrovascular diseases; cervical and other uterine cancers	**Follow-Up:** depends on risk factors and illness **Leading Causes of Death:** cardiovascular diseases; CAD; breast cancer; lung cancer; cerebrovascular diseases, colorectal cancer; COPD; ovarian cancer; diabetes

AIDS, Acquired immune deficiency syndrome; *BSE,* breast self-examination; *CAD,* coronary artery disease; *COPD,* chronic obstructive pulmonary disease; *DRE,* digital rectal examination; *FOB,* fecal occult blood; *FPG,* fasting plasma glucose; *HBV,* hepatitis B vaccine; *HIV,* human immunodeficiency virus; *HRT,* hormone replacement therapy; *IVDU,* intravenous drug user; *MMR,* measles-mumps-rubella; *MVA,* motor vehicle accident; *PPD,* purified protein derivative; *RPR,* rapid plasma reagin; *STD,* sexually transmitted disease; *Td,* tetanus and diphtheria.

Alaskan, Pacific Islander, Native American, and religious communities). Vaccinate women who have male partners who have had sex with men or are IVDUs. Consider vaccination for institutionalized persons and workers in these institutions, for military personnel, and for day care, hospital, and laboratory workers.

- HBV: Vaccinate against HBV in blood product recipients (including hemodialysis clients), persons with frequent occupational exposure to blood or blood products, persons traveling to countries with endemic HBV, household and sexual contacts of HBV carriers, those with multiple recent sex partners or recent sex partners with diagnoses of other recently acquired STDs, prostitutes, and women who have male partners who have had sex with men or are IVDUs.

- MMR: Vaccinate clients born after 1956 and those who lack evidence of immunity to measles (e.g., documented administration of live vaccine on or after the first birthday, laboratory evidence of immunity, or history of diagnosed measles). Ensure women clients are not pregnant before immunizing. Women should not become pregnant for at least 3 months after receiving rubella vaccine.

- Pneumococcal vaccine: Vaccinate clients who have medical conditions that increase the risk of pneumococcal infection (e.g., DM, sickle cell disease, nephrotic syndrome, chronic cardiac or pulmonary disease, Hodgkin's disease, anatomic asplenia, alcoholism, cirrhosis, multiple myeloma, renal disease, and conditions associated with immunosuppression). Vaccinate immunocompetent institutionalized persons who live in high-risk environments or social settings (e.g., certain Native American and Native Alaskan populations). Vaccinate all those older than 65 years.

- Td: Administer Td vaccine every 10 years.

- Varicella: Vaccinate healthy adults without a history of chickenpox or previous immunization. Consider serologic testing for presumed susceptible adults.

REFERENCES

American Academy of Family Physicians. (1997). American Academy of Family Physicians age charts for periodic health examination. In R. B. Murray & J. P. Zentner (Eds.), *Health assessment and promotion strategies* (6th ed., pp. 853-867). Norwalk: Appleton & Lange.

Barry, H. C., & Ebell, M. H. (2000). The woman's health maintenance exam. In M. S. Smith & L. A. Shimp (Eds.), *20 Common problems in women's health care* (pp. 3-20). New York: McGraw-Hill.

Brown, K. M. (2000). *Management guidelines for women's health nurse practitioners.* Philadelphia: Lippincott.

Estes, M. (1998). *Health assessment and physical examination.* New York: Delmar.

Fleischman, C., Honebrink, A., Sherif, K., & Lonmuir, S. (1998). Guidelines for preventive health screening in women. *Women's Health in Primary Care, 1*(5), 413-423.

Johnson, B. E. (1996). Health promotion and disease detection in adult women. In A. A. Johnson, B. E. Johnson, J. L. Murray, & B. S. Apgar (Eds.), *Women's health care handbook* (pp. 7-11). Philadelphia: Hanley & Belfus.

Prevention (1997). *Harvard Women's Health Watch.* 2-4.

Robinson, D., Kidd, P., & Rogers, K. M. (2001). *Primary care across the lifespan.* St. Louis: Mosby.

Youngkin, E. Q., & Davis, M. S. (1997). *Women's health: A primary care clinical guide.* Norwalk: Appleton & Lange.

Review Questions

1. Laurie Hopkins is a 26-year-old clerk at a large grocery store. Which of these comments made by Laurie supports the fact that she is meeting the expected developmental task for her age?
- **a.** "I have several close friends from work; we have lots in common and spend lots of time together."
- **b.** "I date occasionally but I'm really not interested in a steady boyfriend."
- **c.** "I rarely visit my brother and sister; they live too far away."
- **d.** "A friend and I make rag dolls and donate them to a homeless shelter."

2. Which of the following aspects of a plan of care describes primary prevention for a 30-year-old woman?
- **a.** Recommend ibuprofen for menstrual cramps.
- **b.** Advise Tucks for hemorrhoids.
- **c.** Advise use of sunscreen.
- **d.** Advise limiting caffeine to determine its effect on palpitations.

3. Sandy is a 33-year-old woman. Which strategy in a management plan for Sandy is secondary prevention?
- **a.** Pre-conception counseling
- **b.** Contraception counseling
- **c.** Exercises to perform after an ankle sprain
- **d.** Pap smear

4. Which of the following immunizations is appropriate for all women every 10 years?
- **a.** Varicella
- **b.** Td
- **c.** Hepatitis B
- **d.** Influenza

5. Miriam Wilder is a widowed 47-year-old with two adult children. Which factor in Mrs. Wilder's history indicates that she is meeting the expected developmental task for her age?
- **a.** Sexual intimacy within a mutually monogamous relationship
- **b.** Weekly sessions reading on tape for the blind
- **c.** Working as an insurance clerk in a large hospital
- **d.** Visiting twice monthly with her former in-laws

6. Connie Jones is a 26-year-old who presents for an annual examination. History reveals casual sex, use of tanning bed twice weekly, smoking half-pack of cigarettes daily, high-fat diet, and drinking three beers during the weekend. Which action is not essential in assessment of Ms. Jones?

a. STD testing
b. Skin examination
c. Pap smear
d. Mammography

7. Ms. Widener, 45 years old, has a family history positive for cancer. Results of her last mammogram and proctoscopy were negative. How often should these tests be repeated?

a. Repeat mammography in 1 to 3 years and proctoscopy in 3 to 5 years.
b. Repeat mammography every 6 months and proctoscopy every 3 to 5 years.
c. Repeat mammography in 1 to 2 years and proctoscopy in 3 to 5 years.
d. Repeat mammography in 3 years and proctoscopy in 1 year.

Answers and Rationales

1. *Answer:* **a** (assessment)
Rationale: The developmental task of women in this age group is intimacy versus isolation. Intimacy goes beyond heterosexual relationships, including close, meaningful friendships. That this woman has close friendships supports her attainment of the developmental task (Brown, 2000).

2. *Answer:* **c** (implementation/plan)
Rationale: Choices a, b, and d include actions directed at managing existing problems; the goal in choice c is prevention (Robinson, et al. 2001).

3. *Answer:* **d** (implementation/plan)
Rationale: The Pap smear is the only secondary prevention measure (screening measure) listed. Choices a and b involve actions aimed at primary prevention, whereas choice c is a rehabilitative strategy (Robinson, et al. 2001).

4. *Answer:* **b** (implementation/plan)
Rationale: Immunization boosters for Td are recommended at 10-year intervals for adults (Fleischman, et al. 1998).

5. *Answer:* **b** (assessment)
Rationale: Generativity, supporting or leaving a legacy for the next generation, is the developmental task associated with this life stage. Reading for the blind is an excellent example of generativity. The other options do not serve as evidence of generativity (Robinson, et al. 2001).

6. *Answer:* **d** (assessment)
Rationale: Miss Jones's lifestyle places her at risk for several diseases. The NP should definitely assess her skin, screen for STDs, and perform a Pap smear to determine whether there are any problems. Mammography is not indicated by history or by age (Fleischman, et al. 1998).

7. *Answer:* **c** (implementation/plan)
Rationale: Mammography should be repeated in 1 to 2 years and proctoscopy should be repeated in 3 to 5 years (Barry & Ebell, 2000).

WELL CARE DURING PREGNANCY *Cheryl Pope Kish*

PRECONCEPTION CARE

Preconception care provides a systematic approach to identifying medical and behavioral risk factors that have the potential to affect pregnancy and enables preventive and therapeutic interventions before conception to optimize reproductive outcomes and the health of the woman and her children. Preconception care is particularly valuable for women with chronic illnesses or unhealthful lifestyles; organogenesis and early cell differentiation occur during the first weeks of pregnancy, often before the woman suspects she is pregnant. Modifying risks in advance of conception protects fetal development.

Models for Preconception Care (Ratcliffe, et al. 2001):

- Comprehensive visit for the designated purpose of preconception care involves extensive history with risk assessment, physical examination, and laboratory testing that mirrors the initial prenatal visit
- Opportunistic visit in which the elements of the preconception assessment are conducted while the woman is being seen for another reason (e.g., family planning, annual examination)

- Community-based initiatives that include elements of preconceptual care (e.g., screening tests)

Interventions for Preconceptual Care

- Follow up regarding abnormal laboratory or physical examination findings.
- Encourage the following behaviors:
  - Keep a menstrual calendar, eat a well-balanced diet, and decrease caffeine intake.
  - Eat a balanced diet based on the food pyramid.
  - Start taking one prenatal multivitamin and 0.4 mg of folic acid daily (4 mg if client has ever given birth to a child with neural tube defects).
  - Update immunizations and consider smoking cessation.
  - Avoid environmental toxins.
  - Avoid illicit drugs and limit alcohol.
  - Avoid over-the-counter (OTC), prescriptive, and homeopathic medicines until their use has been discussed with the prescribing health care provider.
  - Avoid vitamin A supplements of more than 8000 IU/day.
  - Exercise at least four times per week for 20 to 30 minutes.

- Limit the risk of congenital toxoplasmosis. Cook meat and wash vegetables thoroughly. If the woman has a pet cat that is allowed outside, have someone else empty the litter box.
- Practice safe sexual behaviors.
- Update immunizations.

INITIAL PRENATAL VISIT

This visit should take place as early in the pregnancy as is feasible.

History

- Update preconception, menstrual, contraceptive, social, sexual, and abuse histories.
- Assess medication use, including prescription OTC drugs and herbs.
- Assess habits, including smoking, use of alcohol and illicit drugs, exercise, hours of sleep, and safety.
- Assess readiness for pregnancy and parenthood; confirm pregnancy.
- Assess genetic risk; screen for potential preterm labor.
- Determine estimated date of delivery (EDD) by means of Nägele's rule: Note first day of last menstrual period; subtract 3 months and add 7 days to that date.
- Perform ultrasonography as indicated for the purposes of dating and assessing vaginal bleeding, maternal pelvic masses, uterine abnormalities, ectopic pregnancy, and the presence of multiple gestation.
- Obtain titers for toxoplasmosis, rubella, cytomegalovirus, herpes, and hepatitis as indicated.
- Assess high-risk sexual behavior (e.g., history of STDs, new or multiple partners, and community epidemiology). Perform a *Chlamydia* and gonorrhea screen.

Interventions

- Follow up regarding abnormal laboratory or physical examination findings.
- Encourage the following behaviors:
  - Eat a well-balanced diet and decrease caffeine intake.
  - Start taking one prenatal multivitamin with folic acid.
  - Update immunizations and consider smoking cessation.
  - Avoid environmental toxins, illicit drugs, alcohol, and OTC, prescription, and homeopathic medicines until their use in pregnancy has been discussed with the health care provider.
  - Prevent STDs. Avoid high-risk sexual behavior; use condoms.
  - Exercise at least four times per week for 20 to 30 minutes.

- Limit risk of congenital toxoplasmosis by cooking meat and washing vegetables thoroughly and by having someone else empty the litter box of a pet cat allowed outside.
- Provide the following health education:
  - Discuss prenatal classes and infant feeding (breast versus bottle).
  - Discuss physiologic changes that occur during pregnancy.
  - Note contraindications (if any) for intercourse.
  - Instruct regarding warning signs that require notification of the health care provider, what to avoid, what to do in case of an emergency, and the frequency of prenatal visits.
- Provide psychosocial support and referrals as needed.
- Provide information to relieve discomforts of pregnancy.

Client Teaching Regarding Discomfort during Pregnancy

First Trimester

- Breast tenderness: Wearing a supportive bra may be helpful. Discuss with partner the need for gentleness when touching breasts during lovemaking. Acetaminophen may be used.
- Constipation: Exercise regularly. Increase consumption of water and other liquids. Add fiber to diet, with fresh fruits and whole-grain breads. Drink prune juice. Milk laxatives (milk of magnesia), stool softeners, and bulk producers may be necessary.
- Headaches: Treat with rest; relaxation exercises; warm bath; warm or cold compresses to forehead; face, head, and shoulder massage; and aromatherapy. Acetaminophen may be used.
- Hemorrhoids: Avoid constipation and prolonged sitting. Use warm sitz baths and then application of witch hazel.
- Nausea and vomiting is self-limiting. Take small, frequent meals, with a protein snack at bedtime. Try hard candy, raspberry leaf tea, or 10 drops of peppermint spirits in half of a glass of water. Avoid greasy and spicy foods. Keep dry crackers at the bedside. Drink carbonated beverages. If dehydration, ketosis, or electrolyte abnormalities are present, antiemetics (meclizine, diphenhydramine, and metoclopramide) or pyridoxine may be used.
- Urinary frequency: Decrease caffeine intake. This symptom is limited to early weeks of pregnancy and time after lightening occurs.
- Varicosities: Wear supportive stockings or antiembolism stockings. Rest and elevate legs when possible. Perineal pads may help vulvar varicosities.

Second Trimester

- Backache (musculoskeletal strain): Avoid excessive weight gain, note posture, use good body mechanics, and wear flat or low-heeled shoes. Place a footstool under one foot while standing, a pillow in lumbar area while sitting, and a pillow between the knees while lying on side. Massage and apply ice or heat.

- Backache (sacroiliac dysfunction): Place a wedge-shaped pillow underneath the abdomen while lying on side. Exercise.
- Dizziness and faintness: Avoid lying flat on back, dehydration, and prolonged standing or sitting. Change position slowly. Lie in left lateral position.
- Leukorrhea: Bathe daily; wear cotton underwear and change it frequently.
- Leg cramps: Exercise, including calf stretch exercises and walking. Keep legs warm. Decrease phosphate intake by decreasing milk intake.
- Round ligament pain: Avoid twisting and sudden movements. Bend over or raise knee to chest on affected side. Rest and apply warm compresses.

Third Trimester

- Braxton Hicks contractions: Learn to differentiate between true and false labor. Empty bladder frequently. Increase fluid intake. Resting in a left lateral recumbent position or exercising lightly may help to relieve discomfort. Use relaxation techniques and warm tub baths.
- Edema: Avoid prolonged sitting or standing. Lie in left lateral recumbent position for 1 to 2 hours twice a day and sleep in that position. Elevate legs when possible. Refrain from wearing clothes that constrict the extremities. Increase fluid intake and decrease intake of sugar and fats. Moderate sodium intake.
- Heartburn: Take small, frequent meals. Try eating papaya or raw almonds after meals. Refrain from lying recumbent after eating. Avoid fried, spicy, and gas-producing foods. Sleep with head raised on stacked pillows. Antacids with magnesium hydroxide or magnesium trisilicate (Gaviscon) may be used. Avoid antacids with baking soda, aluminum, or high sodium contents.
- Skin rashes: Apply ice. Diphenhydramine may be used. If relief is not obtained, a dermatologic referral is necessary.

RETURN VISITS
Frequency of Visits

- From 6 to 28 weeks: visits every 4 weeks, or sooner if indicated
- From 28 to 34 weeks: visits every 2 weeks, or sooner if indicated
- From 34 to 41 weeks: visits every week, or sooner if indicated
- If overdue by accurate dating: visits 2 times per week

History

- Fetal movement
- Nausea and vomiting
- Vaginal bleeding or discharge
- Contractions
- Cramping or pelvic pressure
- Dysuria or frequency
- Headaches
- Scotoma or blurred vision
- Edema
- Preterm labor symptoms
- Pain
- Chest
- Abdomen
- Back legs
- Skin changes
- Fever or exposure to infectious disease
- Numbness or tingling of the hands or wrists
- Genital lesions, sores, or growths
- Trauma
- Medications taken
- Assess parental-fetal attachment
- Risk factors for development of family maladaptive behaviors
- Unplanned pregnancy (rape), marital discord or family violence, STD, substance abuse, HIV-seropositive status, adolescence
- Other factors: limited social support and educational background

Laboratory and Diagnostic Procedures

- Proteinuria, glucosuria, ketonuria
- Ultrasonography as indicated
- 9 to 11 weeks: chorionic villi sampling as indicated
- 12 to 14 weeks: early amniocentesis as indicated
- 15 to 16 weeks: traditional amniocentesis as indicated
- 15 to 18 weeks: maternal serum alpha-fetoprotein or maternal serum multiple marker screening
- 24 to 28 weeks: hemoglobin or hematocrit, diabetes screening, and antibody screening, group B streptococcus culture

Physical Examination

- Blood pressure
- Weight
- Fundal height
- Fetal heart rate (FHR)
- Presentation (Leopold's maneuvers)
- Edema
- Other elements as indicated

Interventions

- Fundal height in centimeters should be equal to the number of weeks of gestation plus or minus 2 cm. If fundal height is 3 to 4 cm smaller or larger than the gestational age in weeks, review the dating parameters and the ultrasonograms. Follow up regarding other abnormal laboratory or physical examination findings.

TABLE **4-15** Complications of Pregnancy

COMPLICATION	KEY ASSESSMENT	KEY INTERVENTIONS
Vaginal bleeding second and third trimester	Rule out: • Cervicitis • Cervical polyp • Molar pregnancy (fundal height less than expected for dates; no FHR; possible expulsion of grapelike clear vesicles; excess nausea and vomiting; snowstorm pattern on ultrasonogram) • Leiomyomata (irregular contour uterus) • Placenta previa (painless bleeding; low-lying placenta on ultrasound; avoid vaginal examination) • Placenta abruptio (painful bleeding)	Identify cause. Refer as needed.
Size larger than expected for dates	Assess for: • Polyhydramnios • Multiple pregnancy • Macrosomia • Leiomyoma • Inaccurate dating	Refer as indicated by cause. With fetal macrosomia, assess for gestational diabetes. Note whether client is at risk for postpartum hemorrhage. With polyhydramnios, evaluate newborn for gastrointestinal anomalies. Teach preterm labor prevention strategies.
Size smaller than expected for dates	Assess for: • Inaccurate dating • Incorrect measurement of fundal height • Oligohydramnios • IUGR	Refer as indicated by cause. Conduct fetal surveillance. Advise good nutrition and smoking cessation. If oligohydramnios, evaluate newborn for urinary anomalies.
Multiple pregnancy	Risk factors: • Infertility treatment • Family history of maternal dizygotic twins • Increased parity and maternal age Assess for: • Size/date discrepancy • Increased HCG • Multiple FHR • Extra fetal parts on palpation Complications: • Low birth weight/preterm labor • Gestational diabetes • PIH • IUGR • Anemia • Malpresentation • Twin-to-twin transfusion	Refer to obstetrician. Teach preterm labor prevention strategies. Advise about nutrition adequacy. Conduct fetal surveillance.

Continued

TABLE **4-15** Complications of Pregnancy—Cont'd

COMPLICATION	KEY ASSESSMENT	KEY INTERVENTIONS
Gestational diabetes	Risk factors: • Advanced maternal age • Obesity • Family history diabetes • Black, Hispanic, or Native American ethnicity • Previous fetal macrosomia or unexplained fetal death • Earlier screening indicated with risk factors Complications: • PIH • Polyhydramnios • Fetal macrosomia • Cesarean delivery • Postpartum hemorrhage • Fetal complications Universal prenatal screening at 24 to 28 weeks with 50 g of glucose: • Score higher than 140 indicates need for additional testing 3-hour glucose tolerance test: NPO 8 hours before test • FBS followed by 100 g of glucose; venous blood glucose tested at 1, 2, and 3 hours. Cutoff scores: • FBS, 105 • 1 hour, 190 • 2 hours, 165 • 3 hours, 145 Diagnosis of gestational diabetes requires at least 2 values elevated.	• Refer to or seek co-management by obstetrician and endocrinologist. • Refer to CDE for education. • Dietary prescription: ADA or carbohydrate counting should be used (refer to dietitian as needed). • Use insulin if unable to control with diet. Oral hypoglycemics are contraindicated in pregnancy. • Conduct home blood glucose monitoring several times daily to optimize management. Tight control of blood glucose decreases complications. • Reevaluate postpartum. • 20% to 50% develop chronic diabetes later in life. Risk decreases with maintenance of normal weight.
PIH	Assess for preeclampsia (classic signs at more than 20 weeks gestation) • Hypertension (30 mm Hg systolic or 15 mm Hg diastolic over baseline) • Proteinuria • Edema (face and hands, pitting, excess weight gain) Other signs: • Headache • Blurred vision • Epigastric pain • Oliguria	• Refer or seek co-management with obstetrician. • Conduct close maternal and fetal surveillance. • Increased protein diet and increased fluids are recommended. • Teach client concerning risks. • With increasing severity, may prescribe bed rest and frequent left lateral position to increase perfusion to placenta and kidneys. • May require hospitalization with decreased-stimuli environment. • RUQ or epigastric pain often precedes seizure. • Recommend choice of anti-hypertensive medication, such as alpha methyldopa (Aldomet). • Magnesium sulfate may be needed to prevent seizures.

HELLP syndrome:

Assess for eclampsia—look for seizure activity before, during, or up to 48 hours after delivery. Fetal risk increases with seizures.

Risks factors for PIH:

- Nulliparity
- Family history of PIH
- Chronic HTN
- History of PIH
- Obesity
- Gestational diabetes
- Thrombophilias

Prolonged pregnancy

- Fetal movement counts
- Nonstress testing
- Contraction stress testing
- Biophysical profile

- Give anticipatory guidance related to induction versus expectant management.
- Give psychosocial support and referrals as needed.

ADA, American Diabetes Association diet; *CDE*, certified diabetes educator; *FBS*, fasting blood sugar; *FHR*, fetal heart rate; *HELLP*, hemolysis, elevated liver enzymes, low platelet count; *HCG*, human chorionic gonadotropin; *HTN*, hypertension; *IUGR*, intrauterine growth restriction; *NPO*, nothing by mouth; *PIH*, pregnancy-induced hypertension; *RUQ*, right upper quadrant.

TABLE **4-16** Medications during Pregnancy

GENERAL PRINCIPLES OF MEDICATION ADMINISTRATION DURING PREGNANCY	TERATOGENIC MEDICATIONS
Use FDA pregnancy risk categories (following) when prescribing drugs; select the drug with the safest profile, when choices exist.	ACE inhibitors
A Controlled studies show no risk	Alcohol
B No evidence of risk in humans	Androgens/testosterone
C Risk cannot be ruled out	Carbamazepine
D Positive evidence of risk	Cocaine
X Contraindicated in pregnancy	Coumadin derivatives
For conditions that are self-limited, encourage woman to decline	DES
medications and to use nonpharmacologic management.	Ergotamine
Postpone treatment until after organogenesis during first	Folic acid antagonists (e.g., methotrexate, aminopterin)
trimester when possible.	Lead
Use one agent, if possible.	Lithium
Use the lowest possible dose to achieve desired effect.	Live virus vaccines (MMR, varicella, OPV)
Avoid newly introduced medicines when possible	Phenytoin
Drug dosages may need to be changed during pregnancy	Streptomycin and kanamycin
because of increased volume of distribution and increased	Tetracycline
renal and hepatic clearance.	Trimethadione and paramethadione
At times, serious maternal illness requires medications that	Valproic acid
compromise the fetus. A careful benefit/risk analysis,	Vitamin A and derivatives (isotretinoin, etretinate, retinoids)
including referral to a physician, is essential.	Almost never justified:
	Clarithromycin
	Doxycycline
	Fluoroquinolones
	Oral hypoglycemics

ACE, Angiotensin-converting enzyme; *DES,* diethylstilbestrol; *FDA,* Food and Drug Administration; *MMR,* measles-mumps-rubella; *OPV,* oral polio vaccine.

- Administer Rho(D) immune globulin (RhoGAM) at 28 weeks as indicated.
- Provide information to relieve discomforts of pregnancy.
- Continue encouragement of health promotion activities.
- Provide education on the following topics:
  - Planning for labor and birth
  - Sibling preparation
  - Warning signs of complications
  - Infant car seat
  - Infant feeding and care
  - Postpartum self-care
- Provide psychosocial support and referrals as needed.

See Table 4-15 for a summary of complications in pregnancy and Table 4-16 for a summary of medications in pregnancy.

REFERENCES

American College of Obstetricians and Gynecologists. (1997). *Teratology* (Technical Bulletin #236). Washington, DC: American College of Obstetricians and Gynecologists.

Briggs, G. G., Carson, D. S., & Rayburn, W. F. (2000). Which medications are safe in pregnancy? *Patient Care, December 30,* 19-33.

Brown, K. M. (2000). *Management guidelines for women's health nurse practitioners.* Philadelphia: F. A. Davis.

Cash, J. C., & Glass, C. A. (2000). *Family practice guidelines.* Philadelphia: Lippincott, Williams & Wilkins.

Davis, D. C. (1996). The discomforts of pregnancy. *Journal of Obstetric, Gynecologic, and Neonatal Nursing, 25*(1), 73-81.

Dixon, D., Cobb, T. G., & Clarke, R. W. (2000). The first prenatal visit: A primary care review. *Clinician Reviews, 10*(4), 53-72.

Hawkins, J. W., Roberto-Nichols, D. M., & Stanley-Haney, J. L. (2000). *Protocols for nurse practitioners* (7th ed.). New York: Tiresias.

Helton, M. R. (2000). Prenatal care. In M. A. Smith & L. A. Shimp (Eds.), *20 Common problems in women's health care* (pp. 65-89). New York: McGraw-Hill.

Hueppchen, N. A., & Pressman, E. K. (1999). Preconception care: Planning for a healthy pregnancy. *Women's Health in Primary Care, 2*(4), 259-278.

Powrie, R. O., & Kurl, R. (1999). Prescribing drugs to pregnant women. *Women's Health in Primary Care, 2*(7), 547-554.

Ratcliffe, S. D., Baxley, E. G., Byrd, J. E., & Sakornbut, E. L. (2001). *Family practice obstetrics* (2nd ed.). Philadelphia: Hanley & Belfus.

Smith, M.A, & Shrimp, L.A. (2000). *20 common problems in women's health care.* New York: McGraw-Hill.

Star, W. L., Shannon, M. T., Lommel, L. L., & Gutierrez, Y. M. (1999). *Ambulatory obstetrics* (3rd ed.). San Francisco: USCF Nursing Press.

Walsh, H. J., & Hoody, D. L. (1995). Gestational diabetes: Screening and diagnosis. *ADVANCE for Nurse Practitioners, June*, 37-38, 50.

Youngkin, E. Q., & Davis, M. S. (1998). *Women's health: A primary care clinical guide.* Stamford, CT: Appleton & Lange.

Zamorski, M. A., & Green, M. D. (2001). NHBPEP report on high blood pressure in pregnancy: A summary for family physicians. *American Family Physicians, 64*, 263-270, 273-274.

Review Questions

1. Leslie is a sexually active married 27-year-old whose cycles are regular. She has missed two periods and has objective signs of pregnancy. If her last menstrual period began on July 10 and ended on July 15, what is her EDD?

   a. April 17
   b. April 22
   c. May 17
   d. May 22

2. The NP performs a pelvic examination on Dory at an initial prenatal visit. Which finding of the pelvic examination is inconsistent with a diagnosis of early pregnancy?

   a. Softening of the lower uterine segment
   b. Friability of the cervix
   c. Softening of the cervix
   d. Pale vaginal membranes and cervix

3. At her initial prenatal visit, Kate provides a 24-hour dietary recall, which includes the following data related to breakfast and dinner.

Breakfast	*Dinner*
Orange juice (small glass)	Roast beef
Oatmeal with raisins	Asparagus spears
Milk (1 pint)	Small baked potato with
Decaffeinated	a pat of butter
hot tea (1 cup)	Roll
	Fruit salad
	Milk (1 pint, skim)

In addition to these meals, which lunch menu will best meet Kate's daily nutritional requirements?

   a. Grilled hamburger on a bun, with tomato and lettuce, coleslaw, apple, and pint of milk
   b. Cup of cream of tomato soup, cream cheese and pineapple sandwich, apple pie, and decaffeinated coffee with cream
   c. Cup of beef bouillon, bacon, lettuce, and tomato sandwich, jello, and lemonade
   d. Lettuce, tomato, and cucumber salad with French dressing, prune muffin, slice of melon, and pint of milk

4. Mrs. Jasper's obstetrical history reveals the following:

Pregnant now

1999: Gave birth to full-term male

1996: Gave birth to full-term female

1992: Had miscarriage at 8 weeks

1990: Stillbirth after abruptio placenta at 9 months

1987: Gave birth to female at 30 weeks who died 3 days later Which data would the NP chart?

   a. G4-2-1-2-2
   b. G6-3-1-1-2
   c. G6-2-1-2-2
   d. G5-3-1-1-2

5. Lindy is 7 weeks pregnant when she presents for her initial visit. Which factor in her history is consistent with a risk for toxoplasmosis?

   a. She makes glazed pottery.
   b. She has a pet cockateil.
   c. She eats sushi and steak tartar regularly.
   d. She drinks orange juice whipped with wheat germ and a raw egg.

6. JoBeth asks the NP if she can play tennis during her pregnancy. Which response is most appropriate?

   a. "How much tennis have you played in the past and how long ago?"
   b. "Sure, as long as you don't get overly tired."
   c. "Swimming would be better for you. Do you like to swim?"
   d. "It's best not to engage in active sports; you might fall."

7. Miriam complains of the darkening skin over her nose during pregnancy. In addition to informing her that this is a normal finding associated with pregnancy, the NP should advise Miriam to do which of the following?

   a. Stop using soap on her face.
   b. Use a lubricating cream nightly.
   c. Apply diluted lemon juice twice daily.
   d. Keep the area protected from direct sunlight.

8. Nancy is asked by the NP to keep a record of fetal movements and to bring it to the next clinic visit. One week later, she calls the clinic and anxiously reports that she has not felt the baby move in nearly an hour. Which initial comment by the NP would be best?

   a. "You need to come to the clinic right away for an evaluation."
   b. "Have you been smoking?"
   c. "The baby may be asleep; they take 20- to 30-minute naps."
   d. "Are you having any other problems with your pregnancy?"

9. Susan's glucose screen at 24 weeks' gestation is 160 mg/dL. Which action by the NP is most appropriate in response to that finding?

   a. Notify Susan of the normal finding on the test.
   b. Prescribe a low-carbohydrate diet.
   c. Schedule a 3-hour glucose tolerance test.
   d. Refer her to a diabetologist.

Answers and Rationales

1. *Answer:* **a** (assessment)
   Rationale: To use Nägele rule to determine the woman's EDD, subtract 3 months and add 7 days and a year (Star, et al. 1999).

2. *Answer:* d (assessment)

Rationale: Choice a refers to Hegar's sign and choice c refers to Goodell's sign, both indicative of early pregnancy. The cervix is often friable during pregnancy because of vascular congestion and hormonal changes. The vaginal mucosa and cervix typically have a bluish tint during early pregnancy (Chadwick's sign) as a result of hormonal changes (Ratcliffe, et al. 2001).

3. *Answer:* a (assessment)

Rationale: The partial 24-hour recall indicates limited protein and milk; choice a provides the best source of those nutrients (Ratcliffe, et al. 2001).

4. *Answer:* b (assessment)

Rationale: This woman is in her sixth pregnancy; she has had three full-term deliveries, one premature delivery, and one abortion. She has two living children (Smith & Shimp, 2000).

5. *Answer:* c (assessment)

Rationale: The risk of toxoplasmosis increases with emptying the cat litter pan of a pet allowed outdoors and with eating undercooked meat and poorly washed vegetables (Star, et al. 1999).

6. *Answer:* a (implementation/plan)

Rationale: Assessment always precedes intervention. Pregnant women may play tennis during pregnancy if they are experienced players who play regularly. It would not be appropriate to learn tennis during pregnancy or to restart playing after becoming deconditioned (Star, et al. 1999).

7. *Answer:* d (implementation/plan)

Rationale: The woman is describing melasma (mask of pregnancy), which is a normal hormone-related change that occurs in many pregnancies. It is neither preventable nor treatable; however, it can be minimized by protecting the area from direct sunlight with sunscreen or a hat (Star, et al. 1999).

8. *Answer:* c (implementation/plan)

Rationale: If decreased fetal movement continues, the woman will need to be evaluated. At this point, however, the fetus may be sleeping. The fetus sleeps for 20 to 30 minutes at a time (Star, et al. 1999).

9. *Answer:* c (implementation/plan)

Rationale: A glucose level higher than 140 mg/dL on the glucose screen should be followed up with a 3-hour glucose tolerance test (Star, et al. 1999).

WELLNESS DURING POSTPARTUM   *Cheryl Pope Kish*

HISTORY

- Review clinic or office records for antepartum course, results of laboratory tests, and problem identification and treatment.
- Review hospital records (discharge notes) for intrapartum and postpartum courses. Note duration of labor; type of delivery and anesthesia; episiotomy; sex, Apgar score, weight, and length of newborn; and maternal or newborn complications and treatment. Note discharge hemoglobin and hematocrit levels.
- Inquire about course since discharge (interval history). Include general health, any problems, eating, sleeping, urinary and bowel function, coping, family support, pain, resumption of coitus and birth control method in use or preferred, readmission to hospital, emergency department visits, telephone follow-up for illness, transition to maternal role and adjustment of family to newborn, infant follow-up visit, feeding, and care.
- Review relevant systems as follows.
  - Breasts: pain, integrity of nipples, status of and concerns about breast feeding, if applicable, symptoms of engorgement, milk stasis, or mastitis
  - Abdomen/back: pain, healing of cesarean wound, if applicable, flank pain or paraspinous muscle pain
  - Bladder function: resumption of normal voiding pattern, incontinence, dysuria, signs of urinary tract infection
  - Bowel function: resumption of normal bowel movement pattern, constipation, discomfort (especially with history of third- or fourth-degree perineal laceration), hemorrhoids
  - Perineum: healing of episiotomy site, if applicable, signs of infection, discomfort, topical analgesia or anesthesia in use
  - Lochia or resumption of menses: characteristics of lochia, duration, odor, presence of clots; date menses resumed, duration, amount compared with before pregnancy, associated problems
  - Legs: pain or swelling, varicose veins

PHYSICAL EXAMINATION

- General: Assess affect.
- Assess weight compared with prepregnancy weight.
- Assess vital signs.
- Auscultate heart and lungs.
- Thyroid: Palpate for enlargement.
- Breasts: Note nipple integrity in lactating woman, engorgement, masses, mastitis.
- Abdomen: Note involution of uterus, tenderness, masses, healing of abdominal incision (if applicable), diastasis recti, lymph adenopathy.
- Legs: Note varicosities, swelling, tenderness in calf, Homans' sign, evidence of thrombophlebitis.
- Perineum: Note healing of episiotomy and lacerations.
- Speculum examination: Note presence of rugae, discharge, lesions or lacerations, signs of infection.
- Bimanual examination: Note cervical motion tenderness; status of involution (uterine size); position, mobility, consistency, and tenderness of uterus;

TABLE **4-17**   Common Postpartum Complications

COMPLICATION	CLINICAL FEATURES	MANAGEMENT
Late postpartum hemorrhage: excessive bleeding after first 24 hours postpartum; usually related to subinvolution of placental site or retained placental fragments	Uterine bleeding that continues past normal lochia or is excessive; uterine cramping may be evident. Normal lochia progression: postpartum days 1-3, lochia rubra (bright red); days 4-7, lochia serosa (serous or brown); days 10+, lochia alba (creamy and in decreasing amounts). Normal lochia has fleshy odor and does not contain clots larger than dime-sized.	Generally requires referral to obstetrician for administration of oxytocic agent, such as IV oxytocin (Pitocin) or oral methylergonovine maleate (Methergine, 0.2 mg qid). May require evacuation of uterus to remove placental fragments.
Postpartum depression	Signs of clinical depression beyond 1 to 2 weeks that affects client's ability to function. Suicide ideation is possible. Note: normal postpartum blues during first 1 to 2 weeks are self-limited and include depressed affect, disturbances in eating and sleeping, and difficulties concentrating or making decisions but do not include illogical thought, hallucinations, delusions, or total inability to function, which may occur with postpartum depression.	If suspected, administer screening test for postpartum depression (i.e., Edinburgh Postnatal Depression Scale). Assess suicide and homicide potential. Provide emergency intervention as needed. Consider a no-suicide contract. Refer to mental health provider for antidepressants and individual psychotherapy. Provide anticipatory guidance to family.
Metritis (endometritis): infection of intrauterine cavity, often polymicrobial; can extend to adjacent structures (parametritis)	Risk factors: cesarean delivery, prolonged labor, prolonged rupture of membranes, invasive labor procedures, maternal anemia. Fever higher than 100.4° F; abdominal pain and tenderness; foul lochia	Referral to obstetrician for hospitalization and IV antibiotics may be required. Antibiotic coverage, whether parenteral or oral, is based on culture.
Mastitis: infection of breast tissue in lactating woman secondary to ascending organisms from infant's nasopharynx or hands of staff or nursing mother	Usually preceded by milk stasis. Signs: fever, often higher than 101° F; red, hot, tender wedge of breast tissue. Risk factors: poor hygiene, plastic-lined nursing pads, incorrect positioning to nurse, incorrect pumping technique, restrictive bra, change in number of feedings, failure to empty breasts, lowered maternal defenses (fatigue, stress).	Continue to breast feed. Treat empirically for *Staphylococcus aureus* (usual organism) with 10-day course of penicillinase-resistant antibiotic (i.e., dicloxacillin, 250-500 mg PO q6h) or first- or second-generation cephalosporin (i.e., cephalexin, 250-500 mg PO q6h). Apply moist heat. Use analgesia.

Continued

TABLE **4-17** Common Postpartum Complications—*cont'd*

COMPLICATION	CLINICAL FEATURES	MANAGEMENT
	If pain persists throughout and between feedings, assess newborn for thrush or candidal diaper rash and suspect candida as cause of mastitis and treat accordingly. Without timely or effective treatment, may extend to abscess. Suspect if not improved after 2-3 days of antibiotics.	Abscesses may require surgical incision and drainage. Can continue to breast feed if not too painful or may pump temporarily to maintain lactation.
Transient postpartum thyroiditis: autoimmune; risk factor, family history of thyroid disorders	Initial symptoms of hyperthyroidism at 2-3 months postpartum followed by hypothyroid symptoms Most common symptoms noted: thyroid enlargement, fatigue, palpitations, emotional lability Assess TSH and free T4 levels.	Rarely requires treatment because of transient state. Spontaneous resolution occurs in 70% or more. Others remain hypothyroidal and require replacement therapy. Consider as contributing factor to depression.

TSH, Thyroid-stimulating hormones.

Box 4-1   Important Points about Breast Feeding

Posters and written material about breast feeding support the clinical setting's reputation as a "breast feeding-friendly" practice site.

Inform woman that breast milk is considered nutritionally and immunologically superior. Breast feeding exclusively for 6 months should be recommended. *Advantages of breast feeding for baby* are increased resistance to infectious respiratory and ear infections; enhanced immune response to polio, tetanus, diphtheria, and *Haemophilus influenza*; and decreased chronic illness in childhood. *Advantages for mother* are faster uterine involution, positive bonding with baby, decreased incidence of breast and ovarian cancer, and protection against osteoporosis.

If inverted nipples occur prenatally, breast shells may be recommended during the last 8 weeks of pregnancy. Breast shells are designed to exert gentle negative pressure to draw out the nipple. Worn inside the bra, this flat, soft, silicone or plastic base has a hole for the nipple and a dome to enable air circulation.

Breast feeding extends WIC eligibility. Referral to La Leche League can be helpful for obtaining breast feeding information and support.

Breast milk is contraindicated for infants with mothers who have HIV/AIDS, hepatitis C, and T-cell leukemia virus, Type 1.

Caution breast feeding women to remind all providers that they are nursing so that any necessary medical testing and/or treatment can be modified accordingly. If a medication is essential, the woman may pump her breasts during treatment to sustain lactation. OCPs that contain estrogen are contraindicated; progesterone-only contraception should be delayed until lactation is well established so that the milk supply will not be affected.

The ability of women who have had breast implants or breast augmentation or reduction to breast feed depends on the specifics of the surgical procedure. In some cases, breast feeding is possible; in others, ducts or nerves have been compromised to such an extent that breast feeding is not possible. Implants themselves are not a contraindication to breast feeding.

Women who breast feed need an additional 500 calories per day. Complete vegetarians need to take multivitamins. Drinking to satisfy natural thirst provides the additional physiologic amounts of necessary fluid. Although occasional alcohol is not harmful in small amounts, it is best to delay nursing until the alcohol clears. Women who breast feed should be advised not to smoke; if they cannot quit smoking, they should be advised to decrease the number of cigarettes, wait 2 hours after smoking to nurse, and never smoke while nursing. Caffeine-containing beverages should be limited to two or fewer daily. The infant may experience GI distress with certain foods, such as chocolate or foods that form gas. If this is determined, those foods should be eliminated temporarily from the mother's diet.

The woman can be assured that the baby is getting adequate amounts of breast milk if the baby wets at least six to eight diapers daily.

Cornerstones of preventing/treating nipple soreness and pain:
- Correct latch-on positioning with baby's whole body facing mother, not just baby's head.
- Breaking suction by placing finger in baby's mouth
- Frequent changes of position to change configuration of mouth on nipple (cradling, football hold, side-lying of mother)
- Air-drying between feedings
- Exposure to sunlight or sun lamp for 1 to 2 minutes
- Avoiding drying agents on nipples, such as soap, alcohol, benzoin
- Use of nonallergenic anhydrous lanolin or A&D ointment
- Frequent changes of breast pads and avoiding those with plastic
- Frequent feeding

Suggestions for avoiding engorgement and milk stasis:
- Frequent feedings
- Manual expression of some milk to soften areola to help latch-on
- Moist heat before nursing
- Nursing on least sore side to start to facilitate let-down reflex
- Wearing supportive bra 24 hours a day

Suggestions for women attempting to suppress lactation:
- Wear supportive bra 24 hours daily for 1 week.
- Apply cold compresses or packs for comfort.
- Avoid stimulation of breasts (sexual activity, hot water in shower).
- Use cool, raw cabbage leaves for engorgement (effective for 24 hours); change cabbage leaf when wilted.

AIDS, Acquired immune deficiency syndrome; *GI,* gastrointestinal; *HIV,* human immunodeficiency virus; *OCP,* oral contraceptive pill; *WIC,* Women, Infants, and Children.

adnexa; vaginal muscle tone; evidence of cystocele or rectocele.

- Rectovaginal: Assess integrity of tissues affected by episiotomy and lacerations by palpating along scar; note tenderness of posterior vaginal septum, hemorrhoids.

LABORATORY TESTS

- Hemoglobin or hematocrit: complete blood count (CBC) with documented anemia or postpartum hemorrhage, Pap smear if last examination was more than 1 year ago
- Thyroid function tests with suspected postpartum thyroiditis
- Urinalysis
- Glucose testing: with documented gestational DM or macrosomia in newborn

PLAN

- Provide treatment for any identified problem, seeking consultation or providing referral as needed. (Table 4-17 summarizes common postpartum complications).
- Provide anticipatory guidance related to resumption of sexual activity. Important points include use of water-based lubricant until vagina is fully estrogenized (especially in lactating women); gentle intercourse after arousal; woman-dominant position to decrease pressure against episiotomy site; Kegel exercises several times daily to strengthen pelvic muscles; and for breast feeding mothers, nursing infant before coitus to prevent leakage of milk during foreplay or orgasm.
- Explore contraception options and inform woman about chosen method. Contraceptives containing estrogen are not recommended during the first 3 weeks postpartum because of the risk of thromboembolic disease.
- Provide support and guidance related to breast feeding, if applicable (Box 4-1). Refer to lactation consultant or La Leche League as needed.
- Administer rubella vaccination if woman is not immune and did not receive vaccine during postpartum hospital stay. Remind client that because live-virus vaccine is unsafe during pregnancy, avoiding pregnancy for a minimum of 3 months is essential. Conscientious contraception is critical.
- If hemoglobin level is less than 10 g, supplement iron and advise increase in dietary intake of iron.
- Encourage actions related to health maintenance: healthful diet, Kegel exercise, regular aerobic exercise, adequate rest, no smoking, limited alcohol intake, home, work, driving, and leisure safety factors.
- Recommend monthly BSE and annual gynecologic examinations with Pap smears.

REFERENCES

Bell, K. K., & Rawlings, N. L. (1998). Promoting breast-feeding by managing common lactation problems. *Nurse Practitioner, 23*(6), 102-123.

Berger, D., & Cook, C. L. (1998). Postpartum teaching priorities: The viewpoints of nurses and mothers. *Journal of Obstetric, Gynecologic, and Neonatal Nursing, 27*(2), 161-168.

Brown, K. M. (2000). *Management guidelines for women's health nurse practitioners.* Philadelphia: F. A. Davis.

Cash, J. C., & Glass, C. A. (2000). *Family practice guidelines.* Philadelphia: Lippincott.

Chez, R. A., & Friedman, A. K. (2000). Offering effective breast-feeding advice. *Contemporary Ob/Gyn, 45*(8), 32-50.

Fishbein, E. G., & Burggraf, E. (1998). Early postpartum discharge: How are mothers managing? *Journal of Obstetric, Gynecologic, and Neonatal Nursing, 27*(2), 142-148.

In support of breast-feeding: An action plan. (2001). *Consultant,* February, 295-296.

Kish, C. P. (2002). Postpartum. In D. Robinson (Ed.), *Clinical decision making for nurse practitioners: A case study approach.* Philadelphia: Lippincott.

Kish, C. P. (in press). The postpartum family at risk. In S. B. Olds, M. L. London, & P. A. W. Ladewig (Eds.), *Maternal-newborn nursing: A family- and community-based approach* (7th ed.). Upper Saddle River, NJ: Prentice Hall.

Kish, C. P. (1992). Postpartum home care. In I. Bobak (Ed.), *Maternity and gynecologic care* (5th ed., pp. 735-766). St. Louis: Mosby.

Montgomery, A. M. (2000). Breastfeeding and postpartum maternal care. *Primary Care, 27*(1), 237-250.

Star, W. L., Shannon, M. T., Lommel, L. L., & Gutierrez, Y. M. (1999). *Ambulatory obstetrics.* San Francisco: UCSF Nursing Press.

Stover, A. M., & Marnejon, J. G. (1995). Postpartum care. *American Family Physician, 52*(5), 1465-1472.

Williams, L. R., & Cooper, M. K. (1996). A new paradigm for postpartum care. *Journal of Obstetric, Gynecologic, and Neonatal Nursing, 25*(9), 745-749.

Review Questions

1. Pam Miller is a 25-year-old postpartum woman who plans to formula-feed her newborn. The NP advises Pam regarding ways to suppress lactation. Which behavior by Pam indicates a need for further teaching?

- **a.** She turns her back to running water in the shower to avoid stimulating her breasts.
- **b.** She wears a support bra around the clock the first week after delivery.
- **c.** She increases her fluid intake.
- **d.** She rubs her breasts several times daily with lanolin to promote comfort.

2. Donna Gilbert, a postpartum woman, has a warm, tender, wedge-shaped area in her left breast, low-grade fever, and flu-like symptoms. The NP diagnoses mastitis. In addition to ordering appropriate antibiotics, which action by the NP is appropriate?

- **a.** Advise Donna to continue breast feeding on both sides, starting with the unaffected side to enhance let-down reflex.
- **b.** Recommend that Donna cease breast feeding at once but continue to pump to sustain lactation.
- **c.** Order a drug to suppress lactation and an analgesic for pain relief.

d. Advise Donna to use cold compresses on her affected breast around the clock for comfort.

3. Which finding in a woman's history increases her risk for postpartum metritis?

   a. Precipitated labor and delivery
   b. Epidural anesthesia
   c. Having twins
   d. Prolonged labor

4. Paula Ryan presents for her postpartum follow-up examination after a normal vaginal delivery and postpartum course. Which objective finding of her pelvic examination is consistent with normal findings at 6 weeks' postpartum?

   a. Uterine size, 12-week size
   b. Rugated vagina with pink, moist membranes
   c. Cervical motion tenderness
   d. Reddened gap of 2 mm at episiotomy site

Answers and Rationales

1. *Answer:* **d** (evaluation)
   Rationale: Rubbing the breasts several times daily may provide too much stimulation to adequately suppress lactation (Kish, 2002).

2. *Answer:* **a** (implementation/plan)
   Rationale: Breast feeding is not contraindicated in cases of mastitis; continuing to empty the breasts is an effective treatment. The breast milk is not harmful to the infant; however, it is important that any antibiotics ordered to treat mastitis be safe for infants. The other actions are inappropriate for managing this woman's mastitis (Montgomery, 2000).

3. *Answer:* **d** (assessment)
   Rationale: Prolonged labor and its inherent need for frequent pelvic examinations increases the risk of postpartum metritis. The primary risk is cesarean delivery (Stover & Marnejon, 1995).

4. *Answer:* **b** (assessment)
   Rationale: At 6 weeks, the uterine size should be normal; the vaginal membranes are moist, pink, and rugated; there is no cervical motion tenderness; and the perineum should be well healed (Stover & Marnejon, 1995).

WELLNESS DURING MENOPAUSE   *Cheryl Pope Kish*

DEFINITION

Menopause is part of a natural biologic process that occurs with advancing age and involves a gradual decline in ovarian follicles and decreased responsiveness of the remaining follicles to follicle-stimulating hormone (FSH). Because the major source of estrogen is the ovarian follicle, this process causes a decrease in circulating estrogen and cessation of menstruation. *Menopause* is defined as the absence of menses for 12 consecutive months. The median age for menopause in the United States is 51.4 years; 95% of women experience menopause between ages 44 and 55 (Smith & Shimp, 2000). The average age has remained unchanged over time, despite better nutrition and health care. Because the life expectancy for women in now in the 80s, women spend approximately one-third of their lives in the postmenopausal stage. The age of natural menopause is genetically determined; smokers tend to experience menopause 2 years earlier than nonsmokers. Thin women experience more pronounced vasomotor symptoms. The interval of physiologic change that begins approximately 4 years before the cessation of menstruation and lasts for 1 year afterward is known as *perimenopause.*

   Menopause is said to be premature when it occurs before the age of 40 years. Induced menopause occurs with pelvic radiation, chemotherapy, and surgical removal of both ovaries (bilateral oophorectomy) and contributes to more intense menopausal symptoms because of the precipitous drop in circulating estrogen.

PHYSIOLOGY

Throughout the woman's reproductive life, there is a complex interplay of ovarian-secreted hormones (FSH and luteinizing hormone [LH]) in a feedback loop with estrogen. Ovarian function begins to decline approximately 10 years before menopause. As ovarian follicles decline and estrogen decreases, gonadotropin hormones are no longer inhibited; levels of FSH and LH rise. Over several years, estrogen production decreases to a level too low to initiate the LH surge required for ovulation; ovulation becomes irregular and then ceases. During that interval, many anovulatory cycles occur and women experience irregular menstrual patterns.

HORMONE REPLACEMENT THERAPY

Hormone replacement therapy (HRT) is often prescribed for perimenopausal and postmenopausal women to alleviate many short-term symptoms of estrogen deficiency and to protect against osteoporosis. HRT has been shown to alleviate vasomotor symptoms and symptoms of urogenital atrophy.

   Cardiovascular protection, once claimed as a benefit of HRT, is now uncertain. Recent studies indicate that HRT may not be beneficial for secondary prevention of coronary heart disease (CHD) because of early prothrombotic and proinflammatory effects of HRT.

NOTE: *NHLIB halted the HRT trial early when interim analysis revealed that combined conjugated estrogen/progesterone*

HRT increased the risk for breast cancer (26%), strokes (41%), cardiovascular disease (22%), and thromboembolism (double) in healthy menopausal women compared with a placebo. (Only oral HRT was tested.) No increased risk has been found for estrogen alone in hysterectomized women; that phase of the trial continues. Risk reduction was noted for colorectal cancer (37%) and fractures (24%). Researchers advise that short-term use of the combination HRT for symptom relief poses a small risk; long-term (more than 4 years) therapy is not recommended (Writing Group for the Women's Health Initiative, 2002).

PRE-HRT ASSESSMENT
History

- Note degree of menopausal symptoms, how bothersome they are, and whether they are naturally occurring or induced.
- Medical history: Note diseases that are contraindications for HRT (Table 4-18).
- Social history: Note alcohol and tobacco use.
- Family history: Note maternal age at menopause and presence of osteoporosis, CAD, hypertension, and breast or gynecologic cancer.

TABLE **4-18** Physiologic Changes of Menopause Caused by Decreased Estrogen

SYSTEM	CHANGES	INTERVENTIONS*
Breasts	Atrophy of glandular tissue; nipples become flatter and smaller; size and shape change	Reassure woman that these are normal changes associated with menopause.
Bone	More porous and fragile; increased risk of fracture	Provide safety information to minimize risk of fracture. Encourage therapy to prevent and treat.
Vulva	Atrophy of vulva; decreased subcutaneous tissue; decreased labia majora with some gaping; labia minora almost nonexistent; skin thins; pubic hair becomes sparse; dystrophies and pruritus are common	Reassure of normalcy of changes. Use of estrogen cream is recommended.
Vagina	Increased vaginal pH with increased risk of infections; vagina shorter and narrower, less elastic; some loss of vaginal rugae; membranes pale, thinner, and sensitive to trauma	Vaginal moisturizers (e.g., Replens) and lubricants can be used for intercourse. Use estrogen cream to reverse atrophic changes. Changes in vaginal tissue can be slowed with continuation of regular intercourse.
Uterus	Uterus decreases in size and weight; cervix pales, shrinks, and retracts with loss of fornices; endocervix becomes atrophic	
Ovaries	Shrink; no longer palpable normally	
Pelvic floor musculature	Musculature loses tone; increased incidence of prolapse, cystocele, and rectocele	Pelvic floor (Kegel) exercises maintain muscle tone.
Urinary tract changes	Bladder trigone and urethra atrophy; bladder capacity decreases; incontinence may occur	Recommend Kegel exercises, bladder training, and medication to treat incontinence as needed.
Vasomotor instability	Rapid rises in core temperature experienced by more than 80% of women; flushes/hot flashes, often with profuse perspiration; flashes last 3 to 4 minutes; may occur at night, disrupting sleep	Adjust room temperature; wear breathable fabrics, such as cotton, and layered clothing; use portable fan; limit caffeine, alcohol, warm spicy foods; use stress-management techniques; get regular exercise.
Mood changes	Many women report feeling anxious, irritable, or depressed; relationship with hormone change is unknown; CNS contains cells sensitive to estradiol, and decline of estradiol may have some effect	Exercise, regular diet, stress reduction are important.
Sleep disorders	REM sleep decreases with age and decline of estrogen. Sleep disorder may be exacerbated by hot flashes and night sweats	Evaluate naps, avoid caffeine and smoking, exercise (not before bedtime), maintain comfortable sleep environment, develop nighttime routine, use relaxation techniques, and avoid sleep medications.

*May include systemic HRT.
CNS, Central nervous system; *HRT,* hormone replacement therapy; *REM,* rapid eye movement.

- Note perception of menopause, beliefs about HRT, and feelings about resumption of menses, even temporarily. Note willingness to take medication (2 to 3 years may be adequate for control of menopausal symptoms). A high discontinuation rate exists for HRT because of lack of knowledge of its benefits, intolerance to side effects, and fear of associated cancer, particularly breast cancer.
- Assess for risks of CHD, breast cancer, and osteoporosis to determine appropriateness of prescribing HRT, as follows:
- Risks for CHD:
  - Hypertension
  - Cholesterol profile
  - Left ventricular hypertrophy
  - Smoking
  - DM
- Risks for breast cancer:
  - Family history
  - Age at menarche
  - Age at first live birth
  - Number and results of previous breast biopsies
- Risks for hip fracture (osteoporosis):
  - Maternal hip fracture
  - Hyperthyroidism
  - Current use of benzodiazepines
  - Resting heart rate higher than 80 beats/minute
  - Low bone density
  - Height taller than 165 cm since age 25 years
  - Inability to rise from chair
  - Less than 4 hours of standing daily

Physical Examination

- Vital signs, height, and weight
- Signs of estrogen deficiency (Table 4-18)
- Thyroid
- Cardiovascular and thorax
- Breasts
- Abdomen
- Pelvis

Diagnostic Procedures

- Cholesterol, lipid levels
- CBC
- Chemistry profile
- Serum FSH (higher than 30 to 40 million IU/mL is diagnostic of menopause); check annually beginning at age 50 years
- Bone density testing
- Thyroid profile
- Liver function tests
- Urinalysis
- Pap smear

HORMONE REPLACEMENT OPTIONS
Estrogen Equivalents

- Oral
  - Conjugated equine estrogen, 0.625 mg (e.g., Premarin)
  - Estradiol, 1.0 mg (e.g., Estrace)
  - Estropipate, 0.625 mg (e.g., Ogen, Ortho-Est)
  - Esterified estrogens, 0.625 mg (e.g., Estratab, Menest)
  - 17-Beta-estradiol, 0.5 mg (e.g., Estrace)
- Local vaginal cream for atrophic urogenital changes
- Transdermal (less effective for lipid profile because of liver bypass; less likely to affect clotting function)
  - Transdermal 17-Beta-estradiol, 0.05 mg (e.g., Estraderm, Climara)
- Intramuscular injection (monthly)
  - Estradiol cypionate, 1.5 mg (e.g., Depo-Estradiol)
  - Estrone, 2.5 mg

Progesterone Equivalents: Oral

- Medroxyprogesterone acetate (Provera): most common, 2.5 mg continuous dose or 5 to10 mg cyclic dose

TABLE **4-19** Contraindications to Hormone Replacement Therapy

HORMONE	RELATIVE	ABSOLUTE
Estrogen	Malignant melanoma	Known or suspected breast cancer
	Gallstones	Known or suspected estrogen-dependent cancers
	Hypertension	(e.g., breast, uterus)
	Risk of thromboembolic events	History of active thromboembolism
	Presence of conditions aggravated by fluid retention (CHF, asthma, seizures)	Active liver disease
		Recent MI
	Treatment for breast cancer	Pregnancy
	Endometriosis	Undiagnosed genital bleeding
	Leiomyoma	Unopposed estrogen for women with intact uterus
Progesterone	Liver dysfunction	Pregnancy
	Seizure disorders (raises seizure threshold)	

CHF, Congestive heart failure; *MI,* myocardial infarction.

- Norethindrone acetate (Micronor): 0.15 mg
- Ethinyl estradiol (Estinyl): 0.02, 0.05, or 0.5 mg
- Quinestrol (Estrovis): 100 mcg
- Micronized progesterone (Prometrium): 100 mg continuous dosage (also available as vaginal insert and transdermal cream)

Conjugated Equine Estrogen Combination Products

- Prempro, 0.625 mg estrogen and medroxyprogesterone acetate, 2.5 mg administered orally
- Premphase, 0.625 mg estrogen and medroxyprogesterone acetate, 5 mg (progesterone added to 14 of the 28 tablets in a blister pack)
- Estradiol/norethindrone acetate 0.05/0.14-0.25 combination patch

Other Methods

- Estring is a vaginal ring inserted into the upper third of the vagina that provides slow-release estradiol. Effective for 3 months; requires systemic progesterone with intact uterus.
- Selective estrogen receptor modulator: Raloxifene (Evista), 60 to 120 mg, is a so-called "designer estrogen," which has tissue selectivity; it works as estrogen in selective receptors (bone) but as an antiestrogen in the breast and uterus. It protects against breast cancer but does not relieve hot flashes (may even increase hot flashes) and is not effective for atrophic vaginal tissue.

HRT Regimens

- Continuous estrogen without progesterone can be used only in women who do not have a uterus.
- Continuous cyclic: With uterus intact, progesterone must be added to prevent endometrial carcinoma. Unopposed estrogen is administered for 13 to 16 days, and progesterone is administered the last 10 to 14 days of the cycle. Withdrawal bleeding does occur but is predictable and lighter than a usual period.
- Cyclic/sequential: Administer estrogen daily and progesterone 10 to 14 days of the month; monthly withdrawal bleeding occurs.
- Continuous combined: Administer estrogen daily and progesterone daily; bleeding ceases in most women after 1 year.
- Intermittent progesterone: Administer estrogen daily and progesterone 14 days every 3 months; data are being collected regarding bleeding patterns associated with this newer regimen (bleeding is similar to that experienced with continuous combination regimen).

Principles of HRT

- Begin with lowest effective dose that relieves symptoms.
- Begin as soon as women experience symptoms; less adjustment is required when the body has not been estrogen deficient for long periods.

- Progestins should be added to the regimen for a woman with an intact uterus. For women who have undergone hysterectomy, only estrogen replacement is needed.
- HRT can begin during perimenopause but does not provide contraception. A low-dose oral contraception can be used (caution should be used with smokers older than 35 years). In perimenopausal women, it is advisable to use HRT instead of OCPs because even the lowest dose of oral contraception is 4 times higher in estrogen than standard HRT. Check FSH level on day 6 or 7 of pill-free week. If FSH level is higher than 20 million IU/mL, switch to HRT.
- Once HRT is begun, follow-up is scheduled in approximately 3 months to determine how the therapy is working. Women should be encouraged to call or come in sooner if concerns or problems arise. Once the regimen is well established, yearly follow-up is sufficient.
- Remind the woman that the estrogen-progesterone cycle produces withdrawal bleeding.
- Testosterone can be added if the woman experiences loss of libido. Concerns arise regarding virilization (acne, hirsutism) and adverse effects of androgens on lipid profiles. Esterified estrogen/methyltestosterone, 1.25 mg/2.55 mg (Estratest), or Estratest HS 0.625 mg/1.5 mg are commonly used. NPs may want to consult with physicians concerning adding testosterone to the HRT regimen (Thiedke, 2000).
- Transdermal products have less effect on the lipid profile because the liver is bypassed, but are less likely to affect clotting factors.
- Women receiving monthly intramuscular regimens commonly complain that symptoms recur before the next dose of medication.
- A therapeutic alliance between NP and client is ideal for examining the experience of menopause and treatment options.
- Warn the woman about possible side effects and the need to contact the health provider if they occur. Use the ACHES mnemonic to assess the following possible side effects:
  - **A**bdominal pain
  - **C**hest pain
  - **H**eadaches
  - **E**ye problems
  - **S**evere leg pain
- Other side effects are withdrawal bleeding, bloating, weight gain and fluid retention in extremities, depression, and nausea (may help to take with food or hs).
- With side effects, consider changing dosage of causative agent or type of regimen.

CLIENT EDUCATION

- Encourage the client to explore the meaning of menopause as a life transition and to reframe it positively as an opportunity to capitalize on accumulated life experiences and easing of social roles to reinvest in self and creative expression and to recommit to a healthier lifestyle (Thiedke, 2000).

- Discuss need for annual follow-up.
- Discuss benefits and risks of HRT.
- Emphasize importance of not taking unopposed estrogen because of risk of endometrial hyperplasia. If hormones are not used together, an annual endometrial biopsy is necessary.
- Encourage health promotion actions (stress reduction, smoking cessation, exercise, good nutrition, and safety).
- Discuss the following alternatives to HRT:
  - Phytoestrogens in food sources: apples, carrots, coffee, potatoes, yams, soy products
  - Herbal remedies: ginseng, black cohosh, and dong quai are most widely used for menopausal symptoms
  - Antioxidant vitamins B, C, and E for vasomotor symptom control
  - Vaginal moisturizers and lubricants: remedy vaginal dryness for women who do not want to take HRT
  - Clonidine (Catapres): 0.05 to 0.2 mg PO or transdermally; effective against hot flashes; reevaluate at 3 months and caution regarding possible side effects: orthostatic hypotension, fatigue, sedation, weakness, and dizziness

FOLLOW-UP

- Schedule annual Pap smear and mammogram.
- Encourage client to keep menstrual calendar to evaluate withdrawal bleeding.
- Use strategies to increase compliance with HRT. Fewer than one third of women who receive a prescription for HRT are still taking it 1 year later. This may be because of difficulty being committed to long-term therapy when one is feeling well, fear of cancer, or intolerance for withdrawal bleeding and other side effects. Strategies to encourage compliance with HRT are the following:
  - Acknowledge complexity of decision. The client may have received massive, sometimes inconsistent information.
  - Examine concerns and misgivings about using HRT.
  - Explore options.
  - Indicate willingness to reevaluate decisions and to change dosages and regimens as needed if problems arise (Thiedke, 2000).

REFERENCES

Archer, D. F., & Utian, W. H. (2001). Decisions in prescribing HRT. *Patient Care for the Nurse Practitioner, 4*(5), 45-58.

Battistini, M., & Stanley, H. (2001). Complete care of the older woman. *Patient Care for the Nurse Practitioner, 4*(5), 15-27.

Finkel, M. L., Cohen, M., & Mahoney, H. (2001). Treatment options for the menopausal woman. *The Nurse Practitioner, 26*(2), 5-17.

Hormone replacement therapy: Weighing the hazards and rewards. (1997). *Clinician Reviews, 7*(9), 53-72.

Long, V. E. (1998). Between childbearing and menopause. *Advance for Nurse Practitioners,* December, 52-58.

Moore, A., & Noonan, M. D. (1996). A nurse's guide to hormone replacement therapy. *Journal of Obstetric, Gynecologic, and Neonatal Nursing, 25,* 24-31.

North American Menopause Society (2000). *Menopause core curriculum study guide.* Cleveland: The North American Menopause Society.

Shimp, L. A., & Smith, M. A. (2000). Menopause. In M. A. Smith & L. A. Shimp (Eds.), *20 Common problems in women's health care* (pp. 91-131). New York: McGraw-Hill.

Speroff, L. (2000). Management of the perimenopausal transition. *Contemporary Ob/Gyn, 45*(10), 14-37.

Thiedke, C. C. (2000). Menopause. In C. C. Thiedke & J. A. Rosenfeld (pp. 59-71). *Women's Health.* Philadelphia: Lippincott Williams & Wilkins.

Villablanca, A. C. (2001). HRT and cardiovascular risk in women: Where do we stand? *Women's Health in Primary Care, 4*(2), 121-129.

Writing Group for the Women's Health Initiative. (2002). Risks and benefits of estrogen plus progestin in healthy post menopausal women. *Journal of the American Medical Association, 288*(3), 321–333.

Review Questions

1. Mrs. Lowery, a menopausal woman, is experiencing hot flashes and vaginal dryness that is causing dyspareunia. She is interested in obtaining a prescription for HRT. Which diagnostic test is appropriate before initiating HRT?

- **a.** Mammography
- **b.** Cardiac enzyme panel
- **c.** Chest radiograph
- **d.** Gallbladder ultrasound

2. Which of the following statements is accurate regarding the effects of HRT?

- **a.** HRT decreases the risk of gallbladder disease.
- **b.** HRT produces sleep disturbances.
- **c.** HRT reduces breast cancer risk.
- **d.** HRT protects against osteoporosis.

3. When starting estrogen-progesterone HRT for Mrs. Sullivan, a perimenopausal woman, the NP provides extensive drug information. Which comment made by Mrs. Sullivan indicates a need for further teaching?

- **a.** "So long as I take this medicine everyday, I won't need contraception."
- **b.** "A major effect of this medicine is that it increases libido."
- **c.** "I can expect to have withdrawal bleeding at the end of each month on this medication."
- **d.** "This hormone combination will likely help my vaginal dryness."

4. Mrs. Cooperman is beginning combined transdermal hormonal replacement. When should her initial follow-up visit be scheduled?

   a. 1 week
   b. 1 month
   c. 3 months
   d. 6 months

5. Mrs. Garcia underwent a hysterectomy 10 years ago. She now seeks HRT for symptom relief. Which drug choice is best for Mrs. Garcia?

   a. Progesterone-only pill
   b. Estrogen-only patch
   c. Combination estrogen-progesterone pill
   d. Vaginal cream

Answers and Rationales

1. *Answer:* **a** (analysis/diagnosis)
   Rationale: Because known or suspected breast cancer is a contraindication to HRT, mammogram should precede initiation of HRT (Shimp & Smith, 2000).

2. *Answer:* **d** (implementation/plan)
   Rationale: HRT increases the risk of gallbladder disease and breast cancer and often alleviates sleep disturbances associated with hot flashes and nocturnal sweating; therefore choices a, b, and c are inaccurate. HRT does protect against osteoporosis (North American Menopause Society, 2000).

3. *Answer:* **a** (evaluation)
   Rationale: HRT is not a contraceptive method; this misperception must be clarified immediately. The perimenopausal woman who needs contraception should be started on low-dose OCPs instead of HRT (Long, 1998).

4. *Answer:* **c** (implementation/plan)
   Rationale: The initial follow-up visit for a woman beginning HRT should be scheduled for 2 to 3 months after beginning therapy. (Finkel, et al. 2001).

5. *Answer:* **b** (analysis/diagnosis)
   Rationale: Progesterone protects against endometrial hypertrophy in women with an intact uterus. Because this woman has undergone a hysterectomy, she does not need progesterone. Oral estrogen and the transdermal patch are suitable options (Finkel, et al. 2001).

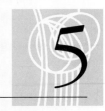

Wellness Promotion: Health Promotion

Denise Robinson

A major role within advanced practice is that of health educator and health promotion advocate. Quality health promotion programs are not created by chance; they are the product of much effort and should be based on sound theoretical models. Theoretical models are the means by which nurse practitioners (NPs) can provide structure and organization to disease prevention and health promotion programs.

DEFINITIONS

To *promote* is to help or encourage to exist or flourish. Pender (1996) defines *health promotion* as being "motivated by the desire to increase well-being and actualize human health potential." Health promotion is not disease or problem specific; it is an approach seeking to expand the positive potential for health. Effective health promotion requires a shift in emphasis from illness to wellness. This kind of change requires that health care providers shift from a paternal approach to a partnership approach, which requires that health care providers be prepared to look beyond traditional treatment modalities and health care delivery systems as they assist clients in achieving optimal health.

Another definition of health promotion is "the process of enabling individuals and communities to increase control over and improve their health" (Green & Raeburn, 1988). The meaning of *health promotion* overlaps considerably with the meaning of *prevention*. The main difference between the concepts of *disease prevention* and *health promotion* seems to be one of focus. Prevention is a disease-related concept; health promotion is health-related. The term *disease prevention* is normally used to represent strategies designed either to reduce risk factors for specific diseases or to enhance personal factors that reduce susceptibility to disease.

Brubaker (1983) believes that health promotion and disease prevention are two sides of the same coin. Health promotion many times incorporates principles of risk appraisal and risk reduction. Information supplied by clients regarding their health behaviors, family health history, personal health history, and personal demographics is compared with data from epidemiologic studies and vital statistics. These comparisons are used to make predictions regarding morbidity and mortality and the strategies that can be used to reduce risks.

Furthermore, preventive services for early detection of disease have resulted in decreased morbidity and mortality from cerebrovascular accidents secondary to untreated hypertension, cervical cancer, phenylketonuria, and congenital hypothyroidism (United States Preventive Services Task Force, 1996). Today, providing immunizations and preventive services continues to be an important part of primary care, and ongoing research has shown the effect of personal lifestyle behaviors on health.

Unfortunately, delivery rates for preventive services in the United States are low, often falling below 50% (United States Public Health Service, 1994). Bergman-Evans and Walker (1996) examined the prevalence of clinical preventive services used by older women. Data regarding 5574 women were obtained from the 1991 *Health Promotion and Disease Prevention Supplement of the National Health Interview Survey.* Of these women, 78% reported having undergone physical examinations during the previous 2 years. However, fewer than 1% reported receiving all the recommended screening services, and only 5.3% of the women were current with recommended immunizations.

Interventions that address a client's personal health practices are crucially important. These areas include the following:

- Tobacco use
- Physical inactivity
- Poor nutrition
- Alcohol and illicit drug use
- Safety measures

Clinicians and clients should discuss and decide on the type of preventive services indicated so that services may be tailored to a client's needs and value system. The risk-to-benefit ratio (known and unknown) for each intervention should be discussed. Clinicians should take every opportunity to deliver preventive services, especially for those with limited access to care. Important points to remember are the following:

- Illness prevention through health promotion is potentially more beneficial than treatment of disease.
- Prevention must be effectively addressed at each client encounter in the office.
- Advanced practice nurses need to focus on health promotion in their practices.
- Incorporate recommended topics into every visit.

There are a number of barriers that may interfere with the incorporation of preventive services into practice, including the following:

- Lack of time
- Lack of reimbursement
- Insufficient staff support
- Insufficient organizational support to keep track of needed services
- Inadequate training and skills
- Emphasis on illness in the health care system
- Numerous recommendations by different organizations, making it difficult to know what preventive services should be performed and when and how often to perform them

Three levels of prevention are currently recognized. *Primary prevention* can be defined as those activities that seek to prevent the initial occurrence of a disease or disorder. Primary prevention is the promotion of health by personal and community-wide efforts, such as improving nutritional status, physical fitness, emotional well being, immunization against infectious diseases, and provision of a safe environment.

Secondary prevention seeks to arrest or retard existing disease through early detection and appropriate treatment. Secondary prevention involves those measures available to persons and populations for early detection and prompt and effective interventions to correct deviations from good health. Annual physical examination incorporating diagnostic procedures for detecting cervical, breast, prostrate, or rectal cancer is an example of secondary prevention.

Tertiary prevention is aimed at reducing complications. Tertiary measures consist of those interventions that reduce impairments and disabilities, minimize suffering caused by existing deviations from good health, and promote a client's adjustment to an altered, chronic condition. The art and science involved in rehabilitation care is an example of tertiary prevention.

HEALTHY PEOPLE 2010

A national health strategy published by the United States Department of Health & Human Services (1991), *Healthy People 2010*, is a platform for action to help Americans ful-

fill their health potential. The report consists of two broad goals: (1) increase quality and years of healthy life and (2) eliminate health disparities (www.healthypeople.gov). To support these goals, *Healthy People 2010* established the following 10 high-priority areas (known as leading health indicators):

- Physical activity
- Overweight and obesity
- Tobacco use
- Substance abuse
- Mental health
- Responsible sexual behavior
- Injury and violence
- Environmental quality
- Immunization
- Access to health care

Most states have developed their own plans addressing these areas. More information can be found at www.healthypeople.gov and at the Office of Disease Prevention and Health Promotion (odphp.osophs.dhhs.gov/).

MODELS OF HEALTH BEHAVIOR

Theories and models should serve as the foundation for planning successful health promotion programs. They can be used to examine the reasons why a specific population may or may not be taking good care of their health. Theories and models can help pinpoint what NPs need to know before developing and planning disease prevention and health promotion programs. They can also provide valuable insight into how NPs might design program strategies to reach a target population so that nursing interventions will make a positive difference.

PIVOTAL HEALTH PROMOTION AND DISEASE PREVENTION THEORETICAL MODELS
Cognitive-Behavioral Models

Contemporary models of health behavior at the individual and interpersonal levels usually fall within the broad category of cognitive-behavioral theories. Two key concepts, following, cut across these theories:

- Behavior is considered to be mediated through cognition (i.e., what we know and think affects how we act).
- Knowledge is necessary but not sufficient to produce behavioral change. Perceptions, motivation, skills, and factors in the social environment also play important roles.

Social Cognitive Theory

The social learning theories presented by Rotter (1954) and Bandura (1977) have been renamed by Bandura (1986) as the *social cognitive theory* (SCT). A fundamental premise of this theory is that people learn not only through their own experiences, but also by observing the actions of others and the results of those actions.

Basic Tenets of Social Cognitive Theory

- Reinforcement combined with a person's expectations of the consequences of behavior determines the specific behavior.
- The environment shapes, maintains, and constrains behavior.
- People are not passive in the process. People can create and change their environments.
- The concept of *reciprocal determinism* states that there is a dynamic interaction among the person, the behavior, and the environment and that change is bidirectional.
- Expectancies are one's beliefs regarding the likely results of an action. SCT proposes that expectancies may be divided into the following three types:
  - Expectancies regarding environmental cues and how events are connected
  - Expectancies regarding how one's own behavior is likely to influence outcomes
  - Expectancies regarding one's own competence to perform the necessary behaviors needed to influence outcomes
- *Incentives* or *reinforcements* have been defined as the value of a particular object or outcome.
- *Self-efficacy* involves beliefs that a person has regarding his or her ability to successfully engage in a desired behavior, also referred to as *perception of self-competence*, are central to SCT. If a person does not expect that a health action will yield a beneficial result, he or she has little reason to attempt it. A person is most likely to perform some behavior when self-efficacy is high and outcome expectations are positive, and persons with positive outcome expectations are more likely to maintain positive behavior change (Skinner & Kreuter, 1997).

Theory of Reasoned Action. The theory of reasoned action (TRA) is relevant in understanding health behavior changes (Fishbein & Ajzen, 1975). Whereas the SCT is concerned with behavior, the TRA provides a model for understanding attitudes toward behaviors:

- Behaviors are mainly determined by intentions. A person's intentions to perform a behavior are a function of his or her attitude toward performing the behavior plus subjective norms.
- This theory suggests that people are likely to engage in behaviors that they intend to do.

Health Behavior Models

The health behavior models address a person's perceptions of the threat of a health problem and the accompanying appraisal of a recommended behavior for preventing or managing the problem.

Health Belief Model. The health belief model (HBM) was one of the first models to adapt theory from the behavioral sciences to health problems. It remains one of the most widely recognized frameworks of health behavior explaining self-care activities, but it has a focus on behavior related to the prevention of disease (Becker, 1974; Rosenstock, 1974). During the 1950s, a group of social psychologists at the United States Public Health Service were influenced to develop the HBM after widespread failure of a program allowing people to participate in low-cost or free-of-charge programs (e.g., chest x-ray examinations for tuberculosis screening, immunizations) to prevent or detect disease. The social psychologists who outlined the model believed that people feared diseases and that health actions were probably motivated by the amount of fear a person has, the amount of fear reduction possible by taking a particular health action, and the obstacles in the way of taking action. They were strongly influenced by Lewin's decision-making model (Lewin, Dembo et al. 1944).

The HBM attempts to explain why people do or do not engage in a particular preventive health action in response to a specific disease threat. Specifically, the HBM contends that whether a person undertakes a recommended health action depends on the following factors:

- Perceptions of the level of personal susceptibility to the particular illness or condition (perceived threat)
- Perceptions of the degree of severity of consequences that might result from contracting the condition (perceived severity)
- Perceptions of the health action's potential benefits in preventing susceptibility (perceived benefits)
- Perceptions of the physical, psychologic, financial, and other barriers related to the advocated behavior (perceived barriers or costs)
- Stimuli or cue to action to trigger appropriate behavior
- Awareness of susceptibility to a disease believed to be serious is thought to provide force leading to action

Health Promotion Model. According to Walker, Sechrist, and Pender (1987), "Health promotion is a multidimensional pattern of self-initiated actions and perceptions that serve to maintain or enhance the level of wellness, self-actualization and fulfillment of the individual."

The Health Promotion Model is proposed as a multivariate model for explaining and predicting the health-promoting components of lifestyle. This model focuses on health promotion without the threat of disease. Factors that influence one's likelihood of engaging in health-promoting behaviors include the following (Pender, 1996):

- Importance of health
- Perceived control of health
- Perceived self-efficacy
- Definition of health
- Perceived health status

- Perceived benefits of health-promoting behaviors
- Perceived barriers to health-promoting behaviors

Definitions

- Health risk appraisal includes screening for disease potential, educating clients regarding unhealthy habits, and stimulating behavioral change.
- Risk factors are characteristics that have been associated with higher risk for a particular disease. Relative risk is determined by the ratio of risk or rate in exposed persons to the risk or rate in unexposed persons.
- Epidemiology is the study of the distribution and determinants of the frequency of disease in humans.
- Mortality refers to death.
- Morbidity refers to illness.

Health Promotion Matrix. The most recent HPM to be developed by nurses focuses on health promotion planning. It is called the Health Promotion Matrix (Gorin & Arnold, 1998). The authors describe this model as a clinical tool to be used by the health professional and the client as partners in health promotion care. The role of the health care professional is to transfer knowledge and skill so that the client can make an informed and deliberate decision regarding taking actions that may enhance health. *Health image* is a central concept.

Precede–Proceed. A discussion of theoretical models for health promotion, disease prevention, and maintenance of function throughout the lifespan is incomplete without including the precede–proceed framework (Green, et al. 1991), which is a popular and comprehensive model developed specifically for health promotion planners. An overriding principle of this model is that most enduring health behaviors are voluntary in nature. This principle is reflected in the model as it seeks to empower persons with understanding, motivation, skills, and active engagement to improve the quality of their lives. The precede–proceed model has nine phases: the first five phases are diagnostic (social, epidemiologic, behavioral and environmental, educational and organizational, and administrative and policy), and the remaining four phases are devoted to implementation and evaluation. The five diagnostic phases serve to identify objectives and set priorities based on importance, immediacy, and changeability. The result of all these diagnoses is a plan with specific objectives and strategies; strategies are based on information learned in the diagnostic phases regarding key causes and factors contributing to the identified problem.

REFERENCES

Ajzen, I. (1988). *Attitudes, personality and behavior.* Chicago: Dorsey Press.

Ajzen, I., & Fishbein, M. (1980). *Understanding attitudes and predicting behavior.* Upper Saddle River, NJ: Prentice Hall.

Bandura, A. (1977). *Social learning theory.* Upper Saddle River: Prentice Hall.

Bandura, A. (1986). *Social foundations of thought and action.* Englewood Cliffs: Prentice Hall.

Becker, M. (1974). The health belief model and personal health behavior. *Health education monographs 2*(4), 324–508.

Becker, M. (1993). A medical sociologist looks at health promotion. *Journal of Health and Social Behavior, 34*(3), 1-6.

Bergman-Evans, B., & Walker, S. (1996). The prevalence of clinical preventive services utilization by older women. *Nurse Practitioner, 21*(4): 88, 90, 99-100.

Brubaker, B. (1983). Health promotion: A linguistic analysis. *Advances in Nursing Science, 5,* 1-14.

Clark, M. (1996). *Nursing in the community* (2nd ed.). Norwalk, CT: Appleton & Lange.

Dines, A., & Cribb, A. (1993). Ottawa Charter for health promotion. In A. Dines & A. Cribb (Eds.), *Health promotion: Concepts and practice.* London: Blackwell Scientific.

Duffy, M. (1988). Determinants of health promotion in midlife women. *Nursing Research, 37,* 358-362.

Epp, J. (1986). *Achieving health for all: A framework for health promotion.* Ottawa, Canada: Department of National Health and Welfare.

Fishbein, M., & Ajzen, I. (1975). *Belief, attitude, intention, and behavior: An introduction to theory and research.* Reading, MA: Addison-Wesley.

Frauman, A., & Nettles-Carlson, B. (1991). Predictors of a health-promoting lifestyle among well adult clients in a nursing practice. *Journal of the American Academy of Nurse Practitioners, 3*(4), 174-179.

Gorin, S., & Arnold, J. (1998). The Health Promotion Matrix. In S. Gorin & J. Arnold (Eds.), *Health promotion handbook* (pp. 91-113). St. Louis: Mosby.

Green, L., & Raeburn, J. (1988). Health promotion: What is it? What will it become? *Health Promotion, 3*(2), 151-159.

Green, L., & Raeburn, J. (1990). Contemporary developments in health promotion: Definitions and challenges. In N. Bracht (Ed.), *Health promotion at the community level* (pp. 29-43). Newbury Park, CA: Sage.

Green, L., Marshall, W., & Kreuter, M. (1991). *Health promotion planning: An educational and environmental approach* (2nd ed.). Mountain View, CA: Mayfield.

Laffrey, S. (1985). Health promotion: Relevance for nursing. *Topics in Clinical Nursing, 7,* 29-38.

Lemley, K., O'Grady, E., Rauckhorst, L., Russell, D., & Small, N. (1994). Baseline preventive data provided by nurse practitioners. *Nurse Practitioner, 19*(5), 57-63.

Lewin, K., Dembo, T., Fesltaper, L., & Sears, P. (1944). Level of aspiration. In J. Hunt (Ed.), *Personality of the Behavior Disorders* (pp. 333-378). New York: Ronald Press.

McKenzie, J., & Smeltzer, J. (1997). *Theories and models commonly used for health promotion interventions: Planning, implementing, and evaluating health promotion programs.* Needham Heights, MA: Allyn & Bacon.

Morgan, I. (2001). Health promotion and disease prevention across the lifespan. In D. Robinson and C. Kish (Eds). *Core concepts in advanced practice* (pp. 567-584). St. Louis: Mosby.

Morgan, I., & Marsh, G. (1998). Historic and future health promotion contexts for nursing. *Image: Journal of Nursing Scholarship, 30*(4), 379-383.

Muhlenkamp, A., Brown, N., & Sands, D. (1985). Determinants of health promotion activities in nursing clinic patients. *Nursing Research, 34,* 327-332.

Nutbeam, D. (1996). Health promotion glossary. In *Health promotion: An anthology* (Scientific Publication No. 557, pp. 343-358). Washington, DC: Pan American Health Organization.

Pender, N. (1996). Health promotion in nursing practice (3rd ed.). Upper Saddle River, NJ: Prentice Hall.

Rosenstock, I. (1974). Historical origins of the health belief model. In M. Becker (Ed.), *The health belief model and personal health behavior.* Thorofare, NJ: Charles B. Slack.

Rosenstock, I. (1990). The health belief model: Explaining behavior through expectancies. In K. Glanz, F. Lewis, & B. Rimer (Eds.), *Health behavior and health education: Theory, research and practice* (pp. 39-59). San Francisco: Josey-Bass.

Rosenstock, I., Strecher, V., & Becker, M. (1988). Social learning theory and the health belief model. *Health Education Quarterly, 15*(2), 175-183.

Rotter, J. (1954). *Social learning theory and clinical psychology.* New York: Prentice Hall.

Skinner, C., & Kreuter, M. (1997). Using theories in planning interactive computer programs. In R. Street, W. Gold, & T. Manning (Eds.), *Health promotion and interactive technology: Theoretical applications and future directions* (pp. 39-65). Mahwah, NJ: Lawrence Erlbaum.

Swanson, J., & Albrecht, M. (1993). *Community health nursing: Promoting the health of aggregates.* Philadelphia: W. B. Saunders.

United States Department of Health and Human Services (1991). *Healthy people 2010: National health promotion and disease prevention objectives.* Washington: Office of Disease Prevention and Health Promotion. Retrieved August 22, 2002, from www.healthypeople.gov.

United States Preventive Services Task Force (1996). *Guide to clinical preventive services* (2nd ed.). Baltimore: Williams & Wilkins.

United States Public Health Service (1994). Put prevention into practice. *Journal of American Academy of Nurse Practitioners, 6*(6), 257-265.

Walker, S., Sechrist, K., & Pender, N. (1987). The health promoting lifestyle in profile: Development and psychometric characteristics. *Nursing Research, 36*(2), 76-80.

Woolf, S., Jonas, S., & Lawrence, R. (1996). *Health promotion and disease prevention in clinical practice.* Baltimore: Williams & Wilkins.

World Health Organization (1986). A discussion document on the concepts and principles of health promotion. *Health Promotion, 1*(1), 73-76.

World Health Organization (1987). Ottawa Charter for health promotion. *Health Promotion, 1*(4), iii-v.

Review Questions

1. Which of the following activities describes primary prevention for men?
   a. Teach testicular self-examination (TSE).
   b. Teach regarding an antihypertensive drug.
   c. Teach a client with gonorrhea regarding the potential for prostatitis later in life.
   d. Educate the client regarding the hazards of substance abuse.

2. Which of the following activities describes primary prevention for Mrs. Cook, an 80-year-old widow?
   a. Encourage Mrs. Cook to work through any grief related to her husband's death.
   b. Refer Mrs. Cook for financial assistance.
   c. Determine whether Mrs. Cook has adequate access to health care.
   d. Contact Mrs. Cook's landlord to install a handrail on the stairs.

3. Ms. Black is a 25-year-old pregnant woman with two small children. Which of the following pertains to secondary prevention?
   a. Prepare the children for the birth of the new child.
   b. Discuss with her the advantages and disadvantages of bottle and breast feeding.
   c. Discuss with her various options for birth control.
   d. Refer her to a women's crisis shelter.

4. Secondary prevention strategies commonly used for women's health care include which of the following?
   a. Pap smear
   b. Contraception counseling
   c. Prepregnancy counseling
   d. Monitoring diabetes and compliance with diabetic regimen

5. To determine the appropriate health promotion activities and screening for a client, it is most important to do which of the following?
   a. Perform a thorough physical examination of the client.
   b. Consider the leading causes of death for that particular age group.
   c. Assess each person's risk factors for morbidity and mortality.
   d. Conduct some laboratory work to assess kidney and liver function.

6. Which of the following indicates that your client is following the health promotion guidelines you suggested?
   a. Weight gain of 2 lbs
   b. Use of the food pyramid as basis for meal planning
   c. Eating a vegetarian diet
   d. Working 50 hours a week as computer programmer

7. Which of the following is considered a goal of *Healthy People 2010*?
   a. Increase self-care activities.
   b. Eliminate health problems.
   c. Increase quality and years of healthy life.
   d. No denial because of finances.

8. Which of the following models might be appropriate to explain to a client the risk and consequences related to a particular condition (i.e., perceived severity)?
   a. Health promotion matrix
   b. Precede–proceed model
   c. HBM
   d. Transtheoretical change model

Answers and Rationales

1. *Answer:* d (implementation/plan)
Rationale: Teaching regarding TSE and antihypertensive drugs implies treatment of existing conditions, whereas teaching regarding gonorrhea and prostatitis is done to prevent complications. Teaching regarding the hazards of substance abuse is the only activity among these choices that promotes prevention of a problem (Clark, 1996).

2. *Answer:* d (implementation/plan)
Rationale: The only activity listed that prevents problems is installing a handrail. The others relate to treating existing conditions or preventing complications (Clark, 1996).

3. *Answer:* d (implementation/plan)
Rationale: Referring Ms. Black to a women's crisis center for spousal violence necessitates the identification of an existing problem. All other options describe primary preventive activities (Clark, 1996).

4. *Answer:* a (implementation/plan)
Rationale: The Pap smear is the only commonly used secondary strategy listed. Contraception and prepregnancy counseling is a primary prevention strategy. Monitoring diabetes is a secondary prevention strategy, but it is not recommended for all women (Swanson & Albrecht, 1993).

5. *Answer:* c (assessment)
Rationale: It is important to consider the leading causes of death for a particular age group to determine what sorts of questions should be included when obtaining the history, but the plan for an individual client is determined by that person's risk for dying as a result of the leading cause of death or any other morbidity or mortality (United States Preventive Services Task Force, 1996).

6. *Answer:* b (evaluation)
Rationale: Using the food pyramid promotes a well-balanced diet according to current nutritional recommendations (Woolf, et al. 1996).

7. *Answer:* c (implementation/plan)
Rationale: The two main goals of *Healthy People 2010* are to increase the quality and years of healthy life and to eliminate health disparities (www.healthypeople.gov).

8. *Answer:* c (implementation/plan)
Rationale: The HBM can be used to explain why people do or do not engage in a particular preventive health action in response to a specific disease threat. The NP can use the notion of perceived severity to emphasize to a client the importance of the prescribed treatment (Morgan, 2001).

EXERCISE   *Denise Robinson*

PHYSICAL ACTIVITY

Physical activity is defined as "any bodily movement produced by skeletal muscles and resulting in calorie expenditure" (Bouchard, et al. 1990). Lifestyle exercise has been characterized as the integration of short bouts of exercise into daily living (Gordon, Kohl, & Blair, 1993).

Goal 1: Increase Quality and Years of Healthy Life

The first goal of *Healthy People 2010* is to help persons of all ages increase life expectancy and improve quality of life. The objectives are to increase the proportion of adolescents who engage in vigorous physical activity that promotes cardiorespiratory fitness 3 or more days per week for 20 or more minutes per occasion; and to increase the proportion of adults who engage regularly, preferably daily, in moderate physical activity for at least 30 minutes per day. Moderate activity is 3 to 6 mets (4 to 7 kcal/min) and includes such activities as brisk walking, leisurely canoeing, swimming, golfing, playing doubles tennis, and cutting the grass.

INCIDENCE

- Twenty-two percent of all people are active.
- Fifty-four percent of all people are somewhat active.
- Forty million people are sedentary.
- Of all deaths, 12% are attributable in part to lack of regular exercise.

- Women generally are less active than men at all ages, and higher rates of inactivity are found among non-Hispanic black women and Mexican-American women.
- People with lower incomes, people with less education, people who are economically disadvantaged, and the elderly are typically not as physically active as others.
- Blacks and Hispanics are generally less physically active than whites.
- Adults in northeastern and southern states tend to be less active than adults in North-Central and Western States.
- People with disabilities are less physically active than people without disabilities.
- By age 75 years, one of three men and one of two women engage in no regular physical activity.
- Physical activity seems to decrease significantly during adolescence (Stephens, Jacobs, & White, 1985), with a decline of almost 50% from childhood through adulthood. Females tend to be more sedentary than males (Rowland, 1990). Because exercise or lack of exercise plays a major role in many disease states, it is imperative that all primary care providers assess and counsel their clients regarding the frequency, duration, and intensity of lifestyle exercise.

BENEFITS OF EXERCISE

- Increase in lean muscle mass
- Increase in bone mass or prevention of bone loss

- Reduction in systolic and diastolic blood pressure (BP)
- Greater high-density lipoproteins (HDLs)
- Reduction in excess body fat
- Lower insulin level and improved glucose tolerance
- Lower incidence of breast cancer and cancer of reproductive tract
- Improved pulmonary function
- Decreased sympathetically mediated cardiovascular response to stress
- Improvement of anxiety and depression
- Reduction of resting heart rate (HR)
- Increased circulating leukocytes; protection against infection
- Enhanced general mood and psychologic well being

BARRIERS TO EXERCISE

The major barriers most people face when trying to increase physical activity are lack of time, lack of access to convenient facilities, and lack of safe environments in which to be active. For more information on *Healthy People 2010* objectives or on physical activity and fitness, visit www.healthypeople.gov.

EXERCISE GUIDELINES

At every visit, promote lifestyle exercise of at least 20 to 30 minutes of vigorous activity three times per week (vigorous activity describes an intensity sufficient enough to produce fatigue in 20 minutes).

Intensity

Exercise to 60% or more of maximum HR, although recent research proposes that moderate exercise can be just as effective in terms of health benefits (Marcus, Selby, & Niaura, 1992). Moderate activity has higher compliance rates, fits better with daily lifestyle, and is well maintained with time (Duncan, Gordon, & Scott, 1991).

- Exercise should include the triad of activities for best health: aerobic activities, flexibility, and muscle training.
- Some exercise is better than none; start simply so that the exercise is enjoyable.
- The person should be able to talk during exercise (known as the *talk test to determine exercise intensity*). This keeps the person exercising at approximately 60% of maximum heart rate.
- Determine the target heart rate as follows:
  - Subtract age from $220 \times .60 =$ minimum heart rate
  - Subtract age from $220 \times .80$ or $.90 =$ maximum heart rate

RISK OF EXERCISE

Most adverse effects are related to injury during exercise. Potential adverse effects include injury, osteoarthritis, myocardial infarction, and, rarely, sudden death. Running or jogging carries a high risk of injury (35% to 65%), as does aerobic dancing, for which risk increases with frequency of classes (United States Preventive Services Task Force, 1996). Injuries can be prevented by avoiding the following:

- Excessive levels of exercise
- Sudden dramatic increases in activity level (especially in those with poor fitness baseline)
- Improper exercise technique or equipment

Intense exercise can cause amenorrhea, bone loss, and an increased fracture risk. Long-term exercise does not seem to increase the prevalence of osteoarthritis in major weight-bearing joints. The risk of adverse cardiovascular events is greater when those who are usually sedentary engage in vigorous activity. The risk of sudden death is lower for those who exercise regularly than for their sedentary counterparts.

CLINICAL INTERVENTIONS

- Promote regular exercise for all children and adults.
- Determine each client's activity level.
- Ascertain barriers to exercise.
- Risk assessment: Men older than 40 years and women older than 50 years with two or more risk factors for coronary artery disease (CAD) should have a resting electrocardiography (ECG) or stress test; others with known risk factors (previous myocardial infarction, pulmonary disease) or possible risk factors (hypertension, cigarette smoking, high blood cholesterol, abuse of drugs, or diabetes) should have a thorough examination before beginning exercise programs (Woolf, Jonas, & Lawrence, 1996).
- Exercise during pregnancy: Women who exercised before pregnancy should be able to continue to exercise during pregnancy. Any pregnant woman who wants to start an exercise program should consult with her obstetrician. Factors that influence exercising during pregnancy include an increased blood volume, cardiac output and resting pulse, increased resting oxygen requirement, change in center of gravity, increased metabolic rate, and increased caloric needs. Pregnant women should stop exercising when fatigued and should choose exercises that minimize the risk of injury (Lee, Rippe, & Wilkinson, 1995).
- Provide information regarding the role of exercise in disease prevention.
- Assist in selecting the appropriate type of exercise (consider factors such as medical limitations and activity characteristics that improve health and enhance compliance).
- Exercise: Regular, moderate-intensity exercise is reasonable for sedentary persons.
- The short-term goal is a small increase from current activity level with progression to achieve cardiovascular fitness. Thirty minutes of brisk walking most days of the week is ideal.
- Sporadic exercise should be discouraged, especially for sedentary persons. Regularity is more important than type of exercise.

- Determine what the person hopes to accomplish with exercise.
- Increase by only 10% each week in terms of time or distance.
- Cut down on sedentary activities, such as TV watching and computer games. Use stairs when possible and make extra steps during the day.
- Provider recommendation is one of the most potent motivators; only 20% of all providers ever talk about exercise.
  - Contracts
  - Maintaining self-monitoring diaries and periodic discussions with provider
  - Providing personalized feedback and praise
  - Setting flexible goals
- Providers who model active lifestyles are more likely to be effective with counseling.
- Encourage the client to "take control."
- It is good to have a system of periodic rewards.
- Gradual change promotes permanent change.

REFERENCES

Barker, L., Burton, J., & Zieve, P. (1999). *Principles of ambulatory medicine* (5th ed.). Baltimore: Williams & Wilkins.

Bouchard, C., Shephard, R., & Stephens, T. (Eds.). (1990). *Exercise, fitness, and health.* Champaign, IL: Human Kinetics Books.

Byrd, J. (1994). Content of prenatal care. In S. D. Ratcliffe, J. E. Byrd, & E. L. Sakornut (Eds.), *Handbook of pregnancy and perinatal care in family practice: Science and practice* (pp. 15-27). Philadelphia: Hanley & Belfus.

Combating childhood obesity. (1996). *Clinician Reviews, 6*(10), 109-110.

Duncan, J., Gordon, N., & Scott, C. (1991). Women walking for health and fitness: How much is enough? *Journal of the American Medical Association, 266,* 3295-3299.

Estes, M. (1998). *Health assessment and physical examination.* New York: Delmar.

Gordon, N., Kohl, H., & Blair, S. (1993). Lifestyle exercise: A new strategy to promote physical activity for adults. *Journal of Cardiopulmonary Rehabilitation, 13,* 161-163.

Johnson, C., Johnson, B., Murray, J., & Apgar, B. (1996). *Women's healthcare handbook.* Philadelphia: Hanley & Belfus, Mosby.

Jones, K., & Jones, J. (1997). Physical activity and exercise. *Clinician Reviews, 7*(13), 81-88, 93-94, 97-98, 101-104.

Lee, I., Rippe, J., & Wilkinson, W. (1995). How much exercise is enough? *Patient Care, 29,* 118-135.

Marcus, B., Selby, V., & Niaura, R. (1992). Self-efficacy and the stages of exercise behavior change. *Research Quarterly Exercise and Sport, 63*(1), 60-66.

Murray, R. B., Zentner, J. P., Pinnell, N. N., & Boland, M. H. (1997). Assessment and health promotion for the person in later maturity. In R. B. Murray & J. P. Zentner (Eds.), *Health assessment and promotion strategies* (6th ed., pp. 693-774). Norwalk, CT: Appleton & Lange.

Norris, R., Carroll, D., & Cochrane, R. (1992). The effects of physical activity and exercise training on psychological stress and well-being in an adolescent population. *Journal of Psychosomatic Research, 36,* 55-65.

Pender, N. (1996). *Health promotion in nursing practice* (3rd ed.). Norwalk, CT: Appleton & Lange.

Remich, M. (1994). Promoting a healthy pregnancy. In E. Q. Youngkin & M. S. Davis (Eds.), *Women's health: A primary care clinical guide* (pp. 383-434). Norwalk, CT: Appleton & Lange.

Rowland, T. (1990). *Exercise and children's health.* Champaign: Human Kinetics.

Sloane, P., & Hicks, M. (1993). Preventive care: An overview. In P. Sloane, L. Slatt, & P. Curtis (Eds.), *Essentials of family medicine.* Baltimore: Williams & Wilkins.

Stephens, T., Jacobs, D., & White, C. (1985). A descriptive epidemiology of leisure-time physical activity. *Public Health Reports, 100,* 147-158.

United States Preventive Services Task Force (1996). *Guide to clinical preventive services* (2nd ed.). Baltimore: Williams & Wilkins.

Will, P., Demko, T., & George, D. (1996). Prescribing exercise for health: A simple framework for primary care. *American Family Physician, 53,* 579-585.

Woolf, S., Jonas, S., & Lawrence, R. (1996). Health promotion and disease prevention in clinical practice. Baltimore: Williams & Wilkins.

Review Questions

1. A client who has started an exercise plan is having minimal success. The NP should consider which of the following?
  a. Contracting with the client
  b. Referral to an exercise physiologist
  c. Implementing dietary changes
  d. Encouraging the client to set a permanent goal

2. To help the client avoid side effects from exercising, the NP should encourage all except which of the following?
  a. Avoiding sudden increases in activity level
  b. Proper use of equipment
  c. An intermittent exercise schedule
  d. Proper technique

3. A 45-year-old man who smokes and has a cholesterol level of 260 g/dL wants to start an exercise program. The NP prescribes which of the following?
  a. Swimming instead of jogging
  b. A stress test
  c. A beta-blocking agent
  d. A fasting blood glucose level

4. Ada, a 60-year-old woman who has been sedentary, is interested in beginning an exercise program. What might be the best form of exercise to begin?
  a. Weight lifting
  b. Swimming
  c. Walking
  d. Jogging

5. Chris currently runs five times a week. He wants to increase his weekly mileage. What recommendation would you give him as how to increase his mileage?
  a. Run as much as he is able each day.
  b. Staying at the same amount is the safest.
  c. He should not increase past 30 miles per week.
  d. Increase by 10% per week.

6. Which of the following is one of the best motivators to promote exercise?

   a. Recommendation from a provider
   b. Written handouts
   c. An offer of exercise classes
   d. Letting the client motivate himself or herself

7. Who is least likely to engage in exercise?

   a. Adolescent male
   b. Adolescent female
   c. Middle aged male
   d. Elderly female

8. Steve is beginning an exercise program. If he is 35 years old, what are the minimum and maximum heart rates you would recommend?

   a. 111 and 166
   b. 150 and 175
   c. 90 and 130
   d. 180 and 200

Answers and Rationales

1. *Answer:* **a** (evaluation)
   Rationale: Contracting has promoted adherence to an exercise plan. Flexible goals promote compliance. Dietary changes should be implemented, with or without success. Referral is not necessary at this time (Marcus, et al. 1992).

2. *Answer:* **c** (implementation/plan)
   Rationale: Regular exercise decreases side effects, as do proper equipment and technique and avoidance of sudden increases in activity level (United States Preventive Services Task Force, 1996).

3. *Answer:* **b** (implementation/plan)
   Rationale: A man older than 40 years with two or more risk factors for CAD should undergo a stress test before initiating an exercise program. Swimming may be detrimental to his health. Beta-blocking agents would decrease his compensatory ability to increase his HR to maintain cardiac output during higher demand (Woolf, et al. 1996).

4. *Answer:* **c** (implementation/plan)
   Rationale: Walking is recommended as a low-impact activity with no special equipment required. It is a particularly good way to get started exercising (Lee, et al. 1995).

5. *Answer:* **d** (implementation/plan)
   Rationale: As a rule of thumb, people should not increase their time or distance by more than 10% per week (Lee, et al. 1995).

6. *Answer:* **a** (implementation/plan)
   Rationale: Most providers do not recommend exercise to their clients. A recommendation to the client can be a good motivator to get started (Jones & Jones, 1997).

7. *Answer:* **d** (assessment)
   Rationale: Women, especially elderly women, are less likely to engage in regular exercise (Jones & Jones, 1997).

8. *Answer:* **a** (implementation/plan)
   Rationale: Using the formula for minimum and maximum heart rates, the rates would be 111 and 166 (Jones & Jones, 1997).

FALLS   *Pamela Kidd*

OVERVIEW
Definition

Falls are injuries sustained from kinetic forces from a loss of balance involving a change in spatial orientation.

Incidence

Hip fractures resulting from falls account for the majority of hospitalizations for fractures and are the second major cause of hospitalization for women who are 85 years of age or older. Sensory impairments are more common in the elderly. Among adults 70 years and older, 18% report vision impairments, 33% report hearing impairments, and 9% report both vision and hearing impairments (Campbell, et al. 1999). Vision loss may occur secondarily to cataracts, glaucoma, and visual field disturbances. Elderly persons with vision impairments report difficulty walking, which is a factor that increases risk of injury. Percentages of fall-related deaths are highest for men in all age categories; this may be because men have a greater number of co-morbid conditions. Approximately 10% of all falls among the elderly occur during acute illness (Mahoney, 1999).

Pathophysiology

● Falls by men often result from slips, whereas women tend to trip and then fall.
● Persons who fall most frequently attribute being in a hurry as the reason for the fall (Berg, Alessio, Mills, & Tong, 1997). Most older adults believe their falls result from internal factors, such as dizziness and poor balance, as opposed to external factors, such as floor rugs and poor lighting.

Factors Increasing Susceptibility. Some evidence exists that once a person has fallen, there is increased anxiety and fear of falling that may lead to increased health care contacts and an overall decreased sense of well being (Gray-Miceli, 1997). Having fallen is a risk factor for future falls because mobility may be limited and function may be decreased. Other risk factors include the following:

   ● Gait disturbance
   ● Physical inactivity
   ● Balance difficulty

- Urinary incontinence
- Change in housing conditions
- Poor pulse rate after standing
- Parkinsonism
- Arthritis
- Divorced, widowed, or unmarried
- Low body mass index
- Incomplete step continuity
- Poor distant visual acuity
- Long-acting benzodiazepines
- Peripheral neuropathy

The changing physiology of aging includes systolic hypertension, susceptibility to hypo- and hyperthermia, decreases in maximal ventilatory capacity, kidney function, and cardiac reserve, and osteoporosis (Baraff, Della-Penna, Williams, & Sanders, 1997). These factors increase the risk of falling by increasing the serum concentration and half-life of some drugs, the incidence of syncope, and the severity of injury.

Polypharmacy is also a risk factor for injury, particularly when the person visits several health care providers, none of whom may have the client's total medication history. Psychotropic agents are associated with falls among the older population. Cardiovascular agents producing peripheral vasodilation are also implicated.

Protective Factors

- Nursing personnel should conduct medication reviews, home safety modifications, and risk factor reductions with elderly clients and family and caregivers.
- No change in the home environment is recommended.
- Tai Chi has been effective in improving strength, balance, and coordination (Kessenich, 1998; Ross & Presswall, 1998). The performance of regular weight-bearing exercises helps maintain joint mobility.

ASSESSMENT: SUBJECTIVE/HISTORY

Although elderly persons may perceive a general increased risk of injury, particularly from falls, as they age and may also perceive that injuries are preventable, they still may not consider themselves to be susceptible for a specific injury event (Braun, 1998).

Symptoms

The acronym SPLATT can help health care providers remember key items to assess, such as **S**ymptoms, **P**revious falls, **L**ocation of fall, **A**ctivity at time of fall, **T**ime of fall, and **T**rauma (both psychologic and physical).

Past Medical History

If the client has a history of previous falls, assess for fear of falling. Signs include the following:

- Anxiety during ambulation
- Sweating or trembling while ambulating (and not before ambulation)
- Clutching objects or people while walking

- Watching own footsteps when walking
- Reluctance to ambulate or change position (Gray-Miceli, 1997)

Medication History

Benzodiazepines and tricyclic antidepressants have been positively related to falls (Cumming, 1998; Leipzid, Cumming, & Tinetti, 1999). The newer selective serotonin reuptake inhibitor (SSRI) agents are also correlated with falls. There are no significant differences between the risk of falls associated with TCAs or SSRIs.

Family History

Not relevant.

Dietary History

Not relevant.

ASSESSMENT: OBJECTIVE/PHYSICAL EXAMINATION
Physical Examination

Assess stability and mobility. Balance limitations can be assessed easily by asking the elderly person to get up from a chair without using his or her arms (the get-up-and-go test). If the person needs to use his or her arms, this indicates a significant weakness in the hip extensors and quadriceps and an increased chance of falling (Mahoney, 1999). Asking the client to walk and talk at the same time can help assess ease of gait and balance. The inability to walk while talking indicates a higher risk of falling and the need to concentrate on motor activities. Falls associated with the greatest injury risk occur in persons with cognitive and neuromuscular deficits and during the actions of climbing stairs, turning around, or reaching for objects.

Heavier persons tend to incur less severe injuries. Falls on hard, non-absorptive ground surfaces, such as tile, wood, and concrete, are more likely to result in injury. Falls are associated not only with hip fractures. Cervical spine injury, for example, occurs with minor energy releases among the elderly. C2 injuries may occur after minor injuries and particularly after falls (Spivak, Weiss, Cotler, & Call, 1994).

Diagnostic Procedures

It is important to explore whether a fall is in itself the primary event or whether it is the result of an undetected decline in health resulting from another health condition. Therefore diagnostic procedures depend on preexisting conditions of the client. Perform the following tests as indicated:

- Complete blood count and basic metabolic panel can rule out anemia, electrolyte imbalances, and hypo- or hyperglycemia as a cause of the fall.
- Radiographs may be indicated based on the extent of the injuries.

- ECG may be needed to rule out dysrhythmia.
- Urinalysis may be used to rule out a common source of infection.

DIAGNOSIS

- Fall related to functional decline
- Fall as primary event (results of diagnostic procedures negative except for those directly related to injuries)

THERAPEUTIC PLAN

Nonpharmacologic Treatment

- Treat fear of falling by helping the client to enroll in a community "roll into a fall" program so that a safe falling technique can be practiced.
- Intervention strategies should also address mitigating the effects of a fall, such as the use of protective hip pads or impact-absorbing floor materials.
- Encourage the use of assistive devices through proper fitting and effective teaching.
- Physical exercise is associated with decreased falls and fracture risk for healthy elderly persons.
- Weight-bearing exercises performed 20 to 30 minutes every day or 60 minutes three times a week is recommended for postmenopausal women. Interventions that focus on dynamic balance rather than static balance (e.g., Tai Chi) may enhance motor and balance control and decrease falls (Lee & Kerrigan, 1999).
- Fall-prevention strategies for skilled nursing facilities include having those personal belongings that are used frequently within adequate reach, keeping furniture in a consistent place, and responding to call lights quickly.

Pharmacologic Treatment

Treatment of osteoporosis decreases the risk of fall-related fractures. Bone density scanning is the best method of assessing bone mineral density. For best effects, antiresorptive therapy using biphosphonates should begin soon after menopause and be continued indefinitely (Beier, Maricic, & Staats, 1998). However, all women, regardless of age, benefit to some degree from biphosphonates. All postmenopausal women should take between 1000 and 1500 mg of calcium and between 400 and 800 IU of vitamin D every day regardless of any prescriptive therapy for osteoporosis (Meiner, 1999).

Client Education

A switch in the living environment of an elderly person (such as moving from a rural community to an urban one or from one house to another) may require reorientation of risk perceptions. Elderly persons who have been living in rural communities may be accustomed to walking in underbrush, around fallen trees, and among animals and may have adapted their movements to accommodate these hazards. However, the same person may not be comfortable crossing a busy street or may underestimate the risk of walking against a crossing light or the speed of an oncoming vehicle.

Referral

A geriatric assessment performed by a geriatric specialist is recommended for an elderly person who has sustained at least one other fall within a 3-month period of the current fall for which the elderly person is seeking care (*ED management of falls in the elderly*, 1998). Also consider referrals to social services, home health care, physical therapy (especially if there is a gait or balance problem assessed), optometric and ophthalmologic examination, and podiatric evaluation (for appropriate footwear).

Prevention

Fall prevention strategies for the home include the following:

- Eliminate household obstacles (floor rugs, books and objects on the floor, furniture that requires walking around).
- Have handrails and lights on all staircases (light switch should be at top and bottom of stairs).
- Eliminate loose tread on stairs.
- Install bathroom grab bars for toilet and tub.
- Use no-slip mats in bathtub and on shower floors.
- Get up slowly from a sitting or lying position.
- Wear shoes with good support and thin nonslip soles.
- Improve the lighting in the home (use 60-watt bulbs or higher and frosted bulbs to reduce glare).
- Keep frequently used kitchen items on lower shelves.
- Get a steady step stool with a bar to hold.
- Light the pathway between the bed and the bathroom.
- Paint door sills a different color to prevent tripping.
- Place a phone near the floor in case the client falls and cannot get up.
- Clinicians are encouraged to perform visual acuity checks, provide mobility counseling, and monitor the use of drugs associated with falls.

EVALUATION/FOLLOW-UP

Each client at each visit should be assessed for fall susceptibility and prevention practices implemented.

COMPLICATIONS

- Undetected internal bleeding leading to shock and death
- Impaired mobility related to fractures and injuries sustained from fall
- Anxiety related to fear of falling

REFERENCES

Baldwin, R., Craven, R., & Dimond, M. (1996). Falls: Are rural elders at greater risk? *Journal of Gerontological Nursing,* August, 14-21.

Baraff, L. J., Della Penna, R., Williams, N., & Sanders, A. (1997). Practice guidelines for the ED management of falls in community-dwelling elderly persons. *Annals of Emergency Medicine, 30*(4), 480-492.

Beier, M., Maricic, M., & Staats, D. (1998). Management of osteoporosis and risk assessment for falls in long-term care. *Annals of Long-term Care, 6* (Suppl. D), 1-16.

Berg, W. P., Alessio, H. M., Mills, E. M., & Tong, C. (1997). Circumstances and consequences of falls in independent community dwelling older adults. *Age and Ageing, 26,* 261-268.

Braun, B. (1998). Knowledge and perception of fall-related risk factors and fall-reduction techniques among community-dwelling elderly individuals. *Physical Therapy, 78*(12), 1262.

Campbell, V. A., Crews, J. E., Moriarty, D. G., Zack, M. M., & Blackman, D. K. (1999). Surveillance for sensory impairments, activity limitation, and health-related quality of life among older adults. *U.S. 1993-1997 MMWR Morbidity & Mortality Weekly Report, 48*(5508), 131-156.

Centers for Disease Control (1999). A tool kit to prevent senior falls. Atlanta: National Center for Injury Prevention and Control.

Chandler, J. M., Duncan, P., Sanders, L., & Studenski, S. (1996). The fear of falling syndrome: Relationship to falls, physical performance, and activities of daily living in frail older persons. *Topics in Geriatric Rehabilitation, 11*(3), 55-63.

Connell, B. R., & Wolf, S. (1997). Environmental and behavioral circumstances associated with falls at home among healthy elderly individuals. *Archives of Physical Medicine and Rehabilitation, 78,* 179-186.

Cumming, R. (1998). Epidemiology of medication-related falls and fractures in the elderly. *Drugs & Aging, 12*(1), 43-53.

ED management of falls in the elderly: Avoiding a downward spiral: Clinical update. (1998). *Journal of Critical Illness, 13*(2), 105-107.

Gray-Miceli, D. (1997). Falling among the aged. *ADVANCE for Nurse Practitioners, 5*(7), 41-42, 44.

Hanlon, J. T., Cutson, T., & Ruby, C. M. (1996). Drug-related falls in the older adult. *Topics in Geriatric Rehabilitation, 11*(3), 38-54.

Hinman, M. R. (1998). Causal attributions of falls in older adults. *Physical & Occupational Therapy in Geriatrics, 15*(3), 71-84.

Kessenich, C. (1998). Tai Chi as a method of fall prevention in the elderly. *Orthopaedic Nursing* (July/August), 27-29.

Koski, K., Luukinen, H., Laippala, P., & Kivela, S. L. (1998). Risk factors for major injurious falls among the home-dwelling elderly by functional abilities: A prospective population-based study. *Gerontology, 44,* 232-238.

Lee, L., & Kerrigan, C. (1999). Identification of kinetic differences between fallers and nonfallers in the elderly. *American Journal of Physical Medicine & Rehabilitation, 78,* 242-246.

Leipzig, R., Cumming, R., & Tinetti, M. (1999). Drugs and falls in older people: A systematic review and meta-analysis: I. Psychotropic drugs. *Journal of the American Geriatric Society, 47,* 30-39.

Luukinen, H., Koski, K., Kivela, S. L., & Laippala, P. (1996). Social status, life changes, housing conditions, health, functional abilities and life-style as risk factors for recurrent falls among the home-dwelling elderly. *Public Health, 110,* 115-118.

Mahoney, J. (1999). Falls in the elderly: Office-based evaluation, prevention, and treatment. *Cleveland Clinic Journal of Medicine, 66*(3), 181-189.

McLean, D., & Lord, S. (1996). Falling in older people at home: Transfer limitations and environmental risk factors. *Australian Occupational Therapy Journal, 43,* 13-18.

Meiner, S. (1999). An expanding landscape: Osteoporosis treatment options today. *Advances for Nurse Practitioners, 7*(7), 27-31, 80.

Ross, M. C., & Presswalla, J. L. (1998). The therapeutic effects of tai chi for the elderly. *Journal of Gerontological Nursing 24*(2), 45-47.

Spivak, J., Weiss, M., Cotler, J., & Call, M. (1994). Cervical spine injuries in patients 65 and older. *Spine 19,* 2302-2306.

Stevens, J., Powell, K., Smith, S., Wingo, P., & Sattin, R. (1997). Physical activity, functional limitations, and the risk of fall related fractures in community-dwelling elderly. *Annals of Epidemiology, 7,* 54-61.

Tinetti, M. E., Baker, D. I., McAvay, G., Claus, E. B., Garrett, P., Gottschalk, M., Koch, M. L., Trainor, K., & Horwitz, R. I. (1994). A multifactorial intervention to reduce the risk of falling among elderly people living in the community. *New England Journal of Medicine, 331,* 821-827.

Vellas, B., Wayne, S., Romero, L., Baumgartner, R., & Garry, P. (1997). Fear of falling and restriction of mobility in elderly fallers. *Age and Ageing, 26,* 189-193.

Wolfson, L., Whipple, R., Derby, C., Judge, J., King, M., Amerman, P., Schmidt, J., & Smyers, D. (1996). Balance and strength training in older adults: Intervention gains and Tai Chi maintenance. *Journal of the American Geriatric Society, 44,* 498-506.

Review Questions

1. After experiencing a fall, a client is seen by the NP. The NP knows she does *not* need to focus on which of the following factors during the assessment?
   a. Symptoms
   b. Previous falls
   c. Activity at time of fall
   d. Exercise history

2. What is the purpose of prescribing Tai Chi as a prevention measure for falls?
   a. It promotes aerobic capacity.
   b. It improves balance and coordination.
   c. It teaches one how to fall correctly.
   d. It creates better concentration.

3. What data support fear of falling as a diagnosis?
   a. Trembling before ambulation
   b. Clutching objects while walking
   c. Not talking to another while walking
   d. Reluctance to wear a different pair of shoes when walking

4. Which of the following categories of medications are associated with falling?
   a. SSRIs
   b. Nonsteroidal anti-inflammatory drugs (NSAIDs)
   c. Antibiotics
   d. Bronchodilators

5. Which of the following assessment data may indicate susceptibility for falling?

    a. Walks and talks at the same time.
    b. Uses arms to get up out of chair.
    c. Needs assistance getting into examination gown.
    d. Asks for assistance in getting onto examination bed.

6. Which of the following should be prescribed to a postmenopausal client to prevent bad consequences as a result of falling?

    a. Biphosphonates
    b. Salmon calcitonin (Miacalcin)
    c. Raloxifene (Evista)
    d. Calcium and vitamin D

Answers and Rationales

1. *Answer:* **d** (assessment)
    Rationale: The acronym SPLATT has been used to remind the provider which areas to assess. These areas are symptoms, previous falls, location of fall, activity at time of fall, time of fall, and trauma resulting from fall. Exercise history is not important at time of assessment.

2. *Answer:* **b** (analysis/diagnosis)
    Rationale: Tai Chi improves muscle strength, balance, and coordination. It has not been proven to improve concentration.

It is not a cardiovascular form of exercise. Correct falling is not taught as part of Tai Chi.

3. *Answer:* **b** (analysis/diagnosis)
    Rationale: Fear of falling is associated with trembling during ambulation and clutching onto people or objects while walking. Not talking to another person may be a person's usual style. It may indicate a need to concentrate but not necessarily fear. It may be wise to wear the same pair of shoes (assuming they are walking shoes) when walking.

4. *Answer:* **a** (assessment)
    Rationale: SSRIs have been correlated with falls. These drugs can impair motor performance as a side effect. The other categories of medications listed have not been implicated.

5. *Answer:* **b** (assessment)
    Rationale: Walking and talking at the same time indicates that a client does not need to concentrate on walking because of comfort with strength and balance. Needing assistance with a gown or bed may be because of lack of knowledge of how the item of clothing should be worn or because of the height of the surface.

6. *Answer:* **d** (implementation/plan)
    Rationale: Only calcium and vitamin D are used as primary preventives of osteoporosis. The other medications listed are usually prescribed in situations of documented osteopenia or osteoporosis using bone density scans.

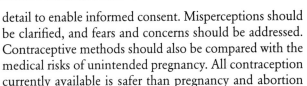

FAMILY PLANNING   *Cheryl Pope Kish*

Approximately 50% of pregnancies in the United States are unintended (Hewitt, 1998). Clients must have access to and education about various forms of contraception.

FACTORS INFLUENCING CHOICE OF CONTRACEPTION

- Lifestyle, including occupation and scheduling that enables compliance
- Relationship status
- Previous experiences with contraceptive methods by both partners
- Religious and cultural beliefs regarding contraception and what is and is not acceptable
- Availability and ease of use
- Readiness to touch genitalia if required (diaphragm, cervical cap, cervical mucus assessment, female condom)
- Cost
- Sexual behaviors (frequency of coitus, number of partners)
- Side effects and risk profile
- Privacy
- Non-contraceptive benefits
- Effectiveness of method
- Reproductive goals

A thorough history and physical examination should precede recommendations regarding contraception. Each method should be examined with the client(s) in enough

detail to enable informed consent. Misperceptions should be clarified, and fears and concerns should be addressed. Contraceptive methods should also be compared with the medical risks of unintended pregnancy. All contraception currently available is safer than pregnancy and abortion (see Table 5-1).

NATURAL FAMILY PLANNING/FERTILITY AWARENESS

The purpose of natural family planning and fertility awareness is to avoid pregnancy by abstaining from intercourse, either totally or during the fertile times of the month. This method, which is suitable for highly motivated couples, has a 1-year failure rate of approximately 20% (Hewitt, 1998). With this method, abstinence is required for approximately 17 days per cycle to compensate for the lack of precision of the method.

For greatest efficacy, the woman should use a variety of measures to plan for appropriately timed periodic abstinence: calendar rhythm, basal body temperature measurement, and cervical mucus assessment. The calendar rhythm method is based on the following three physiologic principles:

- Ovulation occurs 12 to 16 days before the onset of the next menstrual period.
- The ovum can be fertilized for 24 hours after ovulation occurs.

TABLE **5-1** Comparison of Hormonal Methods of Contraception

	COMBINED ORAL CONTRACEPTIVE PILLS	PROGESTIN-ONLY PILL	NORPLANT	DEPO-PROVERA	LUNELLE	ESTROGEN/ PROGESTERONE TRANSDERMAL PATCH (ORTHO EVRA)
Pregnancy with typical use	<5%	<5%	<1%	<1%	<1%	1% (Weight > 198 lb [90 kg] decreases efficacy)
Method requires administration	At approximately the same time daily	Daily (must not delay >3 hours to prevent LH surge and ovulation	Every 5 years	Every 13 weeks	Every 28 to 30 days; not >33 days	New patch every wk × 3 wk followed by 1 patch-free wk
Expected return of fertility after discontinuation	2- to 3-month wait suggested	Immediate	Immediate	4 to 13 months possible; some clients report longer delays	2 to 4 months	Ovulation expected within 6 wk after discontinuing
Anticipated menstrual pattern with method	Spotting with missed pill; usually decreased flow and decreased cramping	Spotting with missed pill; flow and cramping generally less	Unpredictable and sometimes prolonged first year; afterward may become more predictable and lesser amount	Spotting initially; after several doses, may have amenorrhea decreased	Bleed 2 to 3 weeks after first injection, then 22 to 28 days after; flow	Withdrawal bleeding begins during patch-free wk

LH, Leuteinizing hormone.

- Sperm is able to fertilize an ovum for 72 hours after ejaculation.

Women who have regular menstrual cycles are most likely to be successful using this method. It is helpful to document at least three cycles to predict the time of ovulation. The method is not recommended for women with cycles less than 25 days apart or as a sole method of timing periodic abstinence.

Basal body temperature measurement involves a 3-minute temperature assessment on waking, before engaging in any activity or smoking. The temperature increases 0.4° to 0.8° after ovulation because of the thermogenic properties of progesterone. Abstinence is required from the first day of the cycle until the third consecutive day of elevated temperature.

Cervical mucus assessment for planning periodic abstinence is based on the knowledge that the presence and consistency of cervical mucus responds to estrogen and progesterone at different points in the cycle. High levels of unopposed estrogen cause mucus to be copious and slippery. As progesterone levels increase from the corpus luteum, mucus thickens. A simple algorithm can be used to determine timing of coitus. Are secretions noted today? Were secretions noted yesterday? If the answer to both questions is "no," coitus is safe. Familiarity with cervical mucus requires a full cycle without sexual intercourse. Cervical mucus is altered by feminine hygiene products, douching, vaginitis, sexually transmitted diseases (STDs), cervical surgery, lactation, perimenopause, and hormonal contraception.

BARRIER METHODS

Barrier methods decrease the transmission of STDs by 50%. Barrier methods include diaphragms, cervical caps, condoms, contraceptive vaginal film, and spermicides.

Diaphragms

A diaphragm is a round, flat latex device that covers the end of the cervix. Diaphragms are used in conjunction with spermicides and should be left in place for at least 8 hours after coitus but not longer than 24 hours after insertion because of the risk of toxic shock syndrome. One application of spermicide is needed for each act of coitus. Side effects, although few, include increased urinary tract infection (UTI) and irritation from the spermicide. Failure rates average 18%. Diaphragms should be replaced every 2 years and refitted earlier if the woman becomes pregnant or if her weight otherwise changes by 10 to 15 lb. An annual examination and Pap smear and assessment of proper fit are advisable.

Cervical Caps

Cervical caps are similar to diaphragms, except smaller. As a result, they may be more difficult to properly fit and insert. The cervical cap may be left in place for as long as 36 hours. The cap can be used without spermicide. Use of the cap requires negative or normal results of a Pap smear obtained within the preceding year.

Condoms

Most condoms are made of latex and protect against STDs, including human immunodeficiency virus (HIV).

Condoms are available for both men and women; the sheath is placed either over the penis or in the vagina. The failure rate is approximately 12% in 1 year. Oil-based lubricants should not be used with condoms, and the efficacy of the condom may be affected by vaginal medications and by exposure to heat. Condoms for men are less likely to break when a $1/2$-inch reservoir is left at the tip to collect semen. Clients should be reminded that if a condom breaks, emergency contraception is available. Latex allergy precludes use in some couples.

Spermicides

Spermicides are chemicals that inactivate sperm. The most common spermicide is nonoxynol-9. Spermicides are most often used in conjunction with barrier methods, although some protection against pregnancy is provided when used alone. Spermicides have a failure rate of approximately 20%.

Intrauterine Contraceptive Devices

An intrauterine device (IUD) is a sterile artifact placed in the uterus, where it appears to prevent pregnancy primarily by generating a foreign body reaction in the uterus; the resulting inflammatory response is spermicidal. The hormone-releasing IUD (Progestasert) also thickens cervical mucus and inhibits implantation. The failure rate is approximately 2%. The ideal candidate for an IUD is in a stable, mutually monogamous relationship, has at least one child, and has no history of STD. Contraindications include (1) suspected or confirmed pregnancy, (2) abnormalities of the uterine cavity, (3) current or previous pelvic inflammatory disease (PID), (4) postpartum metritis or infected abortion within the previous 3 months, (5) known or suspected uterine malignancy or unresolved abnormal results of a Pap smear, (6) unexplained vaginal bleeding, (7) untreated or uncontrolled cervicitis, (8) history of ectopic pregnancy, (9) woman or partner has multiple sexual partners, (10) genital actinomycosis, (11) increased susceptibility to infection, (12) Wilson's disease (copper IUD, Para-Gard T 380A), and (13) allergy to copper (copper IUD).

Common side effects include menorrhagia and uterine cramping. Early warning signs include the following:

- **P**eriod late (possible pregnancy)
- **A**bdominal pain or dyspareunia
- **I**nfection exposure or abnormal discharge
- **N**ot feeling well, fever, or chills
- **S**tring missing, shorter, or longer than usual

Insertion is scheduled during or immediately after menses in women who have had negative results of a Pap smear within the preceding 6 months, negative results of a chlamydia and gonorrhea tests, and a medical examination that rules out contraindications. A NSAID administered before insertion minimizes cramping.

Although contraception is immediate, abstinence for 24 hours is advisable because of disruption of the cervical mucus barrier. Monthly verification of the IUD string after menstruation or unusual cramping and reporting warning signs immediately are essential points for client education. Follow-up is scheduled shortly after the first menstrual period or no later than 3 months after insertion. The Progestasert IUD is replaced yearly; the Para-Gard T 380A may be left in place for 10 years.

LONG-ACTING PROGESTINS

These preparations prevent contraception by inhibiting ovulation, thickening cervical mucus, and causing the endometrium to become atrophic. Levonorgestrel implants (Norplant) and medroxyprogesterone acetate (Depo-Provera or DMPA) are two such choices.

Levonorgestrel Implants (Norplant)

Levonorgestrel implants consist of six silicone elastomer rods inserted subdermally in the inner aspect of the upper arm. Advantages include contraception for 5 years with a low rate of failure (0.2%). The main disadvantage is the unpredictable vaginal bleeding that occurs in approximately 80% of women during the first year. Other side effects include weight gain, breast tenderness, depression, increased incidence of ovarian cysts, and difficult removal. No protection is provided against STDs. A back-up contraceptive method is needed for the first 7 days after insertion; symptoms of infection should be reported immediately. Follow-up for check of insertion is scheduled for 2 weeks. Contraception effects reverse immediately at the time of removal.

Depo-Provera

This is an injectable method of contraception. The dose is 150 mg every 3 months. Depo-Provera has a failure rate of 0.3% during the first year. Irregular bleeding is also a problem with this product. Other potential side effects include weight gain, breast tenderness, and depression. This is an appropriate contraceptive for postpartum and postabortion clients and may be used by women who are breast feeding once lactation is established. Otherwise, DMPA should be initiated within 5 days after the onset of menses. If the client is more than 1 week late for the injection, pregnancy must be ruled out. The drug should not be administered to a woman whose hematocrit level is lower than 30% without consultation with a physician. The delay to conception after discontinuing the drug is 9 to 22 months.

ORAL CONTRACEPTIVES

Oral contraceptive pills (OCPs) are the most widely used form of reversible birth control in the world. The pharmacologic ingredients in combined OCPs are estrogens (35 µg or less) and progestins. OCPs provide contraception by inhibiting ovulation, inhibiting sperm transport via thickened cervical mucus, and changing the endometrial lining to affect implantation.

Effectiveness ranges from 90% to 96%. In some combination pills, estrogen and progestin may remain constant during 21 days. With biphasics or triphasics, the dose of progestin component varies to duplicate the pattern of ovulatory menstrual cycle. Progestin-only OCPs contain no estrogen and are taken daily at a consistent time; ovulation is not consistently suppressed with the "mini pill" if the dosing schedule varies by more than 3 hours. Use of a back-up method of contraception is advised for the first pill pack. A back-up method is also required when the woman experiences nausea and vomiting or diarrhea or when taking medications that decrease the efficacy of OCPs (antibiotics, anticonvulsants, antifungals, and sedatives). Women are taught that if they miss one pill, they should take it as soon as they remember; if a second pill is missed, an additional method of contraception is necessary.

Noncontraceptive Benefits of Oral Contraceptive Pills

- Regular, predictable menstrual cycles and shorter periods
- Estimated 60% decrease in menstrual flow, which decreases amount of iron loss
- Less dysmenorrhea and, with suppression of ovulation, less mittelschmerz pain
- Decreased fibrocystic breast changes and benign breast disease, ectopic pregnancy, PID, and ovarian and endometrial cancer
- Reduction in symptoms of premenstrual syndrome
- Increased bone density

Absolute Contraindications

- Pregnancy
- Estrogen-dependent neoplasms
- Previous thromboembolism
- Cerebrovascular accident (CVA)
- CAD
- Impaired liver function
- Smoking in a woman older than 35 years

Relative Contraindications

- Elevated BP
- Undiagnosed vaginal bleeding
- Severe headaches
- Diabetes mellitus
- Elevated lipids
- Active gallbladder disease
- Sickle cell anemia

Side Effects

- **A**bdominal pain that is severe
- **C**hest pain, cough, shortness of breath
- **H**eadaches (severe) and dizziness
- **E**ye problems (vision loss or blurring)
- **S**evere leg pain

The client should be reevaluated 3 months after the initiation of OCPs to determine whether there are any problems.

MONTHLY ESTROGEN/PROGESTERONE INJECTION (MPA/E2C)

Medroxyprogesterone acetate (25 mg) and estradiol cypionate (5 mg) (MPA/E2C), marketed as *Lunelle* and ad-ministered as a monthly injection for contraception, is 99% effective. The safety and side effect profiles are similar to those of the combined OCPs, as are the contraindications. As with OCPs, the injection does not protect against STDs. There is commonly a disrupted bleeding pattern when the contraception is initiated, but periods generally become regular after the first month. Reinjection occurs every 28 to 30 days, not to exceed 33 days, but may be administered as early as 23 days to ensure compliance. The initial dose is administered within 5 days after the start of menses. Fertility returns within 2 to 4 months after discontinuation.

ESTROGEN/PROGESTERONE TRANSDERMAL PATCH (ORTHO EVRA)

A transdermal patch is applied to a clean, nonirritated skin surface on the abdomen, upper outer arm, buttock, or torso (excluding breast) on the same day of three consecutive weeks, followed by a patch-free week during which withdrawal bleeding occurs. The mechanism of action and side effects are similar to combined OCPs. If the patch is initiated within 24 hours of the start of menses, no backup is needed; otherwise backup is needed for one cycle. Humidity, heavy perspiration with exercise, temperature change, and immersion in water do not affect adhesion of the patch (Wysocki, 2002).

POSTCOITAL OR EMERGENCY CONTRACEPTION

Pharmacologic postcoital (emergency) contraception disrupts the postovulatory production of progesterone and estradiol, interferes with the passage of the fertilized ovum through the fallopian tube, shortens the luteal phase, and disrupts the cellular structure of the endometrium. This contraceptive method reduces the number of pregnancies by as much as 84%. Side effects include nausea, vomiting, headaches, breast tenderness, dizziness, and alteration of menses onset. The standard dose of 100 mg of ethinyl estradiol and either 0.5 mg of levonorgestrel or 1 mg of norgestrel is followed by a second dose 12 hours later. The first dose should be taken as soon as possible after unprotected intercourse; it must be taken within 72 hours for treatment to be effective. If a dose is vomited within 1 hour, it should be repeated; an antiemetic may be administered. Menses should occur within 21 days; if not, a pregnancy test should be performed. Follow-up in person or by telephone is performed at 3 to 5 weeks to ensure return of menses and to rule out treatment failure. None of the hormonal products used for emergency contraception pose risk to a developing fetus in the event that a pregnancy has occurred.

NONREVERSIBLE CONTRACEPTIVE METHODS
Sterilization

Sterilization is the most common contraceptive method used among married individuals in the United States.

Tubal ligation and vasectomy should be considered permanent. For that reason, the NP should be certain to address possible factors associated with regret and to recommend delaying decisions to allow for additional reflection and counseling when either partner is in doubt. Such factors include the following:

- Young age
- Sterilization decision related to pregnancy outcome or financial crisis
- Marital instability
- Sterilization paid for with public funds (women)
- No or young children at the time of the decision

If Title X (Medicaid) dollars are used to fund sterilization, federal guidelines must be followed. The client must be at least 21 years old and mentally competent, 30 to 180 days must elapse between informed consent and actual procedure, and consent must be given when the woman client is not in labor, facing abortion, or under drug influence.

Complications of tubal ligation are rare, but include bleeding, infection, and risks inherent in any surgery requiring anesthesia. Contraceptive effects are immediate.

Occlusion of the vas deferens to accomplish surgical sterilization of a man, although as effective as tubal ligation, is both safer and less costly. Both surgical and non-scalpel vasectomies are now available; minimal edema and pain are expected. Complications are rare and include hematoma, infection, and granuloma formation. An association between vasectomy and subsequent prostate cancer continues to be studied. Occlusion of the vas deferens has no impact on male hormone production, ability to achieve erection, ejaculation, amount of ejaculate, libido, or physical strength. Contraceptive effectiveness is not immediate; approximately 20 ejaculations (12 weeks) are necessary before sperm are no longer present in semen; a semen analysis validates sterilization.

REFERENCES

Brown, H. P. (2001). Emergency contraceptive pills. *The Female Patient, 26*, 36-42.

Dickerson, V. M. (2001). Contraception in the perimenopause. *The Female Patient, 26*, 12-16.

Grimes, D. A., Hanson, V., & Somdheimer, S. (2001). New approaches to emergency contraception. *Patient Care for the Nurse Practitioner, March*, 44-54.

Hatcher, R. A., Trussell, J., Stewart, F., Cates, W., Stewart, G.K., Guest, F., & Kowal, D. (1998). *Contraceptive technology*. Atlanta: Ardent Media.

Hawkins, J. W., Roberto-Nichols, D. M., & Stanley-Haney, J. L. (2000). Protocols for nurse practitioners in gynecologic settings (7th ed.). New York: Tiresias.

Haws, J. M., Butler, P. G., & Girvin, S. (1997). A comprehensive and efficient process for counseling patients desiring sterilization. *The Nurse Practitioner, 22*(6), 54-66.

Hewitt, G. (1998). Contraception. In F. Zuspan & E. Quillian (Eds.), *Handbook of obstetrics, gynecology, and primary care* (pp. 34-41). St. Louis: Mosby.

Kaunitz, A. M. (1999). Intrauterine devices: Safe, effective, and underutilized. *Women's Health in Primary Care, 2*(1), 39-62.

Kaunitz, A. M. & Jordan, C. W. (1997). Two long-acting hormonal contraceptive options. *Contemporary Nurse Practitioner*, 10-21.

Kupecz, D. (2001). Lunelle: A new contraceptive alternative. *The Nurse Practitioner, 26*(6), 55-59.

National Association of Nurse Practitioners in Women's Health (2001). Oral contraceptives: Beyond contraception. *Supplement to Contemporary OB/GYN, February*. Montvale, NJ: Medical Economics.

Pati, S., Pollack, A. E., & Carnigan, C. (1999). What's new in female sterilization? *Patient Care, March 15*, 118-142.

Pollack, A. E., & Pati, S. (1999). What's new in male sterilization? *Patient Care, March 15*, 143-158.

Rosenfeld, J. A. (2000). Contraception. In C. C. Thedke & J. Rosenfeld (Eds.), *Women's health* (pp. 1-27). Philadelphia: Lippincott, Williams, & Wilkins.

Scoggins, J., & Morgan, G. (1997). *Practice guidelines for obstetrics and gynecology*. Philadelphia: J.B. Lippincott.

Smith, M. A., & Shimp, L. A. (2000). Family planning. In M. A. Smith & L. A. Shimp (Eds.), *20 common problems in women's health care* (pp. 21-64). New York: McGraw-Hill.

Wysocki, S. (2001). Lunelle: A new contraceptive alternative. *The Nurse Practitioner, 26*(6), 55-59.

Wysocki, S., & Moore, A. A. (2002). New developments in contraception: The first transdermal contraceptive system. *Women's Health Care, 1*(3), 9-23.

Review Questions

1. Carol Jean calls to report that she had unprotected sex 96 hours ago and, concerned about pregnancy, is seeking emergency contraception. Which response by the NP is most appropriate?

   a. Advise her that if she becomes pregnant despite taking the drugs, fetal damage is almost certain.

   b. Prescribe one dose stat and another dose in 12 hours of postcoital contraception.

   c. Prescribe a 5-day course of drugs and schedule a follow-up examination.

   d. Explain that it is too late for the drugs to be effective.

2. Betsy is contemplating a cervical cap or a diaphragm; the NP provides comprehensive education regarding each to facilitate Betsy's decision. Which comment Betsy makes indicates that she has understood the information provided?

   a. "The cap cannot be left in as long as a diaphragm; that's a negative."

   b. "With the cap, we won't have to worry about spermicide."

   c. "The cervical cap is much easier to fit and much safer."

   d. "The cervical cap is much less expensive."

3. Which woman would be an appropriate candidate for an IUD?

   a. Maridell, who has a slight rectocele

   b. Elizabeth, who has frequent cystitis

   c. Lana, who is allergic to nonoxynol-9

   d. Peg, who enjoys a monogamous relationship

4. Carla is a 25-year-old mother of two. With her last pregnancy, she experienced thrombophlebitis. Other significant history includes PID. Her periods are regular with moderate flow. Which contraceptive method is most appropriate for Carla?

    a. Medroxyprogesterone acetate and estradiol cypionate (Lunelle)

    b. Combined OCPs

    c. IUD

    d. Medroxyprogesterone acetate (Depo-Provera)

5. Joan is a college student seeking contraception. She will graduate in 1 year and hopes to become pregnant with her first child as soon as possible thereafter. Which contraceptive method is best for Joan?

    a. IUD

    b. OCPs

    c. Medroxyprogesterone acetate

    d. Levonorgestrel implants (Norplant)

6. Which of these women is the best candidate for the progestin-only pill?

    a. Grace, who travels coast to coast twice weekly

    b. Kelly, who often forgets to take prescription drugs

    c. Iris, who wants the pill to help regulate her cycle

    d. Lindsey, who is breast feeding her 8-week-old son

7. The nurse teaches Molly Gunderson how to use a diaphragm for contraception. Which of the following statements made by Molly indicates a need for *further* teaching?

    a. "I should inspect the diaphragm in good light to find any holes before using it."

    b. "I'll need to leave the diaphragm in place for 6 hours after intercourse."

    c. "I should douche before I remove the diaphragm."

    d. "Spermicide makes the diaphragm more effective."

Answers and Rationales

1. ***Answer:* d** (implementation/plan)

    Rationale: Emergency (postcoital) contraception must be administered within 72 hours of unprotected intercourse to be effective (Grimes, Hanson, & Somdheimer, 2001).

2. ***Answer:* b** (evaluation)

    Rationale: The cervical cap can remain in place for up to 48 hours. It is difficult to fit and to insert and remove; the cost is equivalent to that of the diaphragm. Spermicide is not required (Hawkins, et al. 2000).

3. ***Answer:* d** (assessment)

    Rationale: Frequent UTIs, frequent candida, allergy to latex or spermicide, and multiple sexual partners make the diaphragm an inappropriate choice for a woman. A stable monogamous relationship makes her an ideal candidate (Smith & Shimp, 2000).

4. ***Answer:* d** (implementation/plan)

    Rationale: The history of PID in this client makes the IUD a poor choice; her thrombophlebitis serves as a contraindication for both combined OCPs and the medroxyprogesterone acetate and estradiol cypionate combination, which contains estrogen. Medroxyprogesterone acetate (Depo-Provera), a progestin-only contraception, is the best choice (Hatcher, et al. 1998).

5. ***Answer:* b** (implementation/plan)

    Rationale: The IUD is an inappropriate choice because Joan is a nullipara; levonorgestrel implants are a 5-year contraceptive; medroxyprogesterone acetate has been associated with a delayed return to fertility, in some cases up to 22 months. The most appropriate choice is OCPS (Hatcher, et al. 1998).

6. ***Answer:* d** (implementation/plan)

    Rationale: The woman who is breast feeding with established lactation is an appropriate candidate for progestin-only pills; estrogen is contraindicated. Women who have erratic schedules (choice a), forget to take medications (choice b), or need cycle regulation (choice c) are not good candidates (Hatcher, et al. 2000).

7. ***Answer:* c** (evaluation)

    Rationale: Douching before removal of a diaphragm is inappropriate; the woman needs clarification (Hatcher, et al. 2000).

IMMUNIZATIONS   *Denise Robinson*

Recommendations for vaccinating infants, children, and adults are based on characteristics of immunobiologics, scientific knowledge regarding the principles of active and passive immunization and the epidemiology of diseases, and judgments by public health officials and specialists in clinical and preventive medicine. Benefits and risks are associated with the use of all immunobiologics: no vaccine is completely safe or completely effective. Benefits of vaccination range from partial to complete protection against the consequences of infection, ranging from asymptomatic or mild infection to severe consequences, such as paralysis or death. The risks of vaccination range from common, minor, and inconvenient side effects to rare, severe, and life-threatening conditions. Thus recommendations for immunization practices balance scientific evidence of benefits, costs, and risks to achieve optimal levels of protection against infectious disease. These recommendations describe this balance and attempt to minimize risk by providing information regarding dose, route, and spacing of immunobiologics and delineating situations that warrant precautions or contraindicate the use of these immunobiologics. These recommendations are for use only in the United States because vaccines and epidemiologic circumstances often differ in other countries. Individual circumstances may warrant deviations from these recommendations. The relative balance of benefits and risks can change as diseases are controlled or eradicated. For example, because smallpox has been eradicated throughout the world, the risk of complications associated with smallpox vaccine (vaccinia virus) now outweighs any theoretical risk of contracting smallpox or related viruses for the general population. Consequently, smallpox vaccine is no longer recommended routinely for civilians or most military personnel. Smallpox vaccine is now recommended only for selected laboratory and health care workers with certain defined exposures to these viruses.

GENERAL INSTRUCTIONS FOR ADMINISTRATION OF IMMUNIZATIONS

Persons administering vaccines should take the necessary precautions to minimize risk for spreading disease. They should be adequately immunized against hepatitis B, measles, mumps, rubella, and influenza. Tetanus and diphtheria (Td) toxoid immunization is recommended for all persons. Hands should be washed before each new client is treated. Gloves are not required when administering vaccinations, unless the persons administering the vaccine will come into contact with potentially infectious body fluids or has open lesions on his or her hands. Syringes and needles used for injections must be sterile and preferably disposable to minimize the risk of contamination. A separate needle and syringe should be used for each injection. Different vaccines should not be mixed in the same syringe unless specifically licensed for such use. Disposable needles and syringes should be discarded in labeled, puncture-proof containers to prevent inadvertent needle stick injury or reuse.

Routes of administration are recommended for each immunobiologic. To avoid unnecessary local or systemic effects and to ensure optimal efficacy, the practitioner should not deviate from the recommended routes. Injectable immunobiologics should be administered where there is little likelihood of local, neural, vascular, or tissue injury. In general, vaccines containing adjuvants should be injected into the muscle mass; when administered subcutaneously or intradermally, they can cause local irritation, induration, skin discoloration, inflammation, and granuloma formation. Before the vaccine is expelled into the body, the needle should be inserted into the injection site and the syringe plunger should be pulled back. If blood appears in the needle hub, the needle should be withdrawn and a new site selected. The process should be repeated until no blood appears.

Subcutaneous Injections

Subcutaneous injections are usually administered into the thigh of infants and in the deltoid area of older children and adults. A $5/8$- to $3/4$-inch, 23- to 25-gauge needle should be inserted into the tissues below the dermal layer of the skin.

Intramuscular Injections

The preferred sites for intramuscular injections are the anterolateral aspect of the upper thigh and the deltoid muscle of the upper arm. The buttocks should not be used routinely for active vaccination of infants, children, or adults because of the potential risk of injury to the sciatic nerve. In addition, injection into the buttocks has been associated with decreased immunogenicity of hepatitis B and rabies vaccines in adults, presumably because of inadvertent subcutaneous injection or injection into deep fat tissue. If the buttocks is used for passive immunization when large volumes are to be injected or when multiple doses are necessary (e.g., large doses of immunoglobulin [Ig]), the central region should be avoided; only the upper, outer quadrant should be used, and the needle should be directed anteriorly (i.e., not inferiorly or perpendicular to the skin) to minimize the possibility of involvement with the sciatic nerve.

For all intramuscular injections, the needle should be long enough to reach the muscle mass and prevent vaccine from seeping into subcutaneous tissue, but not so long as to endanger underlying neurovascular structures or bone. Vaccinators should be familiar with the structural anatomy of the area into which they are injecting vaccine. A decision regarding needle size and site of injection must be made individually for each person based on age, volume of material to be administered, size of the muscle, and depth below the muscle surface into which the material is to be injected.

Infants (Younger than 12 Months Old). Among most infants, the anterolateral aspect of the thigh provides the largest muscle mass and is therefore the recommended site. However, the deltoid can also be used with the thigh (i.e., when multiple vaccines must be administered at the same visit). In most cases, a $7/8$- to 1-inch, 22- to 25-gauge needle is sufficient to penetrate muscle in the thigh of a 4-month-old infant. The free hand should bunch the muscle, and the needle should be directed inferiorly along the long axis of the leg at an angle appropriate to reach the muscle while avoiding nearby neurovascular structures and bone.

Toddlers and Older Children. The deltoid may be used if the muscle mass is adequate. The needle size can range from 22 to 25 gauge and from $5/8$ to $1/4$ inches, based on the size of the muscle. As with infants, the anterolateral thigh may be used, but the needle should be longer, generally ranging from $7/8$ to $1/4$ inches.

Adults

Multiple Vaccinations. If more than one vaccine preparation is administered or if vaccine and an Ig preparation are administered simultaneously, it is preferable to administer each at a different anatomic site. It is also preferable to avoid administering two intramuscular injections in the same limb, especially if diphtheria-tetanus-pertussis (DTP) vaccine is one of the products administered. However, if more than one injection must be administered in a single limb, the thigh is usually the preferred site because of the greater muscle mass; the injections should be sufficiently separated (i.e., 1 to 2 inches apart) so that any local reactions are unlikely to overlap. See Tables 5-2, 5-3, 5-4, and 5-5.

TABLE **5-2** Recommendations and Minimum Ages and Intervals Between Vaccine Doses*

VACCINE AND DOSE NUMBER	RECOMMENDED AGE FOR THIS DOSE	MINIMUM AGE FOR THIS DOSE	RECOMMENDED INTERVAL TO NEXT DOSE	MINIMUM INTERVAL TO NEXT DOSE
Hepatitis B1†	Birth-2 mo	Birth	1-4 mo	4 wk
Hepatitis B2	1-4 mo	4 wk	2-17 mo	8 wk
Hepatitis B3‡	6-18 mo	6 mo	—	—
DTaP1	2 mo	6 wk	2 mo	4 wk
DTaP2	4 mo	10 wk	2 mo	4 wk
DTaP3	6 mo	14 wk	6-12 mo	6 mo§‖
DTaP4	15-18 mo	12 mo	3 yr	6 mo§
DTaP5	4-6 yr	4 yr	—	—
Hib1§†¶	2 mo	6 wk	2 mo	4 wk
Hib2	4 mo	10 wk	2 mo	4 wk
Hib3#	6 mo	14 wk	6-9 mo	8 wk
Hib4	12-15 mo	12 mo	—	—
IPV1	2 mo	6 wk	2 mo	4 wk
IPV2	4 mo	10 wk	2-14 mo	4 wk
IPV3	6-18 mo	14 wk	3.5 yr	4 wk
IPV4	4-6 yr	18 wk	—	—
PCV1¶	2 mo	6 wk	2 mo	4 wk
PCV2	4 mo	10 wk	2 mo	4 wk
PCV3	6 mo	14 wk	6 mo	8 wk
PCV4	12-15 mo	12 mo	—	—
MMR1	12-15 mo**	12 mo	3-5 yr	4 wk
MMR2	4-6 yr	13 mo	—	—
Varicella††	12-15 mo	12 mo	4 wk	4 wk
Hepatitis A1	≥2 yr	2 yr	6-18 mo	6 mo
Hepatitis A2	≥30 mo	30 mo	—	—
Influenza§§	—	6 mo	1 mo	4 wk
PPV1	—	2 yr	5 yr‖	5 yr
PPV2	—	7 yr‖‖‖	—	—

*Combination vaccines are available. Using licensed combination vaccines is preferred over separate injections of their equivalent component vaccines. (Source: Centers for Disease Control [1999]. Combination vaccines for childhood immunization: Recommendations of the Advisory Committee on Immunization Practices [ACIP], the American Academy of Pediatrics [AAP], and the American Academy of Family Physicians [AAFP]. *MMWR: Morbidity and Mortality Weekly Report, 48*[No. RR-5], 5.) When administering combination vaccines, the minimum age for administration is the oldest age for any of the individual components; the minimum interval between doses is equal to the greatest interval of any of the individual antigens.

†A combination hepatitis B-Hib vaccine is available (Comvex, manufactured by Merck Vaccine Division). This vaccine should not be administered to infants younger than 6 weeks old because of the Hib component.

‡Hepatitis B3 should be administered ≥8 weeks after Hepatitis B2 and 16 weeks after Hepatitis B1, and it should not be administered before age 6 months.

§Calendar months.

‖The minimum interval between DTaP3 and DTaP4 is recommended to be ≥6 months. However, DTaP4 does not need to be repeated if administered ≥4 months after DTaP3.

¶For Hib and PCV, children receiving the first dose of vaccine at age ≥7 months require fewer doses to complete the series (see Centers for Disease Control. [1991]. Haemophilus b conjugate vaccines for prevention of *Haemophilus influenzae,* type b disease among infants and children two months of age and older: Recommendations of the ACIP. *MMWR: Morbidity and Mortality Weekly Report, 40*[No. RR-1], 1-7 and Centers for Disease Control. [2000]. Preventing pneumococcal disease among infants and young children: Recommendations of the ACIP. *MMWR: Morbidity and Mortality Weekly Report, 49*[No. RR-9], 1-35.)

#For a regimen of only polyribosylribitol phosphate-meningococcal outer membrane protein (PRP-OMP, PedvaxHib, manufactured by Merck), a dose administered at age 6 months is not required.

**During a measles outbreak, if cases are occurring among infants aged <12 months, measles vaccination of infants aged ≥6 months can be undertaken as an outbreak countermeasure. However, doses administered at age <12 months should not be counted as part of the series. (Source: Centers for Disease Control. [1998]. Measles, mumps, and rubella—Vaccine use and strategies for elimination of measles, rubella, and congenital rubella syndrome and control of mumps: Recommendations of the ACIP. *MMWR: Morbidity and Mortality Weekly Report, 47*[No. RR-8], 1-57.)

††Children aged 12 months to 13 years require only one dose of varicella vaccine. Persons aged ≥13 years should receive two doses separated by ≥4 weeks.

§§Two doses of inactivated influenza vaccine, separated by 4 weeks, are recommended for children aged 6 months to 9 years who are receiving the vaccine for the first time. Children aged 6 months to 9 years who have previously received influenza vaccine and persons aged ≥9 years require only one dose per influenza season.

‖‖Second doses of PPV are recommended for persons at highest risk for serious pneumococcal infection and those who are likely to have a rapid decline in pneumococcal antibody concentration. Revaccination 3 years after the previous dose can be considered for children at highest risk for severe pneumococcal infection who would be aged <10 years at the time of revaccination (see Centers for Disease Control. [1997]. Prevention of pneumococcal disease: Recommendations of the Advisory Committee on Immunization Practices. *MMWR: Morbidity and Mortality Weekly Report, 46*[No. RR-8], 1-24.)

DTaP, Diphtheria and tetanus toxoids and acellular pertussis; *Hib,* Haemophilus influenza B; *IPV,* inactivated poliovirus vaccine; *PCV,* pneumococcal conjugate vaccine.

TABLE **5-3**   Guidelines for Spacing of Live and Inactivated Antigens

ANTIGEN COMBINATION	RECOMMENDED MINIMUM INTERVAL BETWEEN DOSES
≥2 inactivated	None; can be administered simultaneously or at any interval between doses
Inactivated and live	None; can be administered simultaneously or at any interval between doses
≥2 live parenteral*	4-week minimum interval, if not administered simultaneously

*Live oral vaccines (e.g., Ty21a typhoid vaccine, oral polio vaccine) can be administered simultaneously or at any interval before or after inactivated or live parenteral vaccines.

TABLE **5-4**   Vaccines and Toxoids* Recommended for Adults, by Age Groups, United States

AGE GROUP (YEARS)	VACCINE/TOXOID					
	TD†	MEASLES	MUMPS	RUBELLA	INFLUENZA	PNEUMOCOCCAL POLYSACCHARIDE
18-24	×	×	×	×		
25-64	×	×§	×§	×		
>65	×				×	×

*Refer also to sections in text on specific vaccines or toxoids for indications, contraindications, precautions, dosages, side effects, adverse reactions, and special considerations.
†Td is adsorbed (for adult use), and is a combined preparation containing <2 flocculation units of diphtheria toxoid.
§Indicated for persons born after 1956.
Td, Tetanus and diphtheria.

Longer-than-recommended intervals between doses do not reduce final antibody concentrations. Therefore an interruption in the immunization schedule does not require reinstitution of the entire series of an immunobiologic or the addition of extra doses. However, administering doses of a vaccine or toxoid at less than the recommended minimum intervals may decrease the antibody response and therefore should be avoided. Doses administered at less than the recommended minimum intervals should not be considered part of a primary series.

Some vaccines produce increased rates of local or systemic reactions in certain recipients when administered too frequently (e.g., adult Td, pediatric diphtheria and tetanus toxoid (DT), tetanus toxoid, and rabies vaccines). Such reactions are thought to result from the formation of antigen-antibody complexes. Good record keeping, careful maintenance of client histories, and adherence to recommended schedules can decrease the incidence of such reactions without sacrificing immunity.

SIMULTANEOUS ADMINISTRATION

Experimental evidence and extensive clinical experience have strengthened the scientific basis for administering certain vaccines simultaneously. Many of the commonly used vaccines can safely and effectively be administered simultaneously (i.e., on the same day, not at the same anatomic site). Simultaneous administration is important in certain situations, including imminent exposure to several infectious diseases, preparation for foreign travel, and uncertainty that the person will return for further doses of vaccine.

Killed Vaccines

In general, inactivated vaccines can be administered simultaneously at separate sites. However, when vaccines commonly associated with local or systemic reactions (e.g., cholera, parenteral typhoid, and plague) are administered simultaneously, the reactions might be accentuated. When feasible, it is preferable to administer these vaccines on separate occasions.

Live Vaccines

The simultaneous administration of the most widely used live and inactivated vaccines has not resulted in impaired antibody responses or increased rates of adverse reactions. Administration of combined measles-mumps-rubella (MMR) vaccine yields results similar to the administration of individual measles, mumps, and rubella vaccines at different sites. Therefore there is no medical basis for administering these vaccines separately for routine vaccination instead of the preferred MMR combined vaccine.

Concern has been raised that oral live attenuated typhoid (Ty21a) vaccine theoretically might interfere with the immune response to oral poliovirus (OPV) vaccine when OPV vaccine is administered simultaneously or soon after live oral typhoid vaccine. However, no published data exist to support this theory. Therefore if OPV vaccine and oral live typhoid vaccine are needed at the same time (e.g., when international travel is undertaken on short notice), both vaccines may be administered simultaneously or at any interval before or after each other.

Text continued on p. 795

TABLE **5-5** Immunobiologics* and Schedules for Adults (>18 Years)*†, United States

IMMUNOBIOLOGIC GENERIC NAME	PRIMARY SCHEDULE AND BOOSTER(S)	INDICATIONS	MAJOR PRECAUTIONS AND CONTRAINDICATIONS‡
TOXOIDS			
Td, adsorbed (for adult use)	Two doses IM 4 weeks apart; third dose 6-12 months after second dose; booster every 10 years	All adults	Except in the first trimester, pregnancy is not a contraindication. History of a neurologic reaction or immediate hypersensitivity reaction following a previous dose. History of severe local (Arthus-type) reaction following previous dose. Such individuals should not be given further routine or emergency doses of Td for 10 years.
LIVE-VIRUS VACCINES			
Measles vaccine, live	One dose SC; second dose at least 1 month later, at entry into college or posthigh school education, beginning medical facility employment, or before traveling. Susceptible travelers should receive one dose.	All adults born after 1956 without documentation of live vaccine on or after first birthday, physician-diagnosed measles, or laboratory evidence of immunity; persons born before 1957 are generally considered immune.	Pregnancy; immunocompromised persons§; history of anaphylactic reactions following egg ingestion or receipt of neomycin. (See text.)
Mumps vaccine, live	One dose SC; no booster.	All adults believed to be susceptible can be vaccinated. Adults born before 1957 can be considered immune.	Pregnancy; immunocompromised persons§; history of anaphylactic reaction following egg ingestion. (See text.)
Rubella vaccine, live	One dose SC; no booster.	Indicated for adults, both male and female, lacking documentation of live vaccine on or after first birthday or laboratory evidence of immunity, particularly young adults who work or congregate in places such as hospitals, colleges, and military, as well as susceptible travelers.	Pregnancy; immunocompromised persons§; history of anaphylactic reaction following receipt of neomycin.
Smallpox vaccine (vaccinia virus)	THERE ARE NO INDICATIONS FOR THE USE OF SMALLPOX VACCINE IN THE GENERAL CIVILIAN POPULATION.		
Yellow fever attenuated virus, live (17D strain)	One dose SC 10 days to 10 years before travel; booster every 10 years.	Selected persons traveling or living in areas where yellow fever infection exists.	Although specific information is not available concerning adverse effects on the developing fetus, it is prudent on theoretical grounds to avoid vaccinating a pregnant woman unless she must travel where the risk of yellow fever is high. Immunocompromised persons§; history of hypersensitivity to egg ingestion.

LIVE-VIRUS AND INACTIVATED-VIRUS VACCINES

Vaccine	Schedule/Dosage	Indications	Special Considerations
Polio vaccines: eIPV OPV	eIPV preferred for primary vaccination; two doses SC 4 weeks apart; a third dose 6-12 months after second; for adults with a completed primary series and for whom a booster is indicated, either OPV or eIPV can be administered. If immediate protection is needed, OPV is recommended.	Persons traveling to areas where wild poliovirus is epidemic or endemic. Certain health-care personnel. (See text for recommendations for incompletely vaccinated adults and adults in households of children to be immunized.)	Although there is no convincing evidence documenting adverse effects of either OPV or eIPV on the pregnant woman or developing fetus, it is prudent on theoretical grounds to avoid vaccinating pregnant women. However, if immediate protection against poliomyelitis is needed, OPV is recommended. OPV should not be given to immunocompromised individuals or to persons with known or possibly immunocompromised family members.§ eIPV is recommended in such situations.

INACTIVATED-VIRUS VACCINES

Vaccine	Schedule/Dosage	Indications	Special Considerations
HB inactivated-virus vaccine	Two doses IM 4 weeks apart; third dose 5 months after second; booster doses not necessary within 7 years of primary series. Alternate schedule for one vaccine: three doses IM 4 weeks apart; fourth dose 10 months after the third.	Adults at increased risk of occupational, environmental, social, or family exposure.	Data are not available on the safety of the vaccine for the developing fetus. Because the vaccine contains only noninfectious HBsAg particles, the risk should be negligible. Pregnancy should not be considered a vaccine contraindication if the woman is otherwise eligible.
Influenza vaccine (inactivated whole-virus and split-virus) vaccine	Annual vaccination with current vaccine. Either whole- or split-virus vaccine may be used.	Adults with high-risk conditions, residents of nursing homes or other chronic-care facilities, medical-care personnel, or healthy persons >65 years.	History of anaphylactic hypersensitivity to egg ingestion.
HDCV inactivated, whole-virion; RVA	Preexposure prophylaxis: two doses 1 week apart; third dose 3 weeks after second. If exposure continues, booster doses every 2 years, or an antibody titer determined and a booster dose administered if titer is inadequate (<5). Postexposure prophylaxis: All post-exposure treatment should begin with soap and water. (1) Persons who have (a) previously received postexposure prophylaxis with HDCV, (b) received recommended IM preexposure series of HDCV, (c) received recommended ID preexposure	Veterinarians, animal handlers, certain laboratory workers, and persons living in or visiting countries for >1 month where rabies is a constant threat.	If there is substantial risk of exposure to rabies, preexposure vaccination may be indicated during pregnancy. Corticosteroids and immunosuppressive agents can interfere with the development of active immunity; history of anaphylactic or Type III hypersensitivity reaction to previous dose of HDCV. (See text.)

Continued

TABLE **5-5** Immunobiologics* and Schedules for Adults (> 18 Years)*†, United States—*cont'd*

IMMUNOBIOLOGIC GENERIC NAME	PRIMARY SCHEDULE AND BOOSTER(S)	INDICATIONS	MAJOR PRECAUTIONS AND CONTRAINDICATIONS‡
	series of HDCV in the United States, or (d) have a previously documented rabies antibody titer considered adequate: two doses of HDCV, 1.0 mL IM, one each on days 0 and 3. (2) Persons not previously immunized as noted previously: HRIG 20 IU/kg body weight, half infiltrated at bite site if possible; remainder IM; and five doses of HDCV, 1.0 mL IM one each on days 0, 3, 7, 14, 28.		
INACTIVATED BACTERIA VACCINES			
Cholera vaccine	Two 0.5-mL doses SC or IM or two 0.2-mL doses ID 1 week to 1 month apart; booster doses (0.5 mL IM or 0.2 mL ID) every 6 months.	Travelers to countries requiring evidence of cholera vaccination for entry.	No specific information on vaccine safety during pregnancy. Use in pregnancy should reflect actual increased risk. Persons who have had severe local or systemic reactions to a previous dose.
HbCV	Dosage for adults has not been determined.	May be considered for adults at highest theoretical risk (e.g., those with anatomic or functional asplenia or HIV infection).	No specific information on vaccine safety during pregnancy.
Meningococcal polysaccharide vaccine (tetravalent A, C, W135, and Y)	One dose in volume and by route specified by manufacturer; need for boosters unknown.	Travelers visiting areas of a country that are recognized as having epidemic meningococcal disease.	Pregnancy unless there is substantial risk of infection.
Plague vaccine	Three IM doses; first dose 1.0 mL; second dose 0.2 mL 1 month later; third dose 0.2 mL 5 months after second; booster doses (0.2 mL) at 1- to 2-year intervals if exposure continues.	Selected travelers to countries reporting cases, or in which avoidance of rodents and fleas is impossible; all laboratory and field personnel working with *Yersinia pestis* organisms possibly resistant to antimicrobials; those engaged in *Y. pestis* aerosol experiments or in field operations in areas with enzootic plague where regular exposure to potentially infected wild rodents, rabbits, or their fleas cannot be prevented.	Pregnancy, unless there is substantial and unavoidable risk of exposure; persons with known hypersensitivity to any of the vaccine constituents (see manufacturer's label); patients who have had severe local or systemic reactions to a previous dose.

	Dosage	Indications	Contraindications/Precautions
Pneumococcal polysaccharide vaccine (23 valent)	One dose; revaccination recommended for those at highest risk >6 years after the first dose.	Adults who are at increased risk of pneumococcal disease and its complications because of underlying health conditions; older adults, especially those >65 years of age who are healthy.	The safety of vaccine for pregnant women has not been evaluated; it should not be given during pregnancy unless the risk of infection is high. Previous recipients of any type of pneumococcal polysaccharide vaccine who are at highest risk of fatal infection or antibody loss may be revaccinated >6 years after the first dose. (See text.)
INACTIVATED BACTERIA AND LIVE-BACTERIA VACCINES			
Typhoid vaccine, SC and oral	Two 0.5-mL doses SC 4 or more weeks apart, booster 0.5 mL SC or 0.1 mL ID every 3 years if exposure continues. Four oral doses on alternate days. The manufacturer recommends revaccination with the entire four-dose series every 5 years.	Travelers to areas where there is a recognized risk of exposure to typhoid.	Severe local or systemic reaction to a previous dose. Acetone-killed and acetone-dried vaccines should not be administered ID.
LIVE-BACTERIA VACCINE			
BCG	One dose ID or percutaneously. (See package label.)	For children only, who have prolonged close contact with untreated or ineffectively treated active tuberculosis patients; groups with excessive rates of new infection in which other control measures have not been successful.	Pregnancy, unless there is unavoidable exposure to infective tuberculosis; immunocompromised patients.§
IMMUNE GLOBULINS			
Cytomegalovirus immune globulin (intravenous)	Bone marrow transplant recipients: 1.0 g/kg weekly; kidney transplant recipients: 150 mg/kg initially, then 50-100 mg/kg every 2 weeks.	As prophylaxis for bone marrow and kidney transplant recipients.	
Ig	Hepatitis A prophylaxis: Preexposure: one IM dose of 0.02 mL/kg for anticipated risk of 2-3 months; IM dose of 0.06 mL/kg for anticipated risk of 5 months; repeat appropriate dose at above intervals if exposure continues. Postexposure: one IM dose of 0.02 mL/kg administered within 2 weeks of exposure.	Nonimmune persons traveling to developing countries. Household and sexual contacts of persons with hepatitis A; staff, attendees, and parents of diapered attendees in day care center outbreaks.	

Continued

TABLE **5-5** Immunobiologics* and Schedules for Adults (> 18 Years)†, United States—*cont'd*

IMMUNOBIOLOGIC GENERIC NAME	PRIMARY SCHEDULE AND BOOSTER(S)	INDICATIONS	MAJOR PRECAUTIONS AND CONTRAINDICATIONS‡
HBIg	Measles prophylaxis: 0.25 mL/kg IM (maximum 15 mL) administered within 6 days after exposure.	Exposed susceptible contacts of measles cases.	Ig should not be used to control measles.
	0.06 mL/kg IM as soon as possible after exposure (with HB vaccine started at a different site); a second dose of HBIg should be administered 1 month later (percutaneous/mucous-membrane exposure) or 3 months later (sexual exposure) if the HB vaccine series has not been started. (See text.)	Following percutaneous or mucous-membrane exposure to blood known to be HBsAg positive (within 7 days); following sexual exposure to a person with acute HBV or an HBV carrier (within 14 days).	
TIg	250 U IM.	Part of management of nonclean, nonminor wound in a person with unknown tetanus toxoid status, with less than two previous doses or with two previous doses and a wound more than 24 hours old.	
HRIg	20 IU/kg, up to half infiltrated around wound; remainder IM.	Part of management of rabies exposure in persons lacking a history of recommended preexposure or postexposure prophylaxis with HDCV.	
Vaccinia immune globulin	0.6 mL/kg in divided doses over 24-36 hours; may be repeated every 2-3 days until no new lesions appear.	Treatment of eczema vaccinatum, vaccinia necrosum, and ocular vaccinia.	
VZIg	Persons >50 kg: 125 U/10 kg IM; persons >50 kg: 625 U‖.	Immunocompromised patients known or likely to be susceptible with close and prolonged exposure to a household contact case or to an infectious hospital staff member or hospital roommate.	

*Refer also to sections of text on specific vaccines or toxoids for further details on indications, contraindications, effects and adverse reactions, and special considerations. Refer also to individual ACIP statements (see li Appendix 2). Several other vaccines, toxoids, and immune globulins are licensed and available. These are no the following antitoxins are licensed and available: botulism antitoxin, trivalent equine (ABE) (distrib antitoxin (equine).

†Several vaccines and toxoids are in "Investigational New Drug" (IND) status and available only through the Infectious Diseases. These are: (a) eastern equine encephalitis vaccine (EEE), (b) w (WEE), (c) Venezuelan equine encephalitis vaccine (VEE), and (d) tularemia vaccine. Pentavalent (ABCDE) botul through CDC's Drug Service.

‡When any vaccine or toxoid is indicated during pregnancy, waiting until the second or the third trimester, precaution that minimizes concern about teratogenicity.

§Persons immunocompromised because of immune deficiency diseases, HIV infection (who should primarily not receive fever vaccines) (see text), leukemia, lymphoma, or generalized malignancy or immunosuppressed as a result of alkylating drugs, antimetabolites, or radiation.

‖Some persons have recommended 125 U/10 kg regardless of total body weight.

BCG, Bacille Calmette-Guerin; *eIPV,* enhanced potency inactivated poliovirus vaccine; *HB,* hepatitis B; *HbCV, Haemophilus influenza* B conjugate vaccine; *HBV,* hepatitis B virus; *HDCV,* human diploid cell vaccine; *HIV,* human immunodeficiency virus; *HRIg,* human rabies immunoglobulin; *Ig,* immunoglobulin; *OPV,* oral poliovirus vaccine; *RVA,* rabies vaccine, adsorbed; *Td,* tetanus diphtheria; *TIg,* tetanus immunoglobulin; *VZIg,* varicella zoster immunoglobulin.

Live Viruses

Theoretically, the immune response to one live-virus vaccine might be impaired if administered within 30 days of another live-virus vaccine; however, no evidence exists for currently available vaccines to support this concern. Whenever possible, live-virus vaccines administered on different days should be administered at least 30 days apart.

Routine Childhood Vaccines

Simultaneous administration of all indicated vaccines is important in childhood vaccination programs because it increases the probability that a child will be fully immunized at the appropriate age. During a recent measles outbreak, one study indicated that approximately one third of measles cases among unvaccinated preschool children could have been prevented if MMR had been administered at the same time as another vaccine.

The simultaneous administration of routine childhood vaccines does not interfere with the immune response to these vaccines. When administered at the same time and at separate sites, DTP, OPV, and MMR vaccines have produced seroconversion rates and rates of side effects similar to those observed when the vaccines are administered separately. Simultaneous vaccination of infants with DTP vaccine, OPV vaccine (or inactivated poliovirus [IPV] vaccine), and either *Haemophilus influenzae* B (Hib) vaccine or hepatitis B vaccine has resulted in acceptable response to all antigens. Routine simultaneous administration of DTP vaccine (or diphtheria, tetanus, and acellular pertussis [DTaP] vaccine), OPV (or IPV) vaccine, Hib vaccine, MMR vaccine, and hepatitis B vaccine is encouraged for children who are at the recommended age to receive these vaccines and for whom no specific contraindications exist at the time of the visit, unless, in the judgment of the provider, complete vaccination of the child will not be compromised by administering different vaccines at different visits. Simultaneous administration is particularly important if the child might not return for subsequent vaccinations. Administration of MMR and Hib vaccines at 12 to 15 months of age, followed by DTP vaccine (or DTaP vaccine, if indicated) at 18 months of age remains an acceptable alternative for children with caregivers known to be compliant with other health care recommendations and who are likely to return for future visits; hepatitis B vaccine can be administered at either of these two visits. DTaP vaccine may be used instead of DTP vaccine only for the fourth and fifth dose for children 15 months of age through 6 years (i.e., before the seventh birthday). Individual vaccines should not be mixed in the same syringe unless they are licensed for mixing by the Food and Drug Administration.

Live-virus vaccines can interfere with the response to a tuberculin test. Tuberculin testing, if otherwise indicated, can be performed either on the same day that live-virus vaccines are administered or 4 to 6 weeks later.

BREAST FEEDING AND VACCINATION

Neither killed nor live vaccines affect the safety of breast feeding for mothers or infants. Breastfeeding does not adversely affect immunization and is not a contraindication for any vaccine. Breast-fed infants should be vaccinated according to routine recommended schedules.

Inactivated or killed vaccines do not multiply within the body. Therefore they should pose no special risk for mothers who are breast feeding or for their infants. Although live vaccines do multiply within the mother's body, most have not been shown to be excreted in breast milk. Although rubella vaccine virus may be transmitted in breast milk, the virus usually does not infect the infant, and if it does, the infection is well tolerated. Breastfeeding mothers can receive OPV vaccination without any interruption in the feeding schedule.

PREGNANCY AND VACCINATION

Influenza vaccine should be administered to pregnant women who will be in their second or third trimester of pregnancy during December through March (influenza season). Pregnant women who have not received a three-dose series of Td immunization should receive Td vaccine because short-term immunity is conferred on the fetus, possibly preventing neonatal tetanus.

ROUTINE ADULT VACCINES

Immunizations recommended for adults are based on age, immune status, and exposure risk. To ensure that immunization status is reviewed, providers should review immunizations at age 50 years for the purpose of assessing the need for Td, pneumococcal, and influenza vaccination. Treatment of unexpected injury also provides the opportunity for review of immunizations.

Tetanus-Diphtheria

It is best to administer Td instead of tetanus vaccine alone to adults because diphtheria protection can be helpful, particularly if the adult travels internationally. Regarding wound treatment, for relatively clean wounds, if the adult has completed a three-dose series of Td immunization but has not received a booster within 10 years, administer the Td vaccine. If the wound is severe or contaminated, a booster should be administered if one has not been received within 5 years. A booster should be administered every 10 years.

Measles-Mumps-Rubella

Measles. Adults born in 1957 or later should receive one dose of measles vaccine unless they already received one dose of live measles vaccine on or after their first birthday, have documentation by a physician of having had the disease, or have laboratory evidence (titer) of immunity. College students, health care workers, and international travelers born in 1957 or after should have two doses of measles vaccine or evidence of immunity.

Mumps. Adults born before 1957 are considered immune to mumps. One dose of mumps vaccine is required for adults born in 1957 or after unless they have documented evidence of the disease.

Rubella. Adults born before 1957 are considered immune to rubella. However, female health care workers, regardless of birth year, who may get pregnant should be vaccinated unless they have evidence of immunity.

Hepatitis

Hepatitis A. Adults who travel internationally, adults who live in communities where hepatitis A is considered endemic, homosexual men, intravenous drug users, adults who have occupational risk for infection (e.g., public health sanitarians, food handlers), adults who have chronic liver disease or clotting factor disorders, and members of the armed forces should receive hepatitis A vaccination. Two doses are required, and protection lasts for 20 years.

Hepatitis B. Adults who should be vaccinated are those who are health care and public safety workers, have multiple sex partners, are intravenous drug users, who work with developmentally disabled persons, are hemodialysis and renal failure clients, who receive clotting factors, are international travelers to countries with intermediate or higher rates of hepatitis B, are in close contact with hepatitis B carriers, and are adoptees from countries with endemic hepatitis B. This vaccine is given IM in three doses, with 2 months between the first and second doses and 6 months between the second and third doses. Postvaccination testing (titer assessment) is recommended for persons at occupational risk and for persons who are immunocompromised.

Varicella

Because there is a higher risk that varicella is accompanied by pneumonia or encephalitis in adults, vaccination is recommended for adults who are health care workers who do not know whether they have had the disease (to prevent transmission of virus to clients). The vaccine is given in two 0.5-mL doses SC 4 to 8 weeks apart. If the disease is contracted after vaccination, the severity is diminished.

Haemophilus Influenzae

Adults are who are asplenic as a result of surgery or dysfunction should receive Hib conjugate vaccine. The Advisory Committee on Immunization Practices (ACIP) does not recommend routine vaccination of immunocompromised adults, but some providers choose to immunize these clients.

Meningococcal

Adults are who are asplenic as a result of surgery or dysfunction may receive meningococcal polysaccharide vaccine.

ROUTINE ELDERLY VACCINES
Influenza

Age is not a factor for high-risk adults. Persons at high risk include nursing home residents and clients with cardiopulmonary disorders. These adults should receive annual vaccination regardless of chronologic age. Diabetic clients may also be at higher risk. At age 65 years, vaccination should be received annually regardless of risk factor status. September 1 is considered the first day for administering the vaccine each season.

Pneumococcal

Adults with high-risk conditions defined as chronic heart, lung, or liver disease, alcoholism, diabetes and those who are immunocompromised (have HIV infection, leukemia, myeloma, lymphoma, renal disease or are asplenic or organ recipients), should receive vaccination regardless of age. At age 65 years, immunization should be received regardless of risk status. Immunization is one dose of the 23-valent vaccine. Immunocompromised adults should be revaccinated every 5 years with the 23-valent vaccine. Revaccination should also be used for adults who received the 14-valent vaccine and who are at high risk.

ALTERED IMMUNOCOMPETENCE

The ACIP statement on vaccinating immunocompromised persons summarizes recommendations regarding the efficacy, safety, and use of specific vaccines and Ig preparations for immunocompromised persons. ACIP statements on individual vaccines and Ig preparations contain additional information. Severe immunosuppression can be the result of congenital immunodeficiency, HIV infection, leukemia, lymphoma, generalized malignancy, or therapy with alkylating agents, antimetabolites, radiation, or large amounts of corticosteroids. Severe complications have occurred after vaccination with live, attenuated virus vaccines and live bacterial vaccines among immunocompromised clients. In general, these clients should not receive live vaccines except under certain circumstances as noted in the following. In addition, OPV vaccine should not be administered to any household contact of a severely immunocompromised person. If polio immunization is indicated for immunocompromised clients, their household members, or other close contacts, IPV vaccine should be administered. MMR vaccine is not contraindicated for the close contacts of immunocompromised clients. The degree to which a person is immunocompromised should be determined by a health care provider.

Limited studies of MMR vaccination of HIV-infected clients have not documented serious or unusual adverse events. Because measles may cause severe illness in persons with HIV infection, MMR vaccine is recommended for all asymptomatic HIV-infected persons and should be considered for all symptomatic HIV-infected persons. HIV-infected persons receiving regular Ig therapy via IV

(IgIV) may not respond to MMR vaccine or its individual component vaccines because of the continued presence of passively acquired antibody. However, because of the potential benefit, measles vaccination should be considered approximately 2 weeks before the next monthly dose of IgIV (if not otherwise contraindicated), although an optimum immune response is unlikely to occur. Unless serologic testing indicates that specific antibodies have been produced, vaccination should be repeated (if not otherwise contraindicated) after the recommended interval.

An additional dose of IgIV should be considered for persons receiving routine IgIV therapy who are exposed to measles within 3 weeks after administration of a standard dose (100 to 400 mg/kg) of IgIV.

Killed or inactivated vaccines can be administered to all immunocompromised clients, although response to such vaccines may be suboptimal. All such childhood vaccines are recommended for immunocompromised persons in usual doses and schedules; in addition, certain vaccines such as pneumococcal vaccine or Hib vaccine are recommended specifically for certain groups of immunocompromised clients, including those with functional or anatomic asplenia.

Vaccination during chemotherapy or radiation therapy should be avoided because antibody response is poor. Clients vaccinated while receiving immunosuppressive therapy or during the 2 weeks before starting therapy should be considered unimmunized and should be revaccinated at least 3 months after therapy is discontinued. Clients with leukemia in remission whose chemotherapy has been terminated for 3 months may receive live-virus vaccines.

The exact amount of systemically absorbed corticosteroids and the duration of administration needed to suppress the immune system of an otherwise healthy child are not well defined. Most experts agree that steroid therapy usually does not contraindicate the administration of live-virus vaccine when it is short term (i.e., less than 2 weeks); a low to moderate dose; long-term, alternate-day treatment with short-acting preparations; maintenance physiologic doses (replacement therapy); or administered topically (skin or eyes), by aerosol, or by intraarticular, bursal, or tendon injection. Although of recent theoretical concern, no evidence of increased severe reactions to live vaccines has been reported among persons receiving steroid therapy by aerosol, and such therapy is not in itself a reason to delay vaccination. The immunosuppressive effects of steroid treatment vary, but many clinicians consider a dose equivalent to either 2 mg/kg of body weight or a total of 20 mg per day of prednisone as sufficiently immunosuppressive to raise concerns regarding the safety of vaccination with live-virus vaccines. Corticosteroids used in greater than physiologic doses also can reduce the immune response to vaccines. Health care providers should wait at least 3 months after discontinuation of therapy before administering a live-virus vaccine to clients who have received high systemically absorbed doses of corticosteroids for 2 weeks or more.

STANDARDS FOR PEDIATRIC IMMUNIZATION PRACTICE

National standards for pediatric immunization practices have been established and include true contraindications and precautions to vaccination. True contraindications, applicable to all vaccines, include a history of anaphylactic or anaphylactic-like reactions to the vaccine or a vaccine constituent (unless the recipient has been desensitized) and the presence of a moderate or severe illness with or without a fever. Except as noted previously, severely immunocompromised persons should not receive live vaccines. Persons who develop encephalopathy within 7 days of administration of a previous dose of DTP or DTaP vaccine should not receive further doses of DTP or DTaP vaccine. Persons infected with HIV, those who have household contacts infected with HIV, and those with known altered immunodeficiency should receive IPV vaccine rather than OPV vaccine. Because of the theoretical risk to the fetus, women known to be pregnant should not receive MMR vaccine. Certain conditions are considered precautions rather than true contraindications for vaccination. When faced with these conditions, some providers may elect to administer vaccine if they believe that the benefits outweigh the risks for the client. For example, caution should be exercised when vaccinating a child with DTP vaccine who, within 48 hours of receipt of a previous dose of DTP vaccine, developed fever 40.5° C (105° F) or higher, cried persistently and inconsolably for 3 hours or longer, collapsed or developed a shock-like state, or experienced a seizure within 3 days of receiving the previous dose of DTP vaccine.

Conditions often inappropriately regarded as contraindications to vaccination are also noted. Among the most important are diarrhea and minor upper respiratory illnesses with or without fever, mild to moderate local reactions to a previous dose of vaccine, current antimicrobial therapy, and the convalescent phase of an acute illness. Diarrhea is not a contraindication to OPV.

Febrile Illness

The decision to administer or delay vaccination because of a current or recent febrile illness depends on the severity of symptoms and the cause of the disease.

All vaccines can be administered to persons with minor illnesses, such as diarrhea, mild upper respiratory infection with or without low-grade fever, or other low-grade febrile illness. Studies suggest that failure to vaccinate children with minor illnesses can seriously impede vaccination efforts. Among persons whose compliance with medical care cannot be assured, it is particularly important to take every opportunity to provide appropriate vaccinations.

Most studies from developed and developing countries support the safety and efficacy of vaccinating persons who have mild illnesses. One large ongoing study in the United States has indicated that more than 97% of children with mild illnesses develop measles antibody after vaccination. Only one study has reported a somewhat lower rate of seroconversion (79%) to the measles component of MMR vaccine among children with minor, afebrile upper respiratory infection. Therefore vaccination should not be delayed because of the presence of mild respiratory illness or other illness with or without fever.

Persons with moderate or severe febrile illnesses should be vaccinated as soon as they have recovered from the acute phase of the illness. This precaution avoids superimposing adverse effects of the vaccine on the underlying illness or mistakenly attributing a manifestation of the underlying illness to the vaccine.

Routine physical examinations and measuring temperatures are not prerequisites for vaccinating infants and children who seem to be healthy. Asking the parent or guardian whether the child is ill and then postponing vaccination for those with moderate to severe illnesses or proceeding with vaccination if no contraindications exist are appropriate procedures in childhood immunization programs.

CLIENT INFORMATION

Parents, guardians, legal representatives, and adolescent and adult clients should be informed about the benefits and risks of vaccine in understandable language. Opportunity for questions and answers should be provided before each vaccination.

Vaccine Information Pamphlets

The National Childhood Vaccine Injury Act requires that vaccine information materials be developed for each vaccine covered by the act (DTP vaccine or component antigens, MMR vaccine or component antigens, IPV vaccine, and OPV vaccine). The resulting vaccine information pamphlets must be used by all public and private providers of vaccines, although private providers may elect to develop their own materials. Such materials must contain the specific, detailed elements required by law. Copies of these pamphlets are available from individual providers and from state health authorities responsible for immunization.

IMMUNIZATION RECORDS
Provider Records

Documentation of client vaccinations helps ensure that persons in need of vaccine receive it and that adequately vaccinated clients are not over-immunized, increasing the risk for hypersensitivity (e.g., tetanus toxoid hypersensitivity). Serologic test results for vaccine-preventable diseases (such as those for rubella screening) and episodes of adverse events should be recorded in the permanent medical record of the vaccine recipient.

Health care providers who administer one or more of the vaccines covered by National Childhood Vaccine Injury Compensation Program (NVICP) are required to ensure that the permanent medical record of the recipient (or a permanent office log or file) states the date the vaccine was administered, the vaccine manufacturer, the vaccine lot number, and the name, address, and title of the person administering the vaccine. The term *health care provider* is defined as any licensed health care professional, organization, or institution, whether private or public (including federal, state, and local departments and agencies), under whose authority a specified vaccine is administered. The ACIP recommends that the above information be kept for all vaccines, not only for those required by the National Vaccine Injury act.

Client's Personal Record

Official immunization cards have been adopted by every state and the District of Columbia to encourage uniformity of records and to facilitate the assessment of immunization status by schools and child care centers. The records are also important tools in immunization education programs aimed at increasing parental and client awareness of the need for vaccines. A permanent immunization record card should be established for each newborn infant and maintained by the parent. In many states, these cards are distributed to new mothers before discharge from the hospital. Some states are developing computerized immunization record systems.

Persons without Documentation of Vaccinations

Health care providers frequently encounter persons who have no adequate documentation of vaccinations. Although vaccinations should not be postponed if records cannot be found, an attempt to locate missing records should be made by contacting previous health care providers. If records cannot be located, such persons should be considered susceptible and should be started on the age-appropriate immunization schedule. The following guidelines are recommended: MMR vaccine, OPV vaccine (or IPV vaccine, if indicated), Hib vaccine, hepatitis B vaccine, and influenza vaccine can be administered because no adverse effects of repeated vaccination have been shown to be associated with these vaccines.

Persons who develop serious adverse reactions after the administration of DTP, DTaP, DT, Td, or tetanus toxoid vaccines should be individually assessed before the administration of further doses of these vaccines (see the ACIP recommendations for use of diphtheria, tetanus, and pertussis vaccines).

Pneumococcal vaccine should be administered, if indicated. In most studies, local reactions in adults after revaccination were similar compared with initial vaccination (see the ACIP recommendations for the use of pneumococcal polysaccharide vaccine for further details).

2. When planning care for a client who is trying to stop smoking, the NP should do which of the following?

   a. Ask about tempting situations.
   b. Discuss weight control.
   c. Avoid setting a quit date.
   d. Help the client to find new coping strategies.

3. A client who has been using transdermal nicotine patches calls the NP after experiencing anxiety and restlessness. The NP should do which of the following first?

   a. Prescribe an anti-anxiety agent.
   b. Tell the client that this is a symptom of nicotine withdrawal and that it will go away.
   c. Assess the client's use of drinks containing caffeine.
   d. Prescribe more transdermal nicotine patches.

4. When is preventive education to reduce tobacco in adolescents most effective?

   a. Grades 11 to 12
   b. Grades 7 through 9
   c. For teens as identified as smokers
   d. For teens identified as having alcohol dependence

5. During which phase is the smoker most likely to reject smoking-cessation advice?

   a. Precontemplation
   b. Contemplation
   c. Preparation
   d. Action

6. Which of the following is not part of the 4 A intervention plan for smoking cessation?

   a. Ask all clients if they smoke.
   b. Advise all smokers to stop.
   c. Assist smokers who want to quit.
   d. Advise all smokers to use nicotine patches.

7. Cheryl, an NP, advises all the smokers in her practice to stop smoking. Steve, a client, says that he wants to stop but does not seem committed. Actively pushing the client to quit before he or she is ready may have which of the following results?

   a. Cause the client to really think about stopping.
   b. Set the client up for a failed quit attempt.
   c. Make the client angry.
   d. Have no effect on the cessation process.

8. Which of the following is most descriptive of nicotine withdrawal symptoms?

   a. They are usually mild.
   b. They begin 1 week after stopping.
   c. Symptoms of irritability, restlessness, and increased appetite begin within 24 hours.
   d. Weight gain and somnolence occur.

Answers and Rationales

1. *Answer:* **a** (evaluation)
Rationale: Clients frequently experience relapse during attempts to stop smoking. It does not mean that a referral is needed or that the person cannot stop smoking or is not serious about quitting.

2. *Answer:* **a** (assessment)
Rationale: Asking about tempting situations can help the NP to discuss ways of avoiding these situations as a form of anticipatory guidance. A quit date should be set. Old coping strategies can be used and may be comforting. Discussion regarding weight control may discourage the client from stopping smoking because of fear of weight gain.

3. *Answer:* **c** (evaluation)
Rationale: Although irritability, restlessness, and anxiety are side effects of nicotine withdrawal, the client may be causing an increase in these side effects through the use of caffeine. Non-pharmacologic interventions should be tried first.

4. *Answer:* **b** (implementation/plan)
Rationale: Preventive education for tobacco is most effective when started in grades 7 through 9 (United States Preventive Services Task Force, 1996).

5. *Answer:* **a** (analysis/diagnosis)
Rationale: During the precontemplation phase, smokers are not considering quitting within the next 6 months. They may reject any advice related to quitting (Prochaska & DiClemente, 1992).

6. *Answer:* **d** (implementation/plan)
Rationale: The 4 A plan for smoking cessation includes choices a through c. Advising all smokers to use nicotine patches is not part of the plan (Fiore, 1991).

7. *Answer:* **b** (implementation/plan)
Rationale: Pushing advice on the client before he or she is ready to quit is not a good idea. It may set the client up for a failed attempt to quit and can discourage the client from trying again.

8. *Answer:* **c** (evaluation)
Rationale: Symptoms of nicotine withdrawal begin within 24 hours of smoking cessation; symptoms include increased appetite, irritability, and restlessness (Fiore, 1991).

STRESS MANAGEMENT *Danise Robinson*

Many visits to health care providers are a result of stress-related illnesses; some sources estimate that 60% to 90% of visits may be related to stress (Pelletier & Lutz, 1988). Holmes and Rahe (1967) developed a method to determine the relationships between social readjustment, stress, and susceptibility to illness by means of the Social Readjustment Rating Scale. Strategies for health promotion and reduction of stress are important armamentarium for NPs in primary care.

Stress has been defined as the "non-specific response of the body to any demand made on it" (Selye, 1975). Physiologic responses of the body to stress include the following:

- Dilation of pupils
- Increased RR
- Increased HR
- Peripheral vasoconstriction
- Increased perspiration
- Increased BP
- Increased muscle tension
- Increased gastric motility
- Release of adrenalin
- Increased glucose level

These reactions prepare the body for the "flight or fight" mechanism. Stress is associated with decreased life satisfaction, development of mental disorders, increased incidence of stress-related illnesses, and decreased immunologic function (Pender, 1996). Stressors are interpreted differently by each person. Some stressors are considered positive and challenging, whereas others are viewed as negative and undesirable. Coping strategies assist a person in dealing with stressors. *Coping strategies* can be described as "learned and purposeful cognitive, emotional, and behavioral responses to stressors used to adapt to the environment or to change it" (Lazarus & Folkman, 1984).

Children experience stress and develop coping patterns early in life. Factors such as poverty, chronic illness, and parental dysfunction may influence the child's ability to develop effective coping strategies. Most stress research has been conducted with adults, and the results may not be applicable to children. Five of the most frequent stressors identified by children are feeling sick, having nothing to do, not having enough money to spend, being pressured to get good grades, and feeling left out of the group (Ryan, 1988).

Stressors in adulthood relate to initiating a career, establishing and maintaining a relationship, and child rearing. Work is often cited as a source of stress. Single parents are especially vulnerable to stress as they try to balance child rearing with the demands of a job.

Loss is the primary stressor for the aging adult. Loss of a spouse, loss of a close family member, and even retirement are considered negative life events. Limitations caused by aging, such as decreased visual acuity and decreased inability to perform activities of daily living, may compound the person's reaction to stressors, further compromising the immune system.

STRESS MANAGEMENT

The primary modes of stress management consist of the following goals according to Pender (1996):
- Minimizing frequency of stressors
- Increasing resistance to stress
- Avoiding physiologic arousal from stress

In general, minimizing the frequency of stressors is the first line of defense. If that is not possible, strengthening family and individual coping resources is the next step.

Minimizing Frequency of Stressors
- Change the environment (most proactive approach).
  - Flexible scheduling at work
  - Job sharing
  - Child care at work site
  - Job change
- Avoid excessive change.
- Time block (Girdano & Everly, 1979): Set aside time to focus on a specific change, developing strategies for adjustment by ensuring that necessary time is given to address critical tasks.
- Manage time.
  - Identify and prioritize values and goals.
  - Identify time wasted, overcommitment, and unrealistic expectations.
  - Learn to say "no" to demands that do not match goals.
  - Reduce tasks into smaller parts.
  - Avoiding overload, and delegate responsibilities.
  - Reduce sense of time pressure and urgency.

Increasing Resistance to Stress
- Physical conditioning increases stress resistance.
  - Promote exercise: Exercise seems to provide some stress-resistance benefits (Norris, Carroll, & Cochrane, 1992).
  - Get adequate sleep.
  - Maintain good nutrition.
- Psychologic conditioning increases stress resistance.
  - Enhance self-esteem by engaging in positive verbalization, identifying positive personal aspects.
  - Enhance self-efficacy.
- Undertake tasks that can be successfully completed.
- Mentally rehearse successful completion of task.
  - Increase assertiveness.
  - Greet people by name.
  - Maintain eye contact.

- Comment on positive characteristics of others.
- Take assertiveness training.
- Develop goal alternatives.
- Develop coping resources.
- Self-disclosure reduces stress.
- Self-direction reduces stress.
- Acceptance reduces stress.
- Social support reduces stress.
- Assessment of coping resources through Coping Resources Inventory (Matheny, Aycock, Curlette, 1993)

Avoiding Physiologic Arousal from Stress. The goal of avoiding physiologic arousal from stress is to replace muscle tension and heightened sympathetic nervous system activity with muscle relaxation and increased parasympathetic functioning (Pender, 1996). The following may reduce physiologic reactions to stress:

- Deep breathing exercises
- Relaxation training
- Biofeedback
- Imagery
- Meditation

If the above mechanisms do not work, a crisis may develop. Crisis is psychologic disequilibrium, which is a state that a person, for the time being, can neither escape nor solve with the customary problem-solving resources (Townsend, 1996).

Basic Assumptions of Crisis

- Crisis occurs for all persons; it does not necessarily represent psychopathology.
- Crises are precipitated by specific, identifiable events.
- Crises are personal by nature.
- Crisis is acute, not chronic, and resolves one way or another in a brief period.
- Potential for psychologic growth or deterioration exists.

Phases in Crises

- Vulnerability: emotional, cognitive, or behavioral
- Exposure to precipitating stressor
- Use of previous problem-solving methods
- Increased anxiety when previous coping methods do not work
- All resources tapped to resolve problem
- If crisis not resolved, tension mounting beyond further threshold or increases with time to breaking point
- Major disorganization of individual
- Usually lasts 4 to 6 weeks

Types of Crises

- Situational: acute response to external situational stressor
- Developmental: normal life-cycle transitions
- Posttraumatic stress disorder (PTSD)

Factors Influencing Equilibrium

- Perception of event: realistic or distorted
- Coping mechanisms
- Situational supports

CRISIS INTERVENTION

The goal of crisis intervention is psychologic resolution of the person's immediate crisis and restoration of the level of functioning that existed before crisis.

Phase 1

- Assessment: information gathered regarding precipitating stressor
- Evaluation of risk to life: obvious or potential threat to life or lives of others
- Evidence that person is able or unable to function in his or her usual role

Phase 2

- Planning of therapeutic interventions
  - Determine how much the crisis has disrupted the person's life.
  - Determine whether he or she is able to go to work or school, keep house, and perform other tasks.
  - Determine how this disruption is influencing others in the person's life.

Phase 3

- Intervene with a reality-oriented approach.
- A working relationship is rapidly established and includes unconditional acceptance, active listening, and attending to immediate needs.
- The problem-solving model provides the basis for change and active collaboration with the affected person. The plan must be consistent with the person's culture and lifestyle, must be dynamic, and must be re-negotiable.
  - Listen actively and with concern.
  - Encourage open expression of feelings.
  - Help the person gain an understanding of the crisis.
  - Help the person to gradually accept reality.
  - Help the person to explore new ways of coping with problems.
  - Link the person to a social network.
  - Decision counseling is a technique that is critical to crisis management.
  - Reinforce the newly learned coping methods; provide follow-up after resolution of the crisis (Hoff, 1984).

Phase 4

- Evaluation of crisis resolution and anticipatory planning are developed for recurrence of stressor (Townsend, 1996).
- Follow-up is critical.

REFERENCES

Aguilera, D. (1998). *Crisis intervention: Theory and methodology* (8th ed.). St. Louis: Mosby.

American Psychiatric Association (1994). *Diagnostic and statistical manual of mental disorders* (4th ed.). Washington, DC: American Psychiatric Association.

Barker, L., Burton, J., & Zieve, P. (1995). Principles of ambulatory medicine (4th ed.). Baltimore: Williams & Wilkins.

Clark, M. J. (1996). *Nursing in the community* (2nd ed.). Norwalk, CT: Appleton & Lange.

Girdano, D., & Everly, G. (1979). *Controlling stress and tension.* Englewood Cliffs, NJ: Prentice Hall.

Hobfoll, S. (1988). *The etiology of stress.* Washington, DC: Hemisphere.

Hoff, L. A. (1984). *People in crisis: Understanding and helping* (2nd ed.). Redwood City, CA: Addison-Wesley.

Holmes, T., & Rahe, R. (1967). The social readjustment rating scale. *Journal of Psychosomatic Research, 11,* 213-218.

Lazarus, S., & Folkman, S. (1984). *Stress, appraisal and coping.* New York: Springer.

Matheny, K, Aycock, D., & Curlette, W. (1993). The coping resource inventory for stress: A measure of perceived resourcefulness. *Journal of Clinical Psychology, 49,* 815-829.

Norris, R., Carroll, D., & Cochrane, R. (1992). The effects of physical activity and exercise training on psychological stress and well-being in an adolescent population. *Journal of Psychosomatic Research, 36,* 55-65.

Pelletier, K., & Lutz, R. (1988). Healthy people, healthy business: A critical review of stress management programs in the workplace. *American Journal of Health Promotion, 5,* 12-19.

Pender, N. (1996). *Health promotion in nursing practice* (3rd ed.). Norwalk, CT: Appleton & Lange.

Ryan, N. (1988). The stress-coping process in school-age children: Gaps in the knowledge needed for health promotion. *Advances in Nursing Science, 11,* 1-12.

Selye, H. (1975). *Stress without distress.* New York: NAL Dutton.

Smith, K., Johnson, S., & Mandle, C. (1994). Stress management and crisis intervention. In C. Edelman & C. Mandle (Eds.), *Health promotion throughout the lifespan* (3rd ed., pp. 299-323). St. Louis: Mosby.

Swanson, J., & Albrecht, M. (1993). *Community health nursing: Promoting the health of aggregates.* Philadelphia: W. B. Saunders.

Townsend, M. (1996). *Psychiatric mental health nursing: Concepts of care* (2nd ed.). Philadelphia: F. A. Davis.

United States Preventive Services Task Force (1996). *Guide to clinical preventive services* (2nd ed.). Baltimore: Williams & Wilkins.

United States Public Health Service. (1995). Smoking cessation in adults. *American Family Physician, 51,* 1914-1918.

Wheeler, L. (1997). *Nurse-midwifery handbook: A practical guide to prenatal and postpartum care.* Philadelphia: J. B. Lippincott.

Woolf, S., Jonas, S., & Lawrence, R. (1996). *Health promotion and disease prevention in clinical practice.* Baltimore: Williams & Wilkins.

Review Questions

1. Which of the following is the first priority in stress management?

   a. Minimizing the frequency of stressors

   b. Increasing the client's resistance to stress

   c. Avoiding physiologic arousal from stress

   d. Strengthening family coping mechanisms

2. Which of the following interventions helps to minimize the frequency of stressors?

   a. Promoting exercise

   b. Enhancing self-esteem

   c. Developing assertiveness

   d. Changing the environment

3. When prescribing interventions designed to avoid the physiologic arousal from stress, the NP should do which of the following?

   a. Replace parasympathetic nervous system activity with sympathetic activity

   b. Promote exercise

   c. Discuss time management

   d. Explain the use of imagery

4. What is the difference between a crisis and another anxiety-related event?

   a. A crisis results in emotional deterioration.

   b. A crisis evolves slowly and is not attributed to a specific event.

   c. A crisis is resolvable in a brief period.

   d. A crisis is a psychopathologic event.

5. An NP caring for a client in crisis asks her to describe her daily life. This information will help with which of the following?

   a. Planning therapeutic interventions

   b. Evaluating the person's threat of suicide

   c. Resolving the crisis

   d. Planning for the recurrence of the stressor

6. In helping the client in crisis attain equilibrium, the NP must assess which of the following?

   a. Coping mechanisms

   b. Psychologic history

   c. Response to drug therapy

   d. Medical history

7. An adolescent client is extremely upset about a car crash that she was involved in with an uninsured driver. She is fearful of losing her job because of lack of transportation. What does this reflect?

   a. PTSD

   b. A situational crisis

   c. A developmental crisis

   d. An occupational crisis

8. Which of the following is *not* appropriate when working with a client in crisis?

    a. using active listening
    b. encouraging open expression of feelings
    c. telling the person what is happening in the crisis situation
    d. linking the client to a social network

Answers and Rationales

1. *Answer:* **a** (implementation/plan)
    Rationale: Choices b, c, and d are appropriate in stress management, but the main goal is to decrease the frequency of stressors. If this is accomplished, the need for the other three is also diminished (Pender, 1996).

2. *Answer:* **d** (implementation/plan)
    Rationale: Changing the environment is the most proactive approach to managing stress. It should decrease the amount of stressors, which also decreases the need for choices a, b, and c (Pender, 1996).

3. *Answer:* **d** (implementation/plan)
    Rationale: The aim is to promote parasympathetic stimulation to decrease arousal. Exercise increases sympathetic stimulation. Time management decreases the frequency of stressors, which indirectly decreases sympathetic stimulation. Imagery can reduce physiologic reaction to stress (Pender, 1996).

4. *Answer:* **c** (analysis/diagnosis)
    Rationale: A crisis has the potential for growth, is resolvable in a brief period, is precipitated by a specific event, and can occur in all persons; thus it is not associated with pathology (Townsend, 1996).

5. *Answer:* **a** (assessment)
    Rationale: There are four phases to crisis intervention. Finding out about the amount of disruption in the person's daily life helps in planning therapeutic interventions and targeting resources that the client needs. To assess suicide risk, you need information regarding the precipitating stressor. To prevent recurrence, you must provide anticipatory planning (Townsend, 1996).

6. *Answer:* **a** (assessment)
    Rationale: The client's perception of the event, coping mechanisms, and situational supports are factors that influence equilibrium (Aguilera, 1998).

7. *Answer:* **b** (analysis/diagnosis)
    Rationale: A developmental crisis is a response to a normal life cycle transition. A situational crisis is a response to an external stressor. PTSD occurs later, well after an acute event. (Townsend, 1996).

8. *Answer:* **c** (assessment)
    Rationale: The NP should use active listening and unconditional acceptance and should link the person to a social network. The person should be helped to gradually accept reality and to understand what is happening in the crisis. This may mean letting the person tell the story from his or her perspective. Having the NP tell what is happening in the crisis is judgmental and premature (Hoff, 1984).

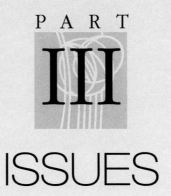

PART

III

ISSUES

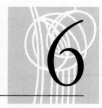

The Nurse Practitioner Role

Cheryl Pope Kish

The nurse practitioner (NP) role was initiated in the mid-1960s because of a physician shortage; Dr. Henry Silva, a pediatrician, and Dr. Loretta Ford, a nursing educator at the University of Colorado, envisioned the NP role as a means to ensure primary health care for children. Education for the role began at the University of Colorado. Initially, NP programs were 1-year certificate programs. Today, a master's degree is required for NP practice; persons who were already practicing as NPs can continue to practice without a master's degree because of the "grandfather" clause.

LICENSURE FOR NURSE PRACTITIONER PRACTICE

The U. S. Constitution delegates to the states the authority to legislate professional practice. Each state has a licensing board that oversees professional nursing practice, including advanced practice, through administration of the state's nurse practice act. The nurse practice act, a legal statute, defines nursing, including advanced practice nursing, delineates the scope and boundary of that practice, and specifies the roles and requirements for practice. A licensing board grants the advanced practice nurse permission to practice in the state and to use the professional title, by licensure, thereby assuring the state's citizens that the practitioner has met minimal competencies for safe practice, in accordance with the state's nurse practice act. Prescriptive authority for NPs varies from state to state regarding the degree of physician oversight and prescription of controlled substances. In some states, the Board of Medicine or the Pharmacy Board has a role in authorizing this aspect of advanced nursing practice. Some states require that NPs prescribe drugs from protocols (similar to standing orders).

CERTIFICATION OF NURSE PRACTITIONERS

Certification is a voluntary process that indicates that the clinician has met some predetermined standard for specialization in a particular area of advanced practice nursing set by a non–governmental agency or association.

Standards usually involve advanced education that includes a designated number of supervised clinical hours and passing a national standardized examination in the specialty area. Certification does not grant the individual any *legal* authority to practice; its primary purpose is to denote that the person holding the certification has met a high standard for competency in a specialty area of nursing practice. Most states do mandate certification as a requirement for NP licensure; some third-party payers require certification for reimbursing NPs for providing care; and certification provides consumers and other providers with additional information about the clinician's competency, but these are not the purposes of certification.

Certification for NPs is granted by the following professional organizations:

- American Academy of Nurse Practitioners (AANP): Certifies adult and family NPs
- American Nurses Credentialing Center (ANCC): Certifies gerontologic, pediatric, adult, family, acute care (in conjunction with the American Association of Critical Care Nurses), and school health NPs
- National Association of Pediatric Nurse Associates and Practitioners (NAPNAP): Certifies pediatric NPs
- National Certification Corporation (NCC): Certifies obstetric and gynecologic, women's health, and neonatal NPs

CREDENTIALING OF NURSE PRACTITIONERS

The NP may seek additional formal recognition of professional standing and clinical competence to obtain clinical privileges to facilitate practice. In this context, credentialing refers to documentation that the NP has met the agency's specified criteria (education, licensure, certification, recommendation/endorsement) for hospital privileges. Some institutions require proof of skill before they allow the NP to perform certain procedures. Whether an NP is eligible for such privileges depends not only on appropriate credentialing, but also on the institutional policy, medical staff bylaws, accreditation standards, and state law.

SCOPE OF PRACTICE

The NP's scope of practice, outlined in the nurse practice act, identifies who the NP is, what the NP can do in that role, and where the NP can legally provide care. Actions that exceed the legal boundaries of practice in a particular state are considered to be violations of the nurse practice act. Familiarity with the state's practice act and associated regulations is critical for legally prudent, safe practice.

Although state practice acts vary, there are similarities in terms of the mission of advanced practice nursing as comprehensive care to clients that is of high quality and based on ethical codes, advanced education, autonomous decision making, and expert skills. NPs are able to perform comprehensive health assessment, determine differential diagnoses, and initiate treatment regimens that involve both pharmacologic and nonpharmacologic measures. For the family NP, the client is defined as a person at any developmental stage of the life cycle, a family, or a community in need of health education, health promotion, restoration, or maintenance.

STANDARDS OF CARE

NPs are expected to practice according to the Standards of Care, the authoritative statements that direct the minimal competent care expected and guide the evaluation of such care. Standards define the NP's accountability to clients. In a court of law, the following questions address whether the Standards of Care were followed (Buppert, 1999):

- Did the NP make the appropriate decision regarding care?
- Was the care effective? Timely?
- Was care provided safely?
- Was the outcome as good as might be expected, considering the client's condition?

The courts will also address whether the NP functioned within the scope of practice as defined by the Nurse Practice Act.

In 1996, the American Nurses Association delineated the Standards of Care for advanced practice nursing in *Scope and Standards of Advanced Practice Registered Nursing*, stating that "the advanced practice registered nurse:

- collects comprehensive client health data.
- critically analyzes the assessment data in determining the diagnoses.
- identifies expected outcomes. . .and individualizes expected outcomes with the client and. . .health care team when appropriate.
- develops a comprehensive plan of care that includes interventions and treatments to attain expected outcomes.
- prescribes, orders, or implements interventions and treatments for the plan of care.
- provides comprehensive clinical coordination of care and case management.

- provides consultation to influence the plan of care for clients, enhance the abilities of others, and effect change in the system.
- employs complex strategies, interventions, and teaching to promote, maintain, and improve health, and prevent illness and injury.
- uses prescriptive authority, procedures, and treatments in accordance with state and federal laws and regulations to treat illness and improve functional health status or provide preventive care.
- identifies the need for additional care and makes referrals as needed.
- evaluates the client's progress in attaining expected outcomes" (p.11-15).

OTHER NURSE PRACTITIONER ROLE EXPECTATIONS

In addition to the role as direct provider of health care, other roles expected of the NP include the following:

- Educator: Includes not only teaching clients and families but also serving as clinical preceptors and mentors for students.
- Leader/manager: Involves leadership behaviors and role modeling for the professional development of peers, colleagues, and others; fostering advancement of the profession; applying critical, creative, and innovative decision making in a care delivery system; political advocacy; and participation in professional organizations.
- Change agent: Uses a deliberate change process to affect care delivery or improve policy, process, or procedural aspects of practice.
- User of nursing theory: Practices advanced nursing according to a nursing model, not according to the medical model.
- Researcher: Uses evidence-based practice, identifies researchable questions from practice, and communicates research findings to expand the professional knowledge base.
- Collaborator: Works with other disciplines to affect client care.
- Evaluator: Performs self-evaluation to ensure adherence to practice standards and state statutes/regulations; maintains currency of practice; evaluates practice structure (setting), processes, and client outcomes.

EMPLOYMENT CONTRACTS AND COLLABORATIVE PRACTICE AGREEMENTS

An employment contract is a written, legally binding agreement between the employer and prospective employee that delineates the terms and conditions of the proposed working relationship that serves to protect the interests of both parties (Buppert, 1999). Virtually any item that is fair and reasonable and makes the NP feel as though he or she has more job security can be placed within a contract, as long as the addition is mutually agreed on by employer. Contracts typically are in effect for 1 year, are re-negotiable, and include the following:

- Scope of services to be provided by the NP (this must be congruent with that defined in the state Nurse Practice Act), including both direct care and non-direct care obligations
- Exact time commitments entailed by the position
- Manner in which the contract can be altered or terminated by either party and for what purposes
- Compensation agreement
- Fringe benefits
- Restrictive covenant clause, which is a non-compete agreement that specifies that if the contract is terminated, the NP cannot engage in a competitive practice within a specified period of time in a defined geographic area
- Specifics of performance evaluation

Collaborative practice agreements as part of the contract or as a separate document are required in some states. This agreement specifies the ways in which the NP and physician agree to work together, capitalizing on the professional roles of both for the mutual benefit of the clients (Sebas, 1994).

MARKETING THE NURSE PRACTITIONER ROLE

Marketing refers to determining the needs and desires of the prospective consumer and designing services, products, or programs to meet those needs (Lachman, 1996). The key elements of marketing include the four Ps: product, price, place, and promotion.

- Product: the unique role of the NP and the way in which an existing practice can be extended by the addition of an NP
- Price: cost advantage in NP-delivered care
- Place: competitive advantage of a practice site or after-hours services
- Promotion: processes devoted to negotiating a position in practice, informing prospective clients about the NP role in general and within a particular practice, and gaining and maintaining clients

REFERENCES

American Nurses Association (1996). *Scope and standards of advanced practice registered nursing.* Washington, DC, American Nurses Association.

Barkley, T. W., Hasking, R. C., & Tejedor, M. A. (2001). Practice issues: Credentialing, prescriptive authority, and liability. *Nurse Practitioner Forum, 12*(2), 106-114.

Buppert, C. (1999). *Nurse practitioner's business and legal guide.* New York: Aspen.

Dunphy, L. M., & Winland-Brown, J. E. (2001). *Primary care: The art and science of advanced practice nursing.* Philadelphia: F. A. Davis.

Lachman, V. D. (1996). Positioning your business in the marketplace. *Advanced Practice Nursing Quarterly, 2*(1), 27-2.

Robinson, D., & Kish, C. P. (2001). *Core concepts in advanced practice nursing.* St. Louis: Mosby.

Sebas. M. (1994). Developing a collaborative practice agreement for the primary care setting. *Nurse Practitioner, 19*(3), 49-51.

Review Questions

1. Which of the following phrases best describes the primary purpose of the advanced practice Standards of Care?

  a. To promote the legal mandates for advanced practice level of care
  b. To regulate the numbers of advanced practice nurses in the United States
  c. To identify criteria for use in evaluating advanced practice nursing
  d. To interpret the legislative intent of the state Nurse Practice Acts

2. Which of the following documents serves as the legal basis for one's practice as an NP?

  a. American Nurses Association Code of Ethics
  b. State nurse practice act
  c. Nightingale Pledge
  d. American Nurses Association Standards of Clinical Practice

3. Which factor served as the impetus for the NP role?

  a. Decision by the Colorado Board of Nursing to expand the role of registered nurses
  b. Shortage of physicians to meet heath care needs of underserved children
  c. Request by the Colorado Secretary of State for nurses who could use the medical model of care
  d. Innovative recruitment strategy by the University of Colorado College of Nursing

4. Bill Green, a family NP, and his prospective employer are discussing a prospective employment contract. The physician mentions the need for a restrictive covenant clause. Bill would correctly understand this clause as doing which of the following?

  a. Restricts his right to compete with the physician within a particular geographic area for a specified length of time if the contract is terminated.
  b. Restricts his right to serve as a preceptor or mentor for NP students for the initial year of practice in the setting.
  c. Restricts his right to collect third-party reimbursement for the care he renders.
  d. Restricts his ability to refer clients to specialists unless they are approved by his collaborative physician.

5. Which comment made by Jill, a newly graduated NP student, indicates a correct understanding of the primary purpose of national certification?

  a. "Unless I pass the certification examination, I cannot be licensed to practice as an NP."
  b. "Becoming certified increases the probability that I can get a job as an NP."

c. "Gaining privileges to admit patients to the hospital demands certification."
d. "National certification demonstrates that I have met the requirements for specialization as an NP."

Answers and Rationales

1. *Answer:* c

Rationale: The Standards of Care identify elements to guide professional practice and to serve as criteria for evaluating that practice (American Nurses Association, 1996).

2. *Answer:* b

Rationale: The particular state's Nurse Practice Act delineates the legal basis for practice as an NP within that state (Buppert, 1999).

3. *Answer:* b

Rationale: A physician shortage that impacted accessibility to primary care for underserved children served as an impetus to the development of the NP role by Dr. Henry Silva and Dr. Loretta Ford in the mid-1960s (Buppert, 1999).

4. *Answer:* a

Rationale: A restrictive covenant is a non-compete clause that is part of most contracts. The statement usually restricts competition for a designated period of time within a specific geographic setting (Buppert, 1999).

5. *Answer:* d

Rationale: Choices a, b, and c are all true statements about the advantages of national certification; however, option d represents the primary purpose for certification: a type of quality assurance that the NP has met predetermined standards for specialization (Robinson & Kish, 2001).

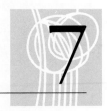

7

Access to Care

Pamela Kidd

DEFINITION

Access to care is defined as a set of factors that affect the potential and actual ability of an individual or group to acquire timely and appropriate health care services (Millman, 1993). Of concern is how a person can access the health care system without insurance. Vulnerable groups include women, children, people of color, poor people, older adults, the chronically ill, the mentally ill, persons with acquired immune deficiency syndrome, substance abusers, homeless persons, immigrants, the uninsured, and the underinsured. The underinsured are those for whom out-of-pocket expenditures for health care exceed 10% of their income (Monheit, Hagin, Berk, et al. 1988).

BARRIERS TO ACCESS

- Inability to pay
  - Uninsured, underinsured
  - Fewer providers willing to serve Medicaid recipients because of low reimbursement rates
- Sociocultural
  - Provider and staff attitudes
  - Language incompatibility
  - Culturally incompetent care
  - Fear of deportation
- Organizational
  - Inadequate capacity
  - Too few public clinics
  - Not enough appointment slots
  - Uneven distribution of health care providers
  - Lack of coordination of services
  - Problems securing Medicaid coverage
  - Transportation barriers
  - Child care problems

STRATEGIES FOR IMPROVING ACCESS

- Establish community health centers.
- Establish migrant health centers.
- National Health Service Corps: Award scholarships to increase the number of providers in underserved areas.
- Increase the number of minority providers.
- Train more primary care providers.

Four Goals for Access Improvement

- Control costs through the use of services.
- Use a business approach to ensure efficiency.
- Ensure quality through the measurement of outcomes.
- Form a partnership to address care across the wellness-illness continuum.

TYPES OF HEALTH CARE DELIVERY SYSTEMS
Primary Care

Four characteristics of primary care are the following:
- First-contact care
- Longitudinal over time
- Comprehensive
- Coordination of client care

Several factors contribute to decreasing access to primary care for the uninsured and underinsured: (1) health care costs continue to rise, (2) fewer people are able to obtain jobs that include health insurance benefits, and (3) there are increased amounts of co-pays (out-of-pocket costs) required to receive services. When people cannot access primary care, they use emergency and urgent care services that further increase health care costs. Primary care providers function as gatekeepers in that they control access to other health care services, such as specialists or testing.

Managed Care

The concept of managed care is congruent with the nursing philosophy of preventive care, cost-effectiveness, efficiency, and evaluation of care. It is the process of the application of standard business practices to the delivery of health care. The goal of managed care is to achieve the best quality product for the least cost, while continuously improving the outcomes. A managed care organization (MCO) is an organization that delivers health services without having to use the services of an insurance company. The employer pays for the MCO, and the MCO assumes all risk.

Types of Managed Care Systems

- Health maintenance organization (HMO): Access to services is based on a fixed monthly fee per enrollee with control for utilization maintained by the HMO. The HMO ensures quality for services provided (must provide evidence), and care can be provided only by participating organizations, physicians, and other service providers.
- Preferred provider organization (PPO): Discounted fees for service are offered instead of capitation. If a client selects a provider outside the network, the difference between the discounted fee and the normal fee is assumed by the client through co-pays or deductible payments. This type of system functions by selling services to organizations (volume principle) versus individuals.
- Point-of-service plan (POS): The client is allowed to use certain providers at a lower cost or to use other providers at a higher cost. Referrals are made by a primary care provider. This plan allows the greatest flexibility in choice of provider.
- Fee-for-service payments: The client sees the physician or other provider of choice, paying the fee out of pocket.
- Health insurance purchasing cooperatives: This system contracts with an MCO to provide standardized packages of medical benefits for fixed per capita rates. Basically, the cooperative acts on behalf of the consumer to secure less expensive rates.

OVERVIEW OF HEALTH CARE DELIVERY
Hospitals

Burden has been placed on family to get the client to the physician instead of the physician coming to see the client in the traditional "house-call." The role of nursing became organized around the gathering of clients in the hospital or other institution. Institutions may be organized into three types: (1) voluntary (not-for-profit), in which profits are turned back into the organization for improvements; voluntary institutions are exempt from taxes and must demonstrate ability to meet their mission; (2) public institutions that are owned by federal, state, or local governments; and (3) proprietary (for-profit) institutions in which the goal is to make a profit for the shareholder.

Health Insurance

During the early 1900s, health care for the poor was financed by charity of the rich. The Great Depression rendered the rich unable to subsidize the poor. The Social Security Act of 1935 was implemented and provided maternal and child health services (Title V) and general public health services (Title VI).

Hospitals began providing health care in return for premiums (advance payment for future services). Blue Cross/Blue Shield (BC/BS) was the first company to offer insurance independent of the hospital. Budgets for services had to be approved by the BC/BS company before the hospital could increase its charges.

After World War II, employers provided health insurance. Employees did not need to pay for health insurance until the 1970s. However, treatment of disease was covered but preventive services were not.

Medicaid/Medicare

Medicaid and Medicare were established in 1965 to alleviate health care access issues for the poor and for older adults and disabled persons, respectively. Often, poor, uneducated persons could not get jobs that included health insurance benefits. Both Medicaid and Medicare offer MCO options. Medicaid is a state-run entitlement program for the poor and uninsured. What Medicaid covers and who is eligible for services differ from state to state.

Medicare is a federally funded program that is financed through employee payroll taxes. Older adults and disabled persons are eligible for benefits. Part A, which is free of charge, covers hospital, nursing home, and home care services. Part B, which is available for a monthly premium, covers physician visits, laboratory fees, and outpatient services. Prescriptions are not covered by either Part A or B.

Health Maintenance Act of 1973

The Health Maintenance act of 1973 provided federal funds for the establishment and expansion of HMOs. Employers with 25 or more employees were required to offer an HMO alternative if one was available in the area.

Consolidated Omnibus Budget Reconciliation Act

The Consolidated Omnibus Budget Reconciliation act (COBRA) allows a person to pay for health insurance at the group rate that was being paid by a previous employer for up to 18 months (29 and 36 months under certain circumstances). This ensures coverage until new employment is found (assuming new employment is begun within 18 months) or until other health insurance coverage is in place. However, frequently, the person cannot afford to pay the premiums between jobs.

State Children's Health Insurance Program

Began in 2000, the State Children's Health Insurance Program (SCHIP) provides health insurance for uninsured children who qualify (200% of federal poverty level). It is important for the NP to know that a child may be eligible for SCHIP even if the family is not eligible for Medicaid based on the state's rules.

Community Health Center Program

Under the Bureau of Primary Health Care, United States Public Health Service, the Community Health Center Program (CHCP) provides services to the poor and underserved in inner-city and rural areas. The Rural Health

Clinic, which requires employment of a midlevel provider and is located in a medically underserved area, is part of this program, as is the Migrant Health Center.

Public Health Care

Public health care was established by law, but services vary dramatically across the country. Most programs are limited to well-baby care, sexually transmitted disease clinics, family planning, tuberculosis screening, and ambulatory mental health services.

REFERENCES

Anderson, M., & Robinson, D. (2001a). Institutions providing health care delivery. In D. Robinson & C. Kish (Eds.), *Clinical concepts for advanced practice nursing*. St. Louis: Mosby.

Anderson, M., & Robinson, D. (2001b). The role of managed care in health care delivery. In D. Robinson & C. Kish (Eds.), *Clinical concepts for advanced practice nursing*. St. Louis: Mosby.

Millman, M. L. (1993). *Access to health care in America: Institute of Medicine (vs) Committee on Monitoring Access to Personal Health Care Services*. Washington, DC: National Academy Press.

Monheit, A., Hagin, M., Berk, M., et al. (1988). The employed uninsured and the role of public policy. *Inquiry, 22,* 348-364.

Review Questions

1. Which of the following best describes primary health care providers?
   a. Gatekeepers to the health care system
   b. Providers who provide care only for acute illnesses
   c. Providers who provide care in rural health settings
   d. Consultants who participate in the plan of care

2. An elderly client needs medication to heal a bleeding ulcer. The client has Medicare Part A insurance. What does the NP tell the client?
   a. Medicare Part A will cover the cost of the medication.
   b. The client needs Medicare Part B to have the medication costs covered.
   c. Neither Medicare Part A or B will cover medications.
   d. Medicare Part A will cover the cost if generic medications are used.

3. Which of the following managed care plans affords the greatest flexibility of choice for the client?
   a. POS
   b. HMO
   c. PPO
   d. MCO

4. An NP provided services for a family that was Medicaid-eligible. Now, the family is no longer Medicaid-eligible. Which of the following is *not* an option for providing services to the children?

   a. Refer the family to the public health department.
   b. Enroll the children in SCHIP.
   c. Consider whether the family may qualify for services through a minority health center.
   d. Refer the children to a PPO plan.

5. An elderly client needs outpatient lab work. The client has Medicare Part A insurance. What should the NP tell the client?
   a. Medicare Part A will cover the outpatient lab work.
   b. Medicare Part A will cover the outpatient lab work if she is diagnosed with a chronic illness.
   c. Medicare Part A will not cover the outpatient lab work.
   d. Medicare Part A will cover the outpatient lab work if the findings are abnormal.

6. What is the main difference among public, proprietary, and voluntary (not-for-profit) hospitals?
   a. The degree of reimbursement provided for nurse practitioners
   b. Whether profits are made
   c. The type of specialty services offered
   d. How profits are distributed

Answers and Rationales

1. Answer: a
Rationale: Primary health care providers are those providers who coordinate the access of clients to other resources within the system. They do not provide care only for acute illnesses or only in rural health settings. Consultants who participate in the plan of care are exactly that: consultants.

2. Answer: c
Rationale: Medicare Part A covers hospital, nursing home, and home care services. Medicare part B covers physician visits and outpatient laboratory testing. Medications are not covered by either Part A or B.

3. Answer: a
Rationale: An HMO requires the use of providers listed within the HMO network. A PPO allows the use of some outside providers at a higher fee. The POS plan allows use of any provider but those included within the managed care plan can be used at a lower fee. An MCO is the company that offers an HMO, POS, or PPO or any combination thereof.

4. Answer: d
Rationale: A PPO plan must be provided through an employer or purchased by individual premium payments, probably not an option for a family that is "on the financial edge" and was recently Medicaid-eligible. The public health department does provide maternal and child services, particularly well care. SCHIP would be an option if the family income were at 200% of the federal poverty level. If the child and/or the family were of a particular ethnic group, services through a minority health center may be available.

5. Answer: c
Rationale: Medicare Part A covers only hospital, nursing home, and home health services. Medicare Part B can be

purchased and covers physician visits, laboratory fees, and outpatient services.

6. *Answer:* d

Rationale: All hospitals need to earn a profit to remain open. Proprietary hospitals share this profit among stockholders. Public and voluntary hospitals reinvest the profits into the hospital. Reimbursement is dictated by federal law and third-party insurer policies. Specialty services are decided by the needs of the population being served, hospital boards, community planning agencies, and, in some cases, stockholders. However, it is possible that all three types of hospitals may offer the same services.

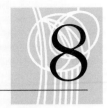

Client Education

Cheryl Pope Kish

Nurse practitioners (NPs) spend an inordinate amount of time educating clients in everyday practice. Educating clients and families is a primary role of the NP. Without engaging the process of client education, the NP could not facilitate management of acute or chronic illness, prevention of illness and injury, or promotion of health. More than 70% of health problems are lifestyle-related, and more than 80% of health problems are handled in the home in this society; these facts serve as a powerful impetus for client education. Presenting oneself at a health care clinic becomes a teachable moment for every client to become an informed consumer of health care. Professional nursing standards, mandates by accrediting bodies, institutional expectations, and governmental regulations have served to emphasize the role and expectations for the nursing profession in educating clients.

PURPOSES OF CLIENT EDUCATION (GREENBERG, 1989)

- To enable clients to assume more responsibility for their health care by being active, not passive, recipients of care
- To facilitate healthier lifestyles through prevention strategies
- To improve clients' abilities to manage acute and chronic illness, cope better, and prevent complications
- To increase compliance with pharmacologic and non-pharmacologic management plans
- To increase client satisfaction, even attracting clients to a practice where education is valued by providers
- To decrease liability by informing clients more thoroughly
- To increase cost-effectiveness of the system

PROCESSES OF CLIENT EDUCATION
Definitions

Education Process. The education process is "a systematic, sequential, planned course of action consisting of two major interdependent operations, teaching and learning, which form a continuous cycle . . . the outcome of which is a mutually desired behavior change." The process engages "two interdependent players, the teacher and the learner. . .in what should always be a participatory approach to teaching and learning" that promotes growth in both (Bastable, 1997).

Teaching. Teaching is a constant stream of deliberate decisions that occur before, during, and after interaction with the learner that increase the likelihood that learning will occur (Hunter, 1984). Teaching can be formal or informal; thoroughly planned and staged or spontaneous; and provided one-on-one, in small groups, and in large groups. The client benefiting from teaching might be an individual, family, group, or entire community. Instruction, the actual interaction with the learner that involves providing information intended to produce learning, is only one aspect of teaching (Bastable, 1997).

Learning. Learning is the conscious or unconscious acquisition of knowledge, skills, or values such that behavior is changed in some way. Learning can occur at any time or at any place in which the learner is exposed to the educational process (Bastable, 1997).

Phases of the Client Education Process

The phases of the client education process parallel those of the nursing process.

Assessment. Assessment involves determining the learning needs, health values, readiness to learn, preferred learning styles, cognitive ability, acuity of senses, developmental ability, level of education and literacy, primary language, and any barriers to learning (e.g., acuity of physical illness, pain, anxiety, hunger, uncomfortable environment). Assessment also includes knowledge of financial and network resources.

Planning. Planning involves mutually setting educational outcomes and objectives and then establishing a method to meet the unique needs of the client. Objectives must be realistic and based on client strengths, limitations, resources, and everyday lifestyle. Standardized learning plans are sometimes available, including some on that can be accessed on the Internet.

Implementation. Implementation involves engaging the learner with specific instructional methods and materials that add to what he or she already knows by relating to information previously learned or to past experience.

Evaluation. Evaluation involves determining the outcomes of instruction based on changes in behavior (knowledge, skills, and/or values).

THE ASSURE MODEL FOR CLIENT EDUCATION (REGA, 1993)

- **A**nalyze the learner.
- **S**tate the objectives.
- **S**elect instructional methods.
- **U**se teaching materials.
- **R**equire learner performance.
- **E**valuate and revise.

OBSTACLES TO LEARNING
Client-Related Factors

Client-related factors include anxiety, stress, pain, sensory deficits, and other symptoms of acute or chronic illness that interfere with engagement in the learning process. Sometimes, a client demonstrates denial and lack of motivation or readiness to learn.

System-Related Factors

System-related factors include lack of privacy, fragmentation of services, time limits on visits, inadequacy of materials that are learner-friendly and culturally sensitive, inconsistency of information being provided (poor coordination of educational process), lack of time and limited motivation on the part of clinicians, and approach of clinicians to teaching.

Content-Related Factors

The complexity and amount of information to learn can seem overwhelming.

LEARNING THEORIES
Behaviorist Theory

Behaviorist theory views learning as the product of stimulus and response and is not concerned with individual internal factors in the learner. Teaching focuses on modifying the stimulus or changing the reinforcement that occurs after the response. This theory values detailed measurable instructional objectives and immediate, positive reinforcement. It recognizes that negative reinforcement slows learning.

Cognitive Theory

Cognitive theory stresses the critical aspects of what is happening "within" the learner (how he or she is perceiving, processing, and structuring information for use). It conceptualizes learning as an active process and the individual's goals, expectations, learning styles, and preferences as being as important to the process as is learning to learn.

Humanistic Theory

Humanistic theory appreciates that learners are unique persons who learn optimally when they are treated with positive regard, when their uniqueness is considered, and when they are involved in decision making.

Andragogy

Andragogy, a theory of adult education, is based on the recognition that adults learn differently from the way children learn and that their instruction should therefore be different. Adults bring rich experience to the learning situation and are generally independent learners. Their impetus to learn something is usually an immediate need or problem; they prefer practical wisdom and do not tolerate time wasting or irrelevant information. Family, work, or other responsibilities often compete for energy and learning time. Adults are vulnerable while learning; they are anxious about their self-image and are often concerned about "looking dumb" (this can make adults hesitant to ask questions about information they believe they should know or to admit that they need help). Approximately 20% of adults are functionally illiterate, which means that they cannot read or write. One should never presume literacy in an adult client.

DOMAINS OF LEARNING

Clients learn in three ways, which are referred to as *learning domains:* cognitive, affective, and psychomotor.

- Cognitive learning involves all those processes related to the intellect: acquiring, storing, and using information. Behaviors in this domain can be leveled in complexity according to the categories of knowing, comprehending, applying, analyzing, synthesizing, and evaluating. Appropriate teaching methods for cognitive learning include lecture, discussion, panel presentations, audiovisuals, handouts and brochures, computer-assisted instruction, games, and simulations.
- Affective learning relates to values, attitudes, feelings, and emotions, beginning with an awareness, willing response, commitment, prioritization, and finally integration into one's lifestyle. Appropriate teaching methods include role play, role modeling, discussions, audiovisuals, and printed materials.
- Psychomotor learning refers to learning fine and gross motor skills and tasks. Individuals learn skills

through demonstration, discussion, audiovisuals, and printed materials. Practice is a significant part of skill learning, depending on the complexity of the behavior to be learned.

Much of learning involves all three domains simultaneously. For example, the diabetic client must learn about the disease process (cognitive), the significance of glycemic control to prevent complications (affective), and how to test blood glucose (psychomotor).

LEARNING PRINCIPLES THAT GUIDE CLIENT EDUCATION

- Good teaching always begins with finding out what the learner already knows.
- Capitalizing on the client's preferred way of learning increases learning.
- Active participation in the learning process increases the likelihood that learning will occur.
- Learning often proceeds best from simple to complex information and from concrete to abstract ideas.
- Use of advanced organizers facilitates learning. For example, tell the person what is to be learned and then cue the learner at each point.
- Applying what is learned immediately afterward helps with retention and transfer.
- Practice and time spent on the task increases the learning of skills.
- Respect for uniqueness, diversity of talents, and preferred ways of learning promotes learning.
- Learning new information is easier when it is related to something already known.
- Learning is enhanced when the information is organized and meaningful.
- Feedback about performance, given as soon as possible, enhances learning.
- A comfortable environment and a facilitative instructor promote learning.

MODELS FOR AFFECTING BEHAVIORAL CHANGES

Transtheoretical Model for Assessing Readiness for Behavioral Change

This model proposes that ceasing high-risk behavior and acquiring health-enhancing behavior involves progressing through five stages of change. Assessing behavior indicative of each stage facilitates planning educational interventions.

Precontemplation. Precontemplation does not involve considering a behavioral change. The role of the NP includes relationship building, consciousness raising (including how disease or behaviors affect self and significant others), and personalizing risk factors based on objective findings. Do not use scare tactics. The

goal is to think about how change might impact life positively.

Contemplation. Contemplation involves considering a behavioral change in the foreseeable future, possibly within 6 months. The role of the NP includes continuing consciousness raising, providing information, praising for considering, and exploring ways to reduce barriers and obstacles to change. The goal is to examine the benefits and obstacles associated with change.

Preparation. Preparation occurs when a client intends to make a change in behavior within the next month and has taken some steps in that direction. The role of the NP is to provide positive reinforcement and offer practical assistance, support, and encouragement. Elicit a target date and anticipated strategy for change.

Action-Engaged in Process of Behavioral Change. The role of the NP is to praise even small successes, reinforce the value of a decision to change, provide help as needed, and refer the client to a support group.

Maintenance. Maintenance occurs when the client has changed behavior and maintained the change for at least 6 months. The role of the NP is to continue to provide positive reinforcement and ask about what has worked and what has been a struggle. Relapse is common. If it occurs, the role of the NP is to help the client learn from the temporary setback and provide encouragement to try again.

Compliance Perspective on Behavioral Change. The compliance perspective represents a traditional view of the clinician-client relationship that is paternalistic. The client is the recipient of care, and the clinician, as an expert, is responsible for the diagnosis, management, and outcome of the disease.

Empowerment Perspective on Behavioral Change. The empowerment perspective assumes that the informed client is the "expert" in his or her own disease and, as such, has the right and responsibility for selecting self-care behaviors consistent with good or better health within the context of daily lifestyle. Efforts to understand the client's perspective, acknowledge feelings, and educate for optimal decision making are cornerstones of this model.

BEHAVIOR STRATEGIES HELPFUL TO LEARNING

- Contracting: developing contract for expected behaviors and realistic goals, including rewards when target goals are reached; acknowledging client's perspective regarding self-care and the feelings engendered by the disease and treatment

- Graduating behavioral change: making small incremental changes over time
- Tailoring: fitting a prescribed behavioral regimen into the client's existing lifestyle with as little disruption as possible
- Self-monitoring: keeping a journal or record of behavioral changes and personal responses
- PLISSIT Model for Providing Sexuality Information (Annon, 1976)
  - **P**ermission: Grant couple permission to raise questions and discuss sexuality comfortably with the care provider; Open a topic with a normalizing statement, such as "We always ask questions about the client's sex life at this clinic" or "Most of the clients I see have questions about _____. I wonder what questions you might have about that?" Permission giving precludes the clinician's imposing a personal value system onto the client.
  - **L**imited **I**nformation: Provide simple, basic facts that relate directly to a client's questions, concerns or problems, diagnosis, or life stage. Such information can be provided by most experienced nurses, not only by advanced practice nurses, and often involves sanctioning particular safe behaviors or informing the unaware client of potential adverse consequences of a particular behavior.
  - **S**pecific **S**uggestions: Provide specific, individualized ideas for what behavioral change(s) can either

TABLE **8-1**   Age-Appropriate Client Education

AGE	GENERAL INFORMATION
Infants and toddlers (0-2 years old)	Cognitive stage: Sensorimotor—learns by exploring self and environment. Play and manipulation of objects helps to learn to differentiate self from the environment. Learning to trust; security needs must be met. Familiar objects can lend security. Depends on parents and others for care; teach parents and other caregivers. Safety is a predominant factor.
Preschoolers (2-6 years old)	Cognitive stage: Preoperational—literal and concrete thinkers unable to generalize. Magical thinking. May believe that he or she caused illness; may believe he or she is being punished by becoming sick. May be fearful of body injury. Believe that objects are "alive." Play is a major way of learning. Curious in exploration of environment, so safety is paramount. Drawing, stories, dolls, puppets, playing with equipment and "acting out" care-giving can be helpful ways to teach.
School agers (7-11 years old)	Cognitive stage: Concrete operations—beginning to understand cause and effect, consequences of actions; needs concrete information in words understandable to them. Play therapy, group activities, drawing/painting, models, dolls, games, audio and videotapes can be used for teaching, as can computers.
Adolescents (12-18 years old)	Cognitive stage: Formal operations—can think abstractly and reason; peer group interaction and acceptance is important. Preoccupied with appearance and how others perceive them. Concerned about looking foolish or "like a baby." Feels invincible: "bad things happen to other people." Learn well with audio and videotapes, reading, group discussions, games/simulations, computers. May resent health education as interference with autonomy or as too authoritative.
Young adulthood (18-40 years old)	More independent and self directed as learner. Makes decisions on basis of past experiences and new information. Desires immediate applicability of learned information. Prefers active participation and inclusion in goal setting and all aspects of learning.
Middle adulthood (40-65 years old)	Often at peak of career; may be at varied stages of parenthood/grandparenthood with myriad competing demands and stressors. Often a time for chronic illness to begin to impact life. Life review and desire to leave a legacy (generativity) prominent goal. Focus; maintaining autonomy.
Older adulthood (>65 years old)	Sensory-motor changes, decreased energy level, decreased short term memory and delayed reaction time may impact learning and must be considered in planning instruction. May feel vulnerable in formal learning situations. Rich past experiences on which educator may capitalize.

be modified or added to remedy the problem or concern.

- **I**ntensive **T**herapy: Conduct comprehensive interventions, generally involving referral to a specialist, possibly for psychotherapy or sexual counseling.

AGE-APPROPRIATE CLIENT EDUCATION

The developmental ability and age of the person must be considered in planning appropriate client education. See Table 8-1.

Selection of Instructional Methods

Decisions regarding which instructional method is appropriate for client education are made on the basis of the following factors:

- Is the method likely to enable the client to meet the desired learning objectives?
- Is the method available?
- Is the method likely to be attractive to the learner? Does it allow active participation? Does it match the learner's cognitive stage, abilities, and preferred method of learning?
- Does the method include materials that are culturally sensitive, at an appropriate reading level, and visually compelling?

Using a variety of methods to capitalize on stimulating multiple senses can be of value. Including the client's significant other is often helpful. Providing written handouts as a follow-up to instruction provides a measure for review at a later time. All instructional methods should include time for questions and answers, clarification as needed, feedback, and reassurance.

QUALITIES OF AN EFFECTIVE CLIENT EDUCATOR

- Knowledge of the subject area
- Ability to assess learner characteristics
- Empathy, concern, and unconditional positive regard for learner
- Good communication skills, including active listening

EVALUATION OF LEARNING

Learning is evaluated by determining whether the objectives for client education were met. Does the client verbalize understanding of the information that is being taught? Is the client able to restate the information? Can he or she answer questions? Does the client's behavior show use of the new information? Can he or she demonstrate the skill taught? If the objectives have not been meet, reassessment for a reason is appropriate and, on the basis of assessment data, the teaching plan can be modified.

Formative Evaluation

Formative evaluation occurs while the educational activity is ongoing and enables adjustments to be made to optimize the likelihood that learning will occur.

Summative Evaluation

Summative evaluation occurs at the end of the educational activity to determine whether the goals have been met. Did change occur as a result of the teaching? Is the change likely to persist over time? Has the client enacted a new way of life that is likely to increase the quality or longevity of life? Change can include a difference in understanding, behavior, attitude, or value.

REFERENCES

Annon, J. (1976). *The behavioral treatment of sexual problems.* Honolulu: Enabling Systems.

Babcock, D. E., & Miller, M. A. (1993). *Client education: Theory and practice.* St. Louis: Mosby.

Bastable, S. B. (1997). *Nurse as educator: principles of teaching and learning.*, Boston: Jones & Bartlett.

Cassidy, C. A. (1999). Using the transtheoretical model to facilitate behavior change in patients with chronic illness. *Journal of the American Academy of Nurse Practitioners, 11*(7), 281-287.

Greenberg, L. (1989). Build your practice with patient education. *Contemporary Pediatrics,* September, 85-106.

Hunter, M. (1984). Knowing, teaching, and supervising. In ASCD Yearbook: *Using what we know about teaching* (pp. 169-192). Alexandria: Association of Supervision and Curriculum Development.

Lustman, P. J., Griffith, L. S., & Clouse, R. E. (1997). Efficacy of cognitive therapy for depression in NIDDM: Results of a controlled clinical trial. *Diabetes, 46* (Suppl), 1.

Muma, R. D., Lyons, B. A., & Newman, T. A. (1996). *Patient education: A practical approach.* Stamford, CN: Appleton & Lange.

Potter, P. A., & Perry, A. G. (1997). *Fundamentals of nursing: Concepts, process, and practice.*, St. Louis: Mosby.

Rega, M. D. (1993). A model approach for patient education. *MEDSURG Nursing, 2*(5), 477-479, 485.

Schrefer, S. (Ed.). (1995). *Mosby's patient teaching tips.* St. Louis: Mosby.

Whitman, N. I., Graham, B. A., & Gleit, C. J. (1992). *Teaching in nursing practice: A professional model* (2nd ed.). Norwalk, CT: Appleton & Lange.

Zimmerman, G. L., Olson, C. G., & Bosworth, M. F. (2000). A "stages of change" approach to helping patients change behavior. *American Family Physician, 61,* 1409-1416.

Review Questions

1. Gwen Monroe is a postpartum client who is breast-feeding. She presents for her 6-week checkup. During the examination, the NP notes dry, atrophic vaginal tissue. In response to a question about whether she has resumed coitus, Gwen responds, "We tried several days ago, but I was too tender." The NP explains the hypoestrogenized vagina associated with breast-feeding and recommends a vaginal lubricant and position change to minimize discomfort during coitus. This is an example of what in the PLISSIT model?

   a. Permission
   b. Limited information

c. Specific suggestion
d. Intensive therapy

2. An NP working with an infertile client teaches her how to assess her basal body temperature. In the PLISSIT model, this is an example of which of the following?

a. Permission
b. Limited information
c. Specific suggestion
d. Intensive therapy

3. A group of NPs in a large practice are interested in adding some special programs for women clients. Considering the risk factors for women, which option is most appropriate?

a. Weight training twice weekly at a local church
b. Seminar for college women on relationship violence
c. Menopause education and support group after hours
d. Seminar on avoiding gallbladder disease

4. Beverly is an NP working with adolescent girls. She wants the clients to appreciate the importance of sexual abstinence during adolescence to their future well being. She plans to teach the girls how to say "no" to premarital sex. Which instructional approach is most likely to accomplish that goal?

a. At frequent intervals, comment with a smile, "Just say no!"
b. Stage a role play in which the girls can practice a "speech" for how to deal with pressure to have sex.
c. Tell the girls that they will be more respected by the young men when they say no to sex.
d. Provide handouts on safe sex and what abstinence means.

5. Chester Jones is a heavy smoker who has been considering quitting. He is interested but has not set a target date, although he would like to quit before his marriage in 6 months. The NP notices Chester reading a brochure about Nicoderm. Which action by the NP would be most appropriate?

a. Cite statistics about lung cancer deaths in men Chester's age.
b. Help Chester examine benefits and obstacles to quitting.
c. Tell Chester that it will be a huge mistake to keep smoking.
d. Tell Chester that unless he quits smoking he will likely die before age 40.

6. Which comment by the NP indicates use of the empowerment model to facilitate behavioral change in a diabetic client?

a. "Lucy, I think it would be in your best interest to monitor your glucose everyday."
b. "Lucy, losing a few pounds would probably mean cutting your injections to twice daily; how might you work at losing a few pounds?"
c. "Lucy, if you don't stop eating sweets, you're going to wind up with an amputated leg, blind, or on a kidney machine."
d. "Lucy, you must start taking this disease more seriously."

7. Tucker Fredrickson is a 17-year-old with newly diagnosed diabetes. Assuming all the following measures are available, which is most effective for teaching Tucker about carbohydrate counting?

a. A handout about diabetic diets with cartoon characters on the margins
b. A one-on-one lecture using food models
c. A group session with other diabetic teens using a Jeopardy game on food choices
d. A book on diabetes from the Joslin Center

Answers and Rationales

1. *Answer:* c
Rationale: Offering specific practical ideas or advice related to the problem or concern is identified by Annon (1976) as specific suggestions.

2. *Answer:* b
Rationale: Simple instruction regarding how to measure basal body temperature is known by most nurses; it is considered limited information in the PLISSIT model.

3. *Answer:* c
Rationale: Although all these options are appropriate for special programs for women, risk assessment and the numerous numbers of aging women in the typical clinic population suggest that any service related to menopause would be appropriate. This option also implies an ongoing enterprise rather than a one-time seminar.

4. *Answer:* b
Rationale: Role play is an extremely effective way for teaching values and attitude changes that are necessary for abstinence in peer pressure situations. Using role play can enable the rehearsal of several messages in response to peer pressure, lending confidence to the adolescent girl who might find herself in the situation. This also offers the NP an opportunity to offer positive feedback.

5. *Answer:* b
Rationale: This client is in the contemplation phase (transtheoretical model) of behavior change. The most appropriate intervention is to examine what can help and hinder him in his intent to quit smoking.

6. *Answer:* b
Rationale: Involving the client in decisions regarding selfcare is a cornerstone of empowering them. The other options posed present a paternalistic, non-empowering approach that tends to be ineffective in affecting behavioral change.

7. *Answer:* c
Rationale: Capitalizing on a peer group and gaming are both appropriate educational strategies for teaching adolescent male clients like Tucker.

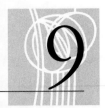

9

Cultural Sensitivity

Cheryl Pope Kish

OVERVIEW
Definition

Culture is a "way of perceiving, behaving, and evaluating the world. It provides a blueprint or guide for determining people's values, beliefs, and practices, including those pertaining to health and illness" (Andrews & Boyle, 1999). The values and beliefs associated with culture are learned within the context of family over time and are generally subconscious yet influence the way in which the person interacts on a day-to-day basis.

In melting pot theory, diverse groups from all over the world gather and are encouraged to forsake their original traditions and to become homogenized as Americans (also known as *enculturation*). The stew pot theory involves an appreciation and acceptance of other cultures. As in stew, each culture is enhanced and becomes more colorful because of exposure to the distinctive traditions of other cultures (Kirkpatrick & Deloughery, 1995).

Cultural factors influence health, not only for the client but also for the family regarding how they perceive illness, identify and interpret symptoms, assume the sick role, manifest pain, approach treatment options, and receive professional support.

Ethnocentrism is the belief that one's own culture is inherently superior to the culture of others. Ethnocentric persons usually try to impose their personal values on others, without taking into account the client's personal perceptions and values.

Transcultural nursing is a term coined by Madeline Leininger, who envisioned blending the disciplines of nursing and anthropology in both theory and practice to enable a cultural perspective for the professional practice of nursing. Although not all advanced practice nurses practice the full scope of transcultural nursing as a specialization, all are encouraged to provide care that is culturally competent (i.e., free of bias and based on cultural diversity). According to Purnell and Paulanka (1998), acquisition of cultural competence involves the following:

"(1) developing an awareness of one's own existence, sensations, thoughts, and environment without letting it have an undue influence on those from other backgrounds; (2) demonstrating knowledge and understanding of the client's culture; (3) accepting and respecting cultural differences; and (4) adapting care to be congruent with the client's culture."

CULTURAL DIFFERENCES

Giger and Davidhizar (1995) suggest that culturally unique persons may differ according to these factors, which can be used for assessment:

- Communication: spoken language and use of silence and nonverbal communication
- Space: degree of comfort observed in conversation, proximity to others, body movements, and perceptions of space
- Social organization: culture, race, ethnicity, family role and function, work, leisure, church, and friends
- Time: use of time, definition of time, social and work time, and time orientation as future, present, or past; some persons who are part of present-focused cultures have difficulty appreciating need for preventive care and may be consistently late for appointments
- Biologic variations: body structure, skin color, hair color, other physical dimensions, enzymatic and genetic existence of diseases specific to populations, susceptibility to illness and disease, nutritional preferences and deficiencies, and psychological characteristics for coping
- Environmental control: cultural health practices, values, and definitions of health and illness; different cultural groups hold differing beliefs about sickness and health, have a different vocabulary related to sickness and health, and often use folk remedies; even when westernized, they may revert to those beliefs and remedies at times of health crisis

ASPECTS OF CULTURAL PROFILE WITH POTENTIAL TO AFFECT HEALTH STATUS: THE CONFHER MODEL (FONG, 1985)

- **C**ommunication: language, dialect, nonverbal, and social customs
- **O**rientation: ethnic identification, acculturation, and values
- **N**utrition: food preferences and taboos
- **F**amily relationships: structure, roles, dynamics, decision-making style, lifestyle, and living accommodations
- **H**ealth beliefs: thoughts on alternative health practices, health beliefs, crisis, and illness beliefs, response to pain and hospitalization, and disease predisposition and resistance
- **E**ducation: learning style, formal and informal education, occupation, and socioeconomic level
- **R**eligion: preferences, beliefs, rituals, and taboos

STRATEGIES FOR CULTURALLY COMPETENT CARE

- Break down language barriers as much as possible, using a translator if necessary. Be sensitive to a family member who is serving as an interpreter when providing information that may cause discomfort for the client or the family member/interpreter.
- Admit when you do not know about a particular aspect of the client's culture, and ask for help in learning about it so that sensitive care can be planned. The client and the family are the nurse practitioner's (NP's) best teachers about culture.
- Explain the rationale for treatment options and the reasons for the suggestions being made.
- Ask how the client wants information to be conveyed and to whom.
- Enlist family members and others (as appropriate) as caregivers.
- Get consent from the appropriate person. In some cultures, this is not just the client.
- Provide language-appropriate written materials.
- Avoid cultural stereotyping. Do not assume that all members of a cultural group hold similar beliefs and values.
- Incorporate dietary preferences into the nutritional plan of care whenever possible.
- Consider findings from the cultural assessment when planning care with the client; if compromise is not possible because of safety factors, make the client/family aware of the reasons without destroying their cultural belief system.

REFERENCES

Andrews, M., & Boyle, J. (1999). Transcultural concepts in nursing care (3rd ed.). Philadelphia: Lippincott.

Fong, C. M. (1985). Ethnicity and nursing practice. *Top Clinical Nursing, 7*(3), 1-10.

Giger, J. N., & Davidhizar, R. E. (1995). Transcultural nursing: Assessment and intervention. St. Louis: Mosby.

Kielich, A. M., & Miller, L. (1996). Cultural aspects of women's health care. *Patient Care, 15,* 60-93.

Kirkpatrick, S., & Deloughery, G. (1995). Cultural influences in nursing. In G. Deloughery (Ed.), *Issues and trends in nursing.* St. Louis: Mosby.

Long, P. (2000). Multicultural care. *Advanced Nurse Practice, May,* 79-80.

Luggen, A. S., & Kish, C. P. (2001). Theories and models of transcultural nursing. In D. Robinson & C. P. Kish (Eds.), *Core concepts in advanced practice nursing* (pp. 467-485). St. Louis: Mosby.

Mattson, S. (2000a). Providing culturally competent care: Strategies and approaches for perinatal clients. *AWHONN Lifelines, 4*(5), 37-39.

Mattson, S. (2000b). Strategies for cultural competence: Providing care for the changing face of the U.S. *AWHONN Lifelines, 4*(3), 49-52.

Purnell, L., & Paulanka, B. (1998). *Transcultural health care.* Philadelphia: F. A. Davis.

Sinclair, B. P. (2000). Putting cultural competence into practice. *AWHONN Lifelines, 4*(2), 7-8.

Review Questions

1. The NP provides health instructions to a client from a culture different from her own. Which evaluation method is most appropriate?

    a. Ask the client if she has understood the instructions.
    b. Ask the client if she has questions.
    c. Ask the client if she needs a family member to be informed as well.
    d. Ask the client to repeat the instructions.

2. Sha Desuwonty, a pregnant woman from another culture, tells the NP, "It is against our customs to eat citrus fruits while we are pregnant. They will make the baby bald. I see that citrus fruits are listed on the sample menu you gave me." Which response from the NP would be best?

    a. Ask her what would happen if she had a bald baby.
    b. Tell her that such beliefs about food are not scientifically based.
    c. Discuss foods that have the same nutritional value as citrus fruits.
    d. Arrange for her to talk with a woman who ate citrus fruits during pregnancy.

3. Maria, age 16, and her family have just moved into the community from another country when she presents with clinical findings of primary dysmenorrhea. She tells the NP that when "my monthly comes and brings its pain, my mother makes me squat down and wash the baseboards of the house; she says it will help the pain." Which response by the NP is most appropriate?

    a. Ask Maria for more details about her mother's remedy and how it affects her cramping.
    b. Tell Maria that this practice is not scientifically based and speak to the mother about it.
    c. Report Maria's mother to the authorities for child neglect.

d. Order NSAIDS and bed rest for the dysmenorrhea; advise Maria not to follow her mother's directions in the future.

4. An NP states that all clients should learn how to read educational materials printed in English. This statement reflects what belief?

- **a.** Stew pot theory
- **b.** Melting pot theory
- **c.** Cultural competence
- **d.** Transcultural nursing theory

5. Beverly is an NP performing a breast assessment and teaching breast self-examination to a young African woman. Beverly uses a breast model with brown skin and written materials with photographs of women with African physical characteristics. This behavior indicates Beverly's value for which cultural approach?

- **a.** Melting pot theory
- **b.** Cultural imposition
- **c.** Cultural blindness
- **d.** Cultural sensitivity

6. Anya has a cultural heritage in which a present-oriented view of time predominates. Which of the following findings is inconsistent with present-oriented health beliefs?

- **a.** Consistent lateness for clinic appointments
- **b.** Showing up for care without an appointment, despite long waits
- **c.** Failure to fully appreciate the necessity for preventive care
- **d.** Demanding to be screened for all common diseases

Answers and Rationales

1. *Answers:* d
Rationale: To determine whether a culturally diverse client has understood the information provided, the clinician should ask the client to repeat the information. Clarification can then be provided as needed (Mattson, 2000a).

2. *Answer:* c
Rationale: Substituting other foods for one against the customs of this woman's cultural group poses no danger to her or her fetus. Hence, the best choice is to discuss other foods of the same nutritional value (Luggen & Kish, 2001).

3. *Answer:* a
Rationale: Assessment precedes decision-making. It is important to determine Maria's perception of the mother's remedy and whether it is effective. As a cultural belief, if it is causing no problem, it can be continued. Additional western medical treatment may also be advised; however, the NP should not speak negatively about a cultural remedy that is not unsafe (Mattson, 2000a).

4. *Answer:* b
Rationale: The stew pot theory involves an appreciation and acceptance of cultural diversity. The melting pot theory supports the process of blending cultures into an indistinguishable, homogenized group (Kirkpatrick & Deloughery, 1995).

5. *Answer:* d
Rationale: Modifying education to reflect the client's beliefs or biological characteristics is a positive method of providing culturally sensitive care. It allows the client to identify with the clients presented in the materials (Andrews & Boyle, 1999).

6. *Answer:* d
Rationale: A present-oriented time view includes aspects related to lack of planning for future health needs but does not include demanding to be screened for all common diseases (Kielich & Miller, 1996).

Ethical and Legal Issues

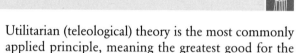

Pamela Kidd

VALUES
Definition

Values are "freely chosen, enduring beliefs or attitudes about the worth of a person, object, idea, or action" (Kozier, Erb, Blais, & Wilkinson, 1998). Values form the basis for behavior and are learned and influenced by the person's sociocultural environment. Professional values are influenced and shaped by personal values. Nurses learn professional values during their socialization into nursing. These values are integrally related to ethical and professional beliefs.

ETHICS
Definition

Ethics is the study of morality. Bioethics is ethics as applied to life. According to Kozier and colleagues (1998, p. 94), "Nurses need to understand their own values related to moral matters and to use ethical reasoning to determine and explain their moral position." A code of ethics is a formal statement or guideline that explains a group's ideals and values. Codes of ethics are usually considered to set a higher standard than legal requirements and expectations.

Ethical Principles
- Ethics is the study of standards of conduct and moral judgment.
- Morality is conforming to a standard of what is considered right and good (Rini, 2001).
- Autonomy means that a client's needs take priority over the needs of society and the health care system.
- Beneficence is to do no harm.
- Justice is the right to fair treatment and the right to privacy, including:
  - Confidentiality: information not publicly reported
  - Anonymity: name cannot be linked to date reported
- Veracity is truthfulness; client must have full, impartial knowledge.

- Utilitarian (teleological) theory is the most commonly applied principle, meaning the greatest good for the greatest number of persons; used as rationale for limiting scarce resources.
- Deontological theory states that norms and rules are based on the duty of one person to another and emphasizes respect for obligations arising from one's role (Rini, 2001).
- Egoism is when the wishes of the care giver are held in higher regard than the wishes of the client; this is to be avoided.
- Respect for human dignity is an ethical principle including the right to self-determination and the right to full disclosure (informed consent).
- Self-determination (autonomy) is the right of sovereignty over one's self; a competent adult has the right to determine whether health care is accepted.

Ethical dilemmas generally involve alternatives that may be in conflict with each other. The choice selected is based on ethical principles.

LEGAL ISSUES
- Laws are constitutions (written or codified), rules, regulations, and ordinances that pertain to a jurisdiction.
- Types of law are the following:
  - Administrative: state boards/State Nurse Practice Acts
  - Civil: private differences between people when redress for damages is sought
  - Criminal: violations deemed to interfere with important social interests
- A tort is a wrongful act against another person or property.
- An unintentional tort is an unintentional wrongful act that produces injury.
- An intentional tort is a civil wrong intentionally committed by a person who desires the result or knows with substantial certainty that a particular result will occur (Rini, 2001). Examples of intentional tort include the following:

- Battery: harmful touching
- Assault: placing a person in apprehension of a harmful contact
- Trespass to personal property: interference denying access by the property owner and causing damage to the property
- Defamation of character: harming someone's reputation by either written word (libel) or spoken word (slander)
- Invasion of privacy: disclosing confidential information to a third party
- False imprisonment: unjustifiably retaining a person without his or her consent
- Fraud: purposefully misrepresenting self, which may cause harm to another person or property
- Negligence is the failure to do something that a reasonable and prudent person would do under similar circumstances or the performance of an action that a reasonable and prudent person would not perform under similar circumstances.
- Negligence in relationship to standard of care is not just a nursing standard but a professional standard of care.
- Malpractice is professional misconduct or lack of skill; it encompasses failure to perform professional skills that a reasonable and prudent professional would perform under similar circumstances or performance of actions that a reasonable and prudent professional would not perform under similar circumstances. This is the specific type of negligence that applies to professionals.

The following four elements of malpractice must be proven:

- Duty owed to the person: To establish duty, the plaintiff must show that the nurse practitioner (NP) and client established a provider-client relationship (Morrison, 1999). The relationship establishes some accountability of one party to the other.
- Breach of duty or standard of care by the professional: Breach of duty is determined by the state nurse practice act, national standards (American Nurses Association [ANA] Code of Ethics, specialty organization), employer policies, or expert testimony. With breach of duty, the required level of expected conduct is violated.
- Proximate cause or direct result is a causal link between the breach and the harm or injury that occurred. An injured party's damage must have a connection to the defendant's breach of duty (Rini, 2001).
- Actual harm or damages: It must be proven that actual harm or damages have occurred.

LIABILITY INSURANCE

The purpose of liability insurance is to shift the risk of liability, which may result in a monetary obligation, to another source (Henry, 1994). There are two types of liability insurance:

- Claims made: Pays damages during the policy's period of coverage.
- Occurrence policy: Pays damages that occurred during the policy's life; the individual no longer has to be carrying the coverage at the time of the litigation.

Damages

Actual (compensatory) damages cover losses sustained by the injured client. These include medical costs, loss of earnings, impairment of future earnings, and pain and suffering (Morrison, 1999).

Punitive damages are designed to punish the defendant (the NP). These may not be allowed in some states and may not be covered by malpractice insurance. Malpractice insurance tends to cover the professional sued for civil violation but not for criminal violation.

The most frequent reason NPs are sued is failure to follow up referrals and abnormal findings on diagnostic tests (Rini, 2001). Ways to prevent this include the following:

- Flagging charts
- Policy requiring review and initialing of charts
- Procedure specifying how client notification will occur
- Process for having abnormal radiographic and laboratory findings faxed to office
- Careful documentation of attempts to follow-up by phone with client
- System that alerts NP to "no show" appointments
- Documentation for all care provided by phone (Rini, 2001)

Good will and effective communication along with a mechanism for allowing clients to voice concerns also prevent litigation.

Informed Consent. All options are explained to the client. The client indicates an understanding of the options and gives permission.

Advance Directives. The client documents instructions (while competent) of what his or her wishes are in case he or she is not competent to make a decision. This avoids the completion of actions and consequences the client did not intend (e.g., ventilator placement for chronic obstructive pulmonary disease).

Double Effect. More than one outcome may occur as the result of the actions of a person. The morality of the action is determined by the intended outcome even if another unintended legally or morally wrong result occurs. This protects the professional in end-of-life care. For example, pain control is administered with the intention of alleviating suffering, even though it may contribute to the death of the person (legally wrong outcome). Respect for self-determination (e.g., advance directives) can allow the professional to commit an act that may have a directly intended outcome and a secondary indirect outcome.

Durable Power of Attorney for Health Care. A durable power of attorney for health care (DPAHC) is a legal document through which a person can name another person (the attorney-in-fact or the DPAHC holder) to make health care decisions for him or her if, and only if, he or she becomes unable to make his or her own health choices (Schooling, 1997). Health care providers who respect the wishes of the attorney-in-fact are protected by law.

PRESCRIPTIVE AUTHORITY

NPs must obtain a Drug Enforcement Administration (DEA) prescriber number before prescribing controlled substances. For safe drug administration, adhere to the following procedures:

- Obtain complete medication history.
- Check for allergies.
- Instruct client about signs and symptoms of possible adverse reactions.
- Document medication and number of refills ordered.

The components of a prescription are the following:
- Client name and address
- Drug name
- Dosage form
- Amount of each dose
- Administration route
- Administration schedule or time
- Total amount of drug to be dispensed
- Number of refills
- Date
- Prescriber's signature and credentials

REFERENCES

Henry, P. (1994). Overview of malpractice insurance. *Nurse Practitioner Forum, 5*(1), 4-6.

Kozier, B., Erb, G., Blais, & Wilkinson, J.M. (1998). Fundamentals of nursing: Concepts, processes, and practice (5th ed.). Menlo Park, CA: Addison-Wesley.

Morrison, C. (1999). A malpractice primer for NPs. *Advanced Nurse Practitioner, 7*(2), 23.

Rini, A. G. (2001). Health care ethics and law. In D. Robinson & C. Kish (Eds.), *Clinical concepts for the advanced practice nurse.* St. Louis: Mosby.

Schooling, J. (1997). Ethical dilemmas: Making life or death decisions. *Advanced Nurse Practitioner, 5*(1), 49-51.

Review Questions

1. The ANA Code of Ethics for nurses provides which of the following?
  a. Legal mandates for advanced practice
  b. Regulations for legal practice
  c. Guidelines for ethical practice
  d. Moral suggestions for ethically compromised situations

2. Which of the following phrases best describes the major purpose of advanced practice standards in nursing?
  a. To promote legal mandates for advanced practice
  b. To regulate the number of advanced practice nurses in the United States
  c. To identify criteria against which advanced practice nursing can be evaluated
  d. To interpret the legislative intent of the state Nursing Practice Act

3. Which of the following statements applies to a situation that constitutes an ethical dilemma?
  a. The problem can be solved with research data.
  b. The information needed is clearly identified.
  c. A decision must be made between undesirable alternatives.
  d. Good outcomes can be obtained if all parties use appropriate ethical theory.

4. What is the legal guide to advanced practice?
  a. ANA Code of Ethics
  b. Hippocratic Oath
  c. State nursing practice act
  d. Nightingale pledge

5. What does it mean for the client to provide informed consent?
  a. The client totally accepts the plan of care.
  b. The client understands the available options.
  c. The client accepts the offer to participate in research.
  d. The client has obtained a second opinion.

6. An employer calls and asks for the diagnosis of a client and whether the client can return to work. Without client permission, the NP tells the employer that the client had low back pain and can return to light duty. Which of the following statements describes the NP's action?
  a. The NP has committed an intentional tort.
  b. The NP has defamed the client's character.
  c. The NP has performed negligently.
  d. The NP was professional in communication.

7. Which of the following is *not* required for malpractice to be present?
  a. Actual damage
  b. Threat of harm
  c. Proximate cause or direct result
  d. Breach of duty

8. What is an action that can be taken to prevent failure to follow up with clients?
  a. Document visits in the medical record.
  b. Document care provided by phone.
  c. Have test results sent directly to the client.
  d. Have a policy and system for flagging charts for review and for initialing.

Answers and Rationales

1. *Answer: c*
  Rationale: The ANA Code of Ethics is a guideline to follow for ethical nursing practice. It has no relationship to legal regu-

lations nor is it mandated for practice. It does not make any moral suggestions.

2. *Answer:* c

Rationale: The standards of care identify criteria by which nursing can be evaluated.

3. *Answer:* c

Rationale: In most dilemmas, the information and decision are not clearly identified; that is what makes it a dilemma. Use of appropriate ethical theory does not guarantee a positive outcome. In many cases, a choice must be made between undesirable alternatives.

4. *Answer:* c

Rationale: Each state nursing practice act delineates the legal guide to practice. The ANA Code of Ethics, the Hippocratic Oath, and the Nightingale pledge are credos that are promoted regarding the care of clients, but they do not have any legal basis for advanced practice.

5. *Answer:* b

Rationale: Informed consent means that the client has had all options explained and has given his or her permission for care. It does not mean that the client totally accepts the plan of care or that a second opinion has been obtained. Although informed consent is obtained while conducting research, it is not reserved for research only.

6. *Answer:* a

Rationale: An intentional tort is a civil wrong intentionally committed by a person who desires a certain result. Types of torts include battery, assault, trespassing, defamation, invasion of privacy, and false imprisonment. Providing information to an employer without the client's permission qualifies as invasion of privacy.

7. *Answer:* b

Rationale: For malpractice to be present, four elements must be proven: (1) Duty owed to the person must be established. To establish duty, the plaintiff must show that the NP and client established a provider-client relationship (Morrison, 1999). The relationship establishes some accountability of one party to the other. (2) Breach of duty or standard of care by the professional must be proven as defined by the state nurse practice act, national standards (ANA Code of Ethics, specialty organization), employer policies, or expert testimony. It must be shown that the required level of expected conduct has been violated. (3) Proximate cause or direct result, which is a causal link between the breach and the harm or injury that occurred, must be demonstrated. An injured party's damage must have a connection to the defendant's breach of duty (Rini, 2001). (4) Actual harm or damages resulting from the breach of duty of standard of care must have occurred.

8. *Answer:* d

Rationale: Having a system in place assures follow-up. Documentation does not guarantee follow-up of abnormal diagnostic tests. Sending results to the client does not ensure that the NP is aware of the results or the need for follow-up.

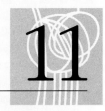

Primary Care

Denise Robinson

The American Nurses Association (ANA) publication *Nursing's Agenda for Health Care Reform* (ANA, 1992) places emphasis on primary care services delivered in workplaces, schools, and other community settings. It identifies the need for ongoing primary care and the delivery of services where people already are. It focuses on primary care and wellness for all, but especially for women and children.

DEFINITION

Primary care includes the following areas:
- Delivery of care at first point of contact with health care system
- Delivery of care that helps resolve health problem for which care is sought
- Continuous and comprehensive care
- Inclusive of health promotion, prevention of disease, and health maintenance
- Inclusive of identification, management, or referral of health problems

Primary care is not the same as primary health care. Primary care addresses personal health services and is not a population-based, public health service, which is considered primary health care. The World Health Organization (WHO) defines primary care as "essential health care based on practical, scientifically sound and socially acceptable methods and techniques made universally accessible to individuals and families in the community through their full participation and at a cost that the community and country can afford to maintain at every stage of their development in the spirit of self-reliance and self-determination. It forms an integral part both of the country's health system, of which it is the central function and main focus, and part of the overall social and economic development of the community" (WHO, 1978). According to Schoultz and Hatcher (1997), "Primary health care looks beyond primary care, and through the collaboration of professionals, community members, and others working in multiple sectors, emphasizes health promotion, development of health policies and prevention of diseases

for all people." Primary care is an essential component of primary health care. Primary health care includes the following five components:
- Equitable distribution
- Appropriate technology
- Focus on health promotion and disease prevention
- Community participation
- Multisectoral approach

Schoultz and Hatcher (1997) call for advanced registered nurse practitioners to take risks, redefine goals, learn how to become partners (not just providers), and work with persons from multiple sectors and the community.

REFERENCES

American Nurses Association. (1992). *A national health program for all of us: The American Health Association's guide to the health care reform debate.* Washington DC: American Public Health Association.

Barnes, D., Eribes, C., Juarbe, T., Nelson, M., Proctor, S., Sawyer, L., Shaul, M., & Meleis, A. (1995). Primary health care and primary care: A confusion of philosophies. *Nursing Outlook, 43*(1), 7-16.

Ellis, J., & Hartley, C. (1995). *Nursing in today's world.* Philadelphia: Lippincott.

Schoultz, J., & Hatcher, P. (1997). Looking beyond primary care to primary health care: An approach to community based action. *Nursing Outlook, 45*(1), 23-26.

World Health Organization. (1978). *Primary health care: Report of the International Conference on Primary Health Care, Alma-Alta, USSR, 6-12 September.* Health for All. Serial No. 1. Geneva: Author.

World Health Organization. (1981). *Global strategy for health for all by the year 2000* (Series No. 3, p. 32) Geneva: World Health Organization Health for All.

Review Questions

1. Which of the following choices best describes primary care providers?

a. Providers who provide care only for acute illness
b. Gatekeepers to the health care system
c. Providers who provide care in rural health settings
d. Consultants who participate in the plan of care

2. When comparing primary care and primary health care, which of the following statements applies to primary health care?
a. Is the broader concept of the two.
b. Is the narrower concept of the two.
c. Deals with personal health issues.
d. Involves "gatekeeping" a person who is accessing the health system.

3. Primary care has a number of characteristics. Which of the following is *not* a component of primary care?
a. Is the first point of contact with the health care system.
b. Provides continuous and comprehensive care.
c. Includes health promotion.
d. Deals with insurance related to care.

4. Misty is an NP in a housing project. She is developing a program called "Girls' Night Out" in which adolescents come to the health center for pizza and discussion of puberty. This is an example of what type of care?
a. Primary health care
b. Primary care
c. Community service
d. Secondary prevention

5. For primary care to be successful, it is important for which of the following to occur?
a. Provider makes all decisions.
b. Client makes all decisions.
c. Client and provider work together to identify best plan for care.
d. Avoid interdisciplinary teams whenever possible.

Answers and Rationales

1. *Answer:* b
Rationale: Primary providers are those providers who coordinate the access of clients to other resources within the system. They do not provide care to acutely ill clients only or in rural settings only. Consultants who participate in the plan of care are exactly that, consultants (Ellis & Hartley, 1995).

2. *Answer:* a
Rationale: Primary health care is the broader concept of the two. It deals with communities and groups of people. Primary care can be thought of as being related more to personal care (Schoutlz & Hatcher, 1997).

3. *Answer:* d
Rationale: Primary care deals with personal care as a person accesses the health care system. Primary care is typically thought of as being the first contact, being continuous and comprehensive, and including health promotion, prevention, and maintenance. Although health insurance, or the lack thereof, certainly impacts primary care, it is generally not identified as being a component of primary care (ANA, 1992).

4. *Answer:* a
Rationale: This is an example of primary health care because it involves the community and is not focused on just one client (Schoultz & Hatchet, 1997).

5. *Answer:* c
Rationale: In the ideal primary care world, the client assumes responsibility for health care and works with the provider to develop a mutually agreed upon plan (Schoultz & Hatchet, 1997).

12

Reimbursement

Pamela Kidd

DEFINITIONS
Current Procedural Terminology

Current procedural terminology (CPT) is a classification system for reporting procedures and services recognized by third-party payers.

International Classification of Diseases

International classification of diseases (ICD) is a classification system that reports the client's diagnosis, symptoms, complaints, and conditions or problems. Each client visit is coded (evaluation and management code). The levels of coding differ regarding the following aspects: (1) number of systems reviewed and number of parameters reviewed for each system, symptoms, degree of history obtained (social, family, medical); (2) number of body systems examined and components of the examination for each system; and (3) complexity of decision making required. Complexity of decision making is based on the following: (1) number of possible diagnoses, (2) number of management options, (3) amount of diagnostic tests and medical records that need to be reviewed, (4) risk of complications, (5) co-morbidities that must be considered in the management plan, and (6) level of risk involved.

Evaluation and Management Codes

- Level 1: service provided by registered nurse
- Level 2: problem focused
- Level 3: expanded problem focused
- Level 4: detailed
- Level 5: comprehensive
  Preventive services (cancer screening procedures, bone density measurements, glucose monitoring, influenza and pneumonia vaccines, and diabetic education) may also be billed.

Resource-Based Relative Value Scale

The resource-based relative value scale determines the level of payment and is based on provider productivity,

malpractice insurance cost, cost of overhead, geographic rates, and the payment rate for nonphysician providers. To bill for a visit, the following must be recorded:
- Face-to-face contact
- ICD code(s)
- CPT code(s)
- Distinction between new and established clients
- Date of service
- Client-identifying information
- Provider-identifying information

Fraud. Fraud is intentional deception or misrepresentation.

Abuse. Abuse includes receiving payment for services when there is no legal entitlement to the payment but there is also no intentional deception. Development of a compliance program (self-audit system) can prevent insurance investigation. A compliance program has the following eight components:
- Learn and stay within payer requirements.
- Follow the rules for assigning a diagnosis and billing code.
- Follow the rules for documenting a client visit.
- Use tools that decrease the time needed for complete documentation (preprinted forms).
- Conduct quarterly audits.
- Show a commitment to detect and correct billing errors.
- Correct errors.
- Conduct legal reviews of contracts and operating procedures.

MEDICARE

There is no restriction for practice setting or geographic area for reimbursement of the nurse practitioner (NP). The NP must apply for a Medicare billing personal identification number.

PRIVATE INSURANCE

Payment is contract-specific and varies across states. Rules for reimbursement vary across payors. The NP must become paneled or credentialed by the payor.

DIRECT BILLING

- The bill is rendered in the name of the NP.
- Payment may be made under the indirect supervision of a physician for services provided to Medicare regardless of setting. The reimbursement rate is 80% of the lesser of the actual charge or 85% of the fee schedule amount for physicians.
- Reimbursement may be made to the employer of the NP. An employer may be a physician, a medical group, a nursing home, or a professional corporation.

Benefits of Direct Reimbursement

- Direct reimbursement puts a price and value on services provided.
- It allows self-employment or enhancement of revenue for employers.
- It provides data regarding services provided and improves the ability to conduct research.
- Direct reimbursement increases the NP's autonomy and authority to act on behalf of clients.
- It empowers NPs within the health system, giving them greater control over practices.

Barriers to Direct Reimbursement

- Organized medicine
- Inability to show cost savings
- Lack of consumer demand for NP services

"INCIDENT TO" SERVICES

"Incident to" services are services rendered by health care professionals employed by a physician and performed under the direct supervision of that physician.

Qualifications of "Incident To" Service

- Service must be an integral part of a physician's diagnosis or treatment.
- Service must be provided under direct supervision of a physician.

NOTE: *Direct supervision in an office setting does not mean that the physician has to be in the same room with the practitioner performing the "incident to" service. The physician must be present in the office suite and immediately available to provide assistance and direction throughout the time that the health care professional is performing the service.*

- Services must be provided by an employee of that physician and must represent an expense incurred by the physician in professional practice.
- Service must be something that is ordinarily performed in a physician's office or clinic.

Billing

Bills are rendered in the name of the physician directly supervising the health care professional as though he or she had personally rendered the service.

Documentation

- The health care professional must write or dictate notes and sign them accordingly.
- State law dictates whether the supervising physician must sign off on the notes made by the health care professional.
- Reimbursement is at 100%. The physician must be on-site, and the client cannot be a new client or an old client with a new problem.
- The physician must provide the initial service for the client and must provide subsequent services frequently enough to reflect his or her active participation in the management of the client's course of treatment.
- Reimbursement is made to the physician.

MEDICAID

Medicaid allows direct billing for Advanced Registered Nurse Practitioners (ARNPs) as follows:

- ARNPs must practice in accordance with established protocols and seek consultation and referral in situations and procedures that are not included in the established protocol. This protocol is a written document jointly approved by the physician and the ARNP at least annually. Included in the protocol should be the scope of diagnostic testing, prescription of medications, and treatments that the ARNP can conduct.
- The ARNP shall have a separate individual provider number and separate clinic or group number, distinct from that of the physician employer.
- If the ARNP is salaried by the facility, fee-for-service billing is not appropriate.
- Payment is made at 75% of the fee schedule designated for physician providers.

REFERENCES

Rapsilber, L., & Anderson, E. (2000). Understanding the reimbursement process. *The Nurse Practitioner, 25*(5), 36, 43, 46, 51-52, 54-56.

Robinson, D. (2001). Reimbursement for advanced practice nursing. In D. Robinson & C. Kish (Eds.), *Core concepts in advanced practice.* St. Louis: Mosby.

Towers, J. (1999). Medicare reimbursement for nurse practitioners. *Journal of the American Academy of Nurse Practitioners, 11*(7), 289-292.

Review Questions

1. Which of the following best describes the purpose of evaluation and management codes?

a. Provides a way of reporting procedures.
b. Allows a listing of client diagnoses.
c. Adjusts for geographic setting where care is provided.
d. Captures the depth and complexity of a client visit.

2. The complexity of clinical decision making varies by all *except* which of the following?
   a. Time spent with the client
   b. Risk of complications
   c. Number of diagnoses
   d. Co-morbidities

3. Which of the following client visits is usually *not* provided by the NP?
   a. Level 5
   b. Level 1
   c. Level 2
   d. Level 3

4. Which of the following characteristics must be present for a visit to be billed for?
   a. The client must have Medicare.
   b. The client must have Medicaid.
   c. Distinction between new or established client is recorded.
   d. Description of the clinic where services were provided.

5. Which of the following statements defines fraud?
   a. Unintentional billing for services when there is no legal entitlement
   b. Intentional misrepresentation
   c. Intent to do harm
   d. Failure to do something that a reasonable and prudent person would do under similar circumstances

6. Which of the following statements describes a compliance program?
   a. Required by Medicaid.
   b. Uses the services of an external evaluator.
   c. Involves quarterly chart audits by the provider.
   d. Is the mechanism used for credentialing.

7. Which of the following is true about direct billing?
   a. Reimbursement is at a higher rate for NPs than physicians for preventive services.
   b. The allowable reimbursement rate is 100%.
   c. Reimbursement is equitable with that for physicians.
   d. The reimbursement rate is less than that for physicians providing the same service.

8. The benefits of direct billing for NPs include all *except* which of the following?
   a. Provides data regarding services provided.
   b. Increases the NP's autonomy.
   c. Allows services to have a value.
   d. Allows for audits.

9. To qualify as an "incident to" service, the service must be which of the following?
   a. Provided with phone contact with the physician.
   b. A procedure usually not performed in the office.

c. Provided to an established client with a new problem.
d. Provided with the physician "on site."

10. Reimbursement for "incident to" services are at what percentage?
   a. 100%.
   b. 80%.
   c. 85%.
   d. 75%.

Answers and Rationales

1. *Answer:* **d**
   Rationale: CPTs are used to report procedures. ICDs are used to report diagnoses. A resource-based relative-value scale allows for geographic variation. Evaluation and management codes capture complexities in decision making.

2. *Answer:* **a**
   Rationale: The complexity of clinical decision making is based on (1) the number of possible diagnoses, (2) the number of management options, (3) the amount of diagnostic tests and medical records that need to be reviewed, (4) the risk of complications, (5) the co-morbidities that must be considered in the management plan, and (6) the level of risk involved.

3. *Answer:* **b**
   Rationale: Level 1 services may be provided by a registered nurse.

4. *Answer:* **c**
   Rationale: Visits may be billed to private insurance payors if the NP is credentialed by the private payor. To bill for a visit, the following must be recorded:
   ● Face-to-face contact
   ● ICD code(s)
   ● CPT code(s)
   ● Distinction between new and established clients
   ● Date of service
   ● Client-identifying information
   ● Provider-identifying information

5. *Answer:* **b**
   Rationale: Negligence is the failure to do something that a reasonable and prudent person would do under similar circumstances. Abuse is unintentional billing for services not rendered. Fraud is intentional deception or misrepresentation. Intent to do harm (such as battery or assault) is an intentional tort.

6. *Answer:* **c**
   Rationale: Some private payors as well as state Medicaid programs may require a compliance program, but not all states do. The purpose of a compliance program is to prevent an external audit. Credentialing ensures that the provider has the correct knowledge and skills to perform services.

7. *Answer:* **d**
   Rationale: Reimbursement is at 80% of the lesser of the actual charge or 85% of the fee schedule amount for physi-

cians. Preventive services are reimbursed using the same criteria as for any other service rendered.

8. *Answer:* d

Rationale: Auditing can occur even when billing through the physician is used because the NP is the documented provider on the client's medical records.

9. *Answer:* d

Rationale: "Incident to" services must be provided under the direct supervision of a physician. The physician must be present in the office suite and immediately available to provide assistance and direction throughout the time that the NP is

performing the service. The service must be something that is ordinarily performed in a physician's office or clinic. The client cannot be a new client or an established client with a new problem.

10. *Answer:* a

Rationale: "Incident to" services are the only services provided by the NP that are reimbursed at 100%. Medicaid services are reimbursed at 75%. Medicare services provided independently by the NP are reimbursed at 80% of the lesser of the actual charge or 85% of the fee schedule amount for physicians.

Research for Nurse Practitioners

Cheryl Pope Kish

Nursing research involves a systematic process of inquiry that helps to expand the science on which the profession of nursing is based. Increasingly, nurse practitioners (NPs) are challenged to use evidenced-based practice to inform their decisions about client care. The ultimate goal of nursing research is improvement of client outcomes. According to the *Standards of Professional Performance* (American Nursing Association, 1996), there is an expectation that advanced practice nurses will use "research to discover, examine, and evaluate knowledge, theories, and creative approaches to health practice" (p. 29). To meet that role expectation, the NP should be able to do the following:

- Critique existing practice for use of evidence-based research findings.
- Identify clinical problems that can be answered with research.
- Share relevant research findings with others.

These role expectations presuppose a basic understanding of research methods and statistics. The current trend toward evidence-based practice involves making decisions through judicious identification, critique, and application of those actions and interactions that are best practices from the most relevant published information. According to Ghosh and Ghosh (2000), this involves a four-step process:

- Formulate a well-balanced question.
- Track down relevant sources.
- Critically appraise the information discovered.
- Determine the applicability of the findings for one's own practice site and client population.

APPROACHES TO RESEARCH

There are two approaches to nursing research: quantitative and qualitative. Both involve rigor that produces credible data for evidence-based practice, and both make significant contributions to nursing science. The approaches may be used independently or in combination in a single study (method triangulation) to enable greater breadth and depth of findings.

Quantitative Approach

The quantitative approach uses numerical data and statistics that are perceived as objective and highly reliable and large samples in an attempt to describe a phenomenon, show relationships between variables, or attempt to detect cause-effect relationships.

Qualitative Approach

The qualitative approach attempts to uncover the personal meaning of subjective experiences by analyzing the words of a small number of participants who provide detailed data regarding their experiences.

ACTION RESEARCH

Action research is a collaborative undertaking that uses the research process to solve a practice-specific clinical problem or to evaluate a particular setting-specific intervention (Norwood, 2000).

ENSURING ETHICAL RESEARCH

Human participants in research studies must be protected from harm and must be informed to the extent necessary to grant their consent for participation. Particular care must be taken when working with vulnerable participants (those whose ability to grant informed consent may be compromised, such as children, prisoners, and the mentally ill). Institutional review boards are a valuable resource for protecting participants' rights by ensuring that proposed research has adhered to ethical principles.

STEPS OF THE RESEARCH PROCESS

1. Identify a researchable problem. A problem is researchable if it can be observed through observable, verifiable, or reproducible data. Ethical or moral problems are not researchable. The problem should also be feasible, subject to ethical study, interesting to the researcher, and of clinical significance.
2. Review related literature to discover what is already known about the research topic and what gaps exist in

current knowledge. Related literature also provides suggestions for how to design an effective study.

3. Place the problem within an organizational framework by associating it with a theory or group of concepts that can give the findings meaning beyond the single, isolated study by linking to a larger body of knowledge.

4. Formulate a hypothesis. The expected relationship between independent and dependent variables should be stated in terms of the following:

   a. Independent variable: cause, treatment, or experimental variable that can be manipulated in a cause-and-effect study

   b. Dependent variable: presumed outcome or effect of manipulated (independent) variable

   c. Extraneous variables: factors that interfere with a clear understanding of the relationship between independent and dependent variables, that offer some competing reason for certain findings; need to be identified, measured, or controlled

5. Select a research design and sampling plan, as follows:

   a. Common quantitative designs

      (1) nonexperimental research–descriptive studies, correlational studies, and longitudinal and cross-sectional studies

      (2) experimental research–highly controlled studies able to yield data regarding cause and effect; requires two groups, manipulation of a variable, and random sampling

      (3) quasi-experimental research–shows cause-effect relationships; lacks either the randomization or control features of true experiments

   b. Common qualitative designs

      (1) phenomenologic–uses interviews and inductive analysis to seek understanding of lived experience

      (2) ethnographic–uses observation, interviews, and document review to seek understanding of a culture or sub-culture

      (3) grounded theory–uses observation, interviews, and document review to develop a theory to explain the phenomenon bring studied

      (4) historical–systematically examines data related to past events to shed light on current behavior or practices

      (5) ideal sample is a random sample–each person in the population of interest has an equal chance of being selected as a research participant

      (6) nonrandom sample, such as volunteer or practice-based sample–limits the conclusions that can be drawn from the study because of possible introduction of bias

6. Collect the data. Data may be collected using interviews, questionnaires, scales, observation, projective techniques, biophysical measures, and existing records. Instruments are evaluated for reliability (consistency)

and validity (degree that it measures what it intends to measure).

7. Analyze the data using statistics. Descriptive statistics are used to describe the subjects and inferential statistics are used to test the hypotheses. Statistical significance lends credibility to research findings. Common statistics used in nursing studies are the following:

   - Mean: arithmetic average
   - Median: mid-value in a set of numbers or 50th percentile
   - Mode: value that recurs most frequently
   - Standard deviation: most frequently used measure for showing variability of scores
   - *t* test: measures differences between two groups by comparing means
   - Analysis of variance: measures differences between two or more groups
   - Chi squared: compares actual frequency in one or more groups with frequency expected if no relationship occurred between two variables

8. Interpret the findings and suggest implications for practice and future research.

9. Communicate the findings so that they may be used to guide practice. Common methods for communicating findings:

   - Publication in professional or lay journals
   - Poster presentation
   - Conference presentations
   - Journal clubs
   - Newsletters
   - Discussion groups
   - Research grand rounds

Barriers to Communicating Research Findings (Norwood, 2000)

- Lack of confidence
- Lack of time

RESEARCH UTILIZATION

Research can influence clinical practice and client outcomes by providing credible evidence on which to base changes in practice, by serving as an impetus for changing one's actions or interactions with clients because of better understanding of a situation, and by serving as justification for examining and modifying policies or procedures or solidifying current practice (Norwood, 2000).

Barriers to the Use of Research Findings in Practice (Norwood, 2000)

- Varying levels of knowledge of research process in general
- Lack of confidence in critiquing research
- Lack of authority to change practice
- Research studies, particularly results sections, that fail to clearly communicate implications of findings for everyday practice

- Acknowledged limitations of studies (i.e., small, non-representative samples, instruments that lack validation, over-use of jargon)
- Lack of time
- Lack of reward and system that operates on tradition as way of knowing and justifying practice decisions

REFERENCES

American Nurses Association. (1996). *Scope and standards of advanced practice registered nursing.*, Washington, DC: American Nurses Association.

Carroll, D. L., Greenwood, R., Lynch, K. E., Sullivan, J. K., Ready, C. H., & Fitzmarie, J. B. (1997). Barriers and facilitators to the utilization of nursing research. *Clinical Nurse Specialist, 11*(5), 207-212.

Gennaro, S. (1994). Research utilization: An overview. *Journal of Obstetric, Gynecologic and Neonatal Nursing, 23*(4), 313-319, 1994.

Ghosh, A. K., & Ghosh, K. (2000). Enhance your practice with evidenced-based medicine. *Patient Care, 29*, 32-56.

Locke, L. F., Silverman, S. J., & Spirduso, W. W. (1998). *Reading and understanding research.* Thousand Oaks: Sage.

Polit, D. F., Beck, C. T., & Hungler, B. P. (2001). *Essentials of nursing research: Methods, appraisal, and utilization* (5th ed.). Philadelphia: Lippincott.

Norwood, S. L. (2000). *Research strategies: The advanced practice nurse.* Upper Saddle River, NJ: Prentice Hall Health.

Shurpin, K. M., Dumas, M. A., & Gallo, K. (1997). Tips for using quantitative research models. *Journal of the American Academy of Nurse Practitioners, 8*(2), 71-74.

Review Questions

1. Which of the following research topics is most appropriately studied using qualitative methods?

   a. Comparison of one-on-one and group instruction to teach self-monitoring of blood glucose

   b. Relationship between length of gestation at time of spontaneous abortion and probability of participating in a grief support group

   c. Attitudes of male NPs related to providing prenatal and postpartal care

   d. Survival skills among college-aged women who experience date rape

2. Josh, a family NP who is considering including a new procedure in his practice with hypertensive clients, has closely examined a report of related research. Which will be the most important consideration in making a decision to include the new procedure?

   a. The findings are statistically significant.

   b. The researcher was a nationally known statistician.

   c. The report appeared in a prestigious publication.

   d. The findings are clinically relevant.

3. Pamela is an NP working in an NP-managed, busy, inner-city clinic. Which factor is most likely to serve as a barrier to Pamela's use of research findings in her practice?

   a. Inner-city clinics differ too much from the controlled settings used for research.

   b. The demands of the practice setting leave little time for using research findings.

   c. Reports of evidence-based practice are inaccessible to the typical NP.

   d. The advanced practice nursing literature has failed to discuss use of research in practice.

4. Ted and Linda, two family NPs, collaborated on a research study related to the best practice for managing pica during pregnancy. There were no statistically significant findings. Which response by Linda is most appropriate?

   a. "I guess we're back to square one on this topic. Bummer!"

   b. "This certainly raises questions for our practice."

   c. "Let's not tell anyone about the lack of success of our study."

   d. "Doing this study was a waste of time and effort."

5. Why are descriptive statistics always used in a quantitative study?

   a. Descriptive statistics form the basis for making inferences about the findings.

   b. Descriptive statistics are used to provide a clearer picture of the participants.

   c. Descriptive statistics may account for unexpected or serendipitous findings.

   d. Descriptive statistics are appropriate for indicating cause-and-effect relationships.

6. Janet is planning a research study to compare the most effective method for orienting new NPs to International Classification of Diseases (ICD)-9 coding. She plans to use a computer program to teach one group while allowing the other group to learn by trial and error. After 1 week, Janet will give a quiz with simulated clients and ask the new NPs to code the visits to assess their learning. What is independent variable in Janet's study?

   a. Simulated clients

   b. Group of new NPs

   c. Quiz to assess ability to use ICD coding

   d. Method of teaching ICD-9 coding

Answers and Rationales

1. *Answer:* **d**
Rationale: Qualitative research is appropriately used to explore the lived experience of persons (Polit, Beck, & Hungler, 2001).

2. *Answer:* **a**
Rationale: Statistically significant findings lend the greatest support for a particular practice (Norwood, 2000).

3. *Answer:* **b**
Rationale: Time is one of the most serious barriers to research utilization in practice (Norwood, 2000).

4. *Answer:* **b**
Rationale: Research efforts are never wasted; one always learns something relevant from questions raised by the study.

Studies often have clinical relevance if not statistical significance in their findings (Polit et al., 2001).

5. *Answer:* b

   Rationale: While inferential statistics are used to test hypotheses, descriptive statistics are used to clearly describe the participants in the study (Norwood, 2000).

6. *Answer:* d

   Rationale: The independent variable is the treatment variable (the variable manipulated) in the study and serves as the presumed cause of the effects seen in the dependent variable. The teaching method (computer program versus trial and error) serves as the independent variable; the quiz evaluating ability at ICD-9 coding is the dependent (outcome) variable (Norwood, 2001).

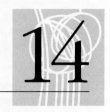

Theories Applicable to Advanced Nursing Practice

Denise Robinson

Nursing has a unique body of knowledge that can serve to guide advanced practice nurses (APNs). Education about holism, prevention, families, communities, caring, and a view of a client as an essential component of health is vital to emphasize the differences between APNs and physicians. Nursing theory, according to Baumann (1998), allows APNs to "structure ideas and interpret information in a way different from the strict biomedical model. It also means being able to consider two views of information, looking at provocative questions and new practice approaches."

The American Association of Colleges of Nursing (1996) identifies theoretical foundations of nursing practice as a core concept for advanced practice. This means graduates should be prepared to critique, evaluate, and use both nursing and nonnursing theory within their practices. The use of theory enables APNs to provide care that focuses on the whole range of a person's health and illness experience and leads to holistic care.

Theory represents a discipline's effort to imbue phenomena of concern with meaning that is unique to that discipline's world view. This meaning allows for an understanding of those phenomena and contributes to the greater purpose of explanation and prediction of future related events; it ultimately allows the discipline to prescribe a course of action that will bring about a desired result. A discipline's efforts in the realm of theory culminate in the development of an integrated larger body of knowledge that underpins and directs the activities of the discipline.

DEFINITIONS

Paradigm reflects the predominant system of philosophy, science, and theory acknowledged by the discipline. The prevailing paradigm makes the phenomena of interest apparent to the discipline and subsequently influences the discipline's research and practice activities. Paradigm is also referred to as *world view* in some literary contexts.

A *philosophy* is constituted by fundamental beliefs about the nature of phenomena. Philosophic beliefs are derived from opinion; because they are not empirically based, they are untestable (Keck, 1998). The prevailing philosophy of the discipline and theorist shapes what subject matter is viewed as appropriate for attention and influences the focus of its theory.

A *phenomenon* is an object, event, or property that constitutes the subject matter of unique concern to a discipline. A phenomenon is identified empirically rather than intuitively and can be the subject of scientific investigation (Keck, 1998).

A *concept* is intended to represent an abstract idea or term that symbolizes a phenomenon and creates mental images of the phenomenon being described (Fawcett & Downs, 1992). Concepts are the foundations for theory.

A *construct* is similar to a concept in that it, too, is an abstraction. However, a construct is not just an abstraction. A construct consists of more than one abstract idea or term and symbolizes the association or interaction of two or more concepts. *Client satisfaction* is an example of a construct; the two concepts are *client* and *satisfaction*. This construct conveys a mental image of the phenomenon that either of the concepts individually fails to achieve. Concepts and constructs are used to generate statements that propose a relationship between or among concepts. This type of statement is called a *proposition*. For example, "Restlessness increases as pain increases" is a propositional statement. Concepts and constructs are also constitutive of *models*. A model is a concrete representation of conceptual and theoretical abstractions. Models are devised to enhance understanding of ideas that cannot be directly observed or visualized and are therefore difficult to grasp (Holder & Chitty, 1997). Models may be represented symbolically through language, although most are commonly communicated graphically.

Concepts, constructs, and propositions come together to constitute a theory. A *theory* is a set of propositions that are logically connected to provide a systematic view of phenomena to describe, explain, predict, or prescribe the phenomena. A *science* is a unified body of knowledge derived from theory that is concerned with a specific focus of interest. The science of a discipline includes the skills and methodologies needed to provide this knowledge (Keck, 1998).

ROLE OF THEORY IN A PRACTICE DISCIPLINE

A theory is a general explanation used to "explain, predict, control, and understand commonly occurring events" (Holder & Chitty, 1997) and is of unique interest to a discipline. Theory organizes and classifies events into a logical, conceptual whole that allows a practitioner to recognize, understand, and manage the phenomenon at hand. For example, a theory of pain encompasses notions of causation and response. Thus a well-defined theory of pain enables a nurse to recognize predictors and indicators of pain. A theory of pain management further facilitates a systematic approach to intervening to achieve goals relative to preventing or minimizing pain.

Characteristics of Theory

Theory functions to provide an internally consistent framework for a discipline's activities considering its goals. The utility of a theory is a function of its ability to consistently guide activities of the discipline congruent with the goals of the discipline. The demonstrated utility of a theory enhances it value to the discipline because it provides a reliable basis for understanding, explaining, and predicting phenomena of interest and concern to the discipline. Continued use and testing of the theory, plus understanding of its ongoing relevance to society, influence its refinement and expansion. Torres (1990) provides the following characteristics that enhance the utility of a theory.

- Theories interrelate concepts in such a way as to create new and more useful ways of looking at a particular phenomenon.
- Theories must be logical in nature.
- Theories must be relatively simple, yet generalizable.
- Theories can be the basis for hypotheses that can be tested.
- Theories contribute to and assist in increasing the general body of knowledge within the discipline through the research implemented to validate them.
- Theories must be consistent with other validated theories, laws, and principles, but they will leave unanswered questions that need to be investigated.

Scope of Theory

Theories differ in their level of scope. The scope of a theory reflects the range of phenomena to which a theory relates or a theory's level of abstraction (Chinn & Kramer, 1995). Theories may be very broad in their range of phenomena of interest and try to portray the larger picture or

they may be very limited in their focus. Although theories are classified according to their level of scope, one should keep in mind that categorization of scope is relative (Chinn & Kramer, 1995). Starting from theory with the broadest scope and moving to the most limited, the different classifications include metatheory, grand theory, midrange theory, and microtheory.

Metatheory is oriented toward philosophic and methodologic issues of theory development. This orientation focuses on concerns related to the nature of theories. Metatheory asks questions about knowledge and about the broader issues within a discipline. It examines questions such as the following: What type or types of theory is or are needed by a discipline? What are appropriate criteria for the analysis and evaluation of theory? What is the nature of theory? (Powers & Knapp, 1990; Chinn & Kramer, 1991; Walker & Avant, 1995).

A *grand theory*, or *broad-range theory*, has within its focus a wide range of phenomena. Its goal is to explain the totality of events related to a discipline. Theoretical formulations within a grand theory are general. In nursing, a grand theory attempts to explain the mission and goals of nursing care (Jacox, 1974; Meleis, 1997). Examples of grand theories include Orem's self-care deficit theory of nursing, Rogers' science of unitary human being, and King's theory of goal attainment (Marriner-Tomey & Alligood, 1998).

Compared with grand theory, *midrange theory* is more limited in scope and level of abstraction. However, the focus of midrange phenomena and concepts can be relevant to all nursing specialties and applicable to a number of nursing care situations. A midrange theory seeks to provide answers to specific nursing questions (Jacox, 1974; Meleis, 1997; Marriner-Tomey & Alligood, 1998). This level of theory may be derived from either earlier nursing theories or disciplines related to nursing. A midrange theory is based on specific practice concepts and is characteristically more concrete than a grand theory. Examples of midrange theories include Peplau's interpersonal relations theory, Leininger's cultural care theory, and Parse's human becoming theory.

Microtheory is also known as *practice theory, empirical generalization*, or *partial theory*. The range of microtheory is more limited and prescribed than that of midrange theory. The goal of microtheory is to provide a nurse with specific desired *client* goals and precise practice directives (Walker & Avant, 1995; Fitzpatrick & Whall, 1996). An example of a microtheory is the physiology of pain phenomena.

Nursing Utilization of Theory

Gortner (1980) has defined *nursing science* as reflecting nursing's understanding of human biology, behavior, health, and illness. In her definition, Gortner includes the process necessary to bring about changes in health status and the behavior patterns associated with normal and critical life events, as well as the principles governing life states and processes. The goal of nursing science is to understand, explain, and represent human nature (Gortner & Schultz, 1988). Nursing science consists of defined concepts describing human responses to health, illness, and therapeutic nursing actions (Hinshaw, 1989). Nursing science in relationship to practice, then, is the body of knowledge with a nursing prospective that produces and tests knowledge gained in nursing work.

Theory and Practice

Chinn and Kramer (1995) define *nursing practice* as the experiences a practicing nurse encounters during the process of caring for people. In nursing, theory is used to enlighten nurses about nursing practice situations and to guide research. The interaction of practice and theory shapes practice and helps in establishing guidelines for practice (Meleis, 1997). These practice experiences are oriented from the views of both nurse and *client*. The experiences are interactive, individual, and framed by the environment.

APNs do not obtain from theory the same structure and guidance they previously obtained from the principles and procedures that exist to standardize practice. Theory challenges existing practice by creating new ways to think and practice (Chinn & Kramer, 1995). From nursing experience and nurses' perceptions of their world, nursing theorists and APNs develop conceptual meanings. These conceptual meanings are arrived at through reflection, discussion, and attempts to make sense of the meanings. APNs and theorists communicating between and among themselves develop language and tools to communicate the meaning of the experiences.

Much has been written about the difficulty of putting theory into practice (Kim, 1993; Kim, 1994; Phillips, Mousseau-Gershman, & Powell, 1998). The individual nurse must bring knowledge to the individual *client* in each nurse-*client* interaction. Or, simply stated, the nurse must choose a nursing intervention that is appropriate for the particular situation. It is at this point that the nurse brings all experience and knowledge to bear; he or she makes a choice of action and then applies the chosen theory (Kim, 1993). It is in this dynamic interaction that theory and practice are integrated for *client* care.

Theories provide a view of a *client* situation that can be accessed by an APN to map the organization of data. Theory helps an APN establish an information and relationship hierarchy for the collected data. From this mapping, care and outcomes can be planned. This systematic collecting and organizing of data leads to working efficiently and purposefully (Raudonis & Acton, 1997).

CONCEPTS IN NURSING THEORIES OR MODELS

Concepts in nursing theories and models include client, environment, health, and nursing action.

Common Nursing Conceptual Models

- Rogers' model of unitary beings: Humans are irreducible. Humans and their environments are mutual and continuous.
- King's central systems model: Humans are open systems that interact with the environment. Goal attainment in nurse-client interactions leads to both nurse and client satisfaction and to effective nursing care.
- Orem's self-care model: The goal of nursing is to help people meet their needs for self-care at a therapeutic level and on a continual basis.
- Roy's adaptation model: People are adaptive systems in constant interaction with changing environments. People adapt to change through coping mechanisms.
- Neuman's system model: The client is composed of five systems: developmental, spiritual, sociocultural, psychologic, and physiologic. The aim of nursing is to promote stability of the client.

Common Nursing Theories of Care

- Leininger's theory of cultural care diversity and universality: Nursing care must be congruent with the client's culture. To achieve congruence, the nurse functions within the areas of cultural care preservation, cultural care negotiation, and cultural care repatterning.
- Watson's theory of caring: Human caring is the moral ideal of nursing. The goal of nursing is to achieve greater harmony of mind, body, and soul. This is achieved through a transpersonal caring process in which nurse and client both participate.

Family Theories

A family is defined as follows:
- Members are united by a bond.
- Members may live together. Members interact and communicate with each other in family roles (e.g., mother-son).
- Members maintain a common culture.

Common Family Theories

- Structural-functional: This theory is concerned with how the family members are arranged, the relationships between the members, and the relationships of members to the family as a whole. Structure serves to facilitate the achievement of family functions.
- Family systems: The focus is on the interactions of the various parts of the family. The family is a system, and a change in one member of the family results in changes for the total family unit.
- Developmental perspective: A family has a life cycle with predictable changes. Tasks are associated with each stage of the cycle. Unpredictable events create needs and require adjustment.
- Interactionist perspective: This theory focuses on the meanings that acts and symbols hold for people. Roles

serve as a means for interaction. The aim is to view situations from the family member's or family's perspective.

- Family ecologic perspective: Broader than the systems theory, this perspective looks at the family's relationship to the environment. Both the environment and the family are constantly changing.
- Social exchange perspective: Family members maintain involvement in relationships on the basis of rewards and costs.
- Family stress perspective (ABCX model): Variability in family response to stress is based on A, hardships; B, resources; C, family's definition of the event; and X, the crisis.

Community Theory

- Epidemiologic perspective: The host is the susceptible person. The agent is the presence or absence of factors that may influence the health of the person. The environment is anything external to the person or agent. A change in any of these factors may change the balance of health.
- Structural-functional perspective: This theory stresses the ability of the community to carry out its functions to attain community goals.
- Systems theory: Emphasis is on the components of the community and the capability of the community to operate as a system for meeting community goals.

Models of Health Behavior

Health Belief Model. The health belief model focuses on an illness prevention-multifactorial model to explain why people make changes to improve their health.

Health Promotion Model. According to Walker, Sechrist, and Pender (1987), "Health promotion is a multidimensional pattern of self-initiated actions and perceptions that serve to maintain or enhance the level of wellness, self-actualization and fulfillment of the individual."

The health promotion model is proposed as a multivariate model for explaining and predicting the health-promoting components of lifestyle. This model focuses on health promotion without the threat of disease. Factors that influence one's likelihood of engaging in health-promoting behaviors include the following (Pender, et al. 1990):

- Importance of health
- Perceived control of health
- Perceived self-efficacy
- Definition of health
- Perceived health status
- Perceived benefits of health-promoting behaviors
- Perceived barriers to health-promoting behaviors

Definitions

- Health risk appraisal includes screening for disease potential, educating clients about unhealthy habits, and stimulating behavior change.

- Risk factors are characteristics that have been associated with higher risk for a particular disease. Relative risk is determined by the ratio of risk or rate in exposed persons to the risk or rate in unexposed persons.
- Epidemiology is the study of the distribution and determinants of the frequency of disease in humans.
- Mortality refers to death.
- Morbidity refers to illness.

Change Theory

Change means a substitution of one thing for another or an alteration in the state or quality of a thing. As a verb, change means to make a thing other than what it was or to become different. Planned change means that one has made choices about how to use theories and methods for the purposes of reaching an identified goal (Tiffany, 1994).

A variety of models and theories describe change. Which model is used depends on the nature of the change and beliefs about the change. Kaluzney and Hernandez (1988) describe three models of change: rational, organizational ecology, and resource dependency.

Teaching Learning Theory

Client Education. Principles of learning include the following (Boyd, 1997):

- Readiness to learn: person's ability and energy to learn
- Assessment of readiness to learn
  - Health status
  - Health values
  - Cognitive, psychologic, and psychomotor abilities
  - Previous learning experiences
  - Developmental characteristics of the learner
- Motivation: person's desire to learn; reinforcements are used to increase or decrease likelihood that behavior will be repeated

Teaching Strategies

- Instructional methods: how the teaching session is structured
- Educational methods: strategies that facilitate learning
  - Progress from simple to complex and from concrete to abstract.
  - Advanced organizers: Tell the learner what is to be learned and then cue the learner to each point.
  - Use specificity and brevity.
  - Repetition strengthens learning.
  - People best remember the first third and the last quarter of information presented; this is known as primacy.
  - Make material relevant.
  - Reinforce learning.

Behavior Strategies

- Contracting: Develop contract of behaviors and rewards.
- Graduating behavioral change: The learner makes small increments of change with time.
- Tailoring: Fit a prescribed regimen into a learner's lifestyle.
- Self-monitoring: The learner analyzes his or her own behavior patterns through "data collection" (e.g., keeping a diary).

Evaluation of Teaching Learning Theory

- Process or formative evaluation: Assess the effectiveness of the teaching process.
- Outcome or impact evaluation: Assess the effectiveness of the teaching process in promoting learning.

REFERENCES

American Association of Colleges of Nursing. (1996). *The essentials of a master's education for advanced practice nursing.* Washington, DC: American Association of Colleges of Nursing.

Baumann, S. (1998). Nursing: the missing ingredient in nurse practitioner education. *Nursing Science Quarterly, 11*(3), 89-90.

Boyd, M. (1997). Health teaching in nursing practice. In D. Caleris, R. Fernandopulle, & B. Mauro (Eds.), *Health care policy.* Cambridge, MA: Blackwell Science.

Chinn, P. L., & Kramer, M. K. (1995). *Theory and nursing: A systematic approach.* St. Louis: Mosby.

Fawcett, J., & Downs, F. (1992). *The relationship of theory and research* (2nd ed.). Philadelphia: F. A. Davis.

Fitzpatrick, J. J., & Whall, A. L. (1996). *Conceptual models of nursing: Analysis and application.* Stamford, CN: Appleton & Lange.

Gortner, S. R. (1980). Nursing science in transition. *Nursing Research, 29*(3), 180-183.

Gortner, S. R., & Schultz, P. (1988). Approaches to nursing science methods. *Image: Journal of Nursing Scholarship, 20*(1), 22-24.

Hinshaw, A. (1989). Nursing science: The challenge to develop knowledge. *Nursing Science Quarterly, 2*(4), 162-171.

Holder, P. J., & Chitty, K. K. (1997). Theory as a basis for professional nursing. In K. K. Chitty (Ed.), *Professional nursing: Concepts and challenges* (pp. 211-231). Philadelphia: W. B. Saunders.

Jacox, A. (1974). Theory construction in nursing: An overview. *Nursing Research, 23*(1), 4-13, 1974.

Kalurney, R., & Hernandez, J. (1988). Studies of change in organizations. In P. Goodman (Ed.), *Change in organization.* San Francisco: Jossey-Bass.

Keck, J. F. (1998). Terminology of theory development. In A. Marriner-Tomey & M. R. Alligood (Eds.), *Nursing theorists and their work* (4th ed.). St. Louis: Mosby.

Kim, H. S. (1993). Putting theory into practice: Problems and prospects. *Journal of Advanced Nursing, 18*(10), 1632-1639.

Kim, H. S. (1994). Practice theories in nursing and a science of nursing practice. *Scholarly Inquiry for Nursing Practice, 8*(2), 145-166.

Marriner-Tomey, A., & Alligood, M. R. (Eds.) (1998). *Nursing theorists and their work* (4th ed.). St. Louis: Mosby.

Meleis, A. I. (1997). Theoretical nursing: development and progress (3rd ed.). Philadelphia: J. B. Lippincott.

Pender, N., Walker, S., & Sechrist. (1990). *The health promotion model: Refinement of validation. Final report to the NCNR, NIH Grant HNR011211.* Dekalb, IL: Northern Illinois University Press.

Phillips, R., Donald, A., Mousseau-Gershman, Y., & Powell, T. (1998). Applying theory to practice: The use of "ripple effect" plans in continuing education. *Nurse Education Today, 18,* 12-19.

Pokorny, B., & Barnard, K. (1992). ANA to revise nursing statement. *American Nurse, 6.*

Powers, B. A., & Knapp, T. R. (1990). *A dictionary of nursing theory and research.* Thousand Oaks: Sage.

Raudonis, B. M., & Acton, G. J. (1997). Theory-based nursing practice. *Journal of Advanced Nursing, 26,* 138-145.

Rawnsley, M. (1999). Response to Fawcett's "The state of nursing science." *Nursing Science Quarterly, 12*(4), 315-318.

Ray, M. (1998). Complexity and nursing science. *Nursing Science Quarterly, 11,* 91-93, 1998.

Rogers, M. (1985). The nature and characteristics of professional education for nursing. *Journal of Professional Nursing, 1,* 382-383.

Rooke, L. (1995). Focusing on King's theory and systems framework in education by using an experiential learning model: A challenge to improve the quality of nursing care. In M. A. Frey & C. Sieloff (Eds.) *Advancing King's Systems Framework and Theory of Nursing.* Newbury Park, CA: Sage.

Rosendahl, P. P., & Ross, V (1982). Does your behaviour affect your patient's response? *Journal of Gerontologic Nursing, 8,* 572-575.

Rutty, J. (1998). The nature of philosophy of science, theory and knowledge relating to nursing and professionalism. *Journal of Advanced Nursing, 28*(2), 243-250.

Sackett, D., Richardson, W., Rosenberg, W. (1998). *Evidence-based medicine: How to practice and teach EBM.* London: Churchill Livingstone.

Sheehy, C., & McCarthy, M. (1998). *Advanced nursing practice.* Philadelphia: F. A. Davis.

Sieloff, C. (Ed.). (1995). *Advancing King's framework and theory for nursing* (pp. 278-293). Newbury Park, CA: Sage.

Silva, M. C. (1986). Research testing nursing theory: State of the art. *Advances in Nursing Science, 9*(1), 1-11.

Simms, L. M., Price, S. A., Ervin, N. E. (1994). The professional practice of nursing administration. Albany: Delmar.

Smith, M. (1993). The contribution of nursing theory to nursing administration practice. *Image: Journal of Nursing Scholarship, 25*(1), 63-67.

Tanner, C., Benner, P., Chesla, C., & Gordon, D. R. (1993). The phenomenology of knowing the patient. *Image: Journal of Nursing Scholarship, 24*(4), 273-280.

Taylor, S. (1988). Nursing theory and nursing process: Orem's theory in practice. *Nursing Science Quarterly, 1*(3), 111-119, 1988.

Taylor, S., & McLaughlin, K. (1991). Orem's general theory of nursing and community nursing. *Nursing Science Quarterly, 4*(4), 153-160.

10. Absent breath sounds are indicative of which of the following?

    a. Pneumothorax
    b. Chronic obstructive pulmonary disease
    c. Pneumonia
    d. Pulmonary embolus

Answers and Rationales

1. *Answer:* **c** (implementation/plan)
    Rationale: It is important that practitioners teach pursed-lip breathing and exercise techniques to maximize oxygen intake. Coping skills help decrease anxiety. Proper use of a metered-dose inhaler helps to deposit medication in the lung, rather than in the device or the mouth. If clients have difficulty with this task, a spacer device can be prescribed.

2. *Answer:* **a** (assessment)
    Rationale: An atrial gallop rhythm may be associated with cor pulmonale.

3. *Answer:* **c** (evaluation)
    Rationale: Serevent or a long acting beta agonist is the best choice to add to Steve's current medications to help control nighttime symptoms (Gross & Ponte, 1998).

4. *Answer:* **c** (analysis/diagnosis)
    Rationale: A transition from a productive cough to a dry, hacking cough suggests that the cough is caused by hyperreactive airways, not necessarily by an infectious process.

5. *Answer:* **b** (assessment)
    Rationale: Decreased appetite and nausea are less likely to be among the clinical presenting symptoms associated with important causes of cough.

6. *Answer:* **a** (assessment)
    Rationale: Headache, facial pain, and halitosis are more indicative of sinusitis, whereas sore throat, fever, nausea, vomiting, and abdominal pain point to streptococcal pharyngitis. Family history of asthma, history of skin rash, and environmental triggers of respiratory distress suggest asthma. Cystic fibrosis commonly has presenting symptoms of steatorrhea, poor weight gain, and recurrent respiratory infections.

7. *Answer:* **c** (assessment)
    Rationale: An examination of the cardiac and respiratory systems, as well as HEENT examination, may narrow the differential diagnosis.

8. *Answer:* **b** (assessment)
    Rationale: Abdominal pain and guarding are more indicative of appendicitis; bronchiolitis is a common problem in children younger than 2 years old and an isolated incident does not suggest more severe pathologic condition; and recurrent vomiting in a 2-month-old in the absence of coughing suggests a gastrointestinal pathologic condition. Cystic fibrosis is the most common cause of rectal prolapse.

9. *Answer:* **b** (analysis/diagnosis)
    Rationale: A history of light-headedness and paresthesias of the perioral area or distal extremities suggest hyperventilation syndrome.

10. *Answer:* **a** (analysis/diagnosis)
    Rationale: The lung is collapsed and thus not against the chest wall; breath sounds therefore will not be heard.

CARDIOVASCULAR SYSTEM

Review Questions

1. What is the most likely cause of chest pain in a 25-year-old new mother?

    a. Myocardial infarction
    b. Pulmonary embolus
    c. Gastroesophageal reflux disease
    d. Angina

2. Which of the following should be ordered for the client who has a history of chest pain and is being sent home?

    a. Digitalis
    b. Penicillin
    c. Amiodarone
    d. Nitroglycerine tablets, SL

3. What is the primary reason to determine the cause of a transient ischemic attack and treat it if possible?

    a. Decrease the number of transient ischemic attacks.
    b. Decrease the number of heart attacks.
    c. Increase function.
    d. Decrease the possibility of stroke.

4. Which of the following diagnoses is important to keep controlled in the client with a transient ischemic attack?

    a. Cataracts
    b. Hypertension
    c. Hypolipidemia
    d. Hypoproteinemia

5. Complete the following sentence: Reversible ischemic neurologic deficit is defined as lasting longer than:

    a. 24 hours and less than 7 days
    b. 2 hours and less than 24 hours
    c. 24 hours and less than 2 days
    d. 20 minutes and less than 3 days

6. All *except* which of the following are important questions to ask the young woman who comes in with left-side weakness?

    a. Use of oral contraceptives

b. Recent delivery
c. History of recent deep venous thrombosis
d. History of pelvic inflammatory disease

7. If the head CT scan results are normal and the client is older, what other radiologic test will likely give the most significant information with respect to a transient ischemic attack?

a. Carotid artery Doppler study
b. Chest x-ray film
c. Pneumoencephalography
d. IV pyelography

8. In most children with congenital heart disease, what is the usual presenting symptom or clinical sign in those children with critical disease?

a. Cough
b. Tachypnea
c. Congestive heart failure
d. Excessive sleeping

9. Why can aortic stenosis lead to syncope?

a. The heart cannot beat properly.
b. The cardiac output is diminished and the brain has decreased blood flow.
c. The cardiac output is increased and the brain is over-perfused.
d. Blood is shunted away from the brain by increased cardiac output.

10. All *except* which of the following laboratory tests may yield useful information in diagnosing the cause of syncope?

a. Complete blood cell count
b. Electrolyte levels
c. Glucose level
d. Liver function tests

Answers and Rationales

1. *Answer:* b (analysis/diagnosis)
Rationale: Young women who have just delivered may produce emboli from the placenta; the most likely place for these to cause occlusion is the lung.

2. *Answer:* d (implementation/plan)
Rationale: Nitroglycerin tablets are ordered so that the client can begin therapy before any damage occurs. It also helps in the diagnosis of coronary chest pain versus noncoronary chest pain.

3. *Answer:* d (implementation/plan)
Rationale: Because a transient ischemic attack is often a precursor of a stroke, it is important to identify and treat the underlying cause in an effort to prevent stroke.

4. *Answer:* b (implementation/plan)
Rationale: Because of the endothelial damage that occurs with prolonged hypertension, it is important to keep this condition controlled.

5. *Answer:* a (analysis/diagnosis)
Rationale: Reversible ischemic neurologic deficits last longer than transient ischemic attacks but are not classified as strokes. By definition, they last less than 7 days, and the neurologic deficit reverses without evidence of stroke.

6. *Answer:* d (assessment)
Rationale: All the other problems can result in emboli traveling to the brain, causing a transient ischemic attack.

7. *Answer:* a (implementation/plan)
Rationale: The most likely site of transient ischemic attack on the list is the carotid artery. The carotid artery study will therefore likely yield the most information.

8. *Answer:* c (assessment)
Rationale: In 80% of children with critical congenital heart disease, they present with congestive heart failure (Saenz, Beebe, Triplett, 1999).

9. *Answer:* b (analysis/diagnosis)
Rationale: Cardiac output is diminished because of the stenosis and the brain has decreased blood flow, causing a syncopal episode.

10. *Answer:* d (implementation/plan)
Rationale: Causes of syncope include anemia (complete blood cell count), hyponatremia (electrolyte levels), and hypoglycemia (glucose level).

GASTROINTESTINAL SYSTEM

Review Questions

1. Which of the following comments by the client indicates a further need for teaching by the NP concerning Giardia?

a. "I need to follow good handwashing techniques after using the toilet."
b. "I can return to my job in the day care after my appointment."
c. "When I go camping I need to drink bottled water."
d. "I need to complete all the prescribed medication."

2. Phyllis is concerned that her younger son may develop encopresis. What teaching is most likely to help prevent this from occurring?

a. Using a toileting diary
b. Eating a well balanced healthy diet
c. Starting toilet training when the child is developmentally ready
d. Using strict consequences if "accidents" occur

3. What objective data must be obtained from a client with suspected irritable bowel syndrome?

a. Height and weight
b. Thorough neurologic evaluation
c. Stool for ova and parasites
d. Current medications

4. What is your most likely diagnosis for a client who reports abdominal pain relieved by bowel movements and constipation alternating with diarrhea for the past 4 months?

a. Diverticulosis
b. Lactose intolerance
c. Appendicitis
d. Irritable bowel syndrome

5. Which of the following statements about hepatitis B viral infections is *false?*

a. It is considered a sexually transmitted disease.
b. At-risk groups are homosexual men, health care workers, and IV drug users sharing needles.
c. It is associated with hepatitis D viral infection.
d. It is treated with interferon on diagnosis.

6. Which of the following hepatitis infections is(are) associated with chronic carrier states?

a. HAV and HBV
b. HBV only
c. HBV and HCV
d. HCV only

7. The NP provides instruction regarding diet for a child with recurrent abdominal pain (RAP). Which comment by the parent indicates a need for *further* instruction?

a. "Steve needs to drink at least four glasses of milk a day."
b. "Sharon should eat foods with increased fiber."
c. "A fast food diet is not helpful for RAP."
d. "Fruit juice should be eliminated or reduced for Steve."

8. Sally is an 8-year-old female who reports a history of abdominal pain for 2 days. Which of the following observations would assist you in concluding that Sally does *not* have an acute surgical abdomen?

a. Sally is lying on the stretcher clutching her abdomen.
b. Sally is able to jump up and down on one foot without difficulty.
c. It is more painful for Sally when you stop palpating her abdomen.
d. Sally is nauseated and has vomited three times.

9. Which of the following symptoms is generally not associated with a medical cause of abdominal pain?

a. Obstipation
b. Constipation
c. Diarrhea
d. Pain after vomiting

10. The most common cause of acute abdominal pain in school-age children is which of the following?

a. Appendicitis
b. Intussusception
c. Testicular torsion
d. Incarcerated hernia

Answers and Rationales

1. *Answer:* b (implementation/plan)
Rationale: Once diagnosed with Giardia, the client cannot return to a job in day care until the disease is resolved (Robinson, Kidd, & Rogers, 2000).

2. *Answer:* c (implementation/plan)
Rationale: Toilet training that is begun before the child is physiologically and developmentally ready may contribute to later toileting problems (Kuhn, Marcus, & Pitner, 1999).

3. *Answer:* a (assessment)
Rationale: Evaluation of weight (and of previous measures) is pertinent to this client. Stool samples for ova and parasites may be justified after you have ruled out other possible causes. Ova and parasite tests are expensive procedures to rule out symptoms caused by parasites; a careful history, physical examination, and preliminary laboratory findings usually precede this laboratory test. Current medications are subjective data. A thorough neurologic examination is not warranted for this client.

4. *Answer:* d (analysis/diagnosis)
Rationale: The client has no indication of an inflammatory process and you do not have a dietary history to determine whether she has a lactose intolerance. Often diverticulosis is seen with left lower quadrant pain. An important point in her history is the relief of pain after defecation. The best choice of diagnosis is irritable bowel syndrome.

5. *Answer:* d (analysis/diagnosis)
Rationale: Treatment is observation for as long as you can, and interferon treatment is not entered readily. All the other choices are true concerning HBV.

6. *Answer:* c (implementation/plan)
Rationale: Hepatitis A never has a chronic carrier state, whereas HBV and HCV do.

7. *Answer:* a (implementation/plan)
Rationale: Decreasing milk and fruit juice can be tried as a means to affect carbohydrate absorption. Fast foods do not help with either the lactose intolerance or constipation. Increased fiber (5 g) has been shown to decrease the incidence of abdominal pain (Stein, 2001).

8. *Answer:* b (assessment)
Rationale: Jumping up and down indicates no peritoneal inflammation and can help rule out an acute surgical abdomen.

9. *Answer:* a (assessment)
Rationale: True obstipation is strongly suggestive of a mechanical bowel obstruction.

10. *Answer:* a (analysis/diagnosis)
Rationale: Intussusception, incarcerated hernia, and testicular torsion occur less frequently in the school age child than does appendicitis.

GENITOURINARY AND REPRODUCTIVE SYSTEMS

Review Questions

1. David, a 7-year-old who is being treated with imipramine (Tofranil) for enuresis, returns for his 2-week follow-up. He is smiling and reports 1 week of consecutive dry nights. What should the family NP do?
   a. Praise David for his success and continue imipramine (Tofranil).
   b. Praise David for his success and begin to taper imipramine (Tofranil).
   c. Discontinue imipramine (Tofranil) and begin antidiuretic hormone on an as-necessary basis.
   d. Discontinue imipramine (Tofranil) and change David's follow-up to an as-necessary basis.

2. A history of hematospermia may be associated with which of the following?
   a. Acute bacterial prostatitis
   b. Benign prostatic hyperplasia
   c. Prostate cancer
   d. Chronic bacterial prostatitis

3. A young man reports urinary urgency, frequency, and abdominal discomfort. Which of the following diagnoses is *not* an appropriate differential diagnosis?
   a. Acute cystitis
   b. Acute prostatitis
   c. Pyelonephritis
   d. Sexually transmitted disease

4. Which of the following factors in a male client's history increases his risk of infertility?
   a. Mitral valve prolapse
   b. Mumps at puberty
   c. Toxoplasmosis in childhood
   d. Surgically-corrected phimosis

5. A man presents with painful hemorrhoids. Which factor in his history increases the risk of this disorder?
   a. Homosexuality with anal receptive sexual practices
   b. Career as a letter carrier
   c. Being underweight and slightly anemic
   d. Preference for high fiber foods

6. What is the ultimate goal of an infertility workup?
   a. A complete evaluation of the female within 6 months
   b. A viable pregnancy and the birth of a healthy infant
   c. A complete evaluation of the couple within 2 years
   d. An adoption plan

7. Which of the following factors in a woman's history decreases the risk of ovarian cysts?
   a. Use of oral contraceptives
   b. Nulliparity
   c. Menarche at 9 years of age
   d. Safe sex practices

8. On physical examination, polycystic ovary syndrome would be characterized by which of the following?
   a. Prominent iliac spines
   b. Hirsutism with male pattern distribution
   c. Large, pendulous breasts
   d. Small, unhooded clitoris

9. Victoria is a 30-year-old symptom-free client in whom a functional ovarian cyst is suspected. When should she be instructed to return for reevaluation?
   a. When her next annual examination is due
   b. In 2 to 3 weeks, just before ovulation
   c. In 36 hours
   d. No follow-up because of lack of symptoms

10. All of the following clients have dysfunctional uterine bleeding. Which client should be referred for immediate evaluation by a gynecologist?
    a. A 17-year-old who began taking a triphasic oral contraceptive pill 3 months ago
    b. A 31-year-old mother of two who uses medroxyprogesterone (Depo-Provera) for contraception
    c. A 29-year-old with an intrauterine device for birth control, abdominal pain, and adnexal mass
    d. A 46-year-old woman who reports saturating four pads per day for 5 days during menses.

Answers and Rationales

1. **Answer: a** (evaluation)
   Rationale: Imipramine (Tofranil) should be continued until 21 consecutive nights of dryness have been achieved.

2. **Answer: d** (assessment)
   Rationale: Hematospermia is not commonly seen in acute bacterial prostatitis, benign prostatic hyperplasia, or prostate cancer.

3. **Answer: c** (analysis/diagnosis)
   Rationale: Cystitis, prostatitis and a sexually transmitted disease need to be considered as differential diagnoses for the symptoms presented here. Not enough information is given to eliminate them from the diagnostic possibilities. Usually with pyelonephritis, the client exhibits fever, chills, and lower back pain. Nausea and anorexia are also common signs of pyelonephritis.

4. **Answer: b** (assessment)
   Rationale: Mumps is associated with infertility in men when it contributes to orchitis. Toxoplasmosis, mitral valve prolapse, and surgically-corrected phimosis are not highly correlated with male infertility.

5. **Answer: a** (assessment)
   Rationale: Anal sex, whether in men or women, is associated with an increased risk of hemorrhoids. Other options include factors that do not increase the risk of hemorrhoids. Choice d, preference for high-fiber foods, lowers the risk.

6. Answer: b (evaluation)
   Rationale: The ultimate goal of an infertility evaluation is a viable pregnancy and the birth of a healthy infant.

7. Answer: a (assessment)
   Rationale: Oral contraceptives and pregnancy modify the risk of ovarian cysts.

8. Answer: b (assessment)
   Rationale: Hirsutism with male distribution pattern, small breasts, and an enlarged clitoris are objective findings in polycystic ovary syndrome.

9. Answer: b (evaluation)
   Rationale: Follow-up in 2 to 3 weeks is appropriate because the functional cyst will have resolved.

10. Answer: c (implementation/plan)
   Rationale: Ectopic pregnancy is one possibility associated with intrauterine device use and warrants emergency intervention by a physician.

MUSCULOSKELETAL SYSTEM

Review Questions

1. What is the *least* likely finding of acute gout on physical examination?
   a. A single, warm, red, tender joint of the lower extremity
   b. Joint effusion with limited range of motion
   c. Low-grade fever with temperature of 99.6° F
   d. Painless tophi with urate deposits on the Achilles tendon

2. In addition to gout, the differential diagnosis for acute monoarthritis is *least* likely to include which of the following?
   a. Septic joint
   b. Bone cancer
   c. Pseudogout
   d. Joint trauma

3. Which of the following is *not* true regarding gamekeeper's thumb?
   a. It is caused by a forced hyperabduction of the thumb.
   b. It is an injury to the ulnar collateral ligament of the thumb.
   c. It is commonly seen in snow skiers.
   d. It is commonly seen in children.

4. Physical findings associated with mallet finger include which of the following?
   a. An extension deformity of the proximal interphalangeal joint
   b. A crush injury of the distal phalanx
   c. Decreased sensation in the distal fingertip
   d. A flexion deformity of the distal interphalangeal joint of the finger

5. Salter-Harris classification is which of the following?
   a. A system to describe long-bone fractures
   b. A classification for distal fibular injuries
   c. A classification of growth plate fractures in children
   d. A classification of wrist injuries

6. Which of the following does *not* require immediate referral to an orthopedic surgeon?
   a. Intraarticular fractures
   b. Fractures with neurovascular compromise
   c. Knee injuries with gross instability
   d. Grade II and III ankle sprains

7. Spinal curves of 20 to 25 degrees require which of the following interventions?
   a. Milwaukee brace
   b. Harrington rod
   c. Range of motion exercises
   d. Observation every 4 to 6 months

8. Lateral S-shaped curvature of the thoracic and lumbar spine is which of the following?
   a. Kyphosis
   b. Scoliosis
   c. Lordosis
   d. Osteoporosis

9. Which of the following applies to nonstructural scoliosis?
   a. Fixed curvature of the spine.
   b. Corrected with front bending.
   c. Treated with a brace.
   d. Requires annual spinal x-ray examinations.

10. Heather, a 37-year-old typist at your office, has initial symptoms of carpal tunnel syndrome. Conservative treatment to initiate includes which of the following?
   a. Steroid injection to the carpal tunnel
   b. Rest of the affected part, ice, and nonsteroidal antiinflammatory drugs
   c. Excision of carpal ligament
   d. Carpal compression

Answers and Rationales

1. Answer: d (assessment)
   Rationale: Tophi are a manifestation of chronic gout, with an average of 10 years of hyperuricemia before development.

2. Answer: b (analysis/diagnosis)
   Rationale: Trauma, infection, and pseudogout can produce acute monoarthritis. Bone cancer is a chronic progressive disease; it is not listed as a differential diagnosis.

3. Answer: d (analysis/diagnosis)
   Rationale: Skier's thumb or gamekeeper's thumb is an injury to the ulnar collateral ligament of the metacarpophalangeal joint of the thumb that occurs with a forced hyperabduction. It is not usually seen in children.

4. *Answer:* **d** (assessment)

Rationale: Mallet deformity is a flexion deformity of the distal interphalangeal joint of the finger. The client cannot actively extend the finger at the distal interphalangeal joint.

5. *Answer:* **c** (analysis/diagnosis)

Rationale: The Salter-Harris classification system is used to describe acute injuries that involve the growth plate. In the individual with an immature skeleton, the growth plate remains open.

6. *Answer:* **d** (implementation/plan)

Rationale: Ankle sprains can be easily managed in the primary care setting. Current treatment involves aggressive functional rehabilitation.

7. *Answer:* **d** (implementation/plan)

Rationale: Spinal curves of 20 to 25 degrees are not severe enough to require intervention other than observation every 4 to 6 months to watch for change.

8. *Answer:* **b** (analysis/diagnosis)

Rationale: The definition of scoliosis is the lateral S- or C-shaped curvature of the thoracic and lumbar spine.

9. *Answer:* **b** (analysis/diagnosis)

Rationale: Functional (nonstrutural) scoliosis is corrected with front bending.

10. *Answer:* **b** (implementation/plan)

Rationale: Conservative treatment is rest, ice, splinting, and nonsteroidal antiinflammatory drugs. Steroid injection and surgery are not conservative treatments.

NEUROLOGIC SYSTEM

Review Questions

1. Which of the following physical findings may be present in a client with a tension-type headache?

  a. Tenderness of pericranial muscles
  b. Unilateral muscle weakness
  c. Ptosis
  d. Eyelid edema

2. Which of the following sets of symptoms is associated with tension-type headache?

  a. Bilateral, mild to moderate, pressing headache lasting 30 minutes to 7 days
  b. Unilateral, moderate to severe, throbbing headache lasting for 4 to 72 hours, aggravated by routine physical activity, with nausea, vomiting, or both; headache preceded by flashing lights
  c. Pounding or dull frontal or occipital pain present when upright and relieved by lying down
  d. More prevalent in men, occurring in attacks of severe unilateral orbital, supraorbital, or temporal pain, lasting 15 to 180 minutes, with miosis

3. Which of the following conditions is linked with a higher risk for Bell's palsy?

  a. Hyperthyroidism
  b. Osteoarthritis
  c. Pregnancy
  d. Crohn's disease

4. What is the *least* likely symptom to suggest Bell's palsy?

  a. Mild tinnitus at onset
  b. Facial weakness progressing during weeks or months
  c. Hypersensitivity to sound
  d. Taste alteration

5. Which finding would cause the NP to consider a diagnosis of Alzheimer's disease?

  a. Acute onset of memory change
  b. Increase episodes of crying
  c. Getting lost in a familiar place
  d. Trouble driving at night

6. In what situation would you consider giving donepezil (Aricept) to a client?

  a. Questionable dementia
  b. Mild to moderate dementia
  c. Severe dementia
  d. Dementia with coexisting depression

7. You place a client on a regimen of tracrine (Cognex). To evaluate the client's response to the medication, what laboratory test would you order weekly initially?

  a. Complete blood cell counts
  b. Alanine aminotransferase levels
  c. Blood glucose levels
  d. Erythrocyte sedimentation rates

8. Which of the following factors in a client's history is *not* a risk factor for Alzheimer's disease?

  a. Smoking
  b. Head injury
  c. Age
  d. Family history

9. Mrs. Johnson has brought her 7-year-old daughter Susie to the office for a follow-up visit. The diagnosis of simple partial seizures was previously made by the pediatric neurologist, and Susie was placed on a regimen of carbamazepine (Tegretol). The follow-up care is to be carried out by the NP. Which of the following is *not* appropriate for the NP to do?

  a. Order an MRI scan for follow-up.

b. Ascertain any untoward side effects that the client may be experiencing.

c. Reinforce education about seizures and antiepileptic drugs.

d. Order complete blood cell counts and liver function tests every 2 to 3 weeks for the first 2 months, then every 3 months.

10. The facial paralysis of Bell's palsy does *not* cause which one of the following?

a. Bilateral forehead wrinkles

b. Incomplete eyelid closure

c. Drooling

d. Flattened nasolabial fold

Answers and Rationales

1. ***Answer:* a** (assessment)

Rationale: Tenderness of pericranial muscles may be present in individuals with tension-type headaches. Unilateral muscle weakness may be associated with a stroke or a neurologic condition, whereas ptosis and eyelid edema are more likely to be identified with a cluster headache.

2. ***Answer:* a** (assessment)

Rationale: Unilateral, moderate to severe, throbbing headache lasting 4 to 72 hours, aggravated by routine physical activity, with nausea, vomiting, or both, headache preceded by flashing lights, is a more suggestive pattern for migraine headache with an aura. Pounding or dull frontal pain, present when upright and relieved by lying down, is likely to occur with a headache after a spinal puncture. Headache that is more prevalent in men, occurs in attacks of severe unilateral orbital, supraorbital, or temporal pain lasting 15 to 180 minutes, with miosis, is a cluster headache.

3. ***Answer:* c** (assessment)

Rationale: Women who are pregnant, especially in the third trimester, are more vulnerable to Bell's palsy. The literature does not list the other conditions as being risk factors.

4. ***Answer:* b** (assessment)

Rationale: Facial weakness progressing over time suggests another cause; Bell's palsy symptoms occur rapidly, during the course of a few hours.

5. ***Answer:* c** (assessment)

Rationale: Acute changes are more indicative of delirium. Decreased night vision is a normal ramification of aging. Crying is associated with depression.

6. ***Answer:* b** (implementation/plan)

Rationale: Donepezil (Aricept) and tacrine (Cognex) are indicated for clients with mild to moderate dementia. These clients still have functioning neurons that can use the acetylcholine that is spared with these drugs.

7. ***Answer:* b** (evaluation)

Rationale: It is important to monitor liver enzymes. Ninety percent of all clinically significant alanine aminotransferase elevations occur within the first 12 weeks of treatment. Alanine aminotransferase elevations resolve with discontinuance of tacrine (Cognex), and many individuals can resume the medication without further sequelae.

8. ***Answer:* a** (assessment)

Rationale: Smoking has been identified as a possible protective factor for Alzheimer's disease. Head injury with loss of consciousness, advancing age, and family history have all been identified as possible risk factors.

9. ***Answer:* a** (evaluation)

Rationale: An MRI is indicated in intractable seizures, focal neurologic abnormalities, and first seizures in adults. The other three choices are appropriate in the follow-up of Mrs. Johnson's daughter.

10. ***Answer:* a** (assessment)

Rationale: Bell's palsy affects the upper and lower portions of the face unilaterally, so the forehead is smooth on the affected side.

ENDOCRINE SYSTEM

Review Questions

1. The NP has completed the examination and diagnosis for an adult with newly diagnosed type 2 diabetes. The fasting plasma glucose level was 250 mg/dL. Which of the following would *not* be included in the plan of care?

a. Insulin

b. Overnight urinary microalbumin test

c. Ophthalmologic examination

d. Hemoglobin A1c

2. A child with diagnosed type 1 diabetes is likely to experience all *except* which of the following?

a. Polydipsia

b. Polyuria

c. Weight gain

d. Fatigue

3. Which of the following would you *not* expect to find in the nutritional history of a person with Cushing's syndrome?

a. Weight gain

b. Vomiting

c. Increased appetite

d. Nausea

4. Ms. Smith is a 45-year-old woman who comes to the NP with reported weight gain, fatigue, and increased appetite. Which of the following would *not* be included in the differential diagnosis?

a. Diabetes mellitus

b. Depression

c. Obesity

d. Hypothyroidism

5. Ms. Taylor brings her 9-year-old daughter to the NP. The daughter has been experiencing polyuria, polydipsia, and weight loss. The nurse practitioner completes a physical examination and orders laboratory tests. Which test will establish the diagnosis of diabetes?

a. Finger-stick blood glucose level
b. Plasma glucose level
c. Urinary glucose level
d. Hemoglobin A1c

6. Which of the following is the best way to assess for the presence of peripheral neuropathy in a client with diabetes?

a. Observation
b. Use of a vibrating tuning fork on toes
c. Use of a monofilament to check sensation on toes, arch, heel and plantar aspect of foot
d. Electromyogram (EMG) test

7. Which of the following lab results can be used to diagnose diabetes?

a. Plasma glucose of 200 mg/dL without symptoms
b. Fasting plasma glucose result higher than 130 mg/dL
c. Plasma glucose level of 180 mg/dL at the 2h mark of an oral glucose tolerance test
d. Fingerstick blood sugar of 120 mg/dL

8. Which of the following are treatment goals in treating a diabetic client?

a. Bedtime plasma glucose between 150 to 200 mg/dL
b. Glycosolated hemoglobin A1c level lower than 7%
c. Preprandial plasma glucose level between 120 and 130 mg/dL
d. Random fingerstick blood glucose level lower than 140 mg/dL

9. A 40-year-old woman was seen by the NP and referred to an endocrinologist for diagnosis and treatment of Addison's disease. Which of the following would *not* be included in the education plan?

a. 1 g sodium diet
b. Self-injection of hydrocortisone
c. Medic-Alert bracelet
d. Signs and symptoms of adrenal insufficiency

10. Which of these diets is recommended in the treatment of type 2 diabetes?

a. Reduced fat intake
b. Follow food pyramid guidelines
c. Low sodium diet
d. High fiber diet

Answers and Rationales

1. *Answer:* a (implementation/plan)
Rationale: Because you do not know if the client has responded to oral hypoglycemic agents, insulin is inappropriate at this time.

2. *Answer:* c (assessment)
Rationale: Children usually experience weight loss. The loss of glucose through the urine results in negative calorie balance and weight loss.

3. *Answer:* b (assessment)
Rationale: Typically individuals with Cushing's syndrome do not have vomiting.

4. *Answer:* d (analysis/diagnosis)
Rationale: Hypothyroidism does not cause appetite changes.

5. *Answer:* b (analysis/diagnosis)
Rationale: The plasma glucose level is the most reliable indicator to establish the diagnosis of diabetes.

6. *Answer:* c (assessment)
Rationale: A monofilament is precalibrated to use 10 g of force when it bends after being pushed into the skin. Clients who cannot feel 75% of points/areas assessed have significant neuropathy. A tuning fork is not as sensitive. Observation will only help with detecting foot ulcerations and deformities. An EMG is used to detect neuromuscular conditions.

7. *Answer:* b (analysis/diagnosis)
Rationale: A fasting blood glucose level of 126 mg/dL or higher is a basis for diagnosing diabetes. A nonfasting plasma glucose level must be 200 mg/dL or higher to diagnose diabetes. At the 2h mark of an oral glucose tolerance test the reading must be 200 mg/dL or higher.

8. *Answer:* b (evaluation)
Rationale: Bedtime plasma glucose should be between 100 and 140 mg/dL. Preprandial and random fingerstick blood glucose levels should be between 80 and 120 mg/dL. Below 7 is the target goal for glycosolated hemoglobin A1c.

9. *Answer:* a (implementation/plan)
Rationale: Salt intake should not be restricted because of the decreased levels of mineralocorticoid therapy causing sodium loss.

10. *Answer:* a (implementation/plan)
Rationale: In type 2 diabetes restriction of calories through reduced fat intake is necessary. In type 1 diabetes following the food pyramid guidelines is recommended. Calorie restriction may not be necessary. High fiber and low sodium diet are not usually needed.

INTEGUMENTARY SYSTEM

Review Questions

1. Which of the following descriptions is characteristic of tinea versicolor lesions?

   a. Small pustules surrounded by erythematous margin
   b. Macerated, scaly plaques with varying vesicles and pustules
   c. Thick, white plaques surrounded by erythema
   d. Round or oval hypopigmented or hyperpigmented macules with fine scales

2. Mark is a 20-year-old college student living in the dormitory. He has itching and burning of both feet. You suspect tinea pedis and examine his feet. You expect to find which of the following?

   a. Macerated, scaly skin between the toes and on the plantar and lateral aspects of feet
   b. Hard nodules and pustules located between the toes
   c. Scales and erythema on the dorsal aspect of the feet and around the ankle
   d. Papules and vesicles on the dorsal and lateral aspects of the feet

3. When viewed under a microscope, the classic "spaghetti and meatballs" pattern seen is characteristic of which tinea infection?

   a. Tinea versicolor
   b. Tinea capitis
   c. Tinea corporis
   d. Tinea pedis

4. Skin lesions most suggestive of scabies are which of the following?

   a. Erythematous papular rashes covering the trunk
   b. Pinpoint, red spots at the nape of the neck
   c. Topical, grayish-white burrows of varying lengths
   d. Thick, crusted plaques varying in size

5. Which of the following is a cardinal symptom of scabies infestation?

   a. A burning sensation on the trunk
   b. Intense itching around the hairline
   c. Generalized itching
   d. Nocturnal itching

6. Steve is a 19-year-old man who has a 3-month history of a sore bump on the sole of his foot. Personal and family histories are unremarkable. Examination shows a small, sharply marginated papule studded with black dots at the metatarsophalangeal junction on the sole of his right foot. What is the most appropriate diagnosis?

   a. Common wart
   b. Plantar wart
   c. Ingrown hair
   d. Callus

7. Jerry has common warts on his hands. The nurse advises him on the various treatments appropriate for warts. Which statement made by Jerry indicates that he understands the instructions?

   a. "I will make an appointment with a dermatologist to get them cut off."
   b. "I will leave these alone and see what happens."
   c. "I should apply a baking soda paste to the warts every night."
   d. "Placing gasoline on the warts will help them go away."

8. Shelly, a 19-year-old woman, just had her annual Pap smear done. The results indicate a low-grade squamous intraepithelial lesion caused by human papillomavirus. When should Shelly have follow-up?

   a. Next year for annual examination
   b. Only when she has problems
   c. Immediate referral for colposcopy
   d. Repeated Pap smear in 6 months

9. Which objective finding is *not* usually associated with herpes zoster?

   a. Scaly, salmon-colored lesions
   b. Painful, vesicular rash
   c. Bullous eruption following the dermatome
   d. Preeruption itching or pain

10. Examination of an 8-year-old boy reveals the following: erythema of lip, with vesicles on the rim of the lip, nasal discharge, and cough. Which diagnosis is most appropriate?

   a. Hand, foot, and mouth disease
   b. Drug eruption
   c. Aphthous stomatitis
   d. Herpes simplex

Answers and Rationales

1. *Answer:* d (assessment)
   Rationale: Tinea versicolor is seen as small, oval or round, hyperpigmented or hypopigmented lesions with fine scales.

2. *Answer:* a (assessment)
   Rationale: Classically, tinea pedis involves the toe webs and the plantar and lateral aspects of the feet. It is usually devoid of vesicular lesions.

3. *Answer:* a (analysis/diagnosis)
   Rationale: Under a Wood's light, tinea versicolor will fluoresce with a characteristic yellow-orange color, and microscopic examination with a potassium hydroxide preparation will reveal hyphae and spores: the classic "spaghetti and meatballs" pattern.

4. *Answer:* c (assessment)
   Rationale: The diagnosis of scabies is suggested by finding topical grayish-white burrows.

5. *Answer:* d (assessment)
   Rationale: A cardinal symptom of scabies is nocturnal itching.

6. *Answer:* **b** (analysis/diagnosis)

Rationale: Plantar warts are frequently painful when pressure is applied over the metatarsal head. Common warts and callus do not usually have black dots, whereas an ingrown hair would be erythematous and would not be located on the sole of the foot.

7. *Answer:* **b** (evaluation)

Rationale: Warts do not need to be treated aggressively because they frequently resolve on their own.

8. *Answer:* **c** (implementation/plan)

Rationale: When a Pap smear reveals a suspicious atypia or squamous epithelial lesion, referral for a colposcopy is indi-cated because of the link of human papillomavirus to cervical cancer.

9. *Answer:* **a** (assessment)

Rationale: All except choice a are commonly seen with herpes zoster. Scaly, salmon-colored lesions are more typical of psoriasis.

10. *Answer:* **d** (analysis/diagnosis)

Rationale: Although the other diseases are considered part of the differential diagnosis, herpetic stomatitis commonly occurs in children, along with the risk factor of a common cold.

PSYCHOSOCIAL SYSTEM

Review Questions

1. Which of the following assessment findings suggests a common behavior problem in a toddler?

   a. Skin—bruises in multiple stages of healing over the body
   b. Neurologic—failed vision and hearing screen results
   c. Neurologic—personal, social and language development delays
   d. Bursts of anger with crying

2. Diagnostic measures helpful to the practitioner in determining whether a behavior problem is minor include which of the following?

   a. Vision screen
   b. Behavior rating scale
   c. Denver II
   d. Hearing screen

3. Sue Smith, a 19-year-old woman, comes to your office for a checkup. On examination, which of the following sets of signs may indicate an eating disorder?

   a. Hypertension, parotid tenderness, and decreased body temperature
   b. Scarring on the dorsa of the hands, excessive dental caries, and orthostasis
   c. Altered mental status, dilated pupils, and tachycardia
   d. Halitosis, increased body temperature, and vertigo

4. A mother brings a child in for a sore throat. She also reports new episodes of misbehavior at school this year. The 8-year-old gets in trouble for talking and showing off, but it really does not affect the child's grades. After treating the sore throat and reinforcing the behavior management system already established in this family, how would the NP best follow up on the behavior problem?

   a. It is a minor behavior problem; no follow-up is needed.
   b. It is a major behavior problem; refer the child to a physician in 3 to 4 weeks.
   c. It is a minor behavior problem; have the child return in 4 to 6 weeks if the behavior is still unmanaged.
   d. It is a minor behavior problem; refer the child to a school counselor.

5. Which of the following sets of diagnostic criteria is used to diagnose anorexic nervosa?

   a. Body weight less than 85% of expected body weight, concern about gaining weight or getting fat, and normal menses
   b. Binge-purging behaviors, body weight normal or slightly below expected body weight, and self-evaluation unduly concerned with weight and shape
   c. Amenorrhea, intense fear of gaining weight or getting fat, and body weight less than 85% of expected body weight
   d. Normal menses, body weight less than 10% of expected body weight, and concern about gaining weight or getting fat

6. In treating a 15-year-old girl with purging-type anorexia nervosa, treatment may include all *except* which of the following?

   a. Antipsychotic medications
   b. Potassium supplementation
   c. Monitoring of pertinent laboratory values
   d. Nutritional consultation

7. Which of the following statements made by the client would indicate a high risk for suicide?

   a. "My husband has asked for a divorce."
   b. "I don't know what happiness is."
   c. "Sometimes I feel that life isn't worth living anymore."
   d. "I sleep all the time and seldom eat."

8. What are the similarities between depression, dysthymia, and bipolar disorder?

   a. They are considered affective/mood disorders.
   b. They are more common in men than in women.
   c. The incidence tends to decrease with age for both men and women.
   d. They are seldom seen in blacks.

9. Which assessment is most appropriate for a teenager who has been drinking for 6 months and is charged with driving while intoxicated?

   a. Alcohol dependence
   b. Dysfunctional family
   c. Adjustment disorder
   d. Alcohol abuse

10. Which primary care clients should be screened for alcohol abuse?

    a. Clients with low incomes
    b. Clients who have not completed high school
    c. Clients who are depressed
    d. All primary care clients (adults and adolescents)

Answers and Rationales

1. *Answer:* **d** (assessment)
    Rationale: Choices a, b, and c all describe physical findings for differential diagnoses of behavioral problems. Bruises in multiple stages of healing and misbehavior signal abuse; failed vision and hearing screens and misbehavior signal sensory deficits or developmental delays; all may occur concomitantly with behavior, but not usually in a toddler.

2. *Answer:* **b** (assessment)
    Rationale: Behavior rating scale is the only possible diagnostic measure offered. Other tools are simply screens to identify deficits. Although sensory and developmental deficits may contribute to or occur with behavior problems, these screens are not diagnostic measures.

NOTE: *Not all behavior rating scales are diagnostic; some serve only as screening tools.*

3. *Answer:* **b** (assessment)
    Rationale: These are possible symptoms of self-induced vomiting and dehydration, which may indicate an eating disorder.

4. *Answer:* **c** (evaluation)
    Rationale: Minor behavior problems that are persistent (longer than 4 weeks in duration) require more in-depth evaluation. Once follow-up contact is made, data may indicate the need for physician referral.

5. *Answer:* **c** (analysis/diagnosis)
    Rationale: Amenorrhea, intense fear of weight gain, and less than 85% expected body weight are criteria used to diagnose anorexia nervosa. Binge-purge behaviors, normal to slightly below expected body weight, and self-evaluation based on body shape are diagnostic criteria.

6. *Answer:* **a** (implementation/plan)
    Rationale: Antipsychotic medications are used to treat thought disorders, such as schizophrenia. Antidepressants are often used for persons with eating disorders related to the comorbidity of affective disorder.

7. *Answer:* **c** (assessment)
    Rationale: All references to suicide need to be taken seriously and require further assessment.

8. *Answer:* **a** (analysis/diagnosis)
    Rationale: All are classified as affective/mood disorders.

9. *Answer:* **d** (analysis/diagnosis)
    Rationale: Alcohol or substance abuse is defined as recurrent use resulting in one or more of the following: failure to fulfill obligations, use of substance in hazardous situations, and legal problems associated with use.

10. *Answer:* **d** (assessment)
    Rationale: Of primary care clients (adults and adolescents), 8% to 20% have drinking problems (abuse or dependence).

MULTISYSTEM DISORDERS

Review Questions

1. When a health history is obtained from a client with edema, it is important to include all *except* which of the following?

    a. "When did the edema begin?"
    b. "Is it affected by position changes?"
    c. "Is it accompanied by shortness of breath?"
    d. "Is the appetite affected?"

2. Which of the following tests is *least* important to perform in a client with edema?

    a. Echocardiography
    b. Fasting liver function test
    c. Chest x-ray examination
    d. Magnetic resonance imaging (MRI)

3. Major findings generally found in congestive heart failure include which of the following?

    a. Electrocardiograph (ECG) changes, weight loss, and hypertension
    b. Weight gain, shortness of breath, and S3
    c. Fever and chills
    d. Bilateral lower extremity edema and brownish pigmentation

4. Which of the following is the most used diagnostic tool for Lyme disease?

    a. Indirect fluorescent antibody
    b. Enzyme-linked immunosorbent assay
    c. Western blot assay
    d. Complete blood cell count with differential

5. Which statement regarding diuretics is *not* true?

    a. Diuretics are most effective for symptomatic relief.
    b. Excessive diuresis can lead to electrolyte imbalance.
    c. Distal, potassium-losing diuretics are used for mild congestive heart failure.
    d. Loop diuretics are used for less severe congestive heart failure.

6. Appropriate palpation for tender points in fibromyalgia includes using which of the following?

a. A rolling motion with the third and fourth fingers on the occiput, trapezius, and lateral epicondyles
b. A rolling motion with the first two fingers on the trapezius, supraspinatus, and second rib
c. Deep, consistent pressure with the thumb on the knees, gluteal area, and second rib
d. A rolling motion with the thumb on the occiput, greater trochanter, and medial malleolus

7. A client with fibromyalgia may initially report which of the following?

a. Low back pain
b. Difficulty falling asleep and frequent awakening
c. Numbness and tingling in the hands, especially at night
d. Fatigue

8. Which of these clients is most likely to have new-onset fibromyalgia?

a. Mr. J., 24 years old, visiting his family practitioner
b. Mrs. S., 84 years old, visiting her internist
c. Mr. R., 62 years old, visiting his family practitioner
d. Mrs. L., 48 years old, visiting her internist

9. Factors that aggravate fibromyalgia symptoms include all *except* which of the following?

a. Humid weather
b. Fatigue
c. Moderate activity
d. Stress

10. A client has widespread pain, fatigue, and depression. Results of complete blood cell count, erythrocyte sedimentation rate, thyroid-stimulating hormone level, and chemistry study results are all normal. Which diagnosis is *least* likely?

a. Major depression
b. Rheumatoid arthritis
c. Fibromyalgia
d. Chronic fatigue syndrome

Answers and Rationales

1. *Answer:* **d** (assessment)
   Rationale: It is important to know how long the edema has been present. A sign of congestive heart failure may be ankle and foot edema at the end of the day, which resolves through nocturia by the following morning.

2. *Answer:* **d** (assessment)
   Rationale: An echocardiogram, a fasting liver function test, and a chest x-ray examination are instrumental in diagnosing the cause of edema.

3. *Answer:* **b** (assessment)
   Rationale: Weight gain, shortness of breath, and S3 are all common signs and symptoms of congestive heart failure.

4. *Answer:* **b** (assessment)
   Rationale: Enzyme-linked immunosorbent assay is the usual method, with Western blot assay used for confirmation of this diagnosis.

5. *Answer:* **d** (implementation/plan)
   Rationale: Clients with more severe heart failure should be treated with one of the loop diuretics (furosemide, bumetanide).

6. *Answer:* **b** (assessment)
   Rationale: The best way to test for tender points is with a rolling pressure by the thumb or first two fingers on the 18 points identified by the American College of Rheumatology. The medial malleolus is not one of those points.

7. *Answer:* **a** (assessment)
   Rationale: Although clients with fibromyalgia do have widespread pain, it is often worse in an axial distribution. The low back pain may be much more severe than the other aches and pains; the client therefore may not mention other symptoms.

8. *Answer:* **d** (analysis/diagnosis)
   Rationale: Only 2% of the general population have fibromyalgia, but those numbers increase 5% to 10% in an internal medicine practice. The most common age at onset is 45 to 55 years, and 73% to 90% of affected individuals are women.

9. *Answer:* **c** (assessment)
   Rationale: Factors that aggravate fibromyalgia include cold, humid weather, physical and mental fatigue, extremes of physical exertion, and stress. Moderate activity is actually helpful.

10. *Answer:* **b** (analysis/diagnosis)
   Rationale: All these diseases can cause pain, fatigue, and depression, but normally rheumatoid arthritis is associated with an elevated erythrocyte sedimentation rate.

COMMUNICABLE DISEASES

Review Questions

1. Which objective finding aids most in diagnosis of lice infestation?

a. Scratched skin on the face, neck, and chest
b. Pus-filled lesions in the scalp
c. Visualization of cream-colored nits on the hair shafts
d. Erythema on pinna of ears

2. Which of the following conditions is *not* appropriate in differential diagnosis with pediculosis?

a. Psoriasis
b. Hair artifact
c. Tinea capitis
d. Lyme disease

3. The practitioner teaches Mrs. Lowe about transmission of lice. Which action on the part of Mrs. Lowe indicates a positive outcome of the instruction?

a. She refuses to let Megan play with the cat.
b. She notifies school authorities about the infestation.
c. She shampoos Megan's hair every other week with lindane.
d. She prohibits Megan from playing near wooded areas.

4. All the following pieces of information should be emphasized during the teaching of a client with mononucleosis *except:*

a. Need for quarantine of family members
b. Need to avoid contact sports
c. Treatment aimed at symptoms
d. Increasing rest and fluids

5. In addition to HEENT, which of the following systems should be included in the physical examination when mononucleosis is suspected?

a. Cardiovascular
b. Abdominal
c. Pelvic
d. Extremities

6. Ed, a Korean war veteran, comes to your office as a new client. During a routine history and physical examination, a chest x-ray film is ordered. Linear calcifications are noted on the ascending aorta. What would your next action be?

a. Order a cardiology consult.
b. Do nothing, because this is an old sign and needs no treatment.
c. Order a venereal disease research laboratory test.
d. Order a stat surgical consultation for an impending dissection.

7. Complications of gonorrhea in the neonate may include which of the following?

a. Urethral stricture
b. Cerebral palsy
c. Mitral valve prolapse
d. Arthritis

8. Which sign exhibited by a 19-year-old woman client would make the nurse practitioner most suspicious of gonorrhea?

a. Odorous, musty vaginal discharge
b. Slow walk, bent over from abdominal pain
c. Strawberry cervix
d. Breast tenderness to palpation

9. Clients with a diagnosis of gonorrhea should be automatically treated for what other infection?

a. Syphilis
b. Trichomoniasis
c. Herpes
d. Chlamydia

10. Because of the high incidence of concurrent infections, the NP should test for what other sexually transmitted disease along with Chlamydia?

a. Syphilis
b. Herpes
c. Gonorrhea
d. Human papillomavirus

Answers and Rationales

1. *Answer:* **c** (assessment)
Rationale: Visualization of lice or nits provides the diagnosis of pediculosis.

2. *Answer:* **d** (analysis/diagnosis)
Rationale: Hair artifact, psoriasis, and tinea capitis must be ruled out in arriving at a diagnosis of pediculosis capitis (Sokoloff, 1994).

3. *Answer:* **b** (evaluation)
Rationale: Pediculosis capitis can be endemic in schools. School authorities must be notified of infestations.

4. *Answer:* **a** (implementation/plan)
Rationale: Family members do not need to be quarantined because they have usually been exposed by the time the diagnosis is made. All other information regarding mononucleosis should be shared with the client and family.

5. *Answer:* **b** (assessment)
Rationale: Because hepatosplenomegaly is present in 50% to 75% of clients, the abdomen should always be examined if mononucleosis is suspected.

6. *Answer:* **c** (assessment)
Rationale: This x-ray finding may be an indication of cardiovascular syphilis (syphilitic aortitis). If the condition is asymptomatic, then a venereal disease research laboratory test should be done. If the condition is symptomatic, then an appropriate referral should be made.

7. *Answer:* **d** (analysis/diagnosis)
Rationale: Gonorrhea may cause urethral stricture in adult males. There is no evidence that gonorrhea causes either mitral valve prolapse or cerebral palsy, although endocarditis and meningitis may occur. Arthritis has been documented as one of the complications of congenitally acquired gonorrhea in the neonate.

8. *Answer:* **b** (assessment)
Rationale: The odorous discharge is typical of bacterial vaginosis; the strawberry cervix is seen in trichomoniasis. Breast tenderness is not a symptom of gonorrhea. The slow walk because of a painful abdomen is seen with pelvic inflammatory disease and is sometimes called the "pelvic inflammatory shuffle."

9. *Answer:* **d** (implementation/plan)
Rationale: Coinfection with Chlamydia is common with gonorrhea, so clients should be treated presumptively with a regimen that is effective for Chlamydia. The practitioner should offer serologic testing for syphilis to anyone who has a positive test result for gonorrhea. There is no clear correlation between gonorrhea and herpes.

10. *Answer:* **c** (implementation/plan)
Rationale: Although sexual practices put one at risk for multiple sexually transmitted diseases, and testing for syphilis should be offered, gonorrhea often coexists with chlamydial infections and has similar symptoms.

REFERENCES

Broderick, P. (1999). Pediatric vision screening for the family physician. *American Family Physician,* September. Retrieved Auguat 23, 2002, from http://www.aafp.org/afp/980901ap/broderic.html.

Gross, K., & Ponte, C. (1998). New strategies in the medical management of asthma. *American Family Physician*, July. Retrieved August 23, 2002, from: http://www.aafp.org/afp/9980700ap/gross.html.

Kuhn, B., Marcus, B., & Pitner, S. (1999). Treatment guidelines for primary nonretentive encopresis and stool toileting refusal. *American Family Physician,* April. Retrieved August 24, 2002, from http://www.aafp./org/afp/990415ap/2171.html.

Robinson, D., Kidd, P., & Rogers, K. M. (2000). *Primary care across the lifespan.* St. Louis: Mosby, Inc.

Saenz, R., Beebe, D. & Triplett, L. (1999). Caring for infants with congenital heart disease and their families. *American Family Physician,* April. Retrieved August 25, 2002 from http://www.aafp.org /afp/990401ap/1857.html.

Sokoloff, F. (1994). Identification and management of pediculosis. *Nurse Practitioner, 19*(8), 62-64.

Stein, M. (2001). Recurrent abdominal pain. *Pediatrics, 107*(4), 935-939.

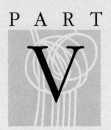

PART

V

SAMPLE
EXAMINATION
QUESTIONS

Sample Examination

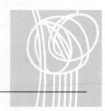

QUESTIONS

1. J.J. is a 2-month-old infant. He is brought to your clinic by his parents with the report that he is not drinking fluids and has been vomiting and having diarrheal stools for 2 days. His mother states that this morning J.J. had an apnea episode. Your examination reveals pink pharyngeal membranes, normal tympanic membranes, and temperature of 100° F. These symptoms are associated with which of the following?

   a. Common cold
   b. Epiglottitis
   c. Croup
   d. Group A streptococcal pharyngitis

2. Signs of right-to-left cardiac shunting include all except which of the following?

   a. Cyanosis
   b. Hepatosplenomegaly
   c. Hypoxemia
   d. Clubbing of the nail beds

3. Important subjective data in a client with chronic obstructive pulmonary disease include all *except* which of the following?

   a. Ability to perform activities of daily living
   b. Weight loss or gain
   c. Urinary frequency
   d. Living will and power of attorney

4. Mr. Greene comes to your office with an acute exacerbation of chronic obstructive pulmonary disease. How often is follow-up needed?

   a. Every 3 to 6 months
   b. As a phone call in 24 to 48 hours
   c. Yearly
   d. Weekly until condition improves

5. Megan, an 8-year-old, is brought in by her mother, Mrs. Lowe, who reports that for the past 3 days Megan has scratched her head and neck almost constantly. Which factor in Megan's history is associated with exposure to lice infestation?

   a. Playing with her dolls in the backyard
   b. Going on a horseback ride with her grandfather
   c. Taking a nap with her grandmother's cat
   d. Trying on hats and coats at a local mall

6. Which of the following is *not* a follow-up plan for a client with allergic conjunctivitis?

   a. Referral to allergist
   b. Follow-up in 1 week for persistent symptoms
   c. Consideration of ophthalmic steroids
   d. Referral to an ophthalmologist

7. Mrs. Jones, a 25-year-old pregnant woman, has been treated for a urinary tract infection for 7 days. She should be instructed to return for follow-up at what time?

   a. On her next prenatal visit
   b. After completion of antibiotics
   c. No follow-up if symptoms resolved
   d. Two days after starting antibiotics

8. A mother brings her 15-year-old daughter to your clinic. Her daughter has lost 15 pounds and reports fatigue and nausea. After completing the physical examination, the nurse practitioner suspects Addison's disease. What should the nurse practitioner do next?

   a. Order a cosyntropin (Cortrosyn) stimulation test.
   b. Order electrolyte levels.
   c. Discuss the findings with the mother.
   d. Consult with a physician.

9. For which of the following reasons would a nurse practitioner appropriately refer a woman who is infertile to a reproductive endocrinologist?

   a. Advice related to assisted reproductive technologies
   b. Advice about a basic infertility work-up
   c. Advice about an adoption plan
   d. Advice about treatment for pelvic inflammatory disease

10. Which of the following drug choices is most appropriate for the woman with primary dysmenorrhea?

   a. Codeine
   b. Acetaminophen
   c. Propoxyphene (Darvon)
   d. Ibuprofen

11. Which of the following symptoms best describes the child with attention-deficit/hyperactivity disorder, hyperactive type?

a. Argues with adults, squirms in seat, and leaves seat in classroom.
b. Makes careless mistakes in schoolwork, is forgetful in daily activities, and talks excessively.
c. Fidgets with hands or feet, talks excessively, and has difficulty waiting for his or her turn.
d. Interrupts others, loses temper, and deliberately annoys others.

12. Which of the following descriptions is most accurate in describing a "herald patch"?
a. Oval, discrete, 2 to 6 cm lesion usually seen on the trunk
b. Round, annular patch with intense itching
c. Oval, discrete, slightly raised patch on the cheek
d. Maculopapular and vesicular erythematous rash on the trunk

13. Mr. Jones, a 35-year-old white man, has severe, boring jabs of pain that started on the right side of his head and now involve the whole right side of his head. Mr. Jones reports that the pain comes in episodes of 10 to 30 minutes' duration and that he has had three attacks in the last 12 hours. Results of Mr. Jones' physical examination are normal except for some redness and tearing of the right eye. Which of the following types of primary headache is Mr. Jones most likely experiencing?
a. Cluster headache
b. Migraine headache
c. Trigeminal neuralgia
d. Tension-type headache

14. What is the rationale for prescribing donepezil (Aricept) in Alzheimer's disease?
a. Stops the progress of the disease.
b. Promotes release of norepinephrine.
c. Produces anticholinergic activity.
d. Prevents degradation of acetylcholine.

15. Which of the following findings suggests that fatigue is related to a systemic disease?
a. Client is having trouble sleeping.
b. The client has lost 3 kg in 1 month.
c. The fatigue has lasted 3 weeks.
d. The client is 5 weeks postpartum.

16. What is the most common postoperative complication of appendectomy?
a. Liver abscess
b. Fecal fistula
c. Wound infection
d. Irritable bowel syndrome

17. A 66-year-old woman seeks treatment for shortness of breath and sharp chest pains for 3 hours. She is recovering from a right knee replacement. You suspect a pulmonary embolism. What plan is most appropriate?
a. Reassure the client that this is a normal occurrence after surgery and will gradually improve.
b. Begin intravenous heparin.
c. Refer or transfer the client immediately for possible ventilation-perfusion scan or angiography.
d. Decrease physical therapy exercises and reevaluate in 24 hours.

18. Scoliosis is most prevalent during which phase of life?
a. Preschool
b. Prepuberty
c. Adolescence
d. Adulthood

19. Which of the following are the best predictor markers for HIV progression?
a. Increasing fatigue and weight loss
b. CD_4 and viral burden
c. Newly diagnosed *Pneumocystis carinii* pneumonia
d. Positive purified protein derivative of tuberculin result

20. It is important to avoid live-virus vaccines in children undergoing chemotherapy because an immunocompromised child could theoretically contract the disease being immunized against. Primary care for such a child and siblings should therefore include all *except* which of the following?
a. Give no measles-mumps-rubella vaccine and no oral polio vaccine to affected child and siblings.
b. Give varicella-zoster immune globulin within 72 to 96 hours of varicella exposure in nonimmune children.
c. Hold all immunizations during chemotherapy treatment.
d. Resume immunizations 2 months after chemotherapy is complete.

21. A history for potential asthma triggers includes information about all *except* which of the following?
a. Concurrent viral infections
b. Concurrent headaches
c. Exercise and physical activity
d. Type of heating in home

22. What is the major determinant of the degree of burn injury?
a. Type of agent producing the burn
b. Age of the client
c. Health status of the client
d. Intensity of the heat released and duration of the exposure

23. A Hispanic client is late for every appointment. Which action by the nurse practitioner is most appropriate?
a. Confront the client and make him or her reschedule.
b. Assess how the client interprets the appointment time.
c. Adjust the appointment schedule to allow for this lateness.
d. Ignore the situation.

24. A nurse practitioner is trying to encourage a client to stop smoking during pregnancy. What should the nurse practitioner tell the client?
a. Smoking produces greater weight gain during pregnancy.
b. Smoking induces iron deficiency anemia during pregnancy.
c. Smoking increases the risk of miscarriage.
d. Smoking produces bigger infants.

25. Matthew, 82 years old, had a complete blood cell count, electrolyte levels, renal profile, and lipid levels drawn before he came to the office. All results are within normal limits. He tells you about a community program that is offering a digital rectal examination and prostate-specific antigen for $10 and asks whether he should have these done. His brother, who is 79, had one done last year. Your comments would include all *except* which of the following?

    a. The digital rectal examination and prostate-specific antigen are tools used to detect prostate cancer at an early stage.

    b. The digital rectal examination and prostate-specific antigen should be used together to detect prostate cancer.

    c. The program is appropriate for him, and he should have it conducted.

    d. The program is not appropriate for him, and he does not need to have it conducted.

26. Which of the following college-age women should have a pregnancy test as part of her clinic visit for treatment of an acute illness?

    a. Marnie, whose menstrual period occurred 3 days ago but was late

    b. Julianne, who has had vaginal spotting for 5 days

    c. Dana, who reports inconsistent use of condoms

    d. Brenda, whose period is due in 2 days

27. A 5-year-old comes in for a kindergarten physical examination. All *except* which of the following is included in your examination?

    a. Height, weight, and blood pressure

    b. Immunizations

    c. Urinalysis

    d. Vision and hearing

28. Elaine is an 80-year-old woman who is seen for melena. You know that this is the most frequent presenting symptom of which of the following conditions?

    a. Stress incontinence

    b. Peptic ulcer disease

    c. Gastroesophageal reflux disease

    d. Constipation

29. The most predictive risk factors for coronary artery disease include all *except* which of the following?

    a. Hypothyroidism

    b. Hypertension

    c. Smoking

    d. Hyperlipidemia

30. Which of the following recommendations should be given to a client receiving treatment for acne with oral tetracycline?

    a. Sunscreen should be applied for all outdoor activities.

    b. Tetracycline should be taken with food.

    c. Tetracycline can be taken with dairy products to decrease gastrointestinal symptoms.

    d. Topical preparations are no longer necessary after systemic treatment begins.

31. What is the treatment of choice for inhibition of platelets?

    a. Aspirin, 81 mg

    b. Warfarin (Coumadin), 5 mg

    c. Aspirin, 1000 mg

    d. Warfarin, 10 mg

32. A 72-year-old reports dyspnea and spitting up blood. Her history indicates that she has recently been recovering from surgical repair of a broken hip and has not been as active as usual. Differential diagnosis must include which of the following?

    a. Tuberculosis

    b. Pulmonary embolism

    c. Pneumonia

    d. Chronic obstructive pulmonary disease

33. How would the nurse practitioner know that a client understood the activity restrictions given for mononucleosis?

    a. Bill returns to work and is lifting 50 pounds of groceries.

    b. Sarah plays golf once per week.

    c. Sylvia is playing in select soccer tournaments.

    d. Todd is playing varsity football.

34. On physical examination for someone with suspected pyelonephritis, which of the following objective findings would you expect?

    a. Suprapubic tenderness

    b. Costovertebral angle tenderness

    c. Mild abdominal pain

    d. Urethral discharge

35. A mother brings her 7-year-old daughter to the nurse practitioner. During the past year, the daughter has gained 20 pounds and noticed an increase in subcutaneous fat. Which of the following is *not* included in the differential diagnosis?

    a. Diabetes mellitus

    b. Depression

    c. Obesity

    d. Hypothyroidism

36. An 18-year-old woman seeks treatment for pelvic pressure and general aching in her left side. She is in the second day of menses and is not sexually active. Which diagnosis is most likely?

    a. Follicular ovarian cyst

    b. Endometrioma

    c. Pelvic inflammatory disease

    d. Ectopic pregnancy

37. Which of the following symptoms in a young woman is consistent with a diagnosis of gonorrhea?

    a. Postcoital bleeding

    b. Severe lower back pain

    c. Thick, white discharge with itching

    d. Fever higher than 101° F

38. The nurse practitioner is helping with a community-wide glaucoma screening effort. Which of the following is most helpful in detecting early glaucoma?

    a. Visual field testing

    b. Schiotz tonometry readings

    c. Vision screening with a Snellen chart

    d. Funduscopic examination of the eye

39. Which of the following findings on physical examination is consistent with a diagnosis of encopresis?

    a. Abdomen is soft and nontender, with no palpable masses.

    b. Rectal vault is empty.

    c. Abdomen is distended, with soft, nontender midline mass.

    d. Rectal vault is filled with soft stool.

40. Your client has been receiving imipramine (Tofranil), 300 mg qd, for the past 3 weeks. When you are evaluating the effectiveness of this medication, your client reports several side effects. Which of the following side effects requires immediate attention?

a. Occasional constipation
b. Dry mouth
c. Urinary retention
d. Blurred vision

41. Which of the following may cause some acnelike eruptions?

a. Trazodone
b. Inhaled steroids
c. Methylphenidate (Ritalin)
d. Lithium

42. Which of the following is a symptom commonly associated with the onset of Bell's palsy?

a. Numbness along the lateral border of the tongue
b. Dizziness
c. Photophobia
d. Pain in or behind the ear

43. Which of the following manifestations is most indicative of chronic Lyme disease?

a. Lymphadenopathy
b. Memory loss
c. Hip and shoulder pain
d. Erythema migrans

44. Pertinent subjective data to obtain from the parents of a 6-month-old who is having diarrhea include all *except* which of the following?

a. History of exposure to animals
b. Number, character, and frequency of stools
c. Any associated symptoms, such as vomiting
d. Number of wet diapers during the past few hours

45. What is the most definitive procedure to diagnose gout?

a. Uric acid level determination
b. Complete blood cell count with differential
c. Joint fluid aspiration
d. X-ray film

46. Which of the following presenting symptoms in a client with an acute musculoskeletal complaint might lead a practitioner to suspect systemic lupus erythematosus?

a. Asymmetric arthritis, peak period of discomfort after prolonged inactivity, inflamed joint, no constitutional symptoms
b. Symmetric arthritis, peak period of discomfort after prolonged inactivity, inflamed joint, presence of constitutional symptoms
c. Symmetric arthritis, peak period of discomfort after prolonged use, no constitutional symptoms
d. Asymmetric arthritis, peak period of discomfort with use, no constitutional symptoms

47. Jimmy's complete blood cell count results are as follows: total white blood cells 35,000 cells/mm³, hemoglobin 7.5, platelets 20,000 cells/mm³, and differential revealing 25% blast cells. Jimmy is immediately referred to a pediatric hematologist-oncologist. Bone marrow aspiration and biopsy confirm a diagnosis of acute lymphocytic leukemia. Induction chemotherapy is started in the hospital, with the plan that his total length of treatment will be 3 years plus a few months. Most of his treatment will be on an outpatient basis. Supportive care guidelines include all *except* which of the following?

a. No intramuscular injections
b. No rectal temperatures or suppositories
c. Use of a soft toothbrush or toothettes for oral care
d. Keeping immunizations up to date

48. Which of the following information is *not* pertinent history helpful for diagnosis for a person with type 2 diabetes mellitus?

a. Nutritional history
b. Pregnancy history
c. Medication history
d. Sexual history

49. During an acute asthma attack, which of the following physical findings is of most concern for the practitioner?

a. Intercostal retractions
b. Tachypnea with end-expiratory wheeze
c. Absence of breath sounds on auscultation
d. Increased capillary refill time

50. Proper care for a client with a developmental delay includes which of the following?

a. Nutritional interventions
b. Family assessment and possible interventions
c. Placing the child in social situations
d. Promoting fine motor skills

51. The client has explained his perception of the problem and his related feelings. If you wish to clarify your understanding of what he meant, what would you say?

a. "Will you repeat what you said from the beginning?"
b. "Am I correct in concluding that you mean . . . ?"
c. "What do you think caused this to happen?"
d. "I'm finding this difficult to believe."

52. A patient wants an HIV test but is concerned about anonymity. What is the best recommendation you can give this patient?

a. Use a special code for HIV testing.
b. Recommend the patient go to an anonymous test site.
c. Tell the patient that only the staff at the office will know.
d. Discuss how nurse practitioners are bound by confidentiality of patient information.

53. Healthy People 2010 nutritional goals include which of the following?

a. Decrease the intake of carbohydrate-containing foods.
b. Increase the number of primary care providers who offer nutritional assessment and referral.
c. Reduce the incidence of anorexia.
d. Increase the number of licensed dietitians available to the public.

54. Healthy People 2010 goals for exercise include which of the following?

a. Daily vigorous activity for 20 minutes
b. An increase in the number of primary care providers who assess and counsel clients regarding physical activity

c. A special emphasis on exercise in older adults

d. Greater exercise levels for females, as compared with males

55. Matthew is an 80-year-old man who is in the office for a regular 3-month check-up. He is feeling well. He is accompanied today by his daughter. Matthew's wife died 2 years ago, and he has adapted well to the loss and he lives with his daughter and her family. His grandchildren often bring Matthew to the office and are attentive. Matthew is receiving a diuretic, potassium supplements, an antihypertensive, a cardiac regulator, a bronchodilator, an antacid, and a sedative for sleep. During your interview, what is the most important issue to look for?

a. Tolerance to medications

b. Compliance with medications

c. Interactive components of medications

d. Schedule on which medications are taken

56. A history of multiple sex partners and subsequent sexually transmitted diseases increases one's risks for which of the following?

a. Acute bacterial prostatitis

b. Benign prostatic hyperplasia

c. Prostate cancer

d. Chronic bacterial prostatitis

57. A healthy 18-year-old man has an appointment with you for a precollege physical examination. He is going to be a trainer for the college football team, and a standardized physical form is required. What information is most pertinent to elicit during the history?

a. Hot water setting at his dwelling, history of varicella, institutionalization, and safe storage of firearms

b. Sexual activity, smoke detector, history of varicella, and tobacco use

c. Regular dental visits, household members trained in cardiopulmonary resuscitation, and injection drug use

d. Motorcycle, bicycle, or all-terrain vehicle helmet; lap and shoulder belts; risk factors for diabetes mellitus; and problem drinking

58. A 3-year-old is at your clinic for a well-child examination. All *except* which of the following are part of your examination?

a. Genital

b. Vision

c. Tuberculosis test

d. Blood pressure

59. Mrs. White is a 32-year-old well woman who needs an eye examination. Which of the following describes the most appropriate eye screening for her?

a. Every 6 months

b. Every year

c. Every 2 years

d. Only when she has a vision problem

60. A young family with a 6-month-old daughter comes in for a well-baby checkup. The parents express concern for future behavior problems after spending a weekend with unruly nieces and nephews. What is the practitioner's best response?

a. Congratulate them on their insight, and suggest a useful parenting book.

b. Initiate a behavior management system so that the family can have practice time.

c. Recommend that parents verbalize expectations to each other and resolve differences before discussing behavior management at their next visit.

d. Emphasize the importance of consistency in discipline and behavior management.

61. Which of the following clients would you suspect as having group A streptococcal pharyngitis?

a. A 6-month-old with fever and barking cough

b. An 8-year-old with fever and sore throat

c. A 29-year-old mother of three with sore throat, low-grade fever, without exudate

d. A 50-year-old man with complaint of sore throat

62. Who of the following is at greatest risk for development of hypertension?

a. A 25-year-old woman who leads a sedentary lifestyle and takes oral contraceptives

b. A 32-year-old black man who smokes and is overweight

c. A 16-year-old boy who has consistent blood pressure readings of 130/80 mm Hg

d. A 5-year-old girl with a heart murmur and blood pressure readings of 90/56 mm Hg

63. Which of the following clients is most likely to need a chest x-ray examination?

a. A 5-year-old with clear nasal drainage and scattered wheezes

b. A 65-year-old with crackles in the left lower lung field

c. A 24-year-old smoker with fever and purulent cough

d. A 40-year-old with cough, headache, and nasal congestion

64. The most important aspects of the history to obtain for children with a chronic cough include all *except* which of the following?

a. Recurrent upper respiratory tract infections

b. Growth patterns

c. Fatty stools

d. Play patterns

65. Tiffany is a 22-year-old woman who had syphilis diagnosed and treated during her pregnancy. Her son Josh was born without problems. During serologic testing 2 days after birth, it is found that Josh has a reactive Venereal Disease Research Laboratory (VDRL). This indicates which of the following?

a. Tiffany had inadequate treatment.

b. Tiffany was treated too late in her pregnancy.

c. Josh has syphilis and should be treated with 2.4 MU penicillin immediately.

d. Josh may have a reactive VDRL test as a result of passive transfer of antibodies from Tiffany.

66. Mr. Quincey is being evaluated for male factor infertility. Which diagnostic test is *not* necessary to this evaluation?

a. Serum testosterone

b. Follicle-stimulating hormone

c. Prolactin

d. Estradiol

67. To minimize side effects, alpha-adrenergic antagonists used in the treatment of benign prostatic hyperplasia, should be given how often?

    a. Every morning
    b. Every evening at dinner
    c. At bedtime
    d. In divided doses

68. Which of the following medications may be best to prescribe to control blood glucose in treating a client with metabolic syndrome (Syndrome X; glucose intolerance, obesity, dyslipidemia, and hypertension)?

    a. Glyburide (Diabeta) 2.5 mg qd
    b. Glimepiride (Amaryl) 2 mg qd
    c. Glucophage (metformin) 500 mg bid
    d. Glipizide (Glucotrol) 5 mg qd

69. Cynthia is a 25-year-old, nulligravid, married woman with the presenting symptom of metrorrhagia for the past 3 months. Which initial question is most appropriate?

    a. What kind of birth control do you use?
    b. How often do you have intercourse?
    c. Do you have any pain with menses?
    d. Have you ever had a uterine biopsy?

70. On the basis of your diagnosis of herpetic conjunctivitis, your plan for treatment should be which of the following?

    a. Cool compresses as needed, sodium sulfacetamide ophthalmic solution 10%
    b. Ophthalmologic referral and ophthalmic steroid drops
    c. Ophthalmologic referral
    d. Bacitracin ophthalmic ointment

71. A 45-year-old married woman has recurrent headaches, episodes of visual disturbance, a history of migraines, and a history of government assistance. Her husband "drinks a lot" and recently lost his job. Which of the following factors does *not* suggest that this woman is at risk for abuse?

    a. Her age is 45 years.
    b. Her husband drinks.
    c. She reports recurring problems with headaches.
    d. She has a low socioeconomic status.

72. Sociocultural factors contribute to the development of eating disorders. These factors include which of the following?

    a. Blurring of generational boundaries
    b. Low self-esteem
    c. Changing roles of women and role destabilization
    d. Affective intolerance

73. Judy is an 18-year-old client visiting your office for evaluation of a plaque on her right shoulder. You diagnose tinea corporis and would like to confirm this diagnosis immediately. Which of the following would you most likely do?

    a. Prepare a slide with potassium hydroxide to visualize hyphae.
    b. Culture a scraping from the center of the lesion in the appropriate medium.
    c. Visualize the fluorescence under a Wood's lamp.
    d. Do a fingernail test to reproduce fine scales.

74. If a client is experiencing delirium, you will expect him or her to demonstrate all *except* which of the following?

    a. History of symptoms occurring within days
    b. Inability to maintain attention
    c. Decline in consciousness
    d. Marked depression

75. Management of a client with increased liver enzymes who is taking a statin should include which of the following?

    a. Repeat liver enzyme panel in 1 week.
    b. Discontinue the drug and repeat liver enzyme panel in 1 week.
    c. Decrease the dose of the drug.
    d. Stop the drug.

76. Which of the following women is most likely to have primary dysmenorrhea?

    a. A 12-year-old who has had two menstrual cycles
    b. A 30-year-old with regular cycles
    c. A 48-year-old with irregular cycles
    d. A 35-year-old taking oral contraceptives

77. All clients with new or recurring peptic ulcers should be tested for which of the following?

    a. Streptococcal infection
    b. Lower esophageal sphincter tone
    c. Increased aspartate aminotransferase and alanine aminotransferase levels
    d. *Helicobacter pylori*

78. What objective information would you obtain from Roger, a 50-year-old man who reports left lower quadrant abdominal pain and constipation?

    a. Deep tendon reflexes
    b. Current medications
    c. History of diarrhea alternating with constipation
    d. Rectal examination and guaiac

79. An infant with a diagnosis at birth of developmental dysplasia of the hip has been in a Pavlik harness for 6 weeks and spontaneous reduction has occurred. When should this harness be removed?

    a. Once reduction has occurred
    b. After several months
    c. After 1 more week
    d. Never

80. A client with stage II lymphoma comes in for a routine physical examination. The nurse practitioner should evaluate all *except* which of the following?

    a. Status of all lymph nodes
    b. Size of the spleen
    c. Weight patterns
    d. Hemoglobin and hematocrit

81. What are the most common types of anemia that can occur during pregnancy and postpartum?

    a. Folic acid deficiency and iron deficiency
    b. Iron deficiency and acute blood loss
    c. Pernicious anemia and acute blood loss
    d. Vitamin B_{12} deficiency and iron deficiency

82. For the adult with persistent nighttime cough, what other respiratory condition should be ruled out as a differential diagnosis?

   a. Pneumonia
   b. Bronchitis
   c. Exercise-induced asthma
   d. Sinusitis

83. Which of the following statements regarding standards of care for nurse practitioners is *not* true?

   a. They are based on the scope of practice.
   b. They are a means to describe and guide practice.
   c. They deal with the phenomena of concern for nurse practitioners.
   d. They are developed by the State Boards of Nursing.

84. Which of the following physician reimbursement figures is correct for nurse practitioners billing Medicare clients?

   a. 100% of the physician charge
   b. 70% of the physician charge
   c. 85% of the physician charge
   d. 50% of the physician charge

85. What is the purpose of an advanced directive?

   a. To promote active euthanasia
   b. To encourage resuscitation of terminally ill clients
   c. To allow the client to direct his or her own care before the need arises
   d. To give power of attorney to the family designee

86. Which of the following clients needs nutritional screening?

   a. An older client
   b. A client with an involuntary loss of 5 pounds within 1 month
   c. A client who is 10% above ideal body weight
   d. A client who is 10% below ideal body weight

87. When explaining the benefits of exercise to a client, the nurse practitioner should discuss which of the following?

   a. Improved fertility
   b. Decreased incidence of diarrhea
   c. Improved glucose tolerance
   d. Increased low-density lipoprotein levels

88. In the interview, Sam, an 87-year-old widower, discloses that he has two firearms in the home. One is a rifle and one is a handgun. What is your next most appropriate question?

   a. Who is able to fire the guns?
   b. Where are the guns stored, and what safety measures are taken?
   c. What are the types of guns and where were they purchased?
   d. Are the firearms legally licensed?

89. What is the focus of the plan for a well-male examination?

   a. Treatment of disease
   b. Prevention of morbidity and mortality
   c. Immunizations
   d. Screening for disease

90. A school-age child comes to your office for a well-child examination. Your anticipatory guidance issues include firearm safety. You know that the most common risk factor associated with injury or death from firearms is which of the following?

   a. Argument with a stranger
   b. Firearm access
   c. Substance use
   d. Peer pressure

91. Mrs. Nance is a 63-year-old woman. Which of the following factors in her history does *not* place her at risk for osteoporosis?

   a. White ethnicity
   b. Total hysterectomy at 38 years
   c. Hormone replacement therapy
   d. Smoking habit, 2 packs/day

92. Symptoms of gallbladder disease may include which of the following?

   a. Diarrhea, bloating, left upper quadrant tenderness
   b. White blood cell counts higher than 40,000 cells/mm^3
   c. Pain with expiration
   d. Right upper quadrant tenderness

93. To prevent deaths from cardiovascular disease among blacks, primary prevention programs for men should target reductions in which of the following?

   a. Cholesterol levels
   b. Glaucoma screening
   c. Diabetes
   d. Hypertension

94. You are seeing a 70-year-old man who reports gradual decrease in his vision. You know that as a result of his age, he is at risk for cataracts. What other symptoms would make you suspect cataracts as the cause of his visual impairment?

   a. Peripheral vision better than central vision
   b. Dull aching behind eyes, particularly in the morning
   c. Improved vision in low light
   d. Occasional floaters in periphery

95. Two days after having a myocardial infarction, a 70-year-old man begins to report substernal chest pain that worsens with deep breathing and movement and is relieved with sitting up and leaning forward. Pericardial friction rub is absent, and no electrocardiogram changes are noted. What is the best differential diagnosis?

   a. Recurrent angina
   b. Pericarditis
   c. Pulmonary embolus
   d. Aortic dissection

96. Megan, a 5-year-old, is brought to the clinic because she has never been able to achieve nighttime dryness. Which of the following physical findings suggests an organic cause for her enuresis?

   a. Height and weight below the fifth percentile and blood pressure of 120/88 mm Hg
   b. Good rectal sphincter tone with no genital anomalies
   c. Abdomen soft and slightly distended, with no masses palpable
   d. Urinalysis results positive for nitrates and leukocytes

97. Which of the following comments by a mother of a child with cystic fibrosis indicates a need for more teaching?

    a. "I will give the pancreatic enzymes with every meal and snack."

    b. "High fat foods should be avoided."

    c. "Adequate fluid intake is important."

    d. "Well child follow-up is needed on a regular basis."

98. Which of the following treatments for gonorrhea is appropriate in the adult client?

    a. Erythromycin

    b. Cefixime

    c. Azithromycin

    d. Acyclovir

99. A complete blood cell count that reveals an elevated white blood cell count is most likely to be associated with which of the following?

    a. Acute bacterial prostatitis

    b. Benign prostatic hyperplasia

    c. Prostate cancer

    d. Chronic bacterial prostatitis

100. A client with previously regular menstrual cycle is experiencing her first episode of amenorrhea. She has normal thyroid-stimulating hormone and prolactin levels. After completing a 5-day course of medroxyprogesterone (Provera), 10 mg, she begins to bleed. The nurse practitioner is able to explain which of the following to the client?

    a. This bleeding is unusual and may indicate a serious pathologic condition.

    b. Her amenorrhea was caused by anovulation and she may need hormonal therapy to initiate menstruation.

    c. Her amenorrhea was caused by ovarian failure and hormone therapy will help to regulate her menses.

    d. She has primary amenorrhea and her menses will regulate themselves in time.

101. Which of the following client reports indicates appropriate attempts to remove environmental triggers to help stop asthma attacks?

    a. "I make my husband smoke in another room, away from me."

    b. "We vacuumed our box springs and mattress to remove dust mites."

    c. "Our dog now gets a weekly bath."

    d. "We put our daughter's stuffed animals on a shelf so that she won't be exposed to their dust."

102. Which information about performing breast self-examination is *inaccurate?*

    a. Breast self-examination is ideally performed 4 to 7 days after the menstrual period.

    b. For oral contraceptive users, breast self-examination can be effectively performed when starting a new pill pack.

    c. Postmenopausal women should select a familiar date and use that day of the month consistently for breast self-examination.

    d. Breast self-examination is unnecessary during pregnancy and lactation.

103. Which of the following is *not* considered a precipitating risk factor for congestive heart failure?

    a. Dietary indiscretion (increased sodium intake)

    b. Cardiac arrhythmia

    c. Appropriate restriction of physical activity

    d. Uncontrolled hypertension

104. Mrs. Jones is a 50-year-old housewife who was seen by you at the clinic with reports of chronic cough and weight loss of 2 months' duration. She insists that there is nothing seriously wrong with her except for this nagging cold. Which defense mechanism is Mrs. Jones using?

    a. Projection

    b. Denial

    c. Rationalization

    d. Sublimation

105. A toddler comes to the clinic for burns on her fingers and the palms of her hands. Her mother states, "She grabbed hold of my curling iron when I had just finished with it. I had turned my back." What objective findings would lead the nurse practitioner to consider abuse?

    a. Linear bullae on palm extending to base of fingers

    b. Circular crusts and erosions on palm and fingertips

    c. From four to five bruises on anterior aspects of lower legs

    d. Anxious appearance with examination and withdrawal from practitioner

106. Jeff's mother has followed instructions for washing the linens and clothes after a scabies infestation. She calls the clinic for advice regarding a new leather jacket that Jeff wore during his infestation. Which of the following is the appropriate advice?

    a. Dry-clean the coat, even though it is new.

    b. Seal the coat in a plastic bag for at least 7 days.

    c. Wipe the coat with an antibacterial solution.

    d. Discard the coat because it cannot be properly cleaned.

107. A 75-year-old man comes to the emergency department with lethargy and suddenly begins to have a tonic-clonic seizure. Of the immediate management steps listed, which is *incorrect?*

    a. Place an oral airway in his tightly closed jaws.

    b. Place a folded blanket on the siderail that his arm keeps hitting.

    c. Attempt to place the client on his side.

    d. Administer oxygen for his cyanosis.

108. Primary management of congestive heart failure includes which of the following?

    a. Use of a beta-blocker

    b. Use of nonsteroidal antiinflammatory drugs

    d. Use of angiotensin converting enzyme (ACE) inhibitor agents

    c. Increased sodium intake

109. How would you manage Ann's care after diagnosis of irritable bowel syndrome?

    a. Stop all milk products.

b. Refer Ann to a surgeon.

c. Increase Ann's fluid and fiber intake.

d. Prescribe cimetidine (Tagamet), 400 mg bid.

110. The family nurse practitioner makes a report of suspected spousal abuse. Appropriate follow-up of the case includes which of the following?

a. Turn the case over to the clinic social worker for monitoring.

b. Periodically contact the client, the case worker, or both until the report has been investigated and the legal process is completed.

c. No follow-up is needed once the report has been made and the case becomes a legal issue.

d. Contact the client daily by phone to ensure her safety.

111. Which of the following best describes the pathophysiologic condition of gastroesophageal reflux disease?

a. Herniations as a result of antireflux barrier defects

b. Reflux as a result of defective esophageal clearance

c. Motility of small intestine affected by pressure

d. Motility diminished as a result of bronchospasms

112. Which best describes Tinel's maneuver?

a. Flex elbows at 90 degrees and hold.

b. Tap on volar surface of wrist at median nerve.

c. Raise arm above head for 60 seconds.

d. Hyperflex wrist for 2 minutes.

113. Which of the following laboratory results is consistent with the diagnosis of microcytic hypochromic anemia in an adult?

a. Decreased mean corpuscular volume (MCV) and mean corpuscular hemoglobin concentration (MCHC) and increased serum iron

b. Increased mean corpuscular volume, mean corpuscular hemoglobin concentration, and serum iron

c. Decreased mean corpuscular volume and increased mean corpuscular hemoglobin concentration and serum iron

d. Decreased mean corpuscular volume, mean corpuscular hemoglobin concentration, and serum iron

114. Client education for a client with a severe seafood allergy is successful when the client does which of the following?

a. Stops swimming in the ocean

b. Uses iodized salt

c. Carries epinephrine with him at all times

d. Agrees to undergo intravenous pyelography for dysuria

115. A young woman comes to the clinic requesting an abortion. The nurse practitioner has negative feelings about abortion. Which of the following actions is most likely to best serve the client?

a. The nurse practitioner sensitively explains her position before asking the woman to speak about her own thoughts on the subject of abortion.

b. The nurse practitioner explains all the options, putting the greatest emphasis on adoption.

c. The nurse practitioner refers her to a provider who feels more comfortable counseling women about abortion.

d. The nurse practitioner refers the woman to a clergyperson.

116. Which of the following is considered primary prevention?

a. Checking for a high blood glucose levels in older clients

b. Discussing how to floss and its importance

c. Providing yearly Pap smears

d. Discussing a low-fat diet with a client with coronary artery disease

117. You have an 82-year-old client with gastrointestinal distress. He is quiet and acquiesces responses to his son, who accompanies him to the office. This client has some bruises on his arms that he cannot explain. He does not make eye contact. You suspect elder abuse. Which of the following statements is *least* appropriate to explore the issue?

a. How have you dealt with problems in the past?

b. What kind of support systems and resources can you draw on?

c. Many people struggle with similar situations. Problems can arise. Are you having problems?

d. These bruises are a sign of abuse, and you cannot go back into that situation.

118. Leslie's last menstrual period began on July 10 and lasted until July 15. Examination findings indicate pregnancy. Which of the following dates is Leslie's expected date of confinement (EDC)?

a. April 8

b. April 17

c. April 22

d. May 17

119. Counseling topics related to safety needs specific for women older than 65 years include which of the following?

a. Abuse and seat belt use

b. Fall prevention and smoke detectors

c. Smoke detectors and hot water heater temperature

d. Fall prevention and hot water heater temperature

120. Which of the following physical findings is consistent with nonpathologic gynecomastia in an adolescent?

a. From 2 to 3 cm, fatty tissue bilaterally beneath the nipples

b. From 1 to 2 cm, unilateral, glandular tissue beneath the nipple

c. Unilateral, hard, ulcerated tissue at the nipple

d. Bilateral inverted nipples

121. Which of the following is the most common systemic antibiotic used in the treatment of severe acne?

a. Isotretinoin

b. Cephalexin (Keflex)

c. Azithromycin

d. Tetracycline

122. Which of the following is *not* true regarding falls in older adults?

a. Acute illness may precipitate falls.

b. Most falls are not caused by normal activities of daily living.

c. Sedatives and antidepressants increase the risk of falls.

    d. Clients should be involved in the falls assessment of the home environment.

123. Sylvia is a 43-year-old woman with a diagnosis of type 2 diabetes. You are preparing to do diabetic teaching for her. What is the first step in this process?

    a. Establish goals.
    b. Assess learner needs.
    c. Choose audio and video materials and client handouts.
    d. Set priorities for learning needs.

124. Mrs. Crawley is 8 months' pregnant. She reports bleeding and swelling of her gums and denies trauma. On the basis of the subjective data, your diagnosis of highest suspicion is which of the following?

    a. Gingivitis
    b. Acute necrotizing ulcerative gingivitis
    c. Canker sore
    d. Oral candidiasis

125. Sue Howard, a 34-year-old woman, has been treated for superficial thrombophlebitis for 7 days. She should be instructed to return for follow-up how often?

    a. Weekly until her symptoms resolve
    b. No follow-up necessary
    c. Only if she experiences chest pain
    d. After completion of antibiotics

126. Which of the following medications is most likely to cause shortness of breath in a client with existing chronic obstructive pulmonary disease or asthma?

    a. Antacids
    b. Beta-blockers
    c. Acetaminophen
    d. Nitrates

127. Tina is a 16-year-old girl who has an appointment for a gynecologic examination and family planning. During the examination the nurse practitioner notes a friable cervix but no discharge. Otherwise, results of her examination are normal. This finding is most consistent with which of the following diagnoses?

    a. Human immunodeficiency virus (HIV)
    b. Syphilis
    c. Candidiasis
    d. Chlamydia

128. Criteria for *Pneumocystis carinii* prophylaxis include which of the following?

    a. CD_4 count 200 cells/mm^3 or less
    b. Known exposure to *P. carinii*
    c. Cough with night sweats
    d. CD_4 count 500 cells/mm^3 or less

129. Which of the following are medications that can precipitate adrenal insufficiency?

    a. Mitotane and phenytoin
    b. Aspirin and erythromycin
    c. Digoxin and hydrochlorathiazide
    d. Furosemide and prednisone

130. Once symptoms have been effectively managed for several months, how often should the client with premenstrual syndrome be seen by the practitioner doing follow-up care?

    a. Every month during the premenstrual phase
    b. Every 3 months
    c. Every 6 months
    d. Every year

131. Your client has decompensated congestive heart failure. Which of the following diuretics will give a more rapid response?

    a. Hydrochlorothiazide
    b. Furosemide
    c. Amiloride
    d. Triamterene-hydrochlorothiazide

132. Primary care clients with alcohol abuse have improved outcomes with which of the following interventions?

    a. Supervised detoxification
    b. Regular urinary drug tests
    c. Brief counseling and regular follow-up
    d. Monthly serum gamma-glutamyl transferase measurement

133. Richard, a 32-year-old man with HIV and a CD_4 count of 312 cells/mm^3, has herpes zoster on his face. He notices one lesion on his nose. What is essential follow-up for this client?

    a. Follow up in 48 hours and begin antiviral therapy immediately.
    b. Immediately refer Richard to an ophthalmologist.
    c. Hospitalize Richard for intravenous antiviral medication.
    d. See Richard in the office in 1 week.

134. Which of the following statements regarding drug therapy for headaches is true?

    a. Rebound headaches result from prophylactic therapy.
    b. Prophylactic therapy is used for clients who have at least one headache a month that interferes with activities of daily living.
    c. Abortive therapy prevents headaches after warning signs appear.
    d. Prescribe the most potent drug to prevent rebound headaches

135. If a client with Parkinson's disease begins having postural hypotension and nausea, which drug is more likely to be the cause?

    a. Pergolide
    b. Bromocriptine
    c. Selegiline
    d. Levodopa

136. Major findings in chronic venous insufficiency include which of the following?

    a. Cyclic abdominal bloating and inability to remove wedding ring
    b. Progressive edema of the leg (particularly lower leg), with thin, shiny, brownish pigmentation often developing
    c. Confusion, weight gain, and arrhythmia
    d. Weight gain, hypotension, and positive Homan's sign

137. Elmer is a 53-year-old truck driver with diagnosis of hepatitis B virus, hepatitis C virus, and superinfection of hepatitis

D virus. He has been followed up in your clinic for the past 6 months. His aspartate aminotransferase and alanine aminotransferase levels have been stable but elevated. What is the most important physical assessment in monitoring Elmer's progress?

    a. General skin examination and general performance status assessment

    b. Abdominal examination to assess liver size and tenderness

    c. Presence of any low-grade fever in the past few weeks

    d. Digital rectal examination to assess for occult blood loss

138. Acute lumbosacral strain occurs most commonly in which of the following age groups?

    a. Those 65 years old or older

    b. Those younger than 20 years

    c. Those between 20 and 40 years old

    d. No particular age group; there is no age discrimination

139. The most common high-dose source of lead exposure for children is which of the following?

    a. Drinking water

    b. Pica

    c. Paint

    d. Soil

140. Which of the following treatments is *not* appropriate first-line management for eczema?

    a. Oatmeal colloidal bath

    b. Topical steroids applied sparingly

    c. Cool compresses with Burow's solution

    d. Tapered course of prednisone

141. Treatment for a client with arthritic changes related to Lyme disease would be:

    a. Doxycycline, 100 mg bid for 30 days

    b. Tetracycline, 500 mg qid for 30 days

    c. Ceftriaxone, 2 g/day IV for 14 days

    d. Erythromycin, 250 mg qid for 21 days

142. Which of the following is true regarding licensure as a nurse practitioner?

    a. Controlled by the Board of Nursing.

    b. Protects the public from incompetence.

    c. Identifies where and how the nurse practitioner provides care.

    d. Controlled by the Board of Medicine and the Board of Nursing.

143. When assessing smoking status, the nurse practitioner should assess all *except* which of the following?

    a. Packs smoked per day

    b. Years as a smoker

    c. Nicotine level of cigarettes used

    d. Previous attempts at stopping and their success

144. Assuming that previous results have been normal, Pap smears should be done every year until 60 years of age; after 60 years of age, how often should a Pap smear be performed.

    a. 1 to 2 years

    b. 1 to 3 years

    c. 2 years

    d. None of the above

145. Which of the following treatments is *not* used for an infant with developmental dysplasia of the hip?

    a. Spica cast

    b. Pavlik harness

    c. Triple diapering

    d. Preliminary traction

146. When can an adolescent with an ankle sprain return to play?

    a. When pain is gone, even with slight limp

    b. After 2 weeks of rest and full range of motion

    c. After resolution of pain, full range of motion, and normal gait

    d. After 1 week with ankle wrap

147. Which of the following pharmacokinetic parameters is increased in older adults?

    a. Drug absorption

    b. Glomular filtration rate

    c. Volume of distribution of water-soluble compounds

    d. Percentage of body fat

148. A 45-year-old woman who has regular menstrual cycles asks whether she is in menopause. Which is the best response for the nurse practitioner to give?

    a. Menopause starts when one is 40 years old and ends at about 50 years.

    b. Menopause is diagnosed with cessation of menstruation for 6 to 12 months.

    c. A diagnosis of menopause is made on the basis of physical findings of hypoestrogenemia.

    d. Only a serum LH level can diagnose menopause in a menstruating woman.

149. Sue Howard, a 34-year-old woman, had acute sinusitis diagnosed today. She should be instructed to return for follow-up in which of the following cases?

    a. There is no improvement in her symptoms within 48 hours.

    b. A cough develops.

    c. Low-grade fever develops.

    d. She has nasal drainage.

150. Which physical finding is most suggestive of hypothyroidism?

    a. Silky hair

    b. Dull facies

    c. Weight loss

    d. Anxious speech

151. A 38-year-old mother of two comes in for a physical examination. The nurse practitioner discovers that the client's mother died at 43 years old of a myocardial infarction. The client eats a low-fat diet and works as a grocery checker. Which of the following factors places her most at risk for coronary artery disease?

a. Her age
b. Her sex
c. Her job
d. Her mother's medical history

152. A client who has frequent recurrence of candidiasis should be evaluated for what other condition?

a. Urinary tract infection
b. Pelvic inflammatory disease
c. Diabetes
d. Lupus

153. Which of the following physical findings is *not* usually found in a child with cystic fibrosis?

a. Hyperinflation and tram lines on chest x-ray examination
b. Steeple sign on chest and lateral neck x-ray examination
c. Wheezes and crackles bilaterally on chest auscultation
d. Digital clubbing and use of accessory muscles with respiration.

154. Mary, a 9-year-old girl, reports "these funny things" on her hand. Which item of the subjective data is *least* important to elicit initially?

a. What changes has she noticed in the "things" since she discovered them?
b. Has she noticed any relationship with anything else?
c. When was her last well physical examination?
d. What does she know about skin cancer?

155. Which of the following descriptions is identified with a migraine with aura headache?

a. Bilateral, mild to moderate, pressing headache lasting 30 minutes to 6 days
b. Unilateral, moderate-to-severe, throbbing headache lasting for 4 to 72 hours, aggravated by routine physical activity, preceded by flashing lights, with nausea, vomiting, or both
c. Pounding or dull frontal or occipital pain present when upright and relieved by lying down
d. More prevalent in men, occurring in attacks of severe unilateral orbital, supraorbital, or temporal pain lasting 15 to 180 minutes and miosis

156. Which of the following objective findings is most specific for Lyme disease?

a. Skin lesion larger than 5 cm in diameter
b. Enlargement of epitrochlear and axillary nodes
c. Decreased range of motion of cervical spine
d. Muscular atrophy

157. The health history should include all *except* which of the following?

a. Information about risk factors
b. Information about reasons for the current visit
c. Review of systems
d. Anticipatory guidance

158. What is the definitive test for osteoarthritis?

a. Erythrocyte sedimentation rate
b. Complete blood cell count

c. Electrolyte levels
d. Physical examination

159. Which of the following illnesses is *not* usually transmitted by the airborne route?

a. Rubella
b. Mumps
c. Tuberculosis
d. Hepatitis

160. A nurse practitioner whose client population includes a large number of depressed people wants to implement a program that is based on a study conducted at another facility. Before implementing the program, what is the first thing the nurse practitioner should do?

a. Examine the study for its scientific integrity.
b. Ask the clients whether they want to participate.
c. Cost out the price of providing the program.
d. Pilot test the program.

161. Healthy People 2010 goals for stress management include which of the following?

a. Increasing the number of worksites with 50 or more employees providing stress-reduction programs
b. Increasing the number of referrals made by primary care providers to psychiatrists for stress control
c. Decreasing the number of primary care visits made for stress management
d. Decreasing the number of stress disorders in children

162. A mother calls regarding implementation of a behavior-management system. The misbehavior of her 3-year-old, who was seen in the office 2 days ago, seems to have increased in frequency and intensity since trying "the system." What is the best response of the provider?

a. Suggest a plan that allows the child to "ease into the system."
b. Tell the mother to call back at the end of 2 weeks to provide a more accurate evaluation of the new system.
c. Reassure the parent that her child is testing limits. Encourage consistency. Keep communication lines open. Follow up 1 to 2 weeks.
d. Ask the mother for specific accounts of misbehavior and the parental response. Consider whether the system has been correctly implemented.

163. Vaginal changes during menopause related to decreased estrogen can be helped by which of the following?

a. Taking a progesterone-only minipill
b. Using a sitz bath
c. Continuing regular sexual intercourse
d. Eating yogurt

164. A client being treated for hyperlipidemia has reached his target goals. The nurse practitioner should do which of the following?

a. Measure total cholesterol at 4 months and perform a full lipid analysis in 1 year.
b. Perform a full lipid profile in 1 month.
c. Measure total cholesterol in 1 year.
d. Check low-density and high-density lipid levels in 6 months.

165. What is the goal of crisis intervention?
- **a.** Enhance a person's level of functioning beyond that before the crisis.
- **b.** Resolve past psychologic stressors.
- **c.** Promote coping strategies used in the past.
- **d.** Resolve the immediate crisis.

166. Expected chemistry laboratory values in a person with Addison's disease would includes which of the following?
- **a.** Hypokalemia, hypernatremia, and hyperglycemia
- **b.** Hypokalemia, hypernatremia, and hypoglycemia
- **c.** Hyperkalemia, hyponatremia, and hyperglycemia
- **d.** Hyperkalemia, hyponatremia, and hypoglycemia

167. To appropriately refer a client with a developmental disability, the nurse practitioner must first assess all *except* which of the following?
- **a.** Gross motor function
- **b.** Language use
- **c.** Social abilities
- **d.** Height and weight

168. What is the appropriate response to the person who comes to the clinic 1 week after treatment with a scabicide and reports continued pruritus?
- **a.** A second treatment is indicated.
- **b.** Pruritus may continue for several days to weeks as a reaction to the mite remains.
- **c.** Pruritus will continue for 1 to 2 weeks as a reaction to the scabicide.
- **d.** Another skin condition is present, and the person should be referred to a dermatologist.

169. Which of the following statements about evaluating blood pressure is true?
- **a.** Blood pressure should be checked in both arms on at least one occasion to verify equivalency.
- **b.** At least three abnormal blood pressure readings 1 month apart are required to document the presence of hypertension.
- **c.** Coffee or cigarettes 5 minutes before a blood pressure check should have no effect on the evaluation.
- **d.** The size and position of the blood pressure cuff have little impact on the accuracy of the reading.

170. Mr. Donaldson, a long-distance runner, was recently diagnosed with acute lumbosacral strain with minimal pain. In instructing on aerobic exercises, the nurse practitioner says that he can do which of the following?
- **a.** Walk or jog lightly.
- **b.** Continue his usual regimen of training.
- **c.** Increase his speed but shorten his distance.
- **d.** Lift weights.

171. Sheila is a 12-month-old child who comes into the office for her well-child check. When you are looking at the immunization records you realize that she got her first measles-mumps-rubella vaccine at 2 weeks less than 12 months. What is your action at this point relative to the measles-mumps-rubella vaccine?
- **a.** She should be revaccinated at 12 to 15 months of age, and an additional vaccine should be given at the time of school entry.
- **b.** This dose is adequate; she just needs one more dose of the measles-mumps-rubella vaccine between 4 and 6 years of age.
- **c.** Sheila should get a dose today and another in 2 weeks, followed by the normal dose at 4 to 6 years of age.
- **d.** Only one dose of the measles-mumps-rubella vaccine is needed.

172. A family nurse practitioner is treating a 10-year-old for chronic constipation. The client has been taking docusate sodium (Colace), 100 mg PO qd, for the past 2 months. He is now having daily soft stools. In evaluating this situation, the family nurse practitioner decides to do which of the following?
- **a.** Reduce the Colace to 50 mg qd, continue diet therapy, and recheck in 1 month.
- **b.** Continue with the same regimen and reevaluate in 6 months.
- **c.** Discontinue the Colace and have the client's parents phone if he has any problems.
- **d.** Discontinue therapy and reevaluate in 3 months.

173. When describing the harmful effects of stress, the nurse practitioner should discuss which of the following?
- **a.** Premature death
- **b.** Higher incidence of alcoholism
- **c.** Decreased immunologic functioning and its consequences
- **d.** Social isolation

174. An adult who is being treated for constipation should be seen for follow-up how often?
- **a.** Every month initially then twice a year
- **b.** Twice a month while constipation persists
- **c.** As needed for problems
- **d.** No follow-up necessary

175. A menopausal woman asks the nurse practitioner how to manage hot flashes. Which suggestion by the practitioner is most appropriate?
- **a.** Limit fluid intake.
- **b.** Limit caffeine intake.
- **c.** Exercise minimally.
- **d.** Avoid hot tubs.

Answers and Rationales

1. *Answer:* **a** (diagnosis/analysis)
Rationale: Infants often show atypical signs and symptoms of the common cold. This presenting picture may be associated with the rhinovirus and respiratory syncytial virus. The client is too young for the other choices.

2. *Answer:* **b** (assessment)
Rationale: Right-to-left shunting is the defining characteristic of the cyanotic heart lesion. This results in hypoxemia as blood returning to the heart passes directly to the systemic circulation without passing through the lungs. This in turn results in cyanosis when the client has 5 mg/dL of blood that is deoxygenated. Clubbing is seen during chronic periods of hypoxemia and is of unknown cause. Hepatosplenomegaly is

associated with right-sided heart failure, which results from fluid overload in left-to-right shunts and pulmonary outflow tract obstructions. This is not seen in right-to-left shunting.

3. *Answer:* c (assessment)

Rationale: It is important to ask questions regarding life (ability to perform activities of daily living), weight loss or gain and during what time, and the client's feelings regarding resuscitation. The practitioner is obligated to provide information on advance directives.

4. *Answer:* b (evaluation)

Rationale: An acute exacerbation can be followed up by phone 24 to 48 hours after the office visit. The follow-up interval for stable chronic obstructive pulmonary disease is 3 to 6 months.

5. *Answer:* d (assessment)

Rationale: Lice live in the seams and linings of clothes and can be transmitted in this manner.

6. *Answer:* c (evaluation)

Rationale: Ophthalmic steroids should be avoided because of the association with increased incidence of glaucoma and cataracts.

7. *Answer:* b (evaluation)

Rationale: Because she is pregnant, Mrs. Jones is considered to have a complicated urinary tract infection. This warrants follow-up with a urine culture once the antibiotic course has been completed. Urinary tract infection has a high correlation with premature labor.

8. *Answer:* d (plan)

Rationale: The nurse practitioner should discuss the findings with an endocrinologist or other physician before discussing the possibility of this diagnosis with the family. The work-up can be completed by the endocrinologist.

9. *Answer:* a (plan/implementation)

Rationale: Referral to a reproductive endocrinologist is appropriate for extensive infertility testing and advice about assisted reproductive options. The nurse practitioner can appropriately address basic infertility testing, adoption plans, and treatment of pelvic inflammatory disease. For additional information on adoption, a referral to a social worker is warranted.

10. *Answer:* d (plan/management)

Rationale: Prostaglandin synthetase inhibitors (nonsteroidal antiinflammatory drugs) are the drugs of choice for primary dysmenorrhea unless there are contraindications or birth control is desired.

11. *Answer:* c (diagnosis/analysis)

Rationale: Making mistakes is an inattentive behavior. Arguing, losing temper, and annoying others are oppositional defiant behaviors.

12. *Answer:* a (assessment)

Rationale: Choice a most accurately describes a herald patch. Herald patches rarely appear on the face and usually do not cause intense itching. There are usually not any vesicles.

13. *Answer:* a (diagnosis)

Rationale: Migraine headache, tension-type headache, and trigeminal neuralgia need to be considered as differential diagnoses for the symptoms presented. Usually cluster headaches occur in men. Severe and boring pain begins on one side of the head and quickly progresses to involve the whole side of the head. Each attack lasts from 10 minutes to 3 hours; the person may experience 1 to 3 attacks per day. The eye on the side with pain turns red and tears.

14. *Answer:* d (implementation)

Rationale: Lack of acetylcholine is thought to be the cause of Alzheimer's disease. Therefore anticholinergics are contraindicated. There is no known drug that stops the progression of the disease.

15. *Answer:* b (assessment)

Rationale: It is unusual for a person with cancer to have a primary presenting symptom of fatigue. Weight changes usually occur. Insomnia may be associated with substance abuse. Duration of the fatigue is not related to a particular disease process. Postpartum fatigue is expected to last for at least 6 weeks.

16. *Answer:* c (evaluation)

Rationale: Wound infection is the most common complication. Liver abscess and fecal fistulas are rare after an appendectomy. Irritable bowel syndrome does not have any association with appendectomy.

18. *Answer:* b (diagnosis/analysis)

Rationale: Scoliosis is most prevalent during the prepubertal growth spurt, occurring in children 10 years old through adolescence.

19. *Answer:* b (evaluation)

Rationale: CD_4 lymphocytes have been viewed as the best predictor of the development of acquired immune deficiency syndrome (AIDS)-related complications such as weight loss, fatigue, and such specific diagnoses as *P. carinii* pneumonia. CD_4 decreases represent immunologic failure, and HIV RNA represents viral aggression. Therapeutic decisions are guided by results of these laboratory tests. A positive purified protein derivative of tuberculin result correlates with exposure to or inadequate previous treatment of tuberculosis.

20. *Answer:* d (plan)

Rationale: Chemotherapy suppresses the ability of the immune system to mount a response to immunizations. Also, live virus immunizations theoretically could cause the very disease that you hope to prevent in the immunocompromised person.

21. *Answer:* b (assessment)

Rationale: Viral respiratory illness, physical exertion, and smoke irritants have all been shown to act as triggers for people with asthma. Although headache may be manifested in some other disease process, it is not currently identified as a trigger.

22. *Answer:* d (assessment)

Rationale: Age, health status, and the type of agent may determine complications from the burn, but not usually severity.

23. *Answer:* b (plan/implementation)

Rationale: Cultures perceive time differently and may place emphasis on the past, present, or future. An appointment may be perceived as a general range of time rather than as a specific clock hour. The client may need care and may not keep a rescheduled appointment. Adjusting the schedule or ignoring the situation will not help the nurse practitioner to understand the client's perspective.

24. *Answer:* c (plan/implementation)

Rationale: Smoking produces low-birth-weight infants, miscarriage, and premature labor. It has no correlation with anemia or weight gain of the mother.

25. *Answer:* c (wellness)

Rationale: Matthew is not having any problems, and his age is a general guideline for discontinuing screening for prostate cancer. Even if cancer is discovered, observation may be the only appropriate therapy.

26. *Answer:* c (diagnosis/analysis)

Rationale: All sexually active women should be considered as being pregnant until proven otherwise. The woman who uses inconsistent barrier contraception is at risk of pregnancy.

27. *Answer:* c (assessment)

Rationale: The American Academy of Pediatrics does not recommend universal urinalysis screening of symptom-free children because research findings reflect the lack of specificity of current urine tests in detecting significant renal or urinary tract disease in these children.

28. *Answer:* b (wellness)

Rationale: Melena is the most frequent presenting symptom of peptic ulcer disease in older adults.

29. *Answer:* a (assessment)

Rationale: The other three choices are most predictive of coronary artery disease.

30. *Answer:* a (plan)

Rationale: Treatment with oral tetracycline, tretinoin, isotretinoin, and doxycycline can result in photosensitivity. Tetracycline must be taken on an empty stomach; dairy products may decrease absorption.

31. *Answer:* a (plan)

Rationale: The actual dose necessary to inhibit platelets is 81 mg of aspirin.

32. *Answer:* b (diagnosis)

Rationale: Pulmonary embolism may be seen with dyspnea and hemoptysis, and it is typically associated with such risk factors as immobility and surgery.

33. *Answer:* b (evaluation)

Rationale: All vigorous lifting, overexertion, and contact sports should be avoided in the first 1 to 2 months after the diagnosis of mononucleosis.

34. *Answer:* b (assessment)

Rationale: Costovertebral angle tenderness is a common finding with pyelonephritis. Suprapubic tenderness is more commonly seen with cystitis, whereas urethral discharge is seen with a sexually transmitted disease. Mild abdominal pain is extremely nonspecific; it may be seen with any number of problems.

35. *Answer:* a (diagnosis)

Rationale: Diabetes usually causes weight loss in children.

36. *Answer:* a (diagnosis/analysis)

Rationale: Follicular ovarian cysts occur during early in the menstrual cycle and cause pelvic pressure, aching, and heaviness.

37. *Answer:* a (assessment)

Rationale: Severe lower back pain is nonspecific for many conditions, including pyelonephritis and back strain. A thick, white discharge with itching is indicative of candidiasis, whereas the discharge associated with gonorrhea is purulent. Postcoital bleeding occurs with cervicitis, which often is present before any noticeable signs and symptoms of gonorrhea.

38. *Answer:* d (assessment)

Rationale: Early glaucoma may be detected by an altered cup-to-disk ratio or bilateral asymmetry in the physiologic cup. Visual field testing is difficult to perform accurately. Schiotz tonometry readings may be falsely low in early disease.

39. *Answer:* c (assessment)

Rationale: Physical findings with encopresis frequently include abdominal distention with a soft, nontender mass in the midline or the lower left quadrant. The rectal vault is usually filled with either liquid or hard stool.

40. *Answer:* c (evaluation)

Rationale: All the listed side effects result from the anticholinergic action of the drug. Only urinary retention requires immediate attention.

41. *Answer:* d (diagnosis/analysis)

Rationale: A variety of medications may cause acnelike lesions. Lithium and any antidepressant compounds containing lithium, phenytoin, trimethadione, systemic corticosteroids, and isoniazid commonly cause acne.

42. *Answer:* d (assessment)

Rationale: Pain in or behind the ear is one of the most common symptoms associated with Bell's palsy.

43. *Answer:* b (assessment)

Rationale: Other responses are common symptoms in the initial acute phase (stages 1 and 2). Loss of memory may occur as a result of cranial neuropathies associated with chronic late manifestations (stage 3).

44. *Answer:* a (assessment)

Rationale: Although in some rare instances diarrhea-causing organisms can be passed from animals to humans, the other three choices are clearly better. Number, character, and quantity of stools must be assessed to determine whether diarrhea exists and to gauge its severity. Urinary output must be assessed to determine the degree of dehydration. Associated symptoms such as vomiting can help lead to a diagnosis and assess the likelihood of dehydration.

45. *Answer:* c (plan)

Rationale: Examination of joint fluid under a polarized microscope is the only definitive means of documenting the presence of monosodium urate crystals. Results of all the other tests may be normal at the time of an acute attack.

46. *Answer:* b (assessment)

Rationale: Constitutional symptoms are diagnostically useful clinical features in the initial evaluation of the client with systemic lupus erythematosus.

47. *Answer:* d (plan/implement)

Rationale: The immune system remains incompetent to mount a response to immunizations for at least 6 months to 1 year after treatment ends. All other responses are appropriate.

48. *Answer:* d (assessment)

Rationale: Sexual history would not provide information useful in establishing the diagnosis and plan.

49. *Answer:* c (assessment)

Rationale: All findings—retractions, tachypnea, decreased breath sounds, and increased capillary refill time—are indicators of respiratory distress. However, of most concern is the absence of breath sounds, which may be an indicator of impending respiratory failure.

50. *Answer:* b (plan)

Rationale: Family dysfunction often occurs because of the strain placed on family resources by caring for a child with a developmental delay. If the delay is in an area other than fine motor or social skills, promoting these two things will not be helpful.

51. *Answer:* b (assessment)

Rationale: This reply facilitates clarification and understanding by both the nurse and the client of what was communicated.

52. *Answer:* b (plan)

Rationale: If the patient wants true anonymity he or she should go to an anonymous test site. Telling the client that nurse practitioners are bound by confidentiality rules may not be enough for the client. All options should be presented.

53. *Answer:* b (plan/implement)

Rationale: Carbohydrates and fiber should be increased. Obesity should be reduced. There are no discussions concerning the number of professionals involved. The goal is to improve nutritional assessment and counseling.

54. *Answer:* b (implement)

Rationale: Vigorous activity should be conducted at least 3 days a week. No groups are given special consideration in relation to exercise. No differences are made for men or women.

55. *Answer:* b (evaluation)

Rationale: Although this is an example of polypharmacy, compliance with medication administration is the most important issue. Only with this assessment can one determine whether there is an interactive element.

56. *Answer:* c (assessment)

Rationale: A link between sexually transmitted diseases and prostate cancer exists, but the exact reason for this is not known.

57. *Answer:* b (assessment)

Rationale: All the topics in choice b are appropriate pieces of information to elicit from a healthy 18-year-old. The other choices include topics that are not appropriate to a healthy 18-year-old. For instance, hot water settings are of concern in a dwelling in which an extremely young or old person lives, and a healthy 18-year-old would neither be institutionalized nor need family members trained in cardiopulmonary resuscitation.

58. *Answer:* c (assessment)

Rationale: A tuberculosis test is usually not recommended unless the child has had a history of exposure or lives in an at-risk population.

59. *Answer:* c (wellness)

Rationale: A well adult needs a vision screening examination every 2 years only. A client with diabetes needs to have an eye examination every year.

60. *Answer:* c (plan)

Rationale: Prevention of behavioral problems through anticipatory guidance is ideal for the nurse practitioner. Analyzing influences of the parents' own upbringing and existing expectations regarding child behavior and management is an important step that is often missed.

The parents have expressed interest and provided a window for teaching. Continuing the process during the next one to two well-child visits allows parental input to personalize a system with guidance by the professional. A recommendation simply to read a book offers only cursory attention to an extremely important issue of childhood.

61. *Answer:* b (diagnosis)

Rationale: The most common age group for group A streptococcal pharyngitis is 5 to 10 years of age. Answer a is the most common presentation for croup. The 29-year-old woman does not have exudate, which is suggestive of a streptococcal pharyngitis. The 50-year-old man is out of the population age group consistent with streptococcal pharyngitis.

62. *Answer:* b (assessment)

Rationale: Risk factors that should be assessed in the history include sedentary lifestyle, obesity, smoking, and dietary history. Medication history that contributes to hypertension includes oral contraceptives. For a 16-year-old boy, a blood pressure reading of 130/80 mm Hg is within normal range. The obese black African-American man who smokes has the most risk factors for hypertension.

63. *Answer:* b (plan)

Rationale: Focal findings such as the crackles in the left lower lobe warrant an x-ray examination for further evaluation.

64. *Answer:* d (assessment)

Rationale: Recurrent upper respiratory infections, changes in growth pattern (weight loss), and fatty stools may be suggestive of cystic fibrosis.

65. *Answer:* **d** (evaluation)
Rationale: If the mother is adequately treated during pregnancy, the infant may still have a reactive VDRL test at birth. This test should be repeated at 1, 2, 4, 6, and 12 months, until it becomes nonreactive.

66. *Answer:* **d** (plan)
Rationale: Serum testosterone, follicle-stimulating hormone, and prolactin levels should be considered when endocrine or chromosomal factors are a possibility. Estradiol levels are applicable to additional female factor testing.

67. *Answer:* **c** (plan)
Rationale: Alpha-adrenergic antagonists often cause symptoms of orthostasis; therefore they should be given at bedtime to minimize the chance of falls related to these side effects.

68. *Answer:* **d** (plan)
Rationale: Glipizide increases insulin secretion in direct response to food and avoids hyperinsulinemia and lipid involvement.

69. *Answer:* **a** (assessment)
Rationale: Spotting or irregular bleeding is common during the first 3 months of contraception by hormonal methods.

70. *Answer:* **c** (plan)
Rationale: A client with a diagnosis of herpes simplex conjunctivitis should be referred to an ophthalmologist because of the potential for damage to sight. Ophthalmic steroids are contraindicated. Sodium sulfacetamide and bacitracin are used in the treatment of bacterial conjunctivitis.

71. *Answer:* **a** (assessment)
Rationale: Age is the only item from the history that does not place this woman at risk for abuse. Clinical signs and symptoms that might be suggestive of domestic violence include chronic headaches and substance abuse (by client or in family). Low socioeconomic status also places this family at increased risk.

72. *Answer:* **c** (assessment)
Rationale: Low self-esteem and affective intolerance are individual factors that may contribute to development of eating disorders. Blurring of generational boundaries is a family factor. Change in women's roles and destabilization of roles have been identified as a sociocultural factor that has contributed to an "atmosphere" in which eating disorders develop.

73. *Answer:* **a** (assessment)
Rationale: Microscopic examination of a scraped specimen of the lesion usually leads to rapid identification of the infective organism.

74. *Answer:* **d** (assessment)
Rationale: Depression is not a characteristic of delirium.

75. *Answer:* **a** (plan)
Rationale: Liver enzymes should be measured at baseline and with increase in dose of statin. Elevation (3 times upper limit of normal on two separate occasions with at least one week between measurements) requires discontinuation of the drug.

76. *Answer:* **b** (assessment)
Rationale: The 30-year-old with regular menstrual periods is assumed to be having ovulatory cycles that are associated with increased prostaglandin release and synthesis. Young girls typically have anovulatory cycles for the first 6 to 12 months. The 48-year-old is most likely premenopausal, and the 35-year-old who is taking oral contraceptives is anovulatory.

77. *Answer:* **d** (diagnosis/analysis)
Rationale: Confirming the presence of *Helicobacter pylori* is important once the diagnosis of ulcer has been made. Elimination of the bacteria is likely to cure the ulcer disease.

78. *Answer:* **d** (assessment)
Rationale: The most relevant objective data to gather for this client are a rectal examination and evaluation of occult blood (guaiac). Deep tendon reflexes generally do not need to be evaluated in someone with gastrointestinal complaints. Current medications and symptoms are examples of subjective data.

79. *Answer:* **b** (plan)
Rationale: Spontaneous reduction of the hips occurs in approximately 90% of affected children in 2 to 6 weeks. The mechanism of this phenomenon is not understood, but the Pavlik harness should be maintained for several months after spontaneous reduction, until the hip has stabilized.

80. *Answer:* **d** (evaluation)
Rationale: When performing a physical examination of a client with a chronic illness, the nurse practitioner must consider the impact of the chronic illness on all body systems. When performing a routine physical examination, clinical signs associated with the chronic disease should be assessed simultaneously. Spleen enlargement, enlargement of multiple lymph nodes, and weight loss are associated with lymphoma. The client's status with respect to the lymphoma should be evaluated. The primary care provider may be able to detect an early progression of the disease, enabling early intervention.

81. *Answer:* **a** (diagnosis/analysis)
Rationale: Folic acid and iron deficiencies are most common during pregnancy. Prenatal vitamins contain iron and folic acid.

82. *Answer:* **d** (diagnosis)
Rationale: Sinusitis may have nighttime cough as a presenting symptom, but most likely it would also have associated sore throat as a result of postnasal drip.

83. *Answer:* **d** (issues)
Rationale: Standards of care are based on the scope of practice and do describe and guide acceptable practice. They are developed by professional organizations, such as the American Nurses Association.

84. *Answer:* **c** (issues)
Rationale: Nurse practitioners are reimbursed at 85% of the physician charge for the same service regardless of practice setting.

85. *Answer:* **c** (issues)
Rationale: Advance directives provide an opportunity for the client to identify his or her wishes regarding resuscitation

and life support before an episode occurs in which it might be needed.

86. *Answer:* a (diagnosis)
Rationale: Older adults are at the highest risk for malnutrition. Nutritional screening should also be conducted for those who are 20% below desirable weight or have had an involuntary weight loss of more than 10 pounds in a month.

87. *Answer:* c (plan)
Rationale: Fertility and diarrhea are not associated with exercise. High-density lipoprotein levels are increased with exercise. Glucose tolerance is improved.

88. *Answer:* b (assessment)
Rationale: Although choice a is important, choice b is the best answer and will provide enough detail for customizing anticipatory guidance in injury prevention. Choices c and d are irrelevant.

89. *Answer:* b (plan)
Rationale: Effective intervention that addresses personal health habits decreases the incidence and severity of the leading causes of death in the United States.

90. *Answer:* b (plan)
Rationale: Injury and death from firearms are a serious problem in the United States. This is a serious issue because some children have easy access to firearms in the home.

91. *Answer:* c (wellness)
Rationale: Hormone replacement therapy helps prevent bone loss, especially after surgically induced menopause.

92. *Answer:* d (assessment)
Rationale: Gallbladder disease is recognized by right upper quadrant pain and tenderness that is more severe with inspiration. Diarrhea is usually not present. White blood cell count is not usually higher than 15,000 cells/mm³. Bloating may be present.

93. *Answer:* d (wellness)
Rationale: Hypertension is the leading cause of cardiovascular death among black men.

94. *Answer:* c (assessment)
Rationale: Persons with nuclear (central) cataracts often have improved vision in low light as a result of the larger viewing area of the crystalline lens caused by pupillary dilatation.

95. *Answer:* b (diagnosis)
Rationale: Pericarditis may develop 2 to 3 days after a myocardial infarction. The type of pain described in the question is most consistent with pericarditis. Associated shortness of breath accompanies the discomfort of a pulmonary embolus. Aortic dissection pain is not relieved with position change. Angina usually does not worsen with deep breathing. Electrocardiogram changes of pericarditis may be masked by the infarction. A pericardial friction rub is not always present.

96. *Answer:* a (diagnosis)
Rationale: Height and weight below the fifth percentile and hypertension are suggestive of chronic occult renal disease. Although the urinalysis is suggestive of a urinary tract infection, the fact that the client has never achieved nighttime dryness

points to a more long-term cause. The other two findings are within normal limits.

97. *Answer:* b (plan)
Rationale: High calorie foods, including those high in fat, should be given to a child with cystic fibrosis. The pancreatic enzyme is used to help the individual tolerate the fat in foods.

98. *Answer:* b (plan)
Rationale: Erythromycin is not indicated for the treatment of gonorrhea in the adult. Azithromycin is the treatment for chlamydia, and acyclovir is the treatment for herpes outbreaks. Cefixime in a single dose is highly effective in treating gonorrhea.

99. *Answer:* a (assessment)
Rationale: With acute bacterial prostatitis, an elevated white blood cell count is usually found; in chronic bacterial prostatitis, a slight elevation may or may not be seen.

100. *Answer:* b (plan/implementation)
Rationale: Bleeding after completing a course of Provera is called "withdrawal bleeding" and is a normal event. It does not indicate a serious pathologic condition. Withdrawal bleeding does not occur with ovarian failure. Because the client had normal menstrual cycles in the past, she does not have primary amenorrhea. Withdrawal bleeding with normal thyroid-stimulating hormone and prolactin levels indicates anovulation, which may persist without hormonal assistance.

101. *Answer:* c (evaluation)
Rationale: For families with pets, regular washing is thought to decrease the animal dander, which acts as a trigger. Smoke is transmitted through air vents and on clothing, so simply moving the smoker to another room will not get rid of the exposure. Vacuuming is not sufficient to remove dust mites. Box springs and mattresses should be sealed in plastic; stuffed animals are dust collectors and should be washed weekly or sealed in plastic.

102. *Answer:* d (plan/implementation)
Rationale: Breast self-examination should be performed throughout the life-cycle. Cancer can occur during pregnancy and lactation, so women should continue to perform breast self-examination at these times.

103. *Answer:* c (diagnosis)
Rationale: Increased sodium intake results in increased water retention and an increase in cardiac workload. Arrhythmias can cause a decrease in ventricular filling (tachycardia) or a decreased cardiac output (severe bradycardia). Uncontrolled hypertension can lead to progressive worsening of left ventricular hypertrophy.

104. *Answer:* b (diagnosis)
Rationale: Denial is the refusal to accept an unpleasant situation as reality based. Projection is the blaming of others for one's own unacceptable thoughts or feelings. Rationalization is making excuses for unacceptable thoughts and behaviors. Sublimation is expressing unacceptable wishes in a more socially acceptable manner.

105. *Answer:* b (assessment)
Rationale: Circular burns with a well-demarcated edge are indicative of cigarette burns. Physical findings do not match

history of cause. Both raise suspicions of abuse. A linear burn matches the history of grabbing a curling iron. Anxiety with examination and bruises on the lower legs are normal findings on a toddler.

106. *Answer:* **b** (plan/implement)
Rationale: An alternate method of destroying the scabies mite in bed linens and clothing is to store them in tightly sealed plastic bags for 7 to 14 days.

107. *Answer:* **a** (implement)
Rationale: Placing an object in the mouth of a person whose jaw is tightly closed may incur injury to the client. The other choices are indicated in the acute management of a seizure.

108. *Answer:* **c** (plan)
Rationale: ACE inhibitors are first-line therapy for symptom control of congestive heart failure.

109. *Answer:* **c** (implement)
Rationale: Increasing fluid and fiber facilitates bowel activity. Referral to a surgeon is not justified. You do not have adequate history or physical findings to recommend a reduction in lactose (an intraluminal factor). Symptoms do not justify using a histamine blocker.

110. *Answer:* **b** (evaluation)
Rationale: Nurse practitioners have the responsibility to follow up closely on all cases of abuse and neglect. The nurse practitioner does not abdicate responsibility once a report has been made to an agency.

111. *Answer:* **b** (diagnosis)
Rationale: Gastrointestinal reflux disease is characterized by reflux of gastric secretions into the esophagus that is caused by an abnormal reflux barrier, defective esophageal clearance, increased gastric secretions, and delayed gastric emptying. Irritable bowel syndrome is characterized by functional disturbances in motor activity, which may be triggered by pressure irritants.

112. *Answer:* **b** (assessment)
Rationale: Tinel's sign is evoked by tapping on the volar wrist at the carpal tunnel.

113. *Answer:* **d** (diagnosis)
Rationale: Microcytic hypochromic anemia has decreased MCV, decreased MCHC, and decreased serum iron.

114. *Answer:* **c** (evaluation)
Rationale: An acute generalized reaction increases the risk of anaphylaxis. Therefore avoiding the allergen is important, but it may not always be possible. Having epinephrine on hand allows action in an emergency. Iodine is the usual cause of allergic reaction to seafood. Therefore other sources of iodine should be avoided.

115. *Answer:* **c** (plan/implementation)
Rationale: It is critical that the nurse practitioner be in touch with his or her beliefs and values to meet the needs of the client. It is difficult for the provider who is negative about induced abortion to present a totally unbiased view. The client deserves to express her honest feelings in a nonjudgmental setting and to learn about all options. Referral to another provider who holds less negative views (if possible in the setting) is the most appropriate option.

116. *Answer:* **b** (wellness)
Rationale: Primary prevention deals with actions that prevent the occurrence of illness. Secondary prevention is an early case finding, as are blood glucose testing and Pap smears. Tertiary prevention deals with teaching and prevention after the fact, as in a client with coronary artery disease.

117. *Answer:* **d** (wellness)
Rationale: All the other answers are nonjudgmental and are phrased to elicit additional information while creating an environment of trust.

118. *Answer:* **b** (diagnosis/analysis)
Rationale: Naegele's rule may be used to calculate the pregnant woman's EDC. To use the rule, 3 months is subtracted from and 7 days are added to the last menstrual period. If the last menstrual period began on July 10 (7/10), the EDC will be April 17 (4/17).

119. *Answer:* **d** (plan/implementation)
Rationale: Injuries from falls and burns caused by dulling of tactile sensation are considered a leading medical problem for women at least 65 years old.

120. *Answer:* **b** (assessment)
Rationale: True gynecomastia consists of glandular tissue. This is distinguishable from adipose tissue when palpated between the thumb and forefinger. The glandular tissue may be either unilateral or bilateral.

121. *Answer:* **d** (implement)
Rationale: Effective topical therapies available for the treatment of acne decrease the need for systemic antibiotic therapy. However, occasionally more severe inflammatory acne does not respond to the topical treatments and a systemic antibiotic may be added to the regimen. Tetracycline is the most common antibiotic agent used for systemic treatment.

122. *Answer:* **b** (wellness)
Rationale: Most falls occur as part of the normal day's activities.

123. *Answer:* **b** (plan)
Rationale: Before the development and implementation of the teaching plan, it is vital to determine what this client currently knows regarding diabetes and to identify what she needs to know about it.

124. *Answer:* **a** (diagnosis/analysis)
Rationale: The symptoms are classic for gingivitis. This is a common complaint in women during the third trimester of pregnancy. It is thought to be an inflammatory response to hormonal changes.

125. *Answer:* **a** (evaluation)
Rationale: There is a small risk of thrombus extension into the deep venous system; therefore the course of superficial thrombophlebitis should be monitored.

126. *Answer:* **b** (implementation/management)
Rationale: Betablockers can stimulate bronchospasm.

127. *Answer:* d (diagnosis/analysis)
Rationale: Chlamydial infection commonly has a friable cervix as its presenting symptom, and the woman frequently does not have any discharge. Syphilis features a chancre, HIV features fatigue as well as other symptoms, and candidiasis usually features a thick, white discharge.

128. *Answer:* a (diagnosis)
Rationale: P. carinii pneumonia is the hallmark AIDS-defining illness and the most common cause of AIDS-related death. Prophylaxis for the prevention of primary or secondary *P. carinii* pneumonia has proved most effective when begun at a CD_4 value 200 cells/mm^3 or less for those with a history of *P. carinii* pneumonia. Prophylaxis should be considered for the client with recurrent oral candidiasis or unexplained fever with temperature higher than 100° F for longer than 2 weeks.

129. *Answer:* a (assessment)
Rationale: Mitotane and phenytoin are associated with adrenal insufficiency.

130. *Answer:* d (evaluation)
Rationale: Clients should be followed monthly for three visits, then annually if symptoms are being managed effectively.

131. *Answer:* b (plan)
Rationale: Loop diuretics (furosemide, bumetanide, and torsemide) cause a more acute diuresis. Loop diuretics should be given intravenously in the presence of pulmonary edema or severe volume overload.

132. *Answer:* c (evaluation)
Rationale: A client with alcohol abuse can reduce alcohol consumption, risk behaviors, and adverse outcomes and improve results of laboratory studies with brief counseling and regular follow-up.

133. *Answer:* b (implement)
Rationale: It is imperative when the trigeminal nerve is involved and a lesion is present on the nose to refer the client immediately to an ophthalmologist. Complications from herpes in the eye can be devastating.

134. *Answer:* c (plan)
Rationale: Abortive therapy is used to treat symptoms once they occur or to prevent headaches.

135. *Answer:* d (evaluation)
Rationale: Levodopa, a dopaminergic drug, produces nausea, postural hypotension, and dyskinesia with prolonged therapy. It is a less effective agent over time.

136. *Answer:* b (assessment)
Rationale: Progressive edema of the lower extremity and thin, shiny, brownish pigmentation are indicative of chronic venous insufficiency.

137. *Answer:* b (evaluation)
Rationale: General examination and general performance are important, but if Elmer is being followed up the most important aspect is to assess his liver size and the presence of tenderness. Low-grade fever is too nonspecific and may be present for a variety of reasons. There is no reason to conduct a digital rectal examination for occult blood loss.

138. *Answer:* c (diagnosis)
Rationale: Older adults are less likely to experience lumbosacral strain than are those younger than 20 years, and back pain is unusual in children.

139. *Answer:* c (diagnosis)
Rationale: The most common source of lead exposure for children is lead in paint.

140. *Answer:* d (plan)
Rationale: Prednisone should be used only in consultation with a physician for a client with severe eczema.

141. *Answer:* a (plan)
Rationale: Doxycycline or amoxicillin is the drug of choice for secondary arthritis associated with Lyme disease. Ceftriaxone is recommended for cardiac or neurologic manifestations.

142. *Answer:* b (issues)
Rationale: The purpose of licensure is to protect the public from incompetence. Although in most states the Board of Nursing controls nurse practitioner practice, in some states it is a combined Board of Medicine and Nursing. The scope of practice describes the how and where of nurse practitioner practice.

143. *Answer:* c (wellness)
Rationale: Pack/years and previous attempts at quitting should be assessed to help develop a plan that has a likelihood of working. Nicotine levels of cigarettes vary, and this information often is not known by the client or readily available to the nurse practitioner. It is assessed indirectly through pack/years.

144. *Answer:* a (plan/implementation)
Rationale: Pap smears may be done every 1 to 2 years after 60 years of age.

145. *Answer:* c (plan)
Rationale: Triple diapering is not recommended because the adductor muscles of the thigh overpower saturated diapers, meaning that abduction cannot be maintained.

146. *Answer:* c (plan)
Rationale: To prevent risk of reinjury to the joint, these guidelines should be used for return to play with any joint injury.

147. *Answer:* d (plan)
Rationale: Drug distribution is one important factor that is affected by the relative increase in body fat and decrease in lean body mass of an older adult. This change causes increased distribution and increased elimination of fat-soluble drugs.

148. *Answer:* b (diagnosis/analysis)
Rationale: The perimenopausal or climacteric period is a 7- to 10-year period of physiologic change before menopause. The average age at menopause is 51 years. Menopause is defined as cessation of menstruation; it is definitely diagnosed by a serum follicle-stimulating hormone level.

149. *Answer:* **a** (evaluation)
Rationale: Cough development is common with sinusitis. Lack of improvement may indicate complications of acute sinusitis or an antibiotic-resistant strain of bacteria.

150. *Answer:* **b** (assessment)
Rationale: Clients with hypothyroidism may have a flat affect and dull facies. Silky hair, weight loss, and anxious speech are more characteristic of hyperthyroidism.

151. *Answer:* **d** (assessment)
Rationale: Age is not a definitive factor. Males are more susceptible than females. A sedentary job places one at risk. History of sudden death or myocardial infarction in a parent or sibling younger than 55 years is a risk factor.

152. *Answer:* **c** (assessment)
Rationale: Diabetes predisposes a woman toward chronic *Candida* infections, as do menopause and a positive HIV status. Urinary tract infections and pelvic inflammatory disease are acute illnesses that do not play a significant part in chronic *candidiasis.* Although a chronic disease, lupus is not known to trigger chronic *candidiasis.*

153. *Answer:* **b** (assessment)
Rationale: Steeple sign on a lateral neck x-ray film is diagnostic for laryngotracheobronchitis (croup). All other findings are consistent with cystic fibrosis.

154. *Answer:* **d** (assessment)
Rationale: Descriptions of the lesion and of its relationship to other things are key diagnostic data. Noting the last well physical examination may help date the appearance of the lesion.

155. *Answer:* **b** (assessment)
Rationale: Bilateral, mild to moderate pressing headache lasting 30 minutes to 7 days is more indicative of a tensiontype headache, whereas pounding or dull frontal or occipital pain present when upright and relieved by lying down is associated with post–spinal puncture headache. Higher prevalence in men, occurrence in attacks of severe unilateral orbital, supraorbital, or temporal pain lasting 15 to 180 minutes, and miosis are associated with cluster headache.

156. *Answer:* **a** (assessment)
Rationale: Erythema migrans lesions 5 cm or larger are most specific for Lyme disease.

157. *Answer:* **d** (assessment)
Rationale: Information gained from the health history is used to provide anticipatory guidance, but the provision of this guidance is not considered a part of the health history.

158. *Answer:* **d** (assessment)
Rationale: Although choices a, b, and c may be considered in rheumatoid arthritis, there is no test specifically for osteoarthritis. The history and physical examination should lead the provider to diagnose osteoarthritis.

159. *Answer:* **d** (diagnosis)
Rationale: Hepatitis is transmitted by oral–fecal or bloodborne routes.

160. *Answer:* **a** (issues)
Rationale: The first step in research use is to make sure that the rigor of the study is sufficient to indicate that the results may be useful. After determining that the study was done correctly, the practitioner can examine the results in light of the new practice setting and client population. A pilot study should be done before offering the program to all clients. Informed consent is always necessary if a program is being offered as part of a research study. Costing out the program is a later step.

161. *Answer:* **a** (plan)
Rationale: Stress-reduction goals focus on adults in Healthy People 2010.The aim is to take steps, including visiting a primary care provider, to control stress. Referrals are not addressed. Worksite programs are emphasized.

162. *Answer:* **c** (evaluation)
Rationale: Implementing a behavior-management system can be trying at the onset. Parents often abandon systems in the early stages because of the difficulty involved. It is critical that the health care provider act as a support to the parents and family throughout the process of adjustment. At 2 days the system has not been enough of a chance to allow accurate assessment of its success. However, a parent who calls deserves a more immediate response for the perceived difficulty.

163. *Answer:* **c** (plan/implementation)
Rationale: Regular intercourse does slow the narrowing and shortening of the vagina. Estrogen supplementation also helps, but progesterone is not useful. Yogurt and sitz baths are not helpful.

164. *Answer:* **a** (plan)
Rationale: Once target goals have been achieved, choice a is correct. It is not necessary to perform a more costly test (full lipid profile) earlier.

165. *Answer:* **d** (implement)
Rationale: A goal is to restore the client to a level of functioning that existed before the crisis by resolving the immediate crisis.

166. *Answer:* **d** (plan)
Rationale: The lack of cortisol causes a decrease in gluconeogenesis and liver glycogen and an increased insulin sensitivity, with resulting hypoglycemia. The decrease in aldosterone leads to hyponatremia and hyperkalemia.

167. *Answer:* **d** (assessment)
Rationale: Height and weight should be recorded for every client, not just those with developmental disabilities. However, the absence of this assessment will not interfere with the referral. Baseline language, fine motor, gross motor, and social skills must be assessed.

168. *Answer:* **b** (evaluation)
Rationale: Pruritus may continue for several days to weeks after the infestation has been treated. This is a temporary reaction to the remains of the mites under the skin.

169. *Answer:* **a** (assessment)
Rationale: Blood pressure readings should be checked in both arms at least once to verify equivalency. At least two

blood pressure readings 2 minutes apart in supine or seated position and after standing for 2 minutes should be used to document hypertension. Coffee, cigarettes, cuff size, and positioning all affect accuracy.

170. *Answer:* **a** (plan)

Rationale: Because Mr. Donaldson has been active, he can continue light jogging, walking, or swimming, but he should not continue the vigor of his usual running until pain subsides. Lifting weights will not affect his aerobic capacity; depending on the weight, it might exceed recommended amounts (20 to 60 pounds, depending on pain level).

171. *Answer:* **a** (evaluation)

Rationale: If the first dose was given before 12 months of age, give No. 1 at 12 to 15 months of age, followed by the second dose between 4 and 6 years.

172. *Answer:* **a** (evaluation)

Rationale: Daily doses of stool softeners should be reduced once soft stools are established. Therapy may need to continue for 2 to 3 months until regular habits are well established. Follow-up should be scheduled every month until the rectal vault is back to a normal size.

173. *Answer:* **c** (plan)

Rationale: Premature death and alcoholism are not directly related to stress. Decreased immunologic function has been correlated with stress levels. Social isolation is not a consequence of stress.

174. *Answer:* **b** (assessment)

Rationale: Adults with chronic constipation should be followed up every 2 weeks until "normal bowel functions" resume. Failure to respond to therapy may indicate a serious underlying pathologic condition.

175. *Answer:* **b** (plan/implementation)

Rationale: Drinking 8 to 10 glasses of water a day does help with vasomotor instability. Regular exercise is also helpful. Caffeine and alcohol intakes should be limited. Hot tubs do not have to be avoided because vasomotor instability is not predictable.

APPENDIX

BETHESDA 2001 TERMINOLOGY FOR REPORTING CERVICAL CYTOLOGY

SPECIMEN TYPE: *Indicate conventional smear (Pap smear) vs. liquid based vs. other*

SPECIMEN ADEQUACY
- Satisfactory for evaluation (*describe presence or absence of endocervical/transformation zone component and any other quality indicators, e.g., partially obscuring blood, inflammation, etc.*)
- Unsatisfactory for evaluation (*specify reason*)
  - Specimen rejected/not processed (*specify reason*)
  - Specimen processed and examined, but unsatisfactory for evaluation of epithelial abnormality because of (*specify reason*)

GENERAL CATEGORIZATION *(optional)*
- Negative for Intraepithelial Lesion or Malignancy
- Epithelial Cell Abnormality: See Interpretation/Result (*specify "squamous" or "glandular" as appropriate*)
- Other: See Interpretation/Result (*e.g., endometrial cells in a woman ≥ 40 years of age*)

AUTOMATED REVIEW
If case examined by automated device, specify device and result.

ANCILLARY TESTING
Provide a brief description of the test methods and report the result so that it is easily understood by the clinician.

INTERPRETATION/RESULT

NEGATIVE FOR INTRAEPITHELIAL LESION OR MALIGNANCY (*when there is no cellular evidence of neoplasia, state this in the General Categorization above and/or in the Interpretation/Result section of the report, whether or not there are organisms or other non-neoplastic findings*)

Organisms
- *Trichomonas vaginalis*
- Fungal organisms morphologically consistent with *Candida* spp
- Shift in flora suggestive of bacterial vaginosis
- Bacteria morphologically consistent with *Actinomyces* spp
- Cellular changes consistent with Herpes simplex virus

Other Non-Neoplastic Findings *(Optional to report; list not inclusive):*
- Reactive cellular changes associated with
  - inflammation (includes typical repair)
  - radiation
  - IUD
- Glandular cells status post hysterectomy
- Atrophy

OTHER
- Endometrial cells *(in a woman ≥ 40 years of age)*
  (Specify if "negative for squamous intraepithelial lesion")

EPITHELIAL CELL ABNORMALITIES
Squamous Cell
- ASC
  - ASC-US
  - cannot exclude HSIL (ASC-H)
- LSIL encompassing: HPV/mild dysplasia/CIN 1
- HSIL encompassing: moderate and severe dysplasia, CIS/CIN 2 and CIN 3
  - with features suspicious for invasion (*if invasion is suspected*)
- Squamous cell carcinoma
Glandular Cell
- Atypical
  - endocervical cells (NOS *or specify in comments*)

Continued

EPITHELIAL CELL ABNORMALITIES—Cont'd
Glandular Cell—Cont'd
- endometrial cells (NOS *or specify in comments*)
- glandular cells (NOS *or specify in comments*)
- Atypical
  - endocervical cells, favor neoplastic
  - glandular cells, favor neoplastic
- Endocervical adenocarcinoma in situ
- Adenocarcinoma
  - endocervical
  - endometrial
  - extrauterine
  - NOS

OTHER MALIGNANT NEOPLASMS: *(specify)*

EDUCATIONAL NOTES AND SUGGESTIONS *(optional)*
Suggestions should be concise and consistent with clinical follow-up guidelines published by professional organizations. (References to relevant publications may be included.)

Retrieved August 18, 2002, from http://bethesda2001.cancer.gov/terminology. *ASC,* Atypical squamous cells; *ASC-US,* atypical squamous cells of undetermined significance; *CIN,* cervical intraepithelial neoplasia; *CIS,* carcinoma in situ; *HPV,* human papilloma virus; *HSIL,* high-grade squamous intraepithelial lesion; *IUD,* intrauterine device; *LSIL,* low-grade squamous intraepithelial lesion; *NOS,* not otherwise specified.

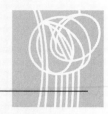

Index